Exploring Medical Language

A STUDENT-DIRECTED APPROACH

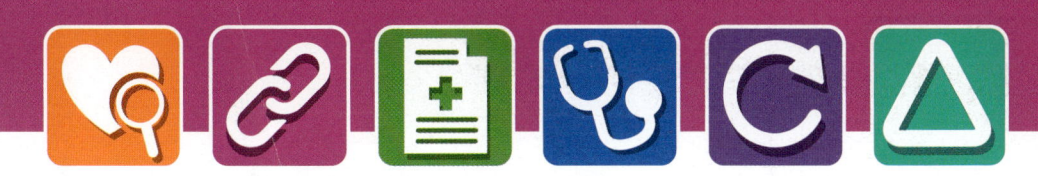

EDITION 12

Danielle LaFleur Brooks, MEd, MA
Coordinator of Teaching & Learning, Allied Health & Science
Faculty, Allied Health & Science
Community College of Vermont
Montpelier, Vermont

Dale Levinsky, MD
Clinical Associate Professor, Family, Community, & Preventative Medicine
University of Arizona College of Medicine
Phoenix, Arizona
Clinical Associate Professor, Family and Community Medicine
University of Arizona College of Medicine
Tucson, Arizona

Author Emeritus Myrna LaFleur Brooks, RN, BEd
Founding President, National Association of Health Unit Coordinators
Faculty Emeritus, Maricopa County Community Colleges
Phoenix, Arizona

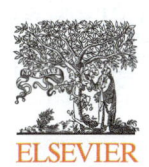

ELSEVIER

Elsevier
3251 Riverport Lane
St. Louis, Missouri 63043

EXPLORING MEDICAL LANGUAGE: A STUDENT-DIRECTED APPROACH, TWELFTH EDITION

ISBN: 978-0-443-34835-8
Set ISBN: 978-0-443-26455-9

Copyright © 2026, Elsevier Inc. All rights reserved, including those for text and data mining, AI training, and similar technologies.

For accessibility purposes, images in electronic versions of this book are accompanied by alt-text descriptions provided by Elsevier. For more information, see https://www.elsevier.com/about/accessibility.

Publisher's note: Elsevier takes a neutral position with respect to territorial disputes or jurisdictional claims in its published content, including in maps and institutional affiliations.

No part of this publication may be reproduced or transmitted in any form or by any means, electronic or mechanical, including photocopying, recording, or any information storage and retrieval system, without permission in writing from the publisher. Details on how to seek permission, further information about the Publisher's permissions policies and our arrangements with organizations such as the Copyright Clearance Center and the Copyright Licensing Agency, can be found at our website: www.elsevier.com/permissions.

This book and the individual contributions contained in it are protected under copyright by the Publisher (other than as may be noted herein).

Permission is hereby granted to reproduce the answer key in this publication in complete pages, with the copyright notice, for instructional use and not for resale.

Although for mechanical reasons some pages of this publication are perforated, only those pages imprinted with an Elsevier Inc. copyright notice are intended for removal.

Notice

Practitioners and researchers must always rely on their own experience and knowledge in evaluating and using any information, methods, compounds or experiments described herein. Because of rapid advances in the medical sciences, in particular, independent verification of diagnoses and drug dosages should be made. To the fullest extent of the law, no responsibility is assumed by Elsevier, authors, editors or contributors for any injury and/or damage to persons or property as a matter of products liability, negligence or otherwise, or from any use or operation of any methods, products, instructions, or ideas contained in the material herein.

Previous editions copyrighted 2022, 2018, 2014, 2012, 2009, 2005, 2002, 1998, 1994, 1989, and 1985.

Content Strategist: Melissa Rawe
Senior Content Development Specialist: Elizabeth McCormac
Publishing Services Manager: Catherine Jackson
Senior Project Manager: Rachel E. McMullen
Design Direction: Renee Duenow

Printed in India

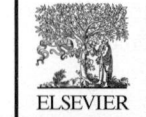

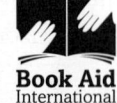

Last digit is the print number: 9 8 7 6 5 4 3 2 1

*For our students,
who continue to inspire us with their dedication
to learning while balancing life's other demands.
Every page is for you.*

Contents

PREFACE Features, vi
Organization of the Textbook, xii
Anatomy of a Chapter, xiii
Online Student Resources, xiv
Online Instructor Resources, xv

PART 1 INTRODUCTION TO WORD PARTS AND HUMAN BODY STRUCTURE
1. Introduction to Medical Language, 1
2. Body Structure, Oncology, and Laboratory Tests, 16
3. Directional Terms, Positions, and Imaging, 60

PART 2 BODY SYSTEMS
4. Integumentary System, 94
5. Respiratory System, 134
6. Urinary System, 188
7. Male Reproductive System, 230
8. Female Reproductive System, 266
9. Obstetrics and Neonatology, 313
10. Cardiovascular, Lymphatic, Immune Systems and Blood, 357
11. Digestive System, 415
12. Eye, 465
13. Ear, 506
14. Musculoskeletal System, 533
15. Nervous System and Behavioral Health, 593
16. Endocrine System, 639

APPENDICES
A. Answer Key, 677
B. Combining Forms, Prefixes, and Suffixes Alphabetized by Word Part, 725
C. Combining Forms, Prefixes, and Suffixes Alphabetized by Definition, 733
D. Abbreviations, 741
E. Pharmacology Terms, 755

ONLINE APPENDICES
F. Additional Combining Forms, Prefixes, and Suffixes, Evolve Resources
G. Health Care Delivery Terms, Evolve Resources
H. Integrative Medicine Terms, Evolve Resources
I. Behavioral Health Terms, Evolve Resources
J. Clinical Research Terms, Evolve Resources
K. Nutrition Terms, Evolve Resources
L. Dental Terms, Evolve Resources
M. Health Information Technology (HIT) Terms, Evolve Resources

Preface

WELCOME TO THE TWELFTH EDITION OF *EXPLORING MEDICAL LANGUAGE*

We are excited to share the new edition of *Exploring Medical Language* with you! The twelfth edition reflects knowledge we have gained through clinical practice and working alongside medical terminology students and instructors. In addition to updating content to reflect current use, we have cross-referenced terms with ICD diagnosis and procedure codes to make sure terms studied are relevant. We have also continued to refine the learning system to more fully utilize learning styles and to support long-term memory. Here is an overview of new and sustaining features:

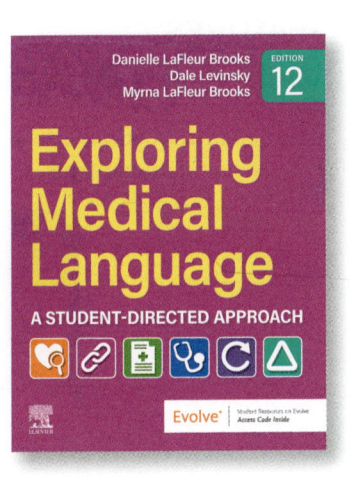

New Content

- Capstone exercise called **Scribe It** concludes the book; students draw on what they have learned from *Exploring Medical Language* to transcribe information from a patient encounter, Chapter 16
- Practical Application exercise called **Use Medical Terms in Clinical Statements**, Chapters 2-16
- Focus on **lab findings**, including a narrative explanation and identification of terms indicating lab findings, Chapters 5-16
- Addition of **phonetic spelling** for abbreviations spoken as whole words, Chapters 2-16
- Introduction of the **SOAP Note** format and associated abbreviations, Chapter 5
- Narrative introduction on **Behavioral Health**, Chapter 15
- More online **Gradable Student Resources** on Evolve

Instructional Strategies

- Word-part learning system used to analyze, define, and build terms
- Body-system organization of content
- Term lists categorized by Terms Built from Word Parts and Terms NOT Built from Word Parts
- Subcategories of terms grouped by topic: Disease and Disorder, Surgical, Diagnostic and Complementary Terms
- Inclusion of medical terms aligned with ICD diagnosis and procedure codes
- Online learning opportunities aligned with the chapter objectives and exercises

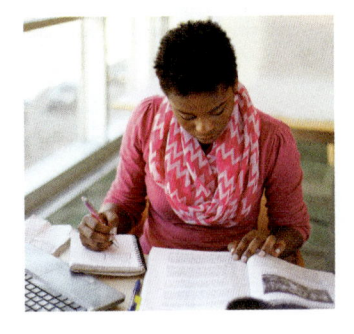

Cornerstone Features

- Paper flashcards
- Illustrations conveying medical concepts
- Historical and informational boxes placed close to corresponding word parts, terms, and abbreviations
- Comprehensive Word Parts Tables that include all word parts used to analyze terms within the chapter
- Label illustration exercises for word parts and terms
- Online Audio Glossary aligned with pronunciation exercises
- Application of terms in medical documents and online EHR Modules
- Chapter at a Glance content summaries

Exploring Medical Language provides an effective introduction to medical language for those entering health professions and related fields, including software development, computer applications and support, insurance, law, equipment supply, pharmaceutical sales, and medical writing. Its hybrid approach of print and electronic learning tools balances hands-on and virtual experiences. Learning activities provided in the textbook, instructor materials, and Evolve offer diverse ways for students to practice recall, make meaning of new information, and demonstrate learning. The learning system offered by *Exploring Medical Language* is designed to appeal to student learning preferences and to support a variety of course formats, including in-person, online, synchronous, and hybrid modalities.

We remain dedicated to supporting instructors and students and invite you to contact us at:

danielle.lafleurbrooks@ccv.edu
dale.levinsky@gmail.com
myrnabrooks@comcast.net

You are also welcome to follow Myrna's educational blog at medicalterminologyblog.com.

Warm regards,
Danielle, Dale, and Myrna

vi Preface

FEATURES

Outline and Objectives

Chapter introductions list sections with page numbers and student learning objectives aligned with chapter content, exercises, and assessments.

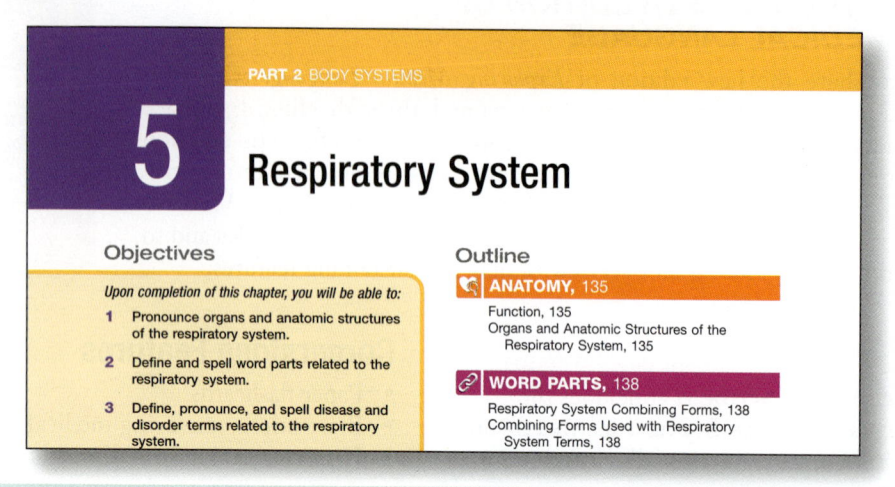

PART 2 BODY SYSTEMS

5 Respiratory System

Objectives

Upon completion of this chapter, you will be able to:
1. Pronounce organs and anatomic structures of the respiratory system.
2. Define and spell word parts related to the respiratory system.
3. Define, pronounce, and spell disease and disorder terms related to the respiratory system.

Outline

ANATOMY, 135
  Function, 135
  Organs and Anatomic Structures of the Respiratory System, 135

WORD PARTS, 138
  Respiratory System Combining Forms, 138
  Combining Forms Used with Respiratory System Terms, 138

Anatomy

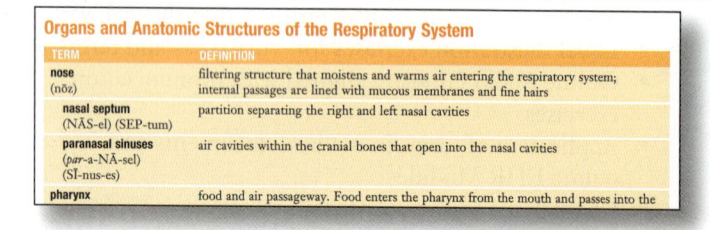

Organs and Anatomic Structures of the Respiratory System

TERM	DEFINITION
nose (nōz)	filtering structure that moistens and warms air entering the respiratory system; internal passages are lined with mucous membranes and fine hairs
nasal septum (NĀS-el) (SEP-tum)	partition separating the right and left nasal cavities
paranasal sinuses (par-a-NĀ-sel) (SĪ-nus-es)	air cavities within the cranial bones that open into the nasal cavities
pharynx	food and air passageway. Food enters the pharynx from the mouth and passes into the

Body-system chapters introduce related anatomy and physiology (A&P). **Pronunciation of organs and anatomical structures** can be practiced using phonetic spelling in the textbook and the Evolve Resources Audio Glossary.

PRONOUNCE ANATOMIC STRUCTURES

Practice saying aloud each of the organs and specific structures on the previous pages.
To hear the terms, go to Evolve Resources at www.evolve.elsevier.com and select:
Student Resources > **Audio Glossary** > Chapter 5 > Anatomic Structures
☐ Check the box when complete.

Word Parts

Word Part Tables present combining forms, suffixes, and prefixes related to chapter content. Textbook exercises, **paper and electronic flashcards,** and online activities reinforce learning.

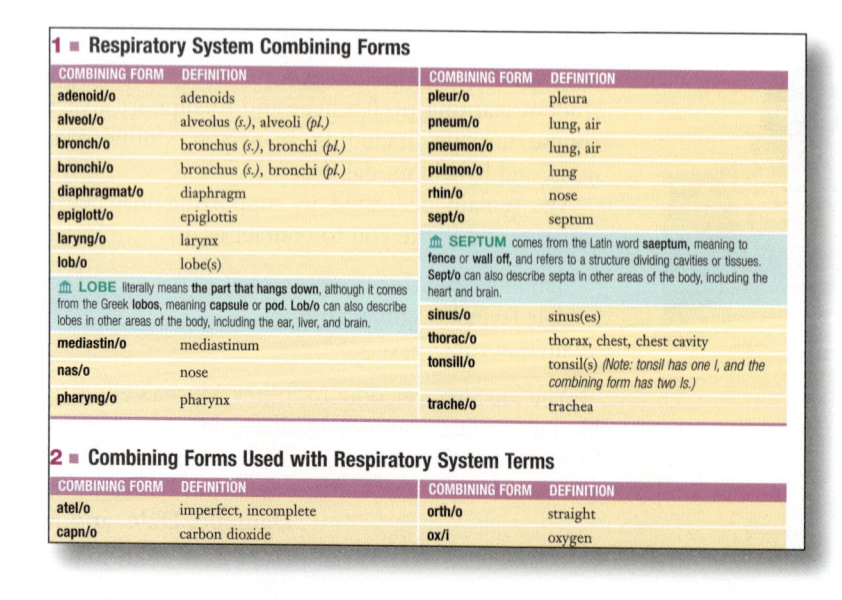

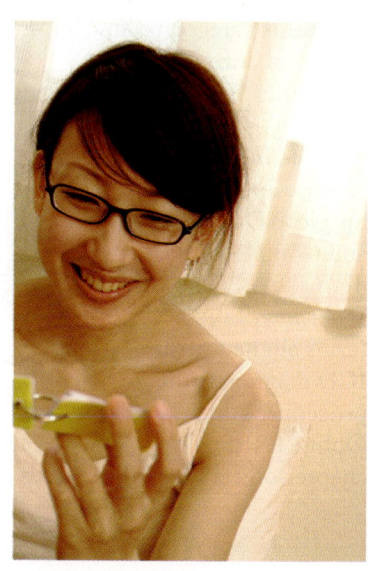

1 ▪ Respiratory System Combining Forms

COMBINING FORM	DEFINITION	COMBINING FORM	DEFINITION
adenoid/o	adenoids	pleur/o	pleura
alveol/o	alveolus (s.), alveoli (pl.)	pneum/o	lung, air
bronch/o	bronchus (s.), bronchi (pl.)	pneumon/o	lung, air
bronchi/o	bronchus (s.), bronchi (pl.)	pulmon/o	lung
diaphragmat/o	diaphragm	rhin/o	nose
epiglott/o	epiglottis	sept/o	septum
laryng/o	larynx	**SEPTUM** comes from the Latin word *saeptum*, meaning to fence or wall off, and refers to a structure dividing cavities or tissues. Sept/o can also describe septa in other areas of the body, including the heart and brain.	
lob/o	lobe(s)		
LOBE literally means **the part that hangs down**, although it comes from the Greek **lobos**, meaning **capsule** or **pod**. Lob/o can also describe lobes in other areas of the body, including the ear, liver, and brain.		sinus/o	sinus(es)
			thorac/o	thorax, chest, chest cavity
mediastin/o	mediastinum	tonsill/o	tonsil(s) (Note: tonsil has one l, and the combining form has two ls.)
nas/o	nose		
pharyng/o	pharynx	trache/o	trachea

2 ▪ Combining Forms Used with Respiratory System Terms

COMBINING FORM	DEFINITION	COMBINING FORM	DEFINITION
atel/o	imperfect, incomplete	orth/o	straight
capn/o	carbon dioxide	ox/i	oxygen

Label Exercises

Interactive illustration exercises help students form connections between word parts and anatomic structures, apply the meaning of word parts, and recall term definitions.

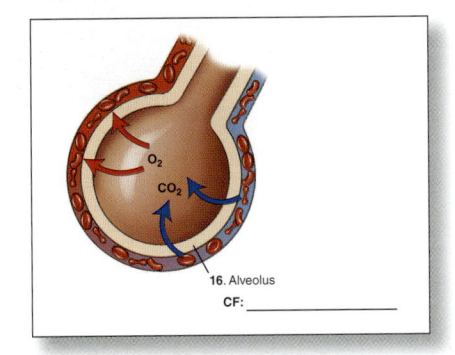

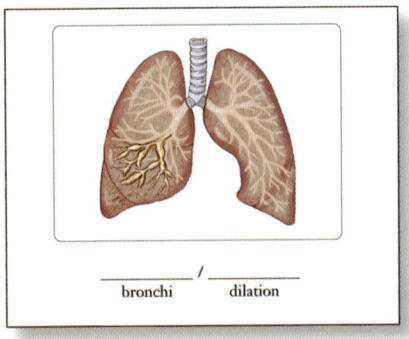

16. Alveolus
CF: _____

_____ / _____
bronchi   dilation

Medical Terms Built from Word Parts

Students **analyze, define,** and **build** medical terms using the meaning of word parts. Learning may be extended through practice with Evolve Student Resources, including online exercises, practice quizzes, and games.

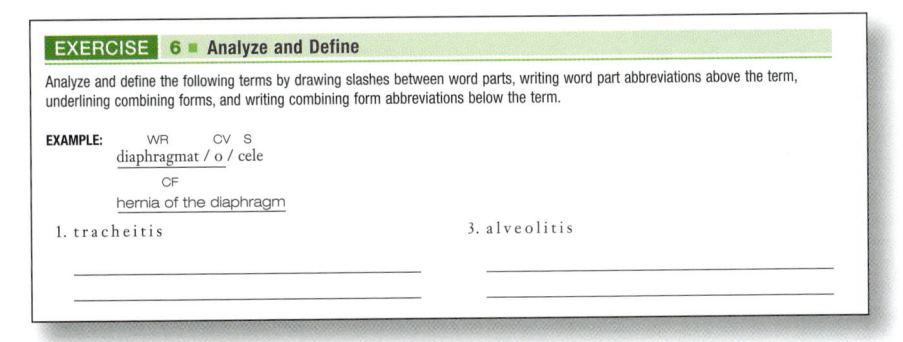

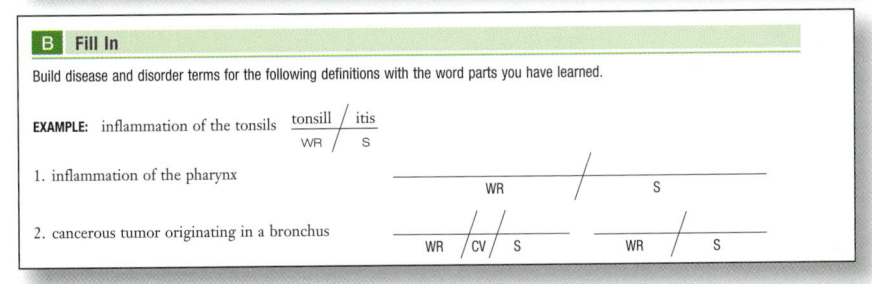

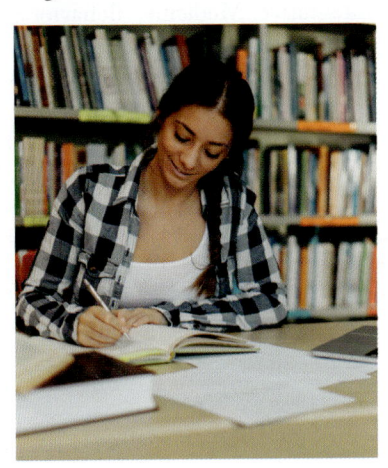

EXERCISE 6 ■ Analyze and Define

Analyze and define the following terms by drawing slashes between word parts, writing word part abbreviations above the term, underlining combining forms, and writing combining form abbreviations below the term.

EXAMPLE: WR   CV   S
         diaphragmat / o / cele
                  CF
         hernia of the diaphragm

1. tracheitis   3. alveolitis
   _____   _____
   _____   _____

B Fill In

Build disease and disorder terms for the following definitions with the word parts you have learned.

EXAMPLE: inflammation of the tonsils tonsill / itis
                                         WR / S

1. inflammation of the pharynx   _____ / _____
                                      WR / S

2. cancerous tumor originating in a bronchus   _____ / _____ / _____ _____ / _____
                                                 WR / CV / S   WR / S

Medical Terms NOT Built from Word Parts

Chapters present tables of Terms NOT Built from Word Parts followed by exercises designed to facilitate memorization. Label exercises match illustrations with terms to form connections between terms and medical concepts.

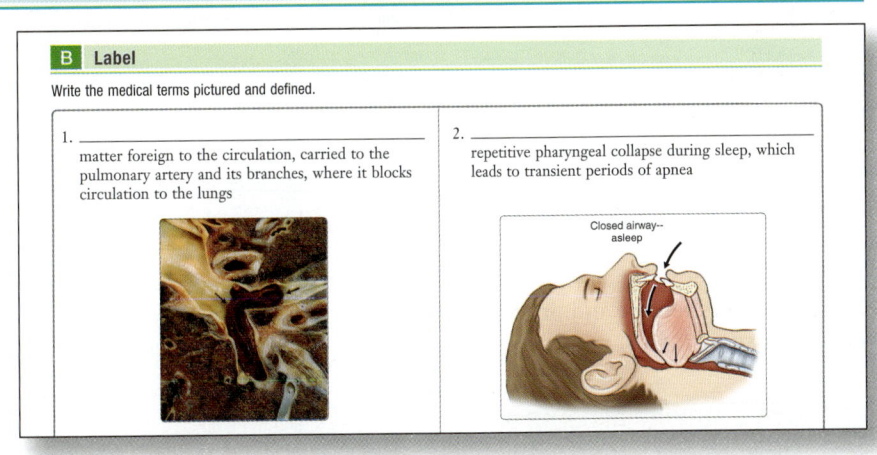

B Label

Write the medical terms pictured and defined.

1. _____
matter foreign to the circulation, carried to the pulmonary artery and its branches, where it blocks circulation to the lungs

2. _____
repetitive pharyngeal collapse during sleep, which leads to transient periods of apnea

Closed airway--asleep

Preface   vii

Pronunciation and Spelling

Pronunciation and spelling exercises may be completed on paper or online. Students may hear terms pronounced and practice spelling online using Evolve Resources.

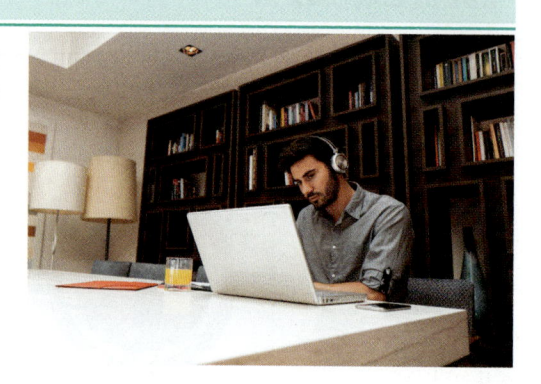

Clinical Categories and Appendices

Body-system chapters present term lists grouped by the categories of **Disease and Disorder, Surgical, Diagnostic,** and **Complementary**. Complementary Terms are categorized by topics, including Signs and Symptoms, Treatments, Equipment, Medical Specialties, and Descriptive Terms. With use of additional appendices in the textbook and online, students may increase their vocabulary in the areas of Pharmacology, Health Care Delivery, Integrative Medicine, Behavioral Health, Clinical Research, Nutrition, Dentistry, and Health Information Technology.

NEW—Identification of terms indicating lab findings.

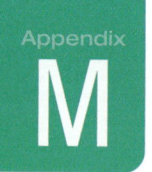

Appendix M: Health Information Technology (HIT) Terms

Health Information Technology (HIT) refers to information management in the healthcare industry and encompasses electronic health records (EHRs), personal health records (PHRs), electronic prescribing (E-prescribing), information privacy, and system security. Health Information Technologists address the technical aspects of health information management.

access levels	security feature that limits access of information to the minimum necessary amount needed to perform required duties
application server provider (ASP)	external company providing computer services over a network, such as an electronic health record system maintained on off-site servers (rather than locally hosted using an on-site server)
algorithm	set of instructions designed to accomplish a task. Algorithms usually take one or more inputs, run them systematically through a series of steps, and provide one or more outputs.
artificial intelligence (AI)	device or product that can imitate intelligent behavior or that mimics human learning and reasoning. Artificial intelligence includes machine learning, neural networks, and natural language processing. Some terms used to describe artificial intelligence include computer-aided detection/diagnosis, statistical learning, deep learning, and smart algorithms.
authentication	verification of the computer user or healthcare provider who is the author of the record, usually a written or electronic signature
bar code medication administration (BCMA)	hardware and software used to provide electronic verification that the "five rights" (right patient, right drug, right dose, right route, and right time) are achieved for the administration of medications; designed for patient safety and to decrease errors.

Complementary Terms

Complementary terms complete the vocabulary presented in the chapter by ... specialists, and related words. A symptom is subjective information reflecti... A sign is objective information detected in the physical examination and in re... tory tests. **Lab findings** are the results of laboratory tests that analyze speci... laboratory tests will be noted in Complementary Term Tables as lab finding...

BUILT FROM WORD PARTS
The following terms can be translated using definitions of word parts. Fu... as needed.

SIGNS AND SYMPTOMS

TERM	DEFINITION	TERM	
1. acapnia (a-CAP-nē-a)	condition of absence (less than normal level) of carbon dioxide (in the blood); (lab finding)	10. hyperpn... (hī-perp...	
2. anoxia (a-NOK-sē-a)	condition of absence (deficiency) of oxygen; (lab finding)	11. hypocap... (hī-pō-...	
ANOXIA literally means **without oxygen** or **absence of oxygen**. The term actually denotes an oxygen deficiency in the body tissues.		12. hypopnea (hī-POP-nē-a)	deficient breathing
3. aphonia (ā-FŌ-nē-a)	condition of absence of voice	13. hypoxemia (hī-pok-SĒ-mē-a)	deficient oxygen in the blood; (lab finding)
4. apnea (AP-nē-a)	absence of breathing	14. hypoxia (hī-POK-sē-a)	condition of deficient oxygen (to the tissues); (lab finding)
5. dysphonia (dis-FŌ-nē-a)	condition of difficult speaking (voice)		The "o" from the prefix **hypo-** is dropped in the terms **hypoxemia** and **hypoxia** because the following word part begins with a vowel.
6. dyspnea (DISP-nē-a)	difficult breathing	15. orthopnea (or-THOP-nē-a)	breathing (more easily) in a straight (upright position) (indicates difficulty breathing in the supine position)
7. eupnea (ŪP-nē-a)	normal breathing		

Historical Perspective and Current Use

Informational boxes anchor medical language in a **historical perspective** and provide details on the **current use of terms.**

🏛 **ATELECTASIS** is derived from the Greek **ateles**, meaning **not perfect**, and **ektasis**, meaning **expansion**. It denotes an incomplete expansion of the lungs.

REACTIVE AIRWAY DISEASE (RAD) is a general term and not a specific diagnosis. It is used to describe a history of wheezing, coughing, and shortness of breath. In some people RAD may lead to **asthma**.

Abbreviations

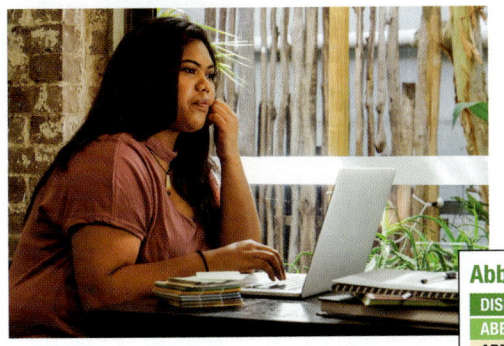

Tables introduce abbreviated medical terms related to chapter content. Textbook exercises, electronic flashcards, online exercises, and practice quizzes reinforce new learning. Students may supplement learning with additional abbreviations and error-prone abbreviations listed in Appendix D.

NEW—Phonetic spellings for abbreviations pronounced as whole words.

Abbreviations

DISEASE AND DISORDERS

ABBREVIATION	TERM	ABBREVIATION	TERM
ARDS	acute respiratory distress syndrome	HAP	hospital-acquired pneumonia
CAP	community-acquired pneumonia	IPF	idiopathic pulmonary fibrosis
CF	cystic fibrosis	LTB	laryngotracheobronchitis
cocci	coccidioidomycosis; spoken as a whole word (KAHK-sē)	OSA	obstructive sleep apnea
		PE	pulmonary embolism
COPD	chronic obstructive pulmonary disease	PE also abbreviates physical examination.	
COVID-19	coronavirus disease; spoken as whole words (CŌ-vid) (NĪN-tēn)	RSV	respiratory syncytial virus
		TB	tuberculosis
flu	influenza; spoken as a whole word (floo)	URI	upper respiratory infection

SOAP Note Format

Medical Record Abbreviations

Documentation of a patient's medical history and health care received is stored in medical records. Medical records are the who, what, when, where, and how of patient care. A common format used to record information from patient encounters is the **SOAP note**. SOAP is an acronym formed from the first letters of the note's section titles, including subjective, objective, assessment, and plan (Table 5.2). In documentation of a visit with a primary care provider, the objective section will include the patient's **vital signs (VS)**, including **temperature (T)**, **blood pressure (BP)**, **pulse (P)** rate, and **respiration (R)** rate.

TABLE 5.2 SOAP Note Format

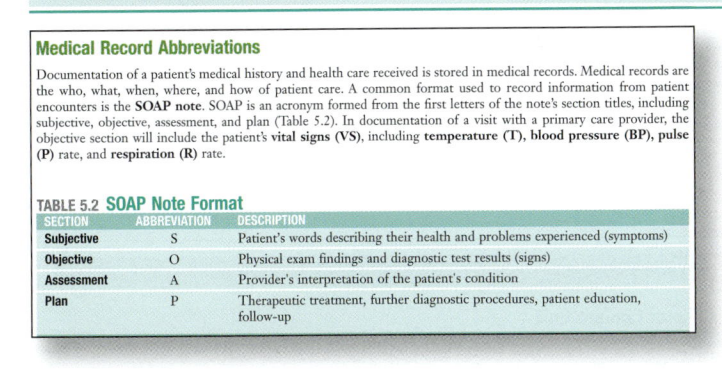

SECTION	ABBREVIATION	DESCRIPTION
Subjective	S	Patient's words describing their health and problems experienced (symptoms)
Objective	O	Physical exam findings and diagnostic test results (signs)
Assessment	A	Provider's interpretation of the patient's condition
Plan	P	Therapeutic treatment, further diagnostic procedures, patient education, follow-up

NEW—Introduction of the SOAP Note documentation style and corresponding abbreviations in Chapter 5

Practical Application

Students apply medical terms to case studies and medical records.

EXERCISE 34 ■ Interact with Medical Documents

A

Read the report and complete it by writing medical terms on answer lines within the document. Definitions of terms to be written appear after the document.

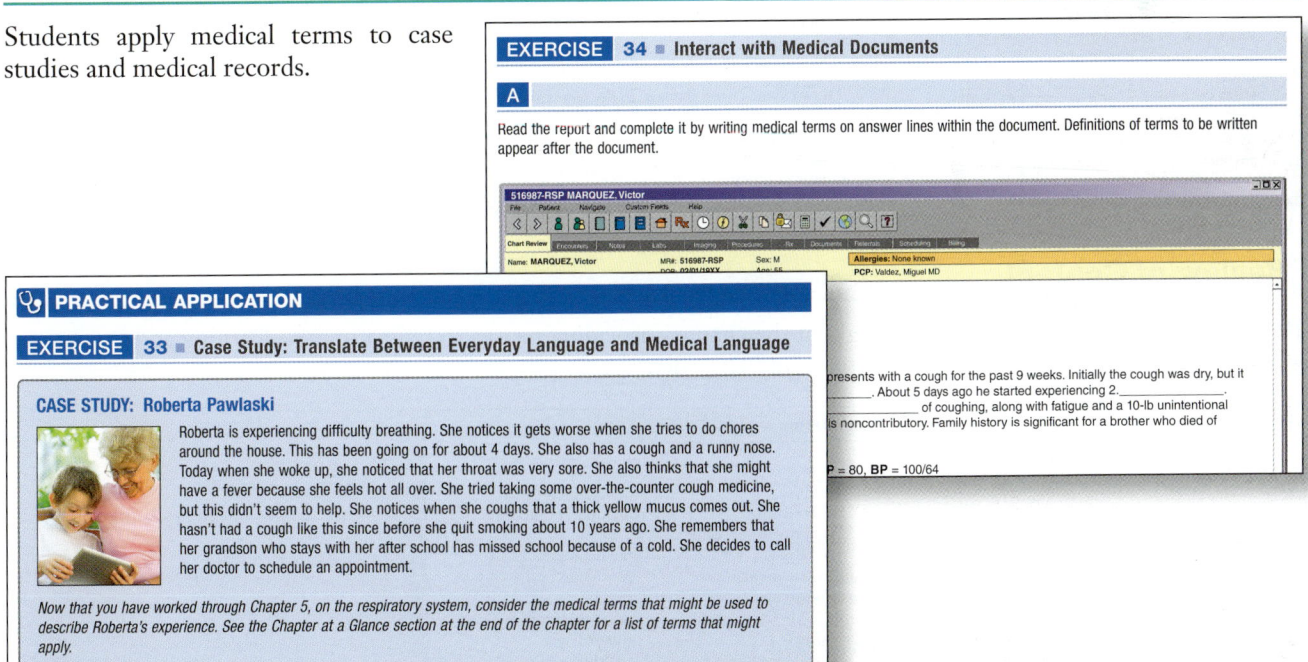

516987-RSP MARQUEZ, Victor

Name: MARQUEZ, Victor   MR#: 516987-RSP   Sex: M
Allergies: None known
PCP: Valdez, Miguel MD

presents with a cough for the past 9 weeks. Initially the cough was dry, but it _____. About 5 days ago he started experiencing 2. _____.
_____ of coughing, along with fatigue and a 10-lb unintentional
is noncontributory. Family history is significant for a brother who died of

P = 80, BP = 100/64

PRACTICAL APPLICATION

EXERCISE 33 ■ Case Study: Translate Between Everyday Language and Medical Language

CASE STUDY: Roberta Pawlaski

Roberta is experiencing difficulty breathing. She notices it gets worse when she tries to do chores around the house. This has been going on for about 4 days. She also has a cough and a runny nose. Today when she woke up, she noticed that her throat was very sore. She also thinks that she might have a fever because she feels hot all over. She tried taking some over-the-counter cough medicine, but this didn't seem to help. She notices when she coughs that a thick yellow mucus comes out. She hasn't had a cough like this since before she quit smoking about 10 years ago. She remembers that her grandson who stays with her after school has missed school because of a cold. She decides to call her doctor to schedule an appointment.

Now that you have worked through Chapter 5, on the respiratory system, consider the medical terms that might be used to describe Roberta's experience. See the Chapter at a Glance section at the end of the chapter for a list of terms that might apply.

Preface

Electronic Health Records (EHR)

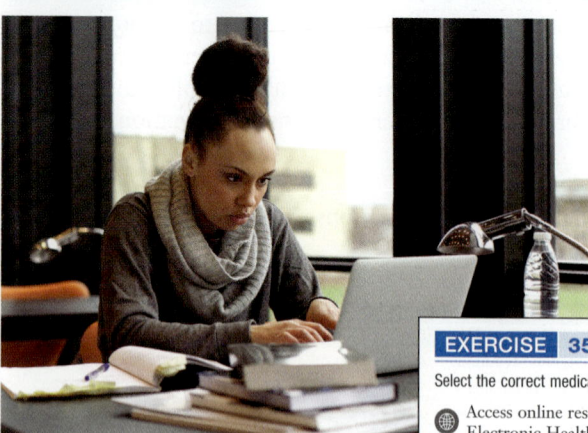

EHR Modules in Practice Student Resources on the Evolve website provide three related medical records for one patient. Students identify medical terms in context while gaining a familiarity with computer applications used in the field.

EXERCISE 35 ■ Use Medical Language in Online Electronic Health Records

Select the correct medical terms to complete three medical records in one patient's electronic file.

Access online resources at evolve.elsevier.com > Evolve Resources > Student Resources > Activities > Chapter 5 > Electronic Health Records

Topic: COPD
Record 1, Chart Review: Progress Note
Record 2, Imaging: Radiology Report
Record 3, Notes: Pulmonary Function Department Note

☐ Check the box when complete.

> Healthcare records are stored and used in an electronic system called **Electronic Health Records (EHR)**. Electronic health records contain a collection of health information of an individual patient; the digitally formatted record can be shared through computer networks with patients, physicians, and other healthcare providers.

Chapter Content Quiz

Designed as formative assessments, Chapter Content Quizzes allow students to test their knowledge by identifying medical terms and abbreviations used in context.

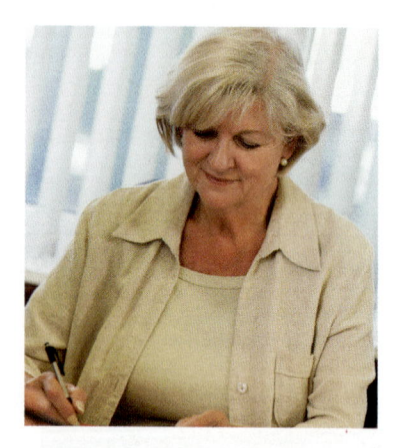

CHAPTER REVIEW

EXERCISE 38 ■ Chapter Content Quiz

Test your understanding of terms and abbreviations introduced in this chapter. Circle the letter for the medical term or abbreviation related to the words in italics

1. The patient was admitted to the emergency department with a *severe nosebleed*.
   a. rhinomycosis
   b. epistaxis
   c. nasopharyngitis
2. The accident caused damage to the *larynx*, necessitating a *surgical repair*.
   a. laryngectomy
   b. laryngostomy
   c. laryngoplasty
5. The physician informed the patient that her *coughing of blood* might be due to tuberculosis.
   a. hemoptysis
   b. pneumothorax
   c. thoracentesis
6. The patient reported dizziness brought on by *ventilation of the lungs beyond normal bodily needs*.
   a. hyperventilation
   b. hypoventilation
   c. dysphonia

Review of Content

Review of Terms exercises appear throughout the chapter, providing pauses to reflect on new learning and to consider all of the terms from a section, such as Disease and Disorder.

EXERCISE 12 ■ Review of Disease and Disorder Terms

Can you define, pronounce, and spell the following terms?

acute respiratory distress syndrome (ARDS)	coccidioidomycosis (cocci)	laryngitis	pulmonary edema
adenoiditis	coronavirus disease (COVID-19)	laryngospasm	pulmonary embolism (PE)
alveolitis	croup	laryngotracheobronchitis (LTB)	pulmonary neoplasm
atelectasis	cystic fibrosis (CF)	lobar pneumonia	pyothorax
asphyxia	deviated septum	nasopharyngitis	rhinitis
asthma	diaphragmatocele	obstructive sleep apnea (OSA)	rhinomycosis
bronchiectasis	diphtheria	pertussis	rhinorrhagia
bronchitis	emphysema	pharyngitis	sinusitis
			tonsillitis

Preface   xi

Chapter at a Glance provides a summary of word parts new to the chapter and terms presented.

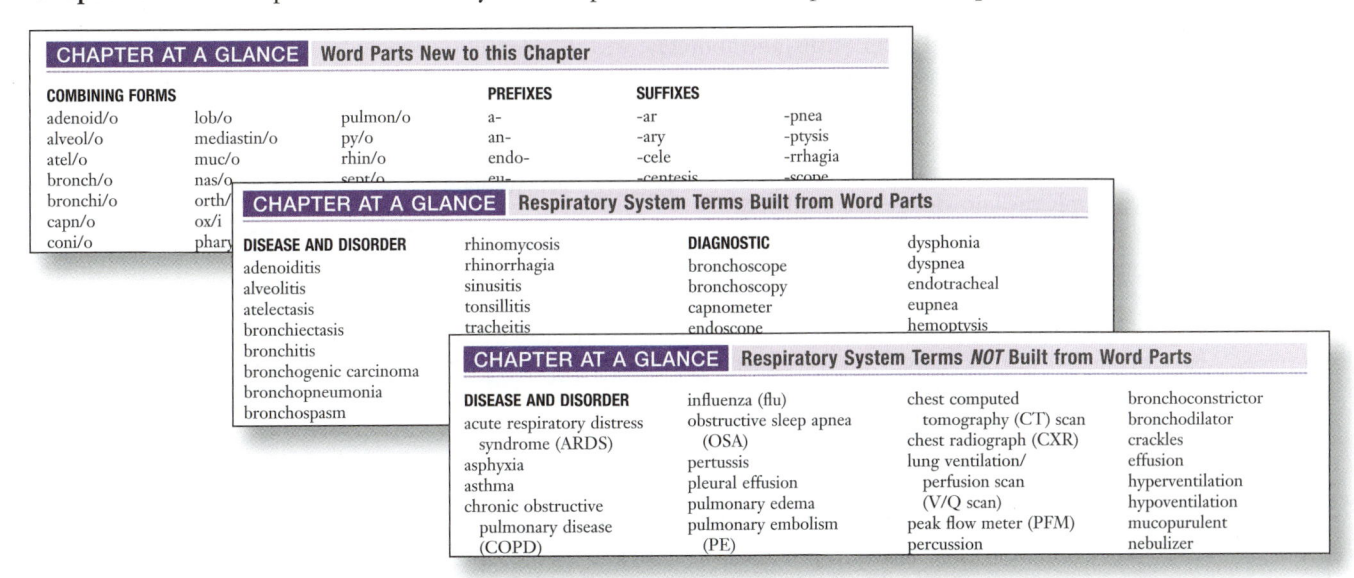

CHAPTER AT A GLANCE Word Parts New to this Chapter

COMBINING FORMS
- adenoid/o
- alveol/o
- atel/o
- bronch/o
- bronchi/o
- capn/o
- coni/o
- lob/o
- mediastin/o
- muc/o
- nas/o
- orth/o
- ox/i
- phary...
- pulmon/o
- py/o
- rhin/o
- sept/o

PREFIXES
- a-
- an-
- endo-
- eu-

SUFFIXES
- -ar
- -ary
- -cele
- -centesis
- -pnea
- -ptysis
- -rrhagia
- -scope

CHAPTER AT A GLANCE Respiratory System Terms Built from Word Parts

DISEASE AND DISORDER
- adenoiditis
- alveolitis
- atelectasis
- bronchiectasis
- bronchitis
- bronchogenic carcinoma
- bronchopneumonia
- bronchospasm
- rhinomycosis
- rhinorrhagia
- sinusitis
- tonsillitis
- tracheitis

DIAGNOSTIC
- bronchoscope
- bronchoscopy
- capnometer
- endoscope
- dysphonia
- dyspnea
- endotracheal
- eupnea
- hemoptysis

CHAPTER AT A GLANCE Respiratory System Terms *NOT* Built from Word Parts

DISEASE AND DISORDER
- acute respiratory distress syndrome (ARDS)
- asphyxia
- asthma
- chronic obstructive pulmonary disease (COPD)
- influenza (flu)
- obstructive sleep apnea (OSA)
- pertussis
- pleural effusion
- pulmonary edema
- pulmonary embolism (PE)
- chest computed tomography (CT) scan
- chest radiograph (CXR)
- lung ventilation/ perfusion scan (V/Q scan)
- peak flow meter (PFM)
- percussion
- bronchoconstrictor
- bronchodilator
- crackles
- effusion
- hyperventilation
- hypoventilation
- mucopurulent
- nebulizer

Capstone Exercise

⚠ CAPSTONE
EXERCISE 32 ▪ Scribe It

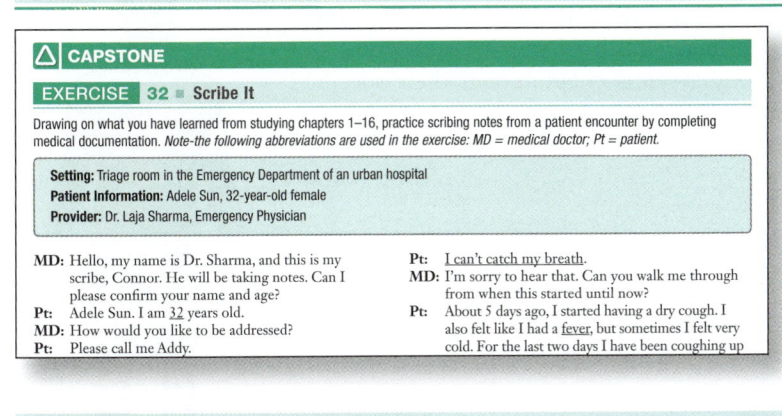

Drawing on what you have learned from studying chapters 1–16, practice scribing notes from a patient encounter by completing medical documentation. Note-the following abbreviations are used in the exercise: MD = medical doctor; Pt = patient.

Setting: Triage room in the Emergency Department of an urban hospital
Patient Information: Adele Sun, 32-year-old female
Provider: Dr. Laja Sharma, Emergency Physician

MD: Hello, my name is Dr. Sharma, and this is my scribe, Connor. He will be taking notes. Can I please confirm your name and age?
Pt: Adele Sun. I am 32 years old.
MD: How would you like to be addressed?
Pt: Please call me Addy.

Pt: I can't catch my breath.
MD: I'm sorry to hear that. Can you walk me through from when this started until now?
Pt: About 5 days ago, I started having a dry cough. I also felt like I had a fever, but sometimes I felt very cold. For the last two days I have been coughing up

NEW—Scribe It, a capstone exercise appearing at the end of Chapter 16, allows students to demonstrate skills acquired during their study of all sixteen chapters of *Exploring Medical Language*.

Online Evolve Resources

Evolve Resources provide multiple ways to practice and assess learning.

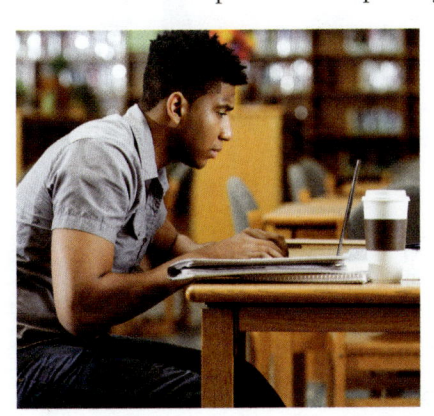

Student Resources
- Audio Glossary
- Flashcards
- Practice Activities
- Spelling Exercises
- Practice Quizzes
- Electronic Health Records
- Games
- Videos

Instructor Resources
- TEACH Handouts
- TEACH Lesson Plans
- TEACH PowerPoints
- Test Bank
- Image Collection
- Sample Course Syllabus and Outline
- Gradable Assessments

Preface

ORGANIZATION OF THE TEXTBOOK

Chapters 1 through 3 provide a foundation for building medical vocabulary. Chapters 4 through 16 organize content by body systems, presenting related word parts, terms, and abbreviations. The textbook concludes with a series of appendices designed to extend student learning as desired.

Introductory Chapters

Chapter 1... may be the most important chapter in the text, because you will apply the knowledge acquired here in the rest of the chapters to learn terms in an easy, quick fashion. The chapter introduces the two categories of terms—those built from word parts and those which are not; each category is accompanied by different types of exercises. Also introduced in this chapter are the **four word parts**—word root, suffix, prefix, and combining vowel, which are the basis of terms built from the word parts category.

EXAMPLE	INTRAVENOUS	
	WORD PART	MEANING
prefix	intra-	within
word root	ven	vein
suffix	-ous	pertaining to
term = p + wr + s	intra/ven/ous	pertaining to within a vein

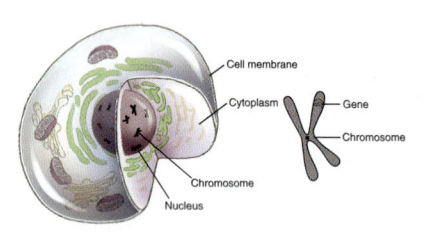

Chapter 2... introduces body structure, oncology, and laboratory tests, while providing immediate practice in recognizing the two categories of terms along with corresponding exercises for each. You will likely be surprised at how fast you learn the meaning and spelling of many medical terms.

Chapter 3... introduces directional terms, positioning, and diagnostic imaging, all of which are relevant to subsequent body systems chapters and their specific medical terms.

Body System Chapters

Chapters 4 through 16... introduce specific body systems with related word parts, terms, and abbreviations and follow a consistent format.

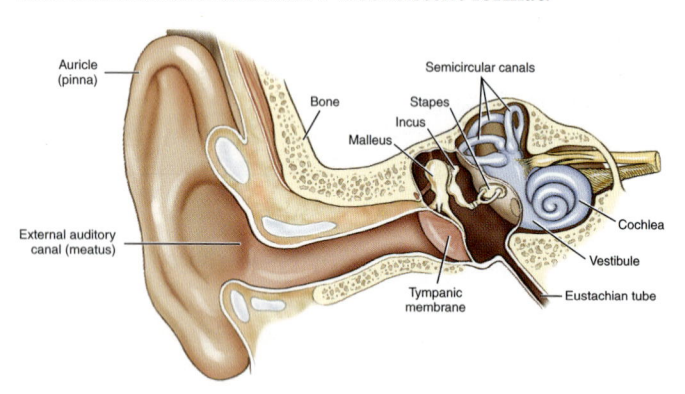

Appendices

Appendices A-E... appear in the textbook and provide an answer key for chapter exercises, comprehensive lists of word parts and abbreviations, a list of error-prone abbreviations, and pharmacology terms.

Appendices F-M... in Practice Student Resources on the Evolve website provide lists of additional word parts, Health Care Delivery Terms, Integrative Medicine Terms, Behavioral Health Terms, Nutrition Terms, Dental Terms, and Health Information Technology Terms.

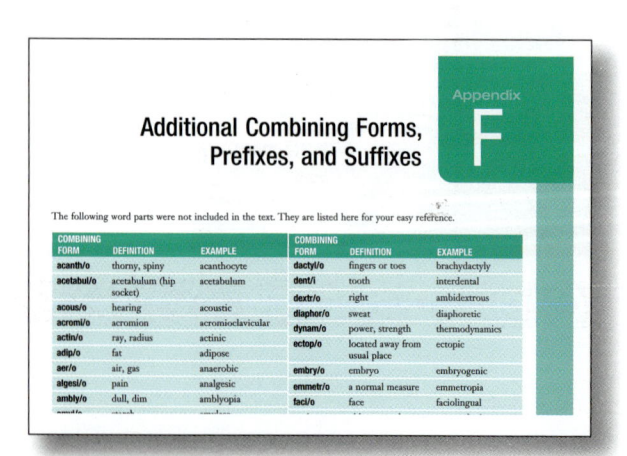

ANATOMY OF A CHAPTER
Let's take a look at the structure of a body system chapter, using Chapter 5 on the respiratory system as an example.

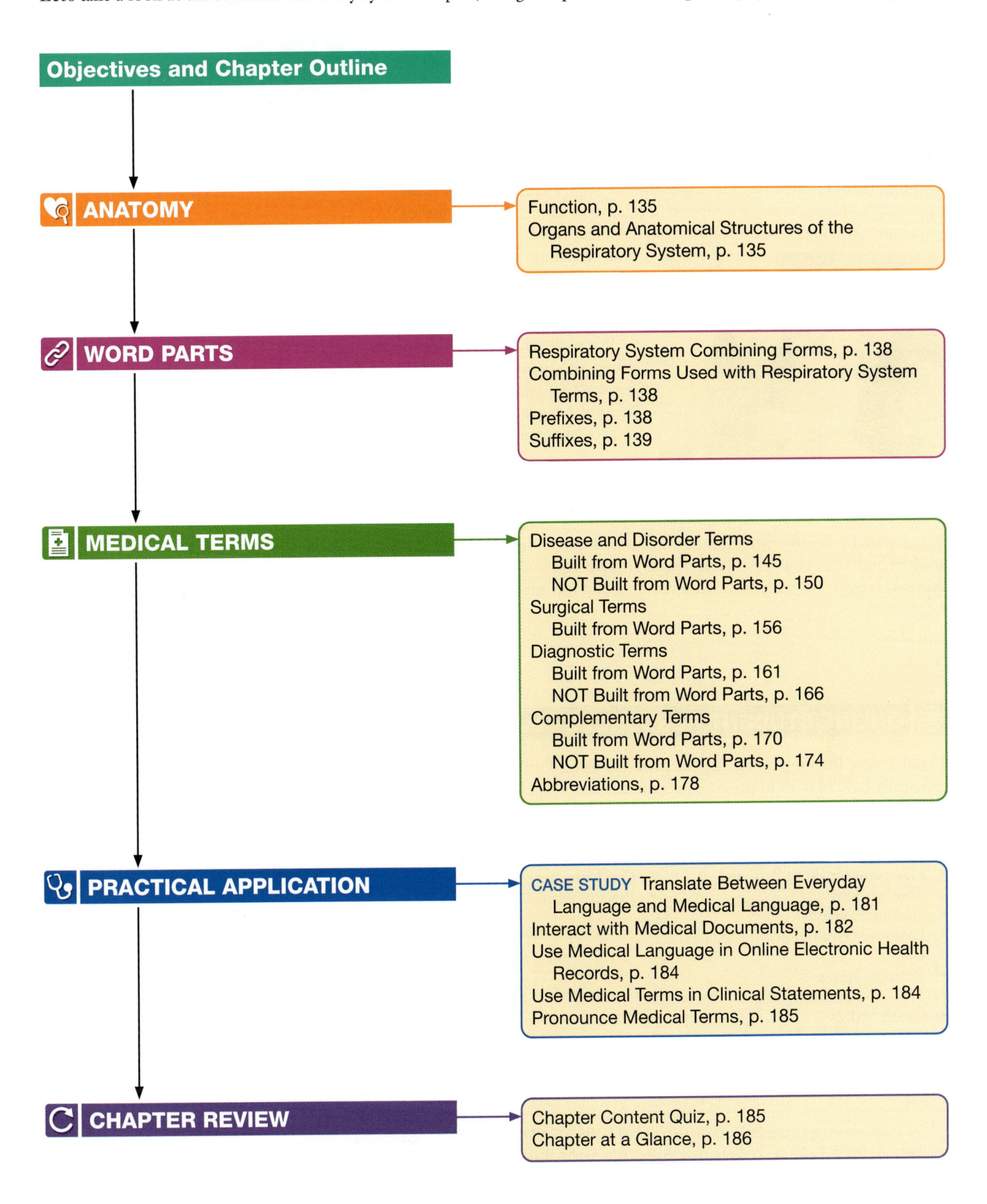

Objectives and Chapter Outline
↓

ANATOMY
- Function, p. 135
- Organs and Anatomical Structures of the Respiratory System, p. 135

↓

WORD PARTS
- Respiratory System Combining Forms, p. 138
- Combining Forms Used with Respiratory System Terms, p. 138
- Prefixes, p. 138
- Suffixes, p. 139

↓

MEDICAL TERMS
- Disease and Disorder Terms
  - Built from Word Parts, p. 145
  - NOT Built from Word Parts, p. 150
- Surgical Terms
  - Built from Word Parts, p. 156
- Diagnostic Terms
  - Built from Word Parts, p. 161
  - NOT Built from Word Parts, p. 166
- Complementary Terms
  - Built from Word Parts, p. 170
  - NOT Built from Word Parts, p. 174
- Abbreviations, p. 178

↓

PRACTICAL APPLICATION
- **CASE STUDY** Translate Between Everyday Language and Medical Language, p. 181
- Interact with Medical Documents, p. 182
- Use Medical Language in Online Electronic Health Records, p. 184
- Use Medical Terms in Clinical Statements, p. 184
- Pronounce Medical Terms, p. 185

↓

CHAPTER REVIEW
- Chapter Content Quiz, p. 185
- Chapter at a Glance, p. 186

Preface

DEAR STUDENT

If you are reading this, you are most likely enrolled in a medical terminology course and preparing for your journey of learning medical language using this textbook. As you flip or scroll through the pages of *Exploring Medical Language*, you may be thinking, "There is so much to learn. How will I do it?" or "Why are there so many exercises?"

Let us assure you that you will acquire the language by completing chapter exercises. While it may seem daunting at first, we encourage you to be as active as possible as you read and work through each chapter.

The exercises approach the terms from all angles: pronunciation, writing, defining, spelling, and application. Chapter content flows from one chapter to the next in a repetitive manner, making the best use of your time. You may build a foundational medical vocabulary by using the textbook alone, or you may choose to extend your learning by utilizing Evolve Resources, which provide supplemental materials online. To register for the *Exploring Medical Language* 12e Evolve Resources, please visit evolve.elsevier.com/LaFleur/exploring or call 1-800-222-9570.

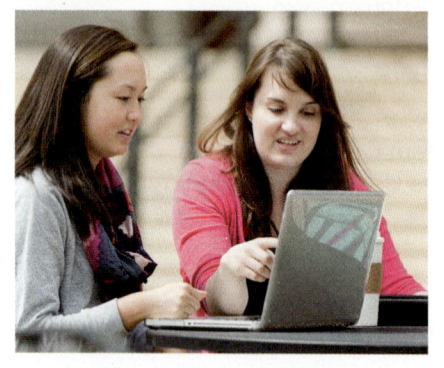

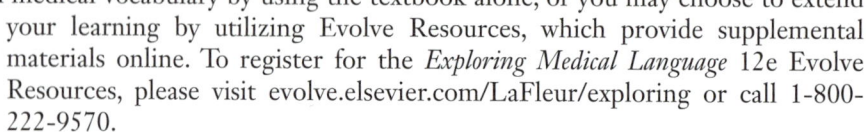

We wish you the best as you embark on this journey. You will join a select group of students who have used *Exploring Medical Language* as a textbook for over 40 years. We would like to hear of your experience with *Exploring Medical Language*, including exercises that were most useful, suggestions for improvement, and so forth. Reach us by e-mail at the following addresses:

danielle.lafleurbrooks@ccv.edu
dale.levinsky@gmail.com
myrnabrooks@comcast.net

We also invite you to visit Myrna's educational blog at **medicalterminologyblog.com**. Follow the blog while you are a student and after you finish your course to help you build on your vocabulary in a fun and engaging way. Posts include quizzes, crosswords, videos, word scrambles, and introduction to emerging medical terms.

Sincerely,
Danielle, Dale, and Myrna

ONLINE STUDENT RESOURCES evolve.elsevier.com/LaFleur/exploring

Practice new learning and test your progress using Evolve Resources. Time spent using the Student Resources can be especially helpful with improving pronunciation and spelling skills, both of which are essential in healthcare professions.

Practice Student Resources
- Audio Glossary
- Flashcards for Word Parts and Abbreviations
- Spelling Exercises
- Electronic Health Record Modules
- Games
- Practice Quizzes
- Medical Animations
- Career Videos
- Additional Appendices with Term Lists by Medical Specialty

Gradable Student Resources
- Exercises
- Quick Quizzes
- Practice Exams

> For assistance in registering for Evolve Resources, call **1-800-222-9570**, visit **service.elsevier.com** and select the link for Evolve, or conduct a browser search for **Evolve Support Center**.

Preface

DEAR INSTRUCTOR

Thank you for choosing *Exploring Medical Language!* We hope you find this learning system supportive of your teaching methods and effective for your students' learning styles. With the purchase of a new textbook, students receive paper flashcards for word parts and pincode access to Evolve Resources for students. You may find the flashcards and online resources, such as pronunciation for term lists and games, useful for class activities and exam preparation.

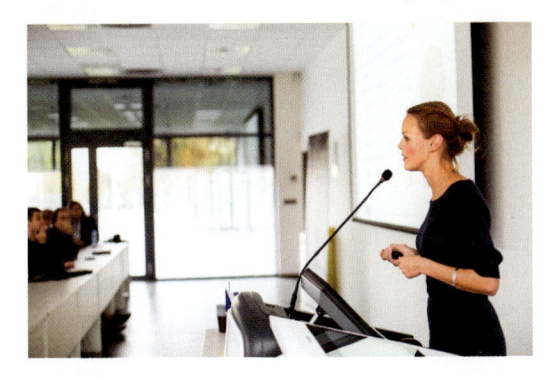

Additional teaching materials are available online using Evolve Resources for Instructors. All resources are objective based, and we recommend beginning with the TEACH Lesson Plans for an overview of how to use the various teaching tools. The first step in accessing teaching materials is to register for the *Exploring Medical Language* 12e Evolve Resources. Once registered, request Evolve Resources and select if you would like to access content only or integrate content into your school's LMS using Content Plus Course Tools. Please visit evolve.elsevier.com/LaFleur/exploring or call 1-800-222-9570 for more information.

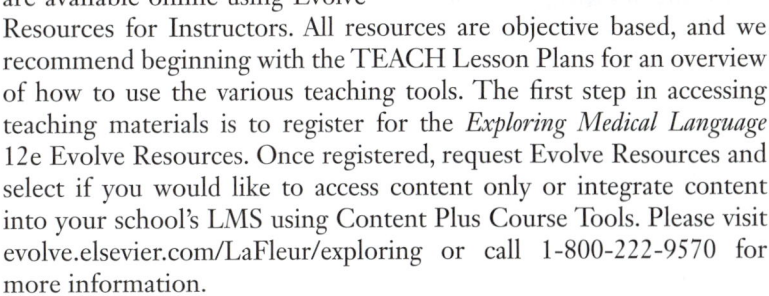

We welcome your comments and questions by email. Danielle, who teaches medical terminology in the traditional classroom, online, and in hybrid formats, is also happy to share ideas and materials. Contact us at:

danielle.lafleurbrooks@ccv.edu
dale.levinsky@gmail.com
myrnabrooks@comcast.net

We also invite you to visit Myrna's educational blog at **medicalterminologyblog.com** to keep up with trends in teaching medical terminology and emerging medical language.

Looking forward to hearing from you,
Danielle, Dale, and Myrna

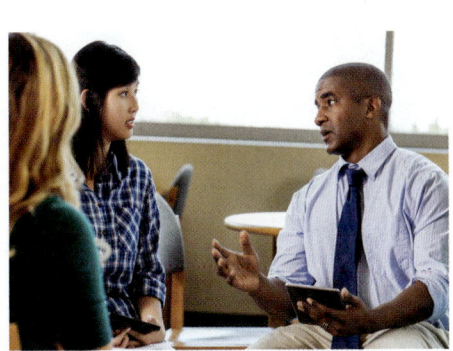

ONLINE INSTRUCTOR RESOURCES evolve.elsevier.com/LaFleur/exploring

Instructor Resources
- Image Collection
- Sample Course Syllabus and Outline
- TEACH Handouts
- TEACH Lesson Plans
- TEACH PowerPoint Slides
- Test Bank

Assessment
- Pretests, TEACH Lesson Plans in Evolve Instructor Resources
- Formative and summative assessment plan for each lesson, TEACH Lesson Plans in Evolve Instructor Resources
- Gradable Exercises, Evolve Student Resources
- Gradable Practice Exams, Evolve Student Resources
- Test Bank to build quizzes and exams, Evolve Instructor Resources

Content Plus Course Tools
- Grades
- Roster & Teams
- Question Bank
- Course Calendar
- Login Report

Access to online course management tools, such as a gradebook and online discussions, is included.

For assistance in registering for Evolve Resources and Content Plus Course Tools, call **1-800-222-9570**, visit **service.elsevier.com** and select the link for Evolve, or conduct a browser search for **Evolve Support Center.**

Contributors, Reviewers, and Advisors

Reviewers and Advisors

Sukriti Bagchi, BS
MD/PhD Candidate
University of Arizona College of Medicine - Phoenix
Phoenix, Arizona

Heather L. Connolly, DC
Certified Medical Examiner
Faculty, Allied Health and Science
Community College of Vermont
Montpelier, VT
South College
Pittsburgh, Pennsylvania

Gregory Labenz, MD
Diagnostic Radiologist, Catalina Radiology, PLC
Nuclear Medicine Medical Director, Northwest Medical Center
Tucson, Arizona

Betsy McLane, MT (ASCP), MEd
Faculty, Allied Health and Science
Community College of Vermont
Winooski, Vermont

Past Contributors, Reviewers, and Advisors

Delena Kay Austin, BTIS, CMA (AAMA)
Health Science Technology Faculty
Macomb Community College
Warren, Michigan

Charo E. Bautista, BSN
Adjunct Faculty
Health Unit Coordinating/Patient Care Associate
GateWay Community College
Maricopa Community Colleges
Phoenix, Arizona

Cynthia Ann Bjerklie, BS
Faculty, Allied Health Science
Community College of Vermont
Montpelier, Vermont

William Bohnert, MD
Past President, American Urological Association
CDI Consultant, Dignity Health
St. Joseph's Hospital
Phoenix, Arizona

Julene Bredeson, CMA (AAMA), PHN, BSN, RN
Medical Assistant Instructor
Ridgewater College
Willmar, Minnesota

Richard K. Brooks, MD, FACP, FACG
Internal Medicine and Gastroenterology (retired)
Mayo Clinic
Clinical Instructor (retired)
Geisel School of Medicine
Dartmouth College
Quechee, Vermont

Sharon A. Brooks, MSN, BA, RN
Practical Nursing Program Director
Sumner College
Portland, Oregon

Ruth Buchner, MEd
Family and Consumer Science / Health Science Educator
Chippewa Falls High School
Chippewa Falls, Wisconsin

Catherine J. Cerulli, MEd
Director, Interwoven Healing Arts
University of Vermont Medical Center
Montpelier, Vermont

Christine Costa, BS, GCM, HUC
Geriatric Care Manager
Tempe, Arizona

Angela Dawson-Walker, CMA, LVN
Apple Valley Unified School District
Apple Valley, California

Ashleigh du Plessis
Student, STEM Studies
Community College of Vermont
Montpelier, Vermont

Carolyn Ehrlich, MSN Psy, NP
Private Practice, Psychiatry (retired)
Phoenix, Arizona

Kelly Eiden, MS, LD, CDS
Interim Dean, Division of Allied Health, Chair of Dietetics
Barnes Jewish College
St. Louis, Missouri

Contributors, Reviewers, and Advisors

Christopher Fields, OD
Optometrist
Fields of Vision Eye Care, Inc.
Lebanon, New Hampshire

Robert L. Fortune, MD
Cardiovascular Surgery (retired)
Scottsdale, Arizona

Janet Funk, MD
Associate Professor of Medicine & Nutritional Sciences
The University of Arizona Cancer Center
Phoenix, Arizona

Deborah Greer, MEd, RT(R)(M)
Program Director-RT Education
Penn Medicine
Philadelphia, Pennsylvania

Erin Hayes, MS, MAT
Foundations of Medicine Instructor
Medicine & Healthcare Strand Leader
Blue Valley Center for Advanced Professional Studies
Overland Park, KS

Cynthia Heiss, PhD, RD
Professor Department of Healthcare Professions
Metropolitan State University of Denver
Denver, Colorado

Jane A. Hlopko, MA, RHIA
Department Chairman, Associate Professor, Health Information Technology
SUNY Broome Community College
Binghamton, New York

Colleen Horan, MD
Gynecologist and Obstetrician
Central Vermont Medical Center
Berlin, Vermont

Marjorie "Meg" Holloway, MS, RN, APRN
Foundations of Medicine Instructor
Medicine & Healthcare Strand Leader
Blue Valley Center for Advanced Professional Studies
Overland Park, Kansas

Bradley D. Johnson, MEd, RT(R)(ARRT)
Faculty, Medical Radiography
Gateway Community College
Phoenix, Arizona

Erinn Kao, PharmD
Pharmacist
RX Outreach, Inc.
St. Louis, Missouri

Sheri Lavadour, RN, BSN, HTP
Sumner College of Nursing, Instructor
Portland, Oregon

Elyse Levinsky, MD, MHSc, FRCSC
Assistant Professor, Obstetrics and Gynaecology
University of Toronto
Toronto, Ontario, Canada

Kara Stuart Lewis, MD
Phoenix Children's Hospital
Phoenix, Arizona

Lynnae Lockett, RN, RMA, CMRS, MSN
Allied Health Program Director
Bryant & Stratton College
Parma, Ohio

Charles Machia
Billing Customer Service
University of Vermont Medical Center
Burlington, Vermont

Melanie Meyer, ND, MS, MPH
Faculty, Allied Health Science
Community College of Vermont
Montpelier, Vermont

Melody Miller, LPN
Medical Assistant Instructor
Lancaster County Career and Technology Center
Willow Street, Philadelphia

Linda A. Mottle, MSN-HAS, RN
Program Director, Clinical Research Program
GateWay Community College
Phoenix, Arizona

Caroline M. Murphy, DDS
General Practice Dentist
Montpelier, Vermont

Bernard S. Nanadiego, MD
Child Psychiatry Fellow, Child and Adolescent Psychiatry Department
University of Arizona
Tucson, Arizona

Veronique M. Parker, MBA
Faculty, Healthcare Management
Maricopa Community Colleges
Phoenix, Arizona

Stephen M. Picca, MD
Internal Medicine and Anesthesiology (retired)
New York, New York

Maynard D. Poland, MD
Internal Medicine (retired)
Milwaukee Medical Clinic;
Medical Director (retired)
Columbia St. Mary's Hospital;
Emeritus Assistant Clinical Professor School of Medicine
University of Wisconsin
Milwaukee, Wisconsin

Toni L. Rodriguez, EdD, RRT, FAARC
Program Director
Respiratory Care Program
GateWay Community College
Phoenix, Arizona

Patricia L. Shinn, PhD, RN
Chair, Nursing Department
River Valley Community College
Claremont, New Hampshire

Charlene Thiessen, MEd, CMT, AHDI-F
Program Director, Medical Transcription
GateWay Community College
Phoenix, Arizona

Sharon Tomkins Luzcu, RN, MA, MBA
Director, Health Services Management Program
GateWay Community College
Phoenix, Arizona

Ann Vadala, BA
Professor, Office Administration
St. Lawrence College
Kingston, Ontario

Cris E. Wells, EdD, MBA, CCRP, RT(R)(M)
Assistant Professor/Director of Interprofessional Programs and the Clinical Research Management Master of Science Program
College of Nursing and Health Innovation
Arizona State University
Phoenix, Arizona

Kari Williams, BS, DC
Program Director
Front Range Community College
Longmont, Colorado

Dokagari Woods, RN, PhD
Assistant Professor of Nursing, Undergraduate Program Director
Tarleton State University
Stephenville, Texas

Acknowledgments

We are incredibly lucky to be supported by a team of skilled professionals who worked tirelessly in creating the twelfth edition of *Exploring Medical Language*. We are grateful for the time, effort, and talents of the following individuals:

Luke Held, Content Strategist, whose support of *Exploring Medical Language* over the years has been instrumental in its success. His ability to listen and advocate for our vision of the textbook was invaluable and made a lasting impact on the work.

Elizabeth McCormac, Senior Content Development Specialist, who guided us through the editorial portion of the project. Her attention to detail, especially with the illustration credits, was very helpful. We appreciated her steady presence and support.

Renee Duenow, Book Designer, who created the beautiful design of the twelfth edition. Her work was instrumental in creating a welcoming and effective learning system. We remain grateful for her attention to detail and the ability to translate our vision to what appears on the page.

Catherine Jackson, Publishing Services Manager, who provided leadership during the production phase of the project.

Rachel McMullen, Senior Project Manager, who expertly guided us through a new production process. Her thoroughness and attention to detail were greatly appreciated.

Babette Morgan, who masterfully copyedited our work, improving its quality and overall consistency.

Prakash Kannan, Digital Media Producer, who facilitated the development of electronic components of the textbook.

Carolyn Kruse and **Andrew Woodard,** who shared their voices on the audio files.

Jeanne Robertson, Medical Illustrator, whose art has brought to life many medical concepts. We have the greatest respect for her attention to detail and ability to bring beauty to technical images.

Winifred K. Starr (1921-1993), who was Myrna's first coauthor and whose creative contributions remain in the text today.

Contributors, Reviewers, and **Advisors** listed on the previous pages who shared their expertise and knowledge.

Faculty, who have adopted the text to teach medical language and have used their valuable time to give us feedback.

Students, who over the years have worn thin the pages of previous editions. Your pursuit of knowledge has been truly inspirational.

Each page of the twelfth edition is better because of your collective contributions.

Thank you.

PART 1 INTRODUCTION TO WORD PARTS AND HUMAN BODY STRUCTURE

Introduction to Medical Language

Outline

INTRODUCTION TO MEDICAL TERMS AND MEDICAL LANGUAGE, 2

Origins of Medical Language, 2
Categories of Medical Terms and Learning Methods, 4

MEDICAL TERMS BUILT FROM WORD PARTS, 4

Four Word Parts, 4
   Word Root, 5
   Suffix, 5
   Prefix, 5
   Combining Vowel, 6
Combining Form, 7
Techniques for Learning Medical Terms Built from Word Parts, 9
   Analyzing Medical Terms, 9
   Defining Medical Terms, 9
   Building Medical Terms, 11

MEDICAL TERMS *NOT* BUILT FROM WORD PARTS, 14

Types of Terms NOT Built from Word Parts, 14
Learning Terms NOT Built from Word Parts, 14

CHAPTER REVIEW, 15

Review of Categories of Medical Terms, 15
Review of Medical Terms Built from Word Parts, 15
Review of Medical Terms NOT Built from Word Parts, 15
Review of Objectives, 15

Answers to Chapter Exercises, Appendix A

Objectives

Upon completion of this chapter, you will be able to:

1. Describe the origins of medical language.
2. Define two categories of medical terms.
3. Identify and define the four word parts and the combining form.
4. Analyze and define medical terms using the meaning of word parts.
5. Build medical terms using the meaning of word parts.

TABLE 1.1 Categories of Medical Terms and Learning Methods, 4
TABLE 1.2 Guidelines for Using Combining Vowels, 7
TABLE 1.3 Word Parts and Combining Form, 8
TABLE 1.4 Word Parts List, 10
TABLE 1.5 Techniques to Learn Medical Terms Built from Word Parts, 12

INTRODUCTION TO MEDICAL TERMS AND MEDICAL LANGUAGE

Medical terms are words used to describe disease, as well as aspects of medicine and health care. Terms built from Greek and Latin word parts, eponyms, acronyms, and modern language are types of medical terms.

Medical language or terminology is the use of medical terms to attain a standardized means of communication within the practice of medicine and in the healthcare industry. The need for fluency in medical language cannot be exaggerated.

Why are many medical terms different from words we use in everyday life? Medical language allows for clear, concise and consistent communication locally, nationally, and internationally. It enables everyone involved in medicine and health care to perform more accurately and efficiently for the patient's benefit. For example, using the medical term **osteoarthritis** (Fig. 1.1), which means **inflammation of the bone and joint,** offers a clear and concise written or verbal communication using one word instead of six. No matter the national language used, the meaning of the medical term does not change.

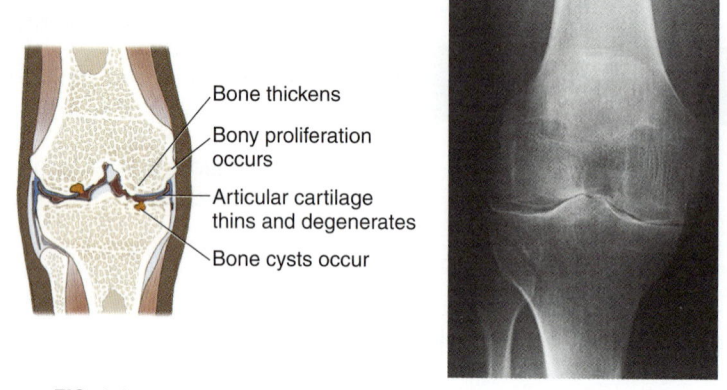

FIG. 1.1 Osteoarthritis of the knee joint, illustration and radiograph.

Origins of Medical Language

The vocabulary of medical language reflects its development over time, beginning with the ancient Greeks. More than 2,000 years ago, Hippocrates and Aristotle were among the first to study and write about medicine. The Romans continued the practice, adopting elements of the Greek language to use alongside Latin. The majority of terms in use today are **built from Greek and Latin word parts**. For learning purposes, these terms are categorized as **Terms Built from Word Parts** in this textbook.

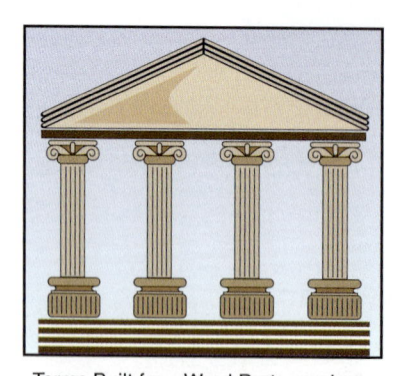

Terms Built from Word Parts, such as arthritis, are of Greek and Latin origin.

Chapter 1 Introduction to Medical Language

As scientific knowledge, medical technology, and medical practice evolved, so did the language of medicine, which now also includes **eponyms, acronyms, and terms from modern language**. Eponyms are terms derived from a name or place. Acronyms are terms formed from the first letters of a phrase. Modern language refers to terms from the English language, which are often descriptive of technology and procedures. For learning purposes, these terms are categorized as **Terms NOT Built from Word Parts** in this textbook.

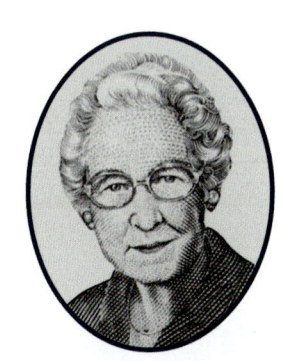

Eponyms are terms derived from the name of a person or place. Examples include **Apgar score**, named after the person who developed it, and **West Nile virus**, named after the first geographical location the virus was identified.

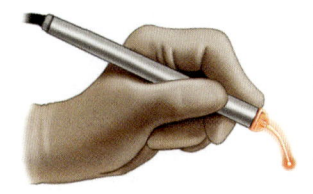

Acronyms, such as **laser** (light amplification by stimulated emission of radiation), are terms formed from the first letters of words in a phrase. Acronyms usually contain a vowel and are spoken as a whole word.

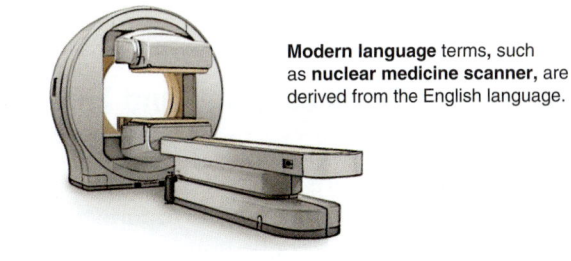

Modern language terms, such as **nuclear medicine scanner**, are derived from the English language.

VIRGINIA APGAR, an obstetric anesthesiologist born in New Jersey, developed the Apgar score in 1952 to measure the physical condition of the newborn.

EXERCISE 1 ■ Origins of Medical Language

Place the letter from the first column to identify the origin of the term in the second column. You may use an answer more than once. *To check your answers to the exercises in this chapter, go to Appendix A at the back of the textbook.*

a. Greek and Latin word parts
b. eponym
c. acronym
d. modern language

_____ 1. Middle Eastern respiratory syndrome
_____ 2. hepatitis
_____ 3. MRSA (methicillin-resistant *Staphylococcus aureus*)
_____ 4. posttraumatic stress disorder
_____ 5. arthritis
_____ 6. cell saver (instrument used during surgery to recover blood lost from the patient)
_____ 7. AIDS (acquired immunodeficiency syndrome)
_____ 8. Alzheimer disease

ALZHEIMER DISEASE VS. ALZHEIMER'S DISEASE The need for clarity and consistency in medical language has resulted in the **modern trend to eliminate the possessive form of eponyms and use instead the nonpossessive form**. The nonpossessive form is observed by the Association for Healthcare Documentation Integrity, the American Medical Association's Manual of Style, in most medical dictionaries, and is the style used throughout this textbook. With either use, the noun that follows is not capitalized.

Categories of Medical Terms and Learning Methods

For the purposes of our studies, medical terms are categorized as *Built from Word Parts* and *NOT Built from Word Parts*. Specific learning methods will be used for each category, as noted in Table 1.1.

EXERCISE 2 ■ Categories of Medical Terms

Complete the following. *To check your answers, go to Appendix A.*

Medical terms _____ _____ _____ _____ can be translated to find their meanings, whereas medical terms _____ _____ _____ _____ _____ cannot be easily translated to find their meanings.

TABLE 1.1 Categories of Medical Terms and Learning Methods

CATEGORY	TYPES OF TERMS	EXAMPLE	LEARNING METHODS
Terms Built from Word Parts (can be translated to find their meanings)	1. Word parts of Greek and Latin origin placed together to form terms that can be translated literally to find their meanings	1. arthr/itis	1. Analyzing terms 2. Defining terms 3. Building terms
Terms NOT Built from Word Parts (cannot be easily translated to find their meanings)	1. Eponyms, terms derived from the name of a person or place 2. Acronyms, terms formed from the first letters of a phrase that can be spoken as a whole word and usually contains a vowel 3. Modern language, terms derived from the English language 4. Terms with Greek and Latin word parts that cannot be easily translated to find their meanings	1. Alzheimer disease 2. MRSA (methicillin-resistant *Staphylococcus aureus*) 3. complete blood count with differential 4. orthopedics	1. Recalling terms 2. Matching terms 3. Defining terms

MEDICAL TERMS BUILT FROM WORD PARTS

Medical terms categorized as Built from Word Parts are composed of Greek and Latin **word roots, prefixes,** and **suffixes** and can be translated to find their meanings. A **combining vowel** is often added to ease pronunciation (Table 1.2 and Table 1.3). Techniques to learn these terms are **analyzing, defining,** and **building** medical terms.

Four Word Parts

Most medical terms categorized as Built from Word Parts consist of some or all of the following components:

1. Word root
2. Suffix
3. Prefix
4. Combining vowel

WORD ROOT

The word root is the word part that is the core of the word. The word root contains the fundamental meaning of the word.

EXAMPLES

In the word	play/er,
	play is the word root.
In the medical term	arthr/itis,
	arthr (which means *joint*) is the word root.
In the medical term	hepat/itis,
	hepat (which means *liver*) is the word root.

> 💡 The word root is the core of the word. All medical terms have at least one word root.

SUFFIX

The suffix is a word part attached to the end of the word root to modify its meaning.

EXAMPLES

In the word	play/er,
	-er is the suffix.
In the medical term	hepat/ic,
	-ic (which means *pertaining to*) is the suffix and *hepat* is the word root for *liver*; therefore, *hepatic* means *pertaining to the liver*.
In the medical term	hepat/itis,
	-itis (which means *inflammation*) is the suffix. The medical term *hepatitis* means *inflammation of the liver*.

> 💡 The suffix is used to modify the meaning of a word. Most medical terms have a suffix.

> **SUFFIXES** frequently indicate:
> - **procedures**, such as -scopy, meaning visual examination, or -tomy, meaning incision
> - **conditions**, such as -itis, meaning inflammation
> - **diseases**, such as -oma, meaning tumor

PREFIX

The prefix is a word part attached to the beginning of a word root to modify its meaning.

EXAMPLES

In the word	re/play,
	re- is the prefix.
In the medical term	sub/hepat/ic,
	sub- (which means *under*) is the prefix, *hepat* is the word root for *liver*, and *-ic* is the suffix for *pertaining to*. The medical term *subhepatic* means *pertaining to under the liver*.
In the medical term	intra/ven/ous,
	intra- (which means *within*) is the prefix, *ven* (which means *vein*) is the word root, and *-ous* (which means *pertaining to*) is the suffix. The medical term *intravenous* means *pertaining to within the vein*.

> 💡 A prefix can be used to modify the meaning of a word. Many medical terms do not have a prefix.

> **PREFIXES** often indicate:
> - **number**, such as bi-, meaning two
> - **position**, such as sub-, meaning under
> - **direction**, such as intra-, meaning within
> - **time**, such as pre-, meaning before
> - **negation**, such as a-, meaning without

EXERCISE 3 ■ Define

Complete the following sentences. *To check your answers, go to Appendix A.*

1. The word root is _____.
2. The suffix is _____.
3. The prefix is _____.

COMBINING VOWEL

The combining vowel is a word part, usually an o, used to ease pronunciation.
The combining vowel is:

- Placed to connect two word roots
- Placed to connect a word root and a suffix
- **Not** placed to connect a prefix and a word root

EXAMPLES:

In the medical term   oste/o/arthr/itis,
o is the combining vowel used between two word roots *oste* (which means *bone*) and *arthr* (which means *joint*).

In the medical term   arthr/o/pathy,
o is the combining vowel used between the word root *arthr* and the suffix *-pathy* (which means *disease*).

In the medical term   sub/hepat/ic,
the combining vowel is not used between the prefix *sub-* (which means *under*) and the word root *hepat* (which means *liver*).

> **VOWELS** are speech sounds represented by the letters a, e, i, o, u, and sometimes y.

> 💡 The combining vowel is used to ease pronunciation; therefore, not all medical terms have combining vowels. Medical terms introduced throughout the text that have combining vowels other than o are highlighted at their introduction.

Four Guidelines for Using Combining Vowels

Learning the four guidelines for using combining vowels will assist you in correctly spelling medical terms categorized as Built from Word Parts. Refer to Table 1.2, as you build terms in the following chapters until the guidelines are second nature to you.

Guideline One
When connecting a word root and a suffix, a combining vowel is used if the suffix does not begin with a vowel.

EXAMPLE
In the medical term   arthr/o/pathy,
the suffix *-pathy* does not begin with a vowel; therefore, a combining vowel is used.

Guideline Two
When connecting a word root and a suffix, a combining vowel is usually not used if the suffix begins with a vowel.

EXAMPLE
In the medical term   hepat/ic,
the suffix *-ic* begins with the vowel *i*; therefore, a combining vowel is not used.

Guideline Three
When connecting two word roots, a combining vowel is usually used even if vowels are present at the junction.

EXAMPLE
In the medical term   oste/o/arthr/itis,
o is the combining vowel used, even though the word root *oste* ends with the vowel *e*, and the word root *arthr* begins with the vowel *a*.

Guideline Four
When connecting a prefix and a word root, a combining vowel is not used.

EXAMPLE
In the medical term sub/hepat/ic,
the combining vowel is not used between the prefix *sub-* and the word root *hepat*.

TABLE 1.2 Guidelines for Using Combining Vowels

COMBINING VOWEL GUIDELINES	Example
1. When connecting a word root and a suffix, a combining vowel is **used** if the suffix **does not begin** with a vowel.	arthr/**o**/pathy
2. When connecting a word root and a suffix, a combining vowel is **usually not used** if the suffix **begins** with a vowel.	hepat/ic
3. When connecting two word roots, a combining vowel is **usually used** even if vowels are present at the junction.	oste/**o**/arthr/itis
4. When connecting a prefix and a word root, a combining vowel is **not used**.	sub/hepat/ic

EXERCISE 4 ■ Combining Vowel

Complete the following. *To check your answers, go to Appendix A.*

1. A combining vowel is _____
   _____.

2. When connecting a word root and a suffix, a combining vowel is _____ if the suffix does not begin with a vowel.

3. When connecting a word root and a suffix, a combining vowel is usually not used if the suffix begins with a _____
   _____.

4. When connecting two _____, a combining vowel is usually used, even if vowels are present at the junction.

5. When connecting a prefix and a word root, a combining vowel is _____ used.

Combining Form

A combining form is a word root with the combining vowel attached, separated by a slash. The combining form is not a word part per se; rather it is the word root and the combining vowel. *For learning purposes, word roots are presented with their combining vowels as **combining forms**.*

EXAMPLES
arthr/o
oste/o
ven/o

> 💡 Word roots are presented as combining forms throughout the text.

EXERCISE 5 ■ Define

Complete the following. *To check your answers, go to Appendix A.*

A combining form is _____
_____
_____.

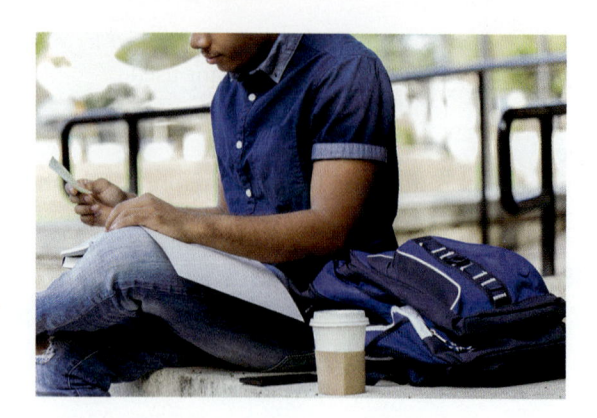

EXERCISE 6 ■ Match

Match the phrases in the first column with the correct terms in the second column. *To check your answers, go to Appendix A.*

_____ 1. attached to the beginning of a word root
_____ 2. usually an *o*
_____ 3. all medical terms built from word parts contain at least one
_____ 4. attached to the end of a word root
_____ 5. word root with combining vowel attached

a. combining vowel
b. prefix
c. combining form
d. word root
e. suffix

EXERCISE 7 ■ True/False

Answer **T** for true and **F** for false. *To check your answers, go to Appendix A.*

_____ 1. There are always prefixes at the beginning of medical terms.
_____ 2. A combining vowel is always used when connecting a word root and a suffix that begins with the letter *o*.
_____ 3. A prefix modifies the meaning of the word.
_____ 4. A combining vowel is used to ease pronunciation.
_____ 5. *I* is the most commonly used combining vowel.
_____ 6. The word root is the core of a medical term.
_____ 7. A combining vowel is used between a prefix and a word root.
_____ 8. A combining form is a word part.
_____ 9. A combining vowel is used when connecting a word root and a suffix if the suffix begins with the letter *g*.

TABLE 1.3 Word Parts and Combining Form

WORD PARTS, COMBINING FORM	DEFINITION	EXAMPLE
Word root	The core of the word	**hepat**/itis
Suffix	Attached to the end of a word root to modify its meaning	hepat/**itis**
Prefix	Attached to the beginning of a word root to modify its meaning	**sub**/hepa/tic
Combining vowel	Usually an *o* used to ease pronunciation	hepat/**o**/megaly
Combining form	Word root with a combining vowel attached, separated by a slash	**hepat/o**

Chapter 1 Introduction to Medical Language

Techniques for Learning Medical Terms Built from Word Parts

The techniques of **analyzing**, **defining**, and **building** are used in this text to learn medical terms categorized as Built from Word Parts. You will use them many times to complete exercises in the following chapters. Refer to Table 1.4 as often as needed, until you become familiar with these techniques.

ANALYZING MEDICAL TERMS

To analyze a medical term, divide it into word parts, and label each word part and each combining form. Follow the procedure below:

1. **Divide the term** into word parts with slashes.

    EXAMPLE: oste / o / arthr / o / pathy

2. **Label each word part** by using the following abbreviations.
    WR   Word Root
    P   Prefix
    S   Suffix
    CV   Combining Vowel

    EXAMPLE: oste / o / arthr / o / pathy
                    WR CV WR CV   S

3. **Identify each combining form** by underlining the word root and combining vowel, and then writing the abbreviation CF below the combining form.

    EXAMPLE: oste / o / arthr / o / pathy
                    WR CV WR CV   S
                    ―――――   ―――――
                    CF   CF

EXERCISE 8 ■ Analyzing Medical Terms

A

Complete the following. *To check your answers, go to Appendix A.*

Three steps to analyze medical terms are:

1. _____
2. _____
3. _____

B

Analyze the following medical term using the three step-procedure. Use Table 1.4 Word Parts List as a reference. *To check your answers, go to Appendix A.*

o s t e o p a t h y

DEFINING MEDICAL TERMS

To define medical terms, apply the meaning of each word part.

Once a term has been analyzed, it is defined using the meanings of word parts identified. Usually, a term's definition starts with the meaning of the suffix, if present, and then shifts to the beginning of the term with the meanings of the word parts and combining forms in the order they appear. Often definitions of terms built from word parts contain additional words, such as articles (the), conjunctions (and), and prepositions (of).

TABLE 1.4 Word Parts List

WORD ROOTS	DEFINITIONS	SUFFIXES	DEFINITIONS	PREFIXES	DEFINITIONS	COMBINING VOWEL
arthr	joint	-itis	inflammation	intra-	within	o
hepat	liver	-ic	pertaining to	sub-	under	
ven	vein	-ous	pertaining to			
oste	bone	-pathy	disease			
		-megaly	enlargement			

EXERCISE 9 ■ Defining Medical Terms

A

Complete the following. *To check your answers, go to Appendix A.*

To define medical terms categorized as Built from Word Parts, _____

_____

B

Define the following medical term. Use Table 1.4 Word Parts List as a reference. *To check your answers, go to Appendix A.*

EXAMPLE: oste/o/arthr/o/pathy

1. Begin by defining the suffix, *-pathy*. Write the definition on the line below.
2. Move to the beginning of the term; define the word roots *oste* and *arthr*. Write the definitions on the line below, continuing the definition of the term.

oste/o/arthr/o/pathy means _____ of the _____ and _____
                                  -pathy   oste   arthr

> 💡 Most medical terms categorized as Built from Word Parts can be defined by beginning with the meaning of the suffix.

EXERCISE 10 ■ Analyze and Define

Using Table 1.4 Word Parts List, analyze and define the following terms. Underline the combining forms. *To check your answers, go to Appendix A.*

EXAMPLE:
```
         WR  CV  WR  CV   S
         oste / o / arthr / o / pathy
          CF         CF
         disease of the bone and joint
```

1. arthritis

2. hepatitis

Chapter 1   Introduction to Medical Language   11

3. subhepatic

_____

_____

4. intravenous

_____

_____

5. arthropathy

_____

_____

6. osteitis

_____

_____

7. hepatomegaly

_____

_____

8. hepatic

_____

_____

BUILDING MEDICAL TERMS

To build medical terms when definitions are provided, place word parts together to form terms.

Building medical terms is a learning technique used to practice the meaning of word parts and to learn definitions of terms built from word parts. In this text, we will build commonly accepted medical terms used in healthcare professions.

EXERCISE 11 ■ Building Medical Terms

A

Complete the following. *To check your answers, go to Appendix A.*

To build medical terms when given definitions means _____

_____.

> Keep in mind that the beginning of the definition usually indicates the suffix.

B

Build the medical term for **disease of a joint.** Use Table 1.4 Word Parts List as a reference, and follow the instructions below. *To check your answers, go to Appendix A.*

1. Find the word part for *disease*. Write the word part in the correct space below.
2. Find the word part for *joint*. Write the word part in the correct space below.
3. Insert the combining vowel *o* in the correct space below. (*A combining vowel is needed because the suffix does not begin with a vowel.*)

_____ / _____ / _____
   WR   CV   S

TABLE 1.5 Techniques to Learn Medical Terms Built from Word Parts

- **Analyzing**
  1. Divide medical terms into word parts
  2. Label each word part
  3. Underline and label each combining form

  oste / o / arthr / o / pathy

  oste / o / arthr / o / pathy
  WR   CV   WR   CV   S

  oste / o / arthr / o / pathy
  WR   CV   WR   CV   S
     CF   CF

- **Defining**
  1. Apply the meaning of each word part contained in the term
  2. Begin by defining the suffix, then move to the beginning of the term

  oste / o / arthr / o / pathy
  WR   CV   WR   CV   S

  disease of the **bone** and **joint**

- **Building**
  1. When given the definition of a term, place word parts together to form the term; the beginning of the definition usually indicates the suffix
  2. Add combining vowels

  disease of the **bone** and **joint**

  oste / _ / arthr / _ / pathy
  WR / CV / WR / CV / S

  oste / o / arthr / o / pathy
  WR / CV / WR / CV / S

EXERCISE 12 ■ Build

Using Table 1.4 Word Parts List as a reference, complete A and B. *To check your answers, go to Appendix A.*

A

Fill in the blanks with word parts defined to label the illustration.

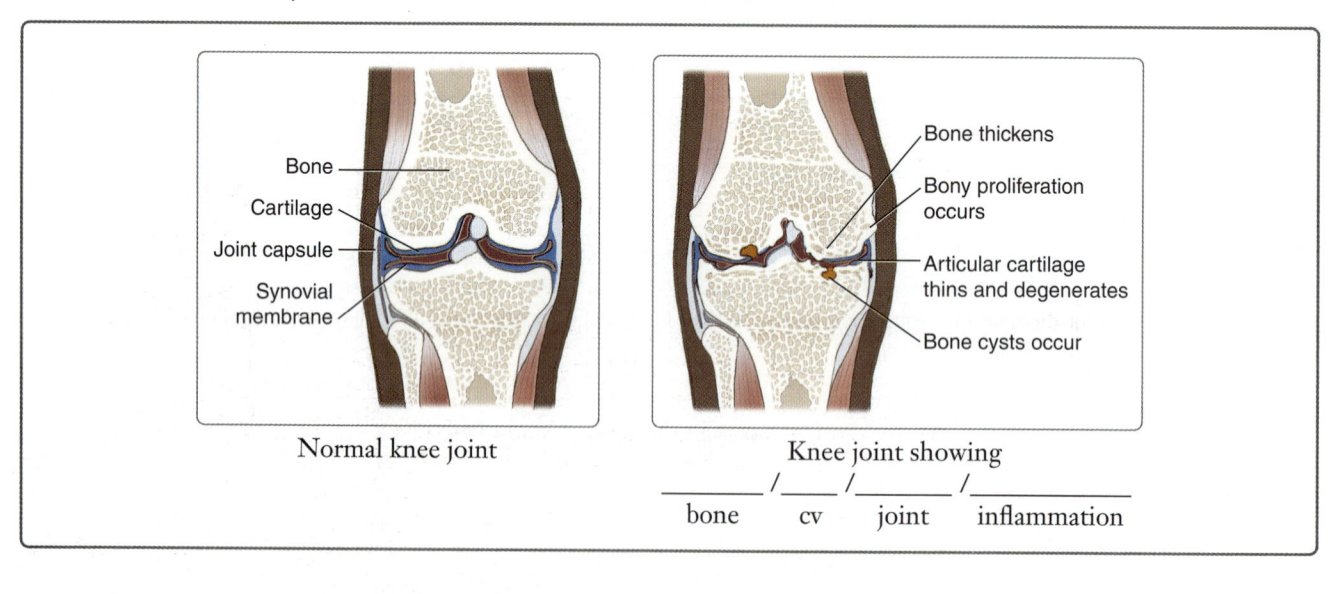

Normal knee joint

Knee joint showing
_____ / ____ / _____ / _____
 bone   cv   joint   inflammation

B

Build medical terms for the following definitions.

EXAMPLE: disease of a joint   arthr / o / pathy
                                    WR / CV / S

> At this time, do not be concerned about which word root goes first when building a term that contains two word roots. The order is usually dictated by common practice; for surgical or diagnostic terms, word roots are sometimes arranged by the order of function or by the order in which an instrument may encounter a structure. As you practice and learn, you will become accustomed to the accepted order.

1. inflammation of a joint — WR / S

2. pertaining to the liver — WR / S

3. pertaining to under the liver — P / WR / S

4. pertaining to within the vein — P / WR / S

5. inflammation of the bone — WR / S

6. inflammation of the liver — WR / S

7. disease of the bone and joint — WR / CV / WR / CV / S

8. enlargement of the liver — WR / CV / S

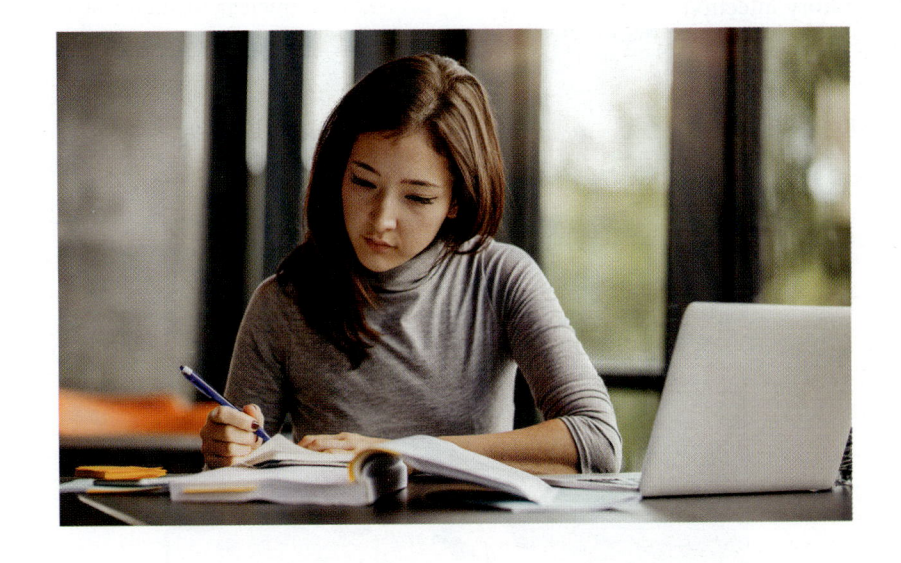

MEDICAL TERMS *NOT* BUILT FROM WORD PARTS

Medical terms categorized as NOT Built from Word Parts are terms that cannot be easily translated to find their meanings. In other words, terms appearing on these lists are not easily understood from the definition of word parts. In some cases, the term is a whole word in English, Greek, or Latin. In some cases, the term is an acronym. And in other instances, the recognizable word parts no longer give an indication of the term's current meaning.

Types of Terms NOT Built from Word Parts

There are several types of terms categorized as NOT Built from Word Parts, including:

1. **Eponyms,** terms derived from the name of a person or place, such as Apgar score and West Nile virus.
2. **Acronyms,** terms formed from the first letter of words in a phrase that can be spoken as a whole word and that usually contain a vowel, such as MRSA (methicillin-resistant *Staphylococcus aureus*).
3. **Modern language,** terms derived from the English language such as complete blood count with differential.
4. **Terms made up of Greek and Latin word parts that cannot be easily translated to find their meaning,** such as orthopedic. Orth/o/ped/ic is made up of three word parts: orth/o meaning straight, ped/o meaning child or foot, and -ic meaning pertaining to. Translated literally, **orthopedic** means **pertaining to a straight child or foot,** whereas its meaning as used today is a **branch of medicine dealing with the study and treatment of diseases and abnormalities of the musculoskeletal system.** Because it cannot be translated from word parts to understand its meaning, the term orthopedic is categorized as NOT Built from Word Parts in this textbook.

> Some terms containing recognizable word parts are categorized as NOT Built from Word Parts because they are difficult to translate for an understanding of their current meanings.

Learning Terms NOT Built from Word Parts

Memorization is the primary method for learning terms NOT Built from Word Parts. A variety of exercises are offered to assist with memorization and cultivation of long-term memory. Label exercises, where the medical concept is depicted with the term's definition, are a student favorite. Writing the correct term to label an image allows for a visual association and provides another way to remember its meaning. Using the learning tools available on Evolve Resources can be particularly effective in learning the meanings of terms NOT Built from Word Parts.

EXERCISE 13 ■ Identify

Place a check mark in the space provided to identify terms NOT Built from Word Parts. This may be the first time you have seen some of these terms. Apply your newly acquired knowledge and see how you do. *To check your answers, go to Appendix A.*

1. _____ arthritis
2. _____ upper respiratory infection
3. _____ Lyme disease
4. _____ AIDS
5. _____ macular degeneration
6. _____ hepatitis
7. _____ nuclear medicine scanner
8. _____ malignant
9. _____ osteopathy
10. _____ Alzheimer disease

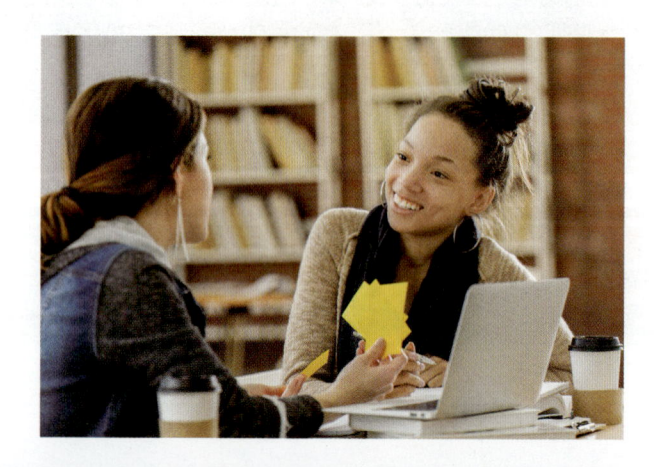

CHAPTER REVIEW

REVIEW OF CATEGORIES OF MEDICAL TERMS

Terms Built from Word Parts—can be translated to find their meaning

Terms NOT Built from Word Parts—cannot be translated easily to find their meaning

REVIEW OF MEDICAL TERMS BUILT FROM WORD PARTS

Word root—core of a word; example, **hepat**

Suffix—attached to the end of a word root to modify its meaning; example, **-ic**

Prefix—attached to the beginning of a word root to modify its meaning; example, **sub-**

Combining vowel—usually an o used between two word roots or a word root and suffix to ease pronunciation; example, hepat **o** pathy

Combining form—word root plus combining vowel separated by a slash; example, **hepat/o**

Analyzing—dividing medical terms into word parts, then labeling each word part and combining form

Defining—applying the meaning of each word part contained in the medical term to derive its meaning

Building—placing word parts together to form terms

REVIEW OF MEDICAL TERMS *NOT* BUILT FROM WORD PARTS

Eponyms—name of a person or place; examples, Apgar score and West Nile virus

Acronyms—from first letter of words; example, MRSA

Modern language—terms derived from the English language; example, complete blood count with differential

Terms made up of Greek and Latin word parts not easily translated; example, orthopedic

REVIEW OF OBJECTIVES

To complete this chapter successfully, you do not need to know what the word parts, such as *arthr*, mean. You will learn these in subsequent chapters. **It is important that you have met these objectives:**

1. Can you describe the origins of medical language?	yes ☐	no ☐
2. Can you define two categories of medical terms?	yes ☐	no ☐
3. Can you identify and define the four word parts and combining form?	yes ☐	no ☐
4. Can you use word parts to analyze and define medical terms?	yes ☐	no ☐
5. Can you use word parts to build medical terms for a given definition?	yes ☐	no ☐

If you answered yes to these questions, you need no further practice because you will be using these concepts repeatedly as you work your way through this text. Refer to this chapter to refresh your memory as needed. Move on to Chapter 2 and begin to build your medical vocabulary.

PART 1 INTRODUCTION TO WORD PARTS AND HUMAN BODY STRUCTURE

2 Body Structure, Oncology, and Laboratory Tests

Objectives

Upon completion of this chapter, you will be able to:

1. Pronounce anatomic structures of the human body.
2. Define and spell word parts related to body structure, color, oncology, and laboratory tests.
3. Define, pronounce, and spell body structure terms.
4. Define, pronounce, and spell oncology terms.
5. Define, pronounce, and spell laboratory terms.
6. Define, pronounce, and spell complementary terms related to body structure, color, oncology, and laboratory tests.
7. Identify and use singular and plural endings.
8. Interpret the meaning of abbreviations related to body structure, oncology, and laboratory tests.
9. Apply medical language in clinical contexts.

TABLE 2.1 Body Systems, 18
TABLE 2.2 Pronunciation Key, 20
TABLE 2.3 Cancer Therapies, 37
TABLE 2.4 Types of Laboratory Tests, 40
TABLE 2.5 Common Plural Endings for Medical Terms, 52

Outline

ANATOMY, 17
Organization of the Body, 17
Body Cavities, 19

WORD PARTS, 20
Body Structure Combining Forms, 20
Combining Forms Used with Body Structure Terms, 21
Color Combining Forms, 21
Prefixes, 21
Suffixes, 21

MEDICAL TERMS, 28
Body Structure Terms, 28
  Built from Word Parts, 28
Oncology, 31
Oncology Terms, 32
  Built from Word Parts, 32
  NOT Built from Word Parts, 36
Laboratory Tests, 40
Laboratory Terms, 41
  Built from Word Parts and
    NOT Built from Word Parts, 41
Complementary Terms, 45
  Built from Word Parts, 45
  NOT Built from Word Parts, 48
Plural Endings for Medical Terms, 51
Abbreviations, 53

PRACTICAL APPLICATION, 54
CASE STUDY Translate Between Everyday Language and Medical Language, 54
Interact with Medical Documents, 55
Use Medical Terms in Clinical Statements, 56
Pronounce Medical Terms in Use, 57

CHAPTER REVIEW, 57
Chapter Content Quiz, 57
Chapter at a Glance, 58

Answers to Chapter Exercises, Appendix A

Chapter 2 Body Structure, Oncology, and Laboratory Tests

ANATOMY

Organization of the Body

The structure of the human body falls into the following four categories: cells, tissues, organs, and systems. Each structure is a highly organized unit of smaller structures.

TERM	DEFINITION
cell (sel)	basic unit of all living things (Fig. 2.1). The human body is composed of trillions of cells, which vary in size and shape according to function.
cell membrane (sel) (MEM-brān)	forms the boundary of the cell
cytoplasm (SĪ-tō-*plas*-em)	gel-like fluid inside the cell
nucleus (NŪ-klē-us)	largest structure within the cell, usually spherical and centrally located. It contains chromosomes for cellular reproduction and is the control center for cellular activity.
chromosomes (KRŌ-ma-sōms)	threadlike structures located in the nucleus of the cell. There are 46 chromosomes in all normal human cells, with the exception of mature sex cells, which have 23.
genes (JĒNS)	regions within the chromosome containing sequences of DNA. Each chromosome has several thousand genes that determine hereditary characteristics.
DNA (D-N-A)	long, complex molecule containing genetic material that regulates the activities of the cell. DNA is the abbreviation for deoxyribonucleic acid.
tissue (TISH-ū)	group of similar cells that performs a specific function
muscle tissue (MUS-el) (TISH-ū)	group of similar cells that has a special ability to contract, usually producing movement
nerve tissue (nurv) (TISH-ū)	group of similar cells that receives and transmits electrochemical signals; found in the nerves, spinal cord, and brain. It is responsible for coordinating and controlling body activities.
connective tissue (ke-NEK-tiv) (TISH-ū)	group of similar cells that attaches, supports, penetrates, and encases various body structures. Adipose (fat), osseous (bone) tissues, and blood are types of connective tissue. Fibrous tissue is a type of connective tissue that provides strength and stability, such as in ligaments and tendons.
epithelial tissue (*ep*-i-THĒ-lē-al) (TISH-ū)	group of similar cells that covers the external surface of the body, forms membranes that line body cavities and organs, and is the primary tissue in glands. Glandular tissue is designed to secrete substances such as digestive enzymes.

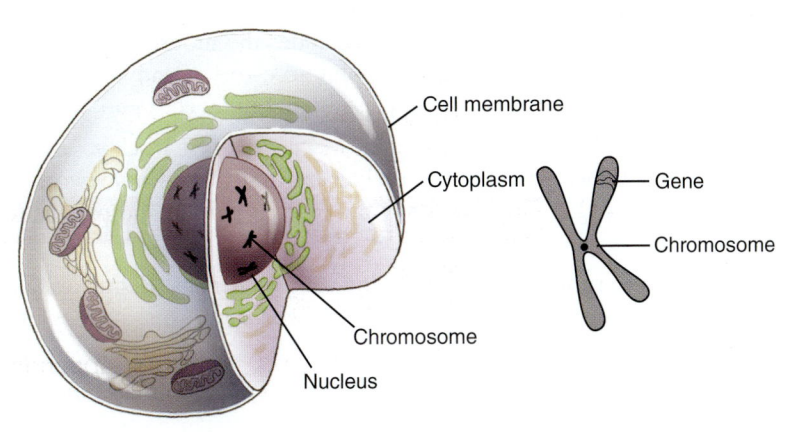

FIG. 2.1 Body cell.

CHROMOSOME is derived from the Greek **chromos**, meaning **color**, and **soma**, meaning **body**. German anatomist Waldeyer first used the term in 1888.

Organization of the Body—cont'd

TERM	DEFINITION
organ (OR-gen)	two or more types of tissues that together perform special body functions. For example, the skin is an organ composed of epithelial, connective, muscle, and nervous tissue.
viscera (VIS-er-a)	large internal organs contained in the body cavities, especially in the abdominal cavity
system (SIS-tem)	group of organs that works together to perform complex body functions. For example, the cardiovascular system consists of the heart, blood vessels, and blood. Its function is to transport nutrients and oxygen to the cells and remove carbon dioxide and other waste products (Table 2.1).

MEDICAL GENOMICS

A **genome** is the complete set of information in the DNA of a specific organism. Experts in **genomics** study the genome to determine its DNA sequences and perform genetic mapping to help understand disease. **Medical genomics** is an emerging discipline that uses a person's individual genome as part of their clinical care. Genomic medicine is being used in areas such as oncology, pharmacology, and infectious disease.

Gene therapy is an experimental procedure to treat or prevent disease. Possible treatments may include replacing a mutated gene with a healthy one, inactivating a mutated gene that doesn't function properly, or introducing a new gene into the body to help fight a disease. The technique remains risky and is currently being tested only for diseases that have no other cures.

TABLE 2.1 Body Systems

BODY SYSTEMS	ORGANS AND FUNCTION
INTEGUMENTARY SYSTEM	Composed of skin, hair, nails, and glands. Forms a protective covering for the body, regulates body temperature, and helps manufacture vitamin D.
RESPIRATORY SYSTEM	Composed of nose, pharynx (throat), larynx (voice box), trachea (windpipe), bronchial tubes, and lungs. Performs respiration, which provides for the exchange of oxygen and carbon dioxide within the body.
URINARY SYSTEM	Composed of kidneys, ureters, bladder, and urethra. Removes waste material (urine) from the body, regulates fluid volume, and maintains electrolyte concentration.
REPRODUCTIVE SYSTEM	Female reproductive system is composed of ovaries, uterine tubes, uterus, vagina, and mammary glands. Male reproductive system is composed of testes, urethra, penis, prostate gland, and associated tubes. Responsible for heredity and reproduction.
CARDIOVASCULAR SYSTEM	Composed of the heart and blood vessels. Pumps and transports blood throughout the body.
LYMPHATIC/IMMUNE SYSTEM	Composed of a network of vessels, ducts, nodes, and organs. Provides for defense against infection and drainage of extracellular fluid.
DIGESTIVE SYSTEM	Composed of the gastrointestinal tract, which includes the mouth, esophagus, stomach, small and large intestines, and anus, plus accessory organs, liver, gallbladder, and pancreas. Prepares food for use by the body cells and eliminates waste.
MUSCULOSKELETAL SYSTEM	Composed of muscle, bones, and joints. Provides movement and framework for the body, protects vital organs such as the brain, stores calcium, and produces red blood cells.
NERVOUS SYSTEM	Composed of the brain, spinal cord, nerves, and sensory organs. Regulates specific body activities by sending and receiving messages. Sensory organs, such as the eye and ear, are also part of the nervous system.
ENDOCRINE SYSTEM	Composed of glands that secrete hormones. Hormones regulate many specific body activities.

Body Cavities

The body is not a solid structure as it appears on the outside, but has five cavities (Fig. 2.2), each containing an orderly arrangement of the internal organs.

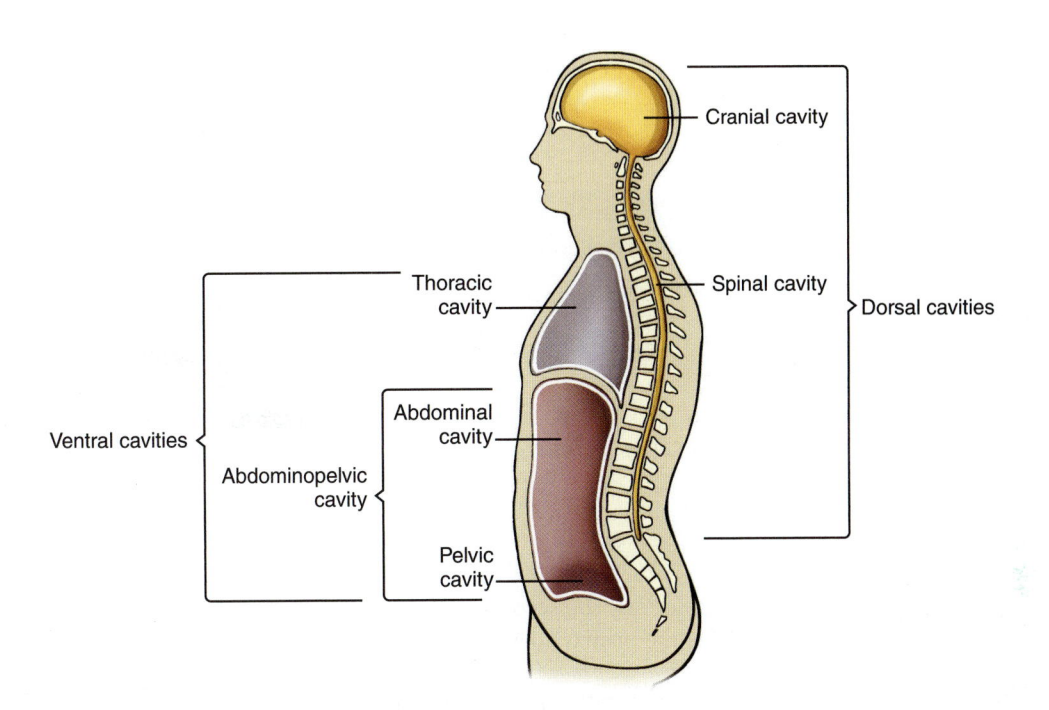

FIG. 2.2 Body cavities.

TERM	DEFINITION
cranial cavity (KRĀ-nē-al) (KAV-i-tē)	space inside the skull (cranium) containing the brain
spinal cavity (SPĪ-nal) (KAV-i-tē)	space inside the spinal column containing the spinal cord
thoracic cavity (thō-RAS-ic) (KAV-i-tē)	space containing the heart, aorta, lungs, esophagus, trachea, bronchi, and mediastinal area
abdominal cavity (ab-DOM-i-nal) (KAV-i-tē)	space containing the stomach, intestines, kidneys, adrenal glands, liver, gallbladder, pancreas, spleen, and ureters
pelvic cavity (PEL-vik) (KAV-i-tē)	space containing the urinary bladder, certain reproductive organs, parts of the small and large intestine, and the anus
abdominopelvic cavity (ab-*dom*-i-nō-PEL-vik) (KAV-i-tē)	both the pelvic and abdominal cavities

PRONOUNCE ANATOMIC STRUCTURES

Practice saying aloud each of the Organization of the Body Terms on the previous pages.

To hear the terms, go to Evolve Resources at www.evolve.elsevier.com and select:
Student Resources > Audio Glossary > Chapter 2 > Anatomic Structures

❏ Check the box when complete.

TABLE 2.2 Pronunciation Key

GUIDELINES	EXAMPLES
1. Words are distorted minimally to indicate proper phonetic sound.	doctor (dok-tor)
2. The macron (¯) indicates the long vowel sound.	donate (dō-nāte) ā as in say ō as in no ē as in me ū as in cute ī as in spine
3. Vowels with no markings should have a short sound.	cell (sel) a as in sad o as in top e as in get u as in cut i as in sit
4. Primary accents are indicated by capital letters; the secondary accent (which is stressed, but not as strongly as the primary accent) is indicated by italics. *There may be geographical variations in pronunciation.*	altogether (*all*-tū-GETH-er) pancreatitis (*pan*-krē-a-TĪ-tis)

WORD PARTS

Use paper flashcards or electronic flashcards on Evolve to assist with memorization of word parts used to analyze, define, and build terms presented in this chapter. To reinforce learning, study one section of the Word Part Table at a time, and then complete the corresponding exercise on the following pages.

1 ■ Body Structure Combining Forms

COMBINING FORM	DEFINITION	COMBINING FORM	DEFINITION
aden/o	gland, glandular tissue	**my/o**	muscle(s), muscle tissue
cyt/o	cell(s)	**neur/o**	nerve(s), nerve tissue
epitheli/o	epithelium, epithelial tissue	**organ/o**	organ
fibr/o	fiber(s), fibrous tissue	**sarc/o**	flesh, connective tissue
hemat/o	blood	**system/o**	system
hist/o	tissue(s)	**viscer/o**	internal organs
lip/o	fat, fat tissue		

2 ■ Combining Forms Used with Body Structure Terms

COMBINING FORM	DEFINITION
aut/o	self
bi/o	life
cancer/o	cancer
carcin/o	cancer
CANCER is a disease characterized by the unregulated, abnormal growth of new cells	
crypt/o	hidden
necr/o	death (cells, body)
eti/o	cause (of disease)

COMBINING FORM	DEFINITION
gno/o	knowledge
iatr/o	physician, medicine (also means treatment)
lei/o	smooth
onc/o	tumor, mass
path/o	disease
rhabd/o	rod-shaped, striated
somat/o	body
vir/o	virus

3 ■ Color Combining Forms

COMBINING FORM	DEFINITION
cyan/o	blue
erythr/o	red
leuk/o	white

COMBINING FORM	DEFINITION
melan/o	black
xanth/o	yellow

4 ■ Prefixes

PREFIX	DEFINITION
dia-	through, complete
dys-	painful, abnormal, difficult, labored
hyper-	above, excessive
hypo-	below, incomplete, deficient, under

PREFIX	DEFINITION
meta-	after, beyond, change
micro-	small
neo-	new
pro-	before

5 ■ Suffixes

SUFFIX	DEFINITION
-al, -ic, -ous	pertaining to
-cyte	cell (Note: the combining form for cell is cyt/o; the suffix for cell is -cyte, ending with an e.)
-gen	substance or agent that produces or causes
-genic	producing, originating, causing
-logist	one who studies and treats (specialist, physician)
-logy	study of
-megaly	enlargement
-oid	resembling
-oma	tumor, swelling

SUFFIX	DEFINITION
-opsy	view of, viewing
-osis	abnormal condition (means *increase* when used with blood cell word roots)
-pathy	disease (Note: the combining form for disease is path/o; the suffix for disease is -pathy, ending with a y.)
-plasia	condition of formation, development, growth
-plasm	growth, substance, formation
-sarcoma	malignant tumor
-sis	state of
-stasis	control, stop, standing

Refer to **Appendix B** and **Appendix C** for alphabetical lists of word parts and their meanings.

Chapter 2 Body Structure, Oncology, and Laboratory Tests

EXERCISE 1 ■ Body Structure Combining Forms

Refer to the first section of the word parts table.

> Reminder: the word root is the core of the word. The combining form is the word root with the combining vowel attached, separated by a vertical slash.

A Label

Fill in the blanks with combining forms in this diagram of types of tissues.
To check your answers, go to Appendix A at the back of the textbook.

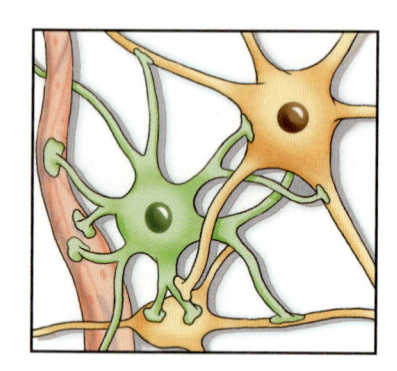

1. Nerve
   CF: _____

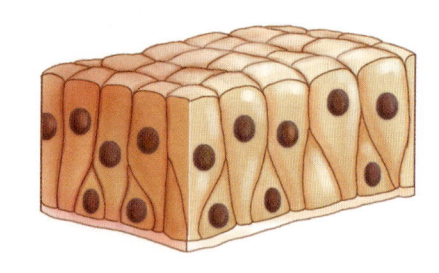

2. Epithelium
   CF: _____

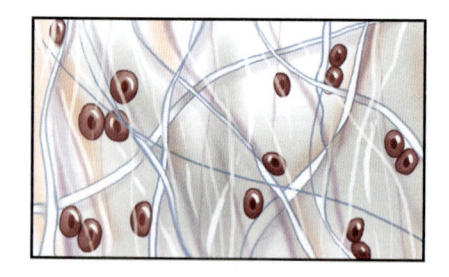

3. Connective
   CF: _____

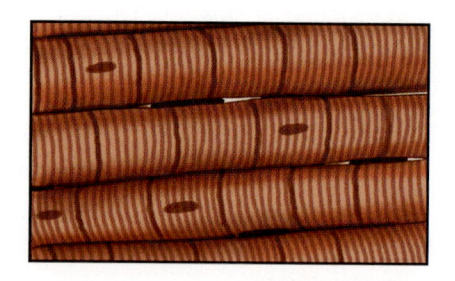

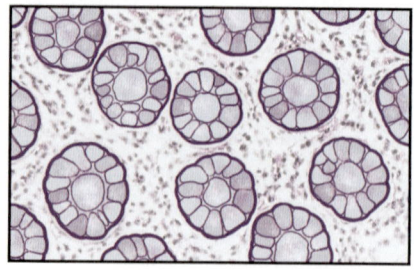

4. Muscle
   CF: _____

5. Gland
   CF: _____

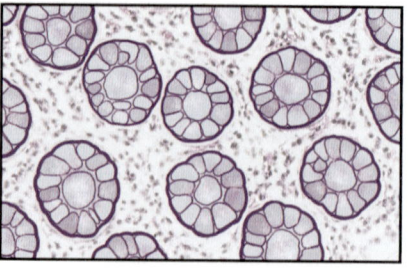

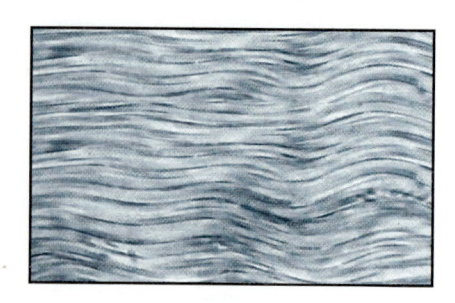

6. Fiber
   CF: _____

Chapter 2 Body Structure, Oncology, and Laboratory Tests   23

B Label

Fill in the blanks with combining forms in this diagram of the organization of the body.

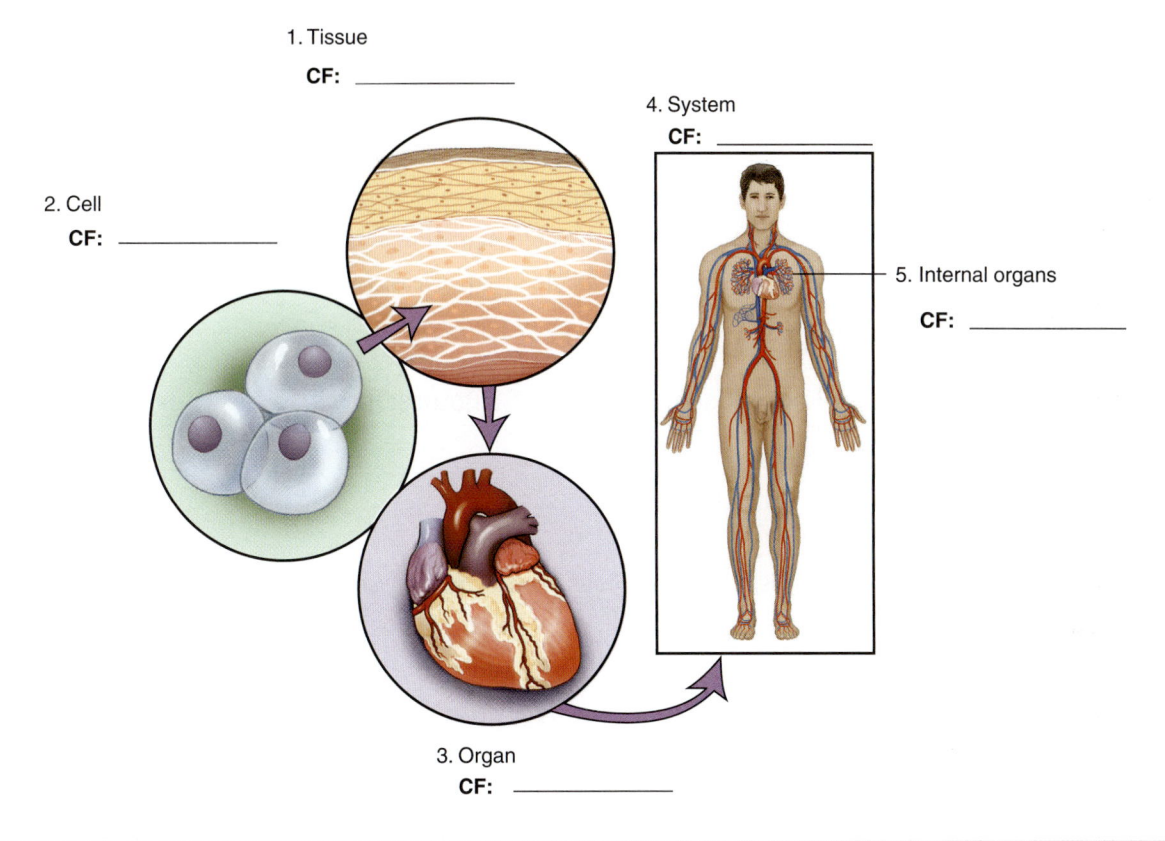

1. Tissue
   CF: _____

2. Cell
   CF: _____

3. Organ
   CF: _____

4. System
   CF: _____

5. Internal organs
   CF: _____

C Define and Match

Step 1: Write the definitions after the following combining forms.
Step 2: Match the descriptions on the right with the combining forms and definitions.

_d_ 1. sarc/o, _flesh, connective tissue_ _____   a. produces movement
____ 2. lip/o, _____   b. group of similar cells
____ 3. viscer/o, _____   c. contained in body cavities
____ 4. cyt/o, _____   d. type of connective tissue
____ 5. hist/o, _____   e. tissue that encases various structures
____ 6. my/o, _____   f. basic unit of all living things

Chapter 2 Body Structure, Oncology, and Laboratory Tests

D Define and Match

Step 1: Write the definitions after the following combining forms.
Step 2: Match the descriptions on the right with the combining forms and definitions.

____c____ 1. neur/o, _nerve_ _____ a. primary tissue in glands
_____ 2. organ/o, _____ b. connective tissue found in ligaments
_____ 3. system/o, _____ c. responsible for coordinating and controlling body activities
_____ 4. epitheli/o, _____ d. group of organs working together
_____ 5. fibr/o, _____ e. tissue designed to secrete something
_____ 6. aden/o, _____ f. made up of at least two kinds of tissues
_____ 7. hemat/o, _____ g. type of connective tissue

EXERCISE 2 ■ Combining Forms Used with Body Structure Terms

Refer to the second section of the word parts table.

A Define

Write the definitions of the following combining forms. *To check your answers, go to Appendix A at the back of the textbook.*

1. onc/o _____
2. carcin/o _____
3. eti/o _____
4. path/o _____
5. somat/o _____
6. cancer/o _____
7. rhabd/o _____
8. lei/o _____
9. gno/o _____
10. iatr/o _____
11. bi/o _____
12. vir/o _____
13. aut/o _____
14. necr/o _____

🏛 CANCER
Carcin and **cancer** are derived from Latin and Greek words meaning **crab**. They originated before the nature of malignant growth was understood. One explanation was that the swollen blood vessels around the diseased area looked like the claws of a crab.

B Identify

Write the combining form for each of the following.

1. disease _____
2. tumor, mass _____
3. cause (of disease) _____
4. cancer a. _____
           b. _____
5. body _____
6. smooth _____
7. rod-shaped, striated _____
8. knowledge _____
9. physician, medicine _____
10. self _____
11. virus _____
12. life _____
13. death _____

Chapter 2   Body Structure, Oncology, and Laboratory Tests   25

EXERCISE 3 ■ Color Combining Forms

Refer to the third section of the word parts table.

A Define

Write the definitions of the following combining forms. *To check your answers, go to Appendix A at the back of the textbook.*

1. cyan/o _____
2. erythr/o _____
3. leuk/o _____
4. xanth/o _____
5. melan/o _____

> **ERYTHR/O** Aristotle noted "two colors of blood" and applied the term **erythros** to the dark red blood.

B Identify

Write the combining form for each of the following.

1. blue _____
2. red _____
3. white _____
4. black _____
5. yellow _____

EXERCISE 4 ■ Prefixes

Refer to the fourth section of the word parts table.

> Reminder: prefixes are placed at the beginning of word roots to modify their meanings.

A Define

Write the definitions of the following prefixes. *To check your answers, go to Appendix A at the back of the textbook.*

1. neo- _____
2. hyper- _____
3. meta- _____
4. hypo- _____
5. dys- _____
6. dia- _____
7. pro- _____
8. micro- _____

B Identify

Write the prefix for each of the following.

1. new _____
2. above, excessive _____
3. below, incomplete, deficient, under _____
4. after, beyond, change _____
5. painful, abnormal, difficult, labored _____
6. through, complete _____
7. before _____
8. small _____

Chapter 2 Body Structure, Oncology, and Laboratory Tests

EXERCISE 5 ■ Suffixes

Refer to the fifth section of the word parts table.

> Reminder: suffixes are placed at the end of word roots to modify their meanings.

A Label

Write the suffixes pictured and defined. *To check your answers, go to Appendix A at the back of the textbook.*

1. _____
   cell

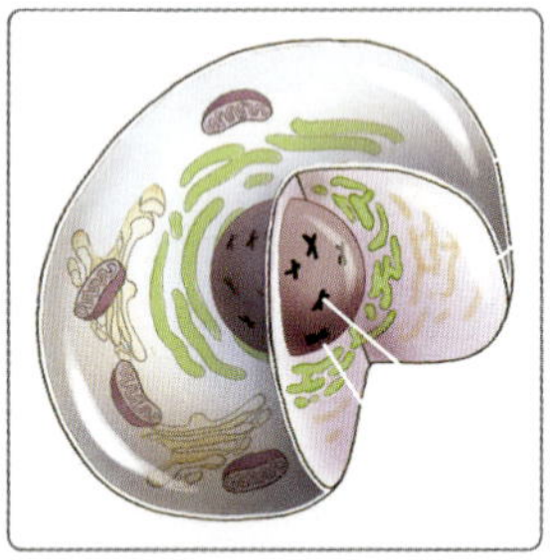

2. _____
   condition of formation, development, growth

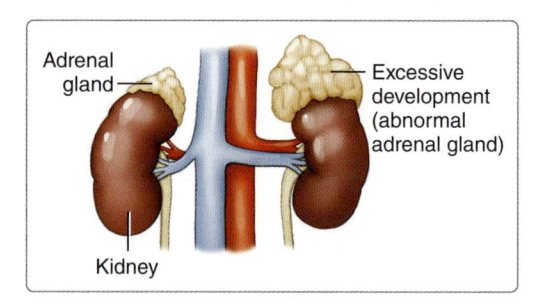

3. _____
   one who studies and treats (specialist, physician)

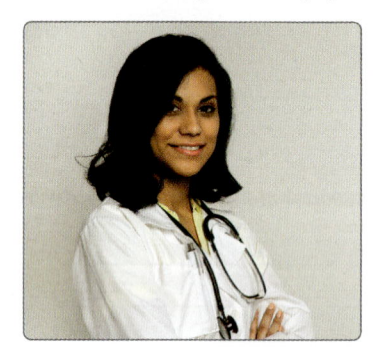

4. _____
   study of

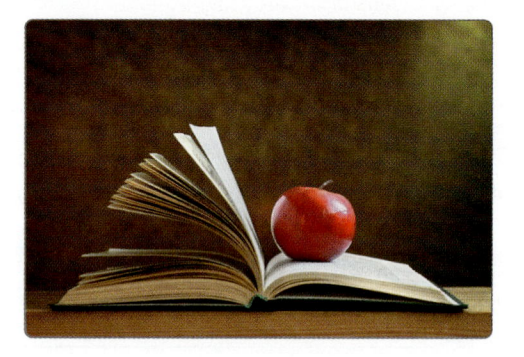

5. _____
   enlargement

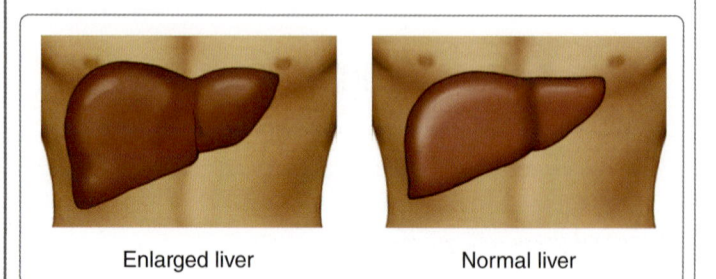

6. _____
   tumor, swelling

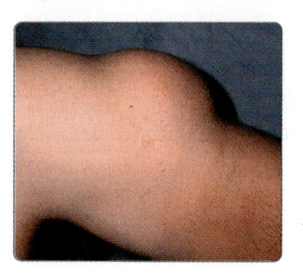

B Match

Match the suffixes in the first column with their correct definitions in the second column.

_____ 1. -osis   a. producing, originating, causing
_____ 2. -pathy   b. growth, substance, formation
_____ 3. -plasm   c. pertaining to
_____ 4. -al, -ic, -ous d. resembling
_____ 5. -stasis   e. control, stop, standing
_____ 6. -oid   f. substance that produces
_____ 7. -gen   g. abnormal condition
_____ 8. -sarcoma   h. state of
_____ 9. -genic   i. malignant tumor
_____ 10. -sis   j. disease
_____ 11. -opsy   k. view of, viewing

> In some instances, suffixes have embedded word roots. For example, the suffix **-pathy** is made up of the word root **path** and the noun ending **-y**. When analyzing medical terms, use the suffix presented in the word parts table. For example, myopathy will be divided as my/o/pathy using the suffix -pathy.

C Define

Write the definitions of the following suffixes.

1. -logist _____   11. -plasia _____
2. -pathy _____   12. -oid _____
3. -logy _____   13. -gen _____
4. -ic _____   14. -genic _____
5. -stasis _____   15. -oma _____
6. -cyte _____   16. -sarcoma _____
7. -osis _____   17. -sis _____
8. -ous _____   18. –megaly _____
9. -plasm _____   19. -opsy _____
10. -al _____

> The suffix **-logist** may indicate a specialist **who is not a physician**, such as a **psychologist**, or a specialist **who is a physician**, such as an **oncologist**. If the specialist is a physician, it will be indicated in the definition. For example, the term **oncologist** is defined as: physician who studies and treats (malignant) tumors.

> Practice two things in your dealings with disease: either help or do not harm the patient.—**Hippocrates** 460–375 BC

MEDICAL TERMS

Medical terms relevant to this chapter have been grouped by topics, such as Body Structure, and are listed in tables designated as Built from Word Parts or NOT Built from Word Parts. The exercises following each table assist with learning term definitions, pronunciations, and spellings.

Body Structure Terms
BUILT FROM WORD PARTS

The following terms can be translated using definitions of word parts. Further explanation is provided within parentheses as needed.

TERM	DEFINITION	TERM	DEFINITION
1. **cytogenic** (sī-tō-JEN-ik)	producing cells	11. **leukocytosis** (lū-kō-sī-TŌ-sis)	increase in the number of white (blood) cells
2. **cytology** (sī-TOL-o-jē)	study of cells	12. **lipoid** (LIP-oid)	resembling fat
3. **dysplasia** (dis-PLĀ-zha)	abnormal development (Fig. 2.4)	13. **myopathy** (mī-OP-a-thē)	disease of the muscle
4. **epithelial** (ep-i-THĒ-lē-al)	pertaining to epithelium	14. **necrosis** (ne-KRŌ-sis)	abnormal condition of cell death (cells and tissue die because of disease)
5. **erythrocyte (RBC)** (e-RITH-rō-sīt)	red (blood) cell	15. **neuropathy** (nū-ROP-a-thē)	disease of the nerves
6. **erythrocytosis** (e-rith-rō-sī-TŌ-sis)	increase in the number of red (blood) cells	16. **organomegaly** (or-ga-nō-MEG-a-lē)	enlargement of an organ
7. **histology** (his-TOL-o-jē)	study of tissue	17. **somatic** (sō-MAT-ik)	pertaining to the body
8. **hyperplasia** (hī-per-PLĀ-zha)	excessive development (number of cells) (Fig. 2.4)	18. **somatogenic** (sō-ma-tō-JEN-ik)	originating in the body (organic as opposed to originating in the mind)
9. **hypoplasia** (hī-pō-PLĀ-zha)	incomplete development (of an organ or tissues)	19. **systemic** (sis-TEM-ik)	pertaining to a (body) system (or the body as a whole)
10. **leukocyte (WBC)** (LŪ-kō-sīt)	white (blood) cell	20. **visceral** (VIS-er-al)	pertaining to the internal organs

💡 **Ellipsis** is the practice of omitting an essential part of a word by common consent. Note this practice in the terms **erythrocyte** (red **blood** cell) and **leukocyte** (white **blood** cell). The word root for blood is omitted.

EXERCISE 6 ■ Pronounce and Spell

Practice pronunciation and spelling on paper and online.

1. **Practice on Paper**
   a. **Pronounce:** Read the phonetic spelling and say aloud the terms listed in the previous table. Refer to Table 2.2 Pronunciation Key as needed.
   b. **Spell:** Have a study partner read the terms aloud. Write the spelling of the terms on a separate sheet of paper.

Chapter 2 Body Structure, Oncology, and Laboratory Tests   29

2. **Practice Online** 🌐
   a. **Access** online learning resources. Go to evolve.elsevier.com > Evolve Resources > Student Resources.
   b. **Pronounce:** Select Audio Glossary > Chapter 2 > Exercise 6. Select a term to hear its pronunciation and repeat aloud.
   c. **Spell:** Select Activities > Chapter 2 > Spell Terms > Exercise 6. Select the audio icon and type the correct spelling of the term.

❑ Check the box when complete.

EXERCISE 7 ■ Analyze and Define

Analyze and define the following body structure terms by drawing slashes between word parts, writing word part abbreviations above the term, underlining combining forms, and writing combining form abbreviations below the term. Refer to Chapter 1 to review analyzing and defining techniques. *This is an important exercise; do not skip any portion of it.* *To check your answers, go to Appendix A at the back of the textbook.*

```
              WR  CV   S
EXAMPLE:    cyt / o / genic
              CF
            producing cells
```

1. cytology

2. histology

3. visceral

4. hypoplasia

5. neuropathy

6. systemic

7. somatic

8. somatogenic

9. epithelial

10. erythrocytosis

11. leukocytosis

12. myopathy

13. erythrocyte

14. leukocyte

EXERCISE 8 ■ Build

A Fill In

Build medical terms for the following body structure definitions by using the word parts you have learned. Refer to Chapter 1 to review medical term building techniques. **This is an integral part of the learning process; do not skip any part of this exercise.**

EXAMPLE: Example: producing cells $\frac{\text{cyt} / \text{o} / \text{genic}}{\text{WR} \quad \text{CV} \quad \text{S}}$

1. disease of the nerves ___ / ___ / ___
   WR / CV / S

2. study of cells ___ / ___ / ___
   WR / CV / S

3. pertaining to the body ___ / ___
   WR / S

4. disease of the muscle ___ / ___ / ___
   WR / CV / S

5. abnormal development ___ / ___
   P / S(WR)

> When analyzing medical terms that have a suffix containing a word root, it may appear, as in the word **dysplasia**, that the term is composed of only a prefix and a suffix. Keep in mind that the word root is embedded in the suffix and is indicated in the *Building Medical Terms* exercises by S(WR).

6. pertaining to the internal organs ___ / ___
   WR / S

7. originating in the body ___ / ___ / ___
   WR / CV / S

8. enlargement of an organ ___ / ___ / ___
   WR / CV / S

9. resembling fat ___ / ___
   WR / S

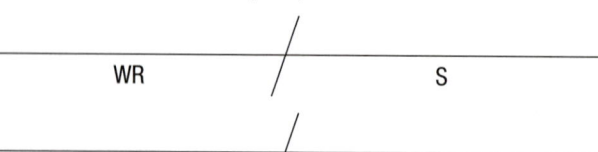

10. pertaining to a (body) system ___ / ___
    WR / S

B Label

Build terms pictured by writing word parts above the definitions.

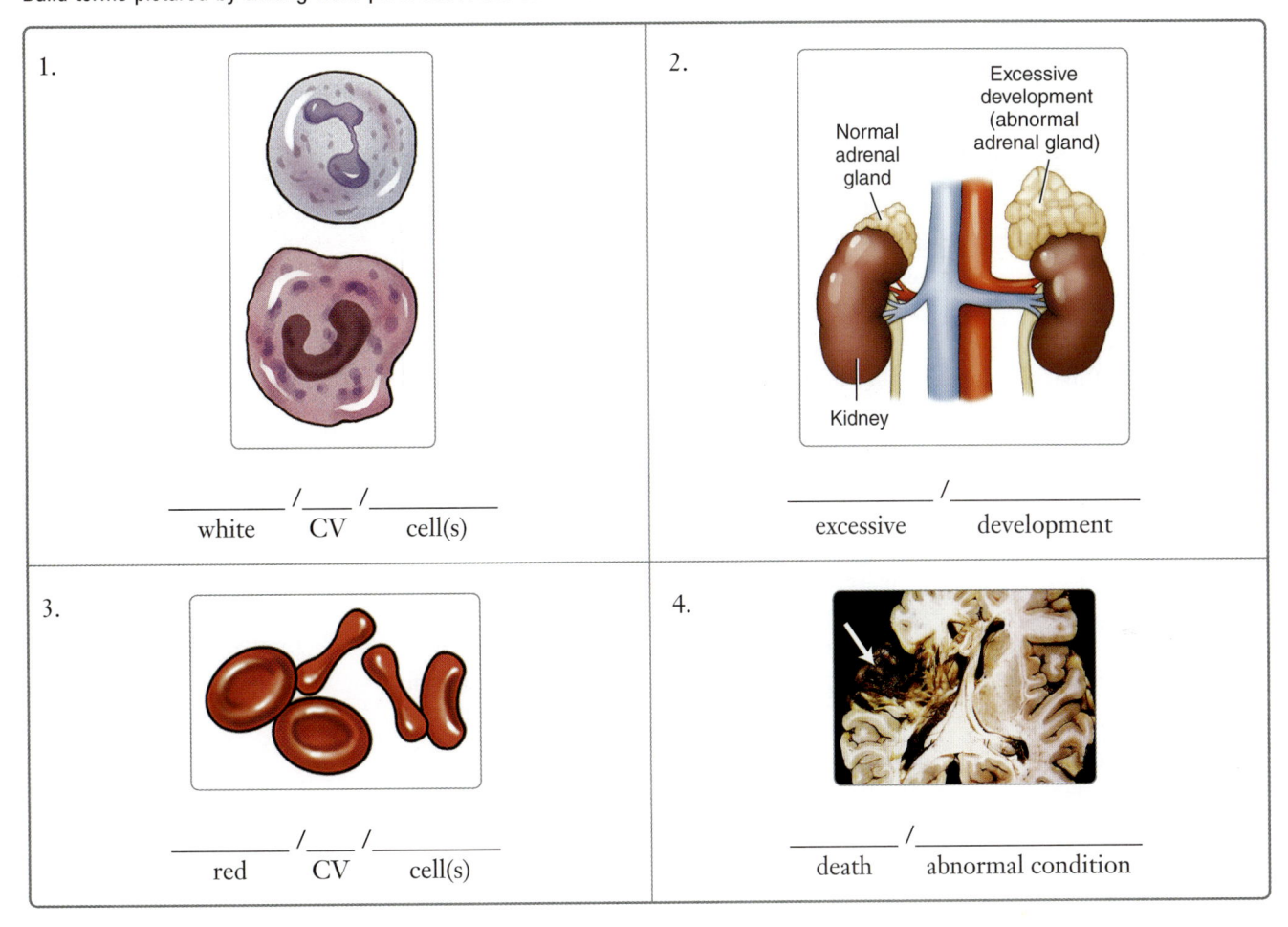

1.

_____ / ___ / _____
white   CV   cell(s)

2.

_____ / _____
excessive   development

3.

_____ / ___ / _____
red   CV   cell(s)

4.

_____ / _____
death   abnormal condition

EXERCISE 9 ■ Review of Body Structure Terms

Can you define, pronounce, and spell the following body structure terms?

cytogenic	erythrocytosis	leukocytosis	organomegaly
cytology	histology	lipoid	somatic
dysplasia	hyperplasia	myopathy	somatogenic
epithelial	hypoplasia	necrosis	systemic
erythrocyte (RBC)	leukocyte (WBC)	neuropathy	visceral

Oncology

Oncology is the study of tumors. Tumors can develop from excessive growth of cells. Tumors, or masses, can be benign (noncancerous) or malignant (cancerous). The names of tumors often include the word root for the body part and the suffix **-oma,** as in the term *my/oma,* which means "tumor composed of muscle." Oncology terms are introduced in this chapter because of their relation to cells and cell abnormalities. This is an introductory list only. **More oncology terms appear in subsequent chapters and are presented with the introduction of the related body systems.**

Oncology Terms
BUILT FROM WORD PARTS

The following terms can be translated using definitions of word parts. Further explanation is provided within parentheses as needed. *At first the list of terms may seem long to you; however, many of the word parts are repeated in many of the terms. You will soon find that knowing parts of the terms makes learning the words easy.* **Analyzing, defining,** and **building exercises** are used to learn these terms.

TERM	DEFINITION	TERM	DEFINITION
1. **adenocarcinoma** (ad-e-nō-*kar*-si-NŌ-ma)	cancerous tumor of glandular tissue	12. **metastasis** (*pl.* **metastases**) (**METS**) (me-TAS-ta-sis) (me-TAS-ta-sēz)	beyond control (transfer of cells from one organ to another, as in malignant tumors) (Fig. 2.3)
2. **adenoma** (ad-e-NŌ-ma)	tumor composed of glandular tissue (benign)		
3. **carcinoma (CA)** (kar-si-NŌ-ma)	cancerous tumor (malignant) (Fig. 2.3)	13. **myoma** (mī-Ō-ma)	tumor composed of muscle tissue (benign)
4. **epithelioma** (ep-i-*thē*-lē-Ō-ma)	tumor composed of epithelial tissue (may be benign or malignant)	14. **neoplasm** (NĒ-ō-plazm)	new growth (of abnormal tissue, benign or malignant)
5. **fibroma** (fī-BRŌ-ma)	tumor composed of fibrous tissue (benign)	15. **neuroma** (nū-RŌ-ma)	tumor composed of nerve tissue (benign)
6. **fibrosarcoma** (fī-brō-sar-KŌ-ma)	malignant tumor composed of fibrous tissue	16. **rhabdomyoma** (rab-dō-mī-Ō-ma)	tumor composed of striated muscle (benign)
7. **leiomyoma** (lī-ō-mī-Ō-ma)	tumor composed of smooth muscle (benign)	17. **rhabdomyosarcoma** (rab-dō-*mī*-ō-sar-KŌ-ma)	malignant tumor of striated muscle
8. **leiomyosarcoma** (lī-ō-*mī*-ō-sar-KŌ-ma)	malignant tumor of smooth muscle	18. **sarcoma** (sar-KŌ-ma)	tumor of connective tissue (such as bone or cartilage; highly malignant)
9. **lipoma** (li-PŌ-ma)	tumor composed of fat tissue (benign tumor)		
10. **liposarcoma** (lip-ō-sar-KŌ-ma)	malignant tumor of fat tissue		
11. **melanoma** (mel-a-NŌ-ma)	black tumor (primarily of the skin)		

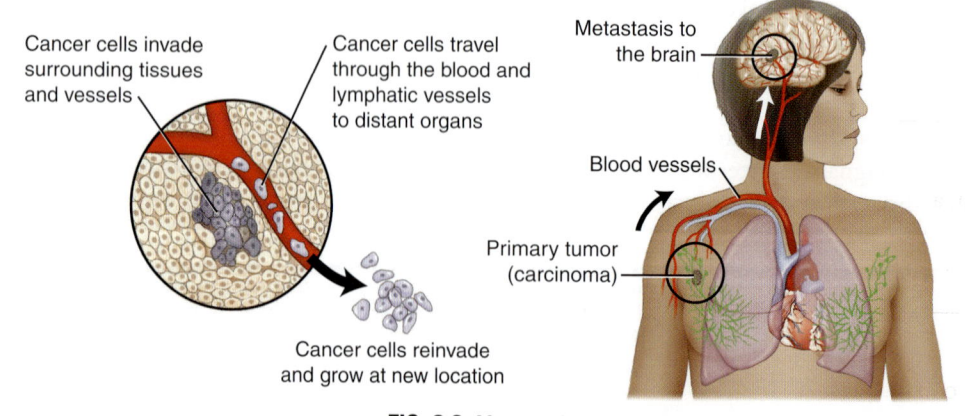

🏛 **SARCOMA** has been used since the time of ancient Greece to describe any fleshy tumor. Since the introduction of cellular pathology, the meaning has become **malignant connective tissue tumor**. Often, an additional word root is used to denote the type of tissue involved, such as **oste** in **osteosarcoma**, which refers to a malignant tumor of the bone.

FIG. 2.3 Metastasis.

Chapter 2 Body Structure, Oncology, and Laboratory Tests   33

TNM STAGING SYSTEM OF CANCER

AJCC (American Joint Committee on Cancer) has devised a classification widely used to stage certain types of cancer properly.
T refers to size and the extent of the primary tumor (ranked 0-4).
N denotes the involvement of the lymph nodes (ranked 0-4).
M defines whether there is metastasis (0 = none; 1 = present).
For example, $T_2 N_1 M_0$
T_2 refers to the primary tumor of 2 cm.
N_1 means spread of tumor to ipsilateral (same side) lymph nodes.
M_0 means no distant metastasis.
This system helps communicate the extent of cancer and is frequently cited by oncologists, surgeons, and radiation oncologists.

EXERCISE 10 ■ Pronounce and Spell

Practice pronunciation and spelling on paper and online.

1. **Practice on Paper**
   a. **Pronounce:** Read the phonetic spelling and say aloud the terms listed in the previous table. Refer to Table 2.2 Pronunciation Key as needed.
   b. **Spell:** Have a study partner read the terms aloud. Write the spelling of the terms on a separate sheet of paper.

2. **Practice Online**
   a. **Access** the online learning resources. Go to evolve.elsevier.com > Evolve Resources > Student Resources.
   b. **Pronounce:** Select Audio Glossary > Chapter 2 > Exercise 10. Select a term to hear its pronunciation and repeat aloud.
   c. **Spell:** Select Activities > Chapter 2 > Spell Terms > Exercise 10. Select the audio icon and type the correct spelling of the term.

❑ Check the box when complete.

EXERCISE 11 ■ Analyze and Define

Analyze and define the following oncology terms by drawing slashes between word parts, writing word part abbreviations above the term, underlining combining forms, and writing combining form abbreviations below the term. *To check your answers, go to Appendix A at the back of the textbook.*

```
              WR  CV   WR  CV   S
EXAMPLE:  lei / o /  my / o / sarcoma
              CF       CF
          malignant tumor of smooth muscle
```

1. sarcoma

2. melanoma

3. epithelioma

4. lipoma

5. neoplasm

6. myoma

Chapter 2 Body Structure, Oncology, and Laboratory Tests

7. neuroma

8. carcinoma

9. adenocarcinoma

10. rhabdomyosarcoma

11. adenoma

12. rhabdomyoma

13. fibroma

14. liposarcoma

15. fibrosarcoma

16. metastasis

EXERCISE 12 ■ Build

A Label

Build terms pictured by writing word parts above the definitions.

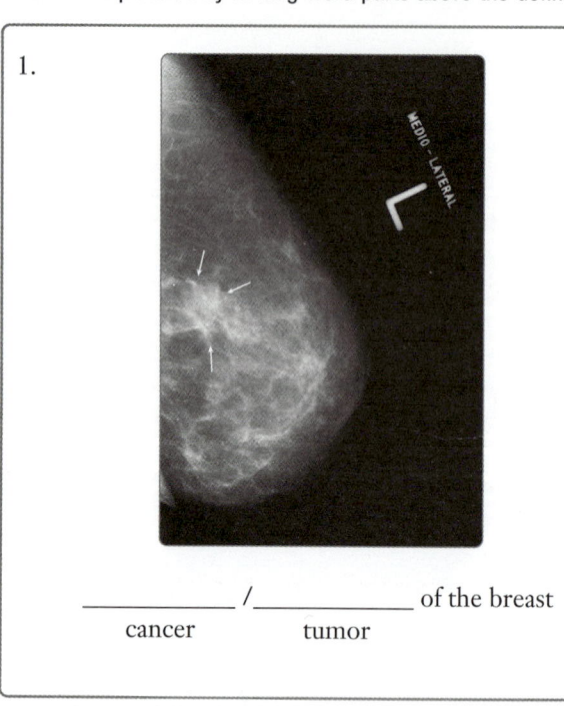

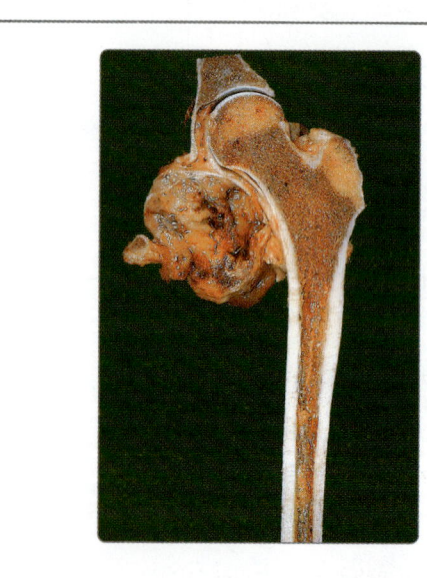

1.

_____ / _____ of the breast
   cancer   tumor

2.

_____ / _____ of the femur
 connective   tumor
   tissue

Chapter 2 Body Structure, Oncology, and Laboratory Tests 35

3.

_____ / _____
black / tumor

4.

_____ / __ / _____ / __ / _____
striated CV muscle CV malignant tumor

5.

_____ / __ / _____ / _____
smooth CV muscle tumor

6.

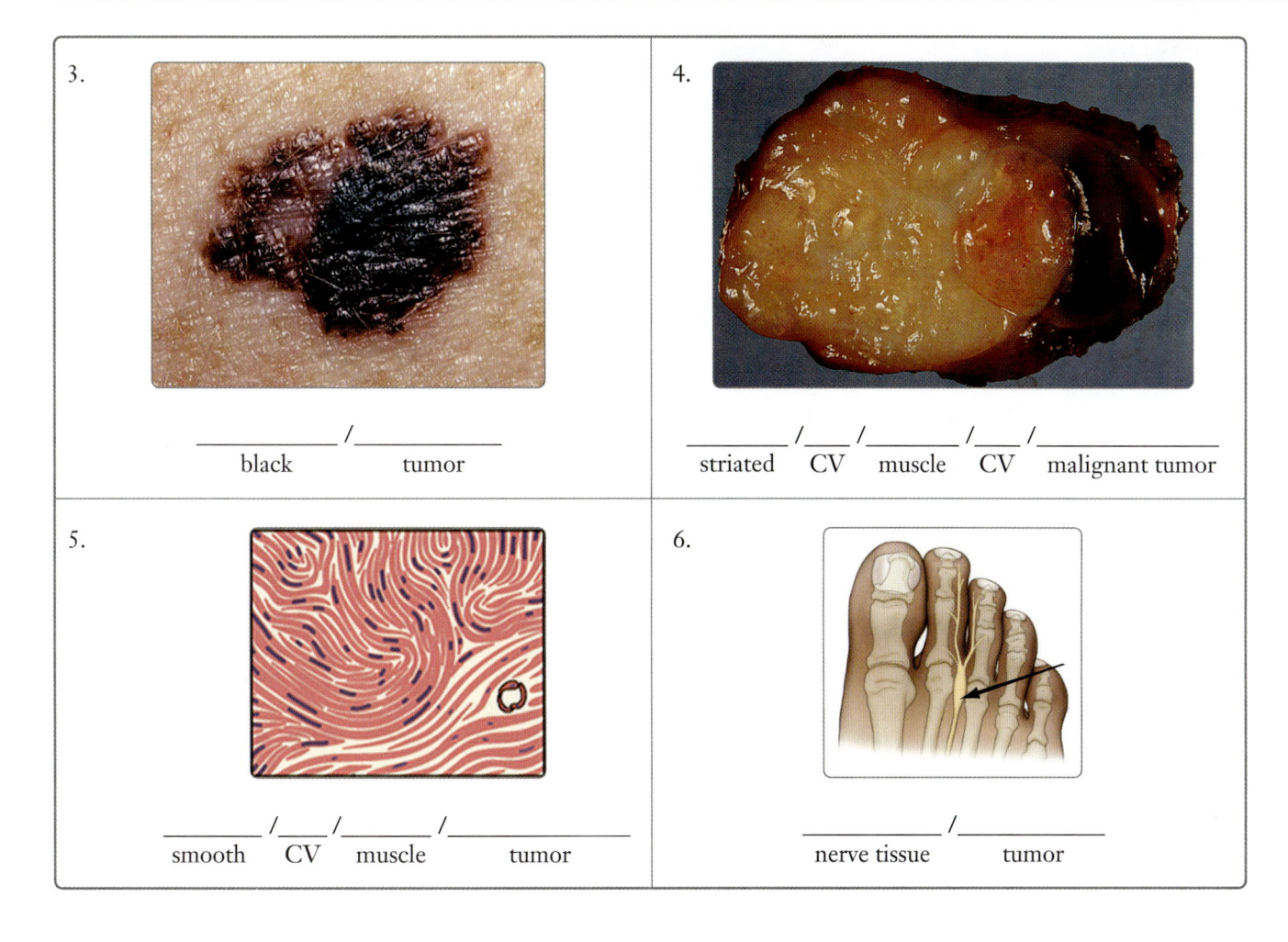

_____ / _____
nerve tissue tumor

B Fill In

Build oncology terms for the following definitions by using the word parts you have learned.

EXAMPLE: tumor composed of fat tissue   lip / oma
                                             WR   S

1. tumor composed of striated muscle   _____ / __ / _____ / __
   WR   CV   WR   S

2. malignant tumor of fat tissue   _____ / __ / _____
   WR   CV   S

3. new growth   _____ / _____
   P   S(WR)

4. tumor composed of epithelial tissue   _____ / _____
   WR   S

5. tumor composed of fibrous tissue   _____ / _____
   WR   S

6. tumor composed of glandular tissue   _____ / _____
   WR   S

7. beyond control _____
   P / S(WR)

8. tumor composed of muscle tissue _____
   WR / S

9. malignant tumor composed of fibrous tissue _____
   WR / CV / S

10. cancerous tumor of glandular tissue _____
    WR / CV / WR / S

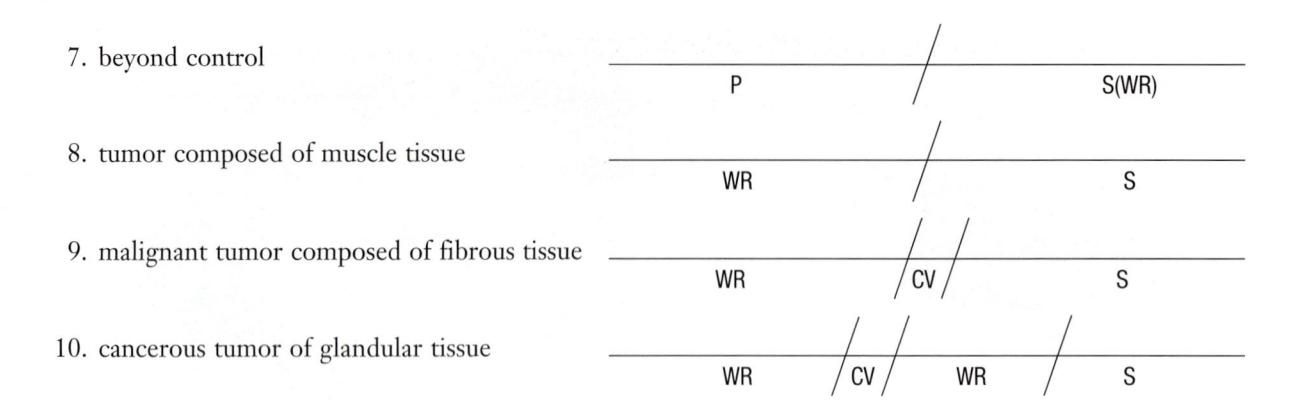

> **INCIDENTALOMA** refers to a lesion that is discovered unexpectedly during diagnostic imaging and has nothing to do with the patient's symptoms or primary diagnosis. The most common organs involved are the adrenal glands; incidentalomas may also be noted in the pituitary and thyroid glands, as well as the lungs, liver, kidneys, pancreas, and ovaries.

Oncology Terms
NOT BUILT FROM WORD PARTS

Though word parts may be present in terms categorized as NOT Built from Word Parts, their meanings are not clear from the definition of word parts. New knowledge may have changed the term's meaning, or the term may be from a Greek or Latin word not easily divided into parts. Other origins for these terms are eponyms, acronyms, or modern language, and some have no apparent explanation for their names.

> Medical terms NOT built from word parts cannot be easily translated to find their meanings. The terms are learned by memorizing the whole word and by using recall and spelling exercises.

TERM	DEFINITION
1. **benign** (be-NĪN)	not malignant, nonrecurrent, favorable for recovery (Fig. 2.5)
2. **biological therapy** (bī-ō-LOJ-i-kel) (THER-a-pē)	treatment of cancer with biological response modifiers (BRM) that work with the immune system (also called **biotherapy** or **immunotherapy**) (Table 2.3)
3. **carcinoma in situ** (kar-si-NŌ-ma) (in) (SĪ-too)	cancer in the early stage before invading surrounding tissue (Fig. 2.4)
🏛 **SITU** is from the Latin term *situs*, which means **position** or **place**. Think of **in situ** as meaning "in place" or "not wandering around."		
4. **chemotherapy (chemo)** (kē-mō-THER-a-pē)	treatment of cancer with medications that target all cells reproducing at a fast rate; destroys both tumor cells and healthy cells that have rapid production rates
5. **encapsulated** (en-KAP-sū-lā-ted)	enclosed within a capsule, as with benign or malignant tumors that have not spread beyond the capsule of the organ in which it originated
6. **hospice** (HOS-pis)	provides palliative or supportive care for terminally ill patients and their families. Usually offered to those who have a prognosis of approximately 6 months or less, when curative forms of treatment are no longer possible or desired. A team-based approach delivers care in a variety of settings, most often in the patient's home.
7. **malignant** (ma-LIG-nant)	tending to become progressively worse and to cause death, as in cancer (Fig. 2.5)
8. **palliative** (PAL-ē-a-tiv)	providing relief but not cure. Symptom management is provided to relieve suffering in all stages of disease, and is not limited to care at the end of life. It can be given with curative or life-prolonging treatment, or with end-of-life (hospice) care. While hospice care includes palliative care, not all of palliative care is hospice care.

TERM	DEFINITION
9. **radiation therapy (XRT)** (rā-dē-Ā-shun) (THER-a-pē)	treatment of cancer with a radioactive substance, x-ray, or radiation (also called **radiation oncology** and **radiotherapy**)
10. **remission** (rē-MISH-un)	improvement or absence of signs of disease

TABLE 2.3 Cancer Therapies

THERAPY	DESCRIPTION
Neoadjuvant therapy	a cancer treatment that precedes other treatment, such as administering chemotherapy or radiation therapy to a patient before surgery.
Adjuvant chemotherapy	the use of chemotherapy after or in combination with another form of cancer treatment, such as administering chemotherapy after surgery or with radiation therapy.
Brachytherapy	the use of radiotherapy, where the source of radiation is placed within or close to the area being treated, such as implantation of radiation sources into the breast to treat cancer (as shown in the illustration).
Biological therapy	the treatment of cancer with the use of man-made biological response modifiers (BRM) that occur naturally in the body. They alter the immune system's interaction with cancer cells to restore, direct, or boost the body's ability to fight disease. For example, an agent called **rituximab (Rituxan),** a monoclonal antibody, is used to treat some lymphomas. Other biological agents are **thalidomide,** which is used to treat multiple myeloma, and **interferon,** which is used in the treatment of lymphomas.

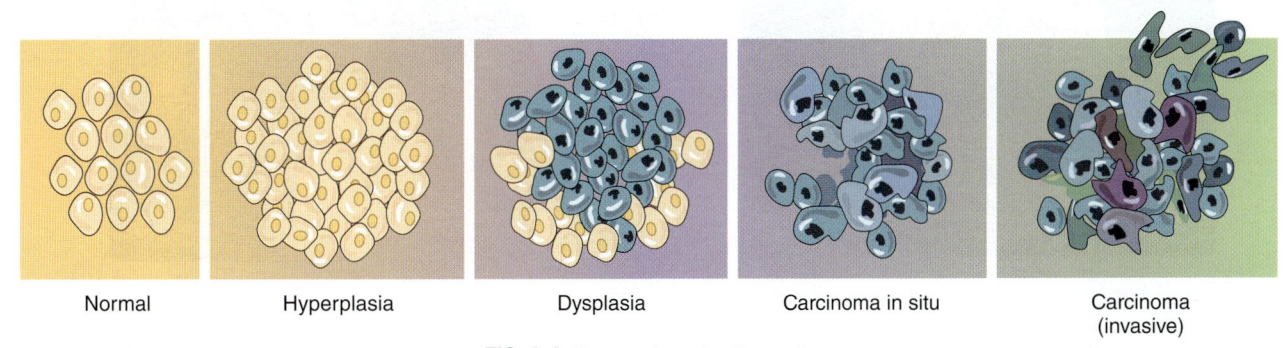

Normal   Hyperplasia   Dysplasia   Carcinoma in situ   Carcinoma (invasive)

FIG. 2.4 Progression of cell growth.

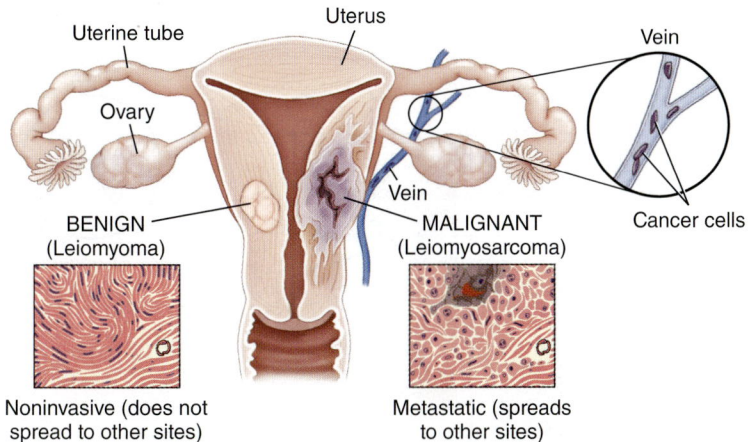

Uterine tube · Uterus · Vein · Ovary · Vein · Cancer cells
BENIGN (Leiomyoma) · MALIGNANT (Leiomyosarcoma)
Noninvasive (does not spread to other sites) · Metastatic (spreads to other sites)

FIG. 2.5 Examples of benign and malignant tumors.

🏛 BENIGN AND MALIGNANT

Benign is derived from the Latin word root **bene**, meaning **well** or **good**, as used in **benefit** or **benefactor**. **Malignant** is derived from the Latin word root **mal** meaning **bad**, as used in **malicious, malaise, malady,** and **malign**.

Chapter 2   Body Structure, Oncology, and Laboratory Tests

EXERCISE 13 ■ Pronounce and Spell

Practice pronunciation and spelling on paper and online.

1. **Practice on Paper**
   a. **Pronounce:** Read the phonetic spelling and say aloud the terms listed in the previous table. Refer to Table 2.2 Pronunciation Key as needed.
   b. **Spell:** Have a study partner read the terms aloud. Write the spelling of the terms on a separate sheet of paper.

2. **Practice Online**
   a. **Access** online learning resources. Go to evolve.elsevier.com > Evolve Resources > Student Resources.
   b. **Pronounce:** Select Audio Glossary > Chapter 2 > Exercise 13. Select a term to hear its pronunciation and repeat aloud.
   c. **Spell:** Select Activities > Chapter 2 > Spell Terms > Exercise 13. Select the audio icon and type the correct spelling of the term.

❏ Check the box when complete.

EXERCISE 14 ■ Fill In

A Label

Write the medical terms pictured and defined. *To check your answers, go to Appendix A at the back of the textbook.*

1. _____
   enclosed within a capsule

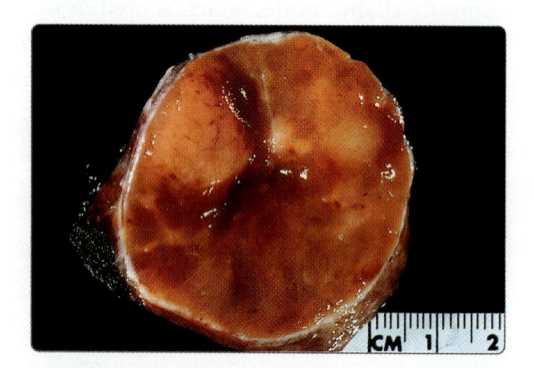

2. _____
   treatment of cancer with a radioactive substance, x-ray, or radiation

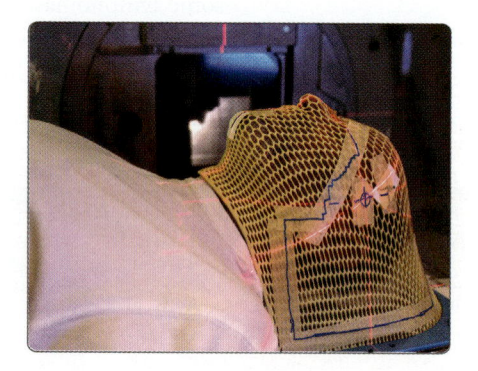

3. _____
   not malignant, nonrecurrent, favorable for recovery

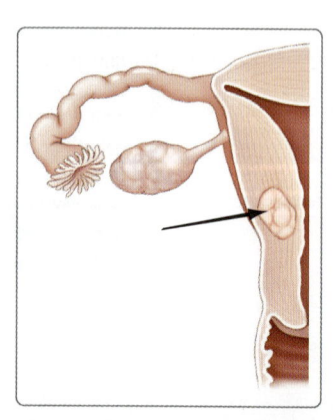

4. _____
   tending to become progressively worse and to cause death

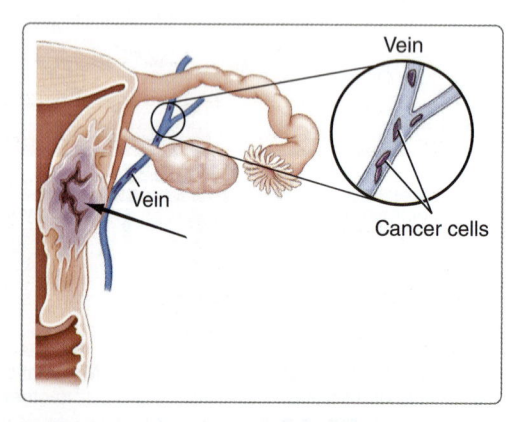

Chapter 2 Body Structure, Oncology, and Laboratory Tests   39

5. _____
treatment of cancer with medications that target all cells reproducing at a fast rate

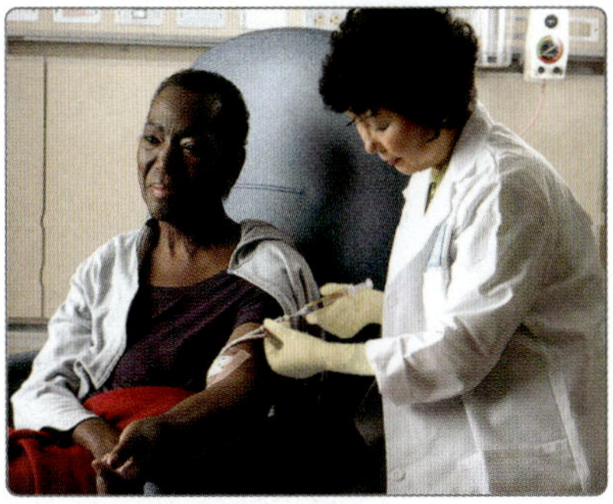

6. _____
cancer in the early stage before invading surrounding tissue

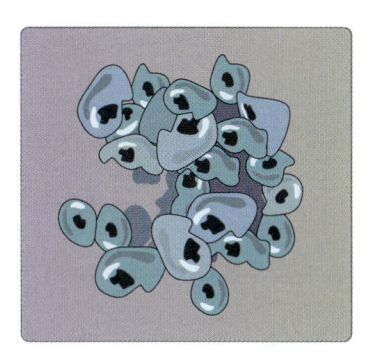

B Identify

Fill in the blanks with the correct terms.

1. **Treatment of cancer with agents that work with the immune system** _____ may be used to treat diseases such as lymphoma and myeloma.
2. **Providing relief but not cure** _____ care may be used at any time during the course of a disease.
3. **Improvement or absence of signs of disease** _____ may last from days to years, or may not occur at all.
4. Although frequently associated with end-of-life treatment for cancer patients, **provides palliative or supportive care for terminally ill patients and their families** _____ can be offered to a person with any type of disease that has a life expectancy of 6 months or less.

C Match

Match the terms in the first column with their correct definitions in the second column.

_____ 1. malignant
_____ 2. remission
_____ 3. carcinoma in situ
_____ 4. benign
_____ 5. hospice
_____ 6. radiation therapy
_____ 7. encapsulated
_____ 8. palliative
_____ 9. chemotherapy
_____ 10. biological therapy

a. provides palliative or supportive care for terminally ill patients and their families
b. not malignant, nonrecurrent, favorable for recovery
c. enclosed within a capsule
d. providing relief but not cure
e. treatment of cancer with medications that target all cells reproducing at a fast rate
f. treatment of cancer with biological response modifiers (BRM) that work with the immune system
g. cancer in the early stage before invading surrounding tissue
h. tending to become progressively worse and to cause death, as in cancer
i. improvement or absence of signs of disease
j. treatment of cancer with a radioactive substance, x-ray, or radiation

> **EXERCISE 15 ■ Review of Oncology Terms**

Can you define, pronounce, and spell the following oncology terms?

adenocarcinoma	epithelioma	malignant	radiation therapy (XRT)
adenoma	fibroma	melanoma	remission
benign	fibrosarcoma	myoma	rhabdomyoma
biological therapy	hospice	metastasis (*pl.* metastases)	rhabdomyosarcoma
carcinoma (CA)	leiomyoma	(METS)	sarcoma
carcinoma in situ	leiomyosarcoma	neoplasm	
chemotherapy (chemo)	lipoma	neuroma	
encapsulated	liposarcoma	palliative	

🔍 Refer to Appendix E for pharmacology terms related to oncology.

Laboratory Tests

Laboratory tests are performed to establish a diagnosis and/or prognosis, and to monitor and evaluate treatment. Specimens that are studied include blood (most common), urine, stool, sputum, sweat, and wound drainage or discharge from body openings, washings, and tissue. General categories are hematology studies, blood chemistry studies, urine studies, and microbiology studies (Table 2.4). Diagnostic laboratories, or labs, are located in hospitals, provider's offices, and in stand-alone facilities. These physical labs are divided into sections according to specialization, such as cytology for the study of cells.

> 💡 The abbreviation **lab**, short for laboratory, can refer to the physical location of the laboratory where specimens are analyzed and for the resulting report providing information on findings.

TABLE 2.4 Types of Laboratory Tests

Hematology studies relate to the physical properties of blood, such as the number of blood cells in the specimen or the clotting and bleeding factors.

Blood chemistry studies measure the amount of certain substances dissolved in the blood, including electrolytes (such as sodium, potassium, and chloride), fats, proteins, glucose (sugar), and enzymes.

Urine studies are performed on urine specimens to diagnose and monitor urinary system diseases and disorders, such as urinary tract infections, kidney stones, and diabetic nephropathy.

Microbiology studies identify the microorganisms that cause disease and infection, and can be divided into traditional and modern methods.

<u>Traditional microbiology studies include:</u>
Culture and sensitivity, a common study performed on almost any specimen. Other microbiology studies include **staining and microscopy** (looking at a sample under a microscope after applying a stain that highlights the suspected microorganism), and **biochemical testing** (using enzymes or other compounds that will cause reactions in a specific pathogen).

<u>Modern microbiology studies include:</u>
Polymerase chain reactions (PCR) work with tiny amounts of DNA from an unknown pathogen in a sample and match it against the DNA of known pathogens, including viruses, bacteria, and parasites. This can be done very quickly (within hours) compared to cultures, which can take days to weeks.

Serology tests depend on antibody/antigen reactions. Antibodies are substances produced by a person's immune system to help defend against infection. Antigens are substances produced by microorganisms that can trigger an immune response in the body. Serology tests are especially helpful for microorganisms that cannot be cultured, including the bacteria that cause syphilis.

Laboratory Terms
BUILT FROM WORD PARTS AND *NOT* BUILT FROM WORD PARTS

The first portion of the table contains laboratory terms that can be translated using definitions of word parts. The second portion of the table contains laboratory terms that cannot be fully understood using the definitions of word parts.

■ Built from Word Parts

TERM	DEFINITION	TERM	DEFINITION
1. autopsy (AW-top-sē)	view of self (postmortem examination to determine the cause of death or obtain evidence)	5. histopathology (his-to-pa-THOL-o-jē)	study of tissue in disease (study of tissue samples taken from patients)
2. biopsy (Bx) (BĪ-op-sē)	view of life (the removal of living tissue from the body to be viewed under the microscope)	6. microbiology (mī-krō-bī-OL-o-jē)	study of small life (study of microorganisms, such as bacteria, fungi, viruses, and parasites)
3. cytopathology (sī-tō-pa-THOL-o-jē)	study of (changes in) cells in disease	7. virology (vi-ROL-o-jē)	study of viruses (branch of microbiology that is concerned with viruses and viral diseases)
4. hematology (hē-ma-TOL-o-jē)	study of blood (branch of medicine that deals with diseases of the blood)		

■ *NOT* Built from Word Parts

TERM	DEFINITION
1. chemistry panel (KEM-is-trē) (PAN-el)	series of tests performed on a blood sample that give information regarding multiple systems, including the kidneys, liver, and lungs; these also provide glucose and protein levels (also called **comprehensive metabolic panel**)
2. complete blood count with differential (CBC with diff) (com-PLĒT) (blud) (kownt) (with) (dif-er-EN-shal)	test for basic blood screening that measures various aspects of erythrocytes (red blood cells), leukocytes (white blood cells), and thrombocytes (platelets); this automated test quickly provides a tremendous amount of information about the blood
3. culture and sensitivity (C&S) (KUL-cher) (and) (sen-si-TIV-i-tē)	test performed on a sample to determine the presence of pathogenic bacteria. The specimen is placed on a medium for growth (culture) and if pathogenic bacteria grow, is then tested for antibiotic sensitivity to identify an antibiotic that will provide the most effective treatment. C&S is used to identify the pathogen present and causing the infection.
4. genetic testing (je-NET-ik) (TEST-ing)	studies generally performed on a blood sample or cheek swab to examine DNA, the chemical database that carries instructions for the body's functions; can reveal changes in genes that may cause illness or disease. Other types of specimens used for testing are amniotic fluid, saliva, skin, and hair.
5. specimen (SPES-i-men)	sample of blood, urine, or body tissue that is taken for medical testing (also called **collection sample**)

42 Chapter 2 Body Structure, Oncology, and Laboratory Tests

EXERCISE 16 ■ Pronounce and Spell

Practice pronunciation and spelling on paper and online.

1. **Practice on Paper**
   a. **Pronounce:** Read the phonetic spelling and say aloud the terms listed in the previous table. Refer to Table 2.2 Pronunciation Key as needed.
   b. **Spell:** Have a study partner read the terms aloud. Write the spelling of the terms on a separate sheet of paper.

2. **Practice Online**
   a. **Access** online learning resources. Go to evolve.elsevier.com > Evolve Resources > Student Resources.
   b. **Pronounce:** Select Audio Glossary > Chapter 2 > Exercise 16. Select a term to hear its pronunciation and repeat aloud.
   c. **Spell:** Select Activities > Chapter 2 > Spell Terms > Exercise 16. Select the audio icon and type the correct spelling of the term.

❏ Check the box when complete.

EXERCISE 17 ■ Laboratory Terms Built from Word Parts

A Analyze and Define

Analyze and define the following laboratory terms by drawing slashes between word parts, writing word part abbreviations above the term, underlining combining forms, and writing combining form abbreviations below the term. *To check your answers, go to Appendix A.*

```
              WR CV  S
EXAMPLE:  hemat / o / logy
              CF
          study of blood
```

1. cytopathology

2. histopathology

3. virology

4. microbiology

5. autopsy

6. biopsy

B Fill In

Build laboratory terms for the following definitions by using the word parts you have learned.

1. study of tissue in disease   ___ / ___ / ___ / ___ / ___
                                       WR CV WR CV S

Chapter 2   Body Structure, Oncology, and Laboratory Tests   43

2. study of viruses _____ / _____ / _____
   WR   CV   S

3. study of (changes in) cells in disease   _____ / ___ / _____ / ___ / _____
   WR   CV   WR   CV   S

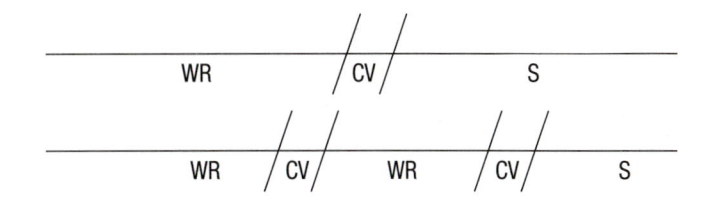

C   Label

Build terms pictured by writing word parts above the definitions.

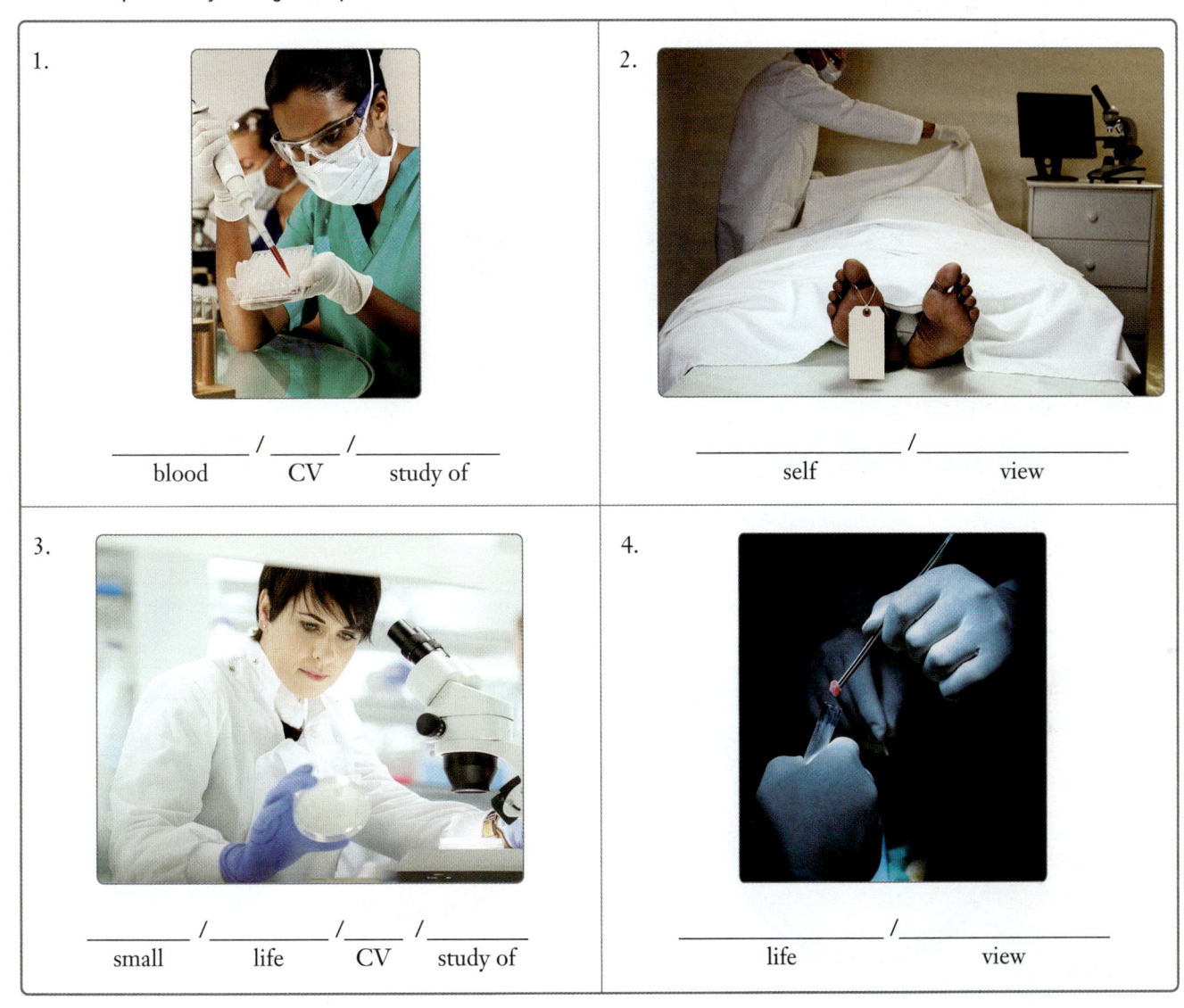

1.
_____ / ____ / _____
blood   CV   study of

2.
_____ / _____
self   view

3.
_____ / _____ / ____ / _____
small   life   CV   study of

4.
_____ / _____
life   view

EXERCISE 18 ■ Laboratory Terms NOT Built from Word Parts

A   Identify

Fill in the blanks with the correct terms.

1. Studies generally performed on a blood sample or cheek swab to examine DNA, the chemical database that carries instructions for the body's functions, are known as _____.

2. _____ is a series of tests performed on a blood sample that gives information regarding multiple systems, including the kidneys, liver, and lungs.

44 Chapter 2 Body Structure, Oncology, and Laboratory Tests

3. A laboratory test for basic blood screening that measures various aspects of erythrocytes, leukocytes, and thrombocytes is a _____

4. _____ is also called a collection sample.

5. The test that places a specimen on a growth medium to check for bacteria and determine the most effective antibiotic is called _____ and _____.

B Label

Write the medical terms pictured and defined.

1. _____
sample of blood, urine, or body tissue that is taken for medical testing

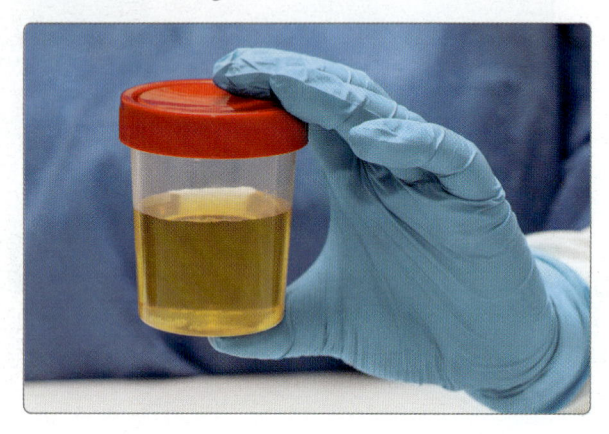

2. _____
series of tests performed on a blood sample that gives information regarding multiple systems

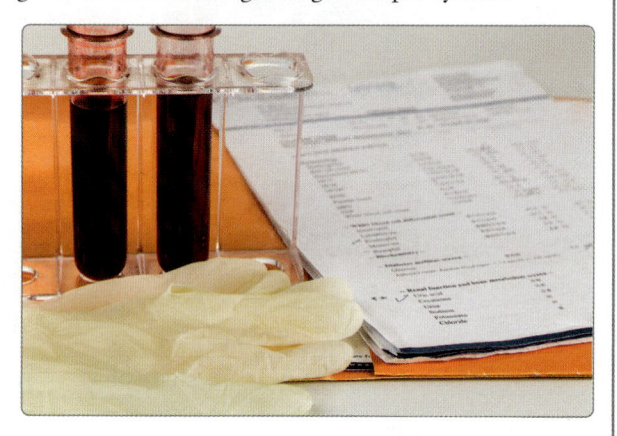

3. _____
can reveal changes in DNA that may cause illness or disease

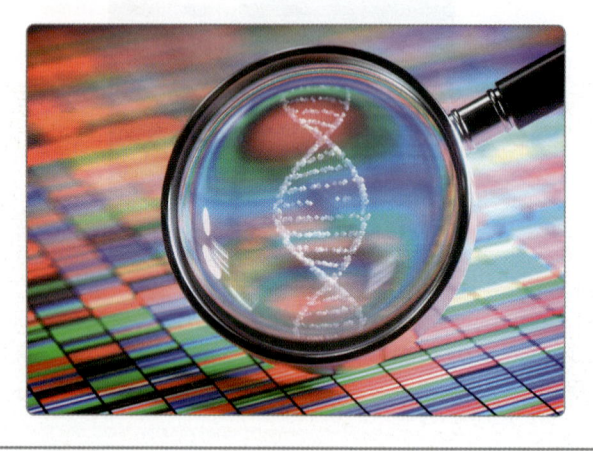

4. _____
test performed on a sample to determine the presence of pathogenic bacteria

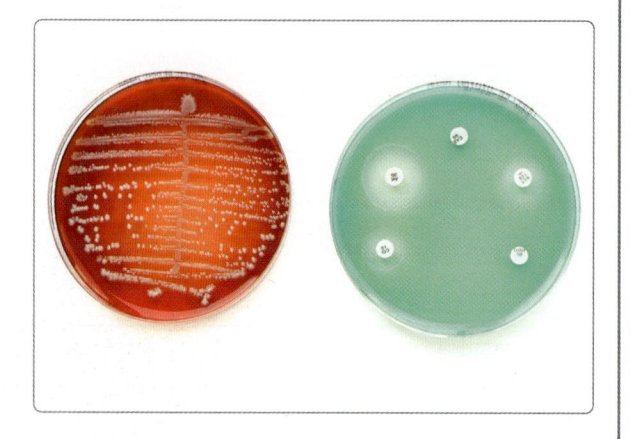

EXERCISE 19 ■ Review of Laboratory Terms

Can you define, pronounce, and spell the following laboratory terms?

autopsy
biopsy (Bx)
chemistry panel
complete blood count with differential (CBC with diff)
culture and sensitivity (C&S)
cytopathology
genetic testing
hematology
histopathology
microbiology
specimen
virology

Chapter 2 Body Structure, Oncology, and Laboratory Tests

Complementary Terms

Complementary terms complete the vocabulary presented in the chapter by describing signs, symptoms, medical specialties, specialists, and related words. A **sign** is objective information and is detected on physical examination, such as an observation that the patient has cyanosis of the nail beds. A **symptom** is subjective and is evidence of disease perceived by the patient, such as stating the feeling of pain in the chest while walking.

■ Built from Word Parts

The following terms can be translated using definitions of word parts. Further explanation is provided within parentheses as needed.

SIGNS & SYMPTOMS

TERM	DEFINITION	TERM	DEFINITION
1. cyanosis (sī-a-NŌ-sis)	abnormal condition of blue (bluish discoloration, especially of the skin, caused by inadequate supply of oxygen in the blood)	2. xanthosis (zan-THŌ-sis)	abnormal condition of yellow (discoloration)

MEDICAL SPECIALTIES AND PROFESSIONS

TERM	DEFINITION	TERM	DEFINITION
3. oncologist (ong-KOL-o-jist)	physician who studies and treats (malignant) tumors	5. pathologist (pa-THOL-o-jist)	physician who studies diseases (examines biopsies and performs autopsies to determine the cause of disease or death)
4. oncology (ong-KOL-o-jē)	study of tumors (a branch of medicine concerned with the study of malignant tumors)	6. pathology (pa-THOL-o-jē)	study of disease (a branch of medicine dealing with the study of the causes of disease and death)

DESCRIPTIVE TERMS

TERM	DEFINITION	TERM	DEFINITION
7. cancerous (KAN-ser-us)	pertaining to cancer	13. iatrogenic (ī-at-rō-JEN-ik)	produced by a physician (the unexpected results from a treatment prescribed by a physician)
8. carcinogen (kar-SIN-o-jen)	substance that causes cancer		
9. carcinogenic (kar-sin-ō-JEN-ik)	producing cancer	14. oncogenic (ong-kō-JEN-ik)	causing tumors
10. carcinoid (KAR-si-noyd)	resembling cancer	15. pathogenic (path-ō-JEN-ik)	producing disease
11. diagnosis (Dx) (dī-ag-NŌ-sis)	state of complete knowledge (the art of identifying a disease based on the patient's signs, symptoms, and test results)	16. prognosis (Px) (prog-NŌ-sis)	state of before knowledge (prediction of the outcome of disease based on the patient's signs, symptoms, and test results)
12. etiology (ē-tē-OL-o-jē)	study of causes (of diseases)		

🏛 **PROGNOSIS** was used by Hippocrates to mean the same then as now: **to foretell the course of a disease**.

46 Chapter 2 Body Structure, Oncology, and Laboratory Tests

EXERCISE 20 ■ Pronounce and Spell

Practice pronunciation and spelling on paper and online.

1. **Practice on Paper**
    a. **Pronounce:** Read the phonetic spelling and say aloud the terms listed in the previous table. Refer to Table 2.2 Pronunciation Key as needed.
    b. **Spell:** Have a study partner read the terms aloud. Write the spelling of the terms on a separate sheet of paper.

2. **Practice Online**
    a. **Access** online learning resources. Go to evolve.elsevier.com > Evolve Resources > Student Resources.
    b. **Pronounce:** Select Audio Glossary > Chapter 2 > Exercise 20. Select a term to hear its pronunciation and repeat aloud.
    c. **Spell:** Select Activities > Chapter 2 > Spell Terms > Exercise 20. Select the audio icon and type the correct spelling of the term.

❏ Check the box when complete.

EXERCISE 21 ■ Analyze and Define

Analyze and define the following complementary terms by drawing slashes between word parts, writing word part abbreviations above the term, underlining combining forms, and writing combining form abbreviations below the term. *To check your answers, go to Appendix A at the back of the textbook.*

```
              WR   CV   S
EXAMPLE:   path / o / genic
              CF
           producing disease
```

1. pathology

2. pathologist

3. diagnosis

4. oncogenic

5. oncology

6. cancerous

7. carcinogenic

8. cyanosis

9. etiology

10. xanthosis

Chapter 2   Body Structure, Oncology, and Laboratory Tests   47

11. carcinoid

_____

_____

12. carcinogen

_____

_____

13. oncologist

_____

_____

14. prognosis

_____

_____

EXERCISE 22 ■ Build

A Label

Build terms pictured by writing word parts above the definitions.

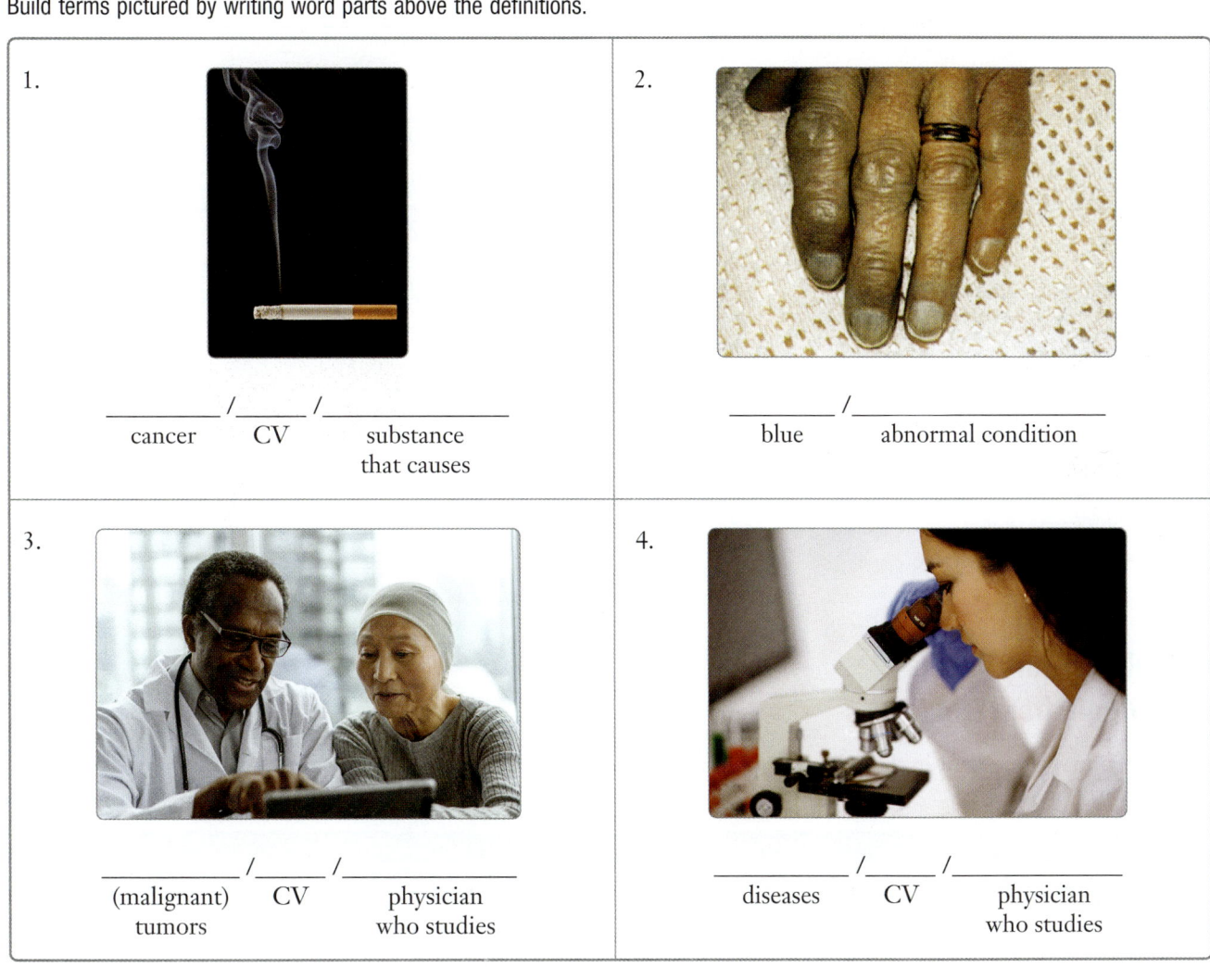

1.

_____ / ____ / _____
cancer   CV   substance
               that causes

2.

_____ / _____
blue   abnormal condition

3.

_____ / ____ / _____
(malignant)   CV   physician
tumors   who studies

4.

_____ / ____ / _____
diseases   CV   physician
                   who studies

48 Chapter 2 Body Structure, Oncology, and Laboratory Tests

B Fill In

Build complementary terms for the following definitions by using the word parts you have learned.

EXAMPLE: producing disease   path / o / genic
                                  WR / CV / S

1. state of complete knowledge   ____ / ____ / ____
                                   P / WR / S

2. produced by a physician   ____ / ____ / ____
                              WR / CV / S

3. study of causes (of diseases)   ____ / ____ / ____
                                    WR / CV / S

4. study of tumors   ____ / ____ / ____
                      WR / CV / S

5. study of disease   ____ / ____ / ____
                       WR / CV / S

6. producing cancer   ____ / ____ / ____
                       WR / CV / S

7. abnormal condition of yellow   ____ / ____
                                   WR / S

8. causing tumors   ____ / ____ / ____
                     WR / CV / S

9. pertaining to cancer   ____ / ____
                           WR / S

10. state of before knowledge   ____ / ____ / ____
                                  P / WR / S

Complementary Terms
■ NOT Built from Word Parts

Word parts may be present in the following terms; however, their full meanings cannot be translated using definitions of word parts alone.

SIGNS & SYMPTOMS			
TERM	**DEFINITION**	**TERM**	**DEFINITION**
1. **afebrile** (ā-FEB-ril)	without fever	4. **febrile** (FEB-ril)	having a fever
2. **erythema** (er-i-THĒ-ma)	redness	5. **inflammation** (in-fla-MĀ-shun)	localized protective response to injury or tissue destruction characterized by redness, swelling, heat, and pain
3. **fatigue** (fa-TĒG)	persistent, excessive tiredness and lack of energy that interferes with daily activities and is unrelated to exertion or lack of sleep		

Chapter 2   Body Structure, Oncology, and Laboratory Tests   49

DESCRIPTIVE TERMS

TERM	DEFINITION	TERM	DEFINITION
6. acute (a-KŪT)	sharp, sudden, short, or severe type of disease	8. exacerbation (eg-zas-er-BĀ-shun)	increase in the severity of a disease or its symptoms
7. chronic (KRON-ik)	disease that continues for a long time	9. idiopathic (id-ē-ō-PATH-ik)	pertaining to disease of unknown origin

OTHER TERMS

TERM	DEFINITION
10. bacteria (*s. bacterium*) (bak-TĒR-ē-a) (bak-TĒR-ē-um)	single-celled microorganisms that reproduce by cell division and may cause infection by invading body tissue
11. fungus (*pl.* fungi) (FUN-gus) (FUN-jī)	organism that feeds by absorbing organic molecules from its surroundings and may cause infection by invading body tissue; single-celled fungi (yeast) reproduce by budding; multi-celled fungi (mold) reproduce by spore formation
12. infection (in-FEK-shun)	invasion of pathogens in body tissue. Types of infection include bacterial, viral, and fungal. An **acute** infection may remain localized if the body's defense mechanisms are effective or may persist to become **subacute** or **chronic**. A **systemic** infection occurs when the pathogen causing a local infection gains access to the vascular or lymphatic system and becomes disseminated throughout the body.
13. microorganism (mī-krō-OR-gan-iz-um)	a form of life that is too small to be seen without a microscope; includes bacteria, fungi, parasites, and viruses
14. parasite (par-ah-SĪT)	organism that feeds from a host it lives on or within. Types of parasites causing human disease include protozoa, single-celled organisms that live inside the host; helminths, worms that live inside the host; and ectoparasites, organisms that live outside the host, attaching or burrowing into the skin.
15. virus (*pl.* viruses) (VĪ-ras) (VĪ-ras-uz)	minute microorganism, much smaller than a bacterium, characterized by a lack of independent metabolism and the ability to replicate only within living host cells; these may cause infection by invading body tissue

EXERCISE 23 ■ Pronounce and Spell

Practice pronunciation and spelling on paper and online.

1. **Practice on Paper**
    a. **Pronounce:** Read the phonetic spelling and say aloud the terms listed in the previous table. Refer to Table 2.2 Pronunciation Key as needed.
    b. **Spell:** Have a study partner read the terms aloud. Write the spelling of the terms on a separate sheet of paper.

2. **Practice Online**
    a. **Access** online learning resources. Go to evolve.elsevier.com > Evolve Resources > Student Resources.
    b. **Pronounce:** Select Audio Glossary > Chapter 2 > Exercise 23. Select a term to hear its pronunciation and repeat aloud.
    c. **Spell:** Select Activities > Chapter 2 > Spell Terms > Exercise 23. Select the audio icon and type the correct spelling of the term.

❏ Check the box when complete.

Chapter 2 Body Structure, Oncology, and Laboratory Tests

EXERCISE 24 ■ Fill In

A Label

Write the medical terms pictured and defined. *To check your answers, go to Appendix A at the back of the textbook.*

1. _____
   having a fever

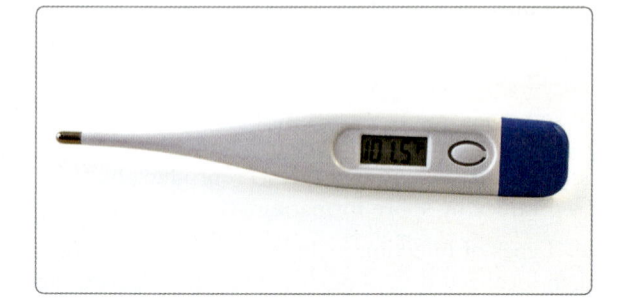

2. _____
   minute microorganism characterized by a lack of independent metabolism

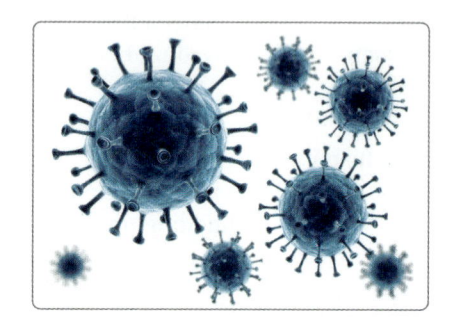

3. _____
   localized protective response characterized by redness, swelling, heat, and pain

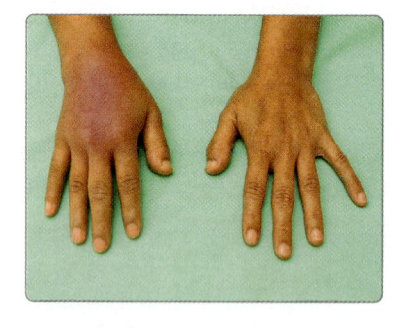

4. _____
   single-celled microorganisms that reproduce by cell division and may cause infection by invading body tissue

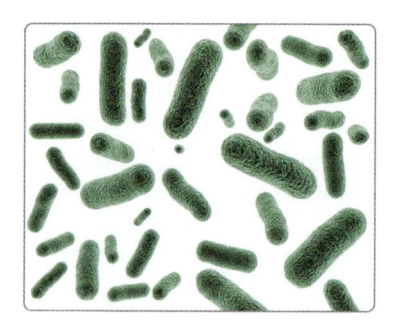

B Identify

Write the definitions for the following terms.

1. parasite _____
2. fungus _____
3. afebrile _____
4. microorganism _____
5. erythema _____
6. infection _____
7. fatigue _____
8. idiopathic _____
9. exacerbation _____
10. chronic _____
11. acute _____

Chapter 2   Body Structure, Oncology, and Laboratory Tests   51

EXERCISE 25 ■ Match

A

Match the complementary terms in the first column with the correct definitions in the second column.

_____ 1. inflammation
_____ 2. fatigue
_____ 3. bacteria
_____ 4. microorganism
_____ 5. exacerbation
_____ 6. febrile
_____ 7. fungus

a. single-celled microorganisms that reproduce by cell division and may cause infection by invading body tissue
b. increase in the severity of a disease or its symptoms
c. a form of life that is too small to be seen without a microscope; includes bacteria, fungi, and viruses.
d. having a fever
e. persistent, excessive tiredness and lack of energy that interferes with daily activities and is unrelated to exertion or lack of sleep
f. localized protective response to injury or tissue destruction characterized by redness, swelling, heat, and pain
g. organism that feeds by absorbing organic molecules from its surroundings; may be single-celled or multi-celled.

B

Match the complementary terms in the first column with the correct definitions in the second column.

_____ 1. infection
_____ 2. erythema
_____ 3. parasite
_____ 4. afebrile
_____ 5. acute
_____ 6. chronic
_____ 7. idiopathic
_____ 8. virus

a. pertaining to disease of unknown origin
b. minute microorganism, characterized by a lack of independent metabolism and the ability to replicate only within living host cells
c. without fever
d. redness
e. organism that feeds from a host it lives on or within
f. invasion of pathogens in body tissue
g. disease that continues for a long time
h. sharp, sudden, short, or severe type of disease

EXERCISE 26 ■ Review of Complementary Terms

Can you define, pronounce, and spell the following complementary terms?

acute	cyanosis	iatrogenic	parasite
afebrile	diagnosis (Dx)	idiopathic	pathogenic
bacteria (s. bacterium)	erythema	inflammation	pathologist
cancerous	etiology	infection	pathology
carcinogen	exacerbation	microorganism	prognosis (Px)
carcinogenic	fatigue	oncogenic	virus (pl. viruses)
carcinoid	febrile	oncologist	xanthosis
chronic	fungus (pl. fungi)	oncology	

Plural Endings for Medical Terms

In the English language plurals are formed by simply adding an "s" or "es" to the end of a word. For example, hand becomes plural by adding an "s" to form hands. Likewise, box becomes boxes by adding "es." In the language of medicine, many terms have Latin or Greek suffixes, and forming plurals for these terms is not quite as easy. Table 2.5, Common Plural Endings for Medical Terms, lists the most common singular and plural endings used in medical terminology. When appropriate, both singular and plural endings are included in the word lists throughout the text, such as metastasis (s.), metastases (pl.).

TABLE 2.5 Common Plural Endings for Medical Terms

SINGULAR ENDINGS	SINGULAR FORMS	PLURAL ENDINGS	PLURAL FORMS
-a	vertebr**a**	-ae	vertebr**ae**
-ax	thor**ax**	-aces	thor**aces**
-is	test**is**	-es	test**es**
-ix	append**ix**	-ices	append**ices**
-ma	carcino**ma**	-mata	carcino**mata**
-nx	lary**nx**	-nges	lary**nges**
-on	gangli**on**	-a	gangli**a**
-sis	metasta**sis**	-ses	metasta**ses**
-um	ov**um**	-a	ov**a**
-us	fung**us**	-i	fung**i**
-y	biops**y**	-ies	biops**ies**

> Because of common usage, some plural forms of medical terms will add an "s" rather than use Greek or Latin plural endings. **Carcinomas** rather than **carcinomata** is frequently seen in medical literature.

EXERCISE 27 ■ Plural Endings

Convert each of the following terms from singular to plural. Refer to Table 2.5 for guidance. Do not be concerned about the meaning of these terms; concentrate only on the plural endings. *To check your answers, go to Appendix A.*

1. etiology _____
2. staphylococcus _____
3. cyanosis _____
4. bacterium _____
5. nucleus _____
6. pharynx _____
7. sarcoma _____
8. carcinoma _____
9. anastomosis _____
10. pubis _____
11. prognosis _____
12. spermatozoon _____
13. fimbria _____
14. thorax _____
15. appendix _____

Chapter 2 Body Structure, Oncology, and Laboratory Tests

EXERCISE 28 ▪ Identify

Circle the correct singular or plural form in each sentence.

1. During a colonoscopy the gastroenterologist noted that the patient had several (**diverticula, diverticulum**) in his transverse colon.
2. Bronchogenic carcinoma was diagnosed in the patient's left (**bronchus, bronchi**).
3. Bilateral (two sides) orchiditis is inflammation of the (**testes, testis**).
4. The light brown mole with notched borders turned out to be a (**melanomata, melanoma**).
5. Multiple (**embolus, emboli**) were observed on the lung scan.
6. Many (**diagnosis, diagnoses**) of benign tumors are picked up during whole-body scanning.
7. Diagnostic studies have shown (**metastasis, metastases**) of the patient's carcinoma of the breast to both her lungs and brain.

Abbreviations

Abbreviations are frequently used verbally and in writing to communicate in the medical and healthcare setting. Abbreviations that are easily misinterpreted and may lead to medication errors are reported to the Institute for Safe Medication Practices. See **Appendix D** for The Joint Commission's "Do Not Use" list of abbreviations. Abbreviations of the terms included in the chapter are listed in the following table.

BODY STRUCTURE

ABBREVIATION	TERM	ABBREVIATION	TERM
RBC	red blood cell (erythrocyte)	WBC	white blood cell (leukocyte)

ONCOLOGY

ABBREVIATION	TERM	ABBREVIATION	TERM
CA	carcinoma	METS	metastasis (*s.*), metastases (*pl.*); spoken as a whole word (metz)

LABORATORY

ABBREVIATION	TERM	ABBREVIATION	TERM
Bx	biopsy	C&S	culture and sensitivity
CBC with diff	complete blood count with differential		

TREATMENTS

ABBREVIATION	TERM	ABBREVIATION	TERM
chemo	chemotherapy; spoken as a whole word (KĒ-mō)	XRT	radiation therapy

DESCRIPTIVE

ABBREVIATION	TERM	ABBREVIATION	TERM
Dx	diagnosis	Px	prognosis

EXERCISE 29 ▪ Abbreviations

Write the term for each of the abbreviations in the following paragraph.

A 55-year-old woman was admitted to the oncology unit after a **Bx** _____ revealed a **Dx** _____ of **CA** _____. She was noted to have **METS** _____ to the lungs and brain. Her **Px** _____ was guarded. Laboratory tests, including **RBC** _____ _____ _____ and **WBC** _____ _____ counts, were ordered. She will receive both **chemo** _____ and **XRT** _____ _____. Her **CBC with diff** _____ _____ _____ with _____ will be monitored to check for any signs of bone marrow suppression. **C&S** _____ and _____ will be obtained if she develops any signs of infection.

PRACTICAL APPLICATION

EXERCISE 30 ■ Case Study: Translate Between Everyday Language and Medical Language

CASE STUDY: Tova Smelkinson

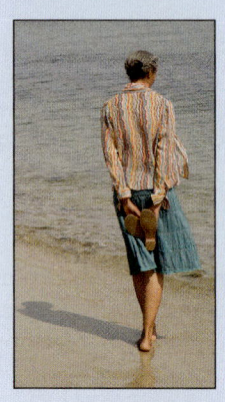

Tova has been having diarrhea. Even worse, she notices blood in it. She had this before when she was younger—and the disease was identified—but she couldn't remember the name. She recalls it was not a cancerous tumor and noted she did not have a fever. She was put on medicine and got better. It looked like a positive outcome. Now it's been going on for 3 weeks. She has pain in her belly with cramps and feels kind of full all the time. She notices she is losing weight, even though she isn't trying. She also feels more tired than usual. Tova makes an appointment with her family doctor to see if she needs to go back on medicine.

Now that you have worked through Chapter 2 on body structure, color, and oncology, consider the medical terms that might be used to describe Tova's experience. See the Chapter at a Glance at the end of the chapter for a list of terms that might apply.

A. Underline phrases in the case study that could be substituted with medical terms.

B. Write the medical term and its definition for three of the phrases you underlined.

MEDICAL TERM	DEFINITION
1.	
2.	
3.	

DOCUMENTATION: Excerpt from Clinical Notation

Tova was able to see her family doctor. The following is a portion of what was noted in her clinical electronic health record (EHR):

A 54-year-old woman presented to the office with 3-week history of bloody diarrhea. She had been diagnosed with ulcerative colitis at the age of 25 years. She was referred for a colonoscopy. The examination revealed a suspicious lesion on the transverse colon. A biopsy was performed and a cytology specimen was obtained. Advanced dysplasia and inflammation were present. The pathologist made a diagnosis of carcinoma of the colon.

C. Underline medical terms presented in Chapter 2 in the previous excerpt from Tova's medical record (EHR).

D. Select and define three of the medical terms you underlined.

MEDICAL TERM	DEFINITION
1.	
2.	
3.	

Chapter 2 Body Structure, Oncology, and Laboratory Tests

EXERCISE 31 ■ Interact with Medical Documents

A

Read the report and complete it by writing medical terms on answer lines within the document. Definitions of terms to be written appear after the document.

830293-ONC GREELEY, Morris

Name: **GREELEY, Morris** MR#: **830293-ONC** Sex: M Allergies: Codeine
DOB: **08/03/19XX** Age: 67 PCP: Seth Barkley MD

Progress Note
Encounter Date: 11/12/20XX
Subjective: Mr. Greeley arrives today for a 1._____ treatment for 2._____ of the sigmoid colon. He had an anterior sigmoid resection in October. 3._____ report revealed 4._____ tumor cells in two of six lymph nodes. The 5FU/Leucovorin protocol is being administered weekly for 6 weeks. Today is his sixth infusion. We plan to start 5._____ _____ after a 2-week hiatus from chemotherapy. The patient continues to do well and is receiving significant support from his family. He has had no hair loss, oral ulcerations, abdominal pain, nausea, or diarrhea.

Objective: Vital signs: Temperature of 98°F. Pulse is 60 beats per minute. Respirations 20. Blood pressure 108/65 mm Hg. His current weight is 183 pounds. HEENT: Tongue and pharynx are normal. PULMONARY: Clear to auscultation. HEART: Regular rate and rhythm without a murmur, rub, or gallop. ABDOMEN: Soft and nontender. No masses or 6._____.
Extremities: No edema or 7._____.

Assessment: 1. Adenocarcinoma of the sigmoid colon with 8._____ to regional lymph nodes.

Plan: 1. 5FU/Leucovorin protocol as outlined above, treatment six of six today, followed by radiation therapy after a 2-week period of rest.

Electronically signed: Brian Smith MD 11/12/20XX 16:30

Definitions of Medical Terms to Complete the Document
Write the medical terms defined on corresponding answer lines in the document.

1. treatment of cancer by using drugs
2. cancerous tumor of glandular tissue
3. study of disease
4. tending to become progressively worse
5. treatment of cancer by using radioactive substance, x-rays, or radiation
6. enlargement of an organ
7. abnormal condition of blue
8. beyond control

B

Read the medical report, and answer the questions below it.

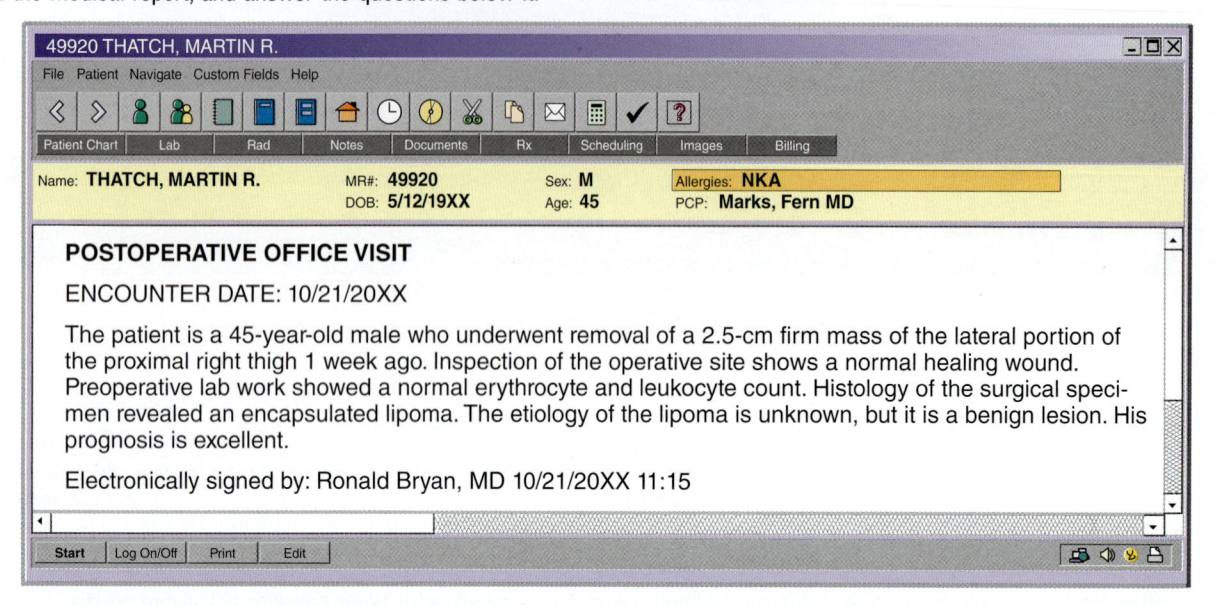

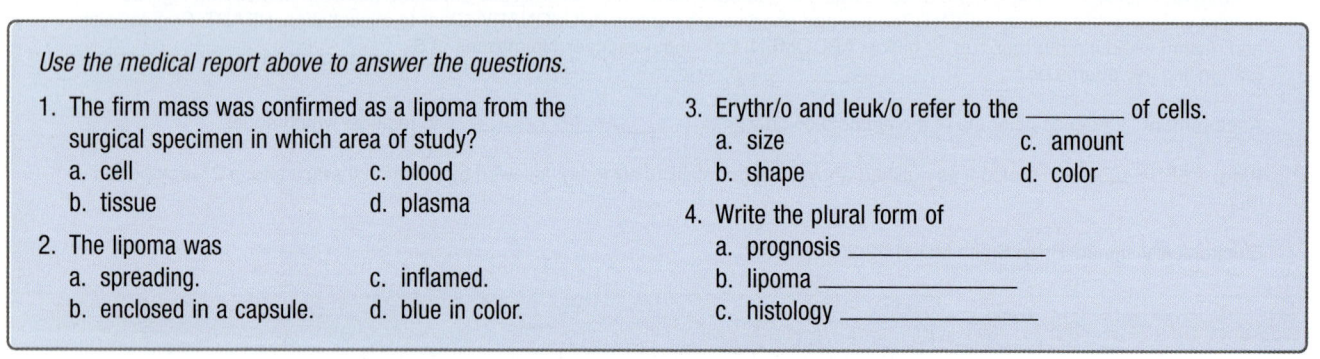

49920 THATCH, MARTIN R.

File Patient Navigate Custom Fields Help

| Patient Chart | Lab | Rad | Notes | Documents | Rx | Scheduling | Images | Billing |

Name: **THATCH, MARTIN R.**   MR#: **49920**   Sex: **M**   Allergies: **NKA**
DOB: **5/12/19XX**   Age: **45**   PCP: **Marks, Fern MD**

POSTOPERATIVE OFFICE VISIT

ENCOUNTER DATE: 10/21/20XX

The patient is a 45-year-old male who underwent removal of a 2.5-cm firm mass of the lateral portion of the proximal right thigh 1 week ago. Inspection of the operative site shows a normal healing wound. Preoperative lab work showed a normal erythrocyte and leukocyte count. Histology of the surgical specimen revealed an encapsulated lipoma. The etiology of the lipoma is unknown, but it is a benign lesion. His prognosis is excellent.

Electronically signed by: Ronald Bryan, MD 10/21/20XX 11:15

Start Log On/Off Print Edit

Use the medical report above to answer the questions.

1. The firm mass was confirmed as a lipoma from the surgical specimen in which area of study?
   a. cell
   b. tissue
   c. blood
   d. plasma

2. The lipoma was
   a. spreading.
   b. enclosed in a capsule.
   c. inflamed.
   d. blue in color.

3. Erythr/o and leuk/o refer to the _____ of cells.
   a. size
   b. shape
   c. amount
   d. color

4. Write the plural form of
   a. prognosis _____
   b. lipoma _____
   c. histology _____

EXERCISE 32 ■ Use Medical Terms in Clinical Statements

For each phrase printed in bold, circle the medical term or abbreviation defined. Answers are listed in Appendix A. For pronunciation practice read the answers aloud.

1. A patient with a(n) **identification of a disease** (diagnosis, prognosis, remission) of **cancer** (chemo, CA, METS) may seek the services of a(n) **physician who studies and treats tumors** (histologist, pathologist, oncologist).

2. The **new growth** (neoplasm, myoma, epithelioma) was biopsied and sent to the laboratory for **study of cells** (pathology, cytology, histology) to determine whether the tumor is **nonrecurring** (malignant, benign, inflammation) or **tending to become progressively worse** (malignant, benign, idiopathic).

3. A urine **sample of blood, urine, or body tissue that is taken for medical testing** (specimen, biopsy, autopsy) was collected from Danisha Scott when she complained of painful urination. It was sent to the **study of small life** (histopathology, hematology, microbiology) department for **test performed on a sample to determine the presence of pathogenic bacteria** (C&S, CBC with diff, WBC).

4. Mrs. Gonzalez' **study of disease** (pathology, cytology, histology) report indicated the presence of **tumor of connective tissue** (carcinoma, sarcoma, lipoma) with **beyond control** (metastasis, remission, neoplasm). She will be transferred to the **study of tumors** (histology, oncology, epithelial) unit of the hospital. The **prediction of a possible outcome of a disease** (Dx, Bx, Px) is poor.

Chapter 2 Body Structure, Oncology, and Laboratory Tests

5. Justin Ang presented to the emergency department with signs and symptoms of a(n) **invasion of pathogens in body tissue** (inflammation, infection, fungus), including **persistent, excessive tiredness and lack of energy that interferes with daily activities** (erythema, infection, fatigue) and a temperature of 101.5° F, indicating that he was **having a fever** (febrile, afebrile, idiopathic). His laboratory results were significant for **increase in the number of white (blood) cells** (erythrocytosis, leukocytosis, necrosis), and he was diagnosed with mononucleosis, which is caused by a **minute microorganism, much smaller than a bacterium, characterized by a lack of independent metabolism and the ability to replicate only within living host cells** (fungus, virus, parasite).

EXERCISE 33 ■ Pronounce Medical Terms in Use

Practice pronunciation of terms by reading aloud the following paragraph. Use the phonetic spellings to assist with pronunciation. The script also contains medical terms not presented in the chapter. If interested, research their meanings using a medical dictionary and reliable online sources.

> A 54-year-old woman presented to the office with a 3-week history of bloody diarrhea. She had been diagnosed with ulcerative colitis at age 25 years. She was referred for a colonoscopy. The examination revealed a suspicious lesion in the transverse colon. A **biopsy** (BĪ-op-sē) was performed and a **cytology** (sī-TOL-o-jē) specimen was obtained. The **pathologist** (pa-THOL-o-jist) made a **diagnosis** (dī-ag-NŌ-sis) of **carcinoma** (kar-si-NŌ-ma) of the colon. Advanced **dysplasia** (dis-PLĀ-zha) and **inflammation** (in-fla-MĀ-shun) existed in the **specimen** (SPES-i-men). The patient underwent surgery and was found to have no evidence of **metastasis** (me-TAS-ta-sis). Her entire colon was removed because of a high risk for developing a **malignant** (ma-LIG-nant) lesion in the remaining colon. She made an uneventful recovery and was referred to an **oncologist** (ong-KOL-o-jist) for consideration of **chemotherapy** (kē-mō-THER-a-pē). Her **prognosis** (prog-NŌ-sis) is generally positive. **Radiation therapy** (rā-dē-Ā-shun) (THER-a-pē) and **biological therapy** (bī-ō-LOJ-i-kel) (THER-a-pē) were not indicated in this case.

CHAPTER REVIEW

EXERCISE 34 ■ Chapter Content Quiz

Test your understanding of terms and abbreviations introduced in this chapter. Circle the letter for the medical term or abbreviation related to the words in italics. *To check your answers, go to Appendix A.*

1. Mr. Roberts was diagnosed as having a *cancerous tumor of connective tissue* or:
   a. sarcoma
   b. melanoma
   c. lipoma

2. The doctor said the tumor was *becoming progressively worse*; that is, it was:
   a. benign
   b. malignant
   c. pathogenic

3. The blood test showed an *increased amount of red blood cells*, or:
   a. erythrocytosis
   b. leukocytosis
   c. cyanosis

4. A *sample of blood, urine, or body tissue that is taken for medical testing* is a:
   a. biopsy
   b. specimen
   c. autopsy

5. The patient was diagnosed with a *tumor composed of fat*, or:
   a. neuroma
   b. carcinoma
   c. lipoma

6. The fatty tumor was *benign*, or:
   a. cancerous
   b. nonrecurrent
   c. recurrent

7. Substances thought to *cause cancer* are called:
   a. carcinoma
   b. carcinogenic
   c. cancerous

8. *Etiology* is the study of:
   a. causes of disease
   b. tissue disease
   c. causes of tumors

9. A *tumor* may be called:
   a. cytoplasm
   b. neoplasm
   c. karyoplasm

10. A *test performed on a sample to determine the presence of pathogenic bacteria* is:
    a. chemistry panel
    b. complete blood count
    c. culture and sensitivity

11. Any *disease of a muscle* is called:
    a. myoma
    b. myopathy
    c. neuropathy

12. The ultrasound revealed marked *abnormal development* on the right kidney or:
    a. hypoplasia
    b. dysplasia
    c. hyperplasia

13. The term that means *produced by a physician* is:
    a. diagnosis
    b. iatrogenic
    c. prognosis

14. The incidence of *black tumor (primarily of the skin)* is increasing.
    a. fibrosarcoma
    b. fibroma
    c. melanoma

15. The *study of tissue in disease* is:
    a. microbiology
    b. histopathology
    c. cytopathology

16. Which of the following is a *malignant tumor*?
    a. sarcoma
    b. fibroma
    c. myoma

17. A *minute microorganism, characterized by a lack of independent metabolism and the ability to replicate only within living host cells*, is a:
    a. bacteria
    b. fungus
    c. virus

18. Which of the following provides *palliative and supportive care for the terminally ill* and their families?
    a. hospice
    b. oncology
    c. biological therapy

19. During an appointment with her oncologist, the patient undergoing chemotherapy reported a *persistent, excessive tiredness and lack of energy* that seemed unrelated to exertion or lack of sleep.
    a. inflammation
    b. fatigue
    c. exacerbation

20. A laboratory test was ordered for a *leukocyte* count or:
    a. WBC
    b. RBC
    c. XRT

CHAPTER AT A GLANCE   Word Parts New to This Chapter

COMBINING FORMS

aden/o	gno/o	onc/o
aut/o	hemat/o	organ/o
bi/o	hist/o	path/o
cancer/o	iatr/o	rhabd/o
carcin/o	lei/o	sarc/o
cyan/o	leuk/o	somat/o
cyt/o	lip/o	system/o
epitheli/o	melan/o	vir/o
erythr/o	my/o	viscer/o
eti/o	necr/o	xanth/o
fibr/o	neur/o	

PREFIXES

dia-
dys-
hyper-
hypo-
meta-
micro-
neo-
pro-

SUFFIXES

-al	-opsy
-cyte	-osis
-gen	-ous
-genic	-pathy
-ic	-plasia
-logist	-plasm
-logy	-sarcoma
-megaly	-sis
-oid	-stasis
-oma	

CHAPTER AT A GLANCE — Medical Terms Built from Word Parts

BODY STRUCTURE
cytogenic
cytology
dysplasia
epithelial
erythrocyte (RBC)
erythrocytosis
histology
hyperplasia
hypoplasia
leukocyte (WBC)
leukocytosis
lipoid
necrosis
myopathy
neuropathy
organomegaly
somatic
somatogenic
systemic
visceral

ONCOLOGY
adenocarcinoma
adenoma
carcinoma (CA)
epithelioma
fibroma
fibrosarcoma
leiomyoma
leiomyosarcoma
lipoma
liposarcoma
melanoma
myoma
metastasis (pl. metastases) (METS)
neoplasm
neuroma
rhabdomyoma
rhabdomyosarcoma
sarcoma

LABORATORY
autopsy
biopsy
cytopathology
hematology
histopathology
microbiology
virology

COMPLEMENTARY
cancerous
carcinogen
carcinogenic
carcinoid
cyanosis
diagnosis (Dx)
etiology
iatrogenic
oncogenic
oncologist
oncology
pathogenic
pathologist
pathology
prognosis (Px)
xanthosis

CHAPTER AT A GLANCE — Medical Terms NOT Built from Word Parts

ONCOLOGY
benign
biological therapy
carcinoma in situ
chemotherapy (chemo)
encapsulated
hospice
malignant
palliative
radiation therapy (XRT)
remission

LABORATORY
chemistry panel
complete blood count with differential (CBC with diff)
culture and sensitivity (C&S)
genetic testing
specimen

COMPLEMENTARY
acute
afebrile
bacteria (s. bacterium)
chronic
erythema
exacerbation
fatigue
febrile
fungus (pl. fungi)
idiopathic
infection
inflammation
microorganism
parasite
virus (pl. viruses)

PART 1 INTRODUCTION TO WORD PARTS AND HUMAN BODY STRUCTURE

3 Directional Terms, Positions, and Imaging

Objectives

Upon completion of this chapter, you will be able to:

1. Define and spell word parts related to directional terms and diagnostic imaging.
2. Define, pronounce, and spell directional terms.
3. Define, pronounce, and spell terms used to describe abdominopelvic regions.
4. Define, pronounce, and spell terms used to describe anatomic planes.
5. Define, pronounce, and spell terms used to describe body positions.
6. Define, pronounce, and spell diagnostic imaging terms.
7. Interpret the meaning of abbreviations presented in this chapter.
8. Apply medical language in clinical contexts.

TABLE 3.1 Usage of Terms with Similar Meanings, 68
TABLE 3.2 Anatomic Planes and Diagnostic Images, 74
TABLE 3.3 Recumbent Positions, 77
TABLE 3.4 Overview of Diagnostic Imaging Procedures, 80

Outline

ANATOMIC POSITION, 61

WORD PARTS, 61
Directional Combining Forms, 61
Diagnostic Imaging Combining Forms, 61
Prefixes, 62
Suffixes, 62

MEDICAL TERMS, 66
Directional Terms, 66
Abdominopelvic Regions, 71
Anatomic Planes, 74
Body Positions, 76
Diagnostic Imaging, 80
Diagnostic Imaging Terms, 81
  Built from Word Parts and
    NOT Built from Word Parts, 81
Abbreviations, 85
  Abdominopelvic Quadrants, 86

PRACTICAL APPLICATION, 88
CASE STUDY Translate Between Everyday Language and Medical Language, 88
Interact with Medical Documents, 89
Use Medical Terms in Clinical Statements, 90
Pronounce Medical Terms in Use, 91

CHAPTER REVIEW, 91
Chapter Content Quiz, 91
Chapter at a Glance, 93

Answers to Chapter Exercises, Appendix A

Types of body movement are presented in Chapter 14, Musculoskeletal System. Terms related to body movement are: *abduction, adduction, inversion, eversion, extension, flexion, pronation, supination,* and *rotation.*

Chapter 3 Directional Terms, Positions, and Imaging   61

ANATOMIC POSITION

When using directional terms, the body is assumed to be in the standard, neutral position of reference, called the **anatomic position** (Fig. 3.1). In this position, the body is viewed as standing erect, arms at the side, palms of the hands facing forward, and feet side by side. The directional terms are the same whether the person is standing or supine (lying face up).

WORD PARTS

Use paper flashcards or electronic flashcards on Evolve to assist with memorization of word parts used to analyze, define, and build terms presented in this chapter. To reinforce learning, study one section of the Word Parts Table at a time, and then complete the corresponding exercise on the following pages.

1 ■ Directional Combining Forms

COMBINING FORM	DEFINITION	COMBINING FORM	DEFINITION
anter/o	front	later/o	side
caud/o	tail (downward)	medi/o	middle
cephal/o	head (upward)	poster/o	back, behind
dist/o	away (from the point of attachment)	proxim/o	near (the point of attachment)
dors/o	back	super/o	above
infer/o	below	ventr/o	belly (front)

2 ■ Diagnostic Imaging Combining Forms

COMBINING FORM	DEFINITION	COMBINING FORM	DEFINITION
radi/o	x-rays, ionizing radiation	tom/o	to cut, section, or slice
son/o	sound		

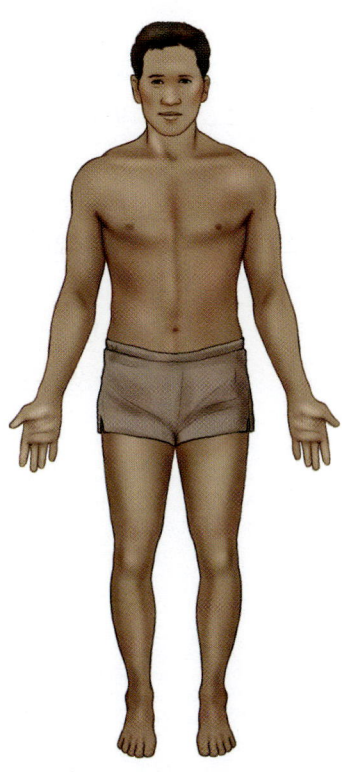

FIG. 3.1 Anatomic position.

3 ■ Prefixes

PREFIX	DEFINITION	PREFIX	DEFINITION
bi-	two	uni-	one

4 ■ Suffixes

SUFFIX	DEFINITION	SUFFIX	DEFINITION
-al	pertaining to	-ic	pertaining to
-gram	the record, radiographic image	-ior	pertaining to
-graph	instrument used to record, the record	-logist	one who studies and treats (specialist, physician)
-graphy	process of recording, radiographic imaging	-logy	study of

> Many suffixes mean **pertaining to**. Three were introduced in Chapter 2: -al, -ic, and -ous. More will be introduced in subsequent chapters. With practice, you will learn which suffix is most commonly used with a particular word root or combining form.

Refer to **Appendix B** and **Appendix C** for alphabetical lists of word parts and their meanings.

EXERCISE 1 ■ Directional Combining Forms

Refer to the first section of the word parts table.

A Define

Write the definitions for the following combining forms. *To check your answers to the exercises in this chapter, go to Appendix A at the back of the textbook.*

1. ventr/o _____
2. cephal/o _____
3. later/o _____
4. medi/o _____
5. infer/o _____
6. proxim/o _____
7. super/o _____
8. dist/o _____
9. dors/o _____
10. caud/o _____
11. anter/o _____
12. poster/o _____

> Do not be concerned about which combining form to use for front or back. As you continue to study and use medical terms, you will become familiar with common usage of each word part.

Chapter 3   Directional Terms, Positions, and Imaging   63

B Label

Fill in the blanks with directional combining forms. *To check your answers, go to Appendix A.*

1. Head
   CF: _____

2. Back
   CF: _____

3. Back, behind
   CF: _____

4. Tail (as in "tail" of the spine)
   CF: _____

5. Front
   CF: _____

6. Belly (front)
   CF: _____

7. Side
   CF: _____

8. Above
   CF: _____

9. Middle
   CF: _____

Leg: point of attachment

10. Near
    CF: _____

11. Away
    CF: _____

12. Below
    CF: _____

HEAD AND TRUNK ONLY Terms built from the combining forms **cephal/o** and **caud/o** are used to describe locations in the head and the trunk of the body.

EXERCISE 2 ■ Diagnostic Imaging Combining Forms

Refer to the second section of the word parts table.

A Match

Match the combining forms in the first column with their correct definitions in the second column. *To check your answers to the exercises in this chapter, go to Appendix A*

_____ 1. tom/o   a. x-rays, ionizing radiation
_____ 2. radi/o   b. sound
_____ 3. son/o   c. to cut, section, or slice

B Label

Write the combining forms pictured and defined.

1. _____
   to cut, section, or slice

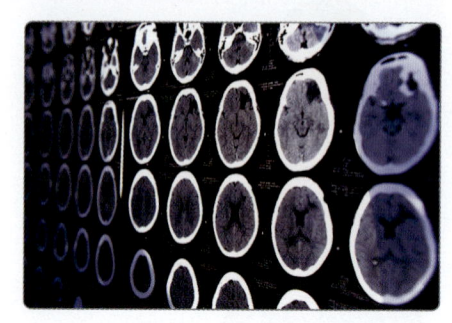

2. _____
   x-rays, ionizing radiation

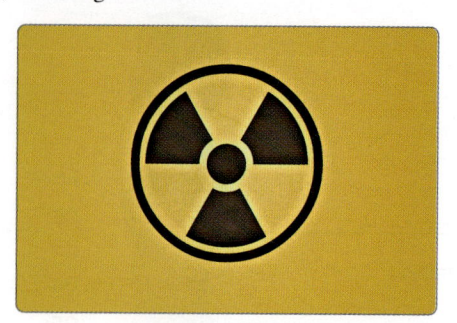

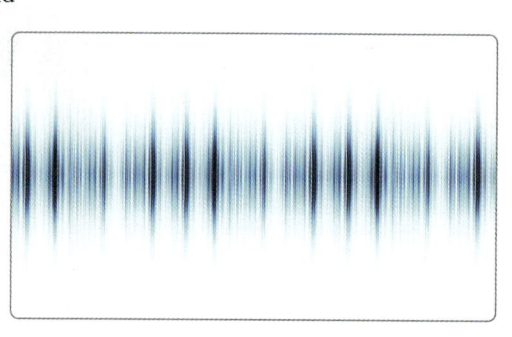

3. _____
   sound

EXERCISE 3 ■ Prefixes

Refer to the third section of the word parts table.

A Label

Write the prefixes pictured and defined.

1. _____
   one

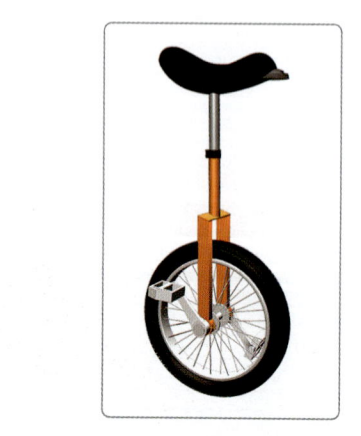

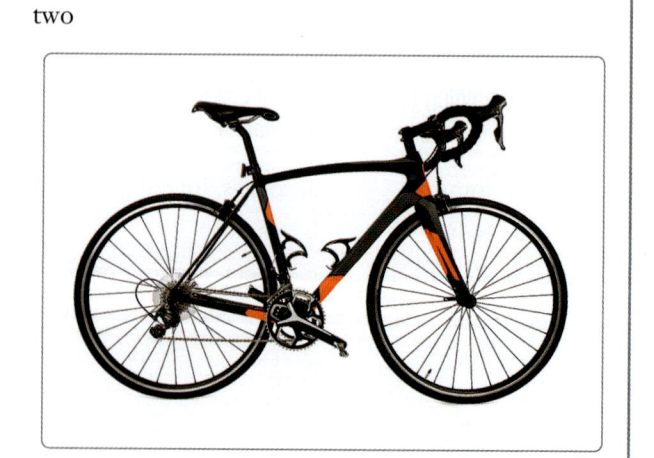

2. _____
   two

Chapter 3 Directional Terms, Positions, and Imaging 65

B Define

Write the definitions of the following prefixes.

1. bi- _____ 2. uni- _____

EXERCISE 4 ■ Suffixes

Refer to the fourth section of the word parts table.

A Label

Write the suffixes pictured and defined.

1. _____
   A. process of recording, or B. radiographic imaging

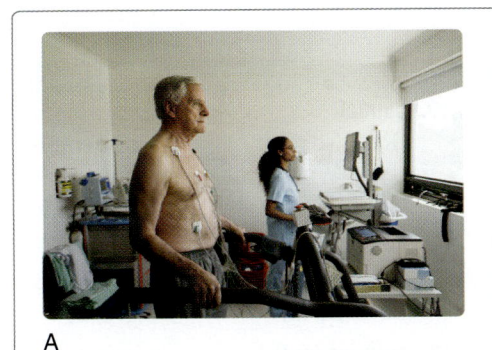

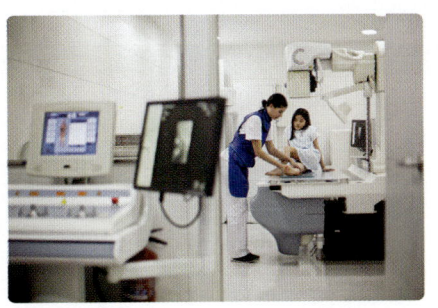

   A   B

2. _____
   A. instrument used to record, or B. the record

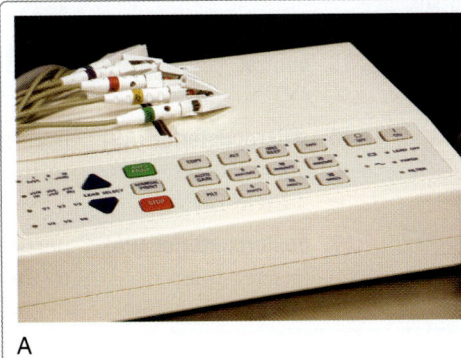

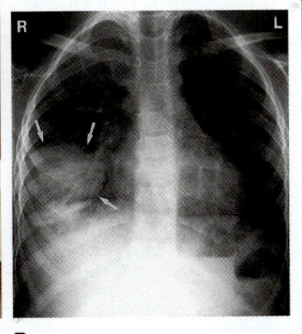

   A   B

3. _____
   A. the record, or B. radiographic image

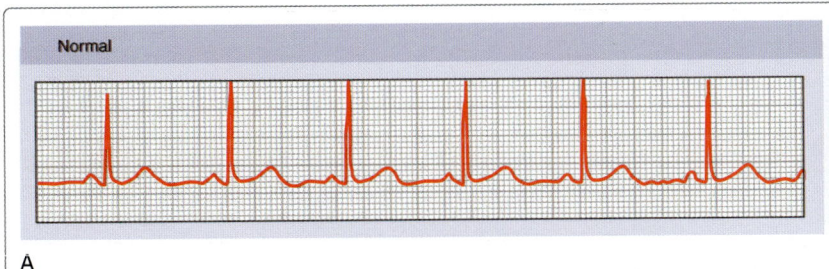

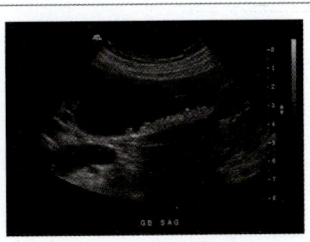

   Normal

   A   B

Chapter 3 Directional Terms, Positions, and Imaging

B Define

Write the definitions of the following suffixes.

1. -graphy _____
2. -graph _____
3. -gram _____
4. -ior _____
5. -ic _____
6. -logist _____
7. -logy _____
8. -al _____

MEDICAL TERMS

Directional Terms

The following terms are built from word parts and can be translated using the definitions of word parts. Further explanation is provided within parentheses as needed.

TERM	DEFINITION	TERM	DEFINITION
1. lateral (lat) (LAT-er-al)	pertaining to the side	10. caudal (KAW-dal)	pertaining to the tail (synonymous with **inferior** in human anatomy when specifying location on the trunk of the body) (Fig. 3.2)
2. medial (med) (MĒ-dē-al)	pertaining to the middle	11. cephalic (se-FAL-ik)	pertaining to the head (Fig. 3.2)
3. unilateral (ū-ni-LAT-er-al)	pertaining to one side (only)	12. anterior (ant) (an-TĒR-ē-or)	pertaining to the front (Fig. 3.2)
4. bilateral (bī-LAT-er-al)	pertaining to two sides	13. posterior (pos-TĒR-ē-or)	pertaining to the back (Fig. 3.2)
5. mediolateral (mē-dē-Ō-LAT-er-al)	pertaining to the middle and to the side	14. dorsal (DOR-sal)	pertaining to the back (Fig. 3.2)
6. distal (DIS-tal)	pertaining to away (from the point of attachment)	15. ventral (VEN-tral)	pertaining to the belly (front) (Fig. 3.2)
7. proximal (PROK-si-mal)	pertaining to near (to the point of attachment)	16. anteroposterior (AP) (an-ter-ō-pos-TĒR-ē-or)	pertaining to the front and to the back
8. inferior (inf) (in-FĒR-ē-or)	pertaining to below (Fig. 3.2)	17. posteroanterior (PA) (pos-ter-ō-an-TĒR-ē-or)	pertaining to the back and to the front
9. superior (sup) (sū-PĒR-ē-or)	pertaining to above (Fig. 3.2)		

EXERCISE 5 ■ Pronounce and Spell

Practice pronunciation and spelling on paper and online.

1. **Practice on Paper**
   a. **Pronounce:** Read the phonetic spelling and say aloud the terms listed in the previous table. Refer to Table 2.2 Pronunciation Key as needed.
   b. **Spell:** Have a study partner read the terms aloud. Write the spelling of the terms on a separate sheet of paper.

2. **Practice Online**
   a. **Access** the online learning resources. Go to evolve.elsevier.com > Evolve Resources > Student Resources.
   b. **Pronounce:** Select Audio Glossary > Chapter 3 > Exercise 5. Select a term to hear its pronunciation and repeat aloud.
   c. **Spell:** Select Activities > Chapter 3 > Spell Terms > Exercise 5. Select the audio icon and type the correct spelling of the term.

❏ Check the box when complete.

EXERCISE 6 ■ Analyze and Define

Analyze and define the following directional terms by drawing slashes between word parts, writing word part abbreviations above the term, underlining combining forms, and writing combining form abbreviations below the term. *To check your answers, go to Appendix A.*

```
              WR  CV  WR   S
EXAMPLE:   medi / o / later / al
                CF
           pertaining to the middle and to the side
```

1. proximal

2. lateral

3. unilateral

4. anteroposterior

5. cephalic

6. superior

7. anterior

8. distal

Chapter 3 Directional Terms, Positions, and Imaging

9. medial

10. bilateral

11. posteroanterior

12. caudal

13. inferior

14. posterior

15. dorsal

16. ventral

TABLE 3.1 Usage of Terms with Similar Meanings

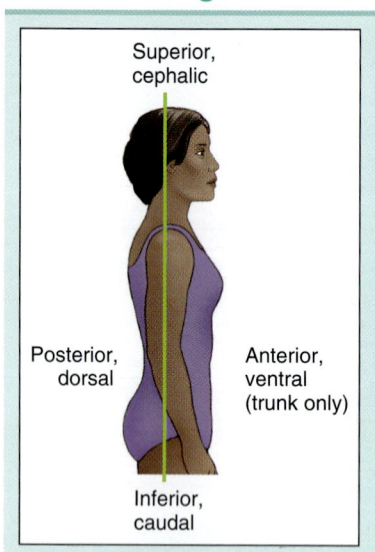

FIG. 3.2 Superior and inferior, cephalic and caudal, posterior and anterior, dorsal, and ventral.

SAME
When describing anatomic structures in the *head* and *trunk* of the body, the following terms are **similar** in meaning and are used interchangeably:
- **Superior** and **cephalic** describe above.
- **Inferior** and **caudal** describe below.
- **Posterior** and **dorsal** describe the back.
- **Anterior** and **ventral** (trunk only) describe the front.

DIFFERENT
Differences in uses of terms include:
- Directional terms ending with **-ior** can indicate spatial relationships of body parts to each other throughout the body. The nose is **anterior** to the ear, and the ear is **posterior** to the nose. The eye is **superior** to the mouth, and the mouth is **inferior** to the eye.
- **Ventral** describes the trunk of the body. The **ventral** cavity is located toward the belly and is made up of the thoracic and abdominopelvic cavities. Ventral may also denote a relationship to the anterior abdominal wall. A **ventral** hernia is a hernia in the anterior abdominal wall.
- **Dorsal** describes the back of the head and trunk. The **dorsal** cavity is located in the posterior portion of the body and is made up of the cranial and spinal cavities. Dorsal also describes the surface of the hand opposite the palm and the top of the foot. The pulse palpable on the **dorsal** surface of the foot is called dorsalis pedis pulse.
- **Cephalic** and **caudal** apply to the head and trunk of the body only, whereas **superior** and **inferior** also apply to limbs. The ankle is **inferior** to the knee.

Chapter 3 Directional Terms, Positions, and Imaging 69

EXERCISE 7 ■ Build

A Label

Build terms pictured by writing word parts above definitions.

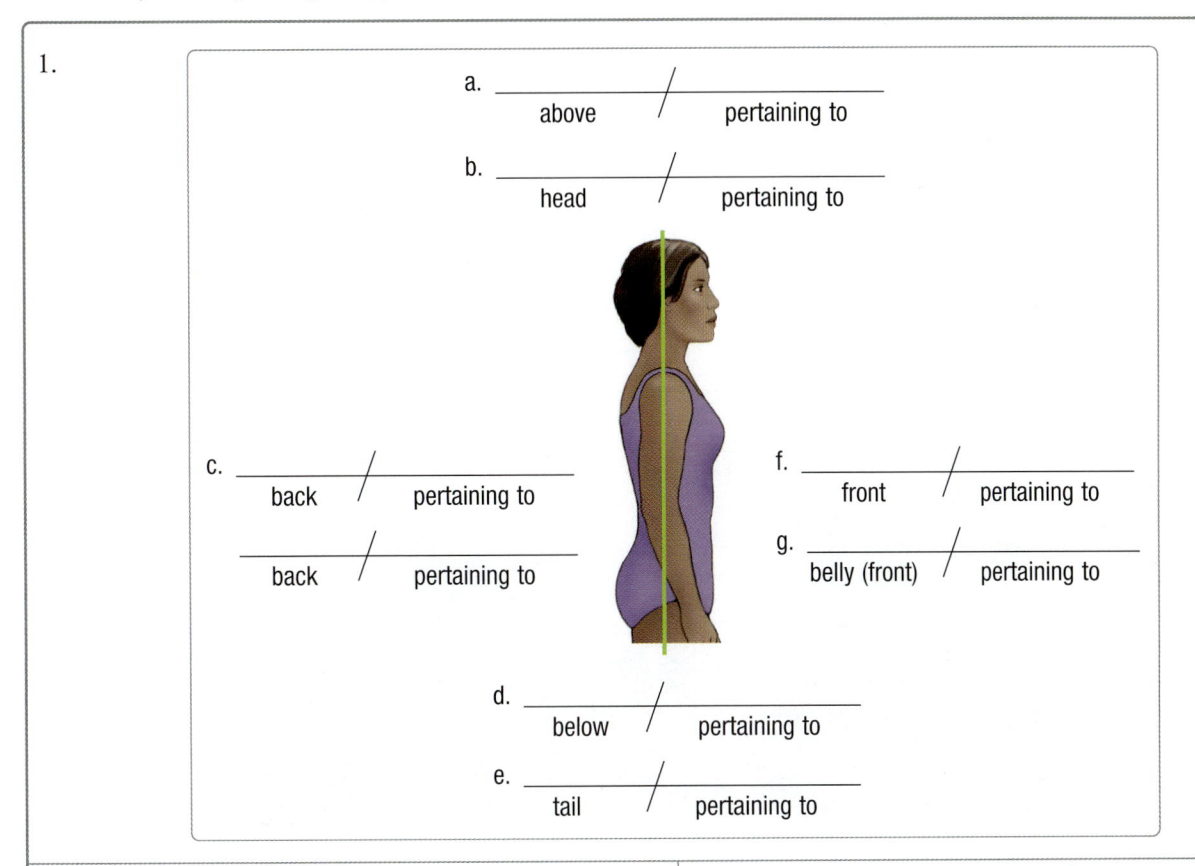

1.
a. _____ / _____
   above / pertaining to

b. _____ / _____
   head / pertaining to

c. _____ / _____
   back / pertaining to

   _____ / _____
   back / pertaining to

f. _____ / _____
   front / pertaining to

g. _____ / _____
   belly (front) / pertaining to

d. _____ / _____
   below / pertaining to

e. _____ / _____
   tail / pertaining to

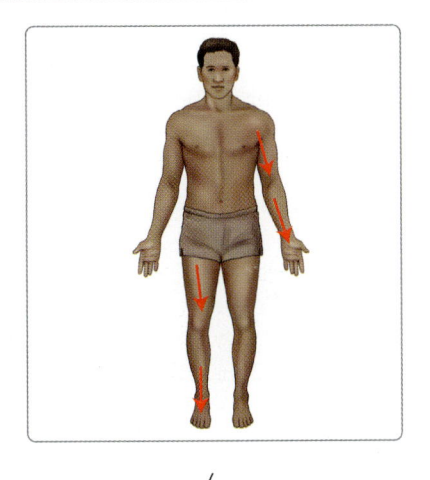

2.
_____ / _____
away from the point of attachment / pertaining to

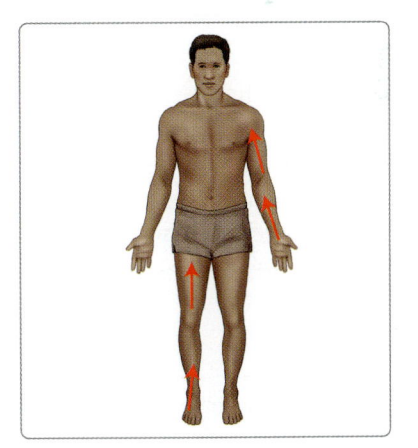

3.
_____ / _____
near the point of attachment / pertaining to

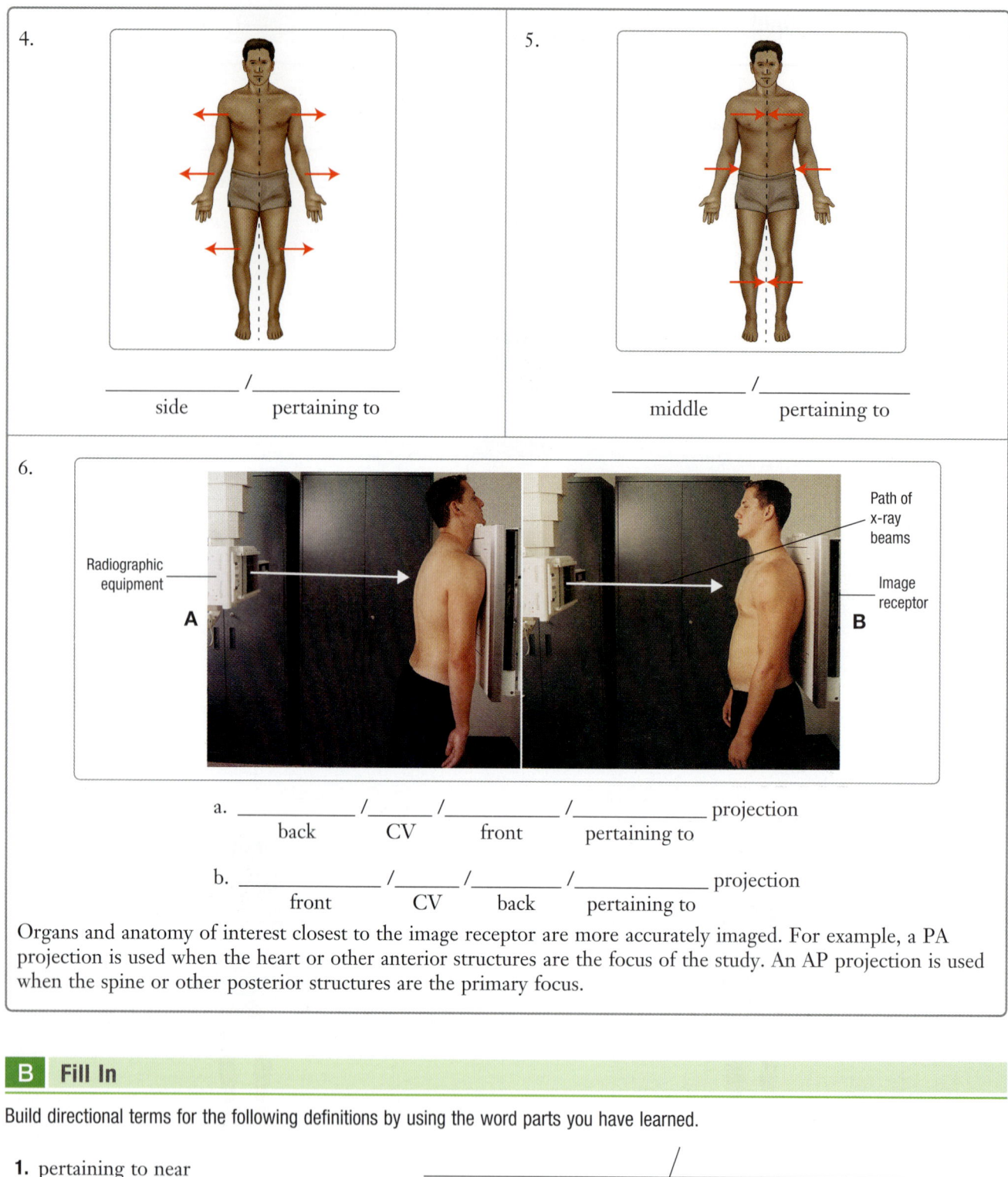

Chapter 3 Directional Terms, Positions, and Imaging

4. _____/_____
    side   pertaining to

5. _____/_____
    middle   pertaining to

6.
   a. _____/___/_____/_____ projection
      back   CV   front   pertaining to

   b. _____/___/_____/_____ projection
      front CV   back   pertaining to

Organs and anatomy of interest closest to the image receptor are more accurately imaged. For example, a PA projection is used when the heart or other anterior structures are the focus of the study. An AP projection is used when the spine or other posterior structures are the primary focus.

B Fill In

Build directional terms for the following definitions by using the word parts you have learned.

1. pertaining to near   _____/_____
                                 WR   S

2. pertaining to away   _____/_____
                                 WR   S

3. pertaining to two sides   _____/_____/_____
                                 P   WR   S

4. pertaining to the middle

___WR___ / ___S___

5. pertaining to the back and to the front

___WR___ / ___CV___ / ___WR___ / ___S___

6. pertaining to the middle and to the side

___WR___ / ___CV___ / ___WR___ / ___S___

7. pertaining to one side (only)

___P___ / ___WR___ / ___S___

8. pertaining to the front and to the back

___WR___ / ___CV___ / ___WR___ / ___S___

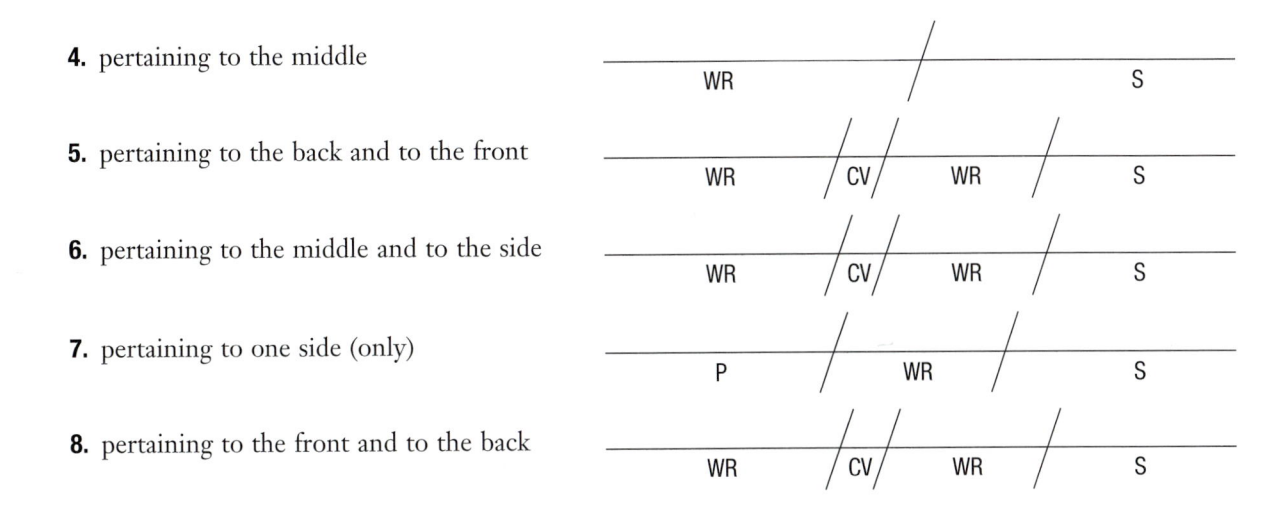

EXERCISE 8 ■ Review of Directional Terms

Can you define, pronounce, and spell the following directional terms?

anterior (ant)	distal	mediolateral	unilateral
anteroposterior (AP)	dorsal	posterior	ventral
bilateral	inferior (inf)	posteroanterior (PA)	
caudal	lateral (lat)	proximal	
cephalic	medial (med)	superior (sup)	

Abdominopelvic Regions

To assist in locating medical problems with greater accuracy and for identification purposes, the abdomen and pelvis are divided into nine regions (Fig. 3.3). Abdominopelvic regions are often used to document the physical examination and medical history to describe signs and symptoms. The number in parentheses indicates the number of regions.

TERM	DEFINITION	TERM	DEFINITION
1. umbilical region (1) (um-BIL-i-kal) (RĒ-jun)	around the navel (umbilicus)	🏛 **HYPOCHONDRIAC** from the Greek **hypo** (meaning under), and **chondros** (meaning cartilage), was used by Hippocrates to refer to the region below rib cartilage. In 1765, it was used to refer to people who had discomfort in this area with no organic findings. Eventually, hypochondriac referred to a person who falsely believed they were ill. More recently, **cyberchondria** emerged as a term describing a pattern of using Internet research to self-diagnose symptoms, causing worry.	
🏛 **UMBILICUS** is a term derived from the Latin **umbo**, which denoted the boss, or protuberant part, of a shield. Around the first century, the term was used to designate either a raised or a depressed spot in the middle of anything.			
2. lumbar regions (2) (LUM-bar) (RĒ-junz)	to the right and left of the umbilical region, near the waist	5. hypogastric region (1) (hī-pō-GAS-trik) (RĒ-jun)	inferior to the umbilical region
3. epigastric region (1) (ep-i-GAS-trik) (RĒ-jun)	superior to the umbilical region	6. iliac regions (2) (IL-ē-ak) (RĒ-junz)	to the right and left of the hypogastric region, near the groin (also called **inguinal regions**)
4. hypochondriac regions (2) (hī-pō-KON-drē-ak) (RĒ-junz)	to the right and left of the epigastric region		

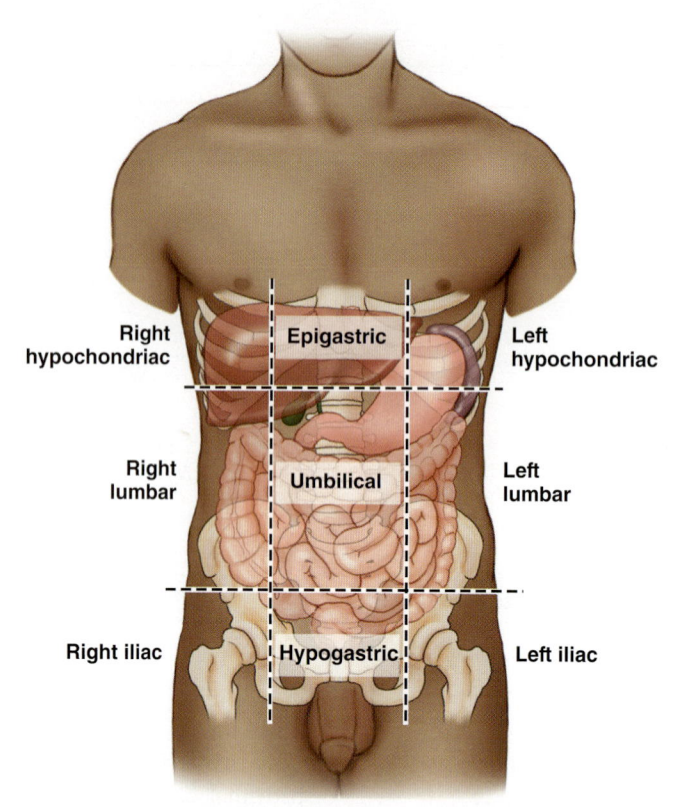

Chapter 3 Directional Terms, Positions, and Imaging

FIG. 3.3 Abdominopelvic regions. References to right and left indicate the right and left of the patient's body.

PREVENTING WRONG-SIDE ERRORS When facing the patient, your right and left will be opposite of the patient's right and left. Confusing the patient's right and left with the provider's right and left can lead to significant errors such as **wrong-sided surgery**.

Tips for preventing wrong-sided errors:

- Remember **"right"** and **"left"** pertain to the right and left of the patient's body.
- Avoid saying **"right"** when **"correct"** is meant.
- When a patient indicates the side choice is **"right,"** confirm the response meant **"correct."**

EXERCISE 9 ▪ Pronounce and Spell

Practice pronunciation and spelling on paper and online.

1. **Practice on Paper**

    a. **Pronounce:** Read the phonetic spelling and say aloud the terms listed in the previous table. Refer to Table 2.2 Pronunciation Key as needed.
    b. **Spell:** Have a study partner read the terms aloud. Write the spelling of the terms on a separate sheet of paper.

2. **Practice Online**

    a. **Access** online learning resources. Go to evolve.elsevier.com > Evolve Resources > Student Resources.
    b. **Pronounce:** Select Audio Glossary > Chapter 3 > Exercise 9. Select a term to hear its pronunciation and repeat aloud.
    c. **Spell:** Select Activities > Chapter 3 > Spell Terms > Exercise 9. Select the audio icon and type the correct spelling of the term.

☐ Check the box when complete.

Chapter 3 Directional Terms, Positions, and Imaging   73

EXERCISE 10 ■ Abdominopelvic Regions

A Label

Fill in the blanks with abdominopelvic regions to label the diagram. *To check your answers, go to Appendix A.*

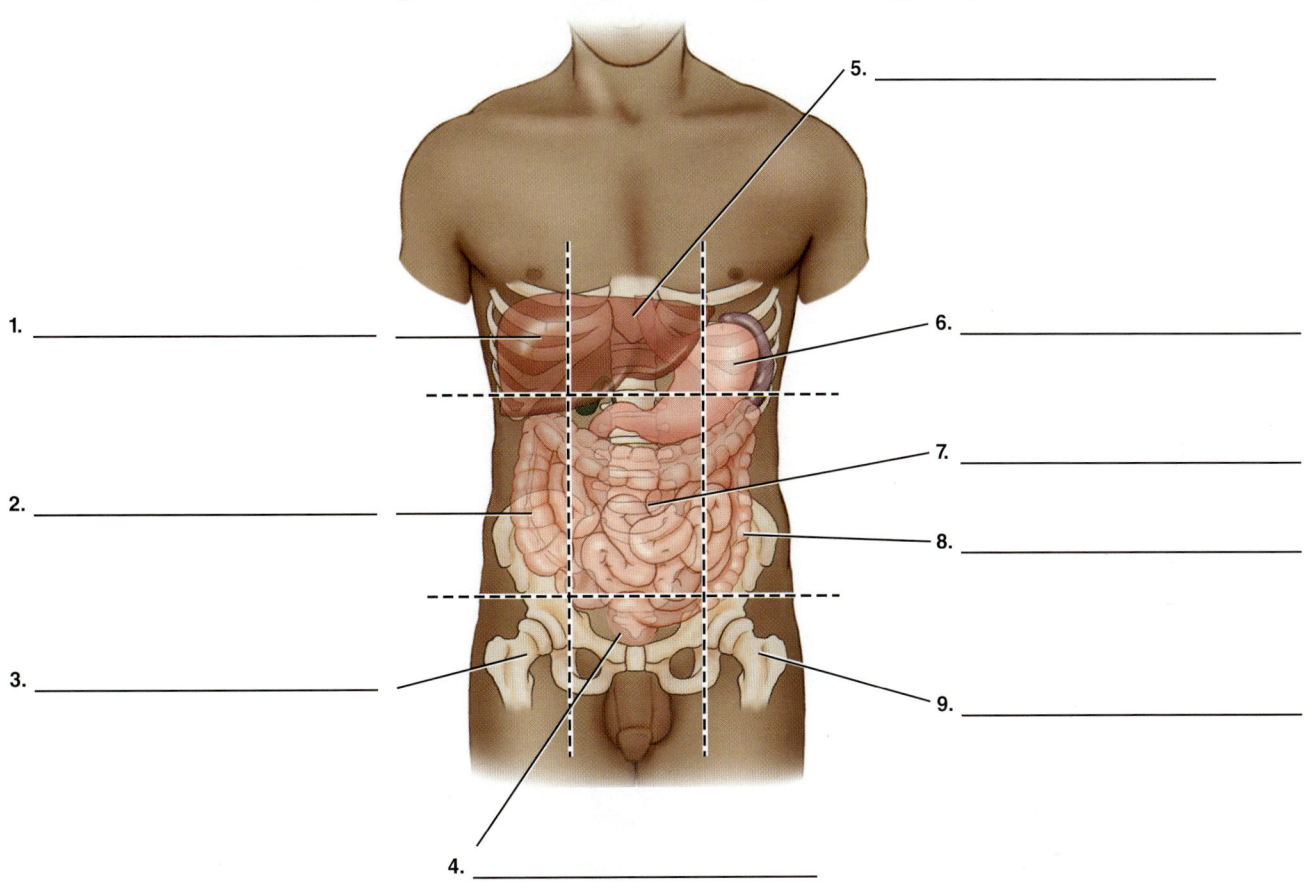

1. _____
2. _____
3. _____
4. _____
5. _____
6. _____
7. _____
8. _____
9. _____

B Match

Match the terms in the first column with their correct definitions in the second column.

_____ 1. epigastric   a. inferior to the umbilical region
_____ 2. hypochondriac   b. superior to the umbilical region
_____ 3. hypogastric   c. right and left of the umbilical region, near the waist
_____ 4. iliac   d. right and left of the epigastric region
_____ 5. lumbar   e. right and left of the hypogastric region, near the groin
_____ 6. umbilical   f. inferior to the epigastric region

EXERCISE 11 ■ Review of Abdominopelvic Regions Terms

Can you define, pronounce, and spell the following abdominopelvic regions?

epigastric region   hypogastric region   lumbar regions
hypochondriac regions   iliac regions   umbilical region

Anatomic Planes

Planes are imaginary flat fields used as points of reference to identify or view the location of organs and anatomic structures. Anatomic planes are frequently used in diagnostic imaging and surgery. The body is assumed to be in the anatomic position unless specified otherwise (Table 3.2).

TERM	DEFINITION	TERM	DEFINITION
1. axial (AK-see-uh-l)	horizontal plane dividing the body into superior and inferior portions (also called **transverse plane** and **horizontal plane**)	4. oblique (ō-BLĒK)	diagonal plane passing through the body at an angle between the horizontal and vertical planes (any plane that is neither vertical nor horizontal)
2. coronal (ko-RŌN-al)	vertical plane passing through the body from side to side, dividing the body into anterior and posterior portions (also called **frontal plane**)	5. parasagittal (*par*-a-SAJ-i-tal)	vertical plane passing through the body from front to back, dividing the body into unequal left and right sides (any plane parallel to the midsagittal plane)
3. midsagittal (mid-SAJ-i-tal)	vertical plane passing through the body from front to back at the midline, dividing the body equally into right and left halves	6. sagittal (SAJ-i-tal)	vertical plane passing through the body from front to back, dividing the body into right and left sides (general term referring to the midsagittal plane and parasagittal planes)

MIDLINE is an imaginary line that separates the body, or body parts, into halves. In medical language, midline is used as a common reference point.

TABLE 3.2 Anatomic Planes and Diagnostic Images

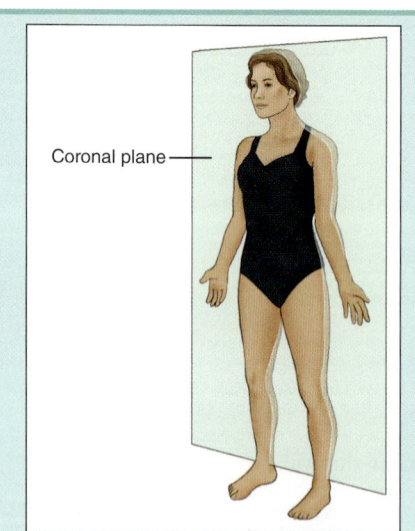

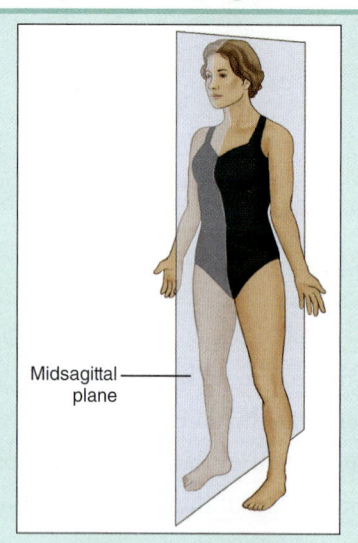

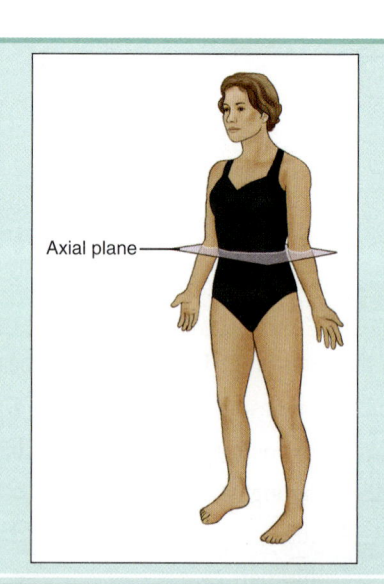

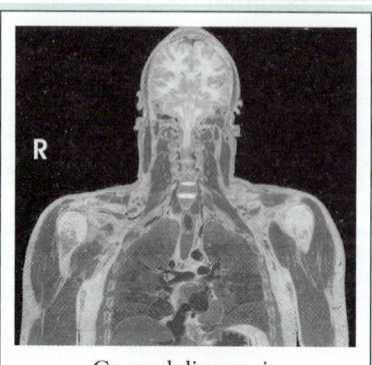

Coronal plane

Midsagittal plane

Axial plane

Coronal diagnostic image (MRI*)

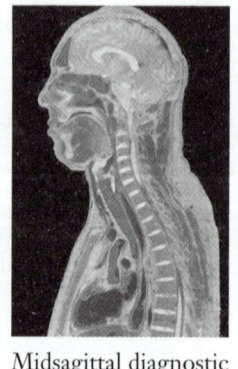

Midsagittal diagnostic image (MRI*)

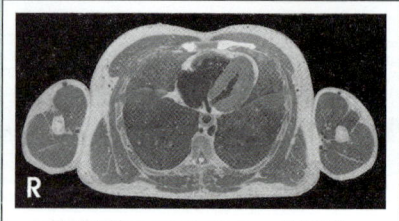

Axial diagnostic image (MRI*)

* MRI abbreviates **magnetic resonance imaging**

Chapter 3   Directional Terms, Positions, and Imaging   75

> **Sagittal** describes vertical planes dividing the body into right and left sides. **Midsagittal** and **parasagittal** planes are both sagittal planes, with the midsagittal plane dividing the body equally into halves and the parasagittal plane dividing the body into unequal sides.

EXERCISE 12 ■ Pronounce and Spell

Practice pronunciation and spelling on paper and online.

1. **Practice on Paper**
   a. **Pronounce:** Read the phonetic spelling and say aloud the terms listed in the previous table. Refer to Table 2.2 Pronunciation Key as needed.
   b. **Spell:** Have a study partner read the terms aloud. Write the spelling of the terms on a separate sheet of paper.

2. **Practice Online**
   a. **Access** online learning resources. Go to evolve.elsevier.com > Evolve Resources > Student Resources.
   b. **Pronounce:** Select Audio Glossary > Chapter 3 > Exercise 12. Select a term to hear its pronunciation and repeat aloud.
   c. **Spell:** Select Activities > Chapter 3 > Spell Terms > Exercise 12. Select the audio icon and type the correct spelling of the term.

❏ Check the box when complete.

EXERCISE 13 ■ Anatomic Planes

A Label

Fill in the blanks with anatomic planes to label the diagram.

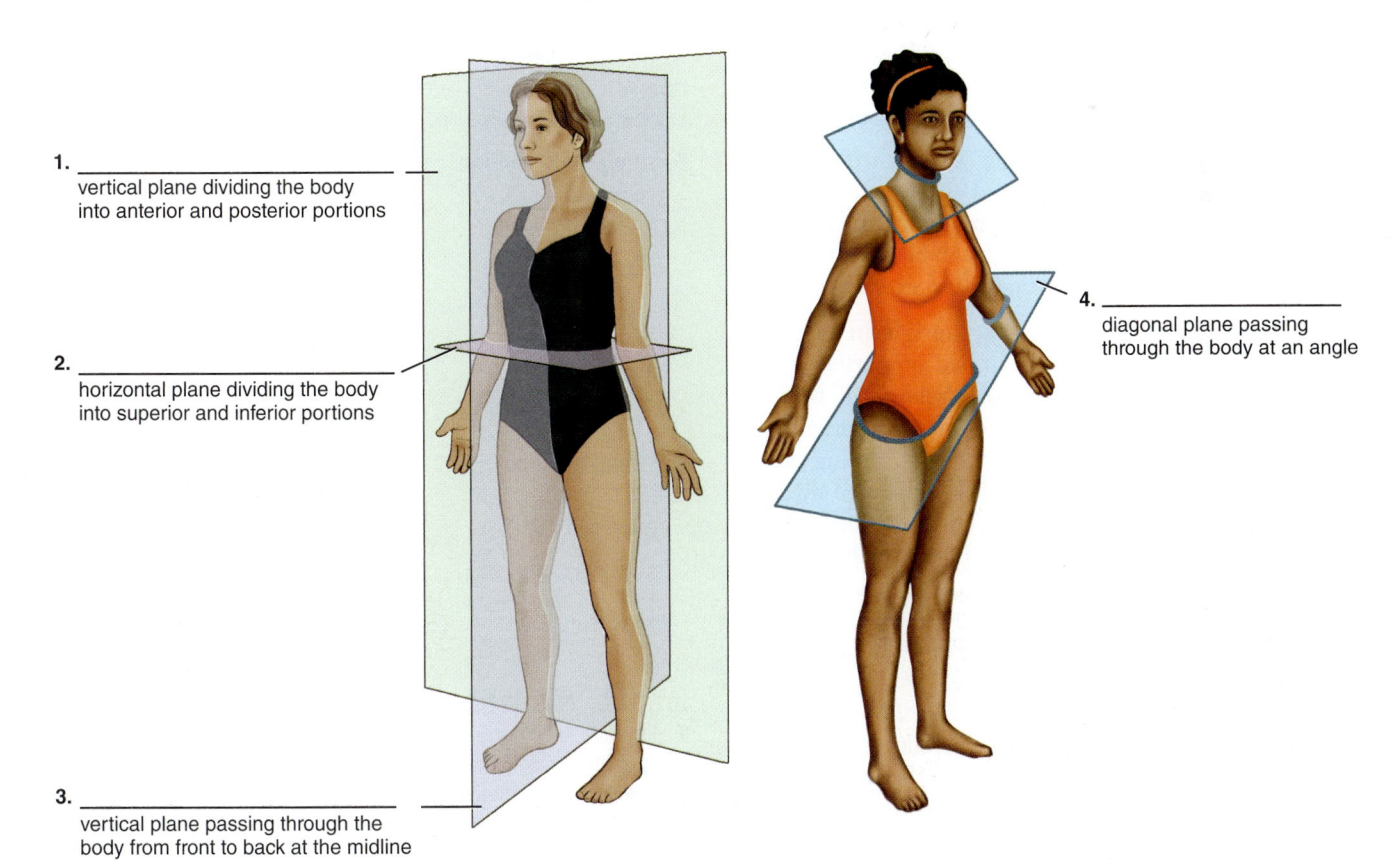

1. _____
   vertical plane dividing the body into anterior and posterior portions

2. _____
   horizontal plane dividing the body into superior and inferior portions

3. _____
   vertical plane passing through the body from front to back at the midline

4. _____
   diagonal plane passing through the body at an angle

B Fill In

Fill in the blanks with the correct terms.

1. The plane that divides the body into superior and inferior portions is the _____ plane.
2. The plane that divides the body **equally** into right and left halves is the _____ plane.
3. The plane that divides the body into anterior and posterior portions is referred to as the _____ plane.
4. Any plane that divides the body into right and left sides is referred to as a(n) _____ plane.
5. The plane that divides the body into **unequal** right and left sides is the _____ plane.
6. Any plane that is neither vertical nor horizontal is a(n) _____ plane.

EXERCISE 14 ■ Review of Anatomic Planes Terms

Can you define, pronounce, and spell the following anatomic planes?

axial plane	midsagittal plane	parasagittal plane
coronal plane	oblique plane	sagittal plane

Body Positions

Position terms are used in health care settings to communicate how the patient's body is placed for physical examination, diagnostic procedures, surgery, treatment, and recovery.

TERM	DEFINITION	TERM	DEFINITION
1. lateral position (LAT-er-al) (pe-ZISH-en)	lying on one side with knees bent; right and left precede the term to indicate the patient's side (also called **side-lying position** and **lateral recumbent position**)	5. recumbent position (rē-KUM-bent) (pe-ZISH-en)	lying down in any position (also called **decubitus position**) (Table 3.3)
		SEMIRECUMBENT POSITION indicates the patient is lying down with the head of the bed raised to a 45° angle. Used in critical care to prevent ventilator-associated pneumonia.	
2. lithotomy position (lith-OT-o-mē) (pe-ZISH-en)	lying on back with legs raised and feet in stirrups, hips and knees flexed, and thighs abducted (away from body) and externally rotated	6. semiprone position (sem-ē-PRŌN) (pe-ZISH-en)	lying on one side between a lateral and prone position with the upper knee drawn up toward the chest and the lower arm drawn behind parallel to the back. "Right" or "left" precede the term to indicate the patient's right or left side.
3. orthopnea position (or-THOP-nē-a) (pe-ZISH-en)	sitting upright in a chair or in bed supported by pillows behind the back. Sometimes the patient tilts forward, resting on a pillow supported by an overbed table. (also called **orthopneic position**)		
		7. sitting position (SIT-ting) (pe-ZISH-en)	bed position with head of the bed elevated at an angle between 15° and 90° and with slight elevation of the knees (also called **Fowler position** and **semisitting position**)
ORTHOPNEA POSITION Orthopnea is built from the combining form **orth/o** meaning straight and the suffix **-pnea** meaning breathing. Patients who need to sit up straight to breathe are placed in the orthopnea position.			
4. prone position (prōn) (pe-ZISH-en)	lying on abdomen, facing downward; head may be turned to one side; also called **ventral recumbent position**	**SITTING POSITION or FOWLER POSITION** indicates the head of the bed is raised between 15° and 90°. Variations in the angle are denoted by **high**, indicating an upright position at approximately 90°; **standard**, indicating an angle between 45° and 60°; **semi**, 30° to 45°; and **low**, in which the head is slightly elevated between 15° and 30°.	

Chapter 3 Directional Terms, Positions, and Imaging 77

TERM	DEFINITION	TERM	DEFINITION
8. supine position (SOO-pine) (pe-ZISH-en)	lying on back, facing upward (also called **dorsal recumbent position**)	**TRENDELENBURG POSITION** Variations include the **modified Trendelenburg position**, in which the torso is flat with the legs raised, and the **reverse Trendelenburg position**, in which the body is tilted so that the feet are lower than the head.	
9. Trendelenburg position (tren-DEL-en-berg) (pe-ZISH-en)	lying on back with body tilted so that the head is lower than the feet; used less often due to risks that include increased pressure within the eyes (intraocular) and within the skull (intracranial)		

TABLE 3.3 Recumbent Positions

Recumbent position (also called **decubitus position**) is a general term indicating the patient is lying down in any position, such as supine, prone, or on one side. The specific position is indicated by additional terms.

dorsal recumbent position... lying on back; the patient is lying down facing upward (also called **supine position**)

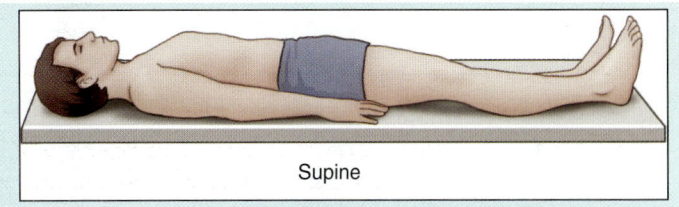

Supine

ventral recumbent position... lying face down; the patient is lying down on the belly. The face may be turned to the right or left. (also called **prone position**)

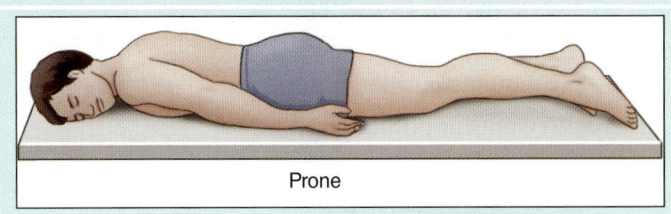

Prone

left lateral recumbent position... lying on the patient's left side (also called **left lateral decubitus position**); right knee may be drawn upward

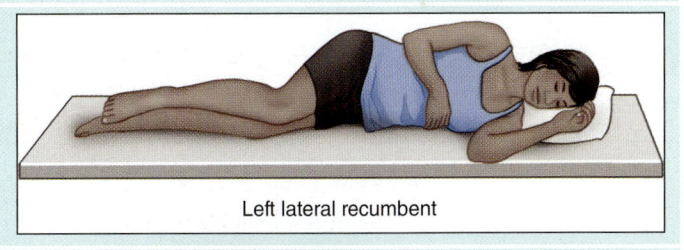

Left lateral recumbent

right lateral recumbent position... lying on the patient's right side; left knee may be drawn upward (also called **right lateral decubitus position**)

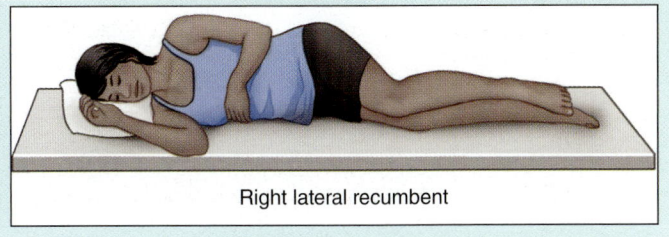

Right lateral recumbent

Chapter 3   Directional Terms, Positions, and Imaging

EXERCISE 15 ■ Pronounce and Spell

Practice pronunciation and spelling on paper and online.

1. **Practice on Paper**
   a. **Pronounce:** Read the phonetic spelling and say aloud the terms listed in the previous table. Refer to Table 2.2 Pronunciation Key as needed.
   b. **Spell:** Have a study partner read the terms aloud. Write the spelling of the terms on a separate sheet of paper.

2. **Practice Online**
   a. **Access** online learning resources. Go to evolve.elsevier.com > Evolve Resources > Student Resources.
   b. **Pronounce:** Select Audio Glossary > Chapter 3 > Exercise 15. Select a term to hear its pronunciation and repeat aloud.
   c. **Spell:** Select Activities > Chapter 3 > Spell Terms > Exercise 15. Select the audio icon and type the correct spelling of the term.

❑ Check the box when complete.

EXERCISE 16 ■ Body Positions

A Match

Match the body position terms in the first column with their descriptions in the second column. *To check your answers, go to Appendix A.*

_____ 1. semiprone position
_____ 2. Trendelenburg position
_____ 3. sitting position
_____ 4. lithotomy position
_____ 5. recumbent position

a. lying on back with body tilted so that the head is lower than the feet; in the modified form the back is flat and the legs are raised
b. lying down in any position
c. lying on back with legs raised and feet in stirrups, hips and knees flexed, and thighs abducted (away from body) and externally rotated
d. also called Fowler position and semisitting position
e. lying on one side between a lateral and prone position

B Label

Write the patient positions pictured and defined.

1. _____ position, lying on back, facing upward (also called **dorsal recumbent position**)

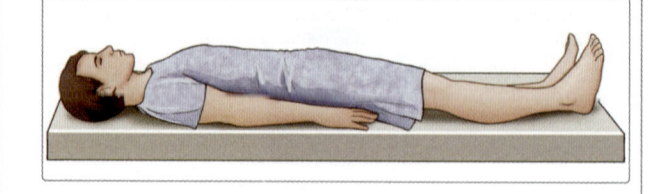

2. _____ position, lying on abdomen, facing downward (also called **ventral recumbent position**)

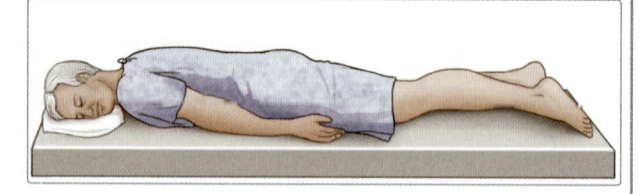

Chapter 3   Directional Terms, Positions, and Imaging   79

3. _____ position, bed position with head of the bed elevated at an angle between 15° and 90° and with slight elevation of the knees

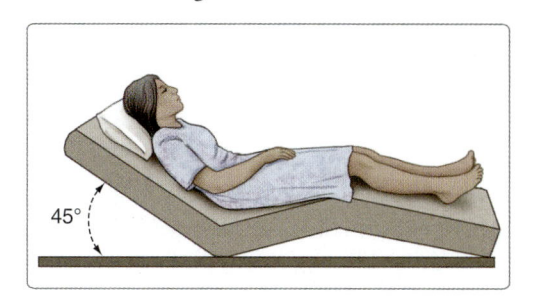

4. _____ position, sitting upright in a chair or in bed supported by pillows behind the back

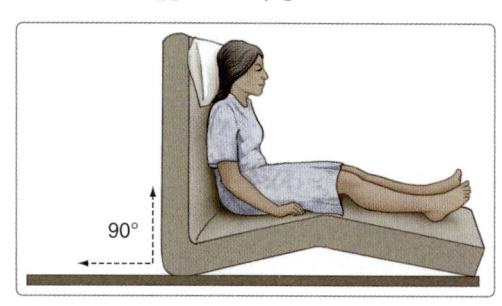

5. _____ position, lying on one side with knees bent

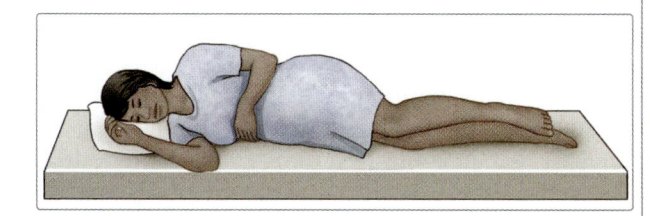

6. _____ position, lying on one side between a lateral and prone position with the upper knee drawn up toward the chest and the lower arm drawn behind parallel to the back

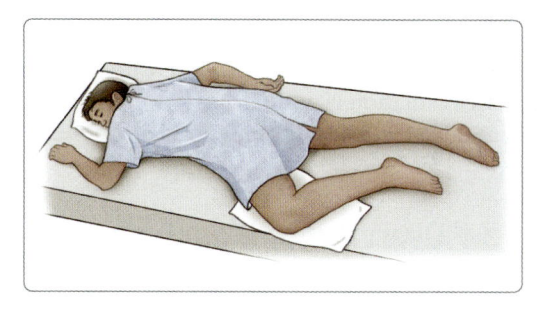

C   Identify

Fill in the blanks with the correct terms.

1. The _____ position, also known as Fowler position, is a bed position where the head of the bed is elevated at an angle between 15° and 90° and is used for a variety of reasons, including aiding breathing, eating, and other activities of daily living in frail patients.
2. An unconscious patient may be placed lying on one side between lateral and prone in the _____ position to avoid choking on fluid draining from the mouth.
3. Primarily used in surgery, the _____ position is a back-lying position in which the body is tilted so that the head is lower than the feet.
4. Patients are placed in the _____ position when undergoing an exam or procedure that requires access to the pelvic cavity, genitals, or rectum.
5. The _____ position, in which the patient sits upright in a chair or bed, is used to improve breathing.

> **EXERCISE 17 ■ Review of Body Position Terms**

Can you define, pronounce, and spell the following body position terms?

lateral position	prone position	sitting position
lithotomy position	recumbent position	supine position
orthopnea position	semiprone position	Trendelenburg position

Diagnostic Imaging

Diagnostic imaging is an important part of the evaluation of patients with a variety of signs and symptoms. The information obtained from imaging generally reveals the presence or absence of abnormalities in the area being studied.

Radiography, or the use of x-rays, was the first form of diagnostic imaging. The process as we know it was discovered in 1895 by Wilhelm Conrad Roentgen in Germany. Because he did not understand the nature of the rays, he named them "x" rays. Today we understand that radiography produces images of internal structures using ionizing radiation emitted from an x-ray tube. An image receptor catches the radiant energy that has been transmitted through the patient. The captured energy is digitally processed to form an image called a **radiograph**, which is stored electronically and displayed on a monitor. Since Roentgen's time, many forms of diagnostic imaging have been developed and are in use today. **Radiology** is the medical specialty dedicated to the use of imaging technology to diagnose and treat disease. See Table 3.4 for an overview of current diagnostic imaging procedures.

Directional terms, abdominopelvic regions, anatomic planes, and body positioning are all important aspects of diagnostic imaging. They are used to ensure that the maximum amount of information is recorded on the image, while unnecessary radiation is minimized. For example, anatomic planes are used in **computed tomography**, **magnetic resonance imaging**, and **sonography** to identify the direction of "cuts" or "slices" demonstrated in the procedure.

TABLE 3.4 Overview of Diagnostic Imaging Procedures

PROCEDURE	VISUALIZES	OFTEN USED TO EXAMINE	USED TO DETECT
Radiography	Dense structures	Bones, lungs	Fractures, tumors, lesions
Fluoroscopy	Deep tissues and hollow structures	Gastrointestinal tract, heart, urinary system, and reproductive systems	Reflux, obstruction, ulcers
Sonography	Soft tissue structures, plus movement of blood, denseness of tissue	Heart, blood vessels, eyes, thyroid, brain, breast, abdominal organs, skin, and muscle	Cysts, tumors, gallstones, vessel blockages, prenatal abnormalities
Magnetic resonance (MR)	Internal organs, spine, joints, blood vessels	Brain, spine, joints, biliary system (gallbladder and bile ducts)	Tumors, torn ligaments, gallstones
Computed tomography (CT)	Internal organs, movement of blood, denseness of tissue	Bones, heart, lungs, vessels, abdominal organs	Disease, injuries, fractures, clots, internal bleeding, tumors
Positron emission tomography (PET)	Cellular and tissue activity	Brain, heart, vessels	Cancer, flow of blood to heart
Single photon emission computed tomography (SPECT)	Blood flow, cellular and tissue activity	Heart, brain, bones	Infection, tumors, blockages

Diagnostic Imaging Terms
BUILT FROM WORD PARTS AND *NOT* BUILT FROM WORD PARTS

The first portion of the table contains Diagnostic Imaging Terms that can be translated using definitions of word parts. The second portion of the table contains Diagnostic Imaging Terms that cannot be fully understood using the definitions of word parts.

■ Built from Word Parts

TERM	DEFINITION
1. **radiograph** (RĀ-dē-ō-*graph*)	record of x-rays
2. **radiography** (rā-dē-OG-rah-fē)	process of recording x-rays
X-RAY Radiography (the procedure) and radiograph (the resulting image) are both also called x-ray.	
3. **radiologist** (rā-dē-OL-o-jist)	physician who specializes in x-rays (specifically the diagnosis and treatment of disease using medical imaging such as x-rays, computed tomography [CT], magnetic resonance imaging [MRI], nuclear medicine [NM], and sonography)
INTERVENTIONAL RADIOLOGISTS guide targeted treatment of disease, including cancer, vascular abnormalities, and reproductive conditions, using diagnostic imaging. Interventional radiologists (IRs) are board-certified physicians who work closely with other medical specialists.	

TERM	DEFINITION
4. **radiology** (ra-dē-OL-o-jē)	study of x-rays (a branch of medicine concerned with the study and application of imaging technology, including x-ray, computed tomography [CT], magnetic resonance imaging [MRI], nuclear medicine [NM], and sonography to diagnose and treat disease)
5. **sonogram** (SON-ō-gram)	record of sound
6. **sonography** (so-NOG-rah-fē)	process of recording sound (also called **ultrasonography [US]**)
7. **tomography** (to-MOG-rah-fē)	process of recording slices (anatomical cross sections)
TYPES OF TOMOGRAPHY include computed tomography (CT), positron emission tomography (PET), and single photon emission computed tomography (SPECT).	

■ *NOT* Built from Word Parts

TERM	DEFINITION
1. **computed tomography (CT)** (kom-PŪ-ted) (to-MOG-rah-fē)	imaging modality that combines x-rays with computer technology to produce detailed, cross-sectional images of the body, called "slices." Oral or intravenous contrast materials may be given to highlight specific regions in the body.
2. **fluoroscopy** (flōr-OS-ka-pē)	imaging of moving body structures, like an x-ray movie. An x-ray beam is passed through the body part being studied, and then the image is transmitted to a monitor in real time so that movement can be seen in detail. Contrast materials are used to help identify and assess the function of different structures.
3. **nuclear medicine (NM)** (NOO-klē-er) (MED-i-sin)	imaging of internal structures using a Gamma camera to detect radiation from different parts of the body after a radioactive material (radioisotope) has been given to the patient
4. **magnetic resonance imaging (MRI)** (mag-NET-ik) (REZ-ō-nans) (IM-a-jing)	high-strength, computer-controlled magnetic fields producing a series of sectional images (slices) that visualize abnormalities such as swelling, infections, tumors, and herniated disks. Contrast materials may be administered.
5. **scan** (skan)	image obtained from diagnostic imaging procedures where data from several angles or sections have been combined; often scans are generated with the use of radioactive materials administered to the patient. Scans are generated by many diagnostic imaging procedures, including but not limited to nuclear medicine, computed tomography, and magnetic resonance imaging.

Chapter 3 Directional Terms, Positions, and Imaging

EXERCISE 18 ■ Pronounce and Spell

Practice pronunciation and spelling on paper and online.

1. **Practice on Paper**
   a. **Pronounce:** Read the phonetic spelling and say aloud the terms listed in the previous table. Refer to Table 2.2 Pronunciation Key as needed.
   b. **Spell:** Have a study partner read the terms aloud. Write the spelling of the terms on a separate sheet of paper.

2. **Practice Online**
   a. **Access** online learning resources. Go to evolve.elsevier.com > Evolve Resources > Student Resources.
   b. **Pronounce:** Select Audio Glossary > Chapter 3 > Exercise 18. Select a term to hear its pronunciation and repeat aloud.
   c. **Spell:** Select Activities > Chapter 3 > Spell Terms > Exercise 18. Select the audio icon and type the correct spelling of the term.

❏ Check the box when complete.

EXERCISE 19 ■ Diagnostic Terms Built from Word Parts

A Analyze and Define

Analyze and define the following diagnostic imaging terms by drawing slashes between word parts, writing word part abbreviations above the term, underlining combining forms, and writing combining form abbreviations below the term. *To check your answers, go to Appendix A.*

```
              WR CV  S
EXAMPLE:   radi / o / logy
               CF
           study of x-rays
```

1. tomography

2. sonogram

3. radiography

4. sonography

5. radiograph

6. radiologist

B Label

Build diagnostic imaging terms pictured by writing word parts above definitions.

1. _____ / _____ / _____ 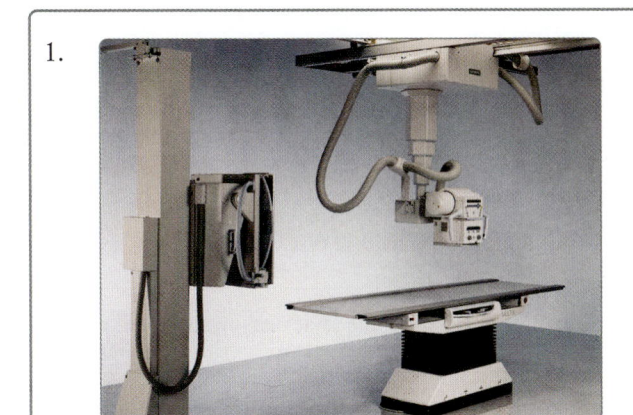
    x-ray   CV   process of recording

2. _____ / _____ / _____ 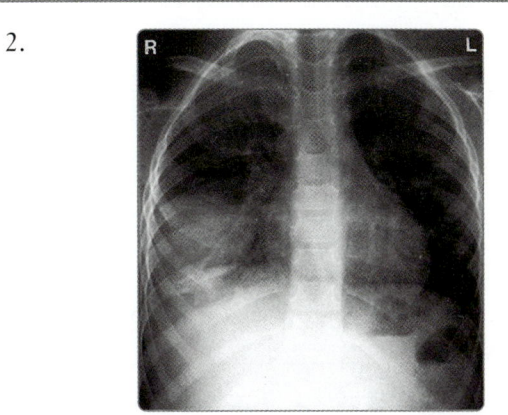
    x-rays   CV   record

3. _____ / _____ / _____ 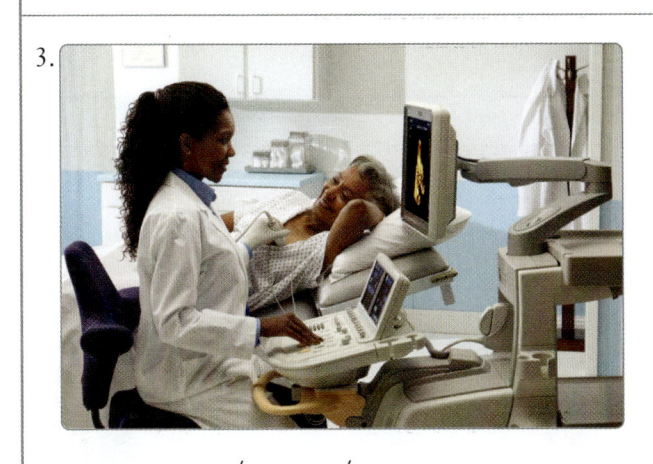
    sound   CV   process of recording

4. _____ / _____ / _____ 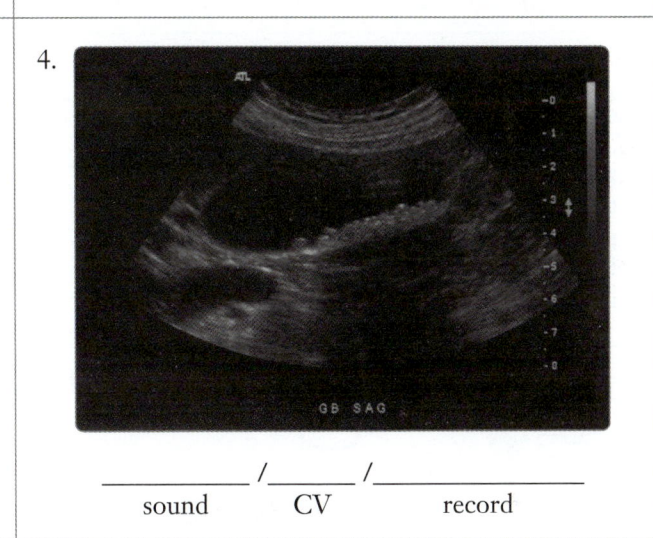
    sound   CV   record

C Fill In

Build diagnostic imaging terms for the following definitions by using the word parts you have learned.

1. process of recording slices   _____ / ___ / _____
                                        WR   CV   S

2. physician who specializes in x-rays   _____ / ___ / _____
                                           WR   CV   S

3. study of x-rays   _____ / ___ / _____
                                        WR   CV   S

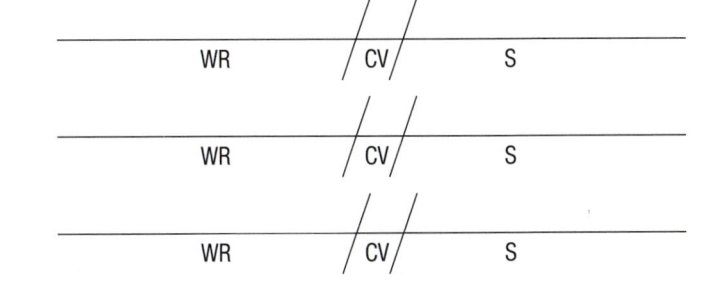

84 Chapter 3 Directional Terms, Positions, and Imaging

EXERCISE 20 ■ Diagnostic Imaging Terms NOT Built from Word Parts

A Identify

Fill in the blanks with the correct terms.

1. The image obtained from a diagnostic imaging procedure where data from several angles or sections have been combined is called a(n) _____.
2. _____ produces images of internal structures using a Gamma camera to detect radiation from different parts of the body after a radioactive material has been given to the patient.
3. Moving x-ray images are produced by _____.
4. The procedure using high-strength, computer-controlled magnetic fields to produce a series of sectional images (slices) is called _____.
5. _____ is the imaging modality combining x-rays with computer technology to produce detailed, cross-sectional images of the body, called "slices."

B Label

Write the diagnostic imaging terms pictured and defined.

1. _____
imaging of moving body structures, like an x-ray movie; an x-ray beam is passed through the body part being studied, and then the image is transmitted to a monitor in real time so that movement can be seen in detail

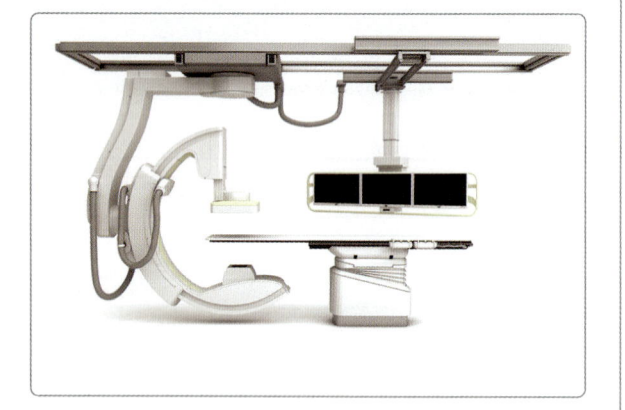

2. _____
imaging modality that combines x-rays with computer technology to produce detailed, cross-sectional images of the body, called "slices"

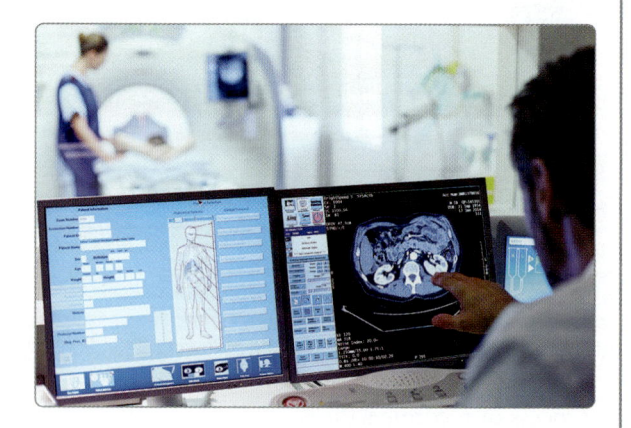

3. _____
imaging of internal structures using a Gamma camera to detect radiation from different parts of the body after a radioactive material has been given to the patient

Posterior   RPO   Rt. lateral   LPO
Perfusion lung scan
Hx: 46-year-old female; history of shortness of breath
Lt. lateral   Anterior
Diacam
Matrix: 128×128
Dose: 3mCi 99mTc-MAA
Counts: 500K/view
Dx: Normal lung study

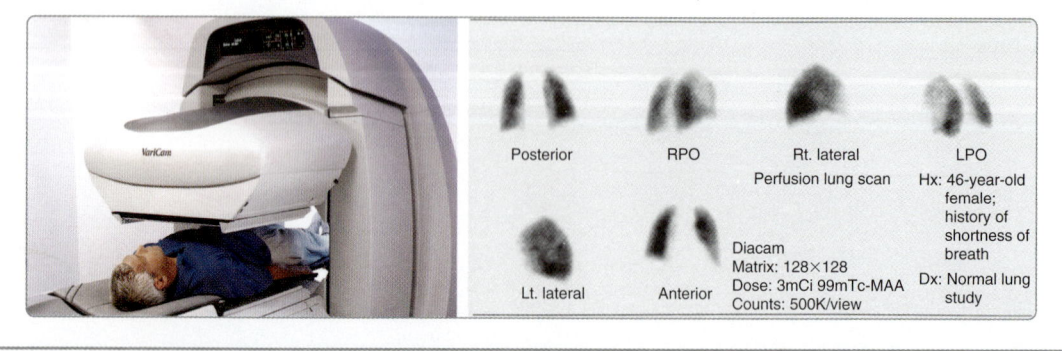

Chapter 3 Directional Terms, Positions, and Imaging   85

4. _____
high-strength, computer-controlled magnetic fields producing a series of sectional images (slices) that visualize abnormalities such as swelling, infections, tumors, and herniated disks

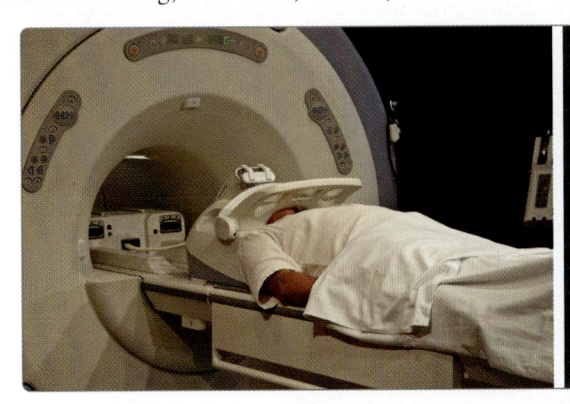

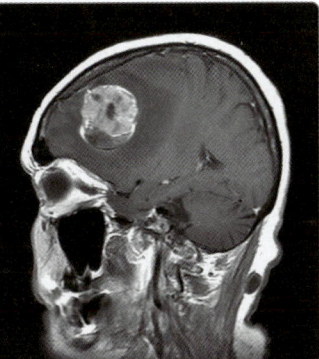

EXERCISE 21 ■ Review of Diagnostic Imaging Terms

Can you define, pronounce, and spell the following diagnostic imaging terms?

computed tomography (CT)	nuclear medicine (NM)	radiologist	sonogram
fluoroscopy	radiograph	radiology	sonography
magnetic resonance imaging (MRI)	radiography	scan	tomography

Abbreviations

DIRECTIONAL TERMS			
ABBREVIATION	TERM	ABBREVIATION	TERM
ant	anterior	med	medial
AP	anteroposterior	PA	posteroanterior
inf	inferior	sup	superior
lat	lateral		

DIAGNOSTIC IMAGING			
ABBREVIATION	TERM	ABBREVIATION	TERM
CT	computed tomography	NM	nuclear medicine
MR	magnetic resonance	US	ultrasonography
MRI	magnetic resonance imaging		

ABDOMINOPELVIC QUADRANTS			
ABBREVIATION	TERM	ABBREVIATION	TERM
LLQ	left lower quadrant	RLQ	right lower quadrant
LUQ	left upper quadrant	RUQ	right upper quadrant

Refer to **Appendix D** for a complete list of abbreviations.

ABDOMINOPELVIC QUADRANTS

The abdominopelvic area can also be divided into four quadrants by using imaginary vertical and horizontal lines that intersect at the umbilicus (Fig. 3.4). These divisions are used by healthcare professionals to specify the location of pain, incisions, markings, lesions, and so forth. The quadrants provide a more general denotation than the abdominopelvic regions, and they are used to describe the location of findings from the physical examination and medical history. The four divisions are:

1. right upper quadrant (RUQ)
2. left upper quadrant (LUQ)
3. right lower quadrant (RLQ)
4. left lower quadrant (LLQ)

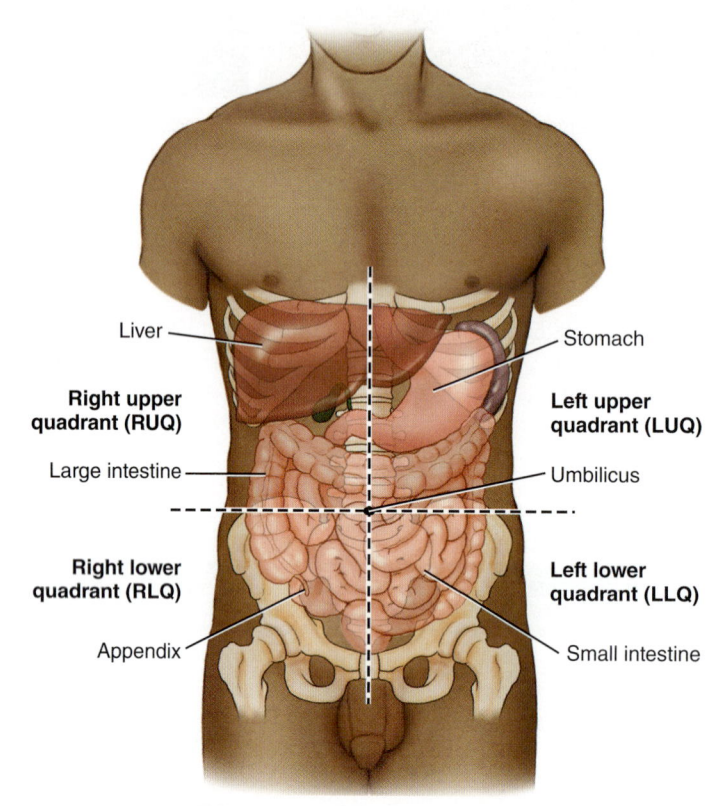

FIG. 3.4 Abdominopelvic quadrants.

Chapter 3 Directional Terms, Positions, and Imaging 87

EXERCISE 22 ■ Abbreviations

A Fill In

Write the terms abbreviated.

1. sup _____
2. ant _____
3. inf _____
4. PA _____
5. AP _____
6. med _____
7. lat _____
8. US _____
9. NM _____
10. MRI _____
11. CT _____
12. MR _____

B Label

Fill in the blanks with abdominopelvic quadrants and abbreviations to label the diagram.

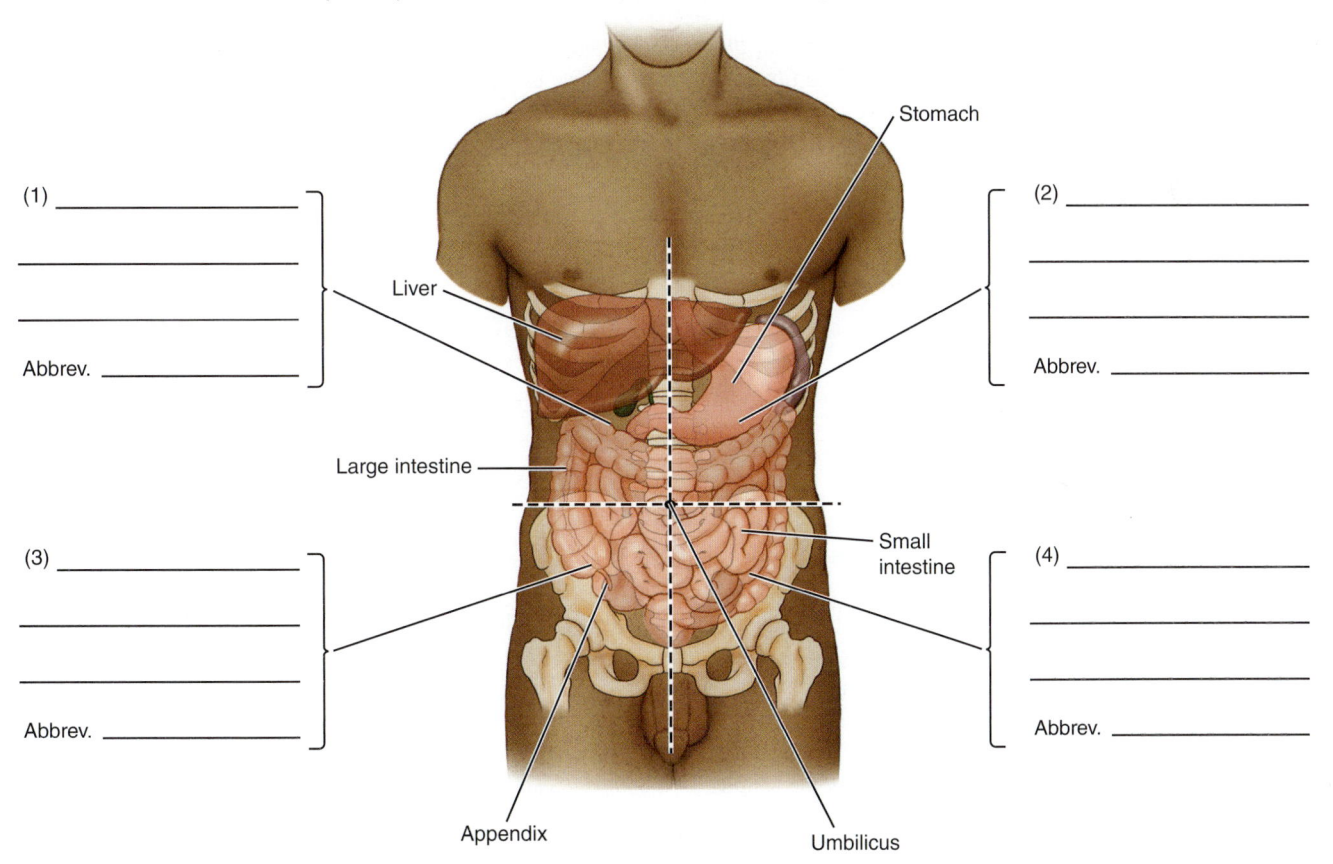

(1) _____
_____
_____
Abbrev. _____

(2) _____
_____
_____
Abbrev. _____

(3) _____
_____
_____
Abbrev. _____

(4) _____
_____
_____
Abbrev. _____

Chapter 3 Directional Terms, Positions, and Imaging

PRACTICAL APPLICATION

EXERCISE 23 ■ Case Study: Translate Between Everyday Language and Medical Language

CASE STUDY: A'idah Khalil

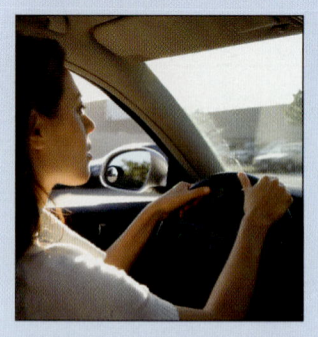

A'idah Khalil was just in a car accident, but luckily, she is awake and knows what is going on around her. The ambulance comes, and the emergency team asks her where she is hurting. Her right foot hurts the most. She has pain in her upper right arm near her shoulder and notices some bleeding there. She also has some pain in her belly near the navel and in her lower back near the waist. The paramedics put her on a hard board on her back facing upward, put some kind of collar around her neck, then load her into the ambulance and take her to the hospital. Upon arrival in the Emergency Department, she is taken to the x-ray department to have pictures taken of her foot. While there, she is also placed into a machine that allows x-ray doctors to view cross sections of her spine and the areas around it.

Now that you have worked through Chapter 3, consider the directional terms, positions, and regions that might be used to describe A'idah's experience. See the Chapter at a Glance section at the end of the chapter for a list of terms that might apply.

A. Underline phrases in the case study that could be substituted with medical terms.

B. Write the medical term and its definition for two of the phrases you underlined.

MEDICAL TERM	DEFINITION
1. _____	_____
2. _____	_____

DOCUMENTATION: Excerpt From Emergency Department Note

The following was documented in the Diagnostic Studies portion of her medical record:

Radiographs (x-rays) of the right lower extremity in the medial and lateral view identify a fracture of the calcaneus with proximal dislocation of the cuboid bone. Radiographs of the cervical spine in AP and oblique projection show no bone injury. CT scan images of the lower back reveal no significant abnormalities.

C. Underline medical terms and abbreviations presented in Chapter 3 in the previous excerpt from A'idah's medical record. See the Chapter at a Glance section at the end of the chapter for a complete list.

D. Select and define two of the medical terms you underlined. To check your answers, go to Appendix A.

MEDICAL TERM	DEFINITION
1. _____	_____
2. _____	_____

Chapter 3 Directional Terms, Positions, and Imaging

EXERCISE 24 — Interact with Medical Documents

A

Read the report and complete it by writing medical terms on answer lines within the document. Definitions of terms to be written appear after the document.

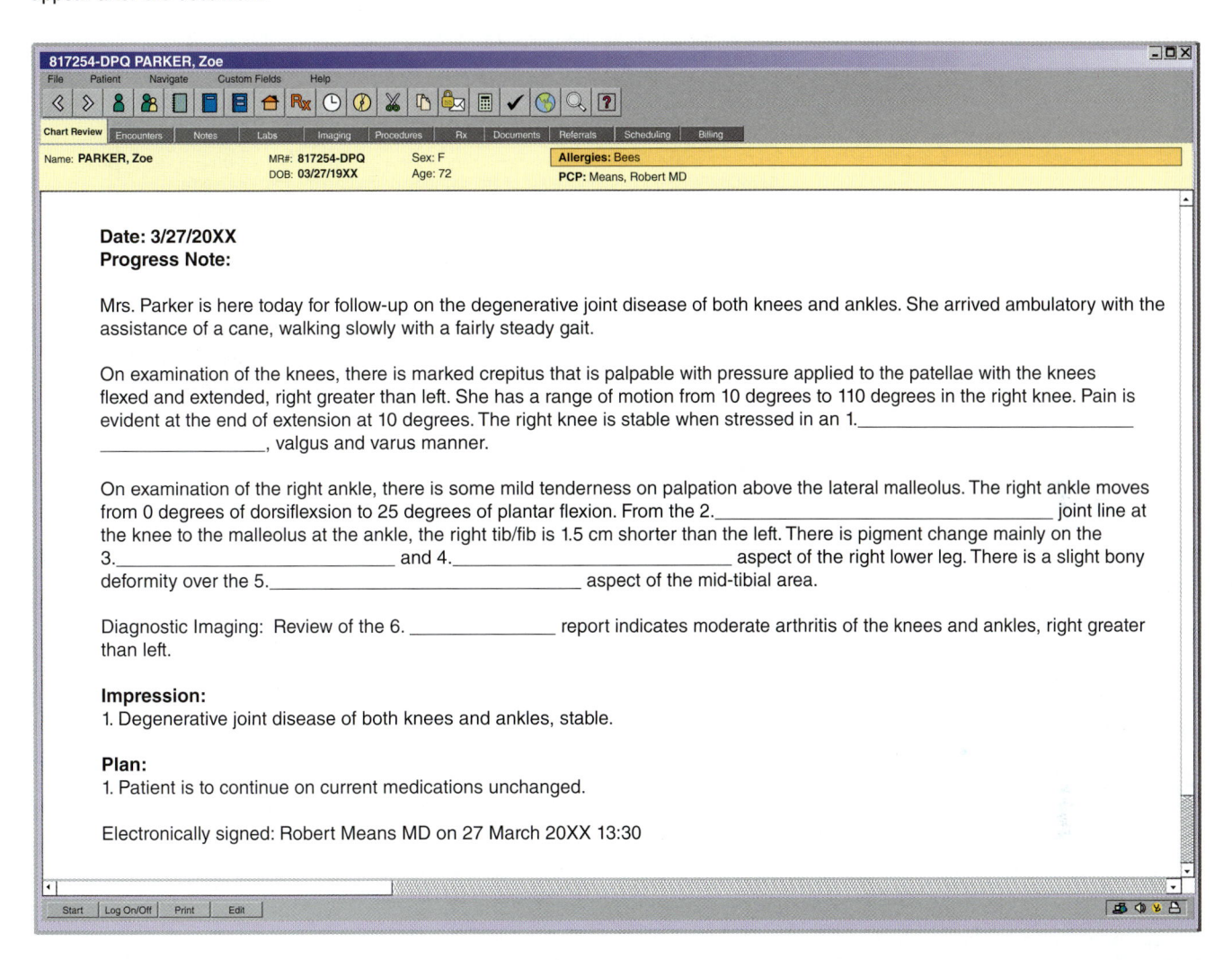

817254-DPQ PARKER, Zoe

Name: PARKER, Zoe MR#: 817254-DPQ Sex: F Allergies: Bees
DOB: 03/27/19XX Age: 72 PCP: Means, Robert MD

Date: 3/27/20XX
Progress Note:

Mrs. Parker is here today for follow-up on the degenerative joint disease of both knees and ankles. She arrived ambulatory with the assistance of a cane, walking slowly with a fairly steady gait.

On examination of the knees, there is marked crepitus that is palpable with pressure applied to the patellae with the knees flexed and extended, right greater than left. She has a range of motion from 10 degrees to 110 degrees in the right knee. Pain is evident at the end of extension at 10 degrees. The right knee is stable when stressed in an 1._____, valgus and varus manner.

On examination of the right ankle, there is some mild tenderness on palpation above the lateral malleolus. The right ankle moves from 0 degrees of dorsiflexion to 25 degrees of plantar flexion. From the 2._____ joint line at the knee to the malleolus at the ankle, the right tib/fib is 1.5 cm shorter than the left. There is pigment change mainly on the 3._____ and 4._____ aspect of the right lower leg. There is a slight bony deformity over the 5._____ aspect of the mid-tibial area.

Diagnostic Imaging: Review of the 6._____ report indicates moderate arthritis of the knees and ankles, right greater than left.

Impression:
1. Degenerative joint disease of both knees and ankles, stable.

Plan:
1. Patient is to continue on current medications unchanged.

Electronically signed: Robert Means MD on 27 March 20XX 13:30

Definitions of Medical Terms to Complete the Document

Write the medical terms defined on corresponding answer lines in the document.

1. pertaining to the front and to the back
2. pertaining to the side
3. pertaining to the back
4. pertaining to the middle
5. pertaining to the front
6. study of x-rays

Chapter 3 Directional Terms, Positions, and Imaging

B

Read the procedure documentation and answer the questions below it.

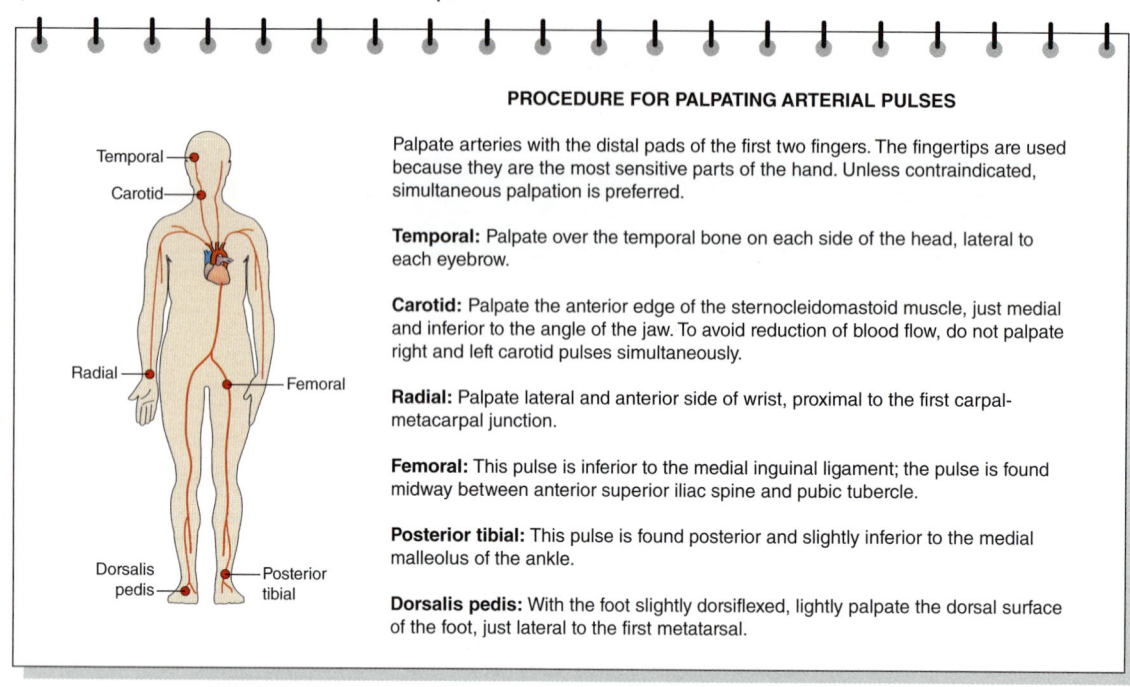

PROCEDURE FOR PALPATING ARTERIAL PULSES

Palpate arteries with the distal pads of the first two fingers. The fingertips are used because they are the most sensitive parts of the hand. Unless contraindicated, simultaneous palpation is preferred.

Temporal: Palpate over the temporal bone on each side of the head, lateral to each eyebrow.

Carotid: Palpate the anterior edge of the sternocleidomastoid muscle, just medial and inferior to the angle of the jaw. To avoid reduction of blood flow, do not palpate right and left carotid pulses simultaneously.

Radial: Palpate lateral and anterior side of wrist, proximal to the first carpal-metacarpal junction.

Femoral: This pulse is inferior to the medial inguinal ligament; the pulse is found midway between anterior superior iliac spine and pubic tubercle.

Posterior tibial: This pulse is found posterior and slightly inferior to the medial malleolus of the ankle.

Dorsalis pedis: With the foot slightly dorsiflexed, lightly palpate the dorsal surface of the foot, just lateral to the first metatarsal.

Use the procedure documentation above to answer the questions. For questions 1-3, circle the correct answer. Use a reference source to answer question 4.

1. The **temporal pulse** is palpated
   a. just above the eyebrow.
   b. to the side of the eyebrow.
   c. below the eyebrow.
   d. to the middle of the eyebrow.

2. The **radial pulse** is palpated
   a. to the side and front of the wrist.
   b. to the side and back of the wrist.
   c. to the middle and back of the wrist.
   d. to the middle and front of the wrist.

3. The **femoral pulse** is located
   a. below the medial inguinal ligament.
   b. above the medial inguinal ligament.
   c. to the front of the medial inguinal ligament.
   d. to the back of the medial inguinal ligament.

4. When used with the foot, *dorsal* has a different meaning. Using a medical dictionary or an online source, describe the dorsal surface of the foot. Hint: try *dorsum* and *dorsalis pedis* as search terms. The dorsal surface of the foot is _____
_____.

EXERCISE 25 ■ Use Medical Terms in Clinical Statements

For each phrase printed in bold, circle the medical term or abbreviation defined. Answers are listed in Appendix A. For pronunciation practice read the answers aloud.

1. In preparation for colonoscopy, the patient was placed in the left **lying on one side with knees bent** (lithotomy, lateral, semiprone) position. During the procedure, a polyp was found in the colon **pertaining to away from the point of attachment** (distal, proximal, medial) to the splenic flexure. A second polyp was found **pertaining to near to the point of attachment** (distal, proximal, medial) to the hepatic flexure.

2. The **study of x-rays** (radiograph, radiology, sonography) uses **diagonal plane passing through the body at an angle** (oblique plane, coronal plane, axial plane) images in the **process of recording x-rays** (sonography, radiologist, radiography) and **imaging of internal structures using a Gamma camera to detect radiation from different parts of the body** (nuclear medicine, magnetic resonance imaging, fluoroscopy) scanning to produce highly accurate images.

Chapter 3 Directional Terms, Positions, and Imaging   91

3. Gallbladder pain frequently occurs in the right **to the right and left of the epigastric** region (lumbar region, hypochondriac region, hypogastric region) and more generally in the **right upper quadrant** (RUQ, URQ, RLQ), while appendicitis pain may start in the **around the navel** (iliac regions, epigastric region, umbilical region) but then settle in the **right lower quadrant** (LRQ, QLR, RLQ).

4. While most patients on respirators are placed in the **lying on back, facing upward** (prone position, supine position, semiprone position), during the COVID-19 pandemic, medical personnel discovered that placing patients in the **lying on abdomen, facing downward** (sitting position, prone position, Trendelenburg position) provided better lung ventilation.

EXERCISE 26 ■ Pronounce Medical Terms in Use

Practice pronunciation of terms by reading aloud the following paragraph. Use the phonetic spellings to assist with pronunciation. The script also contains medical terms not presented in the chapter. If interested, research their meanings by using a medical dictionary or a reliable online source.

> The patient presented to her physician with pain in the right **lumbar region** (LUM-bar)(RĒ-jun) and right **unilateral** (ū-ni-LAT-er-al) leg pain. The pain was felt in the **posterior** (pos-TĒR-ē-or) portion of the leg and radiated to the **distal** (DIS-tal) **lateral** (LAT-er-al) portion of the extremity. There was some **proximal** (PROK-si-mal) muscle weakness reported of the affected leg. A lumbar spine **radiograph** (RĀ-dē-ō-graph) was normal. If the pain does not respond to antiinflammatory medication, she will be referred to an orthopedist.

CHAPTER REVIEW

EXERCISE 27 ■ Chapter Content Quiz

Test your understanding of terms and abbreviations introduced in this chapter. For questions 1-19, circle the letter for the medical term or abbreviation related to the words in italics. For question 20, write medical terms for words in italics.

1. The plane that *divides the body into right and left sides* is a general term used to specify a vertical plane running through the body from the front to back.
   a. coronal plane
   b. axial plane
   c. sagittal plane

2. The *midsagittal plane* more specifically describes the sagittal plane by indicating the body is divided in:
   a. half (equal portions)
   b. unequal portions
   c. anterior and posterior portions

3. Images for computed tomography (CT) scanning can be produced from the sagittal plane, the frontal plane, and the plane *dividing the body into superior and inferior portions* called the:
   a. coronal plane
   b. parasagittal plane
   c. axial plane

4. A polyp was found in the colon *pertaining to away from the point of attachment of a body part* or _____ to the splenic flexure.
   a. distal
   b. proximal
   c. medial

5. The drainage catheter is placed over the right *pertaining to the front* or _____ pelvis.
   a. inferior
   b. posterior
   c. anterior

6. The incision was made at the *pertaining to above* or _____ pole of the lesion.
   a. superior
   b. inferior
   c. lateral

7. The patient complained of *superior to umbilical region* or _____ pain.
   a. hypochondriac region
   b. hypogastric region
   c. epigastric region

8. A *pertaining to a side* or _____ chest radiograph displays the anatomy in the *dividing the body into right and left sides* or _____ plane.
   a. lateral, sagittal
   b. medial, coronal
   c. bilateral, transverse

9. The patient was scheduled for an ultrasound-guided *pertaining to two (both) sides* or _____ thoracentesis.
   a. unilateral
   b. bilateral
   c. mediolateral

10. The doctor's order indicated that the patient with dyspnea (difficulty breathing) was to be placed in the *sitting erect or upright* or _____ position to facilitate breathing.
    a. right semiprone
    b. left recumbent
    c. orthopnea

11. The patient scheduled for lower abdominal surgery was placed in *lying on back with the head lower than the feet* or _____ position.
    a. Trendelenburg
    b. sitting
    c. prone

12. Gallbladder pain is likely to be in the *abbreviated as RUQ* or _____.
    a. lumbar region
    b. right upper quadrant
    c. upper right quadrant

13. The directional term *pertaining to the back* or _____ is often used to describe the back of the hand or upper surface of the foot.
    a. superior
    b. anterior
    c. dorsal

14. Just before birth, the fetus shifted to a *pertaining to the head* or _____ presentation.
    a. cephalic
    b. caudal
    c. ventral

15. A *pertaining to the tail* or _____ epidural steroid injection may be performed to relieve chronic low back pain.
    a. dorsal
    b. caudal
    c. proximal

16. A patient who will be receiving an enema is usually placed in the left *lying on the side with the knee drawn toward the chest and the arm drawn behind* _____ position for gravity to help the fluid flow through the sigmoid colon into the descending colon. This position may also be called left recumbent position.
    a. supine
    b. lithotomy
    c. semiprone

17. *Imaging of moving body structures*, or _____, is frequently used to diagnose abnormalities in the gastrointestinal tract.
    a. magnetic resonance imaging
    b. fluoroscopy
    c. radiography

18. The abbreviation *CT* stands for:
    a. computed topography
    b. commuted tomography
    c. computed tomography
    d. computer tomogramy

19. An interventional *physician who specializes in x-rays*, or _____, may perform procedures such as CT-guided biopsy and radiofrequency ablation of tumors.
    a. radiologist
    b. oncologist
    c. pathologist

20. The pathology report for the patient with a palpable right breast lump included the sections listed below. Fill in the blanks with directional terms indicated by words in italics.

    Right axillary sentinel lymph node biopsy;
    a. Right breast, _____ margin biopsy   (*pertaining to above*)
    b. Right breast, _____ margin biopsy   (*pertaining to below*)

    Right breast, deep margin biopsy;
    c. Right breast, _____ margin biopsy   (*pertaining to the middle*)
    d. Right breast, _____ margin biopsy   (*pertaining to a side*)

CHAPTER AT A GLANCE — Word Parts New to this Chapter

COMBINING FORMS

anter/o	infer/o	son/o
caud/o	later/o	super/o
cephal/o	medi/o	tom/o
dist/o	proxim/o	ventr/o
dors/o	radi/o	

PREFIXES
bi-
uni-

SUFFIXES
-ad
-gram
-graph
-graphy
-ior

CHAPTER AT A GLANCE — Medical Terms Built from Word Parts

DIRECTIONAL TERMS
anterior (ant)
anteroposterior (AP)
bilateral
caudal
cephalic
distal
dorsal
inferior (inf)
lateral (lat)
medial (med)
mediolateral
posterior
posteroanterior (PA)
proximal
superior (sup)
unilateral
ventral

DIAGNOSTIC IMAGING
radiograph
radiography
radiologist
radiology
sonogram
sonography
tomography

CHAPTER AT A GLANCE — Medical Terms NOT Built from Word Parts

ABDOMINOPELVIC REGIONS
epigastric region
hypochondriac regions
hypogastric region
iliac regions
lumbar regions
umbilical region

ANATOMIC PLANES
axial
coronal
midsagittal
oblique
parasagittal
sagittal

BODY POSITIONS
lateral
lithotomy
orthopnea
prone
recumbent
semiprone
sitting
supine
Trendelenburg

DIAGNOSTIC IMAGING
computed tomography (CT)
fluoroscopy
nuclear medicine (NM)
magnetic resonance imaging (MRI)
scan

PART 2 BODY SYSTEMS

4 Integumentary System

Objectives

Upon completion of this chapter, you will be able to:

1. Pronounce anatomic structures of the integumentary system.
2. Define and spell word parts related to the integumentary system.
3. Define, pronounce, and spell disease and disorder terms related to the integumentary system.
4. Define, pronounce, and spell surgical terms related to the integumentary system.
5. Define, pronounce, and spell complementary terms related to the integumentary system.
6. Interpret the meaning of abbreviations related to the integumentary system.
7. Apply medical language in clinical contexts.

TABLE 4.1 Common Skin Infections, 107
TABLE 4.2 Common Skin Lesions, 122

Outline

ANATOMY, 95
Function, 95
Anatomic Structures of the Integumentary System, 95

WORD PARTS, 96
Integumentary System Combining Forms, 96
Combining Forms Used with Integumentary System Terms, 97
Prefixes, 97
Suffixes, 97

MEDICAL TERMS, 101
Disease and Disorder Terms, 101
    Built from Word Parts, 101
    NOT Built from Word Parts, 104
Surgical Terms, 113
    Built from Word Parts and
        NOT Built from Word Parts, 113
Complementary Terms, 116
    Built from Word Parts, 116
    NOT Built from Word Parts, 121
Abbreviations, 126

PRACTICAL APPLICATION, 128
CASE STUDY Translate Between Everyday Language and Medical Language, 128
Interact with Medical Documents, 129
Use Medical Terms in Clinical Statements, 131
Pronounce Medical Terms in Use, 131

CHAPTER REVIEW, 131
Chapter Content Quiz, 131
Chapter at a Glance, 133

Answers to Chapter Exercises, Appendix A

Chapter 4   Integumentary System   95

ANATOMY

The integumentary system is composed of the skin, glands, hair, and nails.

> **INTEGUMENTARY** is derived from the Latin word **tegere**, meaning to **cover**.

Function

The skin forms a protective covering for the body that, when unbroken, prevents entry of bacteria and other invading organisms. The skin also protects the body from water loss and the damaging effects of ultraviolet light. Other functions include regulation of body temperature and synthesis of vitamin D.

Anatomic Structures of the Integumentary System

TERM	DEFINITION
skin (skin)	organ covering the body; made up of layers (also called **cutaneous membrane**) (Fig. 4.1)

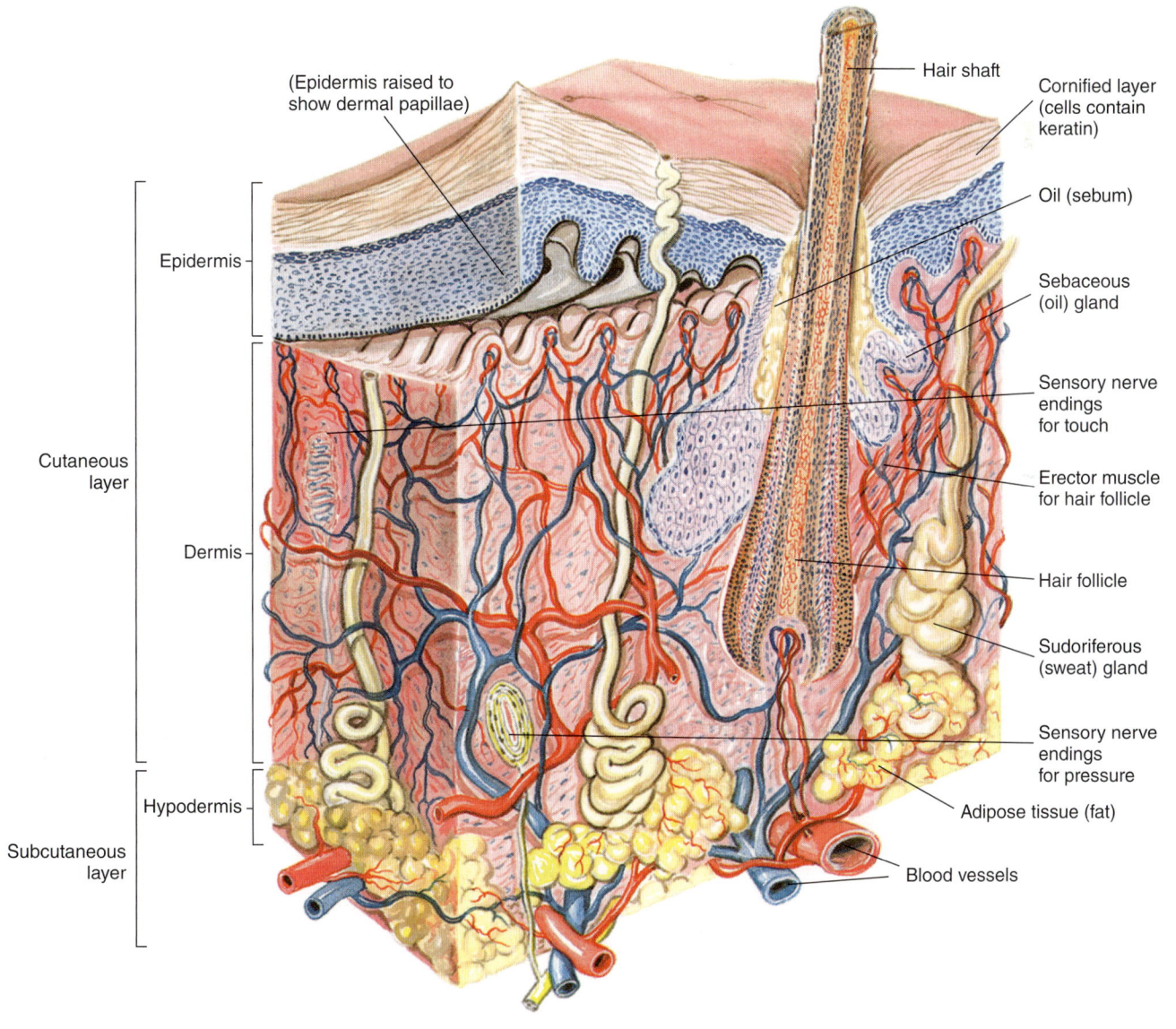

FIG. 4.1 Structure of the skin.

Chapter 4   Integumentary System

TERM	DEFINITION
epidermis (ep-i-DER-mis)	outer layer of skin; protects the body from the external environment
keratin (KAR-a-tin)	scleroprotein component of the hornlike, or cornified, layer of the epidermis. Also, the primary component of the hair and nails
melanin (MEL-a-nin)	dark pigment produced by melanocytes; amount present determines skin color
hair (hār)	compressed, keratinized cells that arise from hair follicles, the sacs that enclose the hair fibers
nails (nālz)	hornlike plates made from flattened epithelial cells; found on the dorsal surface of the ends of the fingers and toes
sebaceous glands (se-BĀ-shas) (glans)	secrete sebum (oil) into the hair follicles where the hair shafts pass through the dermis
sudoriferous glands (soo-da-RIF-er-as) (glans)	tiny, coiled, tubular structures that emerge through pores on the skin's surface and secrete sweat (also called **sweat glands**)
APPENDAGES OF THE SKIN	is a common reference to hair, nails, sudoriferous glands, and sebaceous glands.
dermis (DUR-mis)	inner layer of skin; responsible for its flexibility and mechanical strength
hypodermis (hī-pō-DER-mis)	layer between the dermis and the underlying tissues and organs; contains adipose tissue (fat), connective tissue, nerves, and blood vessels (also called **subcutaneous layer**)

PRONOUNCE ANATOMIC STRUCTURES

Practice saying aloud each of the organs and specific structures on the previous pages.

To hear the terms, go to Evolve Resources at www.evolve.elsevier.com and select:
Student Resources > Audio Glossary > Chapter 4 > **Anatomic Structures**

❏ Check the box when complete.

WORD PARTS

Use paper flashcards or electronic flashcards on Evolve to assist with memorization of word parts used to analyze, define, and build terms presented in this chapter. To reinforce learning, study one section of the Word Parts Table at a time, and then complete the corresponding exercise on the following pages.

1 ■ Integumentary System Combining Forms

COMBINING FORM	DEFINITION	COMBINING FORM	DEFINITION
cutane/o	skin	onych/o	nail
derm/o	skin	seb/o	sebum (oil)
dermat/o	skin	trich/o	hair
hidr/o	sweat	ungu/o	nail
kerat/o	hornlike tissue (keratin), scaly. *Note:* when used with ophthalmology terms, *kerat/o* means cornea.		Do not be concerned about which **combining form** to use for **skin** or **nail**. As you continue to study and use medical terms, you will become familiar with common usage of each word part.

KERAT/O derives from the Greek word keras, meaning horn, and refers to a rough texture like that of an animal's horn.

2 ■ Combining Forms Used with Integumentary System Terms

COMBINING FORM	DEFINITION	COMBINING FORM	DEFINITION
aden/o	gland, glandular tissue	scler/o	hard
crypt/o	hidden	**SCLER/O** When used with ophthalmology terms, **scler/o** refers to the tough outer white portion of the eye called the sclera.	
erythr/o	red
leuk/o	white	staphyl/o	grapelike clusters
myc/o	fungus	strept/o	twisted chains
pachy/o	thick	xanth/o	yellow
phag/o	swallowing, eating	xer/o	dry, dryness
rhytid/o	wrinkles		

3 ■ Prefixes

PREFIX	DEFINITION	PREFIX	DEFINITION
epi-	on, upon, over	para-	beside, around, abnormal
hyper-	above, excessive	per-	through
hypo-	below, incomplete, deficient, under	sub-	under, below
intra-	within	trans-	through, across, beyond

4 ■ Suffixes

SUFFIX	DEFINITION	SUFFIX	DEFINITION
-a	noun suffix, no meaning	-logy	study of
-al	pertaining to	-malacia	softening
-coccus (*pl.* -cocci)	berry-shaped (form of bacterium)	-oma	tumor, swelling
		-osis	abnormal condition (means increase when used with blood cell word roots)
-ectomy	excision, surgical removal
-genic	producing, originating, causing
-ia	diseased state, condition of	-ous	pertaining to
-ic	pertaining to	-plasty	surgical repair
-itis	inflammation	-rrhea	flow, discharge
-logist	one who studies and treats (specialist, physician)		

Refer to **Appendix B** and **Appendix C** for alphabetical lists of word parts and their meanings.

98 Chapter 4 Integumentary System

EXERCISE 1 ■ Integumentary System Combining Forms

Refer to the first section of the word parts table.

A Label

Fill in the blanks with combining forms to label these diagrams. *To check your answers, go to Appendix A at the back of the textbook.*

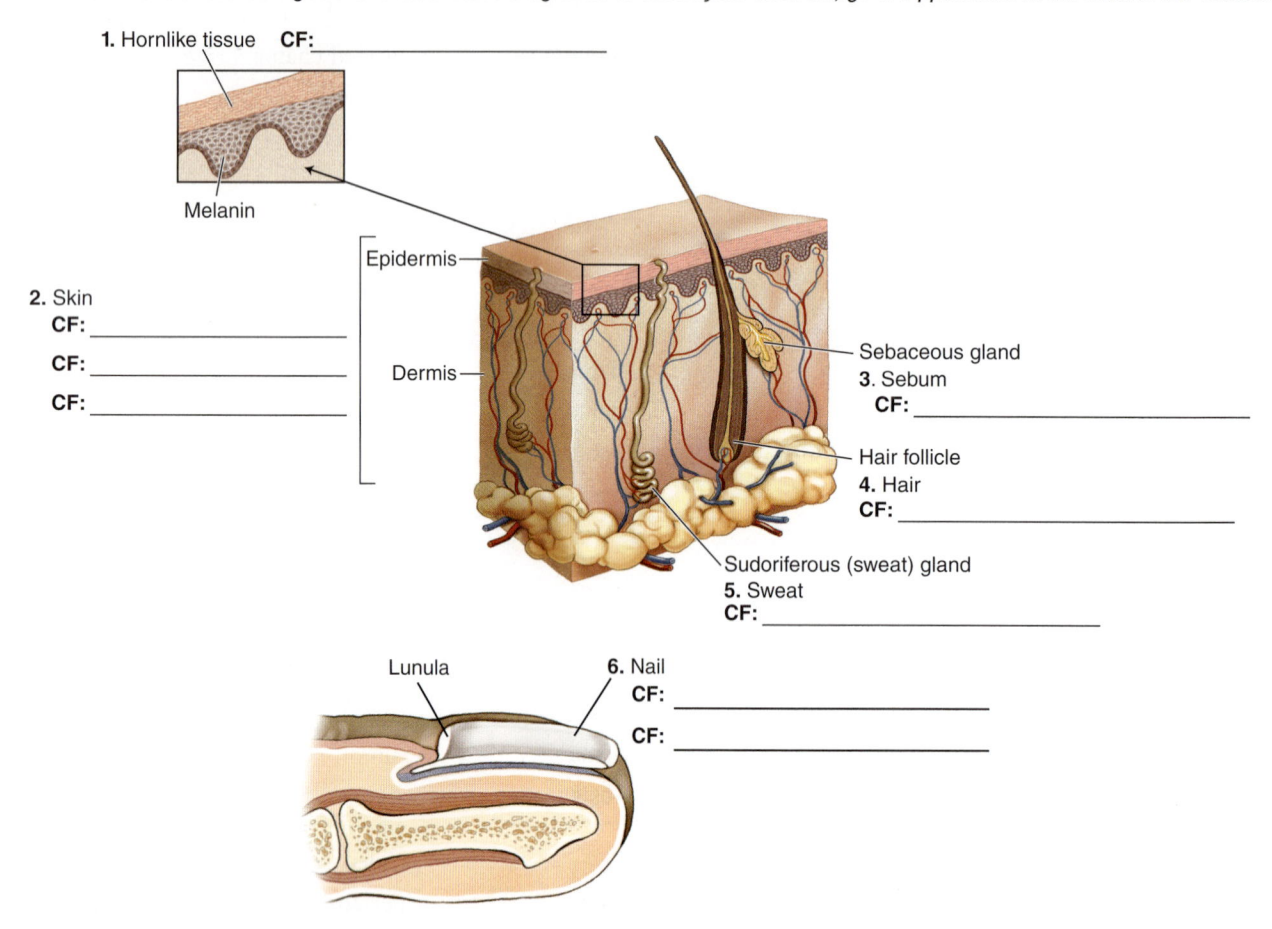

1. Hornlike tissue CF: _____

Melanin

Epidermis

2. Skin
   CF: _____
   CF: _____
   CF: _____

Dermis

Sebaceous gland
3. Sebum
   CF: _____

Hair follicle
4. Hair
   CF: _____

Sudoriferous (sweat) gland
5. Sweat
   CF: _____

Lunula

6. Nail
   CF: _____
   CF: _____

B Define and Match

Step 1: Write the definitions after the following combining forms.
Step 2: Match the descriptions on the right with the combining forms and definitions. Answers may be used more than once.

_____ 1. derm/o _____
_____ 2. seb/o, _____
_____ 3. onych/o, _____
_____ 4. cutane/o, _____
_____ 5. kerat/o, _____
_____ 6. ungu/o, _____
_____ 7. hidr/o, _____
_____ 8. trich/o, _____
_____ 9. dermat/o, _____

a. secreted from sudoriferous glands
b. secreted from sebaceous glands
c. hornlike plates made from flattened epithelial cells
d. organ covering the body; made up of layers
e. scleroprotein component of the hornlike, or cornified, layer of the epidermis
f. compressed, keratinized cells that arise from follicles

Chapter 4 Integumentary System 99

EXERCISE 2 ■ Combining Forms Used with Integumentary System Terms

Refer to the second section of the word parts table.

A Define

Write the definitions of the following combining forms.

1. xanth/o _____
2. staphyl/o _____
3. crypt/o _____
4. pachy/o _____
5. leuk/o _____
6. myc/o _____
7. erythr/o _____
8. scler/o _____
9. strept/o _____
10. xer/o _____
11. rhytid/o _____
12. aden/o _____
13. phag/o _____

B Identify

Write the combining form for each of the following.

1. fungus _____
2. white _____
3. yellow _____
4. dry, dryness _____
5. thick _____
6. twisted chains _____
7. wrinkles _____
8. grapelike clusters _____
9. red _____
10. hidden _____
11. hard _____
12. swallowing, eating _____
13. gland, glandular tissue _____

EXERCISE 3 ■ Prefixes

Refer to the third section of the word parts table.

A Define

Write the definitions of the following prefixes.

1. sub- _____
2. para- _____
3. epi- _____
4. intra- _____
5. per- _____
6. trans- _____
7. hypo- _____
8. hyper- _____

B Identify

Write the prefix for each of the following.

1. within _____
2. under, below _____
3. on, upon, over _____
4. beside, around, abnormal _____
5. through _____
6. through, across, beyond _____
7. above, excessive _____
8. below, incomplete, deficient, under _____

Chapter 4 Integumentary System

EXERCISE 4 ■ Suffixes

Refer to the fourth section of the word parts table.

A Match

Match the suffixes in the first column with their correct definitions in the second column.

_____ 1. -a   a. one who studies and treats (specialist, physician)
_____ 2. -ia   b. producing, originating, causing
_____ 3. -logist   c. diseased state, condition of
_____ 4. -genic   d. tumor, swelling
_____ 5. -oma   e. noun suffix, no meaning

B Label

Write the suffixes pictured and defined.

1. _____
   berry-shaped (form of bacterium)

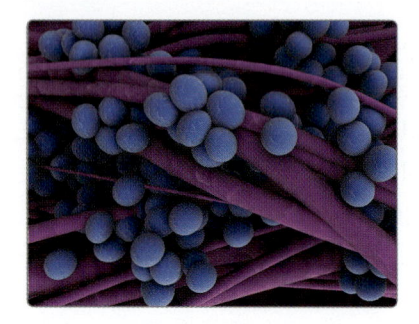

2. _____
   flow, discharge

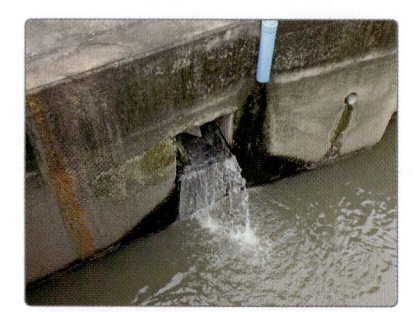

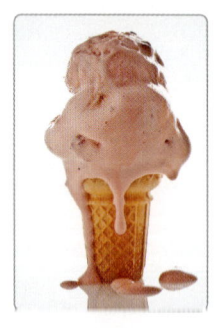

3. _____
   softening

4. _____
   inflammation

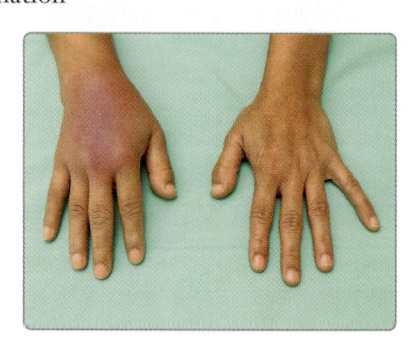

5. _____
   surgical repair

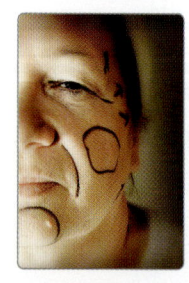

6. _____
   excision, surgical removal

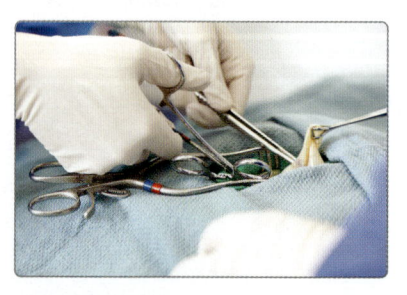

C Define

Write the definitions of the following suffixes.

1. -ous _____
2. -logy _____
3. -al _____
4. -osis _____
5. -ic _____

MEDICAL TERMS

Medical terms relevant to this chapter have been grouped by topics, such as Disease and Disorder, and are listed in tables designated as Built from Word Parts or *NOT* Built from Word Parts. The exercises following each table assist with learning term definitions, pronunciations, and spellings.

Disease and Disorder Terms

BUILT FROM WORD PARTS

The following terms can be translated using definitions of word parts. Further explanation is provided within parentheses as needed.

TERM	DEFINITION	TERM	DEFINITION
1. **dermatitis** (*der*-ma-TĪ-tis)	inflammation of the skin (Fig. 4.2)	10. **paronychia** (*par*-ō-NIK-ē-a)	diseased state around the nail (Note: the a from para- has been dropped.)
2. **dermatofibroma** (*der*-ma-tō-fi-BRŌ-ma)	fibrous tumor of the skin		The final vowel in a prefix may be dropped when the following word root begins with a vowel.
3. **hidradenitis** (*hī*-drad-e-NĪ-tis)	inflammation of a sweat gland	11. **scleroderma** (skle-rō-DER-ma)	hard skin (chronic hardening or induration of the connective tissue of the skin and other organs)
4. **keratosis** (ker-a-TŌ-sis)	abnormal condition (growth) of hornlike tissue (keratin)		
5. **onychocryptosis** (*on*-i-kō-krip-TŌ-sis)	abnormal condition of a hidden nail (also called **ingrown nail**)	12. **seborrhea** (seb-o-RĒ-a)	discharge of sebum (excessive)
6. **onychomalacia** (*on*-i-kō-ma-LĀ-sha)	softening of the nails	**SEBORRHEIC** is the adjective form of **seborrhea** and means pertaining to excessive discharge of sebum.	
7. **onychomycosis** (*on*-i-kō-mī-KŌ-sis)	abnormal condition of a fungus in the nails	13. **xanthoma** (zan-THŌ-ma)	yellow tumor (benign, primarily in the skin)
8. **onychophagia** (*on*-i-kō-FĀ-ja)	condition of eating the nails (nail biting)	14. **xeroderma** (zē-rō-DER-ma)	dry skin (a mild form of a cutaneous disorder characterized by keratinization and noninflammatory scaling)
9. **pachyderma** (*pak*-i-DER-ma)	thickening of the skin		

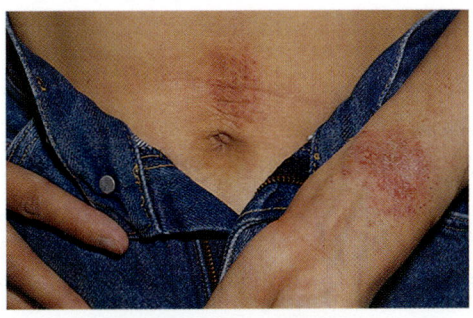

FIG. 4.2 Contact dermatitis.

EXERCISE 5 ■ Pronounce and Spell

Practice pronunciation and spelling on paper and online.

1. **Practice on Paper**
   a. **Pronounce:** Read the phonetic spelling and say aloud the terms listed in the previous table. Refer to Table 2.2 Pronunciation Key as needed.
   b. **Spell:** Have a study partner read the terms aloud. Write the spelling of the terms on a separate sheet of paper.

2. **Practice Online**
   a. **Access** online learning resources. Go to evolve.elsevier.com > Evolve Resources > Student Resources.
   b. **Pronounce:** Select Audio Glossary > Chapter 4 > Exercise 5. Select a term to hear its pronunciation and repeat aloud.
   c. **Spell:** Select Activities > Chapter 4 > Spell Terms > Exercise 5. Select the audio icon and type the correct spelling of the term.

❏ Check the box when complete.

EXERCISE 6 ■ Analyze and Define

Analyze and define the following Disease and Disorder Terms Built from Word Parts by drawing slashes between word parts, writing word part abbreviations above the term, underlining combining forms, and writing combining form abbreviations below the term. If needed, refer to Chapter 1 to review analyzing and defining techniques.

```
              WR   CV  WR   S
EXAMPLE:  onych / o / myc / osis
                  ─────
                   CF
          abnormal condition of a fungus in the nails
```

1. scleroderma

2. hidradenitis

3. dermatitis

4. pachyderma

5. onychomalacia

6. keratosis

7. dermatofibroma

8. paronychia

9. onychocryptosis

10. seborrhea

Chapter 4   Integumentary System   103

11. onychophagia

_____ / _____
_____ / _____

13. xanthoma

_____ / _____
_____ / _____

12. xeroderma

_____ / _____
_____ / _____

EXERCISE 7 ■ Build

A Label

Build terms pictured by writing word parts above definitions.

1.

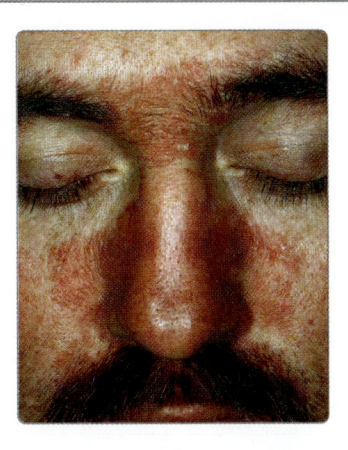

seborrheic _____ / _____
              skin   inflammation

2.

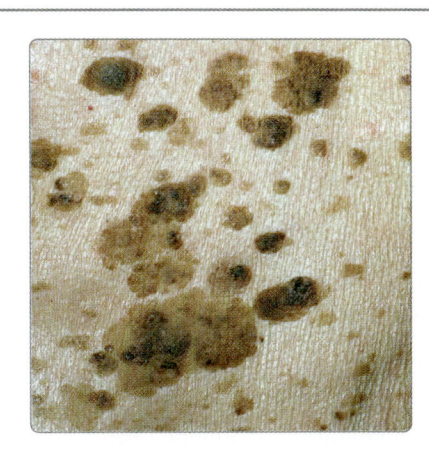

seborrheic _____ / _____
           hornlike tissue   abnormal
                             condition

3.

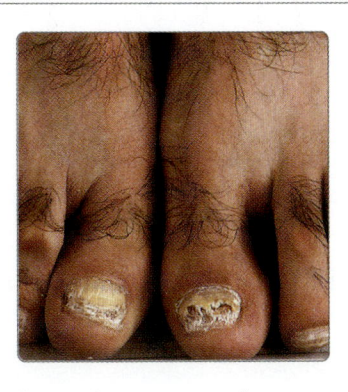

_____ / ____ / _____ / _____
  nail   CV   fungus   abnormal condition

4.

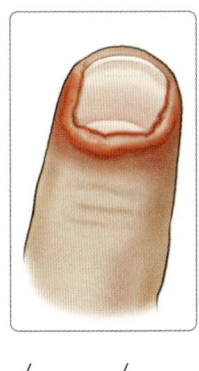

_____ / _____ / _____
 around   nail   diseased state

Chapter 4 Integumentary System

B Fill In

Build disease and disorder terms for the following definitions with the word parts you have learned. If you need help, refer to Chapter 1 to review term-building techniques.

EXAMPLE: abnormal condition (growth) of horny tissue (keratin)   kerat / osis
                                                                      WR / S

1. thickening of the skin   ___ WR ___ / ___ WR ___ / ___ S ___

2. dry skin   ___ WR ___ / ___ CV ___ / ___ WR ___ / ___ S ___

3. discharge of sebum (excessive)   ___ WR ___ / ___ CV ___ / ___ S ___

4. yellow tumor   ___ WR ___ / ___ S ___

5. fibrous tumor of the skin   ___ WR ___ / ___ CV ___ / ___ WR ___ / ___ S ___

6. softening of the nails   ___ WR ___ / ___ CV ___ / ___ S ___

7. inflammation of a sweat gland   ___ WR ___ / ___ WR ___ / ___ S ___

8. abnormal condition of a hidden nail   ___ WR ___ / ___ CV ___ / ___ WR ___ / ___ S ___

9. hard skin   ___ WR ___ / ___ CV ___ / ___ WR ___ / ___ S ___

10. condition of eating the nails   ___ WR ___ / ___ CV ___ / ___ WR ___ / ___ S ___

Disease and Disorder Terms
NOT BUILT FROM WORD PARTS

Word parts may be present in the following terms; however, their full meanings cannot be translated using definitions of word parts alone.

TERM	DEFINITION
1. abrasion (a-BRĀ-zhun)	scraping away of the skin by mechanical process or injury
2. abscess (AB-ses)	localized collection of pus, bacteria, and other material; can occur in the skin (cutaneous abscess) or other locations within the body (internal abscess)
🏛 **ABSCESS** is derived from the Latin *ab*, meaning **from**, and *cedo*, meaning **to go**. The tissue dies and goes away, with the pus replacing it.		
3. acne (AK-nē)	inflammatory disease of the skin involving the sebaceous glands and hair follicles
4. actinic keratosis (ack-TIN-ik) (*ker*-a-TŌ-sis)	precancerous skin condition of hornlike tissue formation that results from excessive exposure to sunlight. It may evolve into a squamous cell carcinoma.

TERM	DEFINITION
5. albinism (AL-bi-niz-um)	congenital hereditary condition characterized by partial or total lack of pigment (melanin) in the skin, hair, and eyes
🏛 **ALBINISM Alb** is a Latin word root meaning **white**. **Leuk** is the Greek word root meaning **white**.	
6. basal cell carcinoma (BCC) (BĀ-sal) (sel) (*kar*-si-NŌ-ma)	malignant epithelial tumor arising from the bottom layer of the epidermis called the basal layer; it seldom metastasizes, but invades local tissue and may recur in the same location. Common in individuals who have had excessive sun exposure. (Fig. 4.3)
7. candidiasis (*kan*-di-DĪ-a-sis)	infection of the skin, mouth (also called **thrush**), or vagina caused by the yeast-type fungus *Candida albicans*. *Candida* is normally present in the mucous membranes; overgrowth causes an infection. Esophageal candidiasis is often seen in patients with acquired immunodeficiency syndrome (AIDS).
🏛 **CANDIDA** comes from the Latin **candidus**, meaning **gleaming white**; **albicans** is from the Latin verb **albicare**, meaning **to make white**. The growth of the fungus is white, and the infection produces a white discharge.	
8. carbuncle (KAR-bung-kl)	infection of skin and subcutaneous tissue composed of a cluster of boils (furuncles, see below) caused by staphylococcal bacteria
9. cellulitis (*sel*-ū-LĪ-tis)	inflammation of the skin and subcutaneous tissue caused by infection; characterized by redness, pain, heat, and swelling
10. contusion (kon-TŪ-zhun)	external injury with no break in the skin, characterized by pain, swelling, and discoloration (also called a **bruise**)
11. eczema (EK-ze-ma)	noninfectious, inflammatory skin disease characterized by redness, blisters, scabs, and itching
12. fissure (FISH-ur)	slit or cracklike sore in the skin
13. furuncle (FER-ung-kl)	painful skin nodule caused by staphylococcal bacteria in a hair follicle (also called a **boil**)

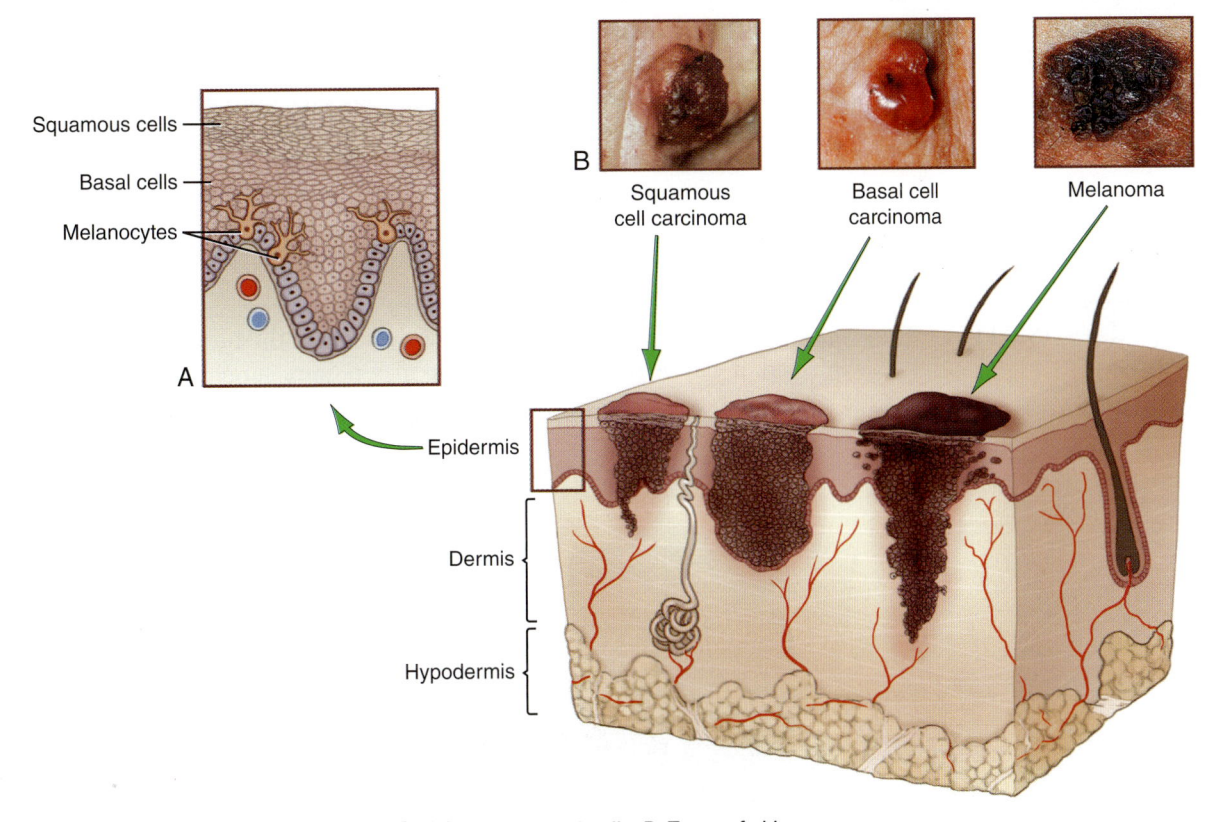

FIG. 4.3 A, Epidermal cells. B, Types of skin cancer.

Disease and Disorder Terms—cont'd
NOT BUILT FROM WORD PARTS

TERM	DEFINITION
14. gangrene (GANG-grēn)	death of tissue caused by loss of blood supply followed by bacterial invasion (a form of necrosis)
15. herpes (HER-pēz)	inflammatory skin disease caused by a herpesvirus and characterized by small blisters in clusters. Many types of herpes exist. Herpes simplex virus type 1, for example, causes fever blisters; herpes zoster, also called shingles, is characterized by painful skin eruptions that follow nerves inflamed by the virus. (see Table 4.1)

🏛 **HERPES** is from the Greek **herpo**, meaning to **creep along**. It is descriptive of the course and type of skin lesion.

16. impetigo (*im*-pe-TĪ-gō)	superficial skin infection characterized by pustules and caused by either staphylococci or streptococci (see Table 4.1)
17. Kaposi sarcoma (KAP-ō-sē) (sar-KŌ-ma)	cancerous condition starting as purple or brown papules that spreads through the skin to the lymph nodes and internal organs; frequently seen with AIDS
18. keloid (KĒ-loyd)	overgrowth of scar tissue
19. laceration (*las*-er-Ā-shun)	torn, ragged-edged wound
20. measles (MĒ-zalz)	highly contagious viral disease characterized by fever, runny nose, cough, and a spreading skin rash. It is a potentially disastrous disease that can lead to pneumonia, severe bleeding, brain infections (which may cause seizures, developmental delay, or chronic brain disease), and sometimes death. Measles is a significant cause of death, despite the availability of a safe, effective vaccine.

🏛 **MEASLES** comes from the Middle English **maselen**, meaning **many little spots**, which are characteristic of the rash.

21. MRSA infection (MER-sah) (in-FEK-shun)	invasion of body tissue by methicillin-resistant *Staphylococcus aureus*, a strain of common bacteria that has developed resistance to methicillin and other antibiotics. It can produce skin and soft tissue infections and sometimes bloodstream infections and pneumonia, which can be fatal if not treated. MRSA is quite common in hospitals and long-term care facilities but is increasingly emerging as an important infection in the general population.
22. pediculosis (pe-*dik*-ū-LŌ-sis)	invasion into the skin and hair by lice
23. pilonidal cyst (*pī*-lō-NĪ-dal) (SIST)	abnormal pocket in the skin that contains hair and skin debris. It is frequently located near the tailbone, at the top of the cleft of the buttocks. If it becomes infected, it can be severely painful and may require surgery. (Fig. 4.4)

🏛 **PILONIDAL** comes from the Latin words **pilus**, meaning **hair**, and **nidus**, meaning **nest**. Pil/o and trich/o are two combining forms for **hair**.

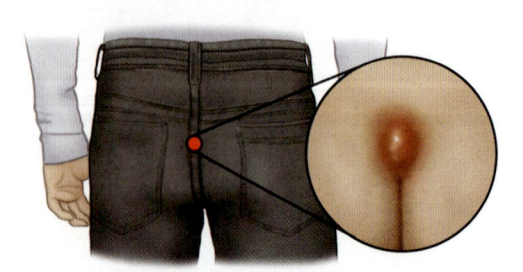

FIG. 4.4 Pilonidal Cyst.

TABLE 4.1 Common Skin Infections

Infections may be caused by a bacterium, fungus, parasite, or virus. Examples of common skin infections include the following:

TYPES	SKIN INFECTIONS	EXAMPLES
Bacterial Infections	carbuncle cellulitis furuncle impetigo MRSA paronychia	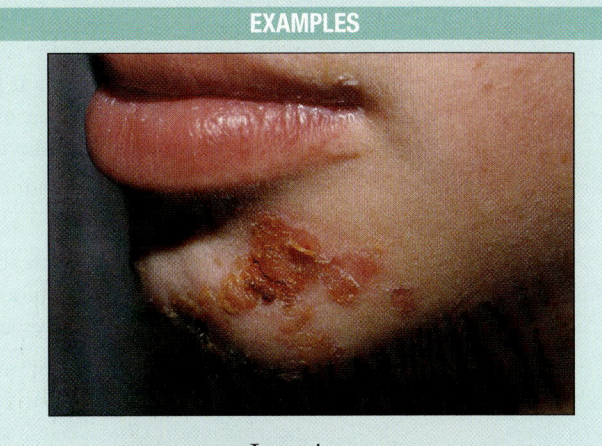 Impetigo
Fungal Infections	candidiasis tinea	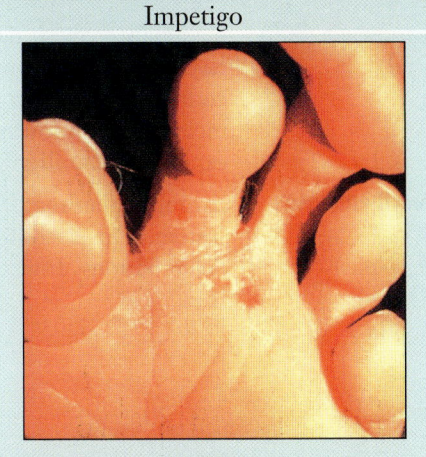 Tinea pedis (also called **athlete's foot**)
Parasitic Infections	scabies pediculosis	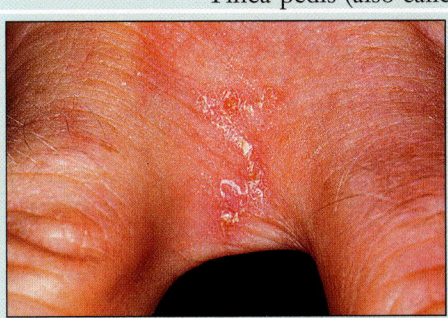 Scabies 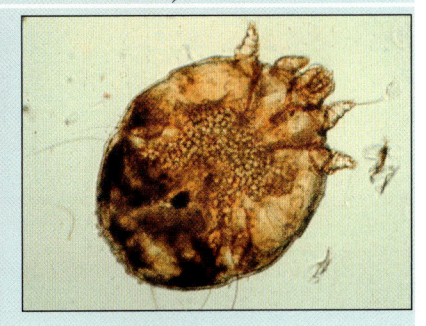 / Scabies mite
Viral Infections	herpes simplex virus type 1; also called fever blister herpes zoster; also called shingles	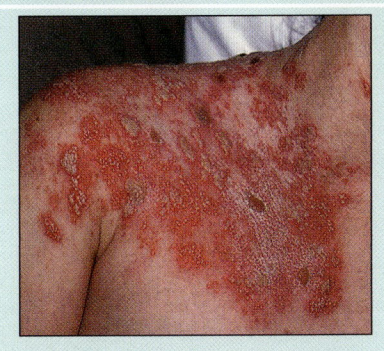 Herpes zoster (vesicles have dried and scabs have begun to form)

Disease and Disorder Terms—cont'd
NOT BUILT FROM WORD PARTS

TERM	DEFINITION
24. **pressure injury** (PRESH-ur) (IN-ja-rē)	damage of the skin and the subcutaneous tissue caused by prolonged pressure, often occurring in bedridden patients; the injury, which may be painful, can present as intact skin or an open ulcer (also called **pressure ulcer** and **bedsore**; formerly called **decubitus ulcer**) (Fig. 4.5)
25. **psoriasis** (so-RĪ-a-sis)	chronic skin condition producing red lesions covered with silvery scales
26. **rosacea** (rō-ZĀ-shē-a)	chronic disorder of the skin that produces erythema, papules, pustules, and abnormal dilation of tiny blood vessels, usually occurring on the central area of the face in people older than 30 years
27. **scabies** (SKĀ-bēz)	skin infection caused by the itch mite, characterized by papule eruptions that are caused by the female burrowing into the outer layer of the skin and laying eggs. This condition is accompanied by severe itching. (Table 4.1)
28. **squamous cell carcinoma (SCC)** (SQWĀ-mus) (sel) (*kar*-si-NŌ-ma)	malignant growth developing from scalelike epithelial tissue of the surface layer of the epidermis; it invades local tissue and may metastasize. While most commonly appearing on the skin, SCC can occur in other parts of the body, including the mouth, lips, and genitals. The most frequent cause is chronic exposure to sunlight. (Fig. 4.3)
29. **systemic lupus erythematosus (SLE)** (sis-TEM-ik) (LŪ-pus) (*e*-ri-*thē*-*ma*-TŌ-sus)	chronic inflammatory disease involving the skin, joints, kidneys, and nervous system. This autoimmune disease is characterized by periods of remission and exacerbations. It also may affect other organs.

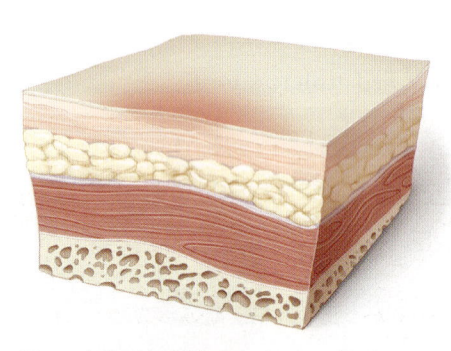

Stage 1 Nonblanching erythema, skin intact.

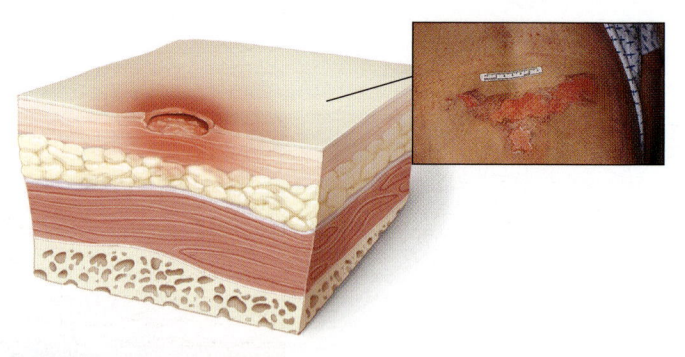

Stage 2 Partial thickness of skin loss involving the epidermis, dermis, or both.

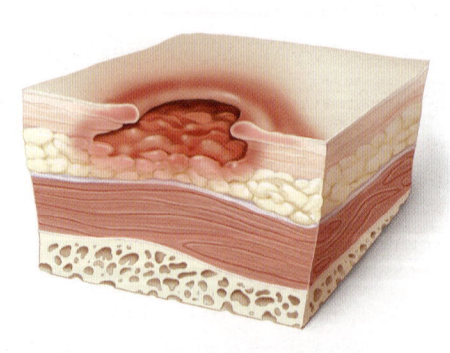

Stage 3 Full thickness of skin loss involving damage or necrosis to subcutaneous tissue.

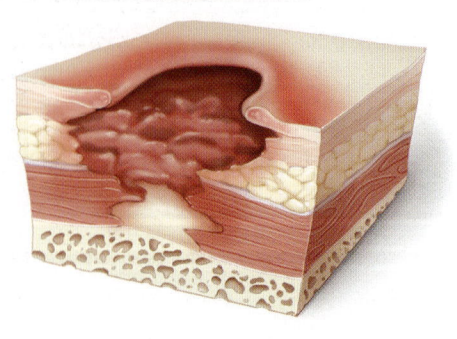

Stage 4 Full thickness of skin loss with extensive destruction, tissue necrosis, possible damage to muscle and bone tissue and other supporting structures.

FIG. 4.5 Pressure injury staging with a photograph of Stage 2.

Chapter 4 Integumentary System 109

TERM	DEFINITION
30. **tinea** (TIN-ē-a)	fungal infection of the skin. The fungi may infect keratin of the skin, hair, and nails. Infections are classified by body regions such as *tinea capitis* (scalp), *tinea corporis* (body), and *tinea pedis* (foot). Tinea in general is also called **ringworm**, and tinea pedis specifically is also called **athlete's foot**. (Table 4.1)
31. **urticaria** (ur-ti-KAR-ē-a)	itchy skin eruption composed of wheals of varying sizes and shapes. Urticaria is sometimes associated with infections and with allergic reactions to food, medicine, or other agents. Other causes include internal disease, physical stimuli, and genetic disorders. (also called **hives**) (Table 4.2)
32. **vitiligo** (vit-i-LĪ-gō)	white patches on the skin caused by the destruction of melanocytes

EXERCISE 8 ■ Pronounce and Spell

Practice pronunciation and spelling on paper and online.

1. **Practice on Paper**
   a. **Pronounce:** Read the phonetic spelling and say aloud the terms listed in the previous table. Refer to Table 2.2 Pronunciation Key as needed.
   b. **Spell:** Have a study partner read the terms aloud. Write the spelling of the terms on a separate sheet of paper.

2. **Practice Online**
   a. **Access** online learning resources. Go to evolve.elsevier.com > Evolve Resources > Student Resources.
   b. **Pronounce:** Select Audio Glossary > Chapter 4 > Exercise 8. Select a term to hear its pronunciation and repeat aloud.
   c. **Spell:** Select Activities > Chapter 4 > Spell Terms > Exercise 8. Select the audio icon and type the correct spelling of the term.

❏ Check the box when complete.

EXERCISE 9 ■ Fill In

A Identify

Fill in the blanks with the correct disease and disorder terms.

1. A chronic inflammatory disease affecting the skin, joints, and other organs is _____ _____.
2. The scraping away of the skin by mechanical process or injury is called a(n) _____.
3. _____ is the name given to the invasion of the skin and hair by lice.
4. An external injury with no break in the skin and characterized by pain, swelling, and discoloration is called a(n) _____.
5. _____ is the name given to tissue death caused by a loss of blood supply followed by bacterial invasion.
6. A cluster of boils caused by staphylococcal bacteria is a _____.
7. An inflammatory skin disease that involves the oil glands and hair follicles is called _____.
8. _____ is the name given to a torn, ragged-edged wound.
9. A(n) _____ _____ is a small hole or tunnel containing hair and skin that can become infected and may require surgery.

10. Damage of the skin and the subcutaneous tissue caused by prolonged pressure, often occurring in bedridden patients, is called _____ _____.
11. A congenital hereditary condition characterized by partial or total lack of pigment (melanin) in the skin, hair, and eyes is _____.
12. _____ _____ is an invasion of methicillin-resistant *Staphylococcus aureus* in the body tissue.
13. A(n) _____ is a localized collection of pus, bacteria, and other material in the skin. It may appear red and feel warm to the touch.

B Label

Write the medical terms pictured and defined.

1. (a) _____, cracklike sore in the skin caused by (b) _____, a noninfectious inflammatory skin disease characterized by redness, blisters, scabs, and itching

2. _____ inflammation of the skin and subcutaneous tissue caused by infection and characterized by redness, pain, heat, and swelling

3. _____ chronic skin condition producing red lesions covered with silvery scales

4. _____ inflammatory skin disease caused by a virus and characterized by small blisters

5. _____ fungal infection of the skin, also known as *ringworm*

6. _____ cancerous condition starting as purple or brown papules

7. _____
hornlike tissue formation that results from excessive exposure to sunlight and is precancerous

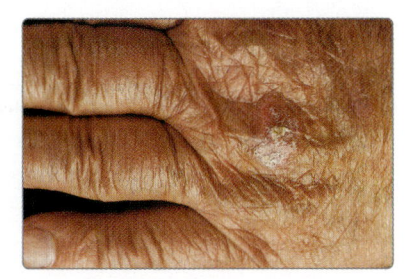

8. _____
painful skin nodule caused by staphylococcal bacteria in a hair follicle

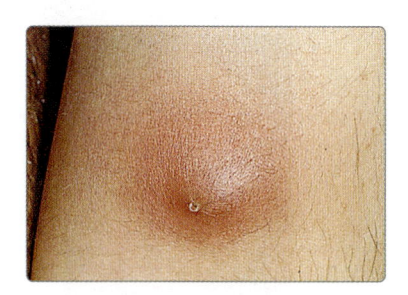

9. _____
malignant growth developing from scalelike epithelial tissue of the surface layer of the epidermis; it invades local tissue and may metastasize

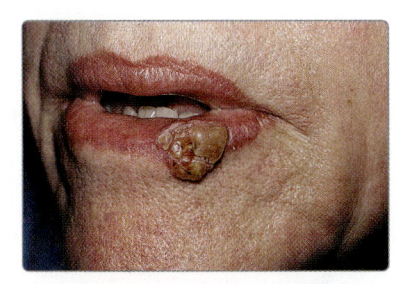

10. _____
malignant epithelial tumor arising from the bottom layer of the epidermis; it seldom metastasizes, but invades local tissue and may recur in the same location

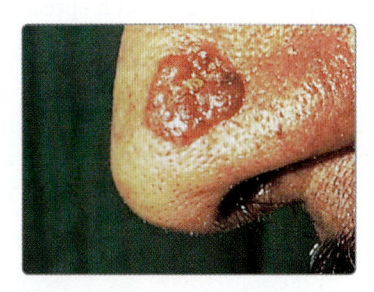

11. _____
superficial skin infection characterized by pustules and caused by either staphylococci or streptococci

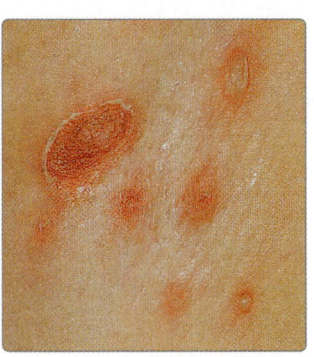

12. _____
skin inflammation caused by the itch mite

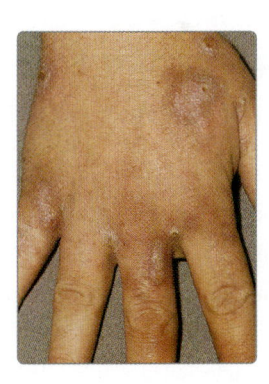

13. _____
itchy skin eruption composed of wheals of varying sizes and shapes

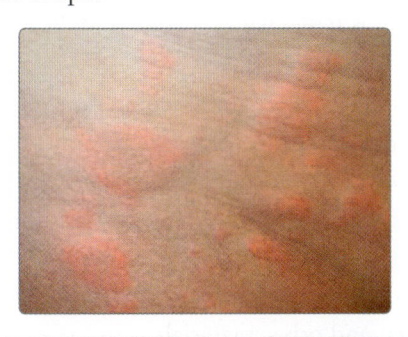

14. _____
infection of the skin, mouth, or vagina caused by *Candida albicans*

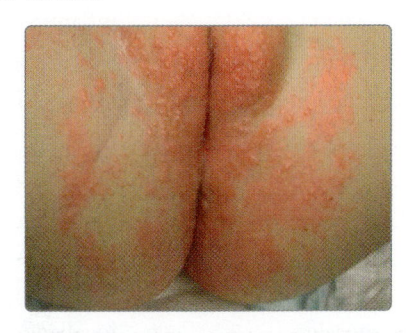

15. _____
white patches on the skin caused by the destruction of melanocytes

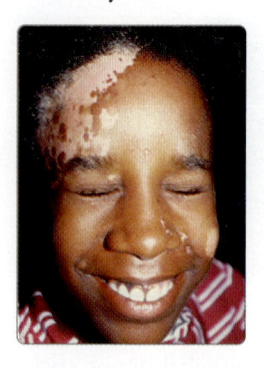

16. _____
chronic disorder of the skin on the central area of the face that produces erythema, papules, pustules, and abnormal dilation of tiny blood vessels

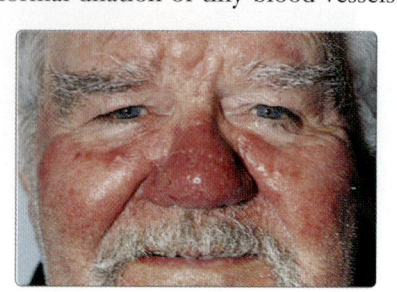

17. _____
a highly contagious viral disease characterized by fever, runny nose, cough, and a spreading skin rash

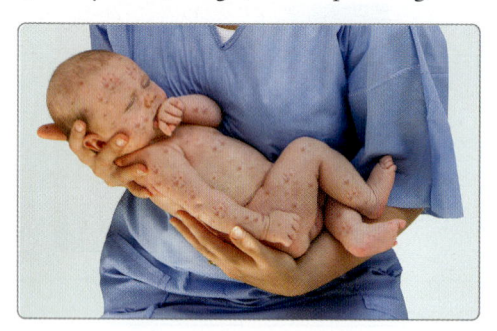

18. _____
overgrowth of scar tissue

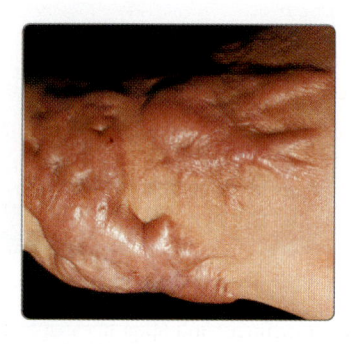

EXERCISE 10 ■ Match

Match the words in the first column with their correct definitions in the second column.

_____ 1. abscess
_____ 2. keloid
_____ 3. furuncle
_____ 4. actinic keratosis
_____ 5. contusion
_____ 6. carbuncle
_____ 7. basal cell carcinoma
_____ 8. fissure
_____ 9. eczema
_____ 10. cellulitis
_____ 11. acne
_____ 12. gangrene
_____ 13. abrasion
_____ 14. rosacea
_____ 15. MRSA infection
_____ 16. measles

a. death of tissue caused by loss of blood supply and entry of bacteria
b. cracklike sore in the skin
c. cluster of boils
d. highly contagious viral disease characterized by fever, runny nose, cough, and a spreading skin rash
e. noninfectious inflammatory skin disease having redness, blisters, scabs, and itching
f. scraped-away skin
g. involves sebaceous glands and hair follicles
h. painful skin nodule caused by staphylococci in a hair follicle
i. inflammation of skin and subcutaneous tissue with redness, pain, heat, and swelling
j. overgrowth of scar tissue
k. external injury characterized by pain, swelling, and discoloration
l. precancerous skin condition caused by excessive exposure to sunlight
m. usually occurring in the central area of the face in people older than 30 years
n. malignant epithelial tumor arising from the bottom layer of the epidermis; it seldom metastasizes, but invades local tissue and may recur in the same location
o. potentially serious infection caused by methicillin-resistant *Staphylococcus aureus*
p. localized collection of pus, bacteria, and other material

EXERCISE 11 ■ Match

Match the words in the first column with their correct definitions in the second column.

_____ 1. herpes
_____ 2. tinea
_____ 3. Kaposi sarcoma
_____ 4. vitiligo
_____ 5. pressure injury
_____ 6. pediculosis
_____ 7. pilonidal cyst
_____ 8. scabies
_____ 9. squamous cell carcinoma
_____ 10. systemic lupus erythematosus
_____ 11. impetigo
_____ 12. urticaria
_____ 13. candidiasis
_____ 14. psoriasis
_____ 15. albinism
_____ 16. laceration

a. skin inflammation caused by the itch mite
b. fungal infection of the skin, hair, and nails
c. red lesions covered by silvery scales
d. inflammatory skin disease having clusters of blisters and caused by a virus
e. chronic inflammatory disease involving the skin, joints, kidney, and nervous system
f. cancerous condition that starts as brown or purple papules
g. composed of wheals
h. torn, ragged-edged wound
i. superficial skin condition having pustules and caused by staphylococci or streptococci
j. characterized by lack of pigment (melanin) in the skin, hair, and eyes
k. infection of the skin, mouth, or vagina caused by a yeast-type fungus
l. invasion of the hair and skin by lice
m. damage of the skin and the subcutaneous tissue caused by prolonged pressure
n. malignant growth developing from scalelike epithelial tissue of the surface layer of the epidermis; it invades local tissue and may metastasize
o. small hole containing hair and skin located at top of buttocks
p. white patches on the skin caused by the destruction of melanocytes

EXERCISE 12 ■ Review of Disease and Disorder Terms

Can you define, pronounce, and spell the following terms?

abrasion	eczema	onychocryptosis	seborrhea
abscess	fissure	onychomalacia	squamous cell carcinoma (SCC)
acne	furuncle	onychomycosis	
actinic keratosis	gangrene	onychophagia	systemic lupus erythematosus (SLE)
albinism	hidradenitis	pachyderma	
basal cell carcinoma (BCC)	herpes	paronychia	tinea
	impetigo	pediculosis	urticaria
candidiasis	Kaposi sarcoma	pilonidal cyst	vitiligo
carbuncle	keloid	pressure injury	xanthoma
cellulitis	keratosis	psoriasis	xeroderma
contusion	laceration	rosacea	
dermatitis	measles	scabies	
dermatofibroma	MRSA infection	scleroderma	

Surgical Terms
BUILT FROM WORD PARTS AND *NOT* BUILT FROM WORD PARTS

The first portion of the table contains Integumentary System Terms that can be translated using definitions of word parts. The second portion of the table contains Integumentary System Terms that cannot be fully understood using the definitions of word parts.

■ Built from Word Parts

TERM	DEFINITION	TERM	DEFINITION
1. **dermatoplasty** (DER-ma-tō-*plas*-tē)	surgical repair of the skin	2. **rhytidectomy** (*rit*-i-DEK-to-mē)	excision of wrinkles (also called **facelift**)

Surgical Terms—cont'd
■ *NOT* Built from Word Parts

TERM	DEFINITION
1. **cauterization** (*kaw*-tur-ī-ZĀ-shun)	destruction of tissue with a hot or cold instrument, electric current, or caustic substance (also called **cautery**)
2. **cryosurgery** (*krī*-ō-SER-jer-ē)	destruction of tissue by using extreme cold, often by using liquid nitrogen (Fig. 4.6)

🏛 **CRYO** comes from the Greek **kruos**, meaning **icy cold** or **frost**.

3. **debridement** (da-BRĒD-ment)	removal of contaminated or dead tissue and foreign matter from an open wound
4. **dermabrasion** (*derm*-a-BRĀ-zhun)	procedure to remove skin scars with abrasive material, such as sandpaper
5. **excision** (ek-SIZH-en)	removal by cutting
6. **incision** (in-SIZH-en)	surgical cut or wound produced by a sharp instrument
7. **incision and drainage (I&D)** (in-SIZH-en) and (DRĀ-nij)	surgical cut made to allow the free flow or withdrawal of fluids from a lesion, wound, or cavity
8. **laser surgery** (LĀ-zer) (SER-jer-ē)	procedure using an instrument that emits a high-powered beam of light used to cut, burn, vaporize, or destroy tissue
9. **Mohs surgery** (mōz) (SER-jer-ē)	technique of microscopically controlled serial excisions of a skin cancer

🏛 **MOHS SURGERY** allows for complete tumor removal while sparing as much normal tissue as possible. Excised tissue is examined for tumor cells during the procedure. Tissue is removed until the biopsy margins are cancer free. The procedure is named after **Dr. Frederic E. Mohs**, Wisconsin, who first used the concept in 1936.

10. **skin graft** (skin) (graft)	skin transplanted to replace a lost portion of the body skin surface; it may be a full-thickness or split-thickness graft.
11. **suturing** (SOO-cher-ing)	to stitch edges of a wound surgically (Fig. 4.7)

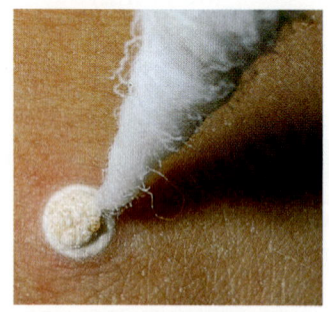

FIG. 4.6 Cryosurgery performed with a nitrogen-soaked, cotton-tipped applicator.

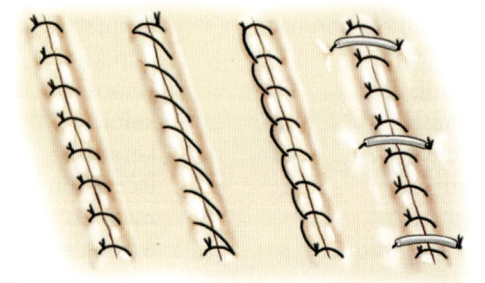

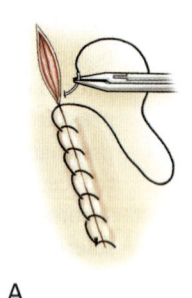

FIG. 4.7 A, Suturing. **B,** Suturing methods. Intermittent   Continuous   Blanket continuous   Retention

EXERCISE 13 ■ Pronounce and Spell

Practice pronunciation and spelling on paper and online.

1. **Practice on Paper**
   a. **Pronounce:** Read the phonetic spelling and say aloud the terms listed in the previous table. Refer to Table 2.2 Pronunciation Key as needed.
   b. **Spell:** Have a study partner read the terms aloud. Write the spelling of the terms on a separate sheet of paper.

Chapter 4 Integumentary System 115

2. **Practice Online**
   a. **Access** online learning resources. Go to evolve.elsevier.com > Evolve Resources > Student Resources.
   b. **Pronounce:** Select Audio Glossary > Chapter 4 > Exercise 13. Select a term to hear its pronunciation and repeat aloud.
   c. **Spell:** Select Activities > Chapter 4 > Spell Terms > Exercise 13. Select the audio icon and type the correct spelling of the term.

❏ Check the box when complete.

EXERCISE 14 ■ Surgical Terms Built from Word Parts

A Analyze and Define

Analyze and define the following Surgical Terms Built from Word Parts by drawing slashes between word parts, writing word part abbreviations above the term, underlining combining forms, and writing combining form abbreviations below the term. *Check your answers in Appendix A.*

1. rhytidectomy

2. dermatoplasty

B Build

Build surgical terms for the following definitions with the word parts you have learned.

1. excision of wrinkles   _____ / _____
                                      WR   S

2. surgical repair of the skin   _____ / _____ / _____
                                      WR   CV   S

EXERCISE 15 ■ Surgical Terms NOT Built from Word Parts

A Identify

Fill in the blanks with the correct surgical terms.

1. _____ _____ is a technique of microscopically controlled serial excisions used for treatment of many skin cancers.
2. A surgical cut or wound produced by a sharp instrument is called a(n) _____.
3. Destruction of tissue with a hot or cold instrument, electric current, or caustic substance is called _____.
4. _____ is to stitch the edges of a wound surgically.
5. A surgical cut made to allow the free flow or withdrawal of fluids from a lesion, wound, or cavity is called _____.
6. _____ is the removal of contaminated or dead tissue and foreign matter from an open wound.
7. Removal by cutting is known as _____.

116 Chapter 4 Integumentary System

8. _____ _____ is a procedure using an instrument that emits a high-powered beam of light used to cut, burn, vaporize, or destroy tissue.
9. The destruction of tissue by using extreme cold, often by using liquid nitrogen, is called _____.
10. _____ is a procedure to remove skin scars with abrasive material.
11. A full-thickness or split-thickness _____ _____ is skin transplanted to replace a lost portion of the body skin surface.

B Match

Match the surgical terms in the first column with their correct definitions in the second column.

_____ 1. suturing
_____ 2. dermabrasion
_____ 3. laser surgery
_____ 4. incision and drainage
_____ 5. cauterization
_____ 6. excision
_____ 7. Mohs surgery
_____ 8. debridement
_____ 9. cryosurgery
_____ 10. incision
_____ 11. skin graft

a. destruction of tissue with a hot or cold instrument, electric current, or caustic substance
b. technique of microscopically controlled serial excisions of a skin cancer
c. surgical cut or wound produced by a sharp instrument
d. surgical cut made to allow the free flow or withdrawal of fluids from a lesion, wound, or cavity
e. removal by cutting
f. removal of contaminated or dead tissue and foreign matter from an open wound
g. procedure using an instrument that emits a high-powered beam of light used to cut, burn, vaporize, or destroy tissue
h. procedure to remove skin scars with abrasive material, such as sandpaper
i. to stitch edges of a wound surgically
j. destruction of tissue by using extreme cold, often by using liquid nitrogen
k. skin transplanted to replace a lost portion of the body skin surface

EXERCISE 16 ■ Review of Surgical Terms

Can you define, pronounce, and spell the following terms?

cauterization	dermatoplasty	incision and drainage (I&D)	rhytidectomy
cryosurgery	excision	laser surgery	skin graft
debridement	incision	Mohs surgery	suturing
dermabrasion			

Complementary Terms
BUILT FROM WORD PARTS

The following terms can be translated using definitions of word parts. Further explanation is provided within parentheses as needed.

SIGNS AND SYMPTOMS			
TERM	**DEFINITION**	**TERM**	**DEFINITION**
1. **erythroderma** (e-*rith*-rō-DER-ma)	red skin (abnormal redness of the skin)	3. **leukoderma** (lū-kō-DER-ma)	white skin (white patches caused by depigmentation)
2. **hypertrichosis** (*hī*-per-tri-KŌ-sis)	abnormal condition of excessive hair (growth) (also called **hirsutism**)	4. **xanthoderma** (*zan*-thō-DER-ma)	yellow skin
		5. **xerosis** (zēr-Ō-sis)	abnormal condition of dryness (of skin, eye, or mouth)

MEDICAL SPECIALTIES

TERM	DEFINITION	TERM	DEFINITION
6. **dermatologist** (*der*-ma-TOL-o-jist)	physician who studies and treats skin (diseases)	7. **dermatology (derm)** (*der*-ma-TOL-o-jē)	study of the skin (branch of medicine that deals with the diagnosis and treatment of skin diseases)

DESCRIPTIVE TERMS

TERM	DEFINITION	TERM	DEFINITION
8. **cutaneous** (kū-TĀ-nē-us)	pertaining to the skin	14. **subcutaneous (subcut)** (*sub*-kū-TĀ-nē-us)	pertaining to under the skin
9. **epidermal** (*ep*-i-DER-mal)	pertaining to upon the skin	15. **subungual** (sub-UNG-gwal)	pertaining to under the nail
10. **hypodermic** (*hī*-pō-DER-mik)	pertaining to under the skin	16. **transdermal (TD)** (trans-DER-mel)	pertaining to through the skin
11. **intradermal (ID)** (*in*-tra-DER-mal)	pertaining to within the skin	**TRANSDERMAL** usually means entering through the skin and refers to the administration of a drug applied to the skin in ointment or patch form. **Percutaneous** usually means performed through the skin, as in the insertion of a needle, catheter, or probe.	
12. **keratogenic** (*ker*-a-tō-JEN-ik)	producing hornlike tissue		
13. **percutaneous** (*per*-kū-TĀ-nē-us)	pertaining to through the skin	17. **ungual** (UNG-gwal)	pertaining to the nail

OTHER TERMS

TERM	DEFINITION	TERM	DEFINITION
18. **staphylococcus** (*pl.* **staphylococci**) **(staph)** (*staf*-il-ō-KOK-us) (*staf*-il-ō-KOK-sī)	berry-shaped (bacterium) in grapelike clusters (these bacteria cause many skin diseases)	19. **streptococcus (*pl.* streptococci) (strep)** (*strep*-tō-KOK-us) (*strep*-tō-KOK-sī)	berry-shaped (bacterium) in twisted chains

EXERCISE 17 ■ Pronounce and Spell

Practice pronunciation and spelling on paper and online.

1. Practice on Paper
   a. **Pronounce:** Read the phonetic spelling and say aloud the terms listed in the previous table. Refer to Table 2.2 Pronunciation Key as needed.
   b. **Spell:** Have a study partner read the terms aloud. Write the spelling of the terms on a separate sheet of paper.
2. Practice Online
   a. **Access** online learning resources. Go to evolve.elsevier.com > Evolve Resources > Student Resources.
   b. **Pronounce:** Select Audio Glossary > Chapter 4 > Exercise 17. Select a term to hear its pronunciation and repeat aloud.
   c. **Spell:** Select Activities > Chapter 4 > Spell Terms > Exercise 17. Select the audio icon and type the correct spelling of the term.

❏ Check the box when complete.

Chapter 4 Integumentary System

EXERCISE 18 ■ Analyze and Define

Analyze and define the following Complementary Terms Built from Word Parts by drawing slashes between word parts, writing word part abbreviations above the term, underlining combining forms, and writing combining form abbreviations below the term. *Check your answers in Appendix A.*

EXAMPLE:
      P   WR   S
intra / derm / al
<u>pertaining to within the skin</u>

1. ungual

2. transdermal

3. streptococcus

4. hypodermic

5. dermatology

6. subcutaneous

7. staphylococcus

8. keratogenic

9. dermatologist

10. cutaneous

11. epidermal

12. xanthoderma

13. erythroderma

14. percutaneous

15. xerosis

16. subungual

17. leukoderma

18. hypertrichosis

Chapter 4 Integumentary System 119

EXERCISE 19 ■ Build

A Label

Build terms pictured by writing word parts above definitions.

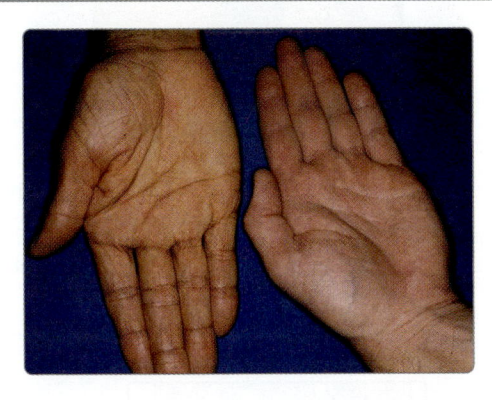

1.
_____ / ____ / _____ /a as seen in jaundice
yellow   CV   skin

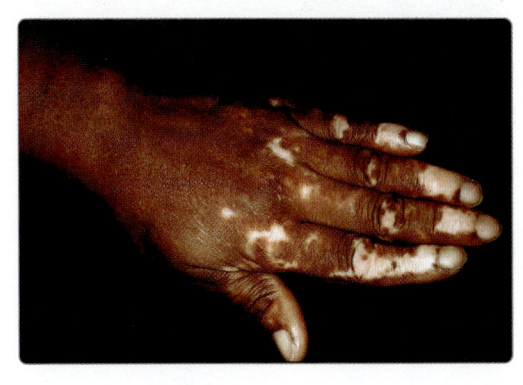

2.
_____ / _____ / _____ /a as seen in vitiligo
white   CV   skin

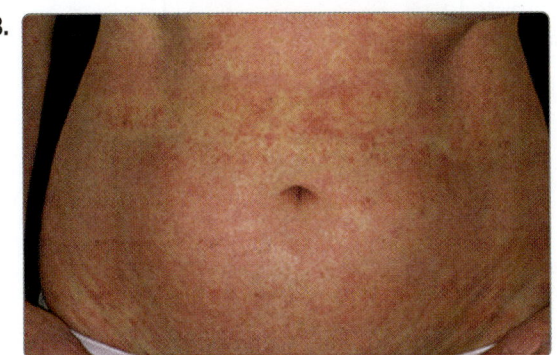

3.
_____ / ___ / _____ /a as seen in exfoliative dermatitis
red   CV   skin

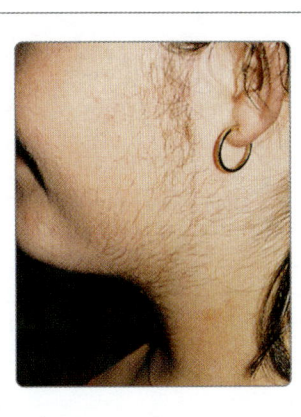

4.
_____ / _____ / _____
excessive   hair   abnormal condition

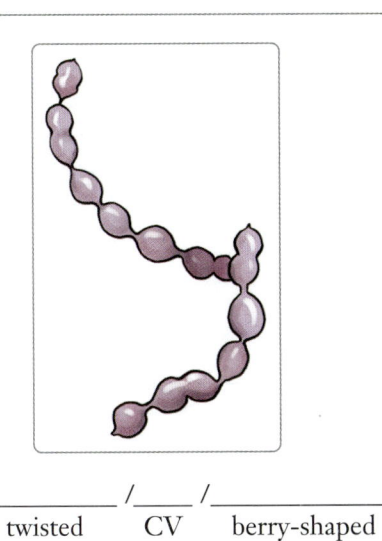

5.
_____ / ____ / _____
   twisted   CV   berry-shaped
                      chains (plural)

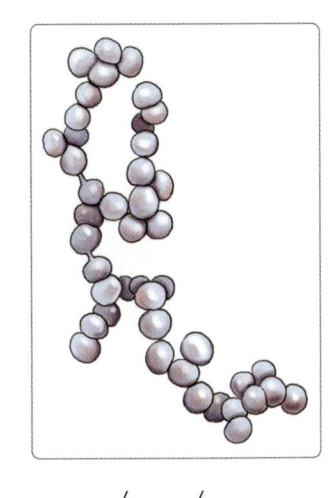

6.
_____ / ____ / _____
  grapelike   CV   berry-shaped
                      clusters (plural)

120 Chapter 4 Integumentary System

7.

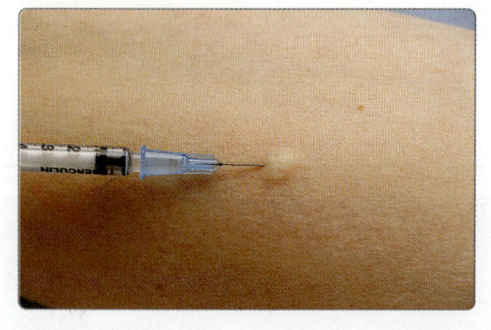

_____ / _____ / _____ injection
within   skin   pertaining to

8.

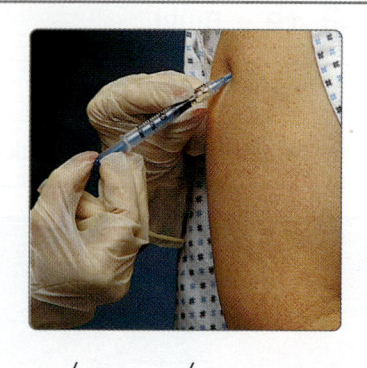

_____ / _____ / _____ injection
under   skin   pertaining to

using a _____ / _____ / _____ needle
         under   skin   pertaining to

9.

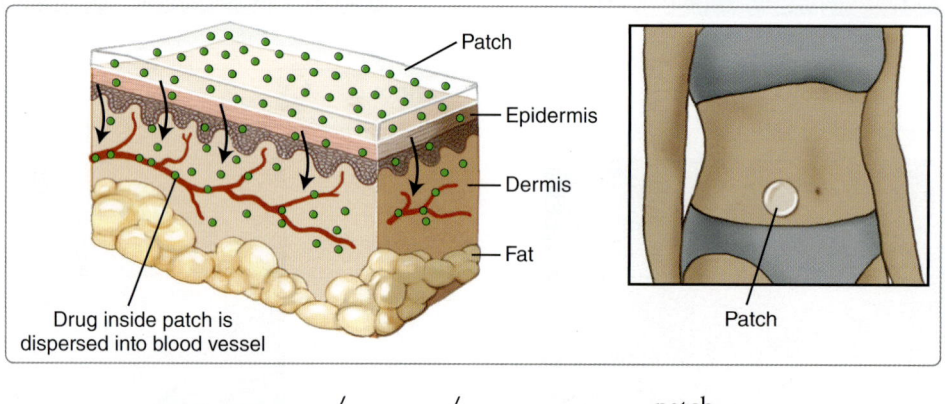

_____ / _____ / _____ patch
through   skin   pertaining to

B Fill In

Build complementary terms with the word parts you have learned.

EXAMPLE: pertaining to under the skin   hypo / derm / ic
                                              P / WR / S

1. study of the skin

   _____ / __ / _____
        WR   CV   S

2. abnormal condition of dryness (of skin, eye, or mouth)

   _____ / _____
        WR   S

3. pertaining to the nail

   _____ / _____
        WR   S

4. pertaining to the skin

   _____ / _____
        WR   S

5. a physician who studies and treats skin (diseases)

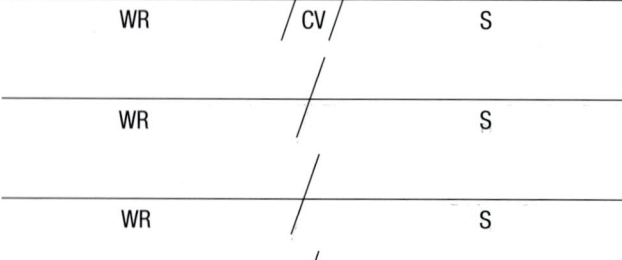

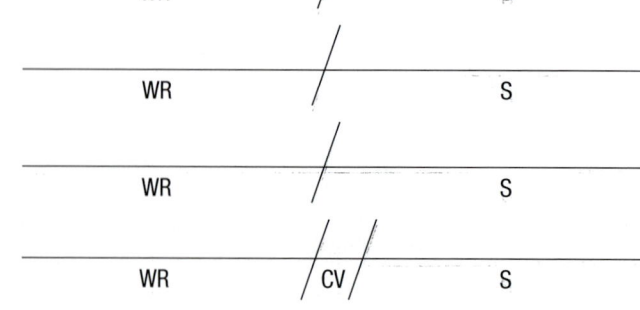

   _____ / __ / _____
        WR   CV   S

Chapter 4 Integumentary System 121

6. pertaining to under the nail

_____ / _____ / _____
P   WR   S

7. pertaining to upon the skin

_____ / _____ / _____
P   WR   S

8. pertaining to through the skin

_____ / _____ / _____
P   WR   S

9. producing hornlike tissue

_____ / _____ / _____
WR   CV   S

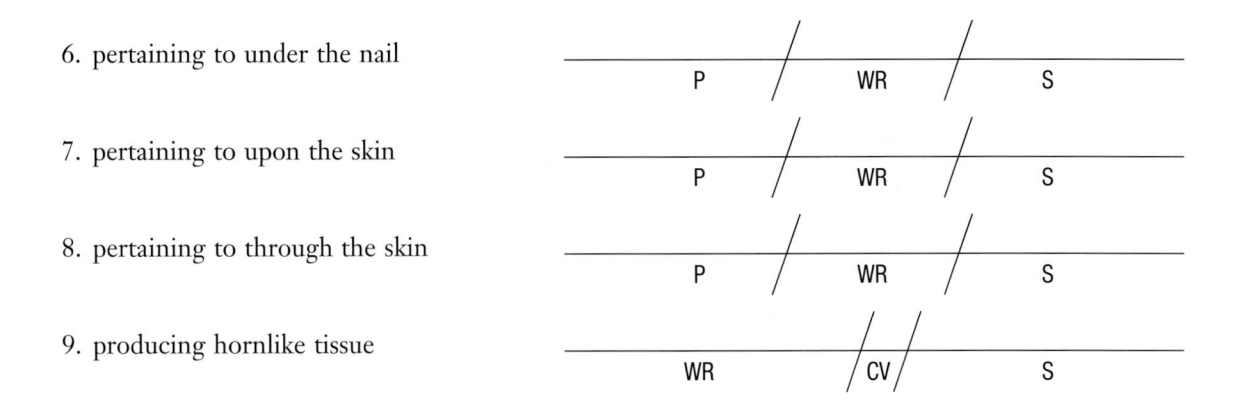

Complementary Terms
NOT BUILT FROM WORD PARTS

Word parts may be present in the following terms; however, their full meanings cannot be translated using definitions of word parts alone.

SIGNS AND SYMPTOMS	
TERM	**DEFINITION**
1. **alopecia** (al-ō-PĒ-sha)	loss of hair; there are multiple types with various causes, including androgenic, areata, and traction
🏛 **ALOPECIA** is derived from the Greek **alopex**, meaning **fox**. One was thought to bald like a mangy fox.	
2. **cyst** (sist)	closed sac containing fluid or semisolid material; can occur in the skin (cutaneous cyst) or other locations within the body (Table 4.2)
3. **diaphoresis** (dī-a-fo-RĒ-sis)	excessive sweating; due to another condition such as a disease, medication, or stress
🏛 **DIAPHORESIS** is derived from Greek **dia**, meaning **through**, and **phoreo**, meaning **carry**. Translated, it means the carrying through of perspiration.	
4. **ecchymosis** (*pl.* **ecchymoses**) (ek-i-MŌ-sis) (ek-i-MŌ-sēz)	large (greater than 1 cm), flat, blue-purple lesion caused by escape of blood into deeper areas of the skin, as may occur when blood is withdrawn by a needle and syringe from an arm vein (Fig 4.8)
ECCHYMOSIS is different from a contusion (bruise) because it can result from mechanisms other than injury, including bleeding disorders, severe kidney disease, and leukemia.	
5. **edema** (e-DĒ-ma)	puffy swelling of tissue from the accumulation of fluid
6. **induration** (in-dū-RĀ-shun)	abnormal hard spot(s) or area of skin; may include underlying tissue
7. **jaundice** (JAWN-dis)	condition characterized by a yellow coloring of the skin, mucous membranes, and sclera (whites of the eyes) caused by the presence of bile (also called **icterus**)
8. **lesion** (LĒ-zhun)	any visible change in tissue resulting from injury or disease. It is a broad term that includes sores, wounds, ulcers, and tumors.
9. **leukoplakia** (lū-kō-PLĀ-kē-a)	condition characterized by white spots or patches on mucous membranes, which may be precancerous
10. **macule** (MAK-ūl)	flat, colored spot on the skin (Table 4.2)
11. **nevus** (*pl.* **nevi**) (NĒ-vus) (NĒ-vī)	circumscribed malformation of the skin, usually brown, black, or flesh colored. A congenital nevus is present at birth and is referred to as a birthmark. (also called a **mole**)
12. **nodule** (NOD-ūl)	small, knotlike mass that can be felt by touch (Table 4.2)

Complementary Terms—cont'd
NOT BUILT FROM WORD PARTS

SIGNS AND SYMPTOMS—CONT'D

TERM	DEFINITION
13. pallor (PAL-or)	paleness
14. papule (PAP-ūl)	small, solid skin elevation (Table 4.2)

TABLE 4.2 Common Skin Lesions

LESION	DEFINITION	CUTAWAY SECTIONS	EXAMPLE
Macule	flat, colored spot on the skin		freckle
Papule	small, solid skin elevation		skin tag / basal cell carcinoma
Nodule	small, knotlike mass		lipoma / metastatic carcinoma / rheumatoid nodule
Wheal	transitory, itchy elevation of the skin		urticaria (hives)
Vesicle	small elevation of epidermis containing liquid		herpes zoster (shingles) / herpes simplex virus type 1 / contact dermatitis
Pustule	elevation of the skin containing pus		impetigo / acne
Cyst	closed sac containing fluid or semisolid material		acne

Chapter 4 Integumentary System   123

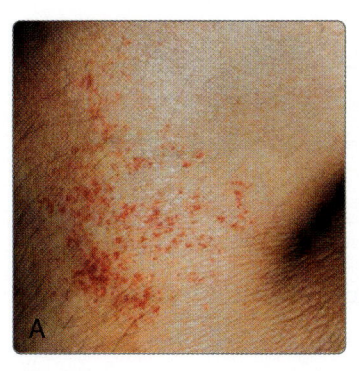

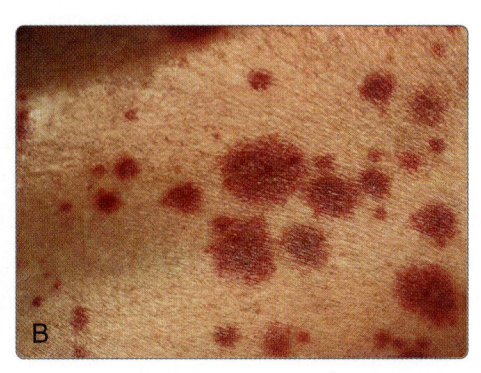

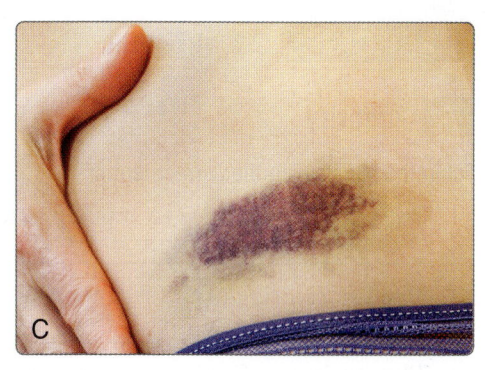

FIG. 4.8 Petechiae, purpura, and ecchymoses are related lesions caused by the escape of blood into the skin and mucous membranes. They vary in size, with petechiae being the smallest in size, up to 0.3 cm; purpura being the next largest, generally from 0.3 cm up to 1 cm; and ecchymoses being the largest, greater than 1 cm. **A,** Petechiae. **B,** Purpura. **C,** Ecchymosis.

TERM	DEFINITION
15. petechiae (*s.* petechia) (pe-TĒ-kē-ē) (pe-TĒ-kē-a)	tiny (0.3 cm or smaller), pinpoint, bright red lesions that result from escape of blood into the skin and mucous membranes (Fig 4.8)
🏛 **PETECHIA** is originally from the Italian **petechio**, meaning **flea bite**. The small hemorrhagic spot resembles the mark made by a flea.	
16. pruritus (prū-RĪ-tus)	itching
17. purpura (PER-pū-ra)	small (between 0.3 cm and 1 cm) reddish-purple lesions caused by escape of blood into skin and mucous membranes (Fig 4.8)
18. pustule (PUS-tūl)	elevation of skin containing pus (Table 4.2)
19. ulcer (UL-ser)	erosion of the skin or mucous membrane
20. verruca (ver-RŪ-ka)	circumscribed cutaneous elevation caused by a virus (also called **wart**)
21. vesicle (VES-i-kl)	small elevation of the epidermis containing liquid (also called **blister**) (Table 4.2)
22. wheal (hwēl)	transitory, itchy elevation of the skin with a white center and a red surrounding area; a wheal is an individual urticaria lesion (hive) (Table 4.2)

🔍 Refer to **Appendix E** for pharmacology terms related to the integumentary system.

EXERCISE 20 ■ Pronounce and Spell

Practice pronunciation and spelling on paper and online.

1. **Practice on Paper**
   a. **Pronounce:** Read the phonetic spelling and say aloud the terms listed in the previous table. Refer to Table 2.2 Pronunciation Key as needed.
   b. **Spell:** Have a study partner read the terms aloud. Write the spelling of the terms on a separate sheet of paper.
2. **Practice Online** 🌐
   a. **Access** online learning resources. Go to evolve.elsevier.com > Evolve Resources > Student Resources.
   b. **Pronounce:** Select Audio Glossary > Chapter 4 > Exercise 20. Select a term to hear its pronunciation and repeat aloud.
   c. **Spell:** Select Activities > Chapter 4 > Spell Terms > Exercise 20. Select the audio icon and type the correct spelling of the term.

❏ Check the box when complete.

124 Chapter 4 Integumentary System

EXERCISE 21 ■ Fill In

A Identify

Fill in the blanks with the correct terms.

1. Excessive sweating due to another condition is called _____.
2. _____ is the name for a flat, colored skin spot.
3. A yellow coloring of the skin, mucous membranes, and sclera caused by the presence of bile is known as _____.
4. The condition of white spots or patches on mucous membranes is called _____.
5. _____ are tiny, pinpoint, bright-red lesions caused by escape of blood.
6. Another name for paleness is _____.
7. Large, flat, blue-purple lesion caused by escape of blood into deeper areas of the skin (as may occur when blood is withdrawn by a needle and syringe) is referred to as _____.
8. A small knotlike mass that can be felt by touch is called a(n) _____.
9. A closed sac containing fluid or semisolid material is called a(n) _____.
10. Itching is called _____.
11. Small (between 0.3 cm and 1 cm) reddish-purple lesions caused by the escape of blood into skin and mucous membranes are known as _____.
12. A small, solid skin elevation is called a(n) _____.
13. A transitory, itchy skin elevation with a white center and a red surrounding area is a(n) _____.
14. A(n) _____ is a skin elevation containing pus.
15. A blister is also called a(n) _____.
16. An abnormal hard spot(s) or area of skin is called _____.
17. _____ is the swelling of tissue.
18. _____ refers to any visible change in tissue resulting from injury or disease.

B Label

Write the medical terms pictured and defined.

1. _____
   erosion of the skin or mucous membrane

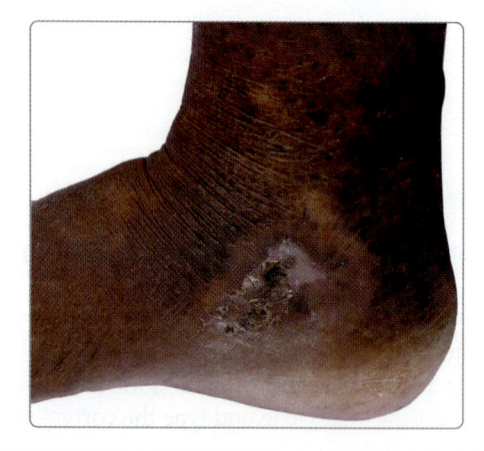

2. _____
   circumscribed malformation of the skin, usually brown, black, or flesh colored (also called a **mole**)

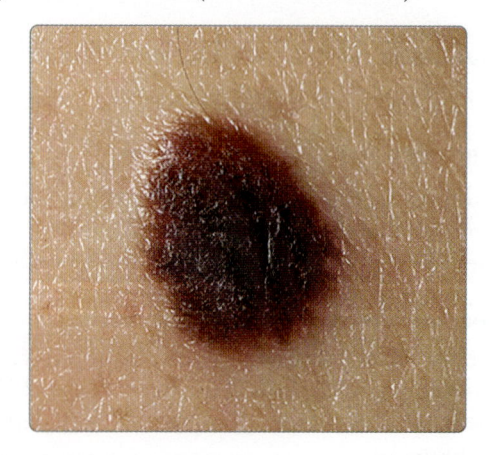

Chapter 4   Integumentary System   125

3. _____
circumscribed cutaneous elevation caused by a virus (also called **wart**)

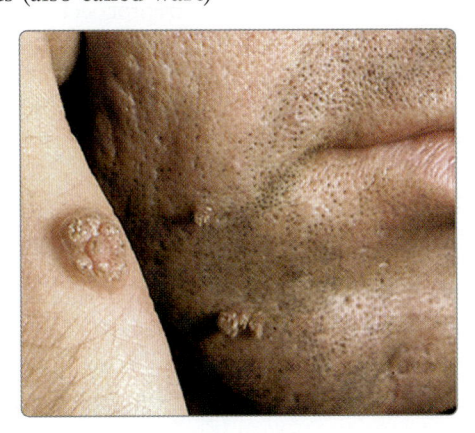

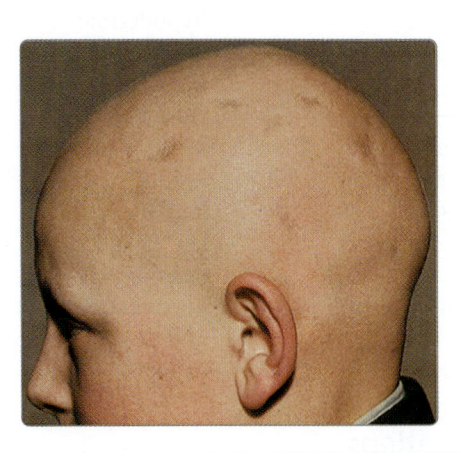

4. _____
loss of hair

EXERCISE 22 ■ Match

Match the words in the first column with their correct definitions in the second column.

_____ 1. lesion
_____ 2. alopecia
_____ 3. induration
_____ 4. nodule
_____ 5. diaphoresis
_____ 6. cyst
_____ 7. ecchymosis
_____ 8. jaundice
_____ 9. edema

a. loss of hair
b. large (greater than 1 cm), flat, blue-purple lesion caused by escape of blood into deeper areas of the skin
c. yellow color to the skin, mucous membranes, and sclera
d. closed sac containing fluid
e. broad term denoting any visible change in tissue, including sores, wounds, ulcers, and tumors
f. small knotlike mass
g. excessive sweating
h. swelling of tissue
i. hard spot(s) or area of skin

EXERCISE 23 ■ Match

Match the terms in the first column with their correct definitions in the second column.

_____ 1. leukoplakia
_____ 2. macule
_____ 3. nevus
_____ 4. pallor
_____ 5. papule
_____ 6. petechiae
_____ 7. pruritus
_____ 8. purpura
_____ 9. pustule
_____ 10. ulcer
_____ 11. verruca
_____ 12. vesicle
_____ 13. wheal

a. mole
b. itching
c. wart
d. condition of white spots or patches on mucous membranes
e. small (between 0.3 cm and 1 cm) reddish-purple lesions
f. skin elevation containing pus
g. small elevation of epidermis containing liquid
h. individual urticaria lesion
i. flat, colored spot on skin
j. small, solid skin elevation
k. paleness
l. tiny (0.3 cm or smaller), pinpoint, bright red lesions
m. erosion of the skin or mucous membrane

EXERCISE 24 ■ Review of Complementary Terms

Can you define, pronounce, and spell the following terms?

alopecia	hypodermic	papule	streptococcus
cutaneous	induration	percutaneous	(*pl.* streptococci)
cyst	intradermal (ID)	petechiae (*s.* petechia)	(strep)
dermatologist	jaundice	pruritus	transdermal (TD)
dermatology (derm)	keratogenic	purpura	ulcer
diaphoresis	lesion	pustule	ungual
ecchymosis	leukoderma	subcutaneous (subcut)	verruca
(*pl.* ecchymoses)	leukoplakia	subungual	vesicle
edema	macule	staphylococcus	wheal
epidermal	nevus (*pl.* nevi)	(*pl.* staphylococci)	xanthoderma
erythroderma	nodule	(staph)	xerosis
hypertrichosis	pallor		

Abbreviations

DISEASE AND DISORDERS

ABBREVIATION	TERM	ABBREVIATION	TERM
BCC	basal cell carcinoma	MRSA	methicillin-resistant *Staphylococcus aureus*; spoken as a whole word (mur-sah)
CA-MRSA	community-associated MRSA infection; spoken as (C-A) (mur-sah)		
HA-MRSA	healthcare-associated MRSA infection; spoken as (H-A) (mur-sah)	SCC	squamous cell carcinoma
		SLE	systemic lupus erythematosus

TREATMENTS

ABBREVIATION	TERM	ABBREVIATION	TERM
FTSG	full-thickness skin graft	STSG	split-thickness skin graft
I&D	incision and drainage		

MEDICAL SPECIALTY

ABBREVIATION	TERM
derm	dermatology; spoken as a whole word (derm)

DESCRIPTIVE

ABBREVIATION	TERM	ABBREVIATION	TERM
ID	intradermal	TD	transdermal
subcut	subcutaneous; spoken as a whole word (sub-KŪT)		

OTHER

ABBREVIATION	TERM	ABBREVIATION	TERM
staph	staphylococcus; spoken as a whole word (staf)	strep	streptococcus; spoken as a whole word (strep)

Refer to **Appendix D** for a complete list of abbreviations.

EXERCISE 25 ■ Fill In

Write the terms abbreviated.

1. The most common form of skin cancer is **BCC** _____ _____ _____.

2. **STSGs** _____ _____ _____ _____ involve taking the epidermis and only a top section of the dermis from the donor site; they rely on the lower dermis at the recipient site to provide nutrients for the healing skin.

3. The entire dermis, along with the epidermis, is taken from the donor site in **FTSGs** _____ _____ _____ _____, which results in less scarring, but also has a higher chance of being unsuccessful.

4. Long-term exposure to sunlight is by far the most frequent cause of **SCC** _____ _____ _____.

5. **SLE** _____ _____ _____ is a chronic relapsing disease, often with long periods of remission.

6. The medication was administered by **subcut** _____ injection.

7. **Staph** _____ bacterium was cultured from the abscess.

8. The culture confirmed a **strep** _____ infection of the throat.

9. **I&D** _____ _____ _____ is used to treat cutaneous abscesses, such as a furuncle.

10. Hormone replacement therapy is available by **TD** _____ administration.

11. The tuberculin test was administered by an **ID** _____ injection.

12. The patient visited the **derm** _____ clinic for a psoriasis follow-up visit.

13. **MRSA** _____ _____ _____ _____ infections originating in a healthcare setting are called **HA-MRSA** _____ _____ _____ _____, whereas MRSA infections in people who have not been in healthcare settings are called **CA-MRSA** _____ _____ _____ _____.

Chapter 4 Integumentary System

PRACTICAL APPLICATION

EXERCISE 26 ■ Case Study: Translate Between Everyday Language and Medical Language

CASE STUDY: Antonne Johnson

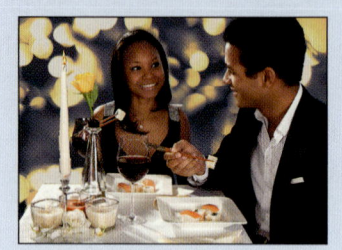

Antonne and his girlfriend were eating out when his mouth began to tingle.

"Hey, are you all right? You look pale," Sasha said.

"My stomach doesn't feel too good." This had happened before, Antonne realized, when he had eaten shellfish. Tonight he had been careful to order sushi made from fish without a shell. He signaled Sasha to call 911. In no time at all, his mouth, face, and arms felt very itchy. As she dialed, Sasha noticed his lips beginning to swell. His cheeks and arms became covered with different-sized red and white bumps. EMTs arrived just as it was becoming difficult for Antonne to breathe. Sasha quickly told them of Antonne's shellfish allergy.

Now that you have worked through Chapter 4 on the integumentary system, consider the medical terms that might be used to describe Antonne's experience. See the Chapter at a Glance section at the end of the chapter for a list of terms that might apply.

A. Underline phrases in the case study that could be substituted with medical terms.

B. Write the medical term and its definition for three of the phrases you underlined.

MEDICAL TERM	DEFINITION
1. _____	_____
2. _____	_____
3. _____	_____

DOCUMENTATION: Excerpt from EMT Notes

CC: Patient says he is having trouble breathing.

History: Ambulance responded to a call from a young woman at a sushi restaurant on behalf of a 27-year-old male. Onset: Patient's symptoms were brought on suddenly while eating; he has experienced one previous episode of anaphylaxis. Medication: Patient has epinephrine injection. Allergies: Patient is allergic to shellfish.

Exam: BP: 90/60 mm Hg, Pulse: 120, O_2: 15L Non-rebreather mask. Pallor of face and hands is present; he appears to be experiencing pruritus and says he might vomit. Patient shows signs of edema around the lips and face and urticaria on his cheeks and arms. Upon auscultation of the lungs, wheezing is present. Assessment/Plan: Anaphylaxis: One dose of epinephrine was delivered by injection.

C. Underline medical terms presented in Chapter 4 in the previous excerpt from Antonne's medical record. See the Chapter at a Glance section at the end of the chapter for a complete list.

D. Select and define three of the medical terms you underlined. To check your answers, go to Appendix A.

MEDICAL TERM	DEFINITION
1. _____	_____
2. _____	_____
3. _____	_____

Chapter 4 Integumentary System

EXERCISE 27 ■ Interact With Medical Documents

A

Read the report and complete it by writing medical terms on answer lines within the document. Definitions of terms to be written appear after the document.

76548-INT WHARTON, Sandra L.

Name: WHARTON, Sandra L. MR#: 76548-INT Sex: F Allergies: None known
DOB: 10/03/19XX Age: 50 PCP: Spring, Lincoln MD

Encounter Date: 7/27/20XX
Operative Report:

History: The patient is a 50-year-old woman presenting to the 1._____ clinic with concerns about a 2._____ _____ located at the 3._____ aspect of her left eyebrow. The patient's medical history is also significant for 4._____, primarily of the scalp and ears, as well as chronic 5._____, primarily of the forearms bilaterally.

Indications for Procedure:
The 6. _____ has been present for approximately 3 months. It measures 1.5 cm × 2.0 cm and has poorly defined borders. Risks, benefits, indications and expectations were discussed with the patient regarding biopsy, and she has agreed to proceed with 7._____ _____.

Preoperative Diagnosis:
Suspicious lesion, left eyebrow.

Anesthesia: Xylocaine 1% with epinephrine.

Procedure: After written consent was obtained, the site was prepped and draped in the usual sterile fashion. Prior to the first stage, the surgical site was injected with anesthesia into the 8._____ layer; the site was tested for anesthesia and re-injected as needed in subsequent stages. In each stage, a(n) 9._____ of a thin layer of abnormal tissue was performed, then immediately coded, cut, and stained for microscopic 10._____ examination. The entire base and margins were examined by the 11. _____/pathologist. 12._____ was used to achieve hemostasis. 13. _____ was performed with 6-0 Vicryl, followed by 6-0 nylon for closure. Pressure dressing was applied.

The patient tolerated the procedure well, without any complications.

Postoperative Diagnosis: 14. _____, with clear margins.

Electronically signed: William Hickman MD on 27 July 20XX 13:30

Definitions of Medical Terms to Complete the Document
Write the medical terms defined on corresponding answer lines in the document.

1. study of the skin
2. small, knotlike mass that can be felt by touch
3. pertaining to the middle
4. precancerous skin condition of hornlike tissue formation
5. noninfectious, inflammatory skin disease characterized by redness, blisters, scabs, and itching
6. any visible change in tissue resulting from injury or disease
7. technique of microscopically controlled serial excisions of skin cancer
8. pertaining to under the skin
9. removal by cutting
10. study of disease
11. physician who studies and treats skin
12. destruction of tissue with a hot or cold instrument, electric current, or caustic substance
13. to stitch edges of a wound surgically
14. malignant epithelial tumor arising from the bottom layer of the epidermis

130 Chapter 4 Integumentary System

B

Read the medical report and answer the questions below it.

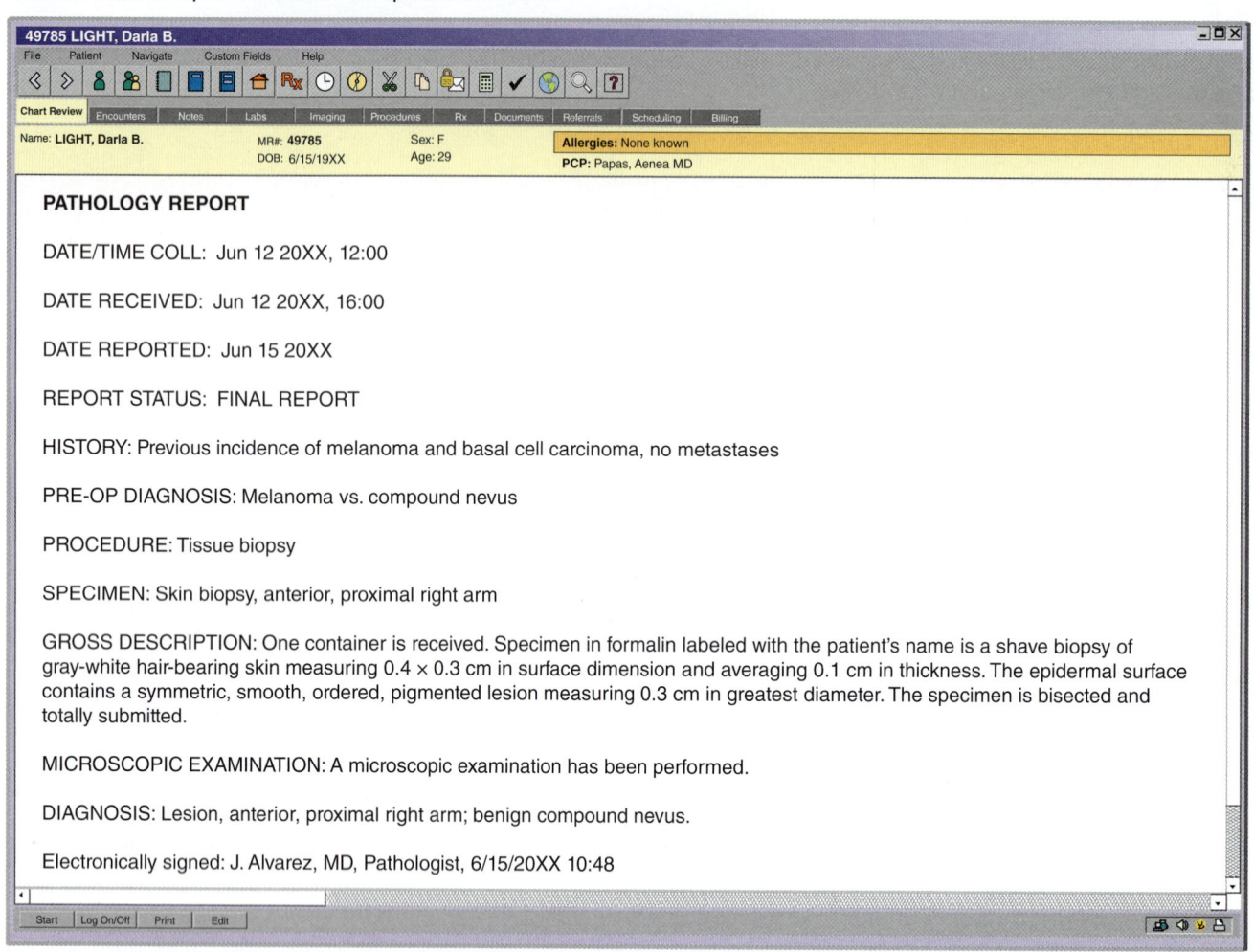

49785 LIGHT, Darla B.

File Patient Navigate Custom Fields Help

Chart Review | Encounters | Notes | Labs | Imaging | Procedures | Rx | Documents | Referrals | Scheduling | Billing

Name: **LIGHT, Darla B.** MR#: **49785** Sex: F Allergies: None known
DOB: 6/15/19XX Age: 29 PCP: Papas, Aenea MD

PATHOLOGY REPORT

DATE/TIME COLL: Jun 12 20XX, 12:00

DATE RECEIVED: Jun 12 20XX, 16:00

DATE REPORTED: Jun 15 20XX

REPORT STATUS: FINAL REPORT

HISTORY: Previous incidence of melanoma and basal cell carcinoma, no metastases

PRE-OP DIAGNOSIS: Melanoma vs. compound nevus

PROCEDURE: Tissue biopsy

SPECIMEN: Skin biopsy, anterior, proximal right arm

GROSS DESCRIPTION: One container is received. Specimen in formalin labeled with the patient's name is a shave biopsy of gray-white hair-bearing skin measuring 0.4 × 0.3 cm in surface dimension and averaging 0.1 cm in thickness. The epidermal surface contains a symmetric, smooth, ordered, pigmented lesion measuring 0.3 cm in greatest diameter. The specimen is bisected and totally submitted.

MICROSCOPIC EXAMINATION: A microscopic examination has been performed.

DIAGNOSIS: Lesion, anterior, proximal right arm; benign compound nevus.

Electronically signed: J. Alvarez, MD, Pathologist, 6/15/20XX 10:48

Use the medical report above to answer the questions.

1. Identify singular and plural forms of medical terms used in the pathology report. Write "p" for plural and "s" for singular next to the terms. Refer to Table 2.5 for plural endings.
   _____ a. melanoma
   _____ b. melanomata
   _____ c. nevi
   _____ d. nevus
   _____ e. metastasis
   _____ f. metastases
   _____ g. biopsy
   _____ h. biopsies

2. The skin biopsy was obtained from:
   a. near the shoulder on the back of the right arm
   b. near the shoulder on the front of the right arm
   c. near the wrist on the back of the right arm
   d. near the wrist on the front of the right arm

3. Use your medical dictionary or a reliable online source to find the meanings of the following terms used in the pathology report:
   a. compound _____
   b. pigmented _____
   c. bisected _____
   d. microscopic _____

EXERCISE 28 ■ Use Medical Terms in Clinical Statements

For each phrase printed in bold, circle the medical term or abbreviation defined. Answers are listed in Appendix A. For pronunciation practice read the answers aloud.

1. The 2-year-old patient who presented with several pimplelike **visible change in tissue resulting from injury or disease** (lesions, lacerations, pressure ulcers) accompanied by erythema was diagnosed with **superficial skin infection characterized by red lesions that progress to blisters and then honey-colored crusts** (herpes, impetigo, jaundice).

2. A **technique of microscopically controlled serial excisions** (cryosurgery, laser surgery, Mohs surgery) was used to treat the patient's recurrent **malignant growth developing from scalelike epithelial tissue of the surface layer of the epidermis** (squamous cell carcinoma, Kaposi sarcoma, basal cell carcinoma).

3. **Strain of common bacteria that has developed resistance to many antibiotics** (SLE, strep, MRSA) is common in hospitals, but is also occurring more frequently in the general population. First symptoms often include **inflammation of the skin and subcutaneous tissue characterized by redness, heat, pain, and swelling** (edema, dermatitis, cellulitis) and a(n) **localized collection of pus accompanied by swelling and inflammation** (abscess, laceration, lesion).

4. **White skin patches caused by depigmentation** (pachyderma, xeroderma, leukoderma), **congenital, hereditary condition characterized by lack of pigment in skin, hair, and eyes** (actinic keratosis, albinism, rosacea) and **white patches on the skin caused by the destruction of melanocytes** (vitiligo, Kaposi sarcoma, systemic lupus erythematosus) are all forms of hypomelanosis, a condition characterized by a deficiency of melanin in the tissues.

5. After clearing out a weedy patch in his front yard, Frank Pisaniello noticed **red skin** (melanoderma, leukoderma, erythroderma) on his forearm that itched quite a bit. He sought treatment from a **physician who studies and treats diseases of the skin** (dermatopathy, dermatologist, dermatopathologist). He was diagnosed as having contact **inflammation of the skin** (dermatitis, erythroderma, dermatopathy), thought to be caused by poison ivy.

EXERCISE 29 ■ Pronounce Medical Terms in Use

Practice pronunciation of terms by reading aloud the following paragraph. Use the phonetic spellings to assist with pronunciation. The script also contains medical terms not presented in the chapter. If interested, research their meanings in a medical dictionary or a reliable online source.

> Emily visited the **dermatology** (der-ma-TOL-o-jē) clinic because of **pruritus** (prū-RĪ-tus) secondary to **dermatitis** (der-ma-TĪ-tis) involving her scalp and areas of her elbows and knees. A diagnosis of **psoriasis** (so-RĪ-a-sis) was made. **Eczema** (EK-ze-ma), **scabies** (SKĀ-bēz), and **tinea** (TIN-ē-a) were considered in the differential diagnosis. An emollient cream was prescribed. In addition the patient showed the **dermatologist** (der-ma-TOL-o-jist) the tender, discolored, thickened nail of her right great toe. Emily learned she had **onychomycosis** (on-i-kō-mī-KŌ-sis), for which she was given an additional prescription for an oral antifungal drug.

CHAPTER REVIEW

EXERCISE 30 ■ Chapter Content Quiz

Test your understanding of terms and abbreviations introduced in this chapter. Circle the letter for the medical term or abbreviation related to the words in italics.

1. *Small (between 0.3 cm and 1 cm) reddish-purple lesions caused by escape of blood into skin and mucous membranes* may be caused by blood disorders, vascular abnormalities, or trauma.
   a. pruritus
   b. purpura
   c. papule

2. The patient required incision and drainage, followed by antibiotics for his infected *abnormal pocket in the skin that contains hair and skin debris*.
   a. pressure injury
   b. pilonidal cyst
   c. pediculosis

3. A *technique of microscopically controlled serial excisions* was used to treat the patient's recurrent *malignant growth developing from scalelike epithelial tissue of the surface layer of the epidermis*.
   a. cryosurgery, STSG
   b. laser surgery, BCC
   c. Mohs surgery, SCC

4. The *localized collection of pus* was incised and drained.
   a. acne
   b. abscess
   c. cyst

5. A culture swab of the wound revealed *invasion of body tissue by methicillin-resistant Staphylococcus aureus*.
   a. MRSA infection
   b. herpes
   c. candidiasis

6. The patient newly diagnosed with a *chronic inflammatory disease involving the skin, joints, kidneys, and nervous system* experienced joint pain with swelling and stiffness, and a butterfly-shaped rash spread over her cheeks and the bridge of her nose.
   a. rosacea
   b. scleroderma
   c. systemic lupus erythematosus

7. *Abnormal condition of excessive hair growth*, also known as hirsutism, may occur in patients who have polycystic ovary syndrome.
   a. hypertrichosis
   b. alopecia
   c. furuncle

8. *Death of tissue caused by loss of blood supply followed by bacterial invasion* may be evidenced by foul-smelling discharge from the infection site.
   a. gangrene
   b. pressure injury
   c. lesion

9. The medical assisting student learned that the medical term for *blister* was:
   a. verruca
   b. keloid
   c. vesicle

10. *Abnormal hard spots or areas of skin* were evident in the patient diagnosed with the *disease characterized by chronic hardening of connective tissue of the skin and other organs*.
    a. lesion, psoriasis
    b. induration, scleroderma
    c. nodule, Kaposi sarcoma

11. *Condition of eating the nails, or nail biting*, can damage skin around the nails and increase chances for infection.
    a. onychophagia
    b. onychomalacia
    c. onychomycosis

12. An injection given *within the skin* is described as:
    a. subcut
    b. TD
    c. ID

13. As a result of the burn to her upper arm, the patient received *skin transplanted to replace a lost portion of the body skin surface*.
    a. laser surgery
    b. dermabrasion
    c. skin graft

14. The *transitory, itchy elevations of the skin with a white center and a red surrounding area* were distributed over the patient's entire body.
    a. nevi
    b. wheals
    c. verrucae

15. *Excessive sweating* without exertion may be a symptom of a serious condition.
    a. diaphoresis
    b. edema
    c. hidradenitis

16. The nursing assistant applied lotion to the patient exhibiting signs of *dry skin*.
    a. xanthoderma
    b. xeroderma
    c. pachyderma

17. *Surgical stitching* was performed to treat the *torn, ragged edged wound*.
    a. cryosurgery, verruca
    b. suturing, laceration
    c. dermabrasion, ulcer

18. Compression of the lateral femoral *pertaining to the skin* nerve results in sensations of aching, burning, stabbing, and/or numbness in the thigh area.
    a. epidermal
    b. cutaneous
    c. intradermal

19. *Superficial skin infection characterized by pustules and caused by either staphylococci or streptococci* is common in young children.
    a. impetigo
    b. measles
    c. herpes

20. Measles vaccine is administered via *subcut* injection, while influenza vaccine is administered via intramuscular or *ID* injection.
    a. subungual, intravasular
    b. subcutaenous, intradermal
    c. sublingual, incisional

Chapter 4 Integumentary System

CHAPTER AT A GLANCE — Word Parts New to this Chapter

COMBINING FORMS

crypt/o	onych/o	staphyl/o
cutane/o	pachy/o	strept/o
derm/o	phag/o	trich/o
dermat/o	rhytid/o	ungu/o
hidr/o	scler/o	xer/o
kerat/o	seb/o	
myc/o		

PREFIXES

epi-
intra-
para-
per-
sub-
trans-

SUFFIXES

-a	-itis
-coccus	-malacia
(*pl.* -cocci)	-plasty
-ectomy	-rrhea
-ia	

CHAPTER AT A GLANCE — Integumentary System Terms Built from Word Parts

DISEASE AND DISORDER

dermatitis
dermatofibroma
hidradenitis
keratosis
onychocryptosis
onychomalacia
onychomycosis
onychophagia
pachyderma
paronychia
scleroderma
seborrhea
xanthoma
xeroderma

SURGICAL

dermatoplasty
rhytidectomy

COMPLEMENTARY

cutaneous
dermatologist
dermatology (derm)
epidermal
erythroderma
hypertrichosis
hypodermic
intradermal (ID)
keratogenic
leukoderma
percutaneous
staphylococcus (*pl.* staphylococci) (staph)
streptococcus (*pl.* streptococci) (strep)
subcutaneous (subcut)
subungual
transdermal (TD)
ungual
xanthoderma
xerosis

CHAPTER AT A GLANCE — Integumentary System Terms NOT Built from Word Parts

DISEASE AND DISORDER

abrasion
abscess
acne
actinic keratosis
albinism
basal cell carcinoma (BCC)
candidiasis
carbuncle
cellulitis
contusion
eczema
fissure
furuncle
gangrene
herpes
impetigo
Kaposi sarcoma
keloid
laceration
measles
MRSA infection
pediculosis
pilonidal cyst
pressure injury
psoriasis
rosacea
scabies
squamous cell carcinoma (SCC)
systemic lupus erythematosus (SLE)
tinea
urticaria
vitiligo

SURGICAL

cauterization
cryosurgery
debridement
dermabrasion
excision
incision
incision and drainage (I&D)
laser surgery
Mohs surgery
skin graft
suturing

COMPLEMENTARY

alopecia
cyst
diaphoresis
ecchymosis (*pl.* ecchymoses)
edema
induration
jaundice
lesion
leukoplakia
macule
nevus (*pl.* nevi)
nodule
pallor
papule
petechiae (*s.* petechia)
pruritus
purpura
pustule
ulcer
verruca
vesicle
wheal

PART 2 BODY SYSTEMS

5 Respiratory System

Objectives

Upon completion of this chapter, you will be able to:

1. Pronounce organs and anatomic structures of the respiratory system.
2. Define and spell word parts related to the respiratory system.
3. Define, pronounce, and spell disease and disorder terms related to the respiratory system.
4. Define, pronounce, and spell surgical terms related to the respiratory system.
5. Define, pronounce, and spell diagnostic terms related to the respiratory system.
6. Define, pronounce, and spell complementary terms related to the respiratory system.
7. Interpret the meaning of abbreviations related to the respiratory system.
8. Apply medical language in clinical contexts.

TABLE 5.1 Endoscopy Suffixes, 162
TABLE 5.2 SOAP Note Format, 178
TABLE 5.3 Other Common Abbreviations Used in Respiratory Care, 180

Outline

ANATOMY, 135
Function, 135
Organs and Anatomic Structures of the Respiratory System, 135

WORD PARTS, 138
Respiratory System Combining Forms, 138
Combining Forms Used with Respiratory System Terms, 138
Prefixes, 138
Suffixes, 139

MEDICAL TERMS, 145
Disease and Disorder Terms, 145
   Built from Word Parts, 145
   NOT Built from Word Parts, 150
Surgical Terms, 156
   Built from Word Parts, 156
Endoscopy, 161
Diagnostic Terms, 161
   Built from Word Parts, 161
   NOT Built from Word Parts, 166
Complementary Terms, 170
   Built from Word Parts, 170
   NOT Built from Word Parts, 174
Medical Record Abbreviations, 178
Abbreviations, 178

PRACTICAL APPLICATION, 181
CASE STUDY Translate Between Everyday Language and Medical Language, 181
Interact with Medical Documents, 182
Use Medical Language in Online Electronic Health Records, 184
Use Medical Terms in Clinical Statements, 184
Pronounce Medical Terms in Use, 185

CHAPTER REVIEW, 185
Chapter Content Quiz, 185
Chapter at a Glance, 186

Answers to Chapter Exercises, Appendix A

Chapter 5   Respiratory System

ANATOMY

The respiratory system comprises the nose, pharynx, larynx, trachea, bronchi, and lungs. The upper respiratory tract includes the nose, pharynx, and larynx. The lower respiratory tract includes the trachea, bronchi, and lungs. (Fig. 5.1)

Function

The function of the respiratory system is the exchange of oxygen (O_2) and carbon dioxide (CO_2) between the atmosphere and body cells. This process is called **respiration** or **breathing**. During **external respiration**, air containing oxygen passes through the respiratory tract, beginning with the nose, pharynx, larynx, and trachea, then into the lungs via the bronchi, and finally into bronchioles (**inhalation** or **inspiration**). There, oxygen passes from the **alveoli**, sacs at the ends of the bronchioles, to the blood in tiny blood vessels called **capillaries**. At the same time, carbon dioxide passes back from the capillaries to the alveoli and is expelled through the respiratory tract (**exhalation** or **expiration**) (Fig. 5.2). During **internal respiration**, the body cells take on **oxygen** from the blood and simultaneously give back **carbon dioxide**, a waste produced when oxygen is used to extract energy from food. Carbon dioxide is transported by the blood back to the lungs for exhalation.

> **RESPIRATION** is also called **breathing** or **ventilation**.

Organs and Anatomic Structures of the Respiratory System

TERM	DEFINITION
nose (nōz)	filtering structure that moistens and warms air entering the respiratory system; internal passages are lined with mucous membranes and fine hairs
nasal septum (NĀS-el) (SEP-tum)	partition separating the right and left nasal cavities
paranasal sinuses (*par*-a-NĀ-sel) (SĪ-nus-es)	air cavities within the cranial bones that open into the nasal cavities
pharynx (FAYR-inks)	food and air passageway. Food enters the pharynx from the mouth and passes into the esophagus. Air enters the pharynx from the nasal cavities or mouth and passes into the larynx. (also called **throat**)
adenoids (AD-e-noids)	lymphoid tissue located on the posterior wall of the nasal cavity (also called **pharyngeal tonsils**)
tonsils (TON-sils)	lymphoid tissue located on the lateral wall at the junction of the oral cavity and oropharynx
larynx (LAYR-inks)	structure housing the vocal cords. Air enters from the pharynx. (also called **voice box**)

> **ADAM'S APPLE** is the largest ring of cartilage in the **larynx** and is also known as the thyroid cartilage. The name came from the belief that Adam, realizing he had sinned when he ate the forbidden fruit, was unable to swallow the apple lodged in his throat.

epiglottis (ep-i-GLOT-is)	flap of cartilage that automatically covers the opening of the larynx and keeps food from entering the larynx during swallowing
trachea (TRĀ-kē-a)	air passageway from the larynx to the bronchi (also called **windpipe**)
mucous membranes (MŪ-kus) (MEM-brānz)	lining of the cavities of the nose, mouth, pharynx, larynx, and trachea that secretes a thin, lubricating fluid (mucus); mucus prevents dehydration and provides protection from pathogens
lungs (lungs)	two spongelike organs in the thoracic cavity. The right lung consists of three lobes, and the left lung has two lobes.
bronchus (*pl.* **bronchi**) (BRONG-kus) (BRONG-ki)	one of two passageways branching from the trachea that conducts air into the lungs, where it divides and subdivides into smaller structures. The branchings resemble a tree; therefore, they are referred to as a **bronchial tree**.

Chapter 5 Respiratory System

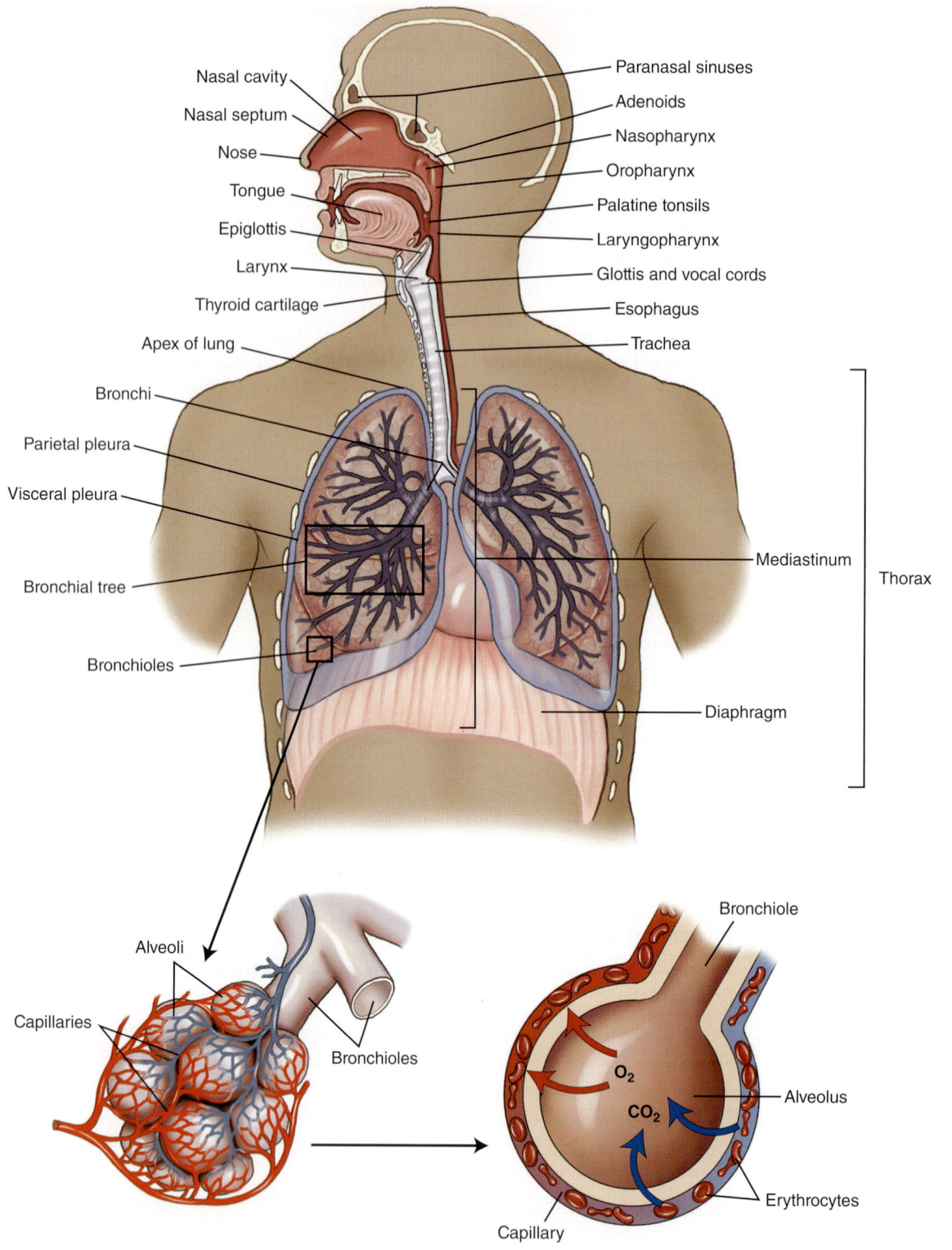

FIG. 5.1 Organs of the respiratory system.

Organs and Anatomic Structures of the Respiratory System—cont'd

TERM	DEFINITION
🏛 **BRONCHI** originated from the Greek **brecho**, meaning **to pour** or **wet**. An ancient belief was that the esophagus carried solid food to the stomach and the bronchi carried liquids.	
bronchioles (BRONG-kē-ōlz)	smallest subdivision of the bronchial tree
alveoli (s. alveolus) (al-VĒ-o-lī) (al-VĒ-o-lus)	air sacs at the end of the bronchioles. Oxygen and carbon dioxide are exchanged through the alveolar walls and the capillaries. (also a term for the sockets in the jaw bones into which the teeth fit)
thorax (THOR-aks)	chest, the part of the body between the neck and the diaphragm encased by the ribs. **Thoracic cavity** is the hollow space between the neck and diaphragm.
pleura (PLOOR-a)	double-folded, serous membrane lining the thoracic cavity (parietal pleura) and covering each lung (visceral pleura). The space between the parietal pleura and visceral pleura, called the pleural cavity, contains serous (watery) fluid.
mediastinum (mē-dē-a-STĪ-num)	space between the lungs. It contains the heart, esophagus, trachea, great blood vessels, and other structures.
🏛 **MEDIASTINUM** literally means **to stand in the middle** because it is derived from the Latin **medius**, meaning **middle**, and **stare**, meaning **to stand**.	
diaphragm (DĪ-a-fram)	muscular partition that separates the thoracic cavity from the abdominal cavity. It aids in the breathing process by contracting and pulling air in, then relaxing and pushing air out.

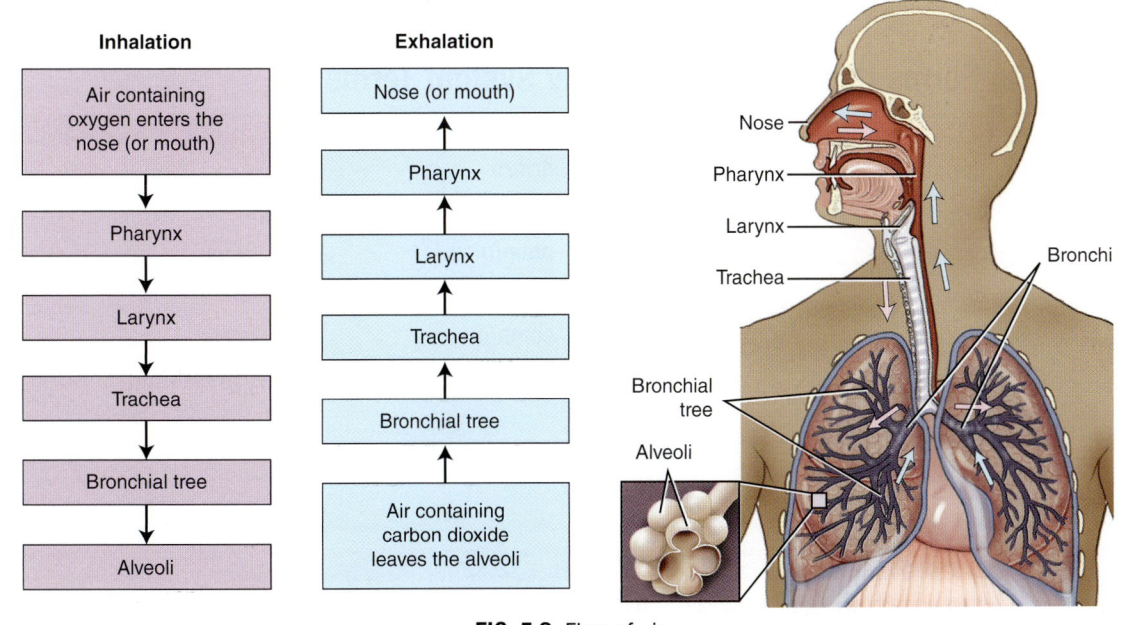

FIG. 5.2 Flow of air.

PRONOUNCE ANATOMIC STRUCTURES

Practice saying aloud each of the organs and specific structures on the previous pages.

To hear the terms, go to Evolve Resources at www.evolve.elsevier.com and select:
Student Resources > **Audio Glossary** > Chapter 5 > Anatomic Structures

❏ Check the box when complete.

Chapter 5 Respiratory System

WORD PARTS

Use paper flashcards or electronic flashcards on Evolve to memorize word parts used to analyze, define, and build medical terms in this chapter. To reinforce learning, study one section of the Word Parts Table at a time, then complete the corresponding exercises on the following pages.

1 ■ Respiratory System Combining Forms

COMBINING FORM	DEFINITION	COMBINING FORM	DEFINITION
adenoid/o	adenoids	pleur/o	pleura
alveol/o	alveolus (s.), alveoli (pl.)	pneum/o	lung, air
bronch/o	bronchus (s.), bronchi (pl.)	pneumon/o	lung, air
bronchi/o	bronchus (s.), bronchi (pl.)	pulmon/o	lung
diaphragmat/o	diaphragm	rhin/o	nose
epiglott/o	epiglottis	sept/o	septum
laryng/o	larynx		
lob/o	lobe(s)		

🏛 **SEPTUM** comes from the Latin word **saeptum,** meaning to **fence** or **wall off,** and refers to a structure dividing cavities or tissues. Sept/o can also describe septa in other areas of the body, including the heart and brain.

🏛 **LOBE** literally means **the part that hangs down**, although it comes from the Greek **lobos**, meaning **capsule** or **pod**. Lob/o can also describe lobes in other areas of the body, including the ear, liver, and brain.

COMBINING FORM	DEFINITION	COMBINING FORM	DEFINITION
		sinus/o	sinus(es)
mediastin/o	mediastinum	thorac/o	thorax, chest, chest cavity
nas/o	nose	tonsill/o	tonsil(s) (Note: tonsil has one l, and the combining form has two ls.)
pharyng/o	pharynx	trache/o	trachea

2 ■ Combining Forms Used with Respiratory System Terms

COMBINING FORM	DEFINITION	COMBINING FORM	DEFINITION
atel/o	imperfect, incomplete	orth/o	straight
capn/o	carbon dioxide	ox/i	oxygen
carcin/o	cancer	phon/o	sound, voice
coni/o	dust	py/o	pus
hem/o	blood	somn/o	sleep
muc/o	mucus	spir/o	breathe, breathing
myc/o	fungus		

3 ■ Prefixes

PREFIX	DEFINITION	PREFIX	DEFINITION
a-, an-	absence of, without (Note: an- is used when the word root begins with a vowel.)	hypo-	below, incomplete, deficient, under
		intra-	within
dys-	painful, abnormal, difficult, labored	neo-	new
endo-	within	poly-	many, much
eu-	normal, good	tachy-	fast, rapid
hyper-	above, excessive		

4 ■ Suffixes

SUFFIX	DEFINITION
-al	pertaining to
-ar, -ary	pertaining to
-cele	hernia, protrusion

HERNIA is protrusion of an organ or tissue through a membrane or cavity wall.

SUFFIX	DEFINITION
-centesis	surgical puncture to aspirate fluid (with a sterile needle)
-desis	surgical fixation, fusion
-eal	pertaining to
-ectasis	stretching out, dilation, expansion
-ectomy	excision, surgical removal
-emia	in the blood
-genic	producing, originating, causing
-ia	diseased state, condition of
-ic	pertaining to
-itis	inflammation
-logist	one who studies and treats (specialist, physician)
-logy	study of
-meter	instrument used to measure
-metry	measurement

SUFFIX	DEFINITION
-oid	resembling
-oma	tumor, swelling
-osis	abnormal condition
-ous	pertaining to
-plasm	growth, substance, formation
-plasty	surgical repair
-pnea	breathing
-ptysis	spitting, coughing
-rrhagia	excessive bleeding

The suffixes **-RRHAGIA** and **-RRHAGE** refer to excessive bleeding and come from the Greek word **rhegynai**, meaning **to burst forth**.

SUFFIX	DEFINITION
-rrhea	flow, discharge
-scope	instrument used for visual examination
-scopic	pertaining to visual examination
-scopy	visual examination
-spasm	sudden, involuntary muscle contraction (spasmodic contraction)
-stenosis	constriction or narrowing
-stomy	creation of an artificial opening
-thorax	chest, chest cavity
-tomy	cut into, incision

EXERCISE 1 ■ Respiratory System Combining Forms

Refer to the first section of the word parts table.

A Define and Match

Step 1: Write the definitions after the following combining forms.
Step 2: Match the descriptions on the right with the combining forms and definitions. Answers may be used more than once.

_____ 1. adenoid/o, _____
_____ 2. diaphragmat/o, _____
_____ 3. epiglott/o, _____
_____ 4. lob/o, _____
_____ 5. nas/o, _____
_____ 6. pharyng/o, _____
_____ 7. pneumon/o, _____
_____ 8. pneum/o, _____
_____ 9. rhin/o, _____
_____ 10. sept/o, _____

a. filtering structure that moistens and warms air entering the respiratory system
b. sections of a lung
c. spongelike organs located in the thoracic cavity
d. lymphoid tissue located on the posterior wall of the nasal cavity
e. flap of cartilage that keeps food out of the larynx
f. partition separating the right and left nasal cavities
g. food and air passageway
h. separates the thoracic cavity from the abdominal cavity

Chapter 5 Respiratory System

B Label

Fill in the blanks with combining forms to label this diagram of the respiratory system.
To check your answers, go to Appendix A at the back of the textbook.

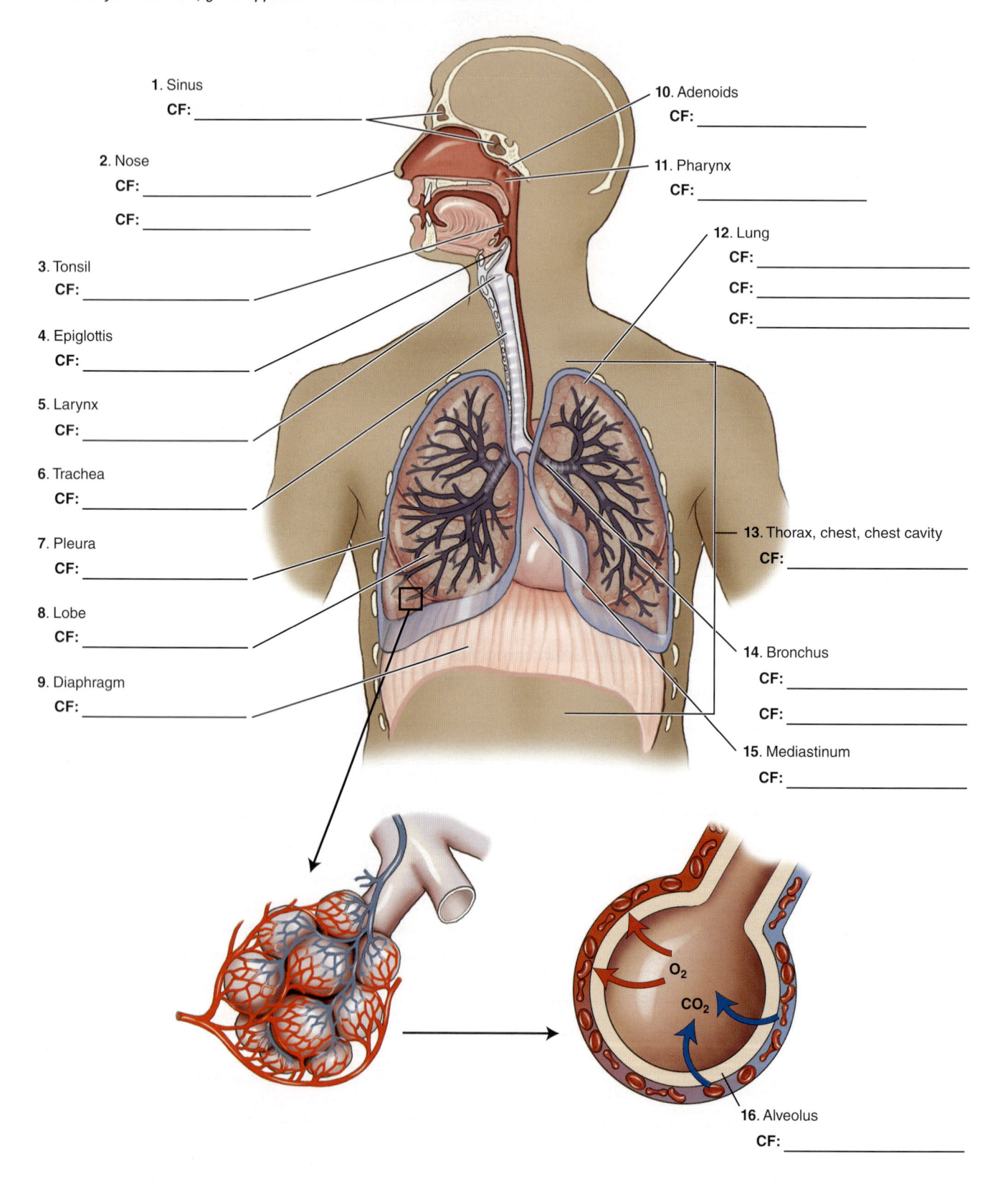

1. Sinus
   CF: _____

2. Nose
   CF: _____
   CF: _____

3. Tonsil
   CF: _____

4. Epiglottis
   CF: _____

5. Larynx
   CF: _____

6. Trachea
   CF: _____

7. Pleura
   CF: _____

8. Lobe
   CF: _____

9. Diaphragm
   CF: _____

10. Adenoids
    CF: _____

11. Pharynx
    CF: _____

12. Lung
    CF: _____
    CF: _____
    CF: _____

13. Thorax, chest, chest cavity
    CF: _____

14. Bronchus
    CF: _____
    CF: _____

15. Mediastinum
    CF: _____

16. Alveolus
    CF: _____

C Define and Match

Step 1: Write the definitions after the following combining forms.
Step 2: Match the descriptions on the right with the combining forms and definitions.

_____ 1. alveol/o, _____
_____ 2. bronch/o, bronchi/o, _____
_____ 3. pulmon/o, _____
_____ 4. laryng/o, _____
_____ 5. pleur/o, _____
_____ 6. thorac/o, _____
_____ 7. trache/o, _____
_____ 8. tonsill/o, _____
_____ 9. sinus/o, _____
_____ 10. mediastin/o, _____

a. space between the lungs containing heart, esophagus, trachea, and other structures
b. air passageway from the larynx to the bronchi
c. spongelike organs located in the thoracic cavity
d. membrane lining the thoracic cavity and covering each lung
e. lymphoid tissue located on the lateral wall at the junction of the oral cavity and oropharynx
f. air cavities within the cranial bones that open into the nasal cavities
g. structure housing the vocal cords
h. air sacs at the end of the bronchioles
i. the part of the body between the neck and diaphragm
j. air passageway from the trachea to the lungs, which divides and subdivides into smaller structures

EXERCISE 2 ■ Combining Forms Used with Respiratory System Terms

Refer to the second section of the word parts table.

A Define

Write the definition of the following combining forms.

1. ox/i _____
2. spir/o _____
3. muc/o _____
4. atel/o _____
5. orth/o _____
6. py/o _____
7. hem/o _____
8. somn/o _____
9. capn/o _____
10. phon/o _____
11. carcin/o _____
12. myc/o _____
13. coni/o _____

B Identify

Write the combining form for each of the following.

1. breathe, breathing _____
2. oxygen _____
3. imperfect, incomplete _____
4. straight _____
5. pus _____
6. mucus _____
7. blood _____
8. sleep _____
9. sound, voice _____
10. carbon dioxide _____
11. dust _____
12. cancer _____
13. fungus _____

🏛 **OXYGEN** was discovered in 1774 by Joseph Priestley. In 1775 Antoine-Laurent Lavoisier, a French chemist, noted that all the acids he knew contained oxygen. Because he thought it was an acid producer, he named it using the Greek **oxys**, meaning **sour**, and the suffix **gen**, meaning **to produce**.

EXERCISE 3 ■ Prefixes

Refer to the third section of the word parts table.

A Define

Write the definitions of the following prefixes.

1. endo- _____
2. a-, an- _____
3. eu- _____
4. poly- _____
5. tachy- _____
6. dys- _____
7. hypo- _____
8. intra- _____
9. hyper- _____
10. neo- _____

B Identify

Write the prefix for each of the following.

1. within   a. _____
             b. _____
2. normal, good _____
3. absence of, without   a. _____
                          b. _____
4. many, much _____
5. fast, rapid _____
6. new _____
7. above, excessive _____
8. below, incomplete, deficient, under _____
9. painful, abnormal, difficult, labored _____

EXERCISE 4 ■ Suffixes

Refer to the fourth section of the word parts table.

A Match

Match the suffixes in the first column with their correct definitions in the second column.

_____ 1. -genic
_____ 2. -ar, -ary, -eal
_____ 3. -cele
_____ 4. -desis
_____ 5. -ectasis
_____ 6. -ia
_____ 7. -thorax
_____ 8. -stenosis
_____ 9. -spasm
_____ 10. -scopic
_____ 11. -centesis
_____ 12. -itis
_____ 13. -pnea

a. stretching out, dilation, expansion
b. pertaining to visual examination
c. pertaining to
d. hernia, protrusion
e. surgical fixation, fusion
f. diseased state, condition of
g. producing, originating, causing
h. surgical puncture to aspirate fluid
i. chest, chest cavity
j. breathing
k. constriction or narrowing
l. sudden, involuntary muscle contraction
m. inflammation

Chapter 5   Respiratory System

B Label

Write the suffixes pictured and defined.

1. _____
   instrument used for visual examination

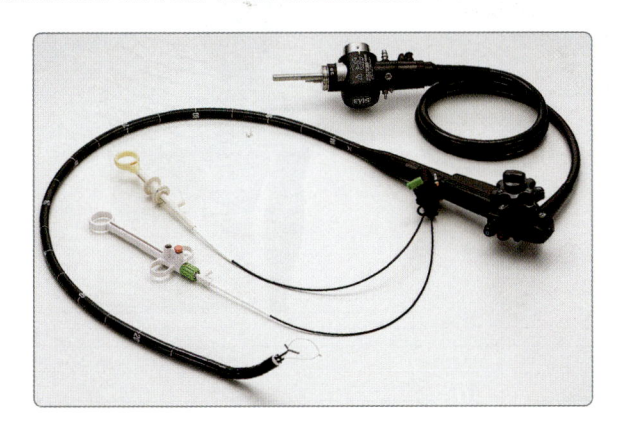

2. _____
   visual examination

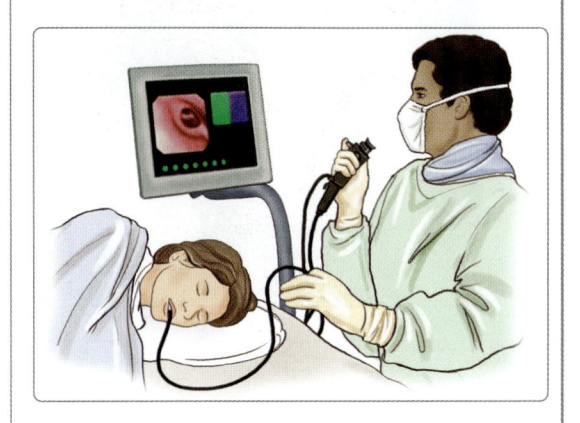

3. _____
   cut into, incision

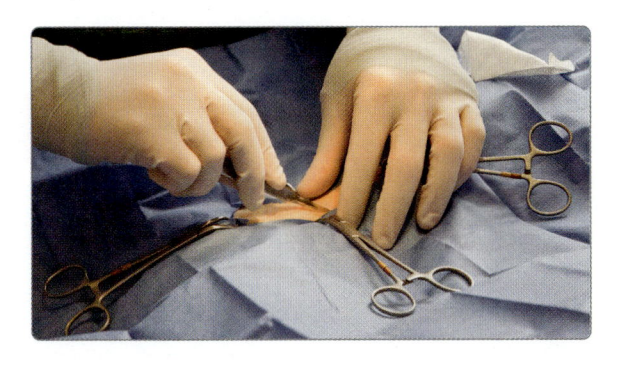

4. _____
   creation of an artificial opening

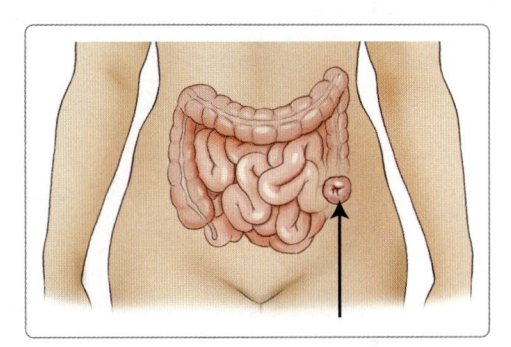

5. _____
   instrument used to measure

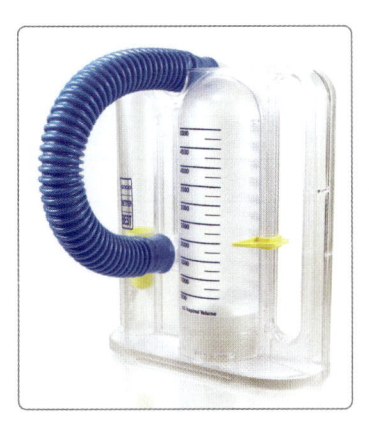

6. _____
   measurement (use of the instrument)

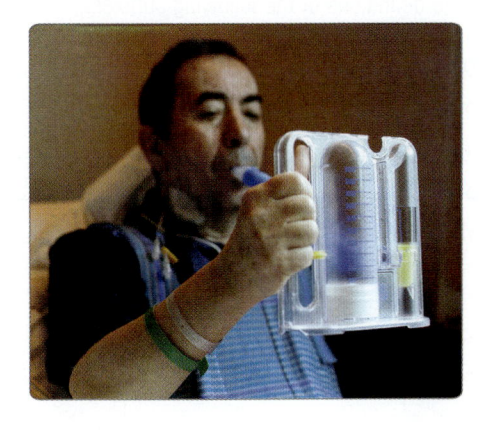

144　Chapter 5　Respiratory System

7. _____
excessive bleeding

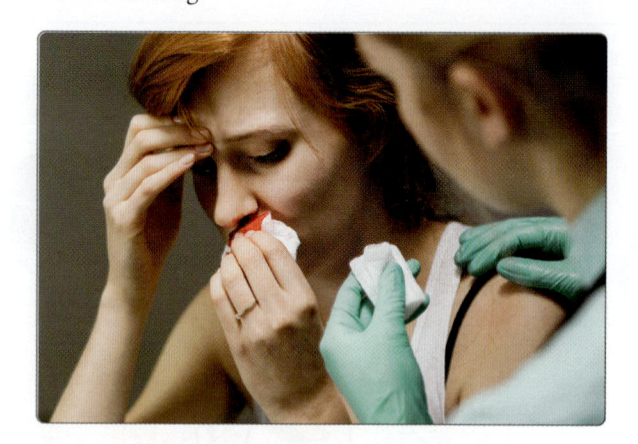

8. _____
spitting, coughing

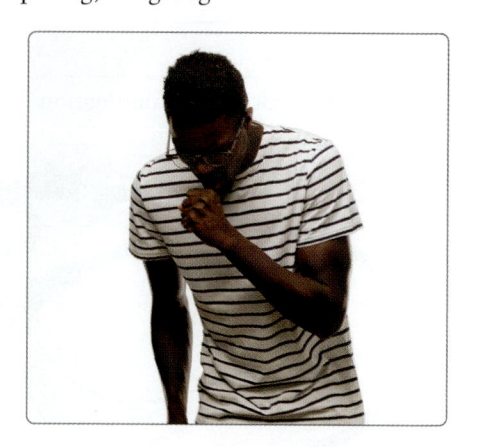

9. _____
excision, surgical removal

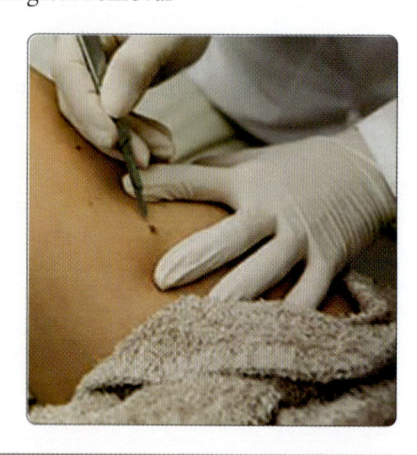

10. _____
in the blood

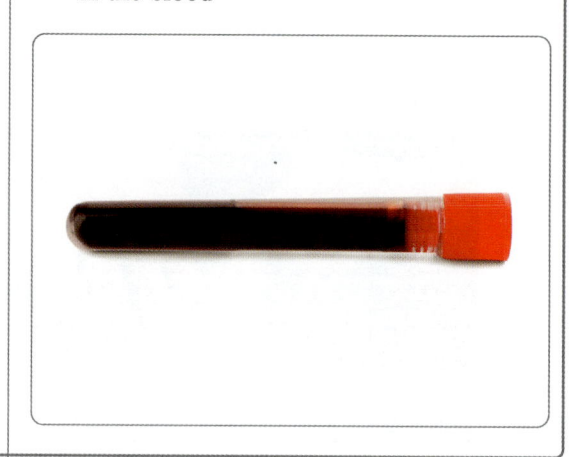

C　Define

Write the definitions of the following suffixes.

1. -rrhea _____
2. -oid _____
3. -logist _____
4. -plasm _____
5. -al, -ic, -ous _____
6. -oma _____
7. -logy _____
8. -plasty _____
9. -osis _____

Chapter 5 Respiratory System

MEDICAL TERMS

Medical terms relevant to this chapter have been grouped by topics, such as Disease and Disorder, and are listed in tables designated as Built from Word Parts or *NOT* Built from Word Parts. The exercises following each table assist with learning term definitions, pronunciations, and spellings.

Disease and Disorder Terms
BUILT FROM WORD PARTS

The following terms can be translated using definitions of word parts. Further explanation is provided within parentheses as needed.

TERM	DEFINITION	TERM	DEFINITION
1. **adenoiditis** (*ad*-e-noyd-Ī-tis)	inflammation of the adenoids	13. **laryngospasm** (la-RING-gō-*spaz*-m)	involuntary muscle contraction of the larynx
2. **alveolitis** (*al*-vē-o-LĪ-tis)	inflammation of the alveoli (pulmonary or dental)	14. **laryngotracheobronchitis (LTB)** (la-*ring*-gō-*trā*-kē-ō-bron-KĪ-tis)	inflammation of the larynx, trachea, and bronchi (the acute form is called **croup**)
3. **atelectasis** (*at*-e-LEK-ta-sis)	incomplete expansion (of the lung or portion of the lung) (Fig. 5.3)	15. **lobar pneumonia** (LŌ-bar) (nū-MŌ-nē-a)	pertaining to the lobe(s); diseased state of the lung (infection of one or more lobes of the lung)
🏛 **ATELECTASIS** is derived from the Greek **ateles**, meaning **not perfect**, and **ektasis**, meaning **expansion**. It denotes an incomplete expansion of the lungs.			
4. **bronchiectasis** (*bron*-kē-EK-ta-sis)	dilation of the bronchi	16. **nasopharyngitis** (*nā*-zō-*far*-in-JĪ-tis)	inflammation of the nose and pharynx
5. **bronchitis** (bron-KĪ-tis)	inflammation of the bronchi (see Fig. 5.5)	17. **pharyngitis** (*far*-in-JĪ-tis)	inflammation of the pharynx
6. **bronchogenic carcinoma** (bron-kō-JEN-ik) (*kar*-si-NŌ-ma)	cancerous tumor originating in a bronchus (also referred to as **lung cancer**) (Fig. 5.4)	18. **pleuritis** (plū-RĪ-tis)	inflammation of the pleura (also called **pleurisy**)
7. **bronchopneumonia** (*bron*-kō-nū-MŌ-nē-a)	diseased state of the bronchi and lungs (an inflammation of the lungs that begins in the terminal bronchioles)	19. **pneumoconiosis** (*nū*-mō-*kō*-nē-Ō-sis)	abnormal condition of dust in the lungs
		PNEUMOCONIOSIS is the general name given for chronic inflammatory disease of the lung caused by excessive inhalation of mineral dust. When the disease is caused by a specific dust, it is named for the dust. For example, the disease caused by silica dust is called **silicosis**.	
8. **bronchospasm** (BRON-kō-*spaz*-m)	involuntary muscle contraction of the bronchi	20. **pneumonia** (nū-MŌ-nē-a)	diseased state of the lung (the infection and inflammation are caused by bacteria such as *Pneumococcus*, *Staphylococcus*, *Streptococcus*, and *Haemophilus*; viruses; and fungi)
9. **diaphragmatocele** (*dī*-a-frag-MAT-ō-sēl)	hernia of the diaphragm (also called **diaphragmatic hernia**)		
10. **epiglottitis** (*ep*-i-glo-TĪ-tis)	inflammation of the epiglottis		
11. **hemothorax** (*hē*-mō-THOR-aks)	blood in the chest cavity (pleural cavity)	21. **pneumonitis** (*nū*-mō-NĪ-tis)	inflammation of the lung
12. **laryngitis** (*lar*-in-JĪ-tis)	inflammation of the larynx		

146 Chapter 5 Respiratory System

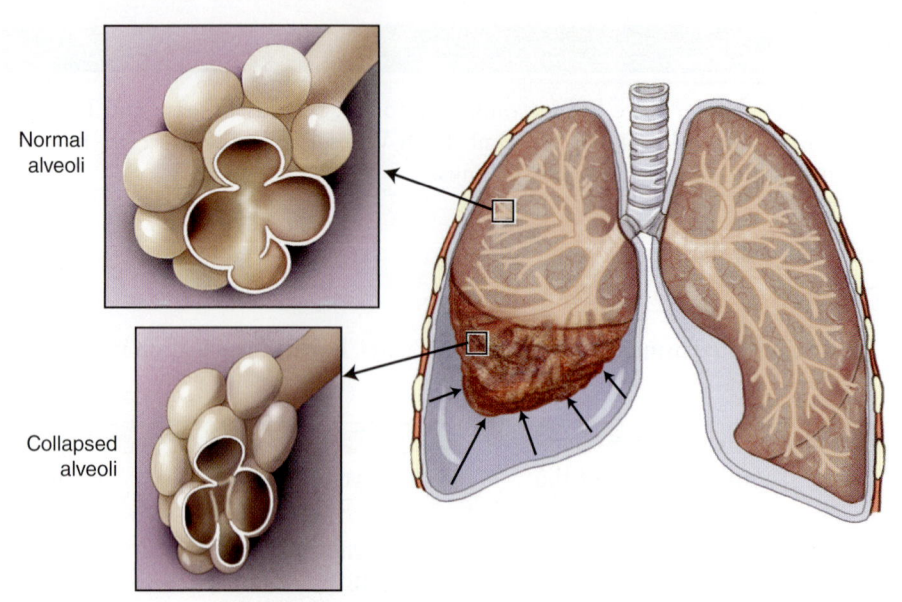

FIG. 5.3 Atelectasis showing the collapsed alveoli.

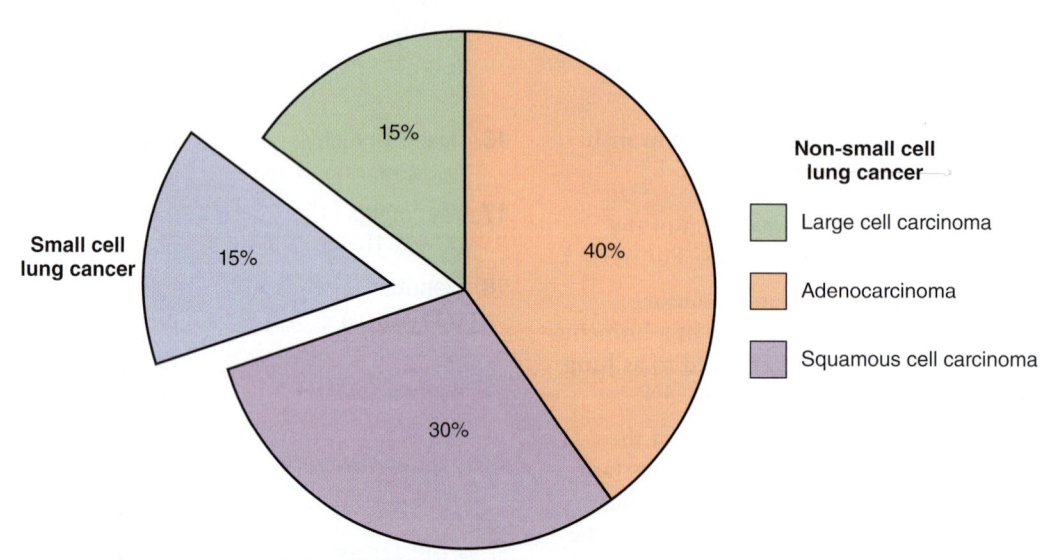

FIG. 5.4 Types of lung cancers. Lung cancer is classified as either small cell or non-small cell. The latter is by far the most common and includes **large cell carcinoma, adenocarcinoma,** and **squamous cell carcinoma**. Lung cancer is one of the most common cancers in the world. It is the deadliest cancer for both men and women. Smoking is the most important risk factor for the development of lung cancer. Symptoms include cough, hemoptysis, chest pain, dyspnea, fatigue, and weight loss. **Thoracentesis, bronchoscopy, chest radiograph, computed tomography (CT),** and **positron emission tomography (PET)** scanning are used for diagnosis. Treatment includes **surgery, chemotherapy,** and **radiation**.

Disease and Disorder Terms—cont'd
BUILT FROM WORD PARTS

TERM	DEFINITION	TERM	DEFINITION
22. **pneumothorax** (nū-mō-THOR-aks)	air in the chest cavity (specifically, the pleural cavity, which causes collapse of the lung and is often a result of an open chest wound)	26. **rhinomycosis** (rī-nō-mī-KŌ-sis)	abnormal condition of fungus in the nose
		27. **rhinorrhagia** (rī-nō-RĀ-ja)	excessive bleeding from the nose (also called **epistaxis**)
23. **pulmonary neoplasm** (PUL-mō-nar-ē) (NĒ-ō-plaz-em)	pertaining to (in) the lung, new growth (tumor)	28. **sinusitis** (sī-nū-SĪ-tis)	inflammation of the sinuses
		29. **tonsillitis** (ton-sil-Ī-tis)	inflammation of the tonsils
24. **pyothorax** (pī-ō-THOR-aks)	pus in the chest cavity (pleural cavity) (also called **empyema**)	30. **tracheitis** (trā-kē-Ī-tis)	inflammation of the trachea
25. **rhinitis** (rī-NĪ-tis)	inflammation of the nose (mucous membranes)	31. **tracheostenosis** (trā-kē-ō-sten-Ō-sis)	narrowing of the trachea

EXERCISE 5 ■ Pronounce and Spell

Practice pronunciation and spelling on paper and online.

1. **Practice on Paper**
   a. **Pronounce:** Read the phonetic spelling and say aloud the terms listed in the previous table. Refer to Table 2.2 Pronunciation Key as needed.
   b. **Spell:** Have a study partner read the terms aloud. Write the spelling of the terms on a separate sheet of paper.

2. **Practice Online**
   a. **Access** online learning resources. Go to evolve.elsevier.com > Evolve Resources > Student Resources.
   b. **Pronounce:** Select Audio Glossary > Chapter 5 > Exercise 5. Select a term to hear its pronunciation and repeat aloud.
   c. **Spell:** Select Activities > Chapter 5 > Spell Terms > Exercise 5. Select the audio icon and type the correct spelling of the term.

❏ Check the box when complete.

EXERCISE 6 ■ Analyze and Define

Analyze and define the following terms by drawing slashes between word parts, writing word part abbreviations above the term, underlining combining forms, and writing combining form abbreviations below the term.

EXAMPLE:
```
          WR       CV  S
     diaphragmat / o / cele
          CF
     hernia of the diaphragm
```

1. tracheitis

_____

_____

2. nasopharyngitis

_____

_____

3. alveolitis

_____

_____

4. pyothorax

_____

_____

5. atelectasis

6. rhinomycosis

7. tracheostenosis

8. epiglottitis

9. laryngitis

10. pulmonary neoplasm

11. pneumonia

12. rhinitis

13. pneumoconiosis

14. bronchopneumonia

15. laryngotracheobronchitis

16. bronchospasm

EXERCISE 7 ■ Build

A Label

Build terms pictured by writing word parts above definitions.

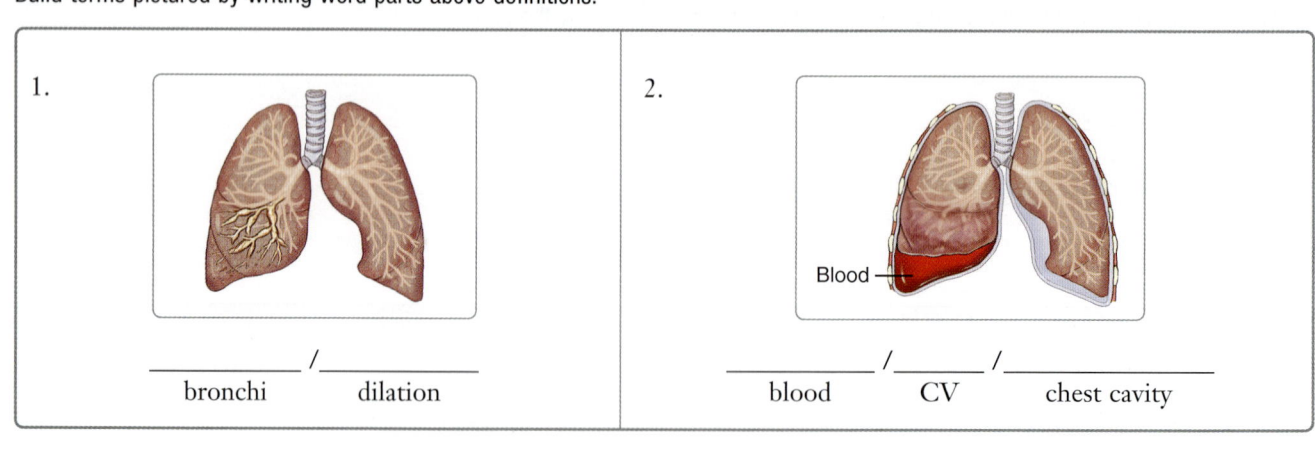

1. _____ / _____
   bronchi   dilation

2. _____ / _____ / _____
   blood   CV   chest cavity

Chapter 5   Respiratory System   149

3.

___ / ___ / ___
air / CV / chest cavity

4.

A. Normal sinuses   B. ___ / ___
                         sinuses inflammation

5.

___ / ___
pleura / inflammation

6.

___ / ___
tonsil / inflammation

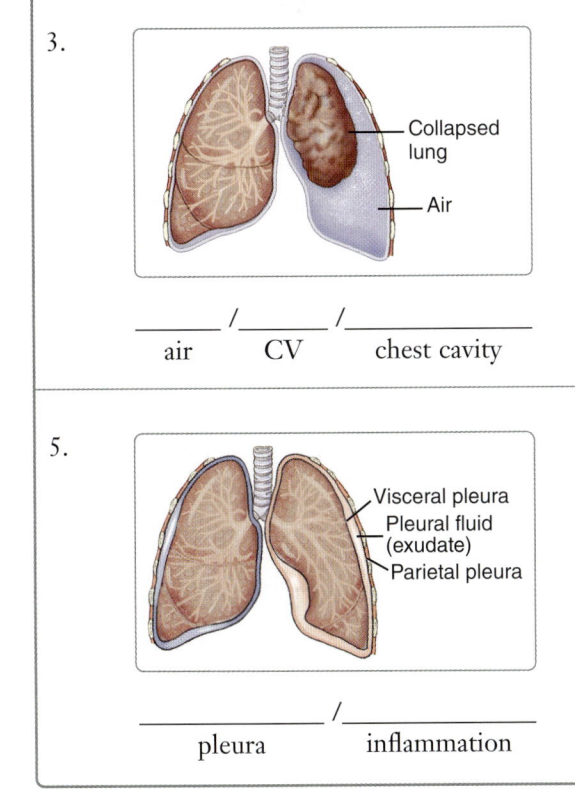

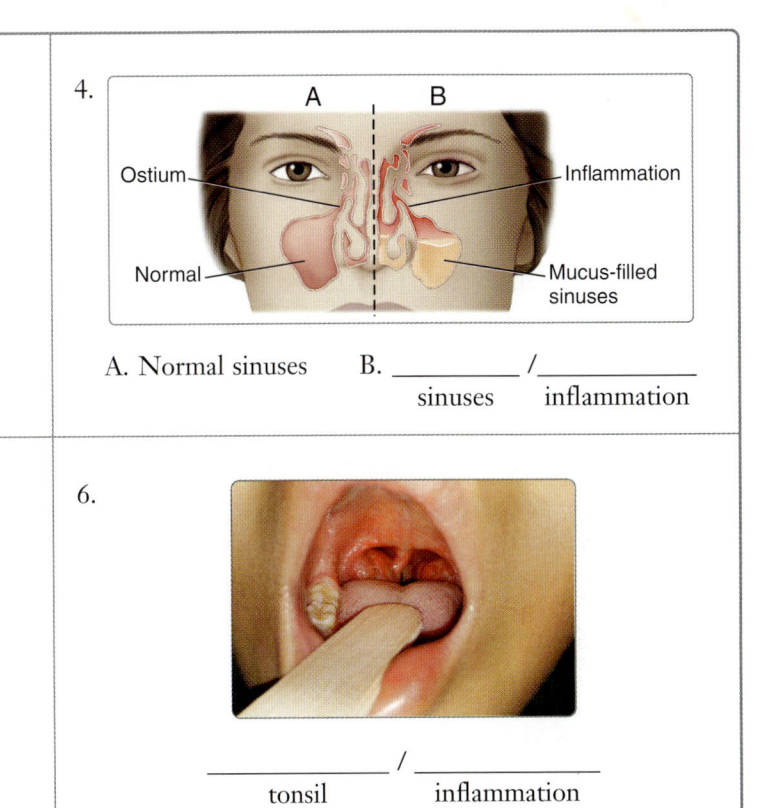

B Fill In

Build disease and disorder terms for the following definitions with the word parts you have learned.

EXAMPLE: inflammation of the tonsils   tonsill / itis
                                              WR / S

1. inflammation of the pharynx   ___ / ___
                                   WR   S

2. cancerous tumor originating in a bronchus   ___ / ___ / ___   ___ / ___
                                                WR / CV / S   WR   S

3. pertaining to the lobe(s); diseased state of the lung   ___ / ___   ___ / ___
                                                            WR   S   WR   S

4. involuntary muscle contraction of the larynx   ___ / ___ / ___
                                                    WR / CV / S

5. hernia of the diaphragm   ___ / ___ / ___
                               WR / CV / S

6. inflammation of the adenoids   ___ / ___
                                    WR   S

7. inflammation of the bronchi   ___ / ___
                                   WR   S

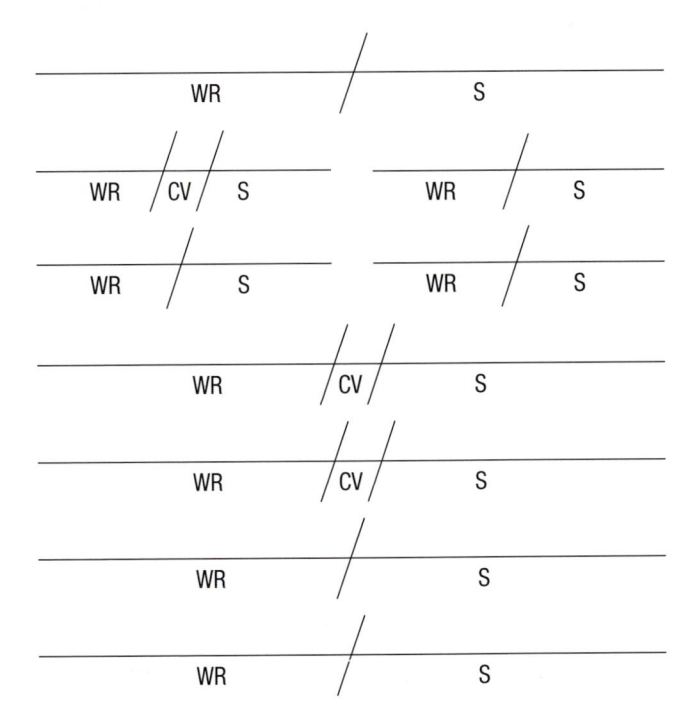

Chapter 5   Respiratory System

8. excessive bleeding from the nose   _____ / _____ / _____
                                                                                                                   WR   CV   S

9. inflammation of the lung   _____ / _____
                                                                                                                          WR   S

Disease and Disorder Terms
NOT BUILT FROM WORD PARTS

Word parts may be present in the following terms; however, their full meanings cannot be translated using definitions of word parts alone.

TERM	DEFINITION
1. **acute respiratory distress syndrome (ARDS)** (a-KŪT) (RES-pi-ra-*tor*-ē) (di-STRES) (SIN-drōm)	life-threatening lung condition caused by disease or injury. Fluid accumulates in the alveoli, resulting in hypoxemia. Symptoms include dyspnea, tachypnea, and cyanosis.
INSIDIOUS/ACUTE/SUBACUTE/CHRONIC are adjectives describing the onset and potential progression of a disease, condition, or syndrome. **Insidious:** gradual and subtle onset of disease **Subacute:** between acute and chronic **Acute:** sharp, sudden, short, or severe type of disease **Chronic:** disease that continues for a long time	
2. **asphyxia** (as-FIK-sē-a)	deprivation of oxygen for tissue use; suffocation
3. **asthma** (AZ-ma)	respiratory disease characterized by coughing, wheezing, and shortness of breath, caused by constriction and inflammation of airways that is reversible between attacks
REACTIVE AIRWAY DISEASE (RAD) is a general term and not a specific diagnosis. It is used to describe a history of wheezing, coughing, and shortness of breath. In some people RAD may lead to **asthma**.	
4. **chronic obstructive pulmonary disease (COPD)** (KRON-ik) (ob-STRUK-tiv) (PUL-mō-*nar*-ē) (di-ZĒZ)	progressive lung disease obstructing air flow, which makes breathing difficult. Chronic bronchitis and pulmonary emphysema are the two main components of COPD. Most COPD is a result of cigarette smoking. (Fig. 5.5)
5. **coccidioidomycosis (cocci)** (kok-*sid*-ē-*oy*-dō-mī-KŌ-sis)	fungal disease affecting the lungs and sometimes other organs of the body (also called **valley fever**)

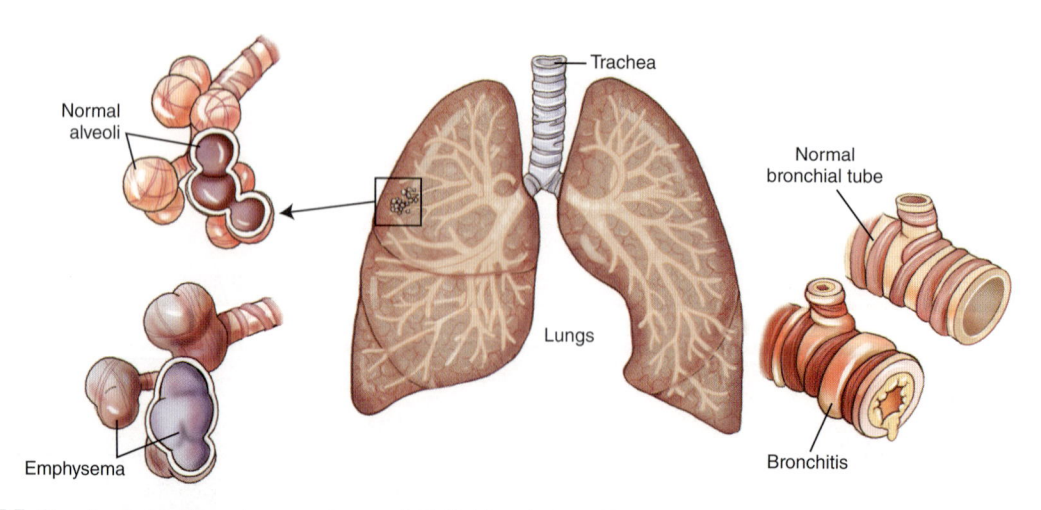

FIG. 5.5 Chronic obstructive pulmonary disease (COPD). Chronic bronchitis and emphysema are both components of COPD.

Chapter 5 Respiratory System 151

TERM	DEFINITION
COCCIDIOIDOMYCOSIS, which occurs in the southwestern portion of the US, is one of several diseases caused by fungal spores found in the soil of specific geographic regions. Other examples include **histoplasmosis**, which occurs in central and eastern states, and **blastomycosis**, which occurs in upper midwestern states. With climate change, fungal diseases such as these are occurring with increasing frequency.	
6. coronavirus disease (COVID-19) (kō-RŌ-na-vī-rus) (di-ZĒZ)	highly contagious respiratory infection caused by the SARS-CoV-2 virus, a strain of the coronavirus; symptoms range from none to severe. Mild symptoms include cough, headache, and muscle aches, while severe symptoms include pneumonia, ARDS, blood clots, and brain disease. Severe illness resulting in hospitalization and death can occur even in healthy people. Post-COVID condition (PCC), frequently called long COVID, will develop in some, including those who experienced a mild disease course.
Several strains of **CORONAVIRUS** exist, including those that cause severe acute respiratory syndrome (SARS), Middle East respiratory syndrome (MERS), and coronavirus disease (COVID-19).	
7. croup (kroop)	condition resulting from acute obstruction of the larynx, characterized by a barking cough, hoarseness, and stridor. It may be caused by viral or bacterial infection, allergy, or foreign body. Occurs mainly in children. (also called **laryngotracheobronchitis**)
8. cystic fibrosis (CF) (SIS-tik) (fī-BRŌ-sis)	hereditary disorder of the exocrine glands characterized by excess mucus production in the respiratory tract, pancreatic deficiency, and other symptoms
9. deviated septum (DĒ-vē-āt-ed) (SEP-tum)	one part of the nasal cavity is smaller because of malformation or injury of the nasal septum
10. diphtheria (dif-THĒR-ē-a)	serious bacterial infection affecting the mucous membranes of the nose and throat. It creates a thick, gray sheet covering the pharynx, which can lead to difficulty breathing, heart failure, paralysis, and even death. It is rare in developed countries due to widespread vaccination against the disease.
11. emphysema (*em*-fi-SĒ-ma)	loss of elasticity of the alveoli resulting in distention causing stretching of the lung. As a result, the body does not receive enough oxygen. (component of COPD) (Fig. 5.5)
12. epistaxis (*ep*-i-STAK-sis)	nosebleed (also called **rhinorrhagia**)
13. idiopathic pulmonary fibrosis (IPF) (id-ē-ō-PATH-ik) (PUL-mō-*nar*-ē) (fī-BRŌ-sis)	chronic progressive lung disorder characterized by increasing scarring, which ultimately reduces the capacity of the lungs; etiology unknown. IPF most often affects adults over the age of 50. Smoking, pollutants, and heredity may play a role in its development. Symptoms include exertional dyspnea and a dry cough. Lung transplant may be indicated in severe cases; there is no cure.
14. influenza (flu) (*in*-flū-EN-za)	contagious respiratory infection caused by an influenza virus; most illness observed in flu season is caused by influenza virus types A and B. Symptoms include fever, runny or stuffy nose, cough, headache, and muscle aches. Severe illness leading to pneumonia and ARDS can occur in older adults, people who are pregnant, infants and young children, and those with underlying medical conditions.
INFLUENZA PANDEMIC is the sudden outbreak of a flu that becomes widespread, affecting a region, a continent, or the world. Examples are H1N1 swine flu and H5N1 avian flu.	
15. obstructive sleep apnea (OSA) (ob-STRUK-tiv) (slēp) (AP-nē-a)	repetitive pharyngeal collapse during sleep, which leads to transient periods of apnea (absence of breathing); can produce daytime drowsiness and elevated blood pressure (Fig. 5.6)
16. pertussis (per-TUS-sis)	highly contagious bacterial infection of the respiratory tract characterized by a severe hacking cough, followed by an acute crowing inspiration, or whoop. It mainly affects infants too young to be vaccinated and adults whose immunity to the vaccine has faded. (also called **whooping cough**)
17. pleural effusion (PLŪ-ral) (e-FŪ-zhun)	fluid in the pleural cavity caused by a disease process or trauma

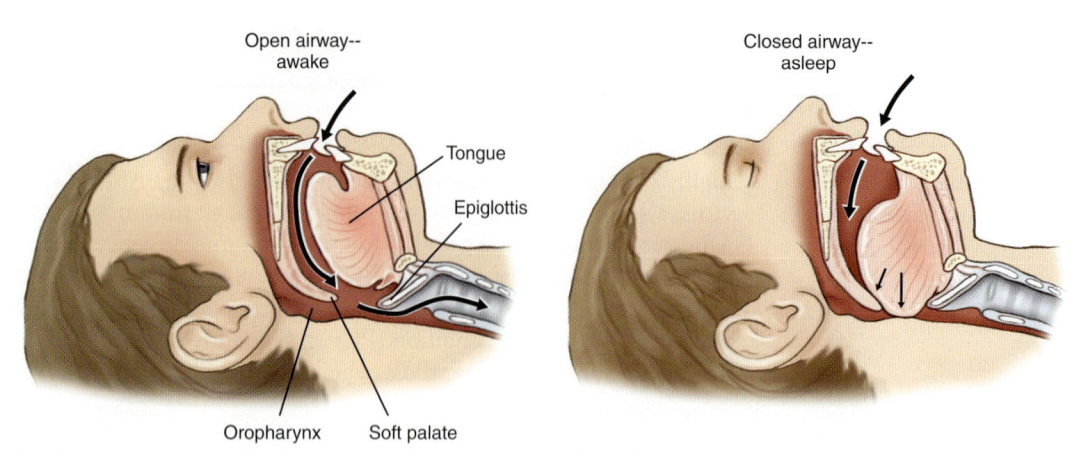

FIG. 5.6 Obstructive sleep apnea (OSA). During sleep, the absence of activity of the pharyngeal muscle structure allows the airway to close. OSA is associated with increased risk for elevated blood pressure, cardiovascular disease, diabetes, and stroke. Obesity is a major risk factor, and weight loss can be an effective treatment. **Polysomnography** is used to diagnose OSA. Treatment includes the use of **CPAP (continuous positive airway pressure)** during sleep and **uvulopalatopharyngoplasty (UPPP)**, a surgical procedure.

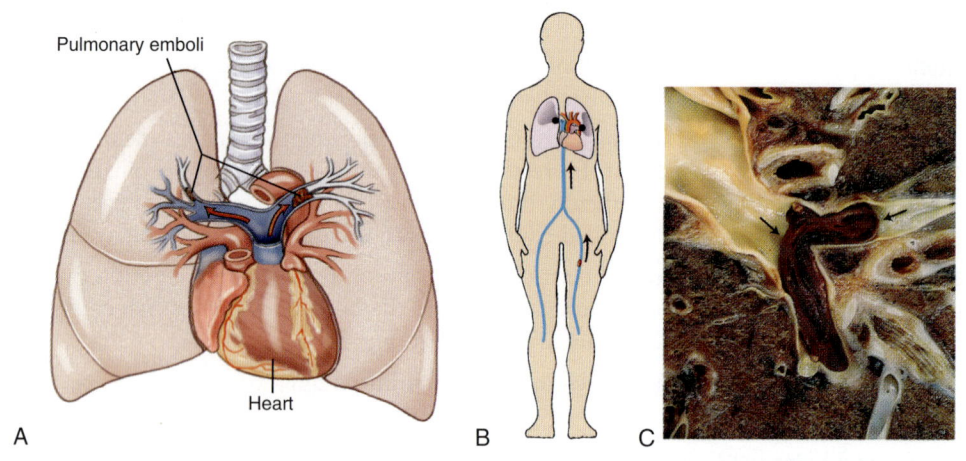

FIG. 5.7 A, Bilateral pulmonary emboli. **B,** Pulmonary emboli usually originate in the deep veins of the lower extremities. **C,** Autopsy specimen of the lung showing a large embolus.

Disease and Disorder Terms—cont'd
NOT BUILT FROM WORD PARTS

TERM	DEFINITION
18. pulmonary edema (PUL-mō-*nar*-ē) (e-DĒ-ma)	fluid accumulation in the alveoli and bronchioles; may be a manifestation of heart failure
19. pulmonary embolism (PE) (PUL-mō-*nar*-ē) (EM-bo-liz-em)	matter foreign to the circulation, carried to the pulmonary artery and its branches, where it blocks circulation to the lungs and can be fatal if of sufficient size or number. Blood clots broken loose from the deep veins of the lower extremities are the most common cause of pulmonary embolism. (Fig. 5.7)
20. tuberculosis (TB) (tū-*ber*-kū-LŌ-sis)	infectious bacterial disease, most commonly spread by inhalation of small particles and usually affecting the lungs; may spread to other organs
TUBERCULOSIS (TB) is one of the most common causes of death worldwide from infectious disease, though it is preventable and curable. The risk for active TB is higher in HIV-infected persons and others with weakened immune systems. The development of multidrug-resistant TB is becoming a problem in treatment of the disease.	
21. upper respiratory infection (URI) (UP-er) (RES-pi-ra-*tor*-ē) (in-FEK-shun)	infection of the nasal cavity, pharynx, or larynx usually caused by a virus (commonly called a **cold**) (Fig. 5.8)

Chapter 5 Respiratory System 153

Upper respiratory tract infection
Common cold
Rhinitis
Sinusitis
Tonsillitis
Pharyngitis
Laryngitis

Nasal cavity
Pharynx
Larynx
Trachea

Lower respiratory tract infection
Tracheitis
Bronchitis
Bronchiolitis
Pneumonia

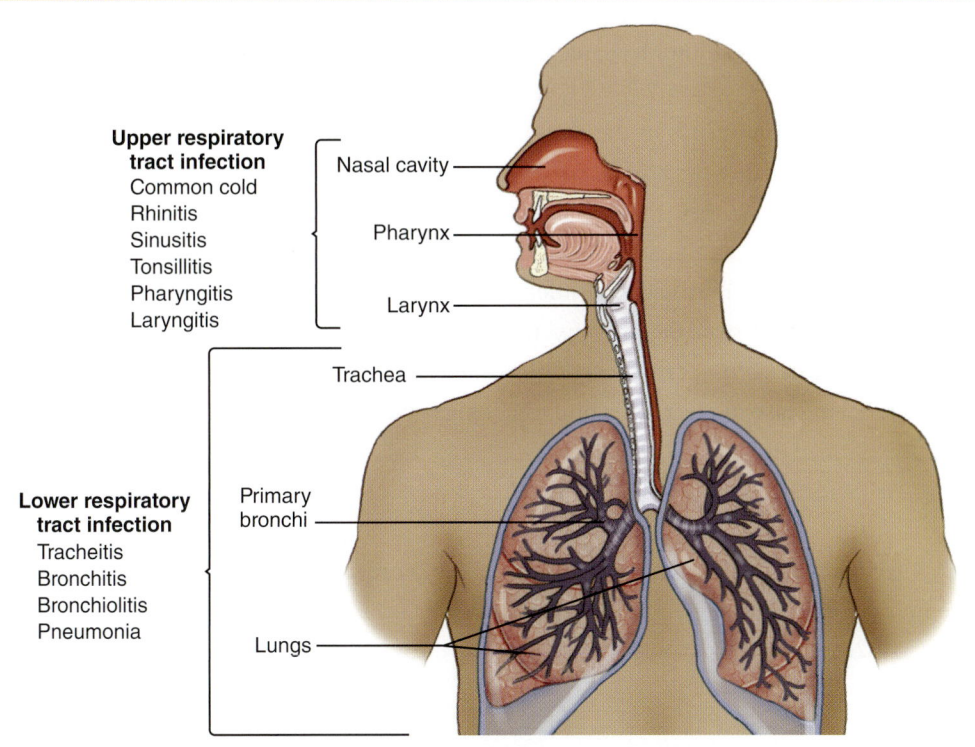

Primary bronchi
Lungs

FIG. 5.8 Upper and lower respiratory tract infections.

EXERCISE 8 ■ Pronounce and Spell

Practice pronunciation and spelling on paper and online.

1. **Practice on Paper**
   a. **Pronounce:** Read the phonetic spelling and say aloud the terms listed in the previous table. Refer to Table 2.2 Pronunciation Key as needed.
   b. **Spell:** Have a study partner read the terms aloud. Write the spelling of the terms on a separate sheet of paper.

2. **Practice Online**
   a. **Access** online learning resources. Go to evolve.elsevier.com > Evolve Resources > Student Resources.
   b. **Pronounce:** Select Audio Glossary > Chapter 5 > Exercise 8. Select a term to hear its pronunciation and repeat aloud.
   c. **Spell:** Select Activities > Chapter 5 > Spell Terms > Exercise 8. Select the audio icon and type the correct spelling of the term.

❏ Check the box when complete.

EXERCISE 9 ■ Fill In

A Identify

Fill in the blanks with the correct terms.

1. _____ _____ is a hereditary disorder characterized by excess mucus production in the respiratory tract.

2. The medical name of a contagious respiratory infection commonly referred to as *flu* is _____.

3. Chronic bronchitis and emphysema are two main components of _____ _____ _____.

4. The medical name for a highly contagious bacterial infection of the respiratory tract characterized by a severe hacking cough followed by a whoop is _____.

154   Chapter 5   Respiratory System

5. _____ is a condition resulting from an acute obstruction of the larynx characterized by a barking cough, hoarseness, and stridor.
6. A condition in which fluid accumulates in the alveoli and bronchioles is _____ _____.
7. _____ is another name for nosebleed.
8. A chronic progressive lung disorder that ultimately reduces the capacity of the lungs is _____ _____.
9. _____ is a serious bacterial infection affecting the mucous membranes of the nose and throat, which creates a thick gray sheet over the pharynx; it is rare in countries with high rates of vaccination.
10. Deprivation of oxygen for tissue use, or suffocation is called _____.
11. An infectious bacterial disease usually affecting the lungs and caused by inhaling infected small particles is _____.
12. _____ _____ _____ _____ is a life-threatening lung condition that results in hypoxemia.
13. The respiratory infection with mild symptoms including cough, headache and muscle aches and with severe symptoms including pneumonia, ARDS, blood clots, and brain disease, or _____ _____, is caused by the virus SARS-CoV-2.

B Label

Write the medical terms pictured and defined.

1. _____
matter foreign to the circulation, carried to the pulmonary artery and its branches, where it blocks circulation to the lungs

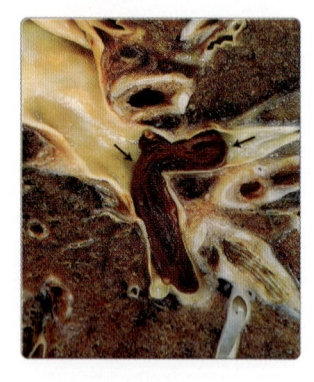

2. _____
repetitive pharyngeal collapse during sleep, which leads to transient periods of apnea

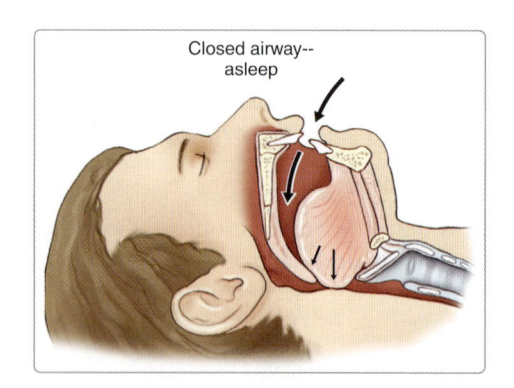

3. _____
one part of the nasal cavity is smaller because of malformation or injury of the nasal septum

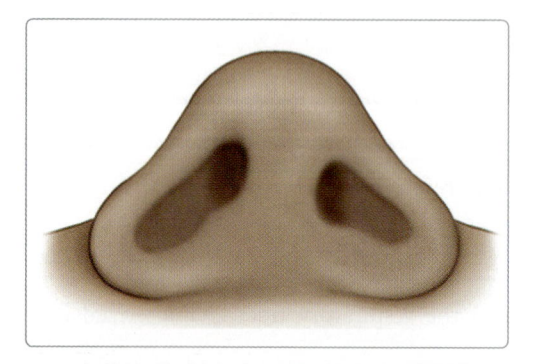

4. _____
fluid in the pleural cavity caused by a disease process or trauma

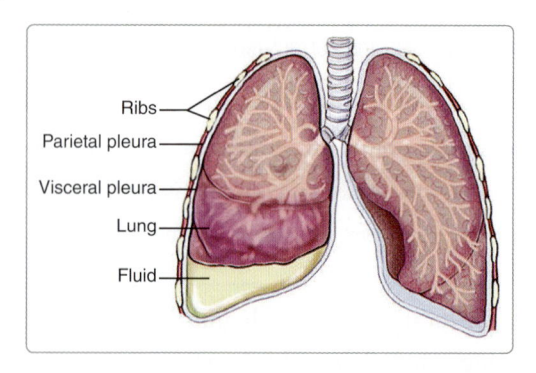

5. _____
respiratory disease characterized by coughing, wheezing, and shortness of breath, caused by constriction and inflammation of airways that is reversible between attacks

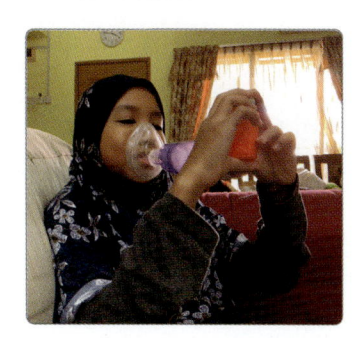

6. _____
fungal disease affecting the lungs and sometimes other organs of the body

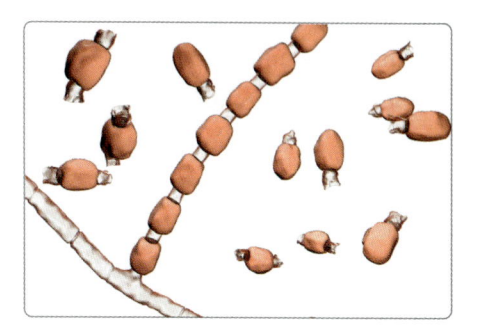

7. _____
loss of elasticity of the alveoli resulting in distention causing stretching of the lung

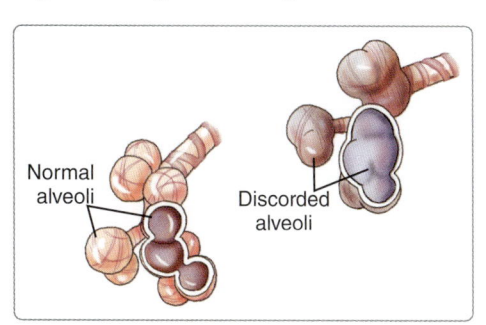

8. _____
infection of the nasal cavity, pharynx, or larynx usually caused by a virus; commonly called a cold

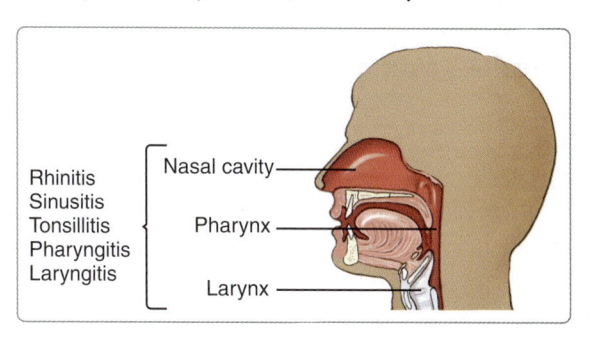

EXERCISE 10 ■ Match

Match the terms in the first column with their correct definitions in the second column.

_____ 1. diphtheria
_____ 2. asthma
_____ 3. chronic obstructive pulmonary disease
_____ 4. coccidioidomycosis
_____ 5. croup
_____ 6. cystic fibrosis
_____ 7. emphysema
_____ 8. epistaxis
_____ 9. influenza
_____ 10. idiopathic pulmonary fibrosis

a. loss of elasticity of alveoli, resulting in stretching of the lung
b. contagious respiratory infection commonly called the flu
c. hereditary disorder characterized by excess mucus in the respiratory system
d. most often caused by cigarette smoking
e. nosebleed
f. condition resulting from acute obstruction of the larynx
g. also called valley fever
h. characterized by scarring of the lung
i. caused by restriction of airways that is reversible between attacks
j. serious bacterial infection that creates a thick gray sheet covering the pharynx

EXERCISE 11 ■ Match

Match the terms in the first column with their correct definitions in the second column.

_____ 1. pertussis
_____ 2. pleural effusion
_____ 3. pulmonary edema
_____ 4. pulmonary embolism
_____ 5. upper respiratory infection
_____ 6. deviated septum
_____ 7. obstructive sleep apnea
_____ 8. tuberculosis
_____ 9. acute respiratory distress syndrome
_____ 10. asphyxia
_____ 11. coronavirus disease

a. life-threatening lung condition caused by disease or injury
b. highly contagious respiratory infection caused by the SARS-CoV-2 virus
c. fluid accumulation in alveoli and bronchioles
d. whooping cough
e. foreign material, carried to the pulmonary artery, where it blocks circulation to the lungs
f. commonly called a cold
g. unequal size of nasal cavities
h. repetitive pharyngeal collapse
i. infectious bacterial disease usually affecting the lungs
j. deprivation of oxygen for tissue use
k. fluid in the pleural cavity

EXERCISE 12 ■ Review of Disease and Disorder Terms

Can you define, pronounce, and spell the following terms?

acute respiratory distress syndrome (ARDS)
adenoiditis
alveolitis
atelectasis
asphyxia
asthma
bronchiectasis
bronchitis
bronchogenic carcinoma
bronchopneumonia
bronchospasm
chronic obstructive pulmonary disease (COPD)
coccidioidomycosis (cocci)
coronavirus disease (COVID-19)
croup
cystic fibrosis (CF)
deviated septum
diaphragmatocele
diphtheria
emphysema
epiglottitis
epistaxis
hemothorax
idiopathic pulmonary fibrosis (IPF)
influenza (flu)
laryngitis
laryngospasm
laryngotracheobronchitis (LTB)
lobar pneumonia
nasopharyngitis
obstructive sleep apnea (OSA)
pertussis
pharyngitis
pleural effusion
pleuritis
pneumoconiosis
pneumonia
pneumonitis
pneumothorax
pulmonary edema
pulmonary embolism (PE)
pulmonary neoplasm
pyothorax
rhinitis
rhinomycosis
rhinorrhagia
sinusitis
tonsillitis
tracheitis
tracheostenosis
tuberculosis (TB)
upper respiratory infection (URI)

Surgical Terms
BUILT FROM WORD PARTS

The following terms can be translated using definitions of word parts. Further explanation is provided within parentheses as needed.

TERM	DEFINITION	TERM	DEFINITION
1. **adenoidectomy** (*ad*-e-noyd-EK-to-mē)	excision of the adenoids	4. **laryngoplasty** (la-RING-gō-*plas*-tē)	surgical repair of the larynx
2. **bronchoplasty** (BRON-kō-*plas*-tē)	surgical repair of a bronchus	5. **laryngostomy** (*lar*-in-GOS-to-mē)	creation of an artificial opening into the larynx
3. **laryngectomy** (*lār*-in-JEK-to-mē)	excision of the larynx	6. **laryngotracheotomy** (la-*ring*-gō-trā-kē-OT-o-mē)	incision into the larynx and trachea

Chapter 5 Respiratory System

TERM	DEFINITION	TERM	DEFINITION
7. **lobectomy** (lō-BEK-to-mē)	excision of a lobe (of the lung) (Fig. 5.9)	13. **thoracentesis** (thor-a-sen-TĒ-sis)	surgical puncture to aspirate fluid from the chest cavity (also called **thoracocentesis**)
8. **pleurodesis** (plū-rō-DĒ-sis)	fusion of the pleura (procedure to close the space between the parietal pleura lining the thoracic cavity and the visceral pleura lining the lungs to prevent the buildup of fluid)		💡 The combining vowel "o" and the "c" in **thorac/o** are dropped in the term **thoracentesis**.
		14. **thoracotomy** (*thor*-a-KOT-o-mē)	incision into the chest cavity (Fig. 5.10)
		15. **tonsillectomy** (*ton*-sil-EK-to-mē)	excision of the tonsils
9. **pneumonectomy** (nū-mō-NEK-to-mē)	excision of a lung (Fig. 5.9)	16. **tracheoplasty** (TRĀ-kē-ō-*plas*-tē)	surgical repair of the trachea
10. **rhinoplasty** (RĪ-nō-*plas*-tē)	surgical repair of the nose	17. **tracheostomy** (*trā*-kē-OS-to-mē)	creation of an artificial opening into the trachea (Fig. 5.11)
11. **septoplasty** (SEP-tō-*plas*-tē)	surgical repair of the (nasal) septum		
12. **sinusotomy** (*sī*-nū-SOT-o-mē)	incision into a sinus	18. **tracheotomy** (*trā*-kē-OT-o-mē)	incision into the trachea (Fig. 5.11)

Pneumonectomy   Segmental resection   Lobectomy   Wedge resection

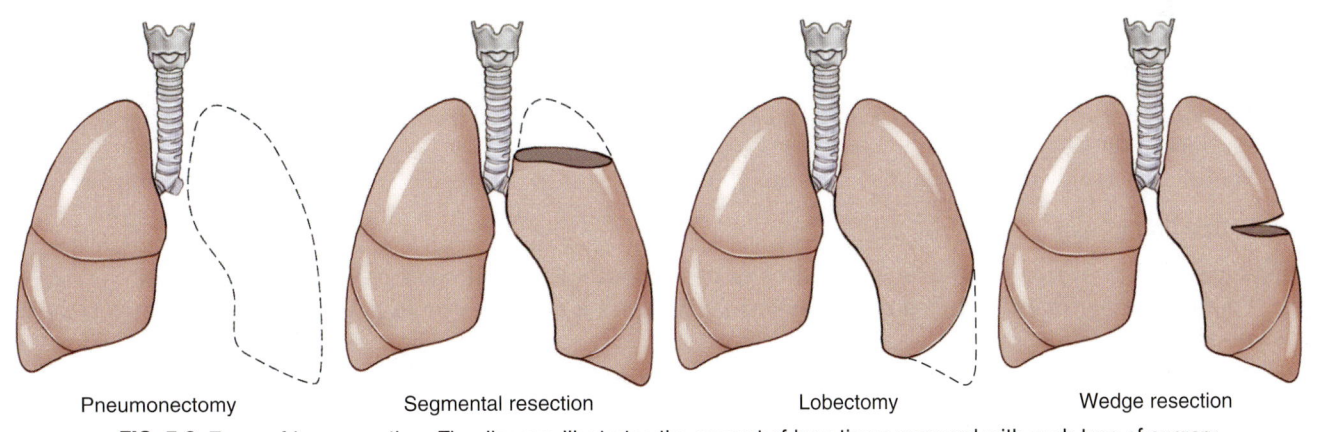

FIG. 5.9 Types of lung resection. The diagram illustrates the amount of lung tissue removed with each type of surgery.

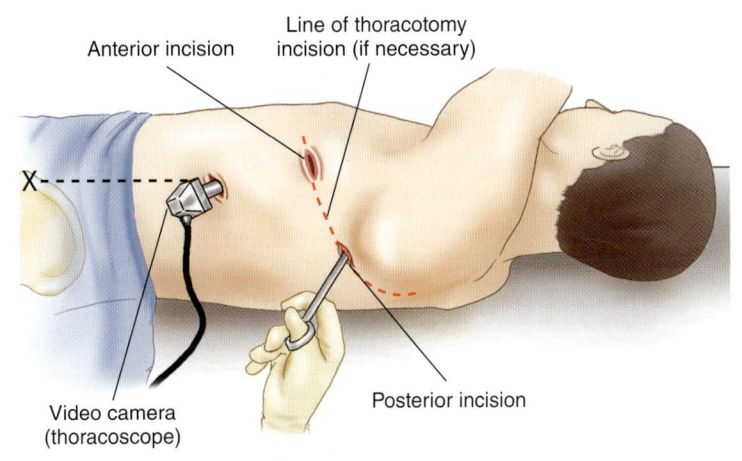

FIG. 5.10 Video-assisted thoracic surgery (VATS) is the use of a **thoracoscope** and video equipment for an endoscopic approach to diagnose and treat thoracic conditions. It often replaces the traditional **thoracotomy**, which required a large incision and greater recovery time.

158 Chapter 5 Respiratory System

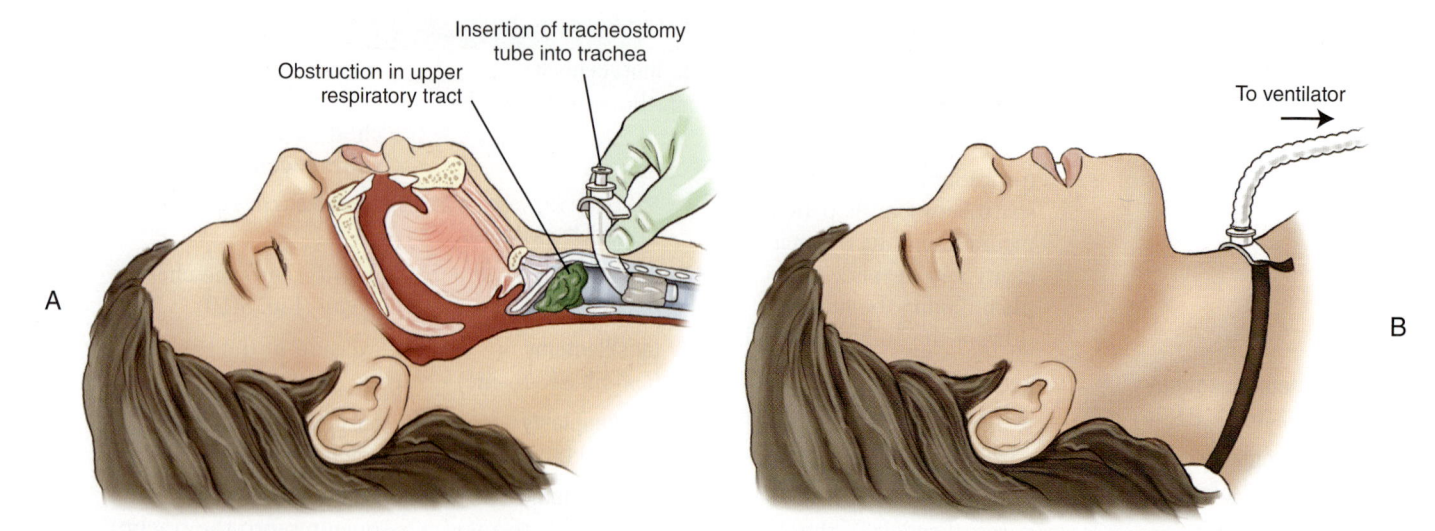

FIG. 5.11 **A,** A **tracheotomy** is performed to establish an airway when normal breathing is obstructed. If the opening needs to be maintained, a tube is inserted, creating a tracheostomy. **B,** A **tracheostomy** may be temporary, as for prolonged mechanical ventilation to support breathing, or it may be permanent, as in airway reconstruction after laryngeal cancer surgery.

EXERCISE 13 ■ Pronounce and Spell

Practice pronunciation and spelling on paper and online.

1. **Practice on Paper**
   a. **Pronounce:** Read the phonetic spelling and say aloud the terms listed in the previous table. Refer to Table 2.2 Pronunciation Key as needed.
   b. **Spell:** Have a study partner read the terms aloud. Write the spelling of the terms on a separate sheet of paper.

2. **Practice Online**
   a. **Access** online learning resources. Go to evolve.elsevier.com > Evolve Resources > Student Resources.
   b. **Pronounce:** Select Audio Glossary > Chapter 5 > Exercise 13. Select a term to hear its pronunciation and repeat aloud.
   c. **Spell:** Select Activities > Chapter 5 > Spell Terms > Exercise 13. Select the audio icon and type the correct spelling of the term.

❑ Check the box when complete.

EXERCISE 14 ■ Analyze and Define

Analyze and define the following terms by drawing slashes between word parts, writing word part abbreviations above the term, underlining combining forms, and writing combining form abbreviations below the term.

EXAMPLE: WR   S
pneumon/ectomy

excision of a lung

1. tracheoplasty

2. septoplasty

Chapter 5 Respiratory System   159

3. laryngostomy

_____

_____

4. sinusotomy

_____

_____

5. laryngoplasty

_____

_____

6. thoracotomy

_____

_____

EXERCISE 15 ■ Build

A Label

Build terms pictured by writing word parts above definitions.

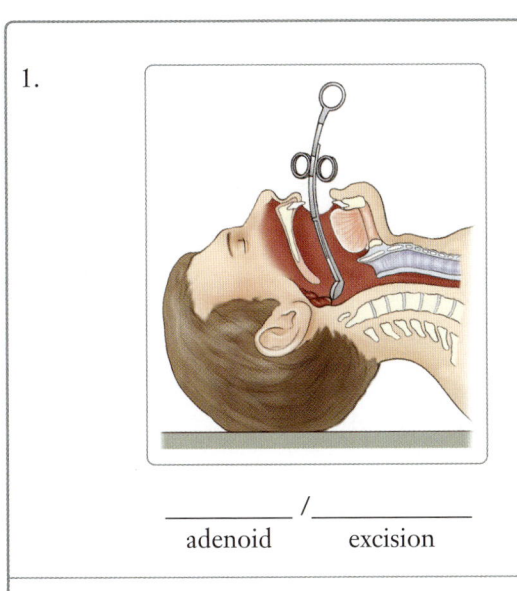

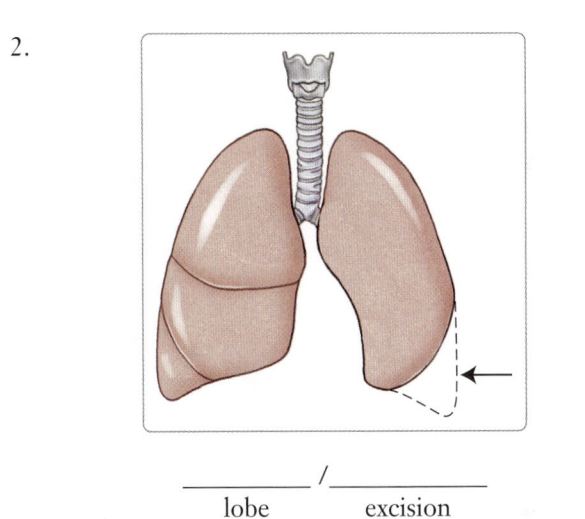

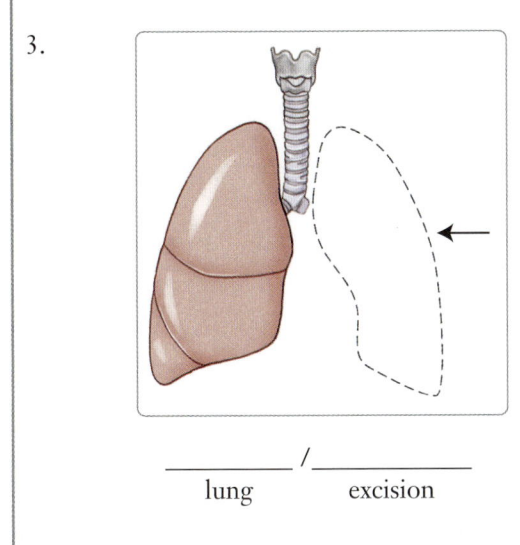

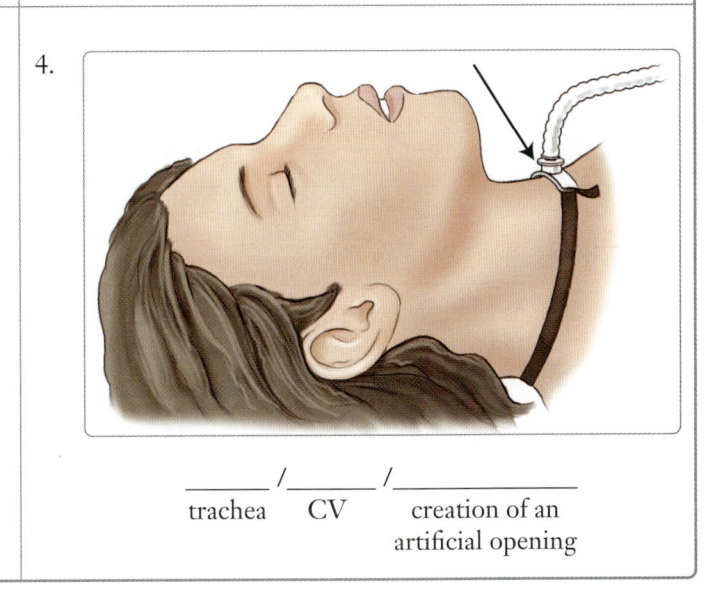

1.

_____/_____
adenoid   excision

2.

_____/_____
lobe   excision

3.

_____/_____
lung   excision

4.

_____/_____/_____
trachea CV creation of an
             artificial opening

160 Chapter 5 Respiratory System

5.

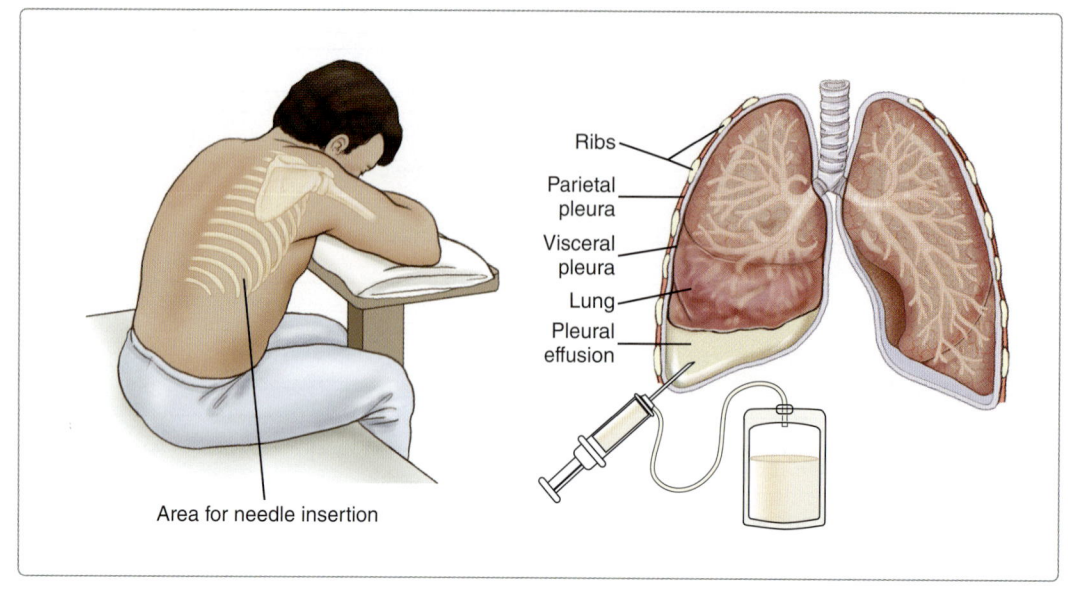

_____ / _____ is used for both diagnosis and treatment.
  chest cavity   surgical puncture
                    to aspirate fluid

6.

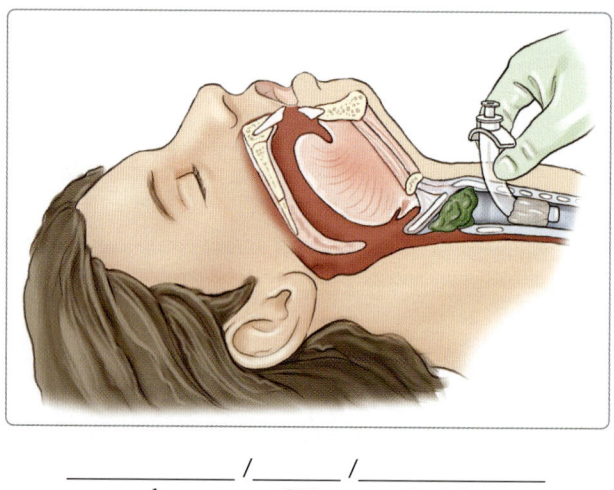

_____ / _____ / _____
    trachea   CV   incision

B Fill In

Build surgical terms for the following definitions by using the word parts you have learned.

EXAMPLE: surgical repair of the larynx   laryng / o / plasty
                                              WR   CV   S

1. incision into the larynx and trachea   _____ / ___ / _____ / ___ / ___
                                             WR   CV   WR   CV   S

2. fusion of the pleura   _____ / ___ / _____
                                                WR   CV   S

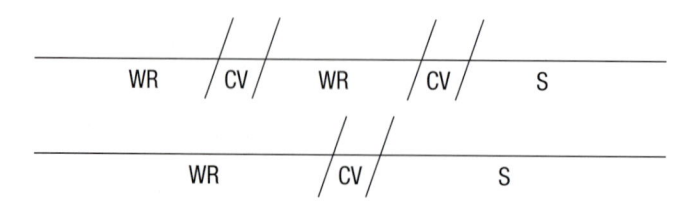

3. excision of the tonsils

　　　　　　　　　　　　WR　　／　　S

4. surgical repair of a bronchus

　　　　　　　　　　　　WR　／CV／　S

5. excision of the larynx

　　　　　　　　　　　　WR　　／　　S

6. surgical repair of the nose

　　　　　　　　　　　　WR　／CV／　S

> **EXERCISE 16 ■ Review of Surgical Terms**

Can you define, pronounce, and spell the following terms?

adenoidectomy	laryngotracheotomy	septoplasty	tracheoplasty
bronchoplasty	lobectomy	sinusotomy	tracheostomy
laryngectomy	pleurodesis	thoracentesis	tracheotomy
laryngoplasty	pneumonectomy	thoracotomy	
laryngostomy	rhinoplasty	tonsillectomy	

Endoscopy

Endoscopy is the general term for direct observation of a hollow body organ or cavity. Endoscopy dates to the time of Hippocrates (460-375 BC) and is translated from the Greek words **"endon"** (**within** or **inward**) and **"skopein"** (to **see** or **view**). By the end of the nineteenth century, cystoscopy, proctoscopy, and esophagoscopy were well established. The original endoscopes were rigid and used for direct observation. Adding lights and lenses to the endoscope allowed visualization of deeper structures.

　　Current endoscopy uses smaller, flexible, tubular instruments and incorporates fiber optics and cameras, which allows images to be viewed on a monitor. Endoscopic procedures and instruments are named after the body part visualized. For example, **bronchoscopy** means **visual examination of the bronchi**, and **bronchoscope** means **instrument used for visual examination of the bronchi** (Fig 5.12).

　　Endoscopes are also used in endoscopic surgery, in which internal organs are reached through natural openings, such as the mouth, or through small incisions. Endoscopic surgery is considered to be **minimally invasive** when compared to the large incisions usually required for traditional surgery. The endoscope allows the surgeon to use the monitor to see inside the body, and to use very small tools at the surgical site.

Diagnostic Terms

The Diagnostic Terms section in this and subsequent chapters presents terms used for tests, labs, and procedures used to diagnose diseases and disorders. Generally, they include laboratory, diagnostic imaging, and endoscopy. In Chapter 5, additional categories have been added to include other diagnostic procedures.

BUILT FROM WORD PARTS

The following terms can be translated using definitions of word parts. Further explanation is provided within parentheses as needed.

ENDOSCOPY

TERM	DEFINITION	TERM	DEFINITION
1. **bronchoscope** (BRON-kō-skōp)	instrument used for visual examination of the bronchi (Fig. 5.12)	2. **bronchoscopy** (bron-KOS-ko-pē)	visual examination of the bronchi (Fig. 5.12)

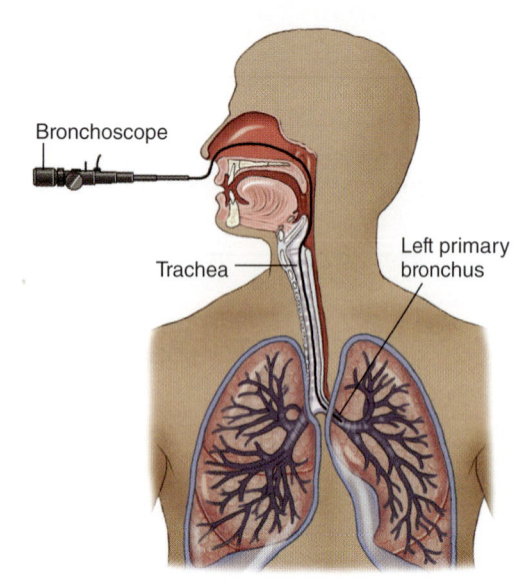

FIG. 5.12 Bronchoscopy. A bronchoscope is inserted through the nostril, pharynx, larynx, and trachea into the bronchus.

TABLE 5.1 Endoscopy Suffixes

Most often the suffixes **-scope**, **-scopy**, and **-scopic** refer to visual examination. An exception is the term **stethoscope**, which is an **instrument used for listening** to body sounds.

Suffix	Names
-scope	the instrument used to view or to examine, such as in the term endoscope; noun
-scopy	visual examination procedure, such as in the term endoscopy; noun
-scopic	means pertaining to visual examination, such as in the term endoscopic; adjective

Diagnostic Terms—cont'd
BUILT FROM WORD PARTS

TERM	DEFINITION	TERM	DEFINITION
3. endoscope (EN-dō-skōp)	instrument used for visual examination within (a hollow organ or body cavity)	7. laryngoscopy (lar-in-GOS-ko-pē)	visual examination of the larynx
4. endoscopic (en-dō-SKOP-ik)	pertaining to visual examination within (a hollow organ or body cavity)	8. mediastinoscopy (mē-dē-a-sti-NOS-ko-pē)	visual examination of the mediastinum
5. endoscopy (en-DOS-ko-pē)	visual examination within (a hollow organ or body cavity)	9. thoracoscope (tho-RAK-ō-skōp)	instrument used for visual examination of the chest cavity (see Fig. 5.10)
6. laryngoscope (la-RING-go-skōp)	instrument used for visual examination of the larynx	10. thoracoscopy (thor-a-KOS-ko-pē)	visual examination of the chest cavity

SLEEP STUDIES

TERM	DEFINITION
11. polysomnography (PSG) (pol-ē-som-NOG-rah-fē)	process of recording many (tests) during sleep (performed to diagnose obstructive sleep apnea [see Fig. 5.6]). Tests include **electrooculography, electrocardiography, electromyography, electroencephalography, air flow monitoring,** and **oximetry**.

PULMONARY FUNCTION

TERM	DEFINITION	TERM	DEFINITION
12. capnometer (kap-NOM-e-ter)	instrument used to measure carbon dioxide (levels in expired gas)	14. spirometer (spī-ROM-e-ter)	instrument used to measure breathing (or lung volumes)
13. oximeter (ok-SIM-e-ter)	instrument used to measure oxygen (saturation in the blood) (Note: the combining vowel is i.)	15. spirometry (spī-ROM-e-trē)	a measurement of breathing (or air flow)

Chapter 5 Respiratory System 163

EXERCISE 17 ■ Pronounce and Spell

Practice pronunciation and spelling on paper and online.

1. **Practice on Paper**
   a. **Pronounce:** Read the phonetic spelling and say aloud the terms listed in the previous table. Refer to Table 2.2 Pronunciation Key as needed.
   b. **Spell:** Have a study partner read the terms aloud. Write the spelling of the terms on a separate sheet of paper.

2. **Practice Online**
   a. **Access** online learning resources. Go to evolve.elsevier.com > Evolve Resources > Student Resources.
   b. **Pronounce:** Select Audio Glossary > Chapter 5 > Exercise 17. Select a term to hear its pronunciation and repeat aloud.
   c. **Spell:** Select Activities > Chapter 5 > Spell Terms > Exercise 17. Select the audio icon and type the correct spelling of the term.

❏ Check the box when complete.

EXERCISE 18 ■ Analyze and Define

Analyze and define the following terms by drawing slashes between word parts, writing word part abbreviations above the term, underlining combining forms, and writing combining form abbreviations below the term.

EXAMPLE:
```
        WR   CV   S
       bronch / o / scopy
            CF
       visual examination of the bronchi
```

1. spirometer

2. laryngoscope

3. capnometer

4. spirometry

5. oximeter

6. laryngoscopy

7. bronchoscope

8. thoracoscope

9. endoscope

10. thoracoscopy

164 Chapter 5 Respiratory System

11. endoscopic

_____

_____

12. endoscopy

_____

_____

13. polysomnography

_____

_____

14. mediastinoscopy

_____

_____

EXERCISE 19 ■ Build

A Label

Build terms pictured by writing word parts above definitions.

1.

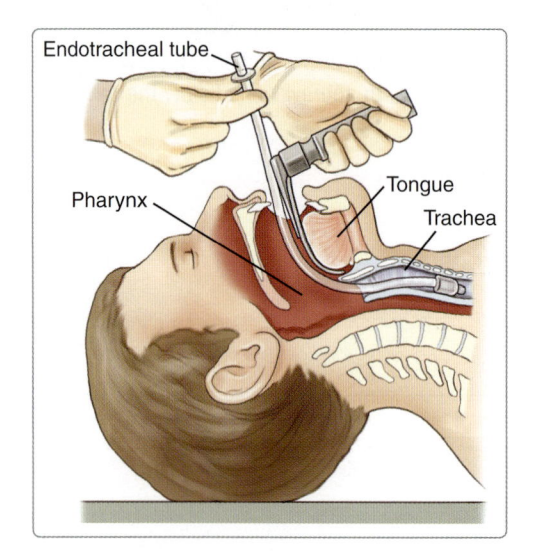

Endotracheal tube
Pharynx
Tongue
Trachea

A _____ / _____ / _____ is used to guide the endotracheal tube into place.
    larynx   CV   instrument used for
                              visual examination

2.

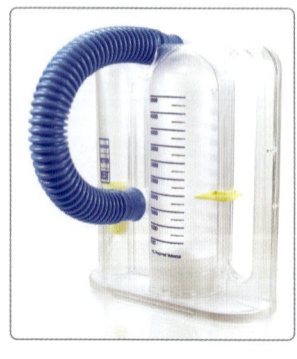

_____ / _____ / _____
breathing CV instrument used
                      to measure

3.

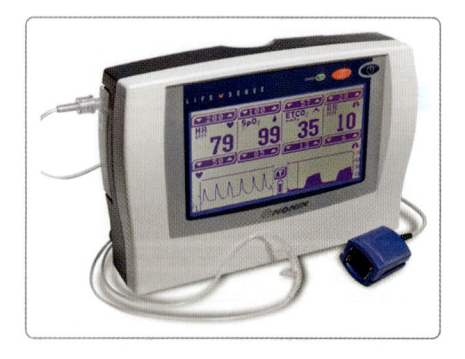

_____ / _____ / _____
carbon   CV instrument used
dioxide   to measure

Chapter 5 Respiratory System 165

4. Pulse _____ / _____ / _____
             oxygen   CV   instrument used to measure

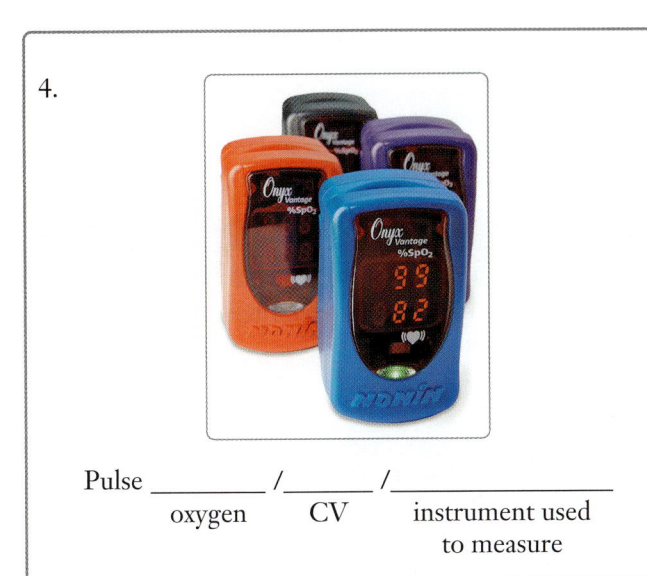

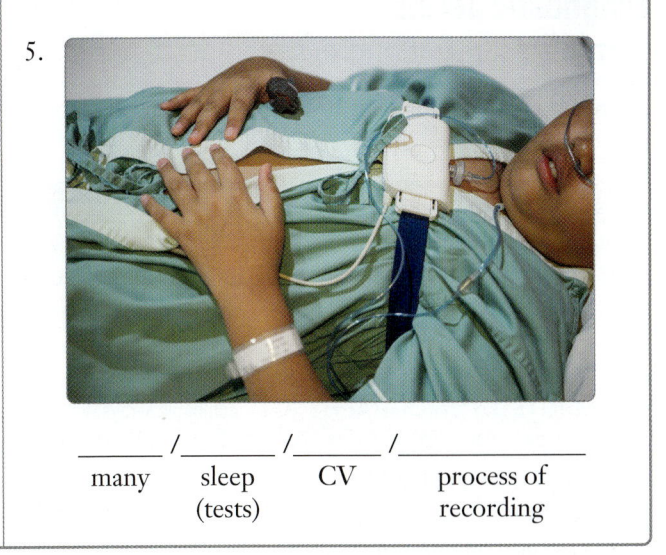

5. _____ / _____ / _____ / _____
      many   sleep   CV   process of
               (tests)   recording

B Fill In

Build diagnostic terms for the following definitions by using the word parts you have learned. *Note: The abbreviation S(WR) indicates the suffix contains a word root.*

EXAMPLE: instrument used to measure oxygen   ox / i / meter
                                                          WR / CV / S

1. visual examination of the larynx   _____ / ____ / _____
                                               WR   CV   S

2. visual examination of the mediastinum   _____ / ____ / _____
                                               WR   CV   S

3. pertaining to visual examination within (a hollow organ or body cavity)   _____ / _____
                                               P   S(WR)

4. visual examination of the chest cavity   _____ / ____ / _____
                                               WR   CV   S

5. visual examination of the bronchi   _____ / ____ / _____
                                               WR   CV   S

6. measurement of breathing   _____ / ____ / _____
                                               WR   CV   S

7. instrument used for visual examination of the bronchi   _____ / ____ / _____
                                               WR   CV   S

8. visual examination within (a hollow organ or body cavity)   _____ / _____
                                               P   S(WR)

9. instrument used for visual examination of the chest cavity   _____ / ____ / _____
                                               WR   CV   S

10. instrument used for visual examination within (a hollow organ or body cavity)   _____ / _____
                                                P   S(WR)

Diagnostic Terms
NOT BUILT FROM WORD PARTS

Word parts may be present in the following terms; however, their full meanings cannot be translated using definitions of word parts alone.

DIAGNOSTIC IMAGING

TERM	DEFINITION
1. chest computed tomography (CT) scan (chest) (kom-PŪ-ted) (tō-MOG-ra-fē) (skan)	computerized radiographic images of the chest performed to diagnose tumors, abscesses, and pleural effusion

COMPUTED TOMOGRAPHY (CT) combines x-rays with computer technology to produce detailed, cross sectional images of the body, called "slices." Oral or intravenous contrast materials may be given to highlight specific regions in the body, resulting in clearer images.

TERM	DEFINITION
2. chest radiograph (CXR) (chest) (RĀ-dē-ō-*graf*)	radiographic image of the chest performed to evaluate the lungs and the heart (also called a **chest x-ray**)
3. lung ventilation/perfusion scan (V/Q scan) (lung) (*ven*-ti-LĀ-shun) (per-FŪ-zhun) (skan)	two nuclear scan tests, one to measure air flow throughout the lungs (ventilation), and one to measure circulation to all areas of the lungs (perfusion). A V/Q scan is used most often to help diagnose or rule out a pulmonary embolism (PE).

LABORATORY

TERM	DEFINITION
4. acid-fast bacilli (AFB) smear (AS-id-fast) (bah-SIL-ī) (smēr)	test performed on sputum to determine the presence of acid-fast bacilli, which cause tuberculosis

ACID-FAST means not easily discolored by acid after staining.

PULMONARY FUNCTION

TERM	DEFINITION
5. arterial blood gas (ABG) (ar-TĒ-rē-al) (blud) (gas)	test performed on arterial blood to determine levels of oxygen (O_2), carbon dioxide (CO_2), and pH (acidity)
6. peak flow meter (PFM) (pēk) (flō) (MĒ-ter)	portable instrument used to measure air flow early in forced exhalation; helps monitor asthma and adjust medication accordingly
7. pulmonary function tests (PFTs) (PUL-mō-*nar*-ē) (FUNK-shun) (tests)	group of tests performed to measure breathing capacity and used to determine external respiratory function; when abnormal, they are useful in distinguishing COPD from asthma. Some tests involve the use of a spirometer.
8. pulse oximetry (puls) (ok-SIM-e-trē)	noninvasive method of measuring oxygen in the blood by using a device that attaches to the fingertip

OTHER

TERM	DEFINITION
9. auscultation (*aws*-kul-TĀ-shun)	the act of listening through a stethoscope for sounds within the body that are abnormal and that suggest abnormalities or disease; used for assessing and diagnosing conditions of the lungs, pleura, heart, arteries, and abdomen
10. percussion (per-KUSH-un)	the act of tapping of a body surface to determine the density of the part beneath by the sound obtained. A dull sound where normally a hollow sound would be elicited indicates displacement of air by fluid or solid waste in a body space or cavity, such as in a potential pleural space.

Chapter 5   Respiratory System

OTHER	
TERM	**DEFINITION**
11. PPD skin test (P-P-D) (skin) (test)	test performed on individuals who may have been exposed to tuberculosis. PPD (purified protein derivative) of the tuberculin bacillus is injected intradermally. Positive tests indicate previous exposure, not necessarily active tuberculosis. (also called **TB skin test**)
12. stethoscope (STETH-ō-skōp)	instrument used to hear internal body sounds; used for performing auscultation and blood pressure measurement

EXERCISE 20 ■ Pronounce and Spell

Practice pronunciation and spelling on paper and online.

1. **Practice on Paper**
   a. **Pronounce:** Read the phonetic spelling and say aloud the terms listed in the previous table. Refer to Table 2.2 Pronunciation Key as needed.
   b. **Spell:** Have a study partner read the terms aloud. Write the spelling of the terms on a separate sheet of paper.

2. **Practice Online**
   a. **Access** online learning resources. Go to evolve.elsevier.com > Evolve Resources > Student Resources.
   b. **Pronounce:** Select Audio Glossary > Chapter 5 > Exercise 20. Select a term to hear its pronunciation and repeat aloud.
   c. **Spell:** Select Activities > Chapter 5 > Spell Terms > Exercise 20. Select the audio icon and type the correct spelling of the term.

❑ Check the box when complete.

EXERCISE 21 ■ Fill In

A Label

Write the medical terms pictured and defined.

1. _____
test performed by intradermal injection on individuals who may have been exposed to tuberculosis

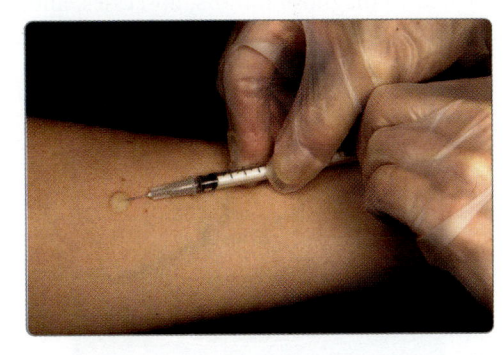

2. _____
portable instrument used to measure air flow in forced exhalation; helps monitor asthma and adjust medication accordingly

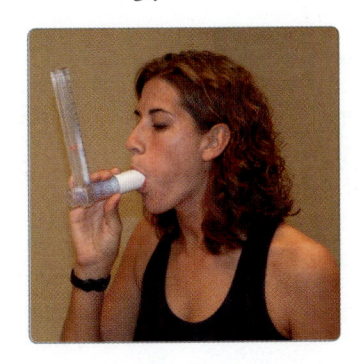

168 Chapter 5 Respiratory System

3. _____
test performed on arterial blood to determine levels of oxygen (O_2), carbon dioxide (CO_2), and pH (acidity)

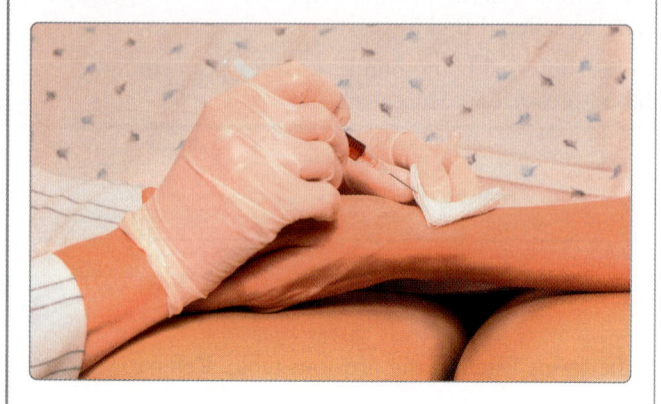

4. _____
noninvasive method of measuring oxygen in the blood by using a device that attaches to the fingertip

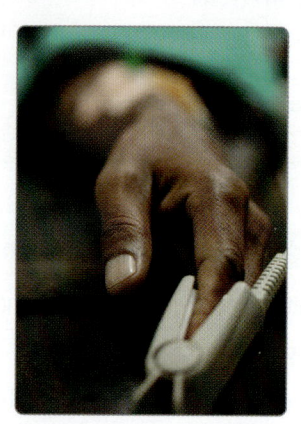

5. _____
instrument used to hear internal body sounds; used for performing auscultation and blood pressure measurement

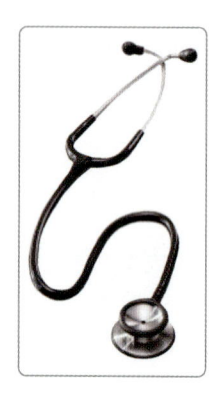

6. _____
two nuclear scan tests used to help diagnose or rule out pulmonary embolism

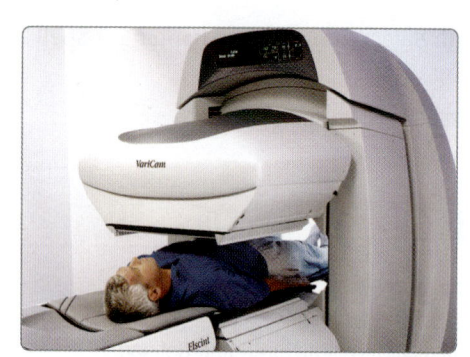

7. _____
radiographic image of the chest performed to evaluate the lungs and the heart

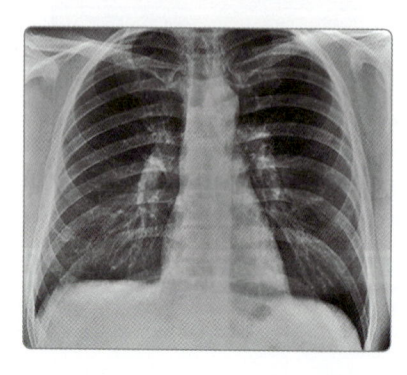

8. _____
computerized radiographic images of the chest performed to diagnose tumors, abscesses, and pleural effusions

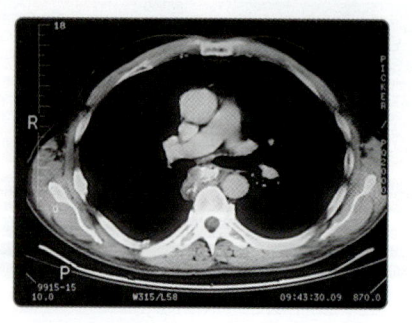

9. _____
the act of listening through a stethoscope for sounds within the body that are abnormal and that suggest abnormalities or disease

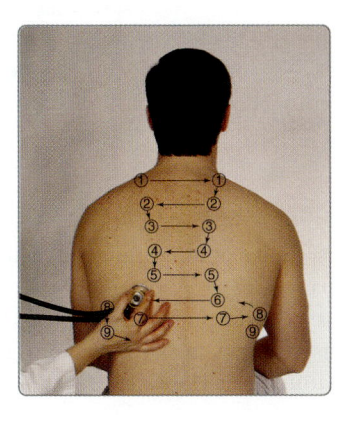

10. _____
the act of tapping of a body surface to determine the density of the part beneath by the sound obtained

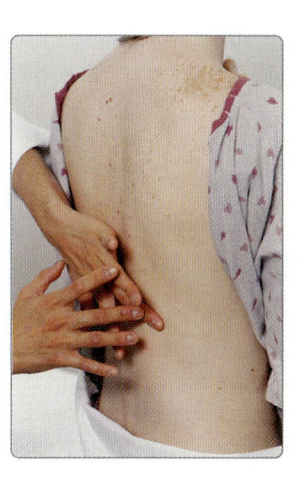

B Identify

Fill in the blanks with the correct terms.

1. A test performed on sputum to diagnose tuberculosis is called _____.
2. _____ is the name of a group of tests performed to measure breathing capacity and to determine external respiratory function or abnormalities.

EXERCISE 22 ■ Match

Match the terms in the first column with their correct definitions in the second column.

_____ 1. lung ventilation/perfusion scan
_____ 2. chest radiograph
_____ 3. chest CT scan
_____ 4. acid-fast bacilli smear
_____ 5. pulse oximetry
_____ 6. arterial blood gas
_____ 7. pulmonary function tests
_____ 8. PPD skin test
_____ 9. auscultation
_____ 10. stethoscope
_____ 11. peak flow meter
_____ 12. percussion

a. computerized images of the chest
b. noninvasive method used to measure oxygen in the blood
c. arterial blood test used to determine levels of oxygen, carbon dioxide, and pH
d. test on sputum for tuberculosis
e. chest x-ray
f. nuclear medicine procedure used to diagnose pulmonary embolism
g. group of tests performed to measure breathing capacity
h. test performed on individuals who may have been exposed to tuberculosis
i. instrument used for auscultation
j. used to help monitor asthma
k. the act of listening for sounds within the body through a stethoscope
l. the act of tapping a body surface to determine density

EXERCISE 23 ■ Review of Diagnostic Terms

Can you define, pronounce, and spell the following terms?

acid-fast bacilli smear (AFB)	chest computed tomography (CT) scan	lung ventilation/perfusion scan (V/Q scan)	pulmonary function tests (PFTs)
arterial blood gas (ABG)	endoscope	mediastinoscopy	pulse oximetry
auscultation	endoscopic	oximeter	spirometer
bronchoscope	endoscopy	peak flow meter (PFM)	spirometry
bronchoscopy	laryngoscope	percussion	stethoscope
capnometer	laryngoscopy	polysomnography (PSG)	thoracoscope
chest radiograph (CXR)		PPD skin test	thoracoscopy

Complementary Terms

Complementary terms complete the vocabulary presented in the chapter by describing signs, symptoms, medical specialties, specialists, and related words. A symptom is subjective information reflecting patient experience as reported by the patient. A sign is objective information detected in the physical examination and in results from diagnostic assessments, such as laboratory tests. **Lab findings** are the results of laboratory tests that analyze specimens of blood, urine, or tissue. Signs detected by laboratory tests will be noted in Complementary Term Tables as lab findings within parentheses following the definition.

BUILT FROM WORD PARTS

The following terms can be translated using definitions of word parts. Further explanation is provided within parentheses as needed.

SIGNS AND SYMPTOMS

TERM	DEFINITION	TERM	DEFINITION
1. acapnia (a-CAP-nē-a)	condition of absence (less than normal level) of carbon dioxide (in the blood); (lab finding)	10. hyperpnea (hī-perp-NĒ-a)	excessive breathing
2. anoxia (a-NOK-sē-a)	condition of absence (deficiency) of oxygen; (lab finding)	11. hypocapnia (hī-pō-KAP-nē-a)	condition of deficient carbon dioxide (in the blood); (lab finding)
ANOXIA literally means **without oxygen** or **absence of oxygen**. The term actually denotes an oxygen deficiency in the body tissues.		12. hypopnea (hī-POP-nē-a)	deficient breathing
3. aphonia (ā-FŌ-nē-a)	condition of absence of voice	13. hypoxemia (hī-pok-SĒ-mē-a)	deficient oxygen in the blood; (lab finding)
4. apnea (AP-nē-a)	absence of breathing	14. hypoxia (hī-POK-sē-a)	condition of deficient oxygen (to the tissues); (lab finding)
5. dysphonia (dis-FŌ-nē-a)	condition of difficult speaking (voice)	💡 The "o" from the prefix **hypo-** is dropped in the terms **hypoxemia** and **hypoxia** because the following word part begins with a vowel.	
6. dyspnea (DISP-nē-a)	difficult breathing	15. orthopnea (or-THOP-nē-a)	breathing (more easily) in a straight (upright position) (indicates difficulty breathing in the supine position)
7. eupnea (ŪP-nē-a)	normal breathing		
8. hemoptysis (he-MOP-ti-sis)	coughing of blood (or blood-stained sputum)	16. rhinorrhea (rī-nō-RĒ-a)	discharge from the nose (as in a cold)
9. hypercapnia (hī-per-KAP-nē-a)	condition of excessive carbon dioxide (in the blood); (lab finding)	17. tachypnea (tak-IP-nē-a)	rapid breathing

MEDICAL SPECIALTIES

TERM	DEFINITION	TERM	DEFINITION
18. pulmonologist (pul-mon-OL-o-jist)	physician who studies and treats diseases of the lung	19. pulmonology (pul-mon-OL-o-jē)	study of the lung (a branch of medicine dealing with diseases of the lung)

Chapter 5 Respiratory System 171

DESCRIPTIVE TERMS

TERM	DEFINITION	TERM	DEFINITION
20. **alveolar** (al-VĒ-ō-lar)	pertaining to the alveolus	27. **mucoid** (MŪ-koyd)	resembling mucus
21. **bronchoalveolar** (*bron*-kō-al-VĒ-o-lar)	pertaining to the bronchi and alveoli	28. **mucous** (MŪ-kus)	pertaining to mucus
22. **diaphragmatic** (*dī*-a-frag-MAT-ik)	pertaining to the diaphragm	**MUCUS** is the noun that describes slimy fluid secreted by the membrane lining cavities that lead outside of the body. **Mucous** is the adjective that means pertaining to mucus. Pronunciation is the same for both terms.	
23. **endotracheal** (*en*-dō-TRĀ-kē-al)	pertaining to within the trachea		
24. **intrapleural** (*in*-tra-PLUR-al)	pertaining to within the pleura (space between the two pleural membranes)	29. **nasopharyngeal** (*nā*-zō-fa-RIN-jē-al)	pertaining to the nose and pharynx
			30. **pulmonary** (PUL-mō-*nar*-ē)	pertaining to the lungs
25. **laryngeal** (lar-IN-jē-al)	pertaining to the larynx	31. **septal** (SEP-tal)	pertaining to the septum
26. **mediastinal** (mē-dē-a-STĪ-nel)	pertaining to the mediastinum	32. **thoracic** (thō-RAS-ik)	pertaining to the chest

EXERCISE 24 ■ Pronounce and Spell

Practice pronunciation and spelling on paper and online.

1. **Practice on Paper**
   a. **Pronounce:** Read the phonetic spelling and say aloud the terms listed in the previous table. Refer to Table 2.2 Pronunciation Key as needed.
   b. **Spell:** Have a study partner read the terms aloud. Write the spelling of the terms on a separate sheet of paper.

2. **Practice Online**
   a. **Access** online learning resources. Go to evolve.elsevier.com > Evolve Resources > Student Resources.
   b. **Pronounce:** Select Audio Glossary > Chapter 5 > Exercise 24. Select a term to hear its pronunciation and repeat aloud.
   c. **Spell:** Select Activities > Chapter 5 > Spell Terms > Exercise 24. Select the audio icon and type the correct spelling of the term.

❏ Check the box when complete.

EXERCISE 25 ■ Analyze and Define

Analyze and define the following terms by drawing slashes between word parts, writing word part abbreviations above the term, underlining combining forms, and writing combining form abbreviations below the term.

```
              P     WR   S
EXAMPLE:  hyper / capn / ia
```
   condition of excessive carbon dioxide (in the blood)

1. mediastinal

2. pulmonology

_____

_____

172 Chapter 5 Respiratory System

3. mucous
_____
_____

4. apnea
_____
_____

5. hypoxia
_____
_____

6. nasopharyngeal
_____
_____

7. intrapleural
_____
_____

8. acapnia
_____
_____

9. dysphonia
_____
_____

10. hypoxemia
_____
_____

11. thoracic
_____
_____

12. diaphragmatic
_____
_____

13. bronchoalveolar
_____
_____

14. hypopnea
_____
_____

EXERCISE 26 ■ Build

A Label

Build terms pictured by writing word parts above definitions.

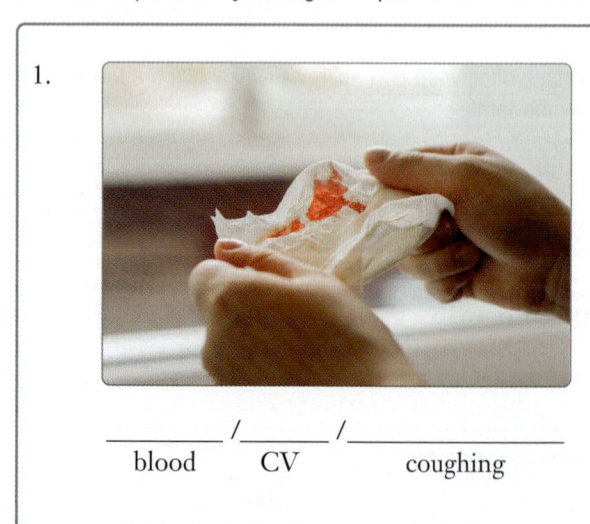

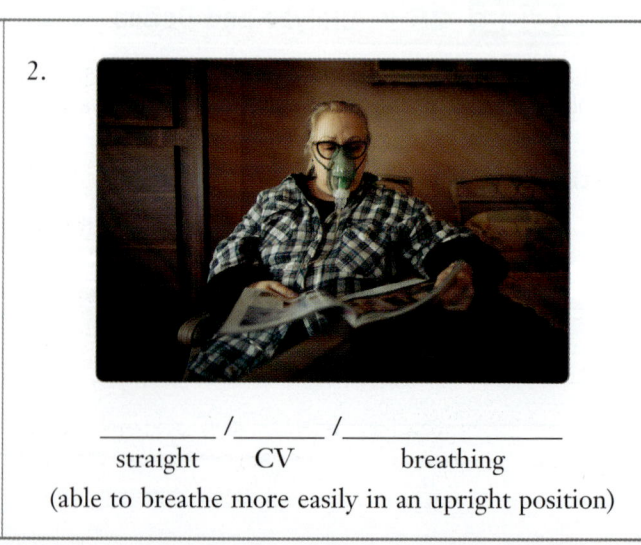

1.
_____ / ____ / _____
blood   CV   coughing

2.
_____ / ____ / _____
straight   CV   breathing
(able to breathe more easily in an upright position)

Chapter 5 Respiratory System   173

3. _____ / ___ / _____
   lung   CV   physician who
                 studies and treats

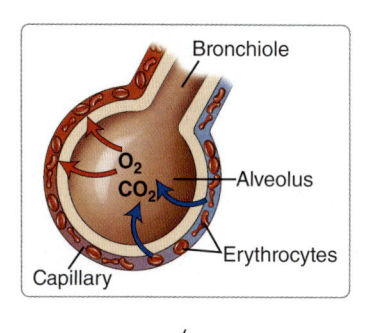

4. _____ / _____
   alveolus   pertaining to

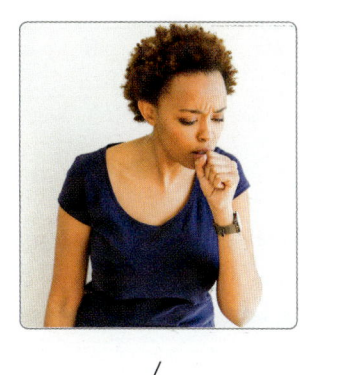

5. _____ / _____
   difficult   breathing

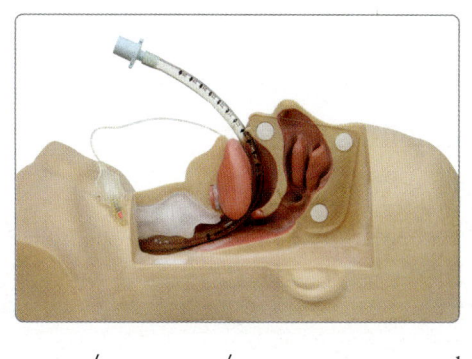

6. _____ / _____ / _____ tube
   within   trachea   pertaining to

B Fill In

Build complementary terms for the following definitions by using the word parts you have learned. *Note: The abbreviation S(WR) indicates the suffix contains a word root.*

EXAMPLE: pertaining to bronchi and alveoli $\frac{bronch}{WR} / \frac{o}{CV} / \frac{alveol}{WR} / \frac{ar}{S}$

1. rapid breathing
   _____ / _____
        P   S(WR)

2. resembling mucus
   _____ / _____
        WR   S

3. discharge from the nose
   _____ / ___ / _____
        WR   CV   S

4. condition of excessive carbon dioxide (in the blood)
   _____ / _____ / _____
        P   WR   S

5. condition of absence of oxygen
   _____ / _____ / _____
        P   WR   S

6. excessive breathing
   _____ / _____
        P   S(WR)

Chapter 5   Respiratory System

7. pertaining to the larynx   ___WR___ / ___S___

8. condition of deficient carbon dioxide (in the blood)   ___P___ / ___WR___ / ___S___

9. normal breathing   ___P___ / ___S(WR)___

10. condition of absence of voice   ___P___ / ___WR___ / ___S___

11. pertaining to the lungs   ___WR___ / ___S___

12. pertaining to the septum   ___WR___ / ___S___

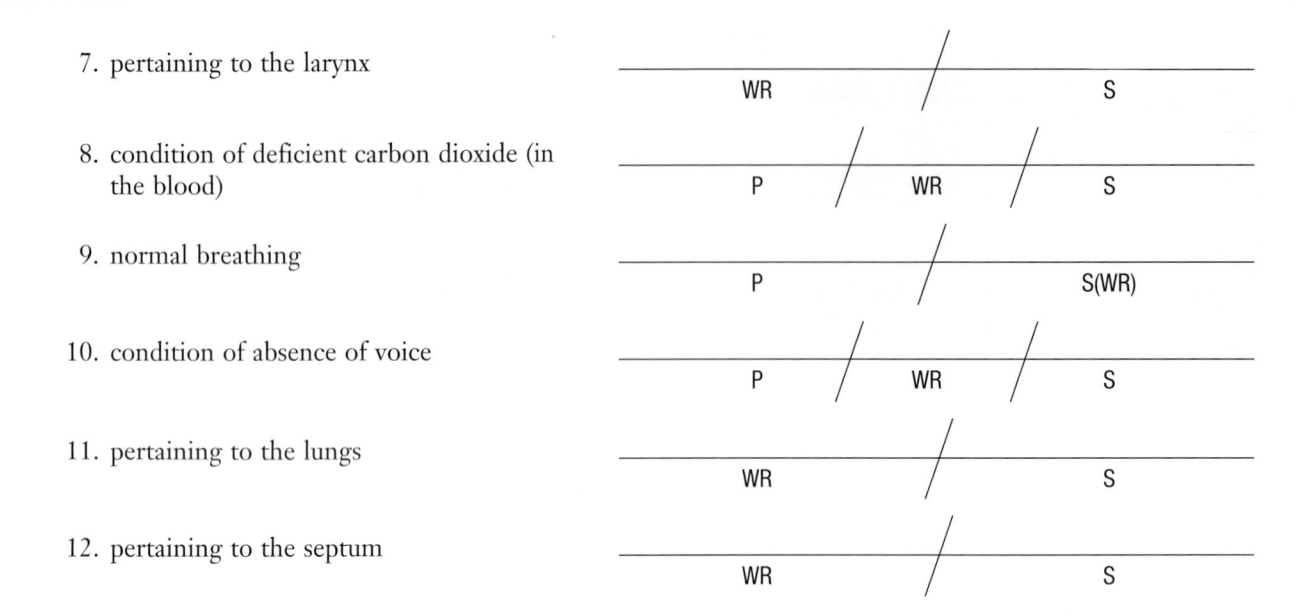

Complementary Terms
NOT BUILT FROM WORD PARTS

Word parts may be present in the following terms; however, their full meanings cannot be translated using definitions of word parts alone.

SIGNS AND SYMPTOMS	
TERM	**DEFINITION**
1. **crackles** (KRAK-els)	discontinuous sounds heard primarily with a stethoscope during inspiration that resemble the sound of the rustling of cellophane; often heard at the base of the lung posteriorly in heart failure, pneumonia, and pulmonary fibrosis (also called **rales**)
2. **effusion** (e-FŪ-zhun)	escape of fluid into tissue or body cavity
3. **hyperventilation** (hī-per-*ven*-ti-LĀ-shun)	ventilation of the lungs beyond normal body needs
4. **hypoventilation** (hī-pō-*ven*-ti-LĀ-shun)	ventilation of the lungs that does not fulfill the body's gas exchange needs
5. **paroxysm** (PAR-ok-siz-em)	periodic, sudden attack
6. **rhonchi** (RONG-kī)	low-pitched, with a snoring quality, breath sounds heard with a stethoscope suggesting secretions in the large airways
7. **stridor** (STRĪD-ir)	harsh, high-pitched breath sound heard on inspiration; indicates an acute laryngeal obstruction
8. **wheeze** (wēz)	whistling noise with a high pitch, caused by air flowing through narrowed airways. Commonly associated with asthma and chronic bronchitis.

TREATMENTS	
TERM	**DEFINITION**
9. **bronchoconstrictor** (*bron*-kō-kon-STRIK-tor)	agent causing narrowing of the bronchi
10. **bronchodilator** (*bron*-kō-dī-LĀ-tor)	agent causing the bronchi to widen

Chapter 5 Respiratory System 175

EQUIPMENT	
TERM	**DEFINITION**
11. **nebulizer** (NEB-ū-lī-zer)	device that creates a mist used to deliver medication for giving respiratory treatment
12. **ventilator** (VEN-ti-lā-tor)	mechanical device used to assist with or substitute for breathing (Fig. 5.13)

DESCRIPTIVE TERMS	
TERM	**DEFINITION**
13. **mucopurulent** (mū-kō-PŪR-ū-lent)	containing both mucus and pus
14. **patent** (PĀ-tent)	open, the opposite of closed or compromised, thus allowing passage of air, as in patent trachea and bronchi (can be applied to any tubular passageway in the body, as in a patent artery, allowing passage of blood)
15. **sputum** (SPŪ-tum)	mucus from the lungs, bronchi, and trachea expelled through the mouth by coughing (also called **phlegm**)

🏛 **SPUTUM** is derived from the Latin **spuere**, meaning **to spit**. In a 1693 dictionary, it is defined as a "secretion thicker than ordinary spittle."

OTHER	
TERM	**DEFINITION**
16. **airway** (ĀR-wā)	passageway by which air enters and leaves the lungs; also a mechanical device used to keep the air passageway open
17. **aspirate** (AS-per-āt)	to withdraw fluid or suction fluid; also to draw foreign material into the respiratory tract
18. **nosocomial infection** (nos-ō-KŌ-mē-al) (in-FEK-shun)	an infection acquired during hospitalization

🔍 Refer to **Appendix E** for pharmacology terms related to the respiratory system.

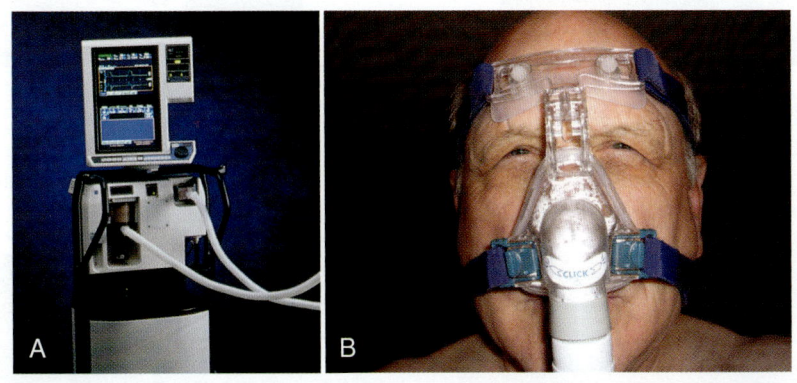

FIG. 5.13 A, Invasive ventilator. Positive pressure ventilator is applied to the patient's airway through an **endotracheal** or **tracheostomy** tube and is used when spontaneous breathing is inadequate to sustain life. **B,** CPAP (continuous positive airway pressure) is a noninvasive ventilation device used for patients who can initiate their own breathing and is often used to treat **obstructive sleep apnea**. BiPAP (bilevel positive airway pressure), not shown, is another noninvasive device that delivers two levels of pressure, one for inspiration and one for expiration, whereas the CPAP machine delivers a predetermined level of pressure.

176 Chapter 5   Respiratory System

EXERCISE 27 ■ Pronounce and Spell

Practice pronunciation and spelling on paper and online.

1. **Practice on Paper**
   a. **Pronounce:** Read the phonetic spelling and say aloud the terms listed in the previous table. Refer to Table 2.2 Pronunciation Key as needed.
   b. **Spell:** Have a study partner read the terms aloud. Write the spelling of the terms on a separate sheet of paper.

2. **Practice Online**
   a. **Access** online learning resources. Go to evolve.elsevier.com > Evolve Resources > Student Resources.
   b. **Pronounce:** Select Audio Glossary > Chapter 5 > Exercise 27. Select a term to hear its pronunciation and repeat aloud.
   c. **Spell:** Select Activities > Chapter 5 > Spell Terms > Exercise 27. Select the audio icon and type the correct spelling of the term.

❑ Check the box when complete.

EXERCISE 28 ■ Fill In

A Label

Write the medical terms pictured and defined.

1. _____
   passageway by which air enters and leaves the lungs; also a mechanical device used to keep the air passageway open

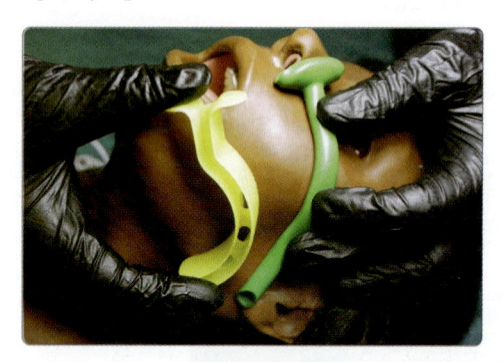

2. _____
   agent causing the bronchi to widen

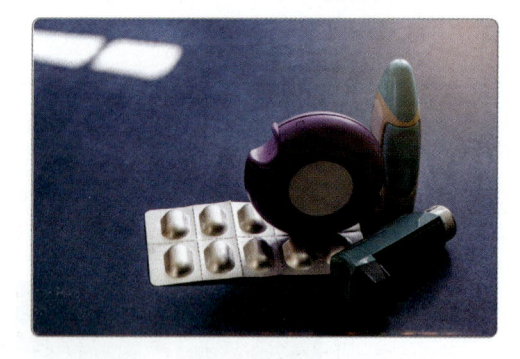

3. _____
   device that creates a mist used to deliver medication for giving respiratory treatment

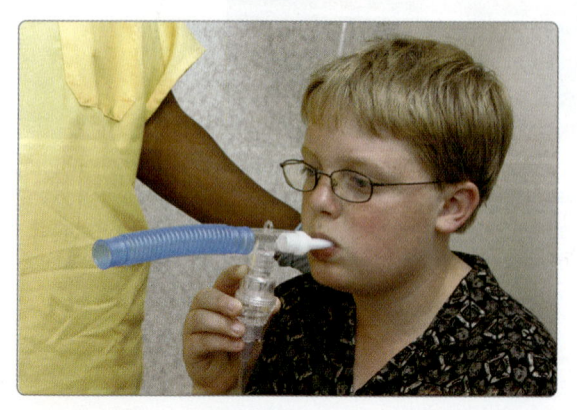

4. _____
   mechanical device used to assist with or substitute for breathing

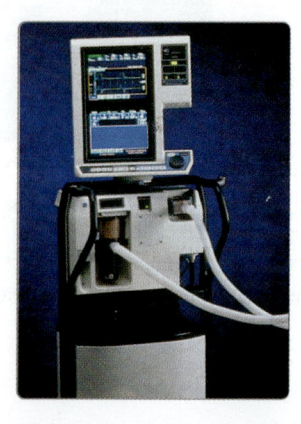

B Identify

Fill in the blanks with the correct terms.

1. Another term for ventilation of the lungs beyond normal body needs is _____.
2. A whistling noise with a high pitch, commonly associated with asthma, is _____.
3. Mucus from the lungs, bronchi, and trachea, expelled through the mouth by coughing, is called _____.
4. To suction or withdraw fluid is to _____.
5. Harsh, high-pitched breath sound heard on inspiration is called _____.
6. Low-pitched breath sounds heard with a stethoscope are called _____.
7. Material containing both mucus and pus is referred to as being _____.
8. _____ is the name given to ventilation of the lungs that does not fulfill the body's gas exchange needs.
9. An infection acquired during hospitalization is called _____.
10. The term that applies to a periodic, sudden attack is _____.
11. An airway must be kept _____ (open) for the patient to breathe.
12. An agent that causes bronchi to narrow is called a(n) _____.
13. _____ is the name given to the escape of fluid into tissue or a body cavity.
14. Resembling the sound of rustling cellophane, _____ may be a presenting sign in pneumonia.

EXERCISE 29 ■ Match

Match the terms in the first column with their correct definitions in the second column.

____ 1. airway
____ 2. aspirate
____ 3. bronchoconstrictor
____ 4. bronchodilator
____ 5. rhonchi
____ 6. crackles
____ 7. hyperventilation
____ 8. effusion
____ 9. stridor

a. low-pitched sounds that suggest secretions in the large airways
b. mechanical device used to keep the air passageway open
c. agent that narrows the bronchi
d. discontinuous sounds heard mainly at the base of the lungs with a stethoscope during inspiration
e. escape of fluid into tissue or body cavity
f. ventilation of the lungs beyond normal body needs
g. to draw foreign material into the respiratory tract
h. agent that widens the bronchi
i. indicates acute laryngeal obstruction

EXERCISE 30 ■ Match

Match the terms in the first column with their correct definitions in the second column.

____ 1. hypoventilation
____ 2. mucopurulent
____ 3. wheeze
____ 4. nebulizer
____ 5. nosocomial infection
____ 6. patent
____ 7. sputum
____ 8. ventilator
____ 9. paroxysm

a. open
b. mucus from lungs, bronchi, and trachea, expelled through the mouth by coughing
c. respiratory treatment device that sends a mist
d. mechanical breathing device
e. ventilation of the lungs that does not fulfill the body's gas exchange needs
f. periodic, sudden attack
g. containing both mucus and pus
h. whistling noise with a high pitch, caused by air flowing through narrowed airways
i. hospital-acquired infection

EXERCISE 31 — Review of Complementary Terms

Can you define, pronounce, and spell the following terms?

acapnia	effusion	mediastinal	rhonchi
airway	endotracheal	mucoid	septal
alveolar	eupnea	mucopurulent	sputum
anoxia	hemoptysis	mucous	stridor
aphonia	hypercapnia	nasopharyngeal	tachypnea
apnea	hyperpnea	nebulizer	thoracic
aspirate	hyperventilation	nosocomial infection	ventilator
bronchoalveolar	hypocapnia	orthopnea	wheeze
bronchoconstrictor	hypopnea	paroxysm	
bronchodilator	hypoxemia	patent	
crackles	hypoxia	pulmonary	
diaphragmatic	hypoventilation	pulmonologist	
dysphonia	intrapleural	pulmonology	
dyspnea	laryngeal	rhinorrhea	

Medical Record Abbreviations

Documentation of a patient's medical history and health care received is stored in medical records. Medical records are the who, what, when, where, and how of patient care. A common format used to record information from patient encounters is the **SOAP note**. SOAP is an acronym formed from the first letters of the note's section titles, including subjective, objective, assessment, and plan (Table 5.2). In documentation of a visit with a primary care provider, the objective section will include the patient's **vital signs (VS)**, including **temperature (T)**, **blood pressure (BP)**, **pulse (P)** rate, and **respiration (R)** rate.

TABLE 5.2 SOAP Note Format

SECTION	ABBREVIATION	DESCRIPTION
Subjective	S	Patient's words describing their health and problems experienced (symptoms)
Objective	O	Physical exam findings and diagnostic test results (signs)
Assessment	A	Provider's interpretation of the patient's condition
Plan	P	Therapeutic treatment, further diagnostic procedures, patient education, follow-up

Abbreviations

DISEASE AND DISORDERS

ABBREVIATION	TERM	ABBREVIATION	TERM
ARDS	acute respiratory distress syndrome	HAP	hospital-acquired pneumonia
CAP	community-acquired pneumonia	IPF	idiopathic pulmonary fibrosis
CF	cystic fibrosis	LTB	laryngotracheobronchitis
cocci	coccidioidomycosis; spoken as a whole word (KAHK-sē)	OSA	obstructive sleep apnea
		PE	pulmonary embolism
COPD	chronic obstructive pulmonary disease	**PE** also abbreviates **physical examination**.	
COVID-19	coronavirus disease; spoken as whole words (CŌ-vid) (NĪN-tēn)	RSV	respiratory syncytial virus
		TB	tuberculosis
flu	influenza; spoken as a whole word (floo)	URI	upper respiratory infection

Chapter 5 Respiratory System

SIGNS AND SYMPTOMS

ABBREVIATION	TERM	ABBREVIATION	TERM
BP	blood pressure	SOB	shortness of breath
P	pulse	T	temperature
R	respirations	VS	vital signs

DIAGNOSTIC

ABBREVIATION	TERM	ABBREVIATION	TERM
ABG	arterial blood gas	PFTs	pulmonary function tests
AFB	acid-fast bacilli	PSG	polysomnography
CXR	chest radiograph (chest x-ray)	VBG	venous blood gas
PFM	peak flow meter	V/Q scan	lung ventilation/perfusion scan

TREATMENTS

ABBREVIATION	TERM
CPAP	continuous positive airway pressure; spoken as a whole word (SĒ-pap)

DESCRIPTIVE

ABBREVIATION	TERM	ABBREVIATION	TERM
LLL	left lower lobe	RLL	right lower lobe
LUL	left upper lobe	RML	right middle lobe
		RUL	right upper lobe

OTHER

ABBREVIATION	TERM	ABBREVIATION	TERM
CO_2	carbon dioxide	O_2	oxygen

🔍 Refer to **Appendix D** for a complete list of abbreviations.

EXERCISE 32 ■ Fill In

Write the terms abbreviated.

1. A variety of tests are used to diagnose **COPD** _____ _____ _____ _____, including:
   - **PFTs** _____ _____,
   - **CXR** _____ _____,
   - **ABG** _____ _____, and
   - **VBG** _____.
2. **SOB** _____ _____ _____ is often a symptom of COPD.
3. A. The lobes of the left lung are:
   - **LUL** _____
   - **LLL** _____

   B. The lobes of the right lung are:
   - **RUL** _____

Chapter 5 Respiratory System

- RML _____
- RLL _____

4. AFB _____ - _____ _____ smear is used to support the diagnosis of TB _____.

5. PSG _____ is used to confirm the diagnosis of OSA _____ _____ _____, which can be treated with CPAP _____ _____ _____.

6. Respiration is the exchange of O_2 _____ and CO_2 _____ _____ between the atmosphere and body cells.

7. Measurements obtained from using a PFM _____ _____ _____ can be used to adjust medication for persons with asthma.

8. The etiology of IPF _____ _____ _____ is unknown.

9. The flu _____ and COVID-19 _____ _____ are serious systemic infections caused by viruses. URIs _____ _____ _____s are most often caused by viruses, though they can also be caused by bacteria.

10. HAP _____ - _____ _____ is one type of nosocomial infection.

11. A V/Q scan _____ _____ / _____ _____ was ordered to rule out PE _____ _____.

12. ARDS _____ _____ _____ _____ is a life-threatening lung condition that usually occurs after a serious illness or injury.

13. CF _____ _____ is a hereditary disorder of the exocrine glands characterized by excess mucus production in the respiratory tract, pancreatic deficiency, and other symptoms.

14. The acute form of LTB _____ _____ is called croup.

15. In CAP _____ - _____ _____ the infection occurs outside of a healthcare setting.

16. Cocci _____ occurs primarily in the southwestern states and is caused by the inhalation of fungal spores growing in the soil that have become airborne through wind or other disturbances.

17. VS _____ _____ are measured to reveal information about the body's basic functions. The four main VS routinely measured by healthcare professionals are: T _____, BP _____ _____, P _____ rate, and R _____ rate.

18. Vaccines are now available to prevent RSV _____ _____ _____ infections for those who are pregnant, infants aged 8 months and younger during RSV season, and people over age 75. RSV generally circulates in the winter and causes cold-like symptoms, which can progress into severe illness in infants and in elders.

TABLE 5.3 Other Common Abbreviations Used in Respiratory Care

ABBREVIATION	TERM	ABBREVIATION	TERM
BiPAP	bilevel positive airway pressure	MDI	metered-dose inhaler
CPT	chest physiotherapy	NIPPV	noninvasive positive-pressure ventilator
DPI	dry powder inhaler	PEP	positive expiratory pressure
HME	heat/moisture exchanger	RT	respiratory therapist
IPPB	intermittent positive-pressure breathing	SVN	small-volume nebulizer
		VAP	ventilator-associated pneumonia

Chapter 5 Respiratory System 181

PRACTICAL APPLICATION

EXERCISE 33 ■ Case Study: Translate Between Everyday Language and Medical Language

CASE STUDY: Roberta Pawlaski

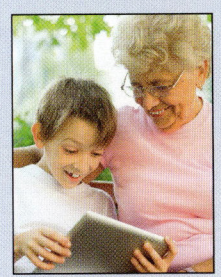

Roberta is experiencing difficulty breathing. She notices it gets worse when she tries to do chores around the house. This has been going on for about 4 days. She also has a cough and a runny nose. Today when she woke up, she noticed that her throat was very sore. She also thinks that she might have a fever because she feels hot all over. She tried taking some over-the-counter cough medicine, but this didn't seem to help. She notices when she coughs that a thick yellow mucus comes out. She hasn't had a cough like this since before she quit smoking about 10 years ago. She remembers that her grandson who stays with her after school has missed school because of a cold. She decides to call her doctor to schedule an appointment.

Now that you have worked through Chapter 5, on the respiratory system, consider the medical terms that might be used to describe Roberta's experience. See the Chapter at a Glance section at the end of the chapter for a list of terms that might apply.

A. Underline phrases in the case study that could be substituted with medical terms.

B. Write the medical term and its definition for three of the phrases you underlined.

MEDICAL TERM	DEFINITION
1. _____	_____
2. _____	_____
3. _____	_____

DOCUMENTATION: Excerpt from Hospital Admission Report

Roberta was able to see her primary care physician later that afternoon. In her electronic health record (EHR), it was noted in the Objective section of the report:

The patient is in no acute distress but exhibits dyspnea when walking. A fair amount of gray mucoid sputum was produced on forced cough. HEENT exam is normal except for erythema and swelling of the pharynx without exudates. Tympanic membranes are clear. There is a moderate amount of purulent rhinorrhea. The nasal mucosa is moderately swollen. Auscultation of the heart reveals a regular rhythm without a murmur, gallop, or rub. The chest is dull to percussion at the right lower base and there are crackles and rhonchi as well.

C. Underline medical terms presented in Chapter 5 used in the previous excerpt from Roberta's medical record. See the Chapter at a Glance section at the end of the chapter for a complete list.

D. Select and define three of the medical terms you underlined. To check your answers, go to Appendix A.

MEDICAL TERM	DEFINITION
1. _____	_____
2. _____	_____
3. _____	_____

Chapter 5 Respiratory System

EXERCISE 34 ■ Interact with Medical Documents

A

Read the report and complete it by writing medical terms on answer lines within the document. Definitions of terms to be written appear after the document.

516987-RSP MARQUEZ, Victor

Name: MARQUEZ, Victor MR#: 516987-RSP Sex: M Allergies: None known
DOB: 02/01/19XX Age: 55 PCP: Valdez, Miguel MD

Date: 01/18/20XX
Family Medicine Clinic Office Visit Note

Chief Complaint: Cough

Subjective: Victor Marquez is a 55-year-old male who presents with a cough for the past 9 weeks. Initially the cough was dry, but it has now become productive with green 1._____. About 5 days ago he started experiencing 2._____. He also complains of 3._____ after 4._____ of coughing, along with fatigue and a 10-lb unintentional weight loss over the last 9 weeks. Past medical history is noncontributory. Family history is significant for a brother who died of AIDs-related 5._____.

Objective: VS: T = 99.5° F, 6._____ = 20, P = 80, BP = 100/64

Examination: General: Thin male, pleasant, slight difficulty with conversation due to 7._____. Head and neck examinations are normal. Pulmonary exam is significant for dullness to percussion suggestive of 8._____ and 9._____ heard on auscultation of the right upper lung fields. Cardiac exam is normal, and examination of the extremities reveals normal pulses and no cyanosis.

Chest radiography reveals a 3 × 3 cm lung mass in the right upper lobe that has irregular margins.

Assessment: Chronic cough accompanied by dyspnea and a 10-lb weight loss and a mass on chest radiograph. Possible diagnoses include 10._____, tuberculosis, or 11._____.

Plan: We will obtain blood tests and refer to 12._____ for a possible lung biopsy.

Mr. Marquez will return here for follow-up after completion of these steps.

Electronically signed: Miguel Valdez, MD, 01/18/20XX 16:45

Definitions of Medical Terms to Complete the Document

Write the medical terms defined on corresponding answer lines in the document.

1. mucus from the lungs, bronchi, and trachea expelled through the mouth by coughing
2. coughing of blood (or blood-stained sputum)
3. difficult breathing
4. periodic, sudden attack (plural)
5. infectious bacterial disease, most commonly spread by inhalation of small particles and usually affecting the lungs
6. respiration (abbreviation)
7. shortness of breath (abbreviation)
8. fluid in the pleural cavity caused by a disease process or trauma
9. discontinuous sounds heard primarily with a stethoscope during inspiration that resemble the sound of the rustling of cellophane
10. cancerous tumor originating in a bronchus
11. fungal disease affecting the lungs and sometimes other organs of the body
12. study of x-rays

Chapter 5 Respiratory System

EXERCISE 34 ■ Interact with Medical Documents—cont'd

B

Read the medical report and answer the questions below it.

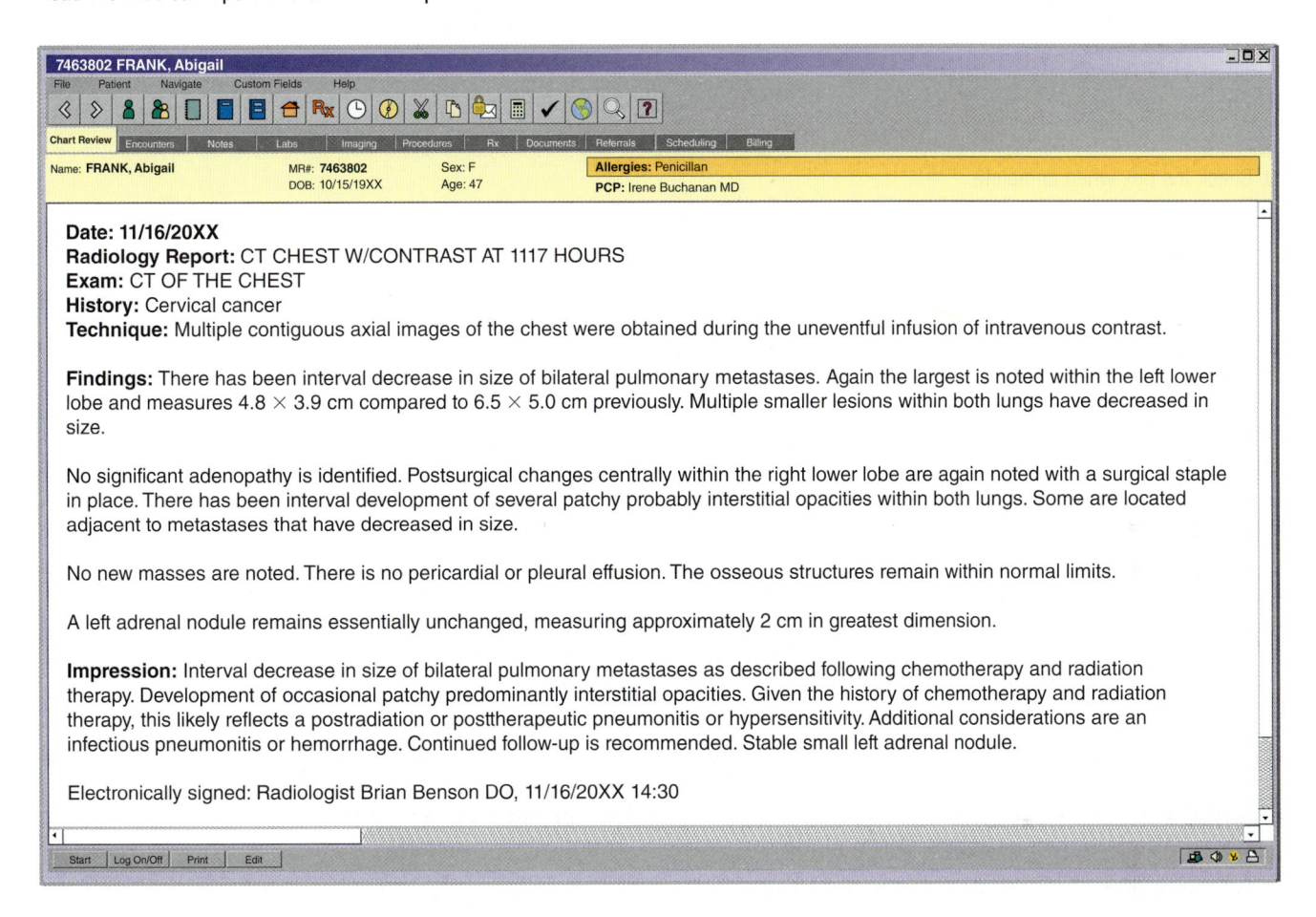

7463802 FRANK, Abigail

Name: FRANK, Abigail **MR#:** 7463802 **Sex:** F **Allergies:** Penicillan
 DOB: 10/15/19XX **Age:** 47 **PCP:** Irene Buchanan MD

Date: 11/16/20XX
Radiology Report: CT CHEST W/CONTRAST AT 1117 HOURS
Exam: CT OF THE CHEST
History: Cervical cancer
Technique: Multiple contiguous axial images of the chest were obtained during the uneventful infusion of intravenous contrast.

Findings: There has been interval decrease in size of bilateral pulmonary metastases. Again the largest is noted within the left lower lobe and measures 4.8 × 3.9 cm compared to 6.5 × 5.0 cm previously. Multiple smaller lesions within both lungs have decreased in size.

No significant adenopathy is identified. Postsurgical changes centrally within the right lower lobe are again noted with a surgical staple in place. There has been interval development of several patchy probably interstitial opacities within both lungs. Some are located adjacent to metastases that have decreased in size.

No new masses are noted. There is no pericardial or pleural effusion. The osseous structures remain within normal limits.

A left adrenal nodule remains essentially unchanged, measuring approximately 2 cm in greatest dimension.

Impression: Interval decrease in size of bilateral pulmonary metastases as described following chemotherapy and radiation therapy. Development of occasional patchy predominantly interstitial opacities. Given the history of chemotherapy and radiation therapy, this likely reflects a postradiation or posttherapeutic pneumonitis or hypersensitivity. Additional considerations are an infectious pneumonitis or hemorrhage. Continued follow-up is recommended. Stable small left adrenal nodule.

Electronically signed: Radiologist Brian Benson DO, 11/16/20XX 14:30

Use the medical report above to answer the questions.

_____ 1. The diagnostic imaging exam performed uses
   a. computerized radiographic images producing "slices"
   b. ionizing radiation produced by a light source
   c. mathematically constructed images and magnetic fields
   d. radiopharmaceuticals

2. **T F** Fluid is present in the pleural space.

3. **T F** Following chemotherapy and radiation, metastases in one lung were decreased.

4. **T F** The patchy interstitial opacities likely reflect a postradiation or posttherapeutic inflammation of the lung.

EXERCISE 35 ■ Use Medical Language in Online Electronic Health Records

Select the correct medical terms to complete three medical records in one patient's electronic file.

🌐 Access online resources at evolve.elsevier.com > Evolve Resources > Student Resources > Activities > Chapter 5 > Electronic Health Records

Topic: COPD
Record 1, Chart Review: Progress Note
Record 2, Imaging: Radiology Report
Record 3, Notes: Pulmonary Function Department Note

❏ Check the box when complete.

> 💡 Healthcare records are stored and used in an electronic system called **Electronic Health Records (EHR)**. Electronic health records contain a collection of health information of an individual patient; the digitally formatted record can be shared through computer networks with patients, physicians, and other healthcare providers.

EXERCISE 36 ■ Use Medical Terms in Clinical Statements

For each phrase printed in bold, circle the medical term or abbreviation defined. Answers are listed in Appendix A. For pronunciation practice read the answers aloud.

1. A symptom is an effect noticed and experienced by the person who has the condition and is part of the subjective portion of a SOAP note. Examples of symptoms include **difficult breathing** (dyspnea, eupnea, apnea), which is sometimes called **shortness of breath** (COPD, SOB, OSA). Another respiratory symptom is **breathing (more easily) in a straight (upright position)** (orthopnea, tachypnea, hyperpnea).

2. Signs are observable findings that can be identified by another person and make up the objective portion of a SOAP note. Signs of an illness can be detected using various tools, including direct observation, auscultation, and laboratory tests. Examples of respiratory signs include **discontinuous sounds heard primarily with a stethoscope during inspiration that resemble the sound of the rustling of cellophane** (wheezes, rhonchi, crackles) and **deficient oxygen in the blood** (hypercapnia, hypopnea, hypoxemia).

3. **Inflammation of the sinus (membranes)** (sinusitis, sinusotomy, nasopharyngitis) is caused by bacteria, viruses, or fungi. It often occurs after an upper respiratory infection or may follow acute allergic **inflammation of the nose (nasal membranes)** (rhinorrhagia, rhinorrhea, rhinitis). Symptoms include **discharge from the nose** (rhinorrhagia, rhinorrhea, rhinitis), malaise, pain, and thick yellow-green drainage. **Pertaining to visual examination within** (endoscope, endoscopic, endoscopy) surgery, drugs, and heat therapy may be used as treatment.

4. **Arterial blood gas** (ABG, BP, PFTs) is a laboratory test performed on a blood sample to measure pH and the amount of **oxygen** (CO_2, O_2, R) and **carbon dioxide** (CO_2, O_2, R) in the blood. The test may be ordered in patients with **progressive lung disease obstructing air flow, which makes breathing difficult** (CF, COPD, ARDS), **life-threatening lung condition caused by disease or injury** (acute respiratory distress syndrome, asthma, croup), or **hereditary disorder of the exocrine glands characterized by excess mucus production in the respiratory tract** (coronavirus disease, cystic fibrosis, diphtheria).

5. A positive result on a **test performed on individuals who may have been exposed to tuberculosis** (pulmonary function test, peak flow meter, PPD skin test) usually leads to a **radiographic image of the chest performed to evaluate the lungs and the heart** (chest radiograph, lung ventilation/perfusion scan, chest computed tomography scan) to determine whether active **infectious bacterial disease, most commonly spread by inhalation of small particles and usually affecting the lungs** (influenza, coccidioidomycosis, tuberculosis) is present.

EXERCISE 37 ■ Pronounce Medical Terms in Use

Practice pronunciation of terms by reading aloud the following paragraph. Use the phonetic spellings to assist with pronunciation. The script also contains medical terms not presented in the chapter. If interested, research their meanings using a medical dictionary and reliable online sources.

> A 24-year-old man visited the emergency department because of **dyspnea** (DISP-nē-a), **hyperpnea** (hī-perp-NĒ-a), and **paroxysms** (PAR-ok-sizms) of cough producing thick, tenacious mucus. He had a history of **asthma** (AZ-ma) since the age of 12 years. A **chest radiograph** (chest) (RĀ-dē-ō-graf) was negative for **pneumonia** (nū-MŌ-nē-a). **Arterial blood gas** (ar-TĒ-rē-al) (blud) (gas) showed **hypoxemia** (hī-pok-SĒ-mē-a) but no **hypercapnia** (hī-per-KAP-nē-a). **Pulmonary function tests** (PUL-mō-ner-ē) (FUNK-shun) (tests) disclosed bronchoconstriction, which was corrected by a **bronchodilator** (bron-kō-dī-LĀ-tor). A **nebulizer** (NEB-ū-lī-zer) was prescribed for treatment. The asthma attack was probably precipitated by an episode of **bronchitis** (bron-KĪ-tis).

CHAPTER REVIEW

EXERCISE 38 ■ Chapter Content Quiz

Test your understanding of terms and abbreviations introduced in this chapter. Circle the letter for the medical term or abbreviation related to the words in italics

1. The patient was admitted to the emergency department with a *severe nosebleed*.
   a. rhinomycosis
   b. epistaxis
   c. nasopharyngitis

2. The accident caused damage to the *larynx*, necessitating a *surgical repair*.
   a. laryngectomy
   b. laryngostomy
   c. laryngoplasty

3. Mr. Garcia was *breathing more easily in a straight, upright position*, so the nurse recorded that he had:
   a. orthopnea
   b. eupnea
   c. dyspnea

4. The *test on arterial blood to determine oxygen, carbon dioxide, and pH levels* indicated that the patient was *deficient in oxygen*, or had:
   a. pulse oximetry, dysphonia
   b. pulmonary functions tests, hypocapnia
   c. arterial blood gas, hypoxia

5. The physician informed the patient that her *coughing of blood* might be due to tuberculosis.
   a. hemoptysis
   b. pneumothorax
   c. thoracentesis

6. The patient reported dizziness brought on by *ventilation of the lungs beyond normal bodily needs*.
   a. hyperventilation
   b. hypoventilation
   c. dysphonia

7. The physician ordered a *device that delivers mist* treatment for her patient with severe asthma symptoms.
   a. airway
   b. nebulizer
   c. ventilator

8. The patient with *blood in the chest cavity* was diagnosed as having:
   a. pneumothorax
   b. pleuritis
   c. hemothorax

9. After surgery, the patient had *foreign matter causing a block in the circulation to the pulmonary artery*.
   a. pleural effusion
   b. pulmonary edema
   c. pulmonary embolism

10. The patient was diagnosed as having *a fungal disease affecting the lung*.
    a. obstructive sleep apnea
    b. coccidioidomycosis
    c. tuberculosis

11. The physician ordered a *radiographic image of the chest* because he suspected *community-acquired pneumonia*.
    a. chest radiograph, CAP
    b. chest CT scan, CPAP
    c. bronchoscopy, HAP

12. The patient received an *intradermal injection* to determine if she had been exposed to TB.
    a. AFB
    b. ABG
    c. PPD skin test

13. The patient was experiencing *rapid breathing*.
    a. hypopnea
    b. tachypnea
    c. eupnea

14. The nurse practitioner heard *discontinuous sounds during respiration that resembled the sound of the rustling of cellophane*.
    a. stridor
    b. rhonchi
    c. crackles

15. *Fusion of the pleura* was performed for the patient with *chronic fluid in the pleural cavity caused by a disease process or trauma* due to untreatable broncho-genic carcinoma.
    a. pneumonectomy, pulmonary edema
    b. pleurodesis, pleural effusion
    c. bronchoplasty, pneumothorax

16. *Serious bacterial infection affecting the mucous membranes of the nose and throat* is less common in developed countries where vaccines are readily available.
    a. idiopathic pulmonary fibrosis
    b. croup
    c. diphtheria

17. Patients with asthma or chronic bronchitis may experience *whistling noise with a high pitch, caused by air flowing through narrowed airways*.
    a. wheeze
    b. rhonchi
    c. crackles

18. A chest CT scan was ordered for the patient with *chronic progressive lung disorder characterized by increasing scarring, which ultimately reduces the capacity of the lungs*.
    a. PE
    b. ARDS
    c. IPF

19. *Escape of fluid into tissue or body cavity* may occur in a variety of locations, including around the lungs (pleural), the heart (pericardial), or the joints.
    a. paroxysm
    b. stridor
    c. effusion

20. *Visual examination of the mediastinum* may be performed in patients with lung cancer to biopsy the lymph nodes and assist with staging of the malignancy.
    a. mediastinoscopy
    b. bronchoscopy
    c. thoracoscopy

CHAPTER AT A GLANCE — Word Parts New to this Chapter

COMBINING FORMS

adenoid/o	lob/o	pulmon/o
alveol/o	mediastin/o	py/o
atel/o	muc/o	rhin/o
bronch/o	nas/o	sept/o
bronchi/o	orth/o	sinus/o
capn/o	ox/i	somn/o
coni/o	pharyng/o	spir/o
diaphragmat/o	phon/o	thorac/o
epiglott/o	pleur/o	tonsill/o
hem/o	pneum/o	trache/o
laryng/o	pneumon/o	

PREFIXES

a-
an-
endo-
eu-
poly-
tachy-

SUFFIXES

-ar	-pnea
-ary	-ptysis
-cele	-rrhagia
-centesis	-scope
-desis	-scopic
-eal	-scopy
-ectasis	-spasm
-ectomy	-stenosis
-emia	-stomy
-meter	-thorax
-metry	-tomy

CHAPTER AT A GLANCE — Respiratory System Terms Built from Word Parts

DISEASE AND DISORDER
adenoiditis
alveolitis
atelectasis
bronchiectasis
bronchitis
bronchogenic carcinoma
bronchopneumonia
bronchospasm
diaphragmatocele
epiglottitis
hemothorax
laryngitis
laryngospasm
laryngotracheobronchitis (LTB)
lobar pneumonia
nasopharyngitis
pharyngitis
pleuritis
pneumoconiosis
pneumonia
pneumonitis
pneumothorax
pulmonary neoplasm
pyothorax
rhinitis
rhinomycosis
rhinorrhagia
sinusitis
tonsillitis
tracheitis
tracheostenosis

SURGICAL
adenoidectomy
bronchoplasty
laryngectomy
laryngoplasty
laryngostomy
laryngotracheotomy
lobectomy
pleurodesis
pneumonectomy
rhinoplasty
septoplasty
sinusotomy
thoracentesis
thoracotomy
tonsillectomy
tracheoplasty
tracheostomy
tracheotomy

DIAGNOSTIC
bronchoscope
bronchoscopy
capnometer
endoscope
endoscopic
endoscopy
laryngoscope
laryngoscopy
mediastinoscopy
oximeter
polysomnography (PSG)
spirometer
spirometry
thoracoscope
thoracoscopy

COMPLEMENTARY
acapnia
alveolar
anoxia
aphonia
apnea
bronchoalveolar
diaphragmatic
dysphonia
dyspnea
endotracheal
eupnea
hemoptysis
hypercapnia
hyperpnea
hypocapnia
hypopnea
hypoxemia
hypoxia
intrapleural
laryngeal
mediastinal
mucoid
mucous
nasopharyngeal
orthopnea
pulmonary
pulmonologist
pulmonology
rhinorrhea
septal
tachypnea
thoracic

CHAPTER AT A GLANCE — Respiratory System Terms NOT Built from Word Parts

DISEASE AND DISORDER
acute respiratory distress syndrome (ARDS)
asphyxia
asthma
chronic obstructive pulmonary disease (COPD)
coccidioidomycosis (cocci)
coronavirus disease (COVID-19)
croup
cystic fibrosis (CF)
deviated septum
diphtheria
emphysema
epistaxis
idiopathic pulmonary fibrosis (IPF)
influenza (flu)
obstructive sleep apnea (OSA)
pertussis
pleural effusion
pulmonary edema
pulmonary embolism (PE)
tuberculosis (TB)
upper respiratory infection (URI)

DIAGNOSTIC
acid-fast bacilli (AFB) smear
arterial blood gas (ABG)
auscultation
chest computed tomography (CT) scan
chest radiograph (CXR)
lung ventilation/perfusion scan (V/Q scan)
peak flow meter (PFM)
percussion
PPD skin test
pulmonary function tests (PFTs)
pulse oximetry
stethoscope

COMPLEMENTARY
airway
aspirate
bronchoconstrictor
bronchodilator
crackles
effusion
hyperventilation
hypoventilation
mucopurulent
nebulizer
nosocomial infection
paroxysm
patent
rhonchi
sputum
stridor
ventilator
wheeze

PART 2 BODY SYSTEMS

6 Urinary System

Objectives

Upon completion of this chapter, you will be able to:

1. Pronounce organs and anatomic structures of the urinary system.
2. Define and spell word parts related to the urinary system.
3. Define, pronounce, and spell disease and disorder terms related to the urinary system.
4. Define, pronounce, and spell surgical terms related to the urinary system.
5. Define, pronounce, and spell diagnostic terms related to the urinary system.
6. Define, pronounce, and spell complementary terms related to the urinary system.
7. Interpret the meaning of abbreviations related to the urinary system.
8. Apply medical language in clinical contexts.

TABLE 6.1 Chronic Kidney Disease Stages, 201

Outline

ANATOMY, 189
Function, 189
Organs and Anatomic Structures of the Urinary System, 189

WORD PARTS, 192
Urinary System Combining Forms, 192
Combining Forms Used with Urinary System Terms, 192
Prefixes, 192
Suffixes, 192

MEDICAL TERMS, 197
Disease and Disorder Terms, 197
    Built from Word Parts, 197
    NOT Built from Word Parts, 201
Surgical Terms, 203
    Built from Word Parts and
        NOT Built from Word Parts, 203
Diagnostic Terms, 209
    Built from Word Parts and
        NOT Built from Word Parts, 209
Complementary Terms, 214
    Built from Word Parts, 214
    NOT Built from Word Parts, 218
Abbreviations, 222

PRACTICAL APPLICATION, 223
CASE STUDY Translate Between Everyday Language and Medical Language, 223
Interact with Medical Documents, 224
Use Medical Language in Online Electronic Health Records, 225
Use Medical Terms in Clinical Statements, 226
Pronounce Medical Terms in Use, 226

CHAPTER REVIEW, 227
Chapter Content Quiz, 227
Chapter at a Glance, 228

Answers to Chapter Exercises, Appendix A

Chapter 6 Urinary System

ANATOMY

Organs of the urinary system are the kidneys, ureters, bladder, and urethra (Figs. 6.1, 6.2, and 6.3).

Function

The urinary system removes waste material from the body, regulates fluid volume, maintains electrolyte concentration in the body fluid, and assists in blood pressure regulation. The kidneys secrete urine formed from water and waste materials such as urea, potassium chloride, sodium chloride, phosphates, and other elements. Urea is the primary compound in human urine. The liver breaks down proteins in the blood to produce ammonia. Because ammonia is toxic, it is combined with other elements to form urea, which is transported in the bloodstream to the kidneys. The kidneys filter the blood and extract urea to form urine. Urine is collected in the renal pelvis of the kidney and is transported through the ureters into the bladder, where it is stored until it can be eliminated. Urine passes from the bladder through the urethra and urinary meatus to the outside of the body (Fig. 6.4).

Organs and Anatomic Structures of the Urinary System

TERM	DEFINITION
kidney (KID-nē)	one of two bean-shaped organs located on each side of the vertebral column on the posterior wall of the abdominal cavity covered anteriorly by the parietal peritoneum. Their function is to remove waste products from the blood and to aid in maintaining water and electrolyte balances.
nephron (NEF-ron)	urine-producing microscopic structure. Approximately 1 million nephrons are located in each kidney.
glomerulus (*pl.* glomeruli) (glō-MER-ū-lus) (glō-MER-ū-lī)	cluster of capillaries at the entrance of the nephron. The process of filtering the blood, thereby forming urine, begins here.

GLOMERULUS is derived from the Latin **glomus**, which means **ball of thread**. It was thought that the rounded cluster of capillary loops at the nephron's entrance resembled thread in a ball.

renal pelvis (RĒ-nal) (PEL-vis)	funnel-shaped reservoir in the kidney that collects the urine and passes it to the ureter
hilum (HĪ-lum)	indentation on the medial side of the kidney where the renal artery, vein, and pelvis are located and the ureter leaves the kidney
ureters (Ū-re-ters)	two slender tubes, approximately 10 to 13 inches (26 to 33 cm) long, that receive the urine from the kidneys and carry it to the posterior portion of the bladder
urinary bladder (Ū-ri-nar-ē) (BLAD-er)	muscular, hollow organ that temporarily holds the urine. As it fills, the thick, muscular wall becomes thinner, and the organ increases in size.

BLADDER is a derivative of the Anglo-Saxon **blaeddre**, meaning a **blister** or **windbag**.

urethra (ū-RĒ-thra)	lowest part of the urinary tract, through which the urine passes from the urinary bladder to the outside of the body. This narrow tube varies in length by sex. It is approximately 1.5 inches (3.8 cm) long in the female and approximately 8 inches (20 cm) in the male, in whom it is also part of the reproductive system. It carries seminal fluid (semen) at the time of ejaculation.
urinary meatus (Ū-ri-nar-ē) (mē-Ā-tus)	opening through which the urine passes to the outside of the body

MEATUS is derived from the Latin **meare**, meaning **to pass** or **to go**. Other anatomic passages share the same name, such as the auditory meatus.

190 **Chapter 6** Urinary System

ORGANS OF THE URINARY SYSTEM

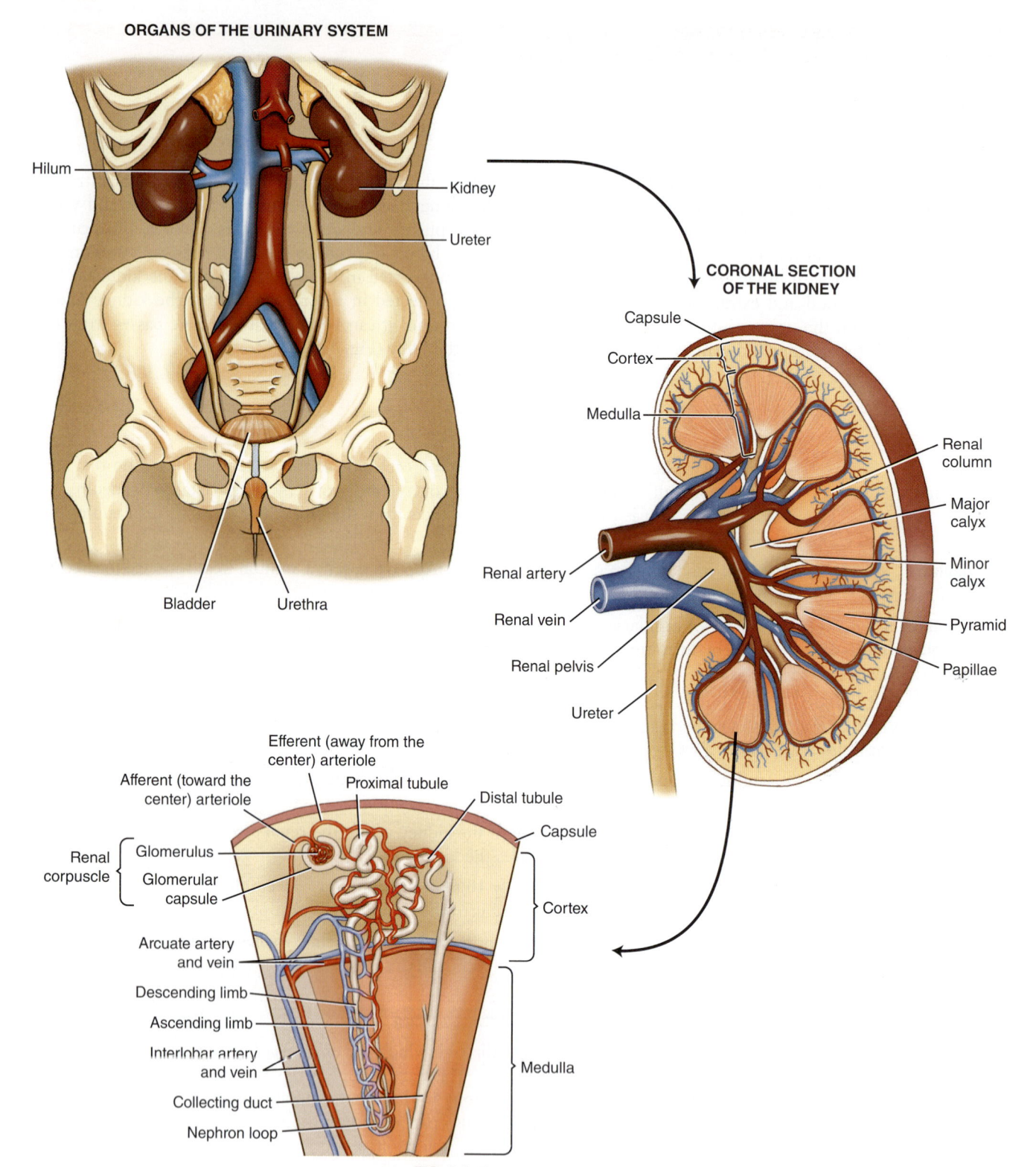

CORONAL SECTION OF THE KIDNEY

FIG. 6.1 The urinary system.

Chapter 6 Urinary System 191

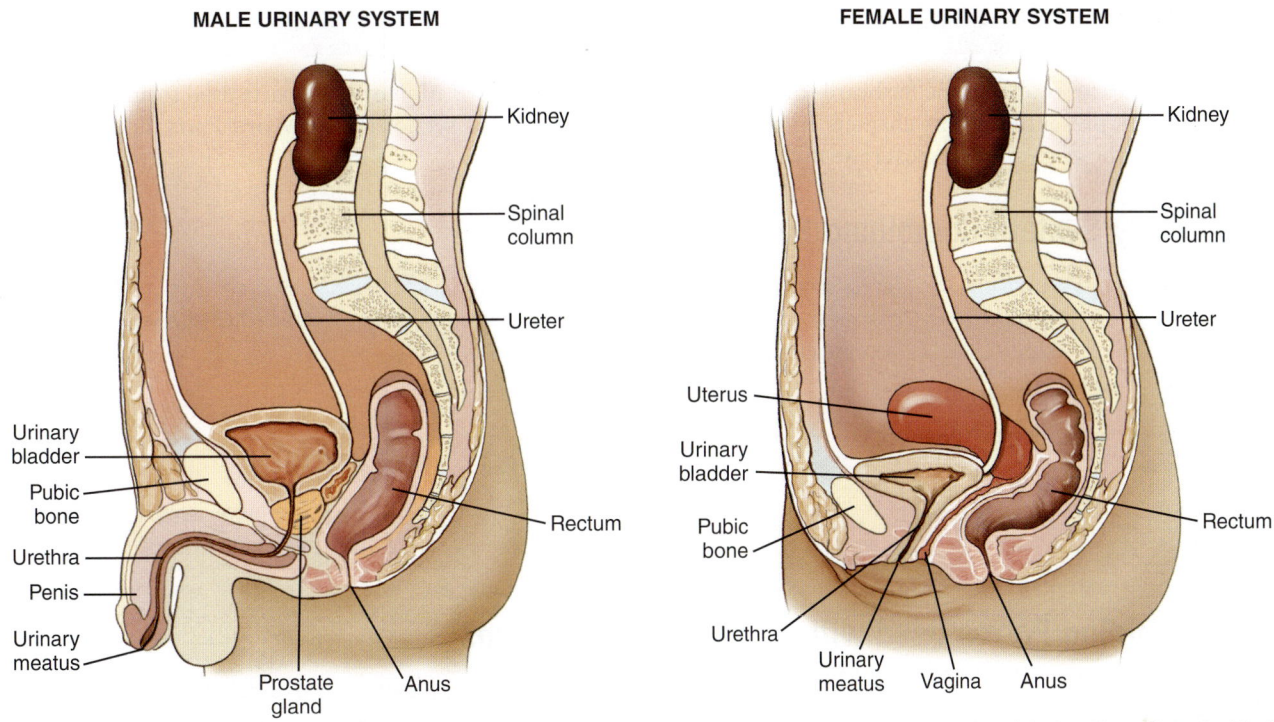

FIG. 6.2 Male and female urinary systems, sagittal view. The male urethra is approximately 8 inches (20 cm) in length compared with the female urethra, which is approximately 1.5 inches (3.8 cm) in length.

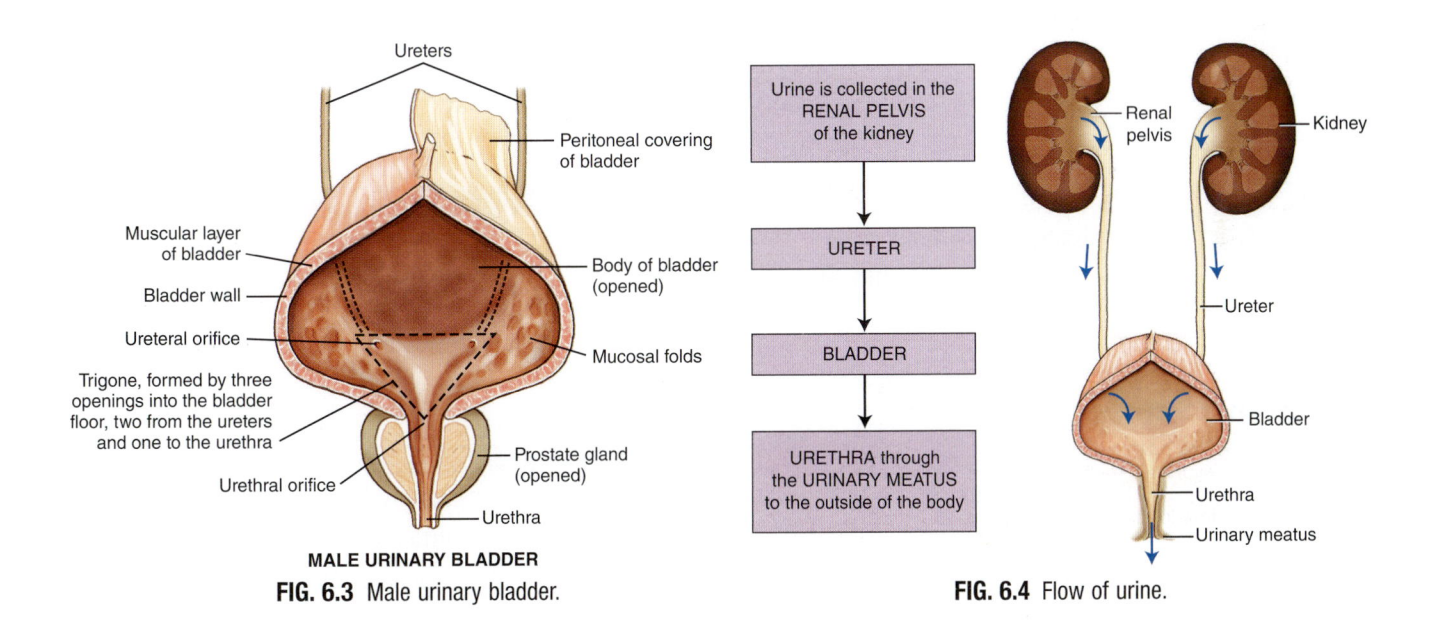

FIG. 6.3 Male urinary bladder.

FIG. 6.4 Flow of urine.

PRONOUNCE ANATOMIC STRUCTURES

Practice saying aloud each of the organs and specific structures on the previous pages.

To hear the terms, go to Evolve Resources at www.evolve.elsevier.com and select:
Student Resources > Audio Glossary > Chapter 6 > **Anatomic Structures**

❑ Check the box when complete.

Chapter 6 Urinary System

🔗 WORD PARTS

Use paper flashcards or electronic flashcards on Evolve to assist with memorization of word parts used to analyze, define, and build terms presented in this chapter. To reinforce learning, study one section of the Word Parts Table at a time, then complete the corresponding exercise on the following pages.

1 ■ Urinary System Combining Forms

COMBINING FORM	DEFINITION	COMBINING FORM	DEFINITION
cyst/o	bladder, sac (*Note:* refers to the urinary bladder unless otherwise identified.)	🏛 **PYELOS** is the Greek word for **tub-shaped vessel**, which describes the renal pelvis shape.	
glomerul/o	glomerulus	ren/o	kidney
meat/o	meatus (opening)	ureter/o	ureter
nephr/o	kidney	urethr/o	urethra
pyel/o	renal pelvis	vesic/o	bladder, sac (*Note:* refers to the urinary bladder unless otherwise identified.)

2 ■ Combining Forms Used with Urinary System Terms

COMBINING FORM	DEFINITION	COMBINING FORM	DEFINITION
albumin/o	albumin	lith/o	stone(s), calculus (*pl.* calculi)
azot/o	urea, nitrogen	noct/i	night (*Note:* the combining vowel is i.)
blast/o	developing cell, germ cell	olig/o	scanty, few
glycos/o	sugar	son/o	sound
hem/o	blood	ur/o	urine, urinary tract
hydr/o	water	urin/o	urine, urinary tract

3 ■ Prefixes

PREFIX	DEFINITION	PREFIX	DEFINITION
a-, an-	absence of, without	intra-	within
dys-	painful, abnormal, difficult, labored	poly-	many, much
		trans-	through, across, beyond

4 ■ Suffixes

SUFFIX	DEFINITION	SUFFIX	DEFINITION
-al	pertaining to	-iasis	condition
-ary	pertaining to	-itis	inflammation
-cele	hernia, protrusion	-lith	stone(s), calculus (*pl.* calculi)
-ectomy	excision, surgical removal	-logist	one who studies and treats (specialist, physician)
-emia	in the blood		
-gram	the record, radiographic image	-logy	study of
-graphy	process of recording, radiographic imaging	-lysis	loosening, dissolution, separating
		-megaly	enlargement

4 ■ Suffixes—cont'd

SUFFIX	DEFINITION	SUFFIX	DEFINITION
-oma	tumor, swelling	-scopy	visual examination
-osis	abnormal condition	-stenosis	constriction or narrowing
-pexy	surgical fixation	-stomy	creation of an artificial opening
-plasty	surgical repair	-tomy	cut into, incision
-ptosis	drooping, sagging, prolapse	-tripsy	surgical crushing
-scope	instrument used for visual examination	-uria	urine, urination

Refer to **Appendix B** and **Appendix C** for alphabetized lists of word parts and their meanings.

EXERCISE 1 ■ Urinary System Combining Forms

Refer to the first section of the word parts table.

A Label

Fill in the blanks with combining forms for this diagram of the urinary system. *To check your answers, go to Appendix A.*

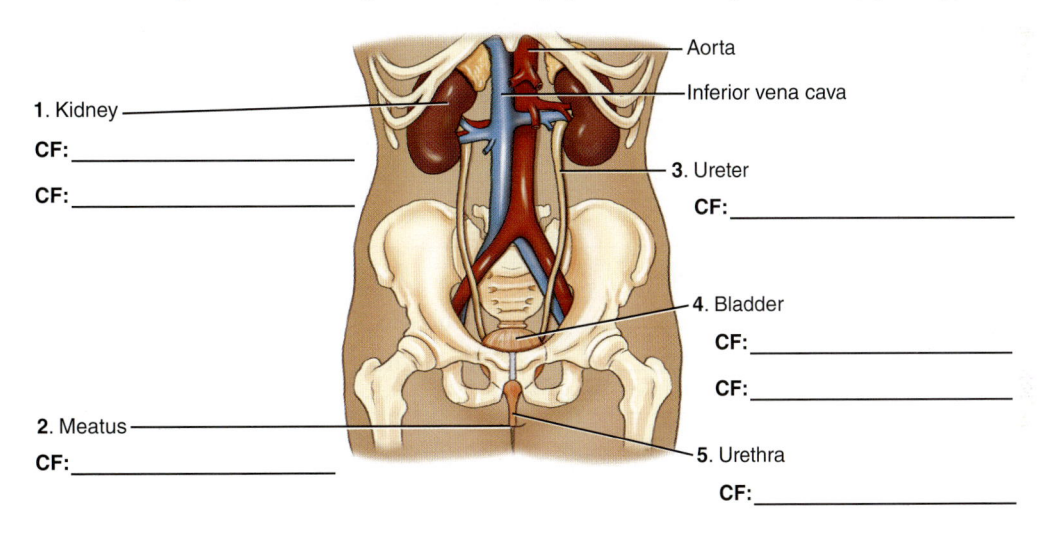

1. Kidney
   CF: _____
   CF: _____

2. Meatus
   CF: _____

3. Ureter
   CF: _____

4. Bladder
   CF: _____
   CF: _____

5. Urethra
   CF: _____

B Define and Match

Step 1: Write the definitions after the following combining forms.
Step 2: Match the descriptions on the right with the combining forms and definitions. Answers may be used more than once.

_____ 1. ren/o, _____
_____ 2. vesic/o, _____
_____ 3. nephr/o, _____
_____ 4. glomerul/o, _____
_____ 5. pyel/o, _____
_____ 6. ureter/o, _____
_____ 7. cyst/o, _____
_____ 8. meat/o, _____
_____ 9. urethr/o, _____

a. stores urine
b. outside opening through which the urine passes
c. carries urine from the kidney to the urinary bladder
d. cluster of capillaries in the kidney where the urine begins to form
e. carries urine from the bladder to the urinary meatus
f. reservoir within the kidney that collects the urine
g. organ that removes waste products from the blood

C Label

Fill in the blanks with combining forms to label these diagrams of the internal kidney structure.

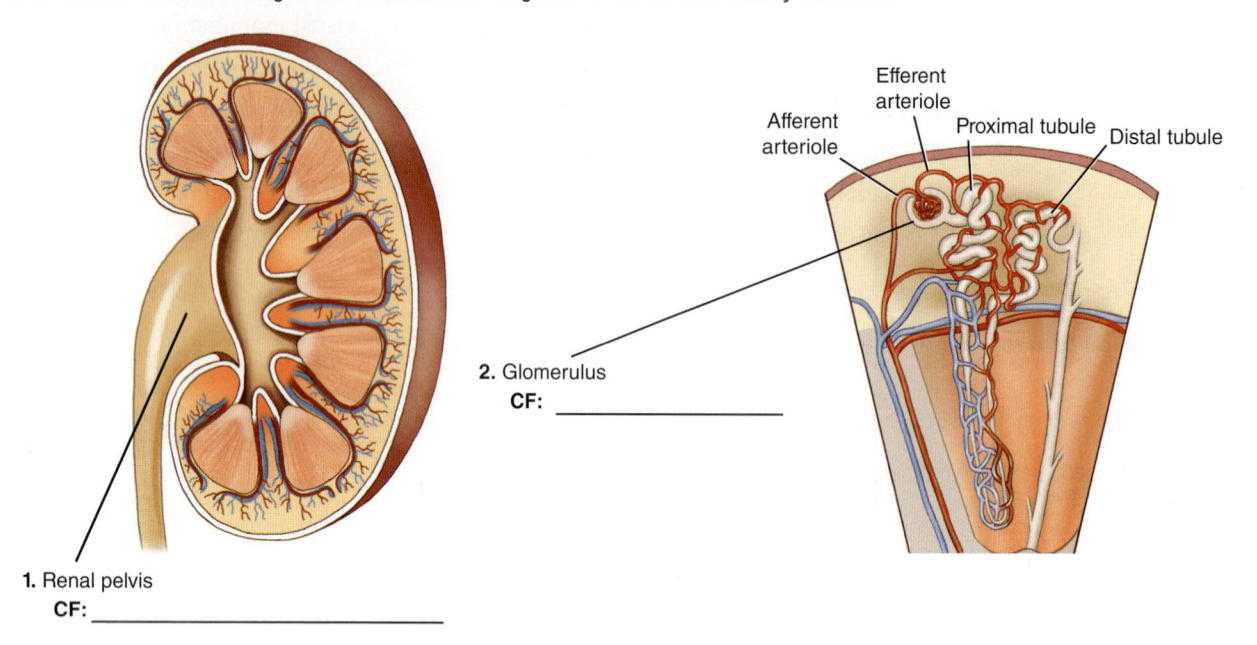

2. Glomerulus
CF: _____

1. Renal pelvis
CF: _____

EXERCISE 2 ■ Combining Forms Used with Urinary System Terms

Refer to the second section of the word parts table.

A Define

Write the definitions of the following combining forms.

1. hydr/o _____
2. azot/o _____
3. noct/i _____
4. lith/o _____
5. albumin/o _____
6. urin/o _____
7. blast/o _____
8. olig/o _____
9. ur/o _____
10. glycos/o _____
11. son/o _____
12. hem/o _____

B Identify

Write the combining form for each of the following.

1. sugar _____
2. urine, urinary tract a. _____
   b. _____
3. water _____
4. developing cell, germ cell _____
5. albumin _____
6. night _____
7. urea, nitrogen _____
8. stone(s), calculus (*pl.* calculi) _____
9. scanty, few _____
10. blood _____
11. sound _____

EXERCISE 3 ■ Prefixes

Refer to the third section of the word parts table.

A Define

Write the definitions of the following prefixes.

1. dys- _____
2. trans- _____
3. a- _____
4. poly- _____
5. intra- _____

B Identify

Write the prefix for each of the following.

1. through, across, beyond _____
2. absence of, without _____
3. painful, abnormal, difficult, labored _____
4. within _____
5. many, much _____

EXERCISE 4 ■ Suffixes

Refer to the fourth section of the word parts table.

A Label

Write the suffixes pictured and defined.

1. _____
   loosening, dissolution, separating

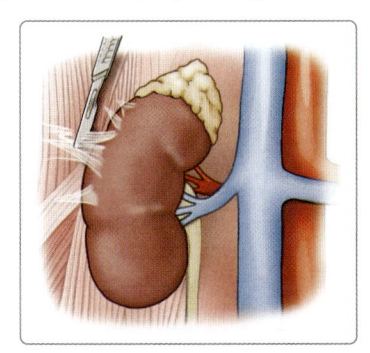

2. _____
   drooping, sagging, prolapse

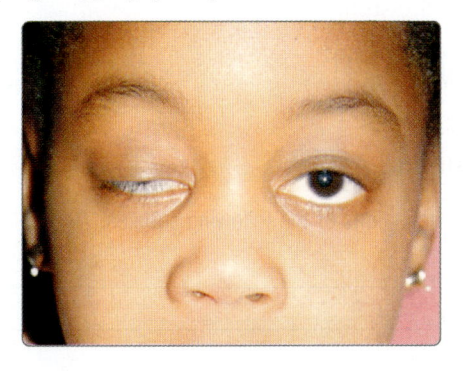

3. _____
   surgical crushing

   Kidney stone being crushed
   Focused shock wave

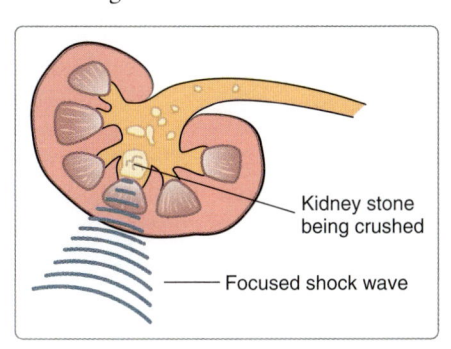

4. _____
   stone(s), calculus (*pl.* calculi)

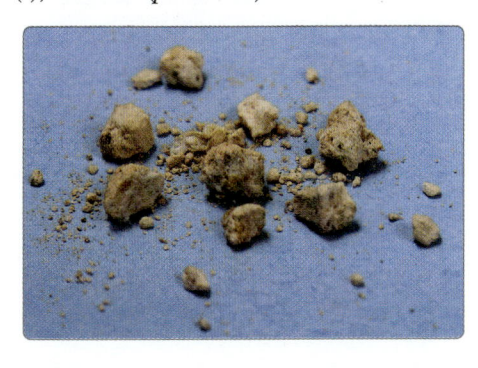

5. _____
surgical fixation

6. _____
urine, urination

B Match

Match the suffixes in the first column with their correct definitions in the second column.

_____ 1. -logist   a. excision, surgical removal
_____ 2. -oma   b. hernia, protrusion
_____ 3. -graphy   c. instrument used for visual examination
_____ 4. -ectomy   d. enlargement
_____ 5. -al   e. pertaining to
_____ 6. -cele   f. one who studies and treats (specialist, physician)
_____ 7. -megaly   g. creation of an artificial opening
_____ 8. -stomy   h. process of recording, radiographic imaging
_____ 9. -plasty   i. tumor, swelling
_____ 10. -scope   j. surgical repair

C Define

Write the definitions of the following suffixes.

1. -stenosis _____
2. -itis _____
3. -iasis _____
4. -logy _____
5. -emia _____

6. -gram _____
7. -ary _____
8. -tomy _____
9. -osis _____
10. -scopy _____

Chapter 6 Urinary System

MEDICAL TERMS

Medical terms relevant to this chapter have been grouped by topics, such as Disease and Disorder, and are listed in tables designated as Built from Word Parts or *NOT* Built from Word Parts. The exercises following each table assist with learning term definitions, pronunciations, and spellings.

Disease and Disorder Terms
BUILT FROM WORD PARTS

The following terms can be translated using definitions of word parts. Further explanation is provided within parentheses as needed.

TERM	DEFINITION	TERM	DEFINITION
1. cystitis (sis-TĪ-tis)	inflammation of the bladder (Fig. 6.5)	7. nephroblastoma (nef-rō-blas-TŌ-ma)	kidney tumor containing developing (germ) cells (malignant tumor) (also called **Wilms tumor**)
2. cystocele (SIS-tō-sēl)	protrusion of the bladder		
3. cystolith (SIS-tō-lith)	stone(s) in the bladder		
4. glomerulonephritis (glō-*mer*-ū-lō-ne-FRĪ-tis)	inflammation of the glomeruli of the kidney	8. nephrolithiasis (*nef*-rō-lith-Ī-a-sis)	condition of stone(s) in the kidney
5. hydronephrosis (*hī*-drō-ne-FRŌ-sis)	abnormal condition of water in the kidney (swelling of the kidney due to a buildup of urine, usually from a blockage in the ureter)	9. nephroma (nef-RŌ-ma)	tumor of the kidney
		10. nephromegaly (*nef*-rō-MEG-a-lē)	enlargement of a kidney
6. nephritis (ne-FRĪ-tis)	inflammation of a kidney		

WILMS TUMOR also called nephroblastoma, is a rare malignancy of the kidney that primarily affects children. Named for German surgeon Dr. Max Wilms who described the disease in 1899, Wilms tumors are generally **unilateral** and can be successfully managed with appropriate surgical and oncological treatment.

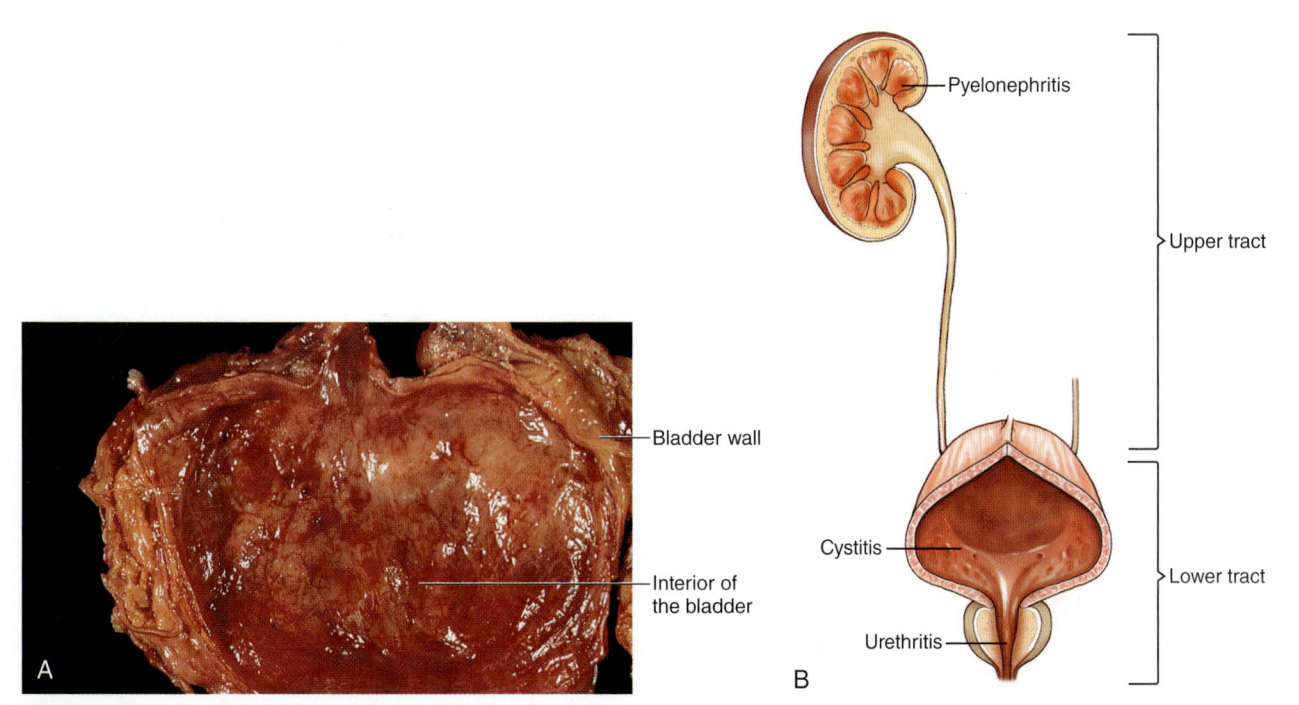

FIG. 6.5 Urinary tract infection. **A,** Acute cystitis. The swollen and red mucosa demonstrates inflammation. Cystitis is more common in women because the urethra is short, allowing easy access of bacteria to the urinary bladder. **B,** Upper and lower urinary tract infections. If cystitis is not treated promptly, the infection can spread to the kidneys, causing pyelonephritis.

Disease and Disorder Terms—cont'd
BUILT FROM WORD PARTS

TERM	DEFINITION	TERM	DEFINITION
11. nephroptosis (*nef*-rop-TŌ-sis)	drooping kidney (also called **floating kidney**)	**UREMIA** was first used by Pierre Piorry, a French physician (1794-1879). He also created the medical terms **toxin, toxemia,** and **septicemia.**	
NEPHROPTOSIS occurs when the kidney is no longer held in place and drops out of its normal position. The kidney is held in place by connective and adipose tissue, so it is susceptible to injury that may also cause the ureter to twist. Truck drivers and horseback riders are prone to this condition		15. ureteritis (ū-*rē*-ter-Ī-tis)	inflammation of a ureter
		16. ureterocele (ū-RĒ-ter-ō-*sēl*)	protrusion of a ureter (distally into the bladder)
12. pyelitis (*pī*-e-LĪ-tis)	inflammation of the renal pelvis	17. ureterolithiasis (ū-*rē*-ter-ō-lith-Ī-a-sis)	condition of stone(s) in the ureter
13. pyelonephritis (*pī*-e-lō-ne-FRĪ-tis)	inflammation of the renal pelvis and the kidney (Fig. 6.5B and Fig. 6.6)	18. urethritis (ū-rē-THRĪ-tis)	inflammation of the urethra
14. uremia (ū-RĒ-mē-a)	urine (urea nitrogen) in the blood (refers the presence of azotemia and a wide range of signs and symptoms associated with chronic kidney disease, including polyuria [excessive urination], polydipsia [excessive thirst], vomiting, and weight loss; associated with renal failure) (also called **uremic syndrome**)	19. ureterostenosis (ū-*rē*-ter-ō-sten-Ō-sis)	narrowing of the ureter
		20. urethrocystitis (ū-*rē*-thrō-sis-TĪ-tis)	inflammation of the urethra and the bladder
		21. **vesicoureteral reflux (VUR)** (ves-i-kō-ū-RĒ-ter-al) (RĒ-fluks)	reflux pertaining to the bladder and ureter (condition in which urine flows backward toward the kidneys. May occur in up to 10% of children, and in some adults)
		REFLUX is the flow of fluid through a vessel or valve in a direction opposite to normal.	

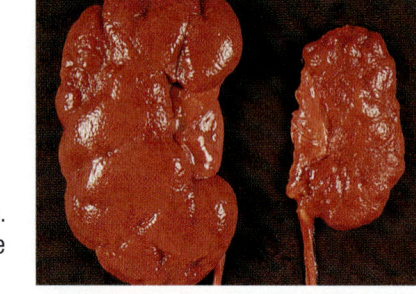

FIG. 6.6 *Kidney on left*, chronic pyelonephritis. *Kidney on right*, normal size with some scarring.

EXERCISE 5 ■ Pronounce and Spell

Practice pronunciation and spelling on paper and online.

1. **Practice on Paper**
   a. **Pronounce:** Read the phonetic spelling and say aloud the terms listed in the previous table. Refer to Table 2.2 Pronunciation Key as needed.
   b. **Spell:** Have a study partner read the terms aloud. Write the spelling of the terms on a separate sheet of paper.

2. **Practice Online**
   a. **Access** online learning resources. Go to evolve.elsevier.com > Evolve Resources > Student Resources.
   b. **Pronounce:** Select Audio Glossary > Chapter 6 > Exercise 5. Select a term to hear its pronunciation and repeat aloud.
   c. **Spell:** Select Activities > Chapter 6 > Spell Terms > Exercise 5. Select the audio icon and type the correct spelling of the term.

❏ Check the box when complete.

EXERCISE 6 ■ Analyze and Define

Analyze and define the following terms by drawing slashes between word parts, writing word part abbreviations above the term, underlining combining forms, and writing combining form abbreviations below the term.

EXAMPLE:
```
        WR    CV   WR    S
   glomerul / o / nephr / itis
        CF
   inflammation of the glomeruli of the kidney
```

1. nephroblastoma

2. ureterostenosis

3. uremia

4. nephroptosis

5. cystocele

6. nephritis

7. pyelitis

8. ureterolithiasis

9. pyelonephritis

10. ureteritis

EXERCISE 7 ■ Build

A Fill In

Build disease and disorder terms for the following definitions by using the word parts you have learned.

EXAMPLE: inflammation of the ureter   ureter / itis
                                          WR / S

1. protrusion of a ureter   _____ / ____ / _____
                                     WR   CV   S

2. inflammation of the urethra and bladder   _____ / ____ / _____ / _____
                                                WR   CV   WR   S

Chapter 6 Urinary System

3. reflux pertaining to the bladder and ureter (condition in which urine flows backward toward the kidneys)

_____ / ___ / _____ / ___ reflux
WR   CV   WR   S

4. inflammation of the glomeruli of the kidney

_____ / ___ / _____ / ___
WR   CV   WR   S

5. tumor of the kidney

_____ / ___
WR   S

B Label

Build terms pictured by writing word parts above definitions.

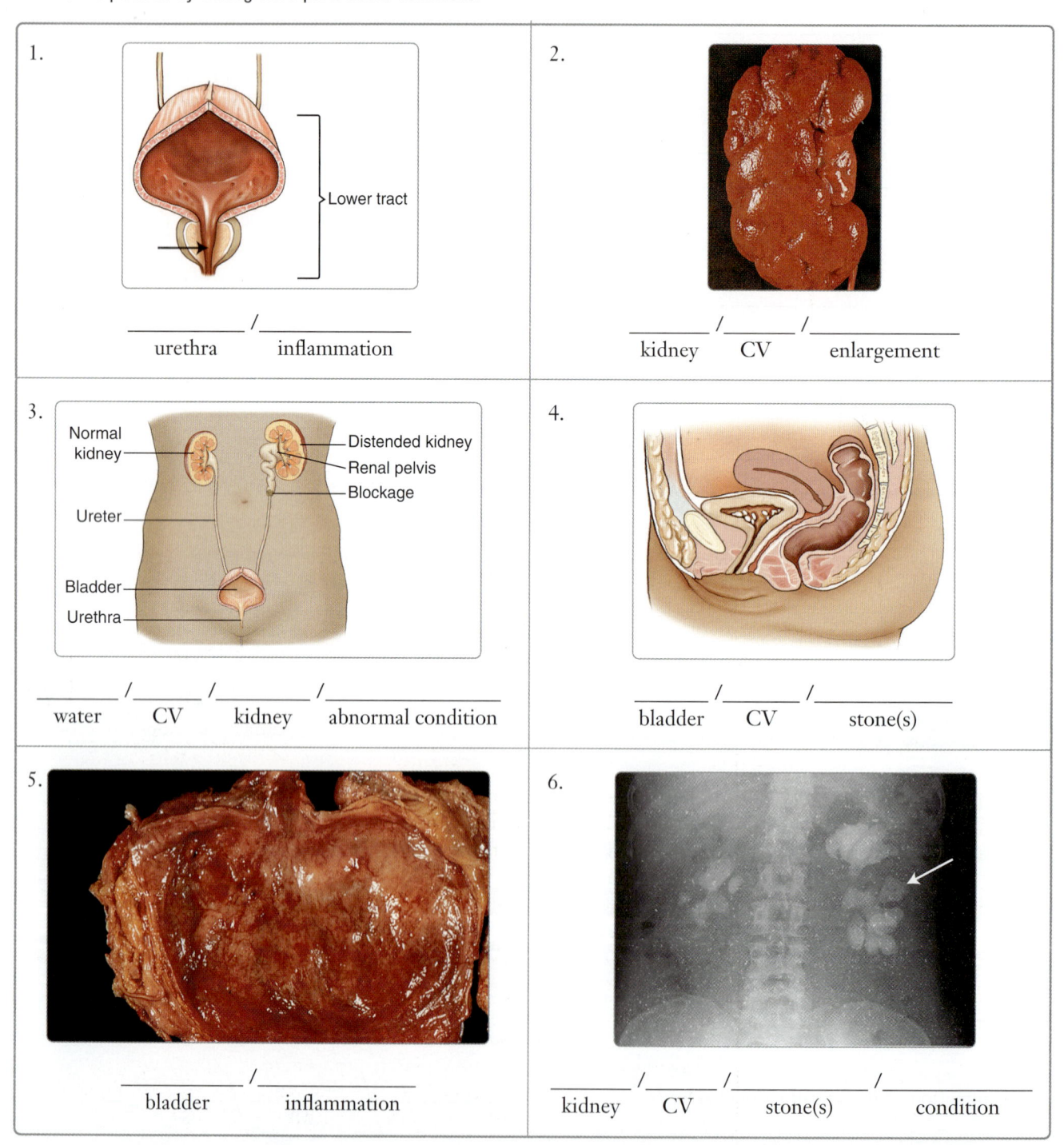

1.

_____ / _____
urethra   inflammation

2.

_____ / ___ / _____
kidney   CV   enlargement

3.

_____ / ___ / _____ / _____
water   CV   kidney   abnormal condition

4.

_____ / ___ / _____
bladder   CV   stone(s)

5.

_____ / _____
bladder   inflammation

6.

_____ / ___ / _____ / _____
kidney   CV   stone(s)   condition

Disease and Disorder Terms
NOT BUILT FROM WORD PARTS

Word parts may be present in the following terms; however, their full meanings cannot be translated using definitions of word parts alone.

TERM	DEFINITION
1. **acute kidney injury (AKI)** (a-KŪT) (KID-nē) (IN-ja-rē)	abrupt decline in kidney function that occurs over hours to days and is usually reversible. Causes include trauma, obstruction, adverse drug reactions, or decreased blood flow from dehydration, burns, hemorrhage, and septic shock. (also called **acute renal failure [ARF]**)
2. **chronic kidney disease (CKD)** (KRON-ik) (KID-nē) (di-ZĒZ)	progressive, irreversible loss of kidney function. Causes include diabetes, hypertension, and autoimmune diseases such as lupus. (also called **chronic renal failure [CRF]**) (Table 6.1)
3. **end-stage kidney disease (ESKD)** (end) (stāj) (KID-nē) (di-ZĒZ)	condition in which kidneys no longer function on their own. Dialysis or kidney transplantation is necessary for survival. (also called **end-stage renal disease [ESRD]**)
4. **epispadias** (ep-i-SPĀ-dē-as)	congenital defect in which the urinary meatus is located on the upper surface of the penis
5. **hypospadias** (hī-pō-SPĀ-dē-as)	congenital defect in which the urinary meatus is located on the underside of the penis. Females may also have a form of hypospadias in which the urinary meatus is unusually located.
6. **polycystic kidney disease (PKD)** (pol-ē-SIS-tik) (KID-nē) (di-ZĒZ)	condition in which the kidney contains many cysts, causing progressive interference with the ability to form urine
7. **renal calculus (pl. calculi)** (RĒ-nal) (KAL-kū-lus), (KAL-kū-lī)	stone(s) in the kidney

TABLE 6.1 Chronic Kidney Disease Stages

Chronic kidney disease (CKD) is divided into 5 stages, which are determined by the **glomerular filtration rate (GFR)**, a measure of kidney function. CKD is NOT reversible, but its progression can be slowed by treating underlying causes.

Stage	GFR Measurement	Meaning	Symptoms
Stage 1	GFR 90 or above (normal)	minor damage to kidneys, presence of protein in the urine; kidneys work normally	usually no symptoms are evident
Stage 2	GFR 60-89	mild damage to kidneys, but they still work well. Protein is present in the urine.	may be asymptomatic, or may have swelling of hands and feet, high blood pressure, or blood in the urine
Stage 3a	GFR 45-59	mild to moderate damage to kidneys, which do not work as well to eliminate waste and fluids	swelling of hands and feet, high blood pressure, or blood in the urine, plus weakness, fatigue, dry or itchy skin, muscle cramps, back pain, difficulties with sleep, and changes in urination
Stage 3b	GFR 30-44	moderate to severe damage to kidneys, which are not working well. Fluid and waste are not fully eliminated.	
Stage 4	GFR 15-29	moderate to severe kidney damage in which they are close to not working at all. Waste products are building up in the blood and include high potassium, high phosphorus, anemia, and acidosis (buildup of acid in the body).	all previously listed symptoms, plus swelling in the arms and legs, nausea, vomiting, and decreased appetite
Stage 5	GFR 15 or below	severe damage: kidneys are failing or have already stopped working. Dialysis or kidney transplant will be necessary to sustain life.	all previously listed symptoms, plus making little or no urine, headaches, difficulty breathing, changes in skin color

Chapter 6 Urinary System

Disease and Disorder Terms—cont'd
NOT BUILT FROM WORD PARTS

TERM	DEFINITION
8. renal hypertension (RĒ-nal) (hī-per-TEN-shun)	elevated blood pressure resulting from kidney disease
9. urinary retention (Ū-rin-ār-ē) (rē-TEN-shun)	abnormal accumulation of urine in the bladder because of an inability to urinate; can be acute (AUR) or chronic (CUR)
10. urinary tract infection (UTI) (Ū-rin-ār-ē) (trakt) (in-FEK-shun)	infection of one or more organs of the urinary tract (Fig. 6.5)

EXERCISE 8 ■ Pronounce and Spell

Practice pronunciation and spelling on paper and online.

1. **Practice on Paper**
   a. **Pronounce:** Read the phonetic spelling and say aloud the terms listed in the previous table. Refer to Table 2.2 Pronunciation Key as needed.
   b. **Spell:** Have a study partner read the terms aloud. Write the spelling of the terms on a separate sheet of paper.

2. **Practice Online**
   a. **Access** online learning resources. Go to evolve.elsevier.com > Evolve Resources > Student Resources.
   b. **Pronounce:** Select Audio Glossary > Chapter 6 > Exercise 8. Select a term to hear its pronunciation and repeat aloud.
   c. **Spell:** Select Activities > Chapter 6 > Spell Terms > Exercise 8. Select the audio icon and type the correct spelling of the term.

❑ Check the box when complete.

EXERCISE 9 ■ Fill In

A Label

Write the medical terms pictured and defined.

1. _____
   congenital defect in which the urinary meatus is located on the underside of the penis

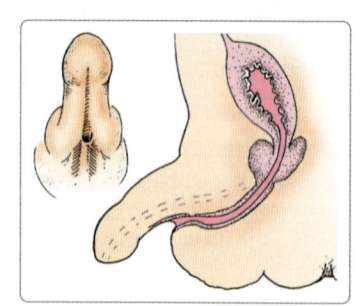

2. _____
   condition in which the kidney contains many cysts, causing progressive interference with the ability to form urine

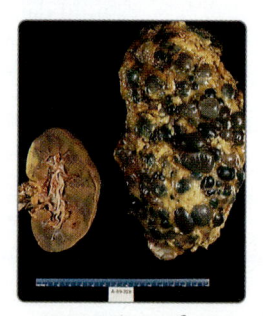

   Kidney on left is a cross-section of normal kidney.

B Identify

Fill in the blanks with the correct terms.

1. Stone in the kidney is also called _____.
2. The inability to urinate, which results in an abnormal amount of urine in the bladder, is known as _____.

Chapter 6 Urinary System   203

3. Elevated blood pressure resulting from kidney disease is _____.
4. _____ is abrupt and usually reversible.
5. _____ is a condition in which the urinary meatus is located on the upper surface of the penis.
6. Infection of one or more organs of the urinary system is called _____.
7. Progressive, irreversible loss of kidney function is called _____
8. _____ is a condition in which the kidneys can no longer function independently.

EXERCISE 10 ■ Match

Match the terms in the first column with their correct definitions in the second column.

_____ 1. end-stage kidney disease   a. kidney with many cysts
_____ 2. hypospadias   b. progressive, irreversible loss of kidney function
_____ 3. acute kidney injury   c. urinary meatus on the upper surface of the penis
_____ 4. renal hypertension   d. kidney stone
_____ 5. polycystic kidney disease   e. abnormal accumulation of urine in the bladder
_____ 6. urinary retention   f. urinary meatus on the underside of the penis
_____ 7. epispadias   g. infection of one or more organs of the urinary system
_____ 8. urinary tract infection   h. characterized by elevated blood pressure
_____ 9. chronic kidney disease   i. condition in which kidneys can no longer function on their own
_____ 10. renal calculus   j. abrupt decline in kidney function that is reversible

EXERCISE 11 ■ Review of Disease and Disorder Terms

Can you define, pronounce, and spell the following terms?

acute kidney injury (AKI)	epispadias	nephroptosis	ureterocele
chronic kidney disease (CKD)	glomerulonephritis	polycystic kidney disease (PKD)	ureterolithiasis
cystitis	hydronephrosis	pyelitis	ureterostenosis
cystocele	hypospadias	pyelonephritis	urethritis
cystolith	nephritis	renal calculus (*pl.* calculi)	urethrocystitis
end-stage kidney disease (ESKD)	nephroblastoma	renal hypertension	urinary retention
	nephrolithiasis	uremia	urinary tract infection (UTI)
	nephroma	ureteritis	vesicoureteral reflux (VUR)
	nephromegaly		

Surgical Terms
BUILT FROM WORD PARTS AND *NOT* BUILT FROM WORD PARTS

The first portion of the table contains Urinary System Terms that can be translated using definitions of word parts. The second portion of the table contains Urinary System Terms that cannot be fully understood using the definitions of word parts.

■ Built from Word Parts

TERM	DEFINITION	TERM	DEFINITION
1. **cystectomy** (sis-TEK-to-mē)	excision of the bladder	4. **lithotripsy** (LITH-ō-trip-sē)	surgical crushing of stone(s) (using shock waves)
2. **cystolithotomy** (*sis*-tō-li-THOT-o-mē)	incision into the bladder to remove stone(s)	5. **meatotomy** (*mē*-a-TOT-o-mē)	incision into the meatus (to enlarge it)
3. **cystostomy** (sis-TOS-to-mē)	creation of an artificial opening into the bladder (for urinary drainage) (also called **vesicostomy**)	6. **nephrectomy** (ne-FREK-to-mē)	excision of the kidney

FIG. 6.7 Percutaneous nephrolithotomy or percutaneous lithotripsy uses a small incision in the back to remove medium or larger-size kidney stones. A nephroscope is passed into the kidney through the incision. In a **nephrolithotomy,** the surgeon removes the stone through the nephroscope. In a **nephrolithotripsy,** the stone is broken into fragments by a lithotripter and then removed through the nephroscope.

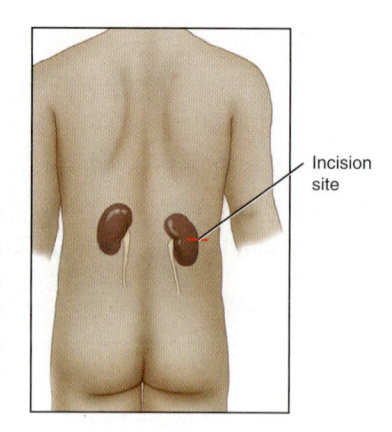

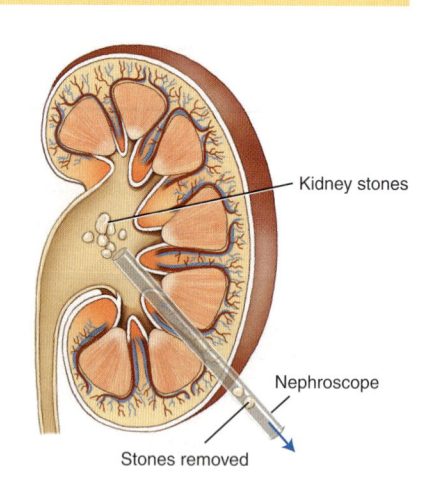

Surgical Terms—cont'd
BUILT FROM WORD PARTS AND *NOT* BUILT FROM WORD PARTS

TERM	DEFINITION
7. nephrolithotomy (nef-rō-li-THOT-o-mē)	incision into the kidney to remove stone(s) (Fig. 6.7)
8. nephrolithotripsy (nef-rō-LITH-o-trip-sē)	surgical crushing of stone(s) in the kidney (using shock waves) (Fig. 6.7)
9. nephrolysis (ne-FROL-i-sis)	separating the kidney (from other body structures)
10. nephropexy (NEF-rō-peks-ē)	surgical fixation of the kidney
11. nephrostomy (ne-FROS-to-mē)	creation of an artificial opening into the kidney
12. pyelolithotomy (pī-el-ō-lith-OT-o-mē)	incision into the renal pelvis to remove stone(s)
13. pyeloplasty (PĪ-el-ō-plas-tē)	surgical repair of the renal pelvis

TERM	DEFINITION
14. ureterectomy (ū-rē-ter-EK-to-mē)	excision of the ureter
15. ureterostomy (ū-rē-ter-OS-to-mē)	creation of an artificial opening into the ureter (for drainage of urine)
16. urethroplasty (ū-RĒ-thrō-plas-tē)	surgical repair of the urethra
17. urostomy (ū-ROS-tō-mē)	creation of an artificial opening into the urinary system
18. vesicourethral suspension (ves-i-kō-ū-RĒ-thral) (sus-PEN-shun)	suspension pertaining to the bladder and urethra

VESICOURETHRAL SUSPENSION with a midurethral sling, called the Marshall-Marchetti Krantz technique, is performed to treat stress incontinence, the involuntary intermittent leakage of urine as a result of pressure from a cough or a sneeze on a weakened area around the urethra and bladder.

■ *NOT* Built from Word Parts

TERM	DEFINITION
1. extracorporeal shock wave lithotripsy (ESWL) (eks-tra-kor-POR-ē-al) (shok) (wāv) (LITH-ō-trip-sē)	noninvasive surgical procedure to crush stone(s) in the kidney or ureter by administration of repeated shock waves. Stone fragments are eliminated from the body in urine. (also called **shock wave lithotripsy [SWL]**)
EXTRACORPOREAL means occurring outside the body.	
2. fulguration (ful-gū-RĀ-shun)	destruction of living tissue with an electric spark (a method commonly used to destroy bladder growths) (Fig. 6.8)
3. renal transplant (RĒ-nal) (TRANS-plant)	surgical implantation of a donor kidney into a patient with inadequate renal function (Fig. 6.9)
RENAL FUNCTION REPLACEMENT THERAPIES • Hemodialysis • Peritoneal dialysis • Renal transplant	

Chapter 6   Urinary System   205

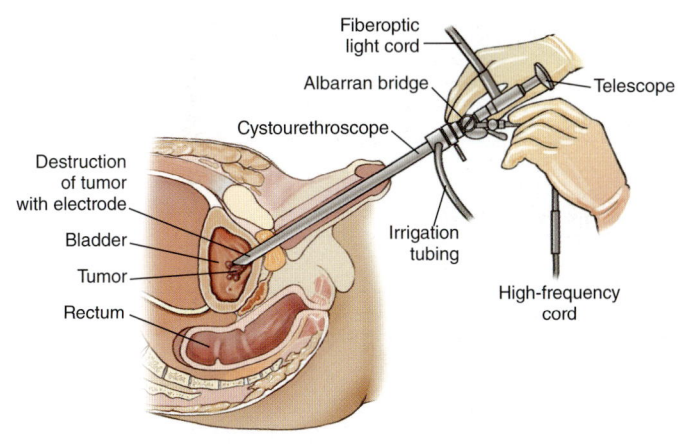

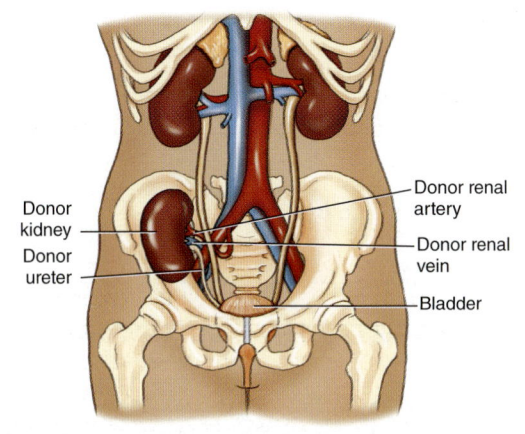

FIG. 6.8 Bladder fulguration.

FIG. 6.9 Renal transplant showing donor kidney and blood vessels in place. Recipient's kidney is not always removed unless it is infected or is a cause of hypertension.

EXERCISE 12 ■ Pronounce and Spell

Practice pronunciation and spelling on paper and online.

1. **Practice on Paper**
   a. **Pronounce:** Read the phonetic spelling and say aloud the terms listed in the previous table. Refer to Table 2.2 Pronunciation Key as needed.
   b. **Spell:** Have a study partner read the terms aloud. Write the spelling of the terms on a separate sheet of paper.

2. **Practice Online**
   a. **Access** online learning resources. Go to evolve.elsevier.com > Evolve Resources > Student Resources.
   b. **Pronounce:** Select Audio Glossary > Chapter 6 > Exercise 12. Select a term to hear its pronunciation and repeat aloud.
   c. **Spell:** Select Activities > Chapter 6 > Spell Terms > Exercise 12. Select the audio icon and type the correct spelling of the term.

❏ Check the box when complete.

EXERCISE 13 ■ Surgical Terms Built from Word Parts

A Analyze and Define

Analyze and define the following terms by drawing slashes between word parts, writing word part abbreviations above the term, underlining combining forms, and writing combining form abbreviations below the term.

1. ureterostomy

2. nephrolithotomy

3. nephrostomy

4. nephrolysis

5. cystectomy

6. pyelolithotomy

206 Chapter 6 Urinary System

7. nephropexy
   _____
   _____

8. cystolithotomy
   _____
   _____

9. nephrectomy
   _____
   _____

10. ureterectomy
    _____
    _____

11. cystostomy
    _____
    _____

12. pyeloplasty
    _____
    _____

13. urostomy
    _____
    _____

14. meatotomy
    _____
    _____

15. lithotripsy
    _____
    _____

16. urethroplasty
    _____
    _____

17. nephrolithotripsy
    _____
    _____

18. vesicourethral suspension
    _____
    _____

B Label

Build terms pictured by writing word parts above definitions.

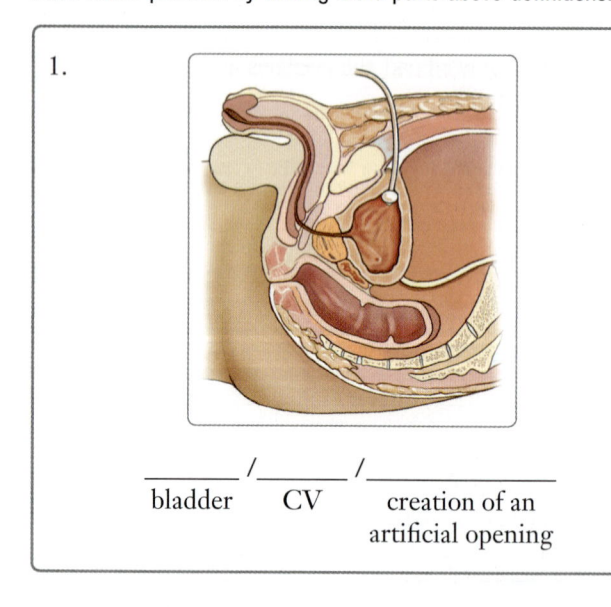

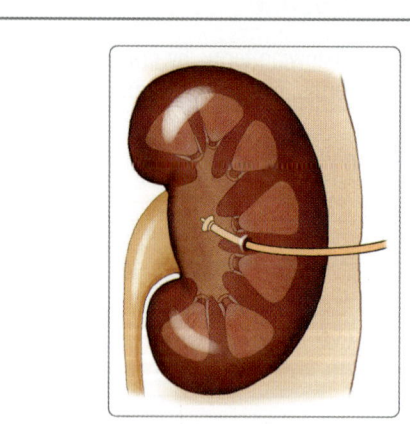

1.

_____ / _____ / _____
bladder   CV   creation of an
                   artificial opening

2.

percutaneous _____ / _____ / _____
              kidney   CV   creation of an
                               artificial opening

Chapter 6 Urinary System 207

3.

_____ / _____ / _____ / _____ / _____
renal   CV   stone   CV   incision
pelvis

4.

Kidney stones
Nephroscope
Stones removed

_____ / _____ / _____ / _____ / _____
kidney   CV   stone   CV   incision

5.

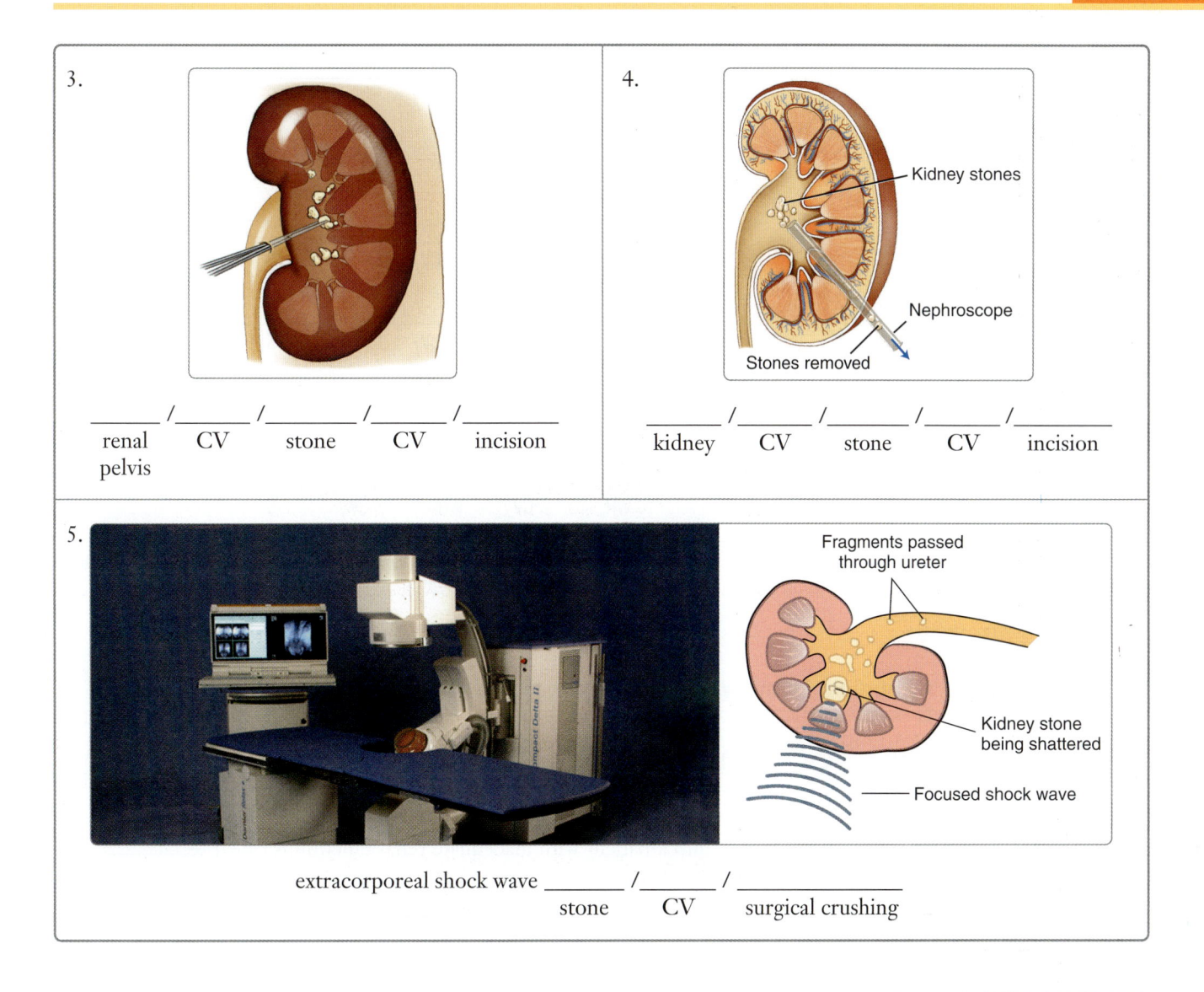

Fragments passed through ureter
Kidney stone being shattered
Focused shock wave

extracorporeal shock wave _____ / _____ / _____
                            stone   CV   surgical crushing

C Fill In

Build surgical terms for the following definitions by using the word parts you have learned.

1. creation of an artificial opening into the ureter

   _____ / _____ / _____
   WR   CV   S

2. excision of the kidney

   _____ / _____
   WR   S

3. surgical crushing of stone(s) in the kidney (using shock waves)

   _____ / _____ / _____ / _____ / _____
   WR   CV   WR   CV   S

4. creation of an artificial opening into the urinary system

   _____ / _____ / _____
   WR   CV   S

5. separating the kidney (from other structures)

   _____ / _____ / _____
   WR   CV   S

6. surgical repair of the renal pelvis

   _____ / _____ / _____
   WR   CV   S

208 Chapter 6 Urinary System

7. surgical repair of the urethra _____ / _____ / _____
   WR   CV   S

8. excision of the bladder _____ / _____
   WR   S

9. incision into the meatus _____ / _____ / _____
   WR   CV   S

10. surgical fixation of the kidney _____ / _____ / _____
    WR   CV   S

11. excision of the ureter _____ / _____
    WR   S

12. incision into the bladder to remove stone(s) _____ / _____ / _____ / _____ / _____
    WR   CV   WR   CV   S

13. suspension pertaining to the bladder and urethra _____ / _____ / _____ / _____ suspension
    WR   CV   WR   S

EXERCISE 14 ■ Surgical Terms NOT Built from Word Parts

A Identify

Fill in the blanks with the correct terms.

1. The surgical implantation of a donor kidney into a patient with inadequate renal function is called _____ _____.

2. The destruction of living tissue with an electric spark is _____.

3. _____ _____ _____ _____ _____ is a noninvasive surgical procedure for removal of kidney or ureteral stones.

B Match

Match the terms in the first column with their correct definitions in the second column.

_____ 1. fulguration   a. implantation of a donor kidney
_____ 2. renal transplant   b. used to destroy bladder growths
_____ 3. ESWL   c. also called shock wave lithotripsy

EXERCISE 15 ■ Review of Surgical Terms

Can you define, pronounce, and spell the following terms?

cystectomy	fulguration	nephrolysis	ureterectomy
cystolithotomy	lithotripsy	nephropexy	ureterostomy
cystostomy	meatotomy	nephrostomy	urethroplasty
extracorporeal shock wave lithotripsy (ESWL)	nephrectomy	pyelolithotomy	urostomy
	nephrolithotomy	pyeloplasty	vesicourethral suspension
	nephrolithotripsy	renal transplant	

Diagnostic Terms
BUILT FROM WORD PARTS AND *NOT* BUILT FROM WORD PARTS

The first portion of the table contains diagnostic terms that can be translated using definitions of word parts. The second portion of the table contains diagnostic terms that cannot be fully understood using the definitions of word parts.

■ Built from Word Parts

DIAGNOSTIC IMAGING

TERM	DEFINITION	TERM	DEFINITION
1. cystogram (SIS-tō-gram)	radiographic image of the bladder	6. retrograde urogram (RET-rō-grād) (Ū-rō-gram)	radiographic image of the urinary tract (retrograde means to move in a direction opposite from normal); contrast material is instilled into the bladder through a urethral catheter, and may extend to the ureters or kidneys in patients with vesicoureteral reflux
2. cystography (sis-TOG-ra-fē)	radiographic imaging of the bladder		
3. nephrosonography (nef-rō-so-NOG-ra-fē)	process of recording the kidney using sound (also called **renal ultrasound**)		
4. pyelogram (PĪ-lō-gram)	radiographic image of the renal pelvis (Fig. 6.11)	7. voiding cystourethrography (VCUG) (VOID-ing) (sis-tō-ū-rē-THROG-ro-fē)	radiographic imaging of the bladder and the urethra (images are taken of the bladder before and during urination using contrast materials [fluoroscopy] or a radioactive material [nuclear medicine]) (Fig. 6.12)
5. renogram (RĒ-nō-gram)	radiographic record of the kidney (an imaging test, used to evaluate kidney function); (also called **nephrogram**) (Fig. 6.10B)		

ENDOSCOPY

TERM	DEFINITION	TERM	DEFINITION
8. cystoscope (SIS-tō-skōp)	instrument used for visual examination of the bladder	10. nephroscopy (ne-FROS-ko-pē)	visual examination of the kidney
9. cystoscopy (sis-TOS-ko-pē)	visual examination of the bladder	11. ureteroscopy (ū-rē-ter-OS-ko-pē)	visual examination of the ureter

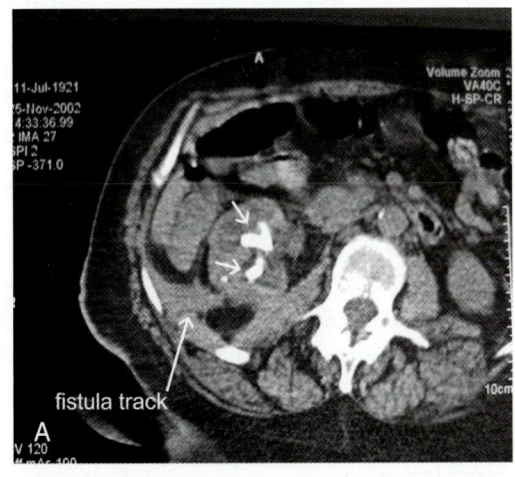

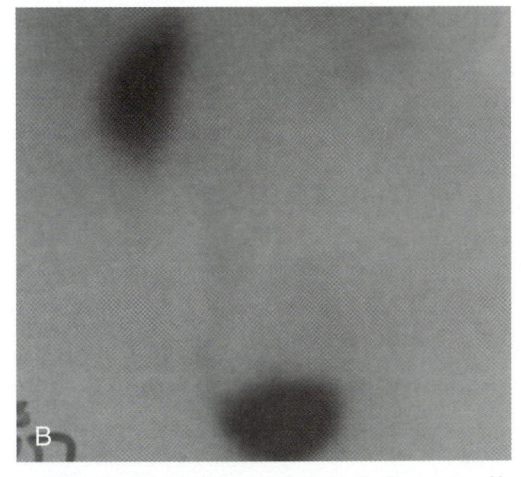

FIG. 6.10 A, CT scan of the kidney. Small arrows point to a large calculus within the renal pelvis (axial view). **B,** Renogram. Nuclear medicine image from the same patient, showing no function of the affected kidney (posterior view).

210 Chapter 6 Urinary System

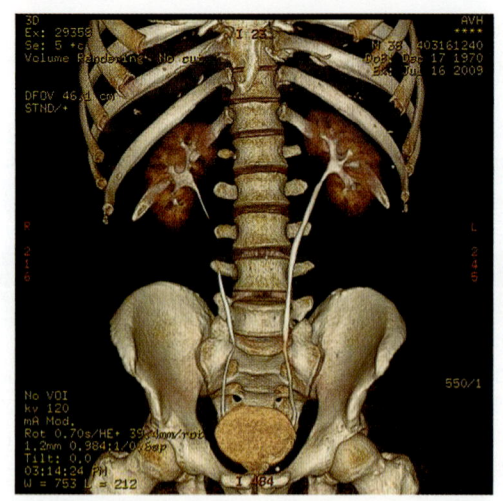

FIG. 6.11 CT pyelogram showing three-dimensional, reconstructed view of the kidneys, renal pelvices, ureters, and bladder. CT pyelogram scans are now the primary diagnostic tool for detecting **urinary tract stones** and **perirenal infections**. Radiographic (plain film) **intravenous pyelograms (IVP)** may still be used to evaluate an obstructing mass.

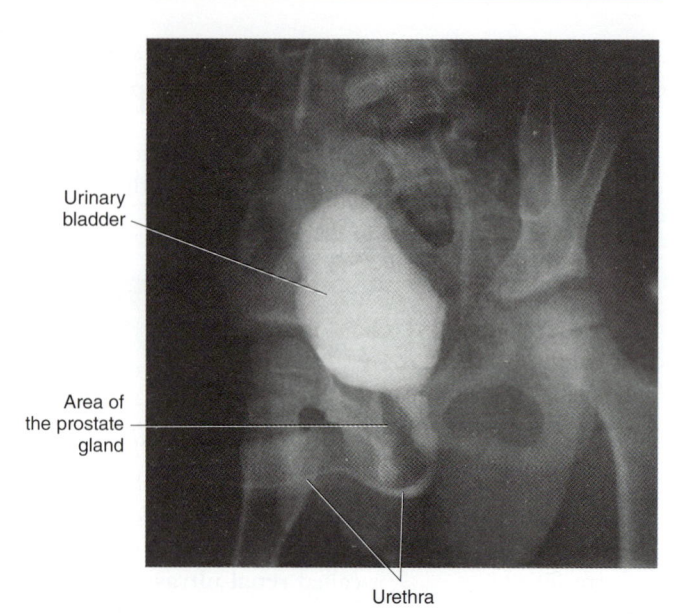

FIG. 6.12 Image obtained by voiding cystourethrography, male (lateral view).

■ NOT Built from Word Parts

DIAGNOSTIC IMAGING	
TERM	**DEFINITION**
1. KUB (K-Ū-B) *each letter is said*	simple radiographic image of the abdomen. It is often used to view the **kidneys**, **ureters**, and **bladder** to determine their size, shape, and location, or to identify radiopaque calculi in these structures. A KUB may also be used to diagnose intestinal obstruction. (also called **flat plate of the abdomen**)

LABORATORY	
TERM	**DEFINITION**
2. blood urea nitrogen (BUN) (blud) (ū-RĒ-a) (NĪ-trō-jen)	test that measures the amount of nitrogen in the blood that comes from urea. An increased BUN detects an abnormality in renal function.
BUN, the abbreviation for blood urea nitrogen, is almost exclusively used to refer to the test. It is pronounced letter by letter, B-Ū-N, not as a whole word.	
3. creatinine (crē-AT-i-nin)	blood test that measures the amount of a waste product in the blood that comes from the normal wear and tear of muscles. An elevated amount may indicate impaired kidney function.
4. glomerular filtration rate (GFR) (gla-MER-yu-ler) (fil-TRĀ-shun) (rāt)	test that measures kidney function by estimating the amount of blood filtered by the kidneys each minute. Higher levels (90 and above) usally reflect normal kidney function, while lower levels indicate various stages of kidney disease. (Table 6.1)
5. specific gravity (SG) (spe-SIF-ik) (GRAV-i-tē)	test performed on a urine specimen to measure the concentrating or diluting ability of the kidneys
6. urinalysis (UA) (ū-rin-AL-is-is)	multiple routine tests performed on a urine specimen. Visual examination and chemical analysis of a urine specimen provide screening for blood, glucose, protein, and other substances in the urine and offer a picture of overall health.
7. urine culture and sensitivity (Ū-rin) (KUL-cher) (and) (sen-si-TIV-i-tē)	test performed on a urine specimen to determine the presence of bacteria and yeast; used to diagnose urinary tract infections
8. urodynamics (ū-rō-dī-NAM-iks)	tests to measure the force and flow of urine in the lower urinary tract (bladder and urethra) by examining the process of voiding; assesses bladder tone, capacity, and pressure. Decreased perineal muscle function, an enlarged prostate, or urethral stricture will affect urine flow rate. (also called **urodynamic studies**)

Chapter 6 Urinary System 211

EXERCISE 16 ■ Pronounce and Spell

Practice pronunciation and spelling on paper and online.

1. **Practice on Paper**
   a. **Pronounce:** Read the phonetic spelling and say aloud the terms listed in the previous table. Refer to Table 2.2 Pronunciation Key as needed.
   b. **Spell:** Have a study partner read the terms aloud. Write the spelling of the terms on a separate sheet of paper.

2. **Practice Online**
   a. **Access** online learning resources. Go to evolve.elsevier.com > Evolve Resources > Student Resources.
   b. **Pronounce:** Select Audio Glossary > Chapter 6 > Exercise 16. Select a term to hear its pronunciation and repeat aloud.
   c. **Spell:** Select Activities > Chapter 6 > Spell Terms > Exercise 16. Select the audio icon and type the correct spelling of the term.

❑ Check the box when complete.

EXERCISE 17 ■ Diagnostic Terms Built from Word Parts

A Analyze and Define

Analyze and define the following terms by drawing slashes between word parts, writing word part abbreviations above the term, underlining combining forms, and writing combining form abbreviations below the term.

1. (voiding) cystourethrography

2. cystography

3. nephrosonography

4. cystoscope

5. cystogram

6. cystoscopy

7. pyelogram

8. renogram

9. nephroscopy

10. ureteroscopy

B Label

Build terms pictured by writing word parts above definitions.

1. _____ / _____ / _____
   bladder   CV   radiographic image

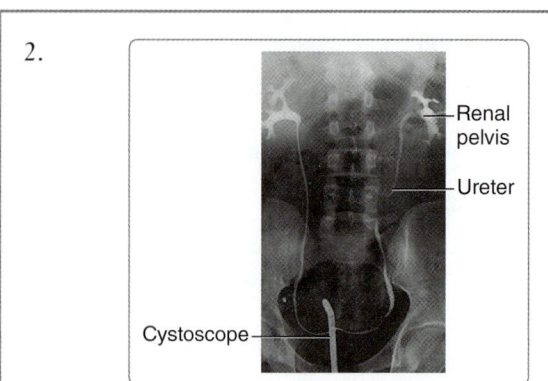

2. retrograde _____ / _____ / _____
   urinary tract   CV   radiographic image

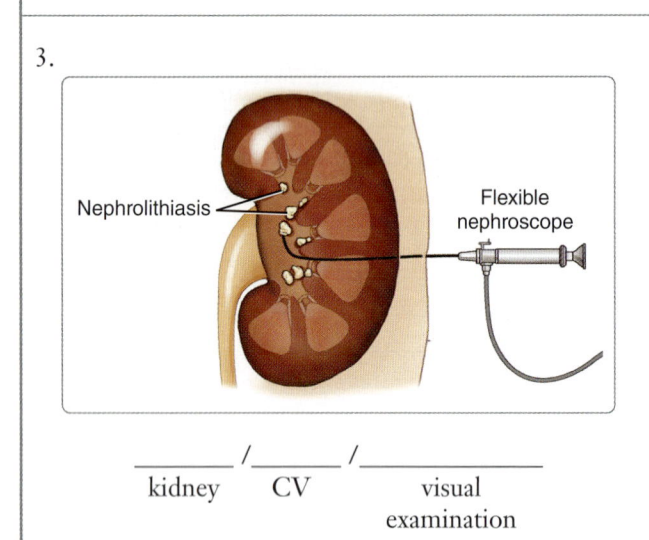

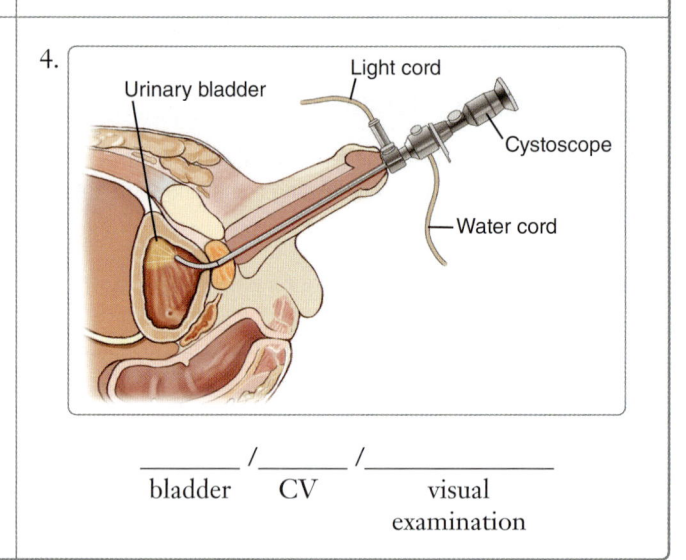

3. _____ / _____ / _____
   kidney   CV   visual examination

4. _____ / _____ / _____
   bladder   CV   visual examination

C Fill In

Build diagnostic terms that correspond to the following definitions by using the word parts you have learned.

1. visual examination of the ureter
   _____ / _____ / _____
   WR   CV   S

2. radiographic image of the renal pelvis
   _____ / _____ / _____
   WR   CV   S

3. process of recording the kidney using sound
   _____ / ___ / _____ / ___ / _____
   WR   CV   WR   CV   S

4. instrument used for visual examination of the bladder
   _____ / _____ / _____
   WR   CV   S

Chapter 6   Urinary System   213

5. radiographic imaging of the bladder and the urethra

voiding _____ / ___ / _____ / ___ / ___
          WR   CV   WR   CV   S

6. radiographic imaging of the bladder

_____ / ___ / ___
  WR   CV   S

7. radiographic record of the kidney, used to evaluate kidney function

_____ / ___ / ___
  WR   CV   S

EXERCISE 18 ■ Diagnostic Terms NOT Built from Word Parts

A Label

Write the medical terms pictured and defined.

1. _____
test that measures the amount of nitrogen in the blood that comes from urea

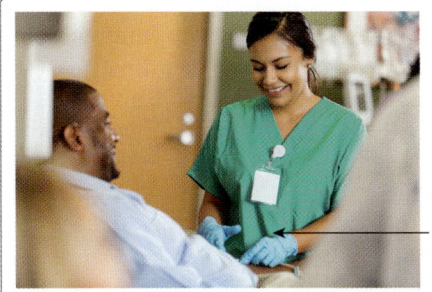

Phlebotomist preparing to withdraw a blood sample

2. _____
multiple tests performed on a urine specimen

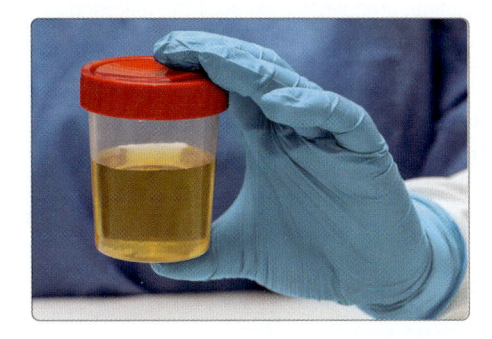

3. _____
radiographic image of the abdomen to view kidneys, ureters, and bladder

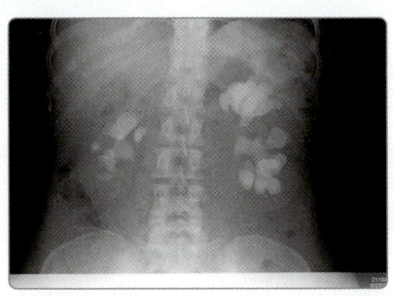

Note the bilateral calculi that fill the renal pelvis. Due to their distinctive shape, these are called **staghorn calculi** because of their resemblance to the antlers of a stag.

4. _____
test on urine specimen to measure the concentrating and diluting abilities of the kidneys

Laboratory results

URINE
COLOR_____
APPEARANCE_____
PH_____
SG_____
ACETONE_____
GLUCOSE_____
BACTERIA_____
WBC_____
RBC_____
CASTS_____
OCCULT BLOOD_____
OTHER_____

B Match

Match the terms in the first column with their correct definitions in the second column.

_____ 1. specific gravity
_____ 2. urodynamics
_____ 3. urinalysis
_____ 4. KUB
_____ 5. creatinine
_____ 6. blood urea nitrogen
_____ 7. urine culture and sensitivity
_____ 8. glomerular filtration rate

a. radiographic image of the kidneys, ureters, and bladder
b. test that measures the amount of nitrogen in the blood that comes from urea
c. urine test to measure concentrating or diluting abilities of the kidneys
d. multiple routine tests performed on a urine sample
e. test that measures kidney function by estimating the amount of blood filtered by the kidneys each minute
f. test performed on a urine specimen to determine the presence of bacteria and yeast
g. tests to measure the force and flow of urine in the lower urinary tract
h. test that measures the amount of a waste product in the blood that comes from the normal wear and tear of muscles

EXERCISE 19 ■ Review of Diagnostic Terms

Can you define, pronounce, and spell the following terms?

blood urea nitrogen (BUN)
creatinine
cystogram
cystoscope
cystoscopy
glomerular filtration rate (GFR)
KUB
nephrography
nephroscopy
nephrosonography
pyelogram
renogram
retrograde urogram
specific gravity (SG)
ureteroscopy
urinalysis (UA)
urine culture and sensitivity
urodynamics
voiding cystourethrography (VCUG)

Complementary Terms
BUILT FROM WORD PARTS

The following terms can be translated using definitions of word parts. Further explanation is provided within parentheses as needed.

SIGNS AND SYMPTOMS

TERM	DEFINITION	TERM	DEFINITION
1. albuminuria (al-bū-min-Ū-rē-a)	albumin in the urine (albumin is an important protein in the blood, but when found in the urine, may indicate kidney disease; small amounts may be present in the absence of kidney disease); (lab finding)	4. dysuria (dis-Ū-rē-a)	difficult or painful urination
		5. glycosuria (glī-kō-SŪ-rē-a)	sugar (glucose) in the urine; (lab finding)
		6. hematuria (hēm-a-TU-rē-a)	blood in the urine; (symptom and lab finding)
2. anuria (an-Ū-rē-a)	absence of urine (failure of the kidney to produce urine)	7. nocturia (nok-TŪ-rē-a)	night urination
3. azotemia (az-ō-TĒ-mē-a)	nitrogen in the blood (laboratory abnormality indicating an increase in nitrogen-containing compounds, including urea and creatinine; one of many signs and symptoms of uremia); (lab finding)	8. oliguria (ol-i-GŪ-rē-a)	scanty urine (amount)
		9. polyuria (pol-ē-Ū-rē-a)	much (excessive) urine
		10. pyuria (pī-Ū-rē-a)	pus in the urine; (lab finding)

MEDICAL SPECIALTIES

TERM	DEFINITION	TERM	DEFINITION
11. **nephrologist** (ne-FROL-o-jist)	physician who studies and treats diseases of the kidney	13. **urologist** (ū-ROL-o-jist)	physician who studies and treats diseases of the urinary tract
12. **nephrology** (ne-FROL-o-jē)	study of the kidney (a branch of medicine dealing with diseases of the kidney)	14. **urology** (ū-ROL-o-jē)	study of the urinary tract (a branch of medicine dealing with diseases of the male and female urinary systems and the male reproductive system)

UROLOGIST/NEPHROLOGIST A **urologist** treats diseases of the male and female urinary system and the male reproductive system both medically and surgically. A **nephrologist** treats kidney diseases and prescribes and manages dialysis therapy.

DESCRIPTIVE TERMS

TERM	DEFINITION	TERM	DEFINITION
15. **intravesical** (*in*-tra-VES-i-kal)	pertaining to within the (urinary) bladder	17. **transurethral** (*trans*-ū-RĒ-thral)	pertaining to through the urethra
16. **meatal** (mē-Ā-tal)	pertaining to the meatus	18. **urinary** (Ū-rin-*ār*-ē)	pertaining to urine

EXERCISE 20 ■ Pronounce and Spell

Practice pronunciation and spelling on paper and online.

1. **Practice on Paper**
    a. **Pronounce:** Read the phonetic spelling and say aloud the terms listed in the previous table. Refer to Table 2.2 Pronunciation Key as needed.
    b. **Spell:** Have a study partner read the terms aloud. Write the spelling of the terms on a separate sheet of paper.
2. **Practice Online**
    a. **Access** online learning resources. Go to evolve.elsevier.com > Evolve Resources > Student Resources.
    b. **Pronounce:** Select Audio Glossary > Chapter 6 > Exercise 20. Select a term to hear its pronunciation and repeat aloud.
    c. **Spell:** Select Activities > Chapter 6 > Spell Terms > Exercise 20. Select the audio icon and type the correct spelling of the term.

❏ Check the box when complete.

EXERCISE 21 ■ Analyze and Define

Analyze and define the following terms by drawing slashes between word parts, writing word part abbreviations above the term, underlining combining forms, and writing combining form abbreviations below the term.

1. nocturia

2. urologist

3. oliguria

4. nephrologist

216   **Chapter 6**   Urinary System

5. hematuria
   _____
   _____

6. urology
   _____
   _____

7. polyuria
   _____
   _____

8. albuminuria
   _____
   _____

9. anuria
   _____
   _____

10. azotemia
    _____
    _____

11. pyuria
    _____
    _____

12. urinary
    _____
    _____

13. glycosuria
    _____
    _____

14. dysuria
    _____
    _____

15. nephrology
    _____
    _____

16. intravesical
    _____
    _____

17. meatal
    _____
    _____

18. transurethral
    _____
    _____

EXERCISE 22 ■ Build

A Fill In

Build complementary terms for the following definitions by using the word parts you have learned. *Note: The abbreviation S(WR) indicates the suffix contains a word root.*

1. night urination   _____ WR _____ / _____ S _____

2. scanty urine   _____ WR _____ / _____ S _____

3. pus in the urine   _____ WR _____ / _____ S _____

Chapter 6 Urinary System 217

4. physician who studies and treats diseases of the urinary tract

_____ / _____ / _____
WR   CV   S

5. much (excessive) urine

_____ / _____
P   S(WR)

6. study of the kidney

_____ / _____ / _____
WR   CV   S

7. pertaining to urine

_____ / _____
WR   S

8. nitrogen in the blood

_____ / _____
WR   S

9. study of the urinary tract

_____ / _____ / _____
WR   CV   S

10. pertaining to through the urethra

_____ / _____ / _____
P   WR   S

11. sugar (glucose) in the urine

_____ / _____
WR   S

12. pertaining to within the (urinary) bladder

_____ / _____ / _____
P   WR   S

13. absence of urine

_____ / _____
P   S(WR)

14. albumin in the urine

_____ / _____
WR   S

B Label

Build terms pictured by writing word parts above definitions.

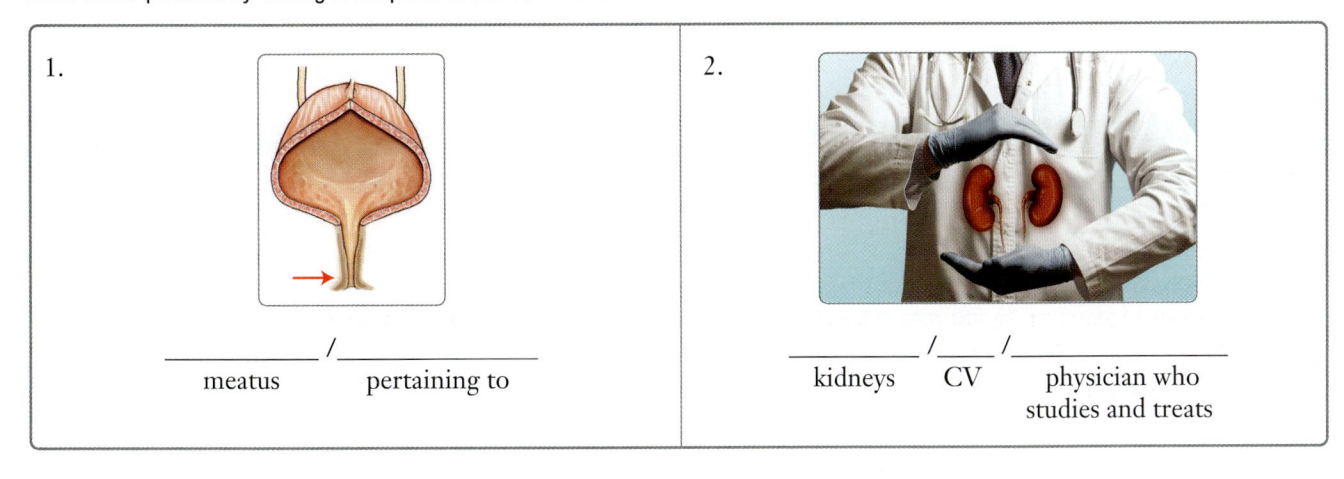

1.

_____ / _____
meatus   pertaining to

2.

_____ / _____ / _____
kidneys   CV   physician who studies and treats

3.

_____ / _____
difficult   urination
or painful

4.

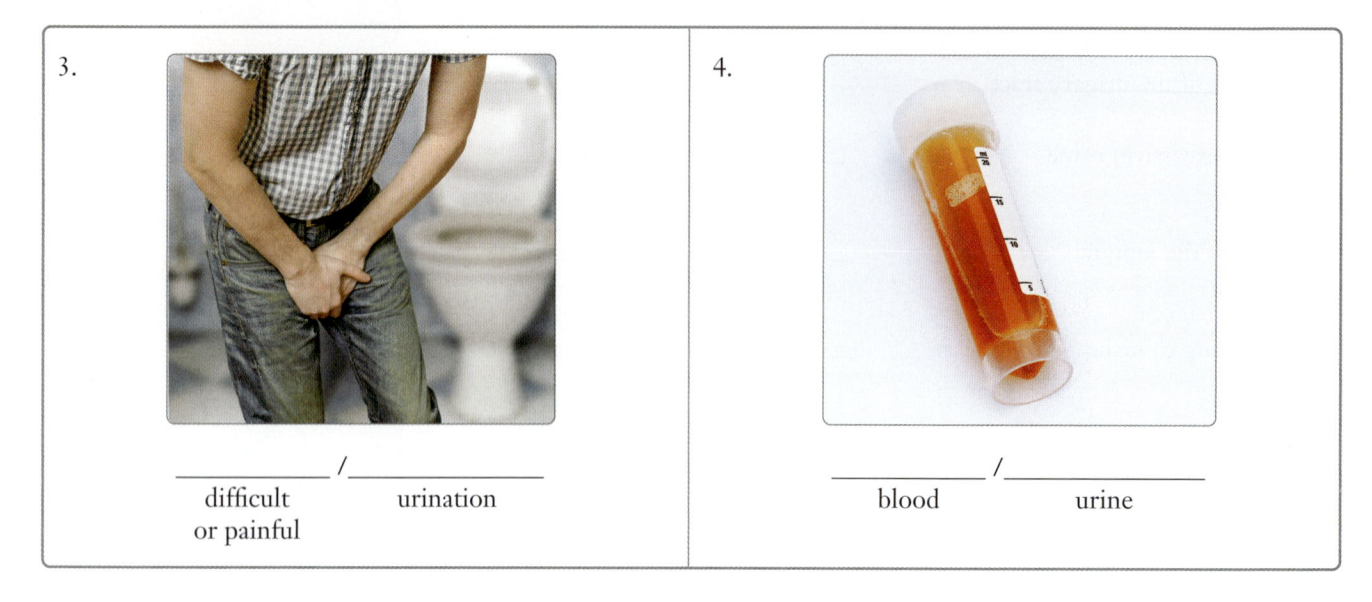

_____ / _____
blood   urine

Complementary Terms
NOT BUILT FROM WORD PARTS

Word parts may be present in the following terms; however, their full meanings cannot be translated using definitions of word parts alone.

SIGNS AND SYMPTOMS	
TERM	**DEFINITION**
1. enuresis (*en*-ū-RĒ-sis)	involuntary urination. **Nocturnal enuresis**, or bed-wetting, has been described in early literature and continues to be a problem affecting 15% to 20% of school-aged children. There is no one cause for bed-wetting. **Diurnal enuresis** is daytime wetting, which may be caused by a small bladder. Various treatments are used to treat diurnal enuresis. Children generally outgrow daytime wetting.
2. prolapse (prō-LAPS)	displacement of an organ or anatomic structure from its normal position (also called **ptosis**)
3. stricture (STRIK-chūr)	abnormal narrowing, such as a urethral stricture
4. urinary incontinence (Ū-rin-ār-ē) (in-KON-ti-nens)	inability to control the bladder, causing leakage of urine

TREATMENTS	
TERM	**DEFINITION**
5. diuretic (*dī*-ū-RET-ik)	agent that promotes the formation and excretion of urine
6. hemodialysis (HD) (*hē*-mō-dī-AL-i-sis)	procedure that uses a machine to withdraw blood, filter out waste and excess fluid, and return clean blood to the body; used as a kidney replacement therapy when the kidneys stop working (Fig. 6.13A)
7. peritoneal dialysis (*par*-i-tō-NĒ-al) (dī-AL-i-sis)	procedure that uses blood vessels inside the abdominal lining (peritoneum) to filter waste and excess fluid from the blood with the aid of a cleansing solution that contains water, salt, and other additives. An alternative to hemodialysis. (Fig. 6.13B)
8. urinary catheterization (Ū-rin-ār-ē) (*kath*-e-ter-i-ZĀ-shun)	passage of a tubelike device (catheter) into the urinary bladder to withdraw urine

Chapter 6 Urinary System 219

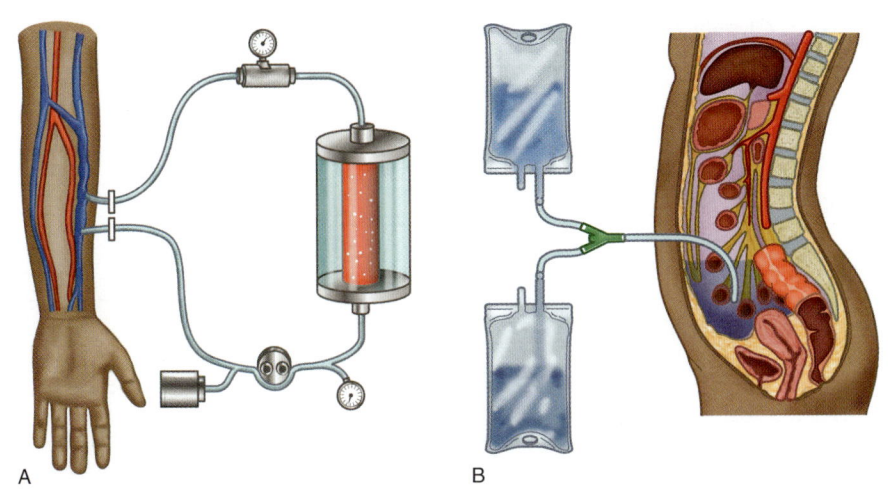

FIG. 6.13 Types of dialysis. **A,** Hemodialysis. A fistula (passageway) is surgically created between an artery and a vein in the arm; blood is removed, filtered by a machine, then replaced at this site. **B,** Peritoneal dialysis. A catheter is surgically inserted into the abdominal cavity; a sterile cleansing solution is instilled by gravity and then drained from the same catheter once filtering is complete.

EQUIPMENT	
TERM	**DEFINITION**
9. **catheter (cath)** (KATH-e-ter)	flexible, tubelike device, such as a urinary catheter, for withdrawing or instilling fluids
🏛 **CATHETER** is derived from the Greek **katheter,** meaning a **thing let down.** A catheter lets down the urine from the bladder.	
10. **urinal** (Ū-rin-al)	receptacle for urine

OTHER	
TERM	**DEFINITION**
11. **distended** (dis-TEN-ded)	stretched out (a bladder is distended when filled with urine)
12. **electrolytes** (ē-LEK-trō-lītz)	minerals in the body, such as sodium and potassium, that carry an electric charge. Electrolyte balance is necessary for the body to function normally and is maintained by the kidneys.
13. **void** (voyd)	to empty or evacuate waste material, especially urine

🔍 Refer to Appendix E for pharmacology terms related to the urinary system.

EXERCISE 23 ▪ Pronounce and Spell

Practice pronunciation and spelling on paper and online.

1. **Practice on Paper**

    a. **Pronounce:** Read the phonetic spelling and say aloud the terms listed in the previous table. Refer to Table 2.2 Pronunciation Key as needed.

    b. **Spell:** Have a study partner read the terms aloud. Write the spelling of the terms on a separate sheet of paper.

2. **Practice Online** 🌐

    a. **Access** online learning resources. Go to evolve.elsevier.com > Evolve Resources > Student Resources.

    b. **Pronounce:** Select Audio Glossary > Chapter 6 > Exercise 23. Select a term to hear its pronunciation and repeat aloud.

220 Chapter 6 Urinary System

  c. **Spell:** Select Activities > Chapter 6 > Spell Terms > Exercise 23. Select the audio icon and type the correct spelling of the term.

❑ Check the box when complete.

EXERCISE 24 ■ Fill In

A Label

Write the medical terms pictured and defined.

1. _____
procedure that uses a machine to withdraw blood, filter out waste and excess fluid, and return clean blood to the body

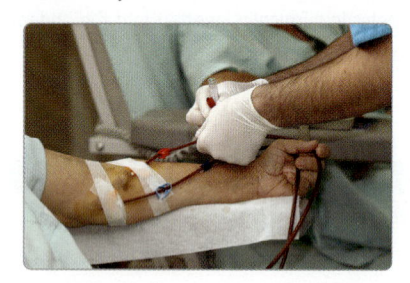

2. _____
flexible, tubelike device for withdrawing or instilling fluids

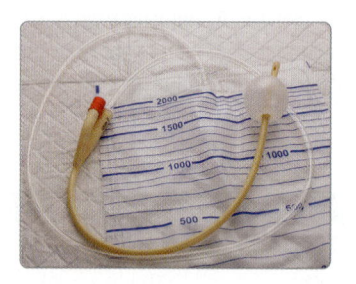

3. _____
stretched out

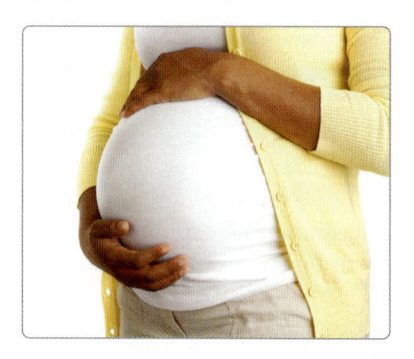

4. _____
involuntary urination

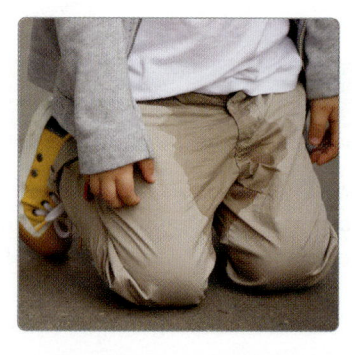

5. _____
receptacle for urine

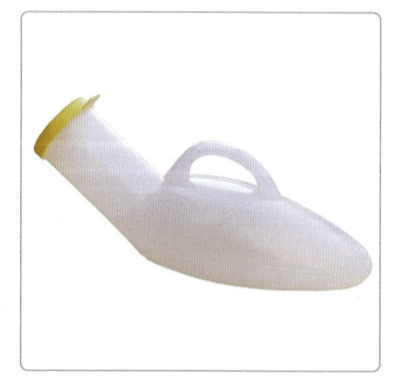

6. _____
procedure that uses blood vessels inside the abdominal lining (peritoneum) to filter waste and excess fluid from the blood with the aid of a cleansing solution

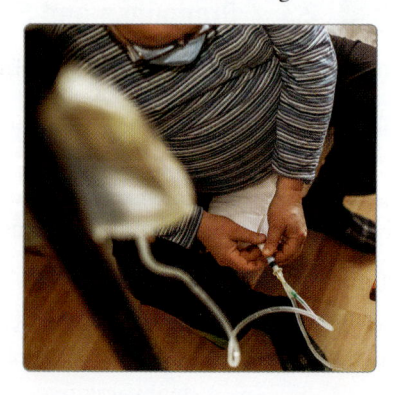

B Identify

Fill in the blanks with the correct terms.

1. Minerals in the body, such as sodium and potassium, are called _____.
2. A(n) _____ agent promotes the formation and excretion of urine.
3. Ptosis is another name for _____, which is displacement of an organ or anatomic structure from its normal position.
4. The inability to control the bladder, causing leaking of urine, is called _____.
5. The passage of a tubelike device into the urinary bladder to withdraw urine is _____.
6. To evacuate waste material, especially urine, is to _____.
7. A(n) _____ is an abnormal narrowing.

EXERCISE 25 ■ Match

A

Match the terms in the first column with their correct definitions in the second column.

_____ 1. catheter
_____ 2. urinary catheterization
_____ 3. distended
_____ 4. void
_____ 5. hemodialysis
_____ 6. urinary incontinence

a. to evacuate or empty waste material, especially urine
b. inability to control the bladder, causing leakage of urine
c. procedure that uses a machine to filter out waste and excess fluid
d. flexible, tubelike device for withdrawing or instilling fluids
e. stretched out
f. passage of a tubelike device into the urinary bladder to remove urine

B

Match the terms in the first column with their correct definitions in the second column.

_____ 1. prolapse
_____ 2. peritoneal dialysis
_____ 3. stricture
_____ 4. urinal
_____ 5. enuresis
_____ 6. diuretic
_____ 7. electrolytes

a. displacement of an organ or anatomic structure from its normal position
b. receptacle for urine
c. agent that promotes the formation and excretion of urine
d. procedure that uses blood vessels inside the abdominal lining to filter waste and excess fluid
e. balance is necessary for the body to function normally
f. involuntary urination
g. abnormal narrowing

EXERCISE 26 ■ Review of Complementary Terms

Can you define, pronounce, and spell the following terms?

albuminuria	enuresis	nocturia	urinary
anuria	glycosuria	oliguria	urinary incontinence
azotemia	hematuria	peritoneal dialysis	urinary catheterization
catheter (cath)	hemodialysis (HD)	polyuria	urinal
distended	intravesical	prolapse	urologist
diuretic	meatal	pyuria	urology
dysuria	nephrologist	stricture	void
electrolytes	nephrology	transurethral	

Abbreviations

DISEASE AND DISORDERS

ABBREVIATION	TERM	ABBREVIATION	TERM
AKI	acute kidney injury	ESKD	end-stage kidney disease
ARF	acute renal failure	ESRD	end-stage renal disease
AUR	acute urinary retention	OAB	overactive bladder
CKD	chronic kidney disease	PKD	polycystic kidney disease
CRF	chronic renal failure	UTI	urinary tract infection
CUR	chronic urinary retention	VUR	vesicoureteral reflux

DIAGNOSTIC

ABBREVIATION	TERM	ABBREVIATION	TERM
BUN	blood urea nitrogen	SG	specific gravity
GFR	glomerular filtration rate	UA	urinalysis
KUB	kidneys ureters (and) bladder	VCUG	voiding cystourethrography

TREATMENT AND EQUIPMENT

ABBREVIATION	TERM	ABBREVIATION	TERM
cath	catheterization, catheter; spoken as a whole word (kath)	ESWL	extracorporeal shock wave lithotripsy
		HD	hemodialysis

Refer to Appendix D for a complete list of abbreviations.

EXERCISE 27 ■ Fill In

Write the terms abbreviated.

1. When imaging is used to diagnose obstructive uropathy, a **KUB** _____ (and) _____ is usually performed first. A urogram may be used for confirming or excluding obstruction and determining its level and cause. For further examination, **VCUG** _____ may be performed to evaluate the posterior urethra and check for **VUR** _____.
2. **SG** _____ is one of many tests performed on the urine specimen during a **UA** _____. It measures the concentration of particles, including water and electrolytes in the urine.
3. **BUN** _____ is a laboratory test done on a blood sample that measures nitrogen that comes from urea. **GFR** _____ reflects normal kidney function if it is above 90, and severe kidney disease at levels of 30 and below.
4. The number, size, and type of stones are important in determining whether **ESWL** _____ _____ is the best method for treating renal calculi.
5. Bladder **cath** _____ may be used for either **AUR** _____ or **CUR** _____, but carries the risk of **UTI** _____.
6. Peritoneal dialysis, **HD** _____, and renal transplant are known as renal replacement therapies.
7. The more current term for **ARF** _____ is **AKI** _____. Onset is sudden and full recovery can occur with prompt treatment. **CKD** _____ is a more modern term for **CRF** _____. It is irreversible and progressive. **ESKD** _____, sometimes referred to as **ESRD** _____, is when kidney function will not sustain life. A kidney transplant or dialysis may be used as treatment.
8. Urge incontinence is another name for **OAB** _____ and involves a sudden, strong need to urinate. As the bladder contracts, leakage of urine occurs.
9. Nephrosonography, or renal ultrasound, may be used to help diagnose **PKD** _____, which is usually hereditary, and may be accompanied by renal hypertension, hematuria, or nephrolithiasis.

Chapter 6 Urinary System 223

PRACTICAL APPLICATION

EXERCISE 28 ■ Case Study: Translate Between Everyday Language and Medical Language

CASE STUDY: Tyrone Parker

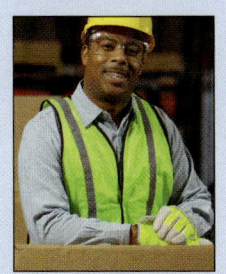

Tyrone Parker was feeling fine until about 3 days ago. He was at his job at a warehouse when he noticed pain in his back, but only on the left side. At first he thought maybe he pulled something when he was moving inventory. He took some over-the-counter pain medicine, but this didn't really seem to help. In the past when he had back pain, it got better after a night of sleep. When he woke up the next morning, the pain was worse and had spread into the lower part of his belly and his groin, still on the left side. He also noticed blood when he urinated. He was worried that he might have an infection of his bladder. He did not experience difficulty urinating but decided to make an appointment to see a physician who treats diseases of the urinary tract.

Now that you have worked through Chapter 6, on the urinary system, consider the medical terms that might be used to describe Tyrone's experience. See the Chapter at a Glance section at the end of the chapter for a list of terms that might apply.

A. Underline phrases in the case study that could be substituted with medical terms.

B. Write the medical term and its definition for three of the phrases you underlined.

MEDICAL TERM	DEFINITION
1. _____	_____
2. _____	_____
3. _____	_____

DOCUMENTATION: Excerpt from the Urgent Care Visit

Tyrone decided to go to Urgent Care because he could receive care right away. The following was noted in the Subjective section of the Electronic Health Record (EHR).

The patient is a 38-year-old man who was in his usual state of good health when he began to experience left-sided flank pain accompanied by gross hematuria 3 days ago. He denies chills or fever. He has no prior history of renal calculi but was treated for UTI 1 year ago. His father had end-stage kidney disease requiring hemodialysis.

C. Underline medical terms presented in Chapter 6 in the previous excerpt from Tyrone's medical record. See the Chapter at a Glance section at the end of the chapter for a complete list.

D. Select and define three of the medical terms you underlined. To check your answers, go to Appendix A.

MEDICAL TERM	DEFINITION
1. _____	_____
2. _____	_____
3. _____	_____

Chapter 6 Urinary System

EXERCISE 29 — Interact with Medical Documents

A

Read the report and complete it by writing medical terms on answer lines within the document. Definitions of terms to be written appear after the document.

83658 OLIVER, Bruno

Name: OLIVER, Bruno   MR#: 7463802   Sex: M   Allergies: NKDA
DOB: 07/30/19XX   Age: 32   PCP: Betsy Bathilde MD

Date of Admssion: 09/20/20XX
Date of Discharge: 09/23/20XX

Discharge Summary: Bruno Oliver is a 32-year-old male, appearing his stated age, who was admitted to the hospital after presenting to the emergency department on 09/20/20XX in acute distress. He complained of intermittent pain in the right posterior lumbar area, radiating to the right flank. He has a family history of 1. _____ and has been treated for this condition two other times in the past 10 years.

The white blood count, hemoglobin, and hematocrit were normal. The urinalysis showed microscopic 2. _____ .

This patient was admitted to the 3. _____ Unit and was administered intravenous morphine sulfate for pain control. VITAL SIGNS: Low-grade temperature of 99.4°F. Initial blood pressure was 146/92 mm Hg.

A 4. _____ revealed 5. _____ in the region of the right renal pelvis. A 6. _____ with a CT 7. _____ confirmed the presence of the three stones in the right kidney. Significant ureteral obstruction was present.

A percutaneous 8. _____ was completed with no complications. A ureteral stent was inserted as was an indwelling Foley 9. _____. Drainage from the right kidney was pale yellow in 48 hours. The Foley catheter was removed 3 days postoperatively.

At discharge, the patient is voiding without difficulty. The stones were sent to the laboratory for analysis. The report indicated that they were calcium oxalate.

The patient is to follow up with his urologist in a week to have his ureteral stent removed.

Electronically signed: Evan Landis, DO 09/23/20XX 09:18

Definitions of Medical Terms to Complete the Document

Write the medical terms defined on corresponding answer lines in the document.

1. condition of stones in the kidney
2. blood in the urine
3. study of the urinary tract
4. radiographic image of the abdomen
5. stones
6. visual examination of the bladder
7. radiographic image of the renal pelvis
8. incision into the kidney to remove a stone
9. flexible, tubelike device

B

Read the medical report and answer the questions below it.

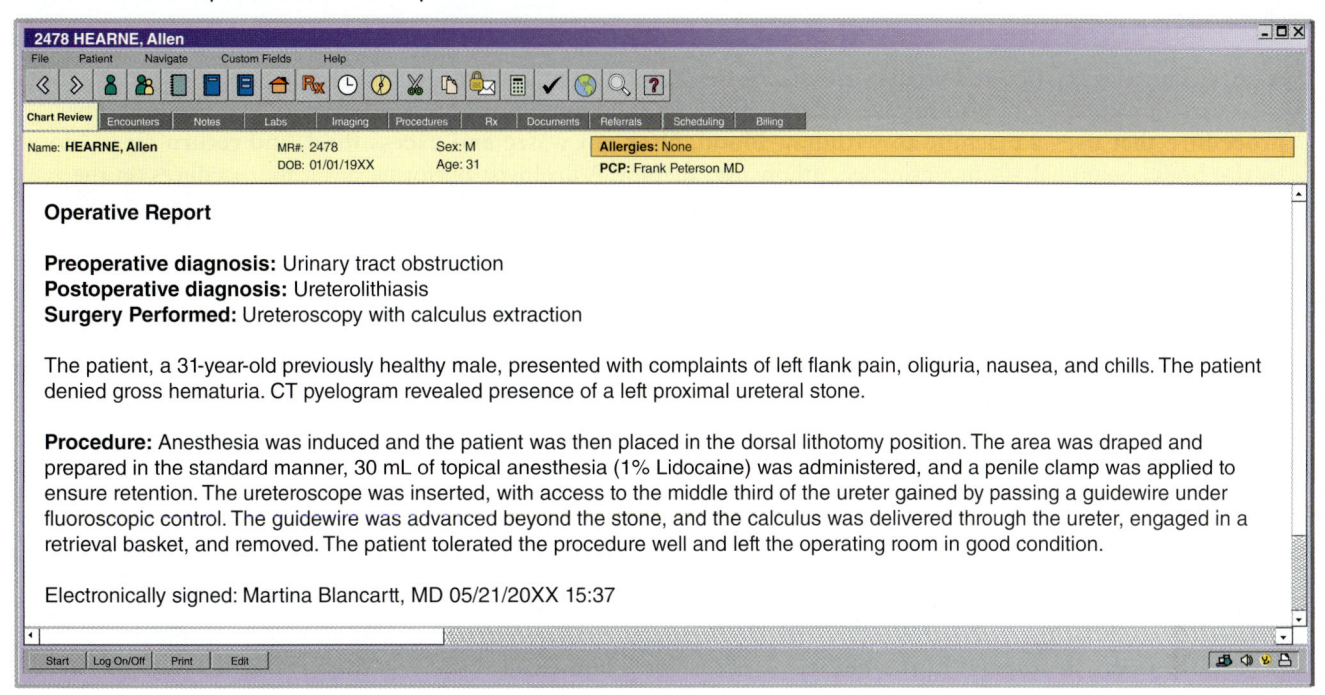

2478 HEARNE, Allen

Name: HEARNE, Allen MR#: 2478 Sex: M Allergies: None
DOB: 01/01/19XX Age: 31 PCP: Frank Peterson MD

Operative Report

Preoperative diagnosis: Urinary tract obstruction
Postoperative diagnosis: Ureterolithiasis
Surgery Performed: Ureteroscopy with calculus extraction

The patient, a 31-year-old previously healthy male, presented with complaints of left flank pain, oliguria, nausea, and chills. The patient denied gross hematuria. CT pyelogram revealed presence of a left proximal ureteral stone.

Procedure: Anesthesia was induced and the patient was then placed in the dorsal lithotomy position. The area was draped and prepared in the standard manner, 30 mL of topical anesthesia (1% Lidocaine) was administered, and a penile clamp was applied to ensure retention. The ureteroscope was inserted, with access to the middle third of the ureter gained by passing a guidewire under fluoroscopic control. The guidewire was advanced beyond the stone, and the calculus was delivered through the ureter, engaged in a retrieval basket, and removed. The patient tolerated the procedure well and left the operating room in good condition.

Electronically signed: Martina Blancartt, MD 05/21/20XX 15:37

Use the medical report above to answer the questions.

1. The patient presented with a complaint of
   a. difficult or painful urination.
   b. excessive urine.
   c. scanty urine.
   d. pus in the urine.

2. The presence of a ureteral stone was revealed by
   a. radiographic imaging.
   b. magnetic resonance imaging.
   c. ultrasound.
   d. computed tomography.

3. T F More than one stone was removed from the ureter.

4. Ureteroscope and ureteral are terms not included in the chapter. Using your knowledge of the meaning of word parts, define these terms.
   a. ureteral _____
   b. ureteroscope _____
   _____

EXERCISE 30 ■ Use Medical Language in Online Electronic Health Records

Select the correct medical terms to complete three medical records in one patient's electronic file.

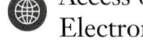

🌐 Access online resources at evolve.elsevier.com > Evolve Resources > Student Resources > Activities > Chapter 6 > Electronic Health Records

Topic: Renal Calculus
Record 1, Encounters: Office Visit
Record 2, Procedures: Operative Report
Record 3, Notes: Postoperative Office Visit

❏ Check the box when complete.

EXERCISE 31 ■ Use Medical Terms in Clinical Statements

For each phrase printed in bold, circle the medical term or abbreviation defined. Answers are listed in Appendix A. For pronunciation practice read the answers aloud.

1. A **physician who studies and treats diseases of the kidney** (dermatologist, oncologist, nephrologist) takes care of patients with **progressive, irreversible loss of kidney function** (UTI, AKI, CKD) and prescribes **procedure that uses a machine to withdraw blood, filter out waste and excess fluid, and return clean blood to the body** (hemodialysis, incontinence, lithotripsy) therapy. A urologist performs surgical procedures on the male and female urinary systems, including **creation of an artificial opening into the ureter** (ureteroplasty, ureterostomy, ureterectomy), and treats diseases of the male reproductive system.

2. Mr. Garcia complained of **difficult or painful urination** (dysuria, anuria, oliguria). The **multiple routine tests done on a urine specimen** (cystogram, cystoscopy, urinalysis) revealed **pus in the urine** (nocturia, pyuria, enuresis). He was diagnosed and treated for **inflammation of the bladder** (cystitis, nephritis, pyelonephritis).

3. Tassiana Smith, a 10-year-old girl, has had recurrent (chronic) **inflammation of the urethra and bladder** (urethrocystitis, pyelonephritis, hydronephrosis). To determine the cause, the physician ordered a **radiographic image of the urinary tract** (retrograde urogram, pyelogram, renogram) to be followed by voiding **radiographic imaging of the bladder and urethra** (cystourethrography, nephrosonography, ureteroscopy) if necessary.

4. David Chang presented to the emergency department with visible **blood in the urine** (hematuria, nocturia, glycosuria) along with back and groin pain. A renal ultrasound revealed right proximal **condition of stone(s) in the ureter** (ureterocele, ureteritis, ureterolithiasis). He was treated with antiinflammatory medication and referred to **study of the urinary tract** (nephrology, urology, cytology) to schedule **noninvasive surgical procedure to crush stone(s) in the kidney or ureter by administration of repeated shock waves** (ESKD, VCUG, ESWL).

EXERCISE 32 ■ Pronounce Medical Terms in Use

Practice pronunciation of terms by reading aloud the following paragraph. Use the phonetic spellings to assist with pronunciation. The script also contains medical terms not presented in the chapter. If interested, research their meanings in a medical dictionary or a reliable online source.

A 76-year-old woman consulted with her primary care physician because of **hematuria** (hēm-a-TŪ-rē-a) and **dysuria** (dis-Ū-rē-a). She was referred to a **urologist** (ū-ROL-o-jist). **Urinalysis** (ū-rin-AL-is-is) disclosed 1+ albumin and mild **pyuria** (pī-Ū-rē-a) in addition to the hematuria. A spiral CT scan was obtained. Mild **nephrolithiasis** (nef-rō-lith-Ī-a-sis) was observed but no **hydronephrosis** (hī-drō-ne-FRŌ-sis). Finally a **cystoscopy** (sis-TOS-ko-pē) was performed, which showed mild **cystitis** (sis-TĪ-tis). A **urinary tract infection** (Ū-rin-ār-ē) (trakt) (in-FEK-shun) was diagnosed and the patient responded favorably to antibiotics. The urologist did not advise **lithotripsy** (LITH-ō-trip-sē) for the **renal calculi** (RĒ-nal) (KAL-kū-lī).

Chapter 6 Urinary System 227

CHAPTER REVIEW

EXERCISE 33 ■ Chapter Content Quiz

Test your understanding of terms and abbreviations introduced in this chapter. Circle the letter for the medical term or abbreviation related to the words in italics.

1. The patient was diagnosed with a *drooping kidney*, or:
   a. nephromegaly
   b. nephroblastoma
   c. nephroptosis

2. The patient's radiographic image showed *condition of stones in the ureter*, or a condition known as:
   a. ureterocele
   b. ureterolithiasis
   c. ureterostenosis

3. The patient was scheduled for a right ureteral pelvic junction *ESWL*, a surgical procedure to:
   a. separate tissue
   b. create an artificial opening
   c. remove a stone

4. The physician first suspected diabetes when told of the *excessive amounts of urine* voided, or:
   a. oliguria
   b. polyuria
   c. dysuria

5. The urologist told the patient with the drooping kidney that it is necessary to *secure the kidney in place* by performing a:
   a. nephropexy
   b. nephrolysis
   c. nephrolithotripsy

6. A *test that measures kidney function by estimating the amount of blood filtered by the kidneys* was ordered for the patient with bilateral edema of the lower legs, ankles, and feet:
   a. GFR
   b. UA
   c. BUN

7. The patient was scheduled for a *radiographic image of the urinary bladder*, or:
   a. cystoscopy
   b. cystogram
   c. cystography

8. The patient's mother informed the doctor of her son's *involuntary urination*, or:
   a. diuresis
   b. dysuria
   c. enuresis

9. The patient presented with a(n) *abnormal accumulation of urine in the bladder because of an inability to urinate*, or:
   a. polycystic kidney disease
   b. urinary retention
   c. urinary tract infection

10. The nurse practitioner ordered a *UA* on the patient or:
    a. urine
    b. urinary
    c. urinalysis

11. *Albuminuria* indicates a kidney problem because of albumin in the:
    a. blood
    b. urine
    c. urea

12. In the term nephrolithotripsy, *which word part indicates surgery*?
    a. first combining form
    b. second combining form
    c. suffix

13. When the bladder is *stretched out* because of urine, it is considered to be:
    a. distended
    b. contracted
    c. flexible

14. What is the procedure that uses the abdominal lining and a cleansing solution to filter waste in patients with Stage 5 chronic kidney disease?
    a. hemodialysis
    b. peritoneal dialysis
    c. renal transplant

15. A ureteral *stricture* means the ureter is:
    a. ballooning
    b. narrowing
    c. blocked

16. The patient with *urine (urea nitrogen) in the blood* presented with polyuria, polydipsia, vomiting, and weight loss.
    a. azotemia
    b. hematuria
    c. uremia

17. A *creation of an artificial opening into the urinary system* was required for the patient who had a cystectomy due to carcinoma of the bladder.
    a. urostomy
    b. ureterostomy
    c. urethroplasty

18. Two types of *inability to control the bladder causing leakage of urine* are stress, caused by sneezing, coughing, or bearing down, and urge, which results when patients have to rush to get to the bathroom.
    a. urinary incontinence
    b. stricture
    c. prolapse

19. A(n) *pertaining to within the (urinary) bladder* treatment with mitomycin may be used to treat bladder cancer.
    a. meatal
    b. transurethral
    c. intravesical

20. Furosemide is a common *agent that promotes the formation and excretion of urine* that is used to treat edema and congestive heart failure.
    a. urinary catheterization
    b. diuretic
    c. peritoneal dialysis

CHAPTER AT A GLANCE — Word Parts New to This Chapter

COMBINING FORMS

albumin/o	glycos/o	noct/i	ureter/o	
azot/o	hydr/o	olig/o	urethr/o	
blast/o	lith/o	pyel/o	urin/o	
cyst/o	meat/o	ren/o	vesic/o	
glomerul/o	nephr/o	ur/o		

SUFFIXES

-iasis	-ptosis	
-lith	-tripsy	
-lysis	-uria	
-pexy		

CHAPTER AT A GLANCE — Urinary System Terms Built from Word Parts

DISEASE AND DISORDER
cystitis
cystocele
cystolith
glomerulonephritis
hydronephrosis
nephritis
nephroblastoma
nephrolithiasis
nephroma
nephromegaly
nephroptosis
pyelitis
pyelonephritis
uremia
ureteritis
ureterocele
ureterolithiasis
urethritis
ureterostenosis
urethrocystitis
vesicoureteral reflux (VUR)

SURGICAL
cystectomy
cystolithotomy
cystostomy
lithotripsy
meatotomy
nephrectomy
nephrolithotomy
nephrolithotripsy
nephrolysis
nephropexy
nephrostomy
pyelolithotomy
pyeloplasty
ureterectomy
ureterostomy
urethroplasty
urostomy
vesicourethral suspension

DIAGNOSTIC
cystogram
cystography
cystoscope
cystoscopy
nephroscopy
nephrosonography
pyelogram
renogram
retrograde urogram
ureteroscopy
voiding cystourethrography (VCUG)

COMPLEMENTARY
albuminuria
anuria
azotemia
dysuria
glycosuria
hematuria
intravesical
meatal
nephrologist
nephrology
nocturia
oliguria
polyuria
pyuria
transurethral
urinary
urologist
urology

CHAPTER AT A GLANCE: Urinary System Terms *NOT* Built from Word Parts

DISEASE AND DISORDER
acute kidney injury (AKI)
chronic kidney disease (CKD)
end-stage kidney disease (ESKD)
epispadias
hypospadias
polycystic kidney disease (PKD)
renal calculus (*pl.* calculi)
renal hypertension
urinary retention
urinary tract infection (UTI)

SURGICAL
extracorporeal shock wave lithotripsy (ESWL)
fulguration
renal transplant

DIAGNOSTIC
blood urea nitrogen (BUN)
creatinine
glomerular filtration rate (GFR)
KUB
specific gravity (SG)
urinalysis (UA)
urine culture and sensitivity
urodynamics

COMPLEMENTARY
catheter (cath)
distended
diuretic
electrolytes
enuresis
hemodialysis (HD)
peritoneal dialysis
prolapse
stricture
urinal
urinary catheterization
urinary incontinence
void

PART 2 BODY SYSTEMS

7 Male Reproductive System

Objectives

Upon completion of this chapter, you will be able to:

1. Pronounce organs and anatomic structures of the male reproductive system.
2. Define and spell word parts related to the male reproductive system.
3. Define, pronounce, and spell disease and disorder terms related to the male reproductive system.
4. Define, pronounce, and spell surgical terms related to the male reproductive system.
5. Define, pronounce, and spell diagnostic terms related to the male reproductive system.
6. Define, pronounce, and spell complementary terms related to the male reproductive system.
7. Interpret the meaning of abbreviations related to the male reproductive system.
8. Apply medical language in clinical contexts.

TABLE 7.1 Prostate Cancer, 240
TABLE 7.2 Types of Prostatectomies, 243
TABLE 7.3 Surgical Treatments for Benign Prostatic Hyperplasia, 250

Outline

ANATOMY, 231
Function, 231
Organs and Anatomic Structures of the Male Reproductive System, 231

WORD PARTS, 233
Male Reproductive System Combining Forms, 233
Combining Forms Used with Male Reproductive System Terms, 233
Prefixes, 233
Suffixes, 233

MEDICAL TERMS, 236
Disease and Disorder Terms, 236
  Built from Word Parts, 236
  NOT Built from Word Parts, 239
Surgical Terms, 243
  Built from Word Parts, 243
  NOT Built from Word Parts, 247
Diagnostic Terms, 253
  NOT Built from Word Parts, 253
Complementary Terms, 255
  Built from Word Parts and
    NOT Built from Word Parts, 255
Abbreviations, 258

PRACTICAL APPLICATION, 260
CASE STUDY Translate Between Everyday Language and Medical Language, 260
Interact with Medical Documents, 261
Use Medical Language in Online Electronic Health Records, 262
Use Medical Terms in Clinical Statements, 263
Pronounce Medical Terms in Use, 263

CHAPTER REVIEW, 264
Chapter Content Quiz, 264
Chapter at a Glance, 265

Answers to Chapter Exercises, Appendix A

230

Chapter 7   Male Reproductive System

ANATOMY

The organs of the male reproductive system include external genitalia and internal structures (Fig. 7.1). The male external genitalia include the penis and scrotum, which contains the testes and an initial section of each vas deferens. Internal structures, located within the male pelvis, include a major portion of each vas deferens, the seminal vesicles, and the prostate gland. The penis and urethra are shared between the male reproductive and urinary systems.

Function

The function of the male reproductive system is to produce, sustain, and transport sperm, the male reproductive germ cells, and to secrete the hormone testosterone (Fig. 7.2).

Organs and Anatomic Structures of the Male Reproductive System

TERM	DEFINITION
testis (*pl.* testes) (TES-tis), (TES-tēs)	primary male sex organ, paired, oval-shaped, and enclosed in a sac called the **scrotum**. The testes produce spermatozoa (sperm cells) and the hormone testosterone. (also called **testicle**)
seminiferous tubules (*sem*-i-NIF-er-es) (TOO-bū-elz)	approximately 900 coiled tubes within the testes in which spermatogenesis occurs
sperm (spurm)	the microscopic male germ cell, which, when united with the ovum, produces a zygote (fertilized egg) that with subsequent development becomes an embryo (also called **spermatozoon,** *pl.* **spermatozoa**) (Fig. 7.2)
testosterone (tes-TOS-te-rōn)	the principal male sex hormone. Its chief function is to stimulate the development of the male reproductive organs and secondary sex characteristics such as facial and pubic hair.
epididymis (*pl.* **epididymides**) (*ep*-i-DID-a-mis) (*ep*-i-DID-i-mē-dēz)	coiled tube attached to each testis that provides for storage, transit, and maturation of sperm; continuous with each vas deferens

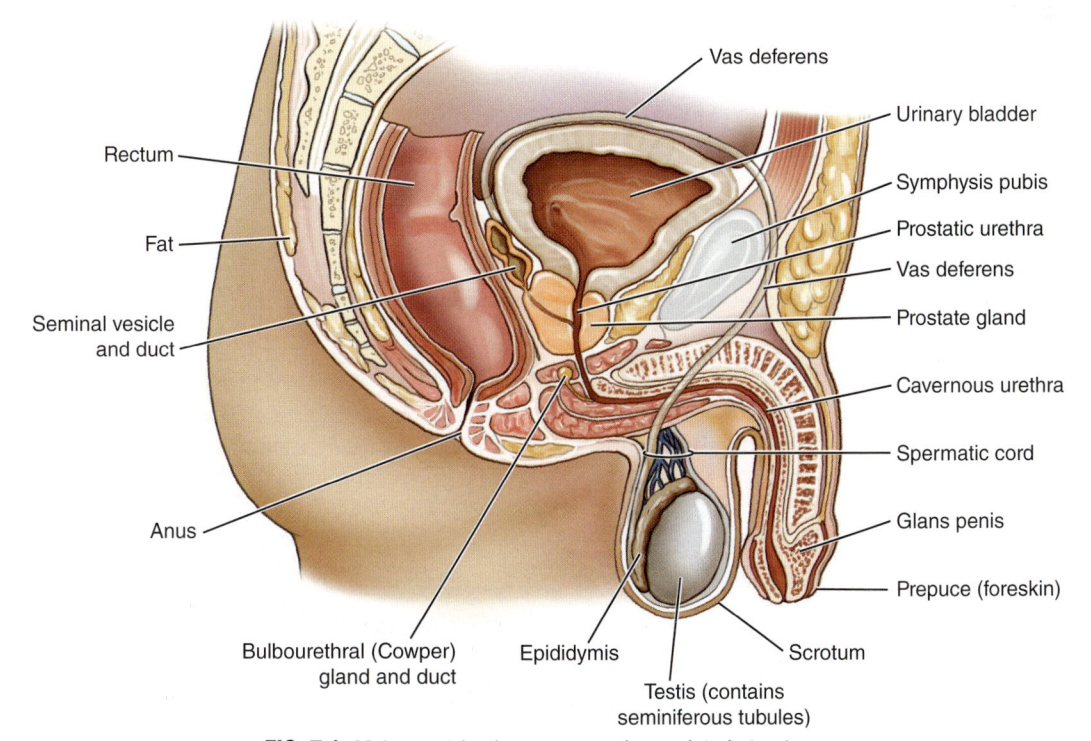

FIG. 7.1 Male reproductive organs and associated structures.

232 Chapter 7 Male Reproductive System

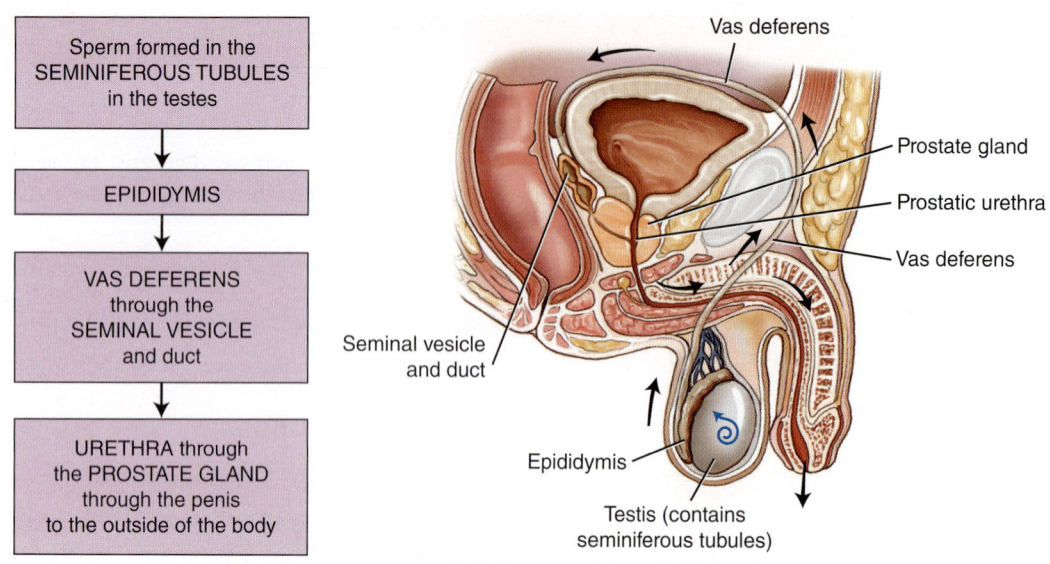

FIG. 7.2 Origination and transportation of sperm.

TERM	DEFINITION
vas deferens (vas) (DEF-ar-enz)	duct (tube) carrying the sperm from the epididymis to the urethra. The **spermatic cord** encloses each vas deferens with nerves, lymphatics, arteries, and veins. The urethra also connects with the urinary bladder and carries urine outside the body. A circular muscle constricts during intercourse to prevent urination. (also called **ductus deferens**)
seminal vesicles (SEM-e-nel) (VES-i-kelz)	two accessory glands located posterior to the base of the bladder that open into the vas deferens. The glands secrete a thick fluid that forms part of the semen.
prostate gland (PROS-tāt) (gland)	walnut-shaped gland that encircles the proximal section of the urethra. The prostate gland secretes a fluid that aids in the movement of the sperm and ejaculation.
🏛 **PROSTATE** is derived from the Greek *pro*, meaning **before**, and **statis**, meaning **standing** or **sitting**. Anatomically it is the gland standing before the bladder.	
semen (SĒ-men)	substance composed of sperm, seminal fluids, and other secretions
scrotum (SKRŌ-tem)	sac containing the testes and their corresponding epididymides, from which each vas deferens begins. The scrotum is suspended on both sides of and posterior to the penis.
penis (PĒ-nis)	male organ of urination and coitus (sexual intercourse)
glans penis (glanz) (PĒ-nis)	enlarged tip on the end of the penis
prepuce (PRE-pūs)	fold of skin covering the glans penis in uncircumcised males (foreskin of the penis)
genitalia (jen-i-TĀ-lē-a)	reproductive organs (male or female); includes internal and external reproductive organs (also called **genitals**)
gonads (GŌ-nadz)	primary reproductive organs; testes in males, ovaries in females

PRONOUNCE ANATOMIC STRUCTURES

Practice saying aloud each of the organs and specific structures on the previous pages.

To hear the terms, go to Evolve Resources at www.evolve.elsevier.com and select:
Student Resources > Audio Glossary > Chapter 7 > Anatomic Structures

❑ Check the box when complete.

Chapter 7 Male Reproductive System

WORD PARTS

Use paper flashcards or electronic flashcards on Evolve to memorize word parts used to analyze, define, and build medical terms in this chapter. To reinforce learning, study one section of the Word Parts Table at a time, then complete the corresponding exercise on the following pages.

1 ■ Male Reproductive System Combining Forms

COMBINING FORM	DEFINITION	COMBINING FORM	DEFINITION
andr/o	male	prostat/o	prostate gland
balan/o	glans penis	sperm/o	sperm, spermatozoon (*pl.* spermatozoa)
epididym/o	epididymis	spermat/o	sperm, spermatozoon (*pl.* spermatozoa)
orch/o	testis, testicle	vas/o	vessel, duct (vas deferens in terms describing the male reproductive system)
orchi/o	testis, testicle		
orchid/o	testis, testicle	vesicul/o	seminal vesicle(s)

2 ■ Combining Forms Used with Male Reproductive System Terms

COMBINING FORM	DEFINITION	COMBINING FORM	DEFINITION
cyst/o	bladder, sac	lith/o	stone(s), calculus (*pl.* calculi)
crypt/o	hidden	olig/o	scanty, few

3 ■ Prefixes

PREFIX	DEFINITION	PREFIX	DEFINITION
a-	absence of, without	hyper-	above, excessive
an-	absence of, without		

4 ■ Suffixes

SUFFIX	DEFINITION	SUFFIX	DEFINITION
-algia	pain	-tomy	cut into, incision
-ectomy	excision, surgical removal	-pexy	surgical fixation
-ia	diseased state, condition of	-pathy	disease
-ic	pertaining to	-plasia	condition of formation, development, growth
-ism	state of		
-itis	inflammation	-plasty	surgical repair
-lith	stone(s), calculus (*pl.* calculi)	-rrhea	flow, discharge
		-stomy	creation of an artificial opening

Refer to **Appendix B** and **Appendix C** for alphabetized word parts and their meanings.

Chapter 7 Male Reproductive System

EXERCISE 1 ■ Male Reproductive System Combining Forms

Refer to the first section of the Word Parts Table.

A Label

Fill in the blanks with combining forms for this diagram of the male reproductive system. *To check your answers, go to Appendix A.*

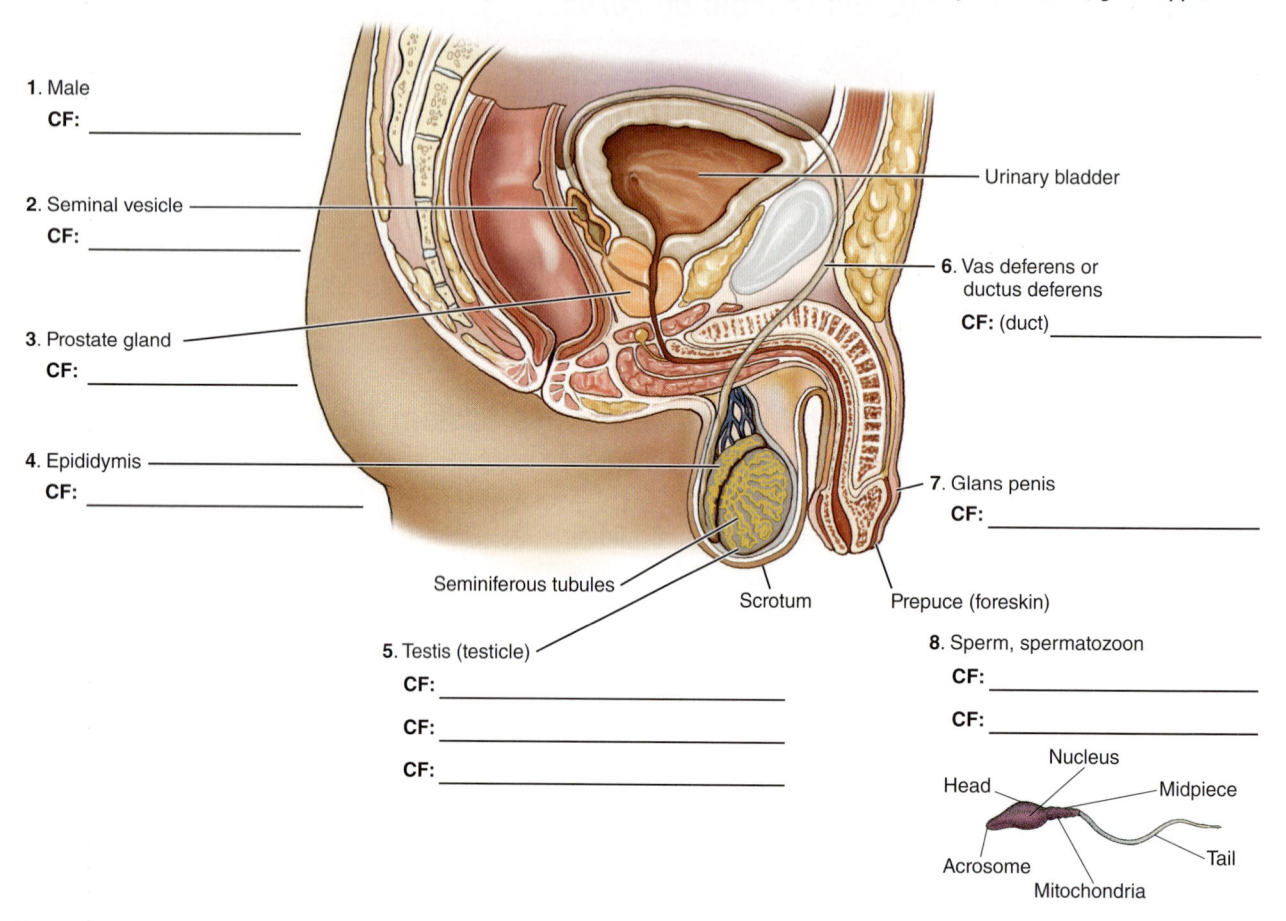

1. Male
   CF: _____

2. Seminal vesicle
   CF: _____

3. Prostate gland
   CF: _____

4. Epididymis
   CF: _____

5. Testis (testicle)
   CF: _____
   CF: _____
   CF: _____

6. Vas deferens or ductus deferens
   CF: (duct) _____

7. Glans penis
   CF: _____

8. Sperm, spermatozoon
   CF: _____
   CF: _____

B Define and Match

Step 1: Write the definitions after the following combining forms.
Step 2: Match the descriptions on the right with the combining forms and definitions. Answers may be used more than once; no answer line appears for those not described in a lettered item.

_____ 1. sperm/o, _____
_____ 2. vas/o (vas deferens), _____
_____ 3. spermat/o, _____
_____ 4. balan/o, _____
_____ 5. prostat/o, _____
_____ 6. orch/o, _____
_____ 7. vesicul/o, _____
_____ 8. orchi/o, _____
_____ 9. epididym/o, _____
_____ 10. orchid/o, _____
_____ 11. andr/o, _____

a. duct (tube) carrying the sperm from the epididymis to the urethra
b. enlarged tip on the end of the penis
c. two accessory glands located posterior to the base of the bladder that open into the vas deferens
d. primary male sex organ, paired, oval-shaped, and enclosed in a sac
e. coiled tube attached to each testis that provides for storage, transit, and maturation of sperm
f. walnut-sized gland that encircles a proximal section of the urethra; secretes fluid that aids in the movement of the sperm and ejaculation
g. microscopic male germ cell, which, when united with the ovum, produces a zygote

EXERCISE 2 ■ Combining Forms Used with Male Reproductive System Terms

Refer to the second section of the Word Parts Table.

A Define

Write the definitions of the following combining forms.

1. olig/o _____
2. crypt/o _____
3. lith/o _____
4. cyst/o _____

B Identify

Write the combining forms for the following definitions.

1. stone(s), calculus (*pl.* calculi) _____
2. bladder, sac _____
3. hidden _____
4. scanty, few _____

EXERCISE 3 ■ Prefixes

Refer to the third section of the Word Parts Table.

A Identify

Write the prefixes for the following definitions.

1. absence of, without a. _____
                              b. _____
2. above, excessive _____

B Define

Write the definitions of the following prefixes.

1. hyper- _____
2. an- _____
3. a- _____

EXERCISE 4 ■ Suffixes

Refer to the fourth section of the Word Parts Table.

A Match

Match the suffixes in the first column with the correct definitions in the second column. A definition may be used more than once.

_____ 1. -plasia   a. flow, discharge
_____ 2. -algia   b. cut into, incision
_____ 3. -ia   c. disease
_____ 4. -tomy   d. condition of formation, development, growth
_____ 5. -rrhea   e. pertaining to
_____ 6. -ic   f. diseased state, condition of
_____ 7. -pathy   g. pain

B Match

Match the suffixes in the first column with the correct definitions in the second column. A definition may be used more than once.

_____ 1. -stomy   a. surgical repair
_____ 2. -ectomy   b. stone(s), calculus (*pl.* calculi)
_____ 3. -pexy   c. surgical fixation
_____ 4. -itis   d. state of
_____ 5. -plasty   e. inflammation
_____ 6. -ism   f. excision, surgical removal
_____ 7. -lith   g. creation of an artificial opening

Chapter 7 Male Reproductive System

MEDICAL TERMS

Medical terms relevant to this chapter have been grouped by topics, such as Disease and Disorder, and are listed in tables designated as Built from Word Parts or *NOT* Built from Word Parts. The exercises following each table assist with learning term definitions, pronunciations, and spellings.

Disease and Disorder Terms
BUILT FROM WORD PARTS

The following terms can be translated using definitions of word parts. Further explanation is provided within parentheses as needed.

TERM	DEFINITION	TERM	DEFINITION
1. andropathy (an-DROP-a-thē)	disease of the male (specific to the male, such as orchitis)	5. cryptorchidism (krip-TOR-ki-diz-em)	state of hidden testis (during fetal development, testes are located in the abdominal area near the kidneys. Before birth they move down into the scrotal sac. Failure of one or both of the testes to descend from the abdominal cavity into the scrotum before birth results in cryptorchidism). (also called **undescended testicle** and **undescended testicles**) (Fig. 7.4)
2. anorchism (an-OR-kizm)	state of absence of testis (unilateral or bilateral)		
3. balanitis (bal-a-NĪ-tis)	inflammation of the glans penis		
4. benign prostatic hyperplasia (BPH) (be-NĪN) (pros-TAT-ik) (hī-per-PLĀ-zha)	excessive development pertaining to the prostate gland (non-malignant enlargement of the prostate gland; causes narrowing of the urethra, which interferes with the passage of urine. Symptoms include frequency of urination, nocturia, urinary retention, and incomplete emptying of the bladder). (also called **benign prostatic hypertrophy**) (Fig. 7.3)	6. epididymitis (ep-i-did-i-MĪ-tis)	inflammation of the epididymis
		7. orchiepididymitis (or-kē-ep-i-did-i-MĪ-tis)	inflammation of the testis and the epididymis
		8. orchitis (or-KĪ-tis)	inflammation of the testis (also called **orchiditis**)
		9. prostatitis (pros-ta-TĪ-tis)	inflammation of the prostate gland
		10. prostatocystitis (pros-ta-tō-sis-TĪ-tis)	inflammation of the prostate gland and the (urinary) bladder
PROSTATIC HYPERPLASIA refers to tissue changes resulting from an abnormal increase in the number of cells as may occur with age. While **benign prostatic hyperplasia** is the correct term for the pathologic process, **benign prostatic hypertrophy** is sometimes used to describe this condition.		11. prostatolith (pros-TAT-ō-lith)	stone(s) in the prostate gland

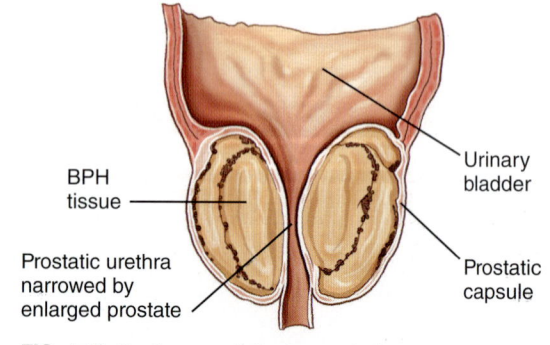

FIG. 7.3 Benign prostatic hyperplasia grows inward, causing narrowing of the urethra.

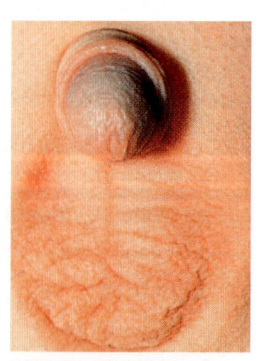

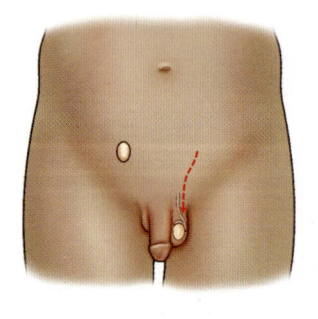

FIG. 7.4 A, Bilateral cryptorchidism. **B,** The arrow indicates the descent of the testis into the scrotal sac, which occurs before birth.

Chapter 7 Male Reproductive System   237

TERM	DEFINITION	TERM	DEFINITION
12. **prostatorrhea** (*pros*-ta-tō-RĒ-a)	discharge from the prostate gland	13. **prostatovesiculitis** (*pros*-ta-tō-ves-*ik*-ū-LĪ-tis)	inflammation of the prostate gland and the seminal vesicles

EXERCISE 5 ■ Pronounce and Spell

Practice pronunciation and spelling on paper and online.

1. **Practice on Paper**
   a. **Pronounce:** Read the phonetic spelling and say aloud the terms listed in the previous table. Refer to Table 2.2 Pronunciation Key as needed.
   b. **Spell:** Have a study partner read the terms aloud. Write the spelling of the terms on a separate sheet of paper.

2. **Practice Online**
   a. **Access** online learning resources. Go to evolve.elsevier.com > Evolve Resources > Student Resources.
   b. **Pronounce:** Select Audio Glossary > Chapter 7 > Exercise 5. Select a term to hear its pronunciation and repeat aloud.
   c. **Spell:** Select Activities > Chapter 7 > Spell Terms > Exercise 5. Select the audio icon and type the correct spelling of the term.

❏ Check the box when complete.

EXERCISE 6 ■ Analyze and Define

Analyze and define the following terms by drawing slashes between word parts, writing word part abbreviations above the term, underlining combining forms, and writing combining form abbreviations below the term.

1. prostatolith

2. balanitis

3. orchitis

4. prostatovesiculitis

5. prostatocystitis

6. orchiepididymitis

7. prostatorrhea

8. epididymitis

9. (benign) prostatic hyperplasia

10. cryptorchidism

238   Chapter 7   Male Reproductive System

11. prostatitis

_____

_____

12. anorchism

_____

_____

13. andropathy

_____

_____

EXERCISE 7 ■ Build

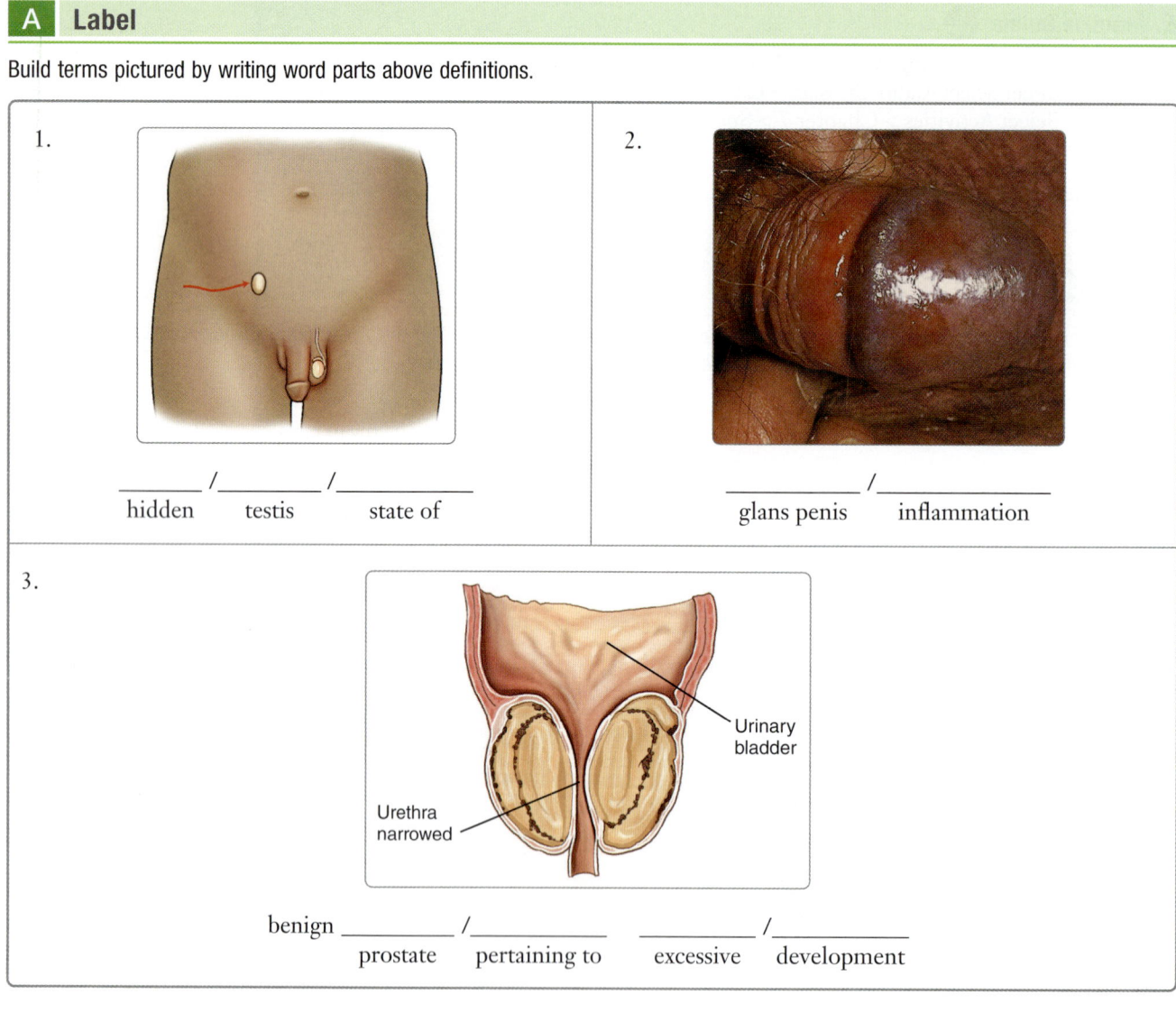

A Label

Build terms pictured by writing word parts above definitions.

1.

_____ / _____ / _____
hidden   testis   state of

2.

_____ / _____
glans penis   inflammation

3.

benign _____ / _____   _____ / _____
        prostate   pertaining to   excessive   development

B Fill In

Build disease and disorder terms for the following definitions with the word parts you have learned.

EXAMPLE: inflammation of the glans penis balan / itis
                                                WR / S

1. inflammation of the prostate gland and the (urinary) bladder
   ___ WR / CV / WR / S

2. stone(s) in the prostate gland
   ___ WR / CV / S

3. inflammation of the testis
   ___ WR / S

4. inflammation of the epididymis
   ___ WR / S

5. discharge from the prostate gland
   ___ WR / CV / S

6. inflammation of the prostate gland and the seminal vesicles
   ___ WR / CV / WR / S

7. state of absence of testis
   ___ P / WR / S

8. inflammation of the prostate gland
   ___ WR / S

9. inflammation of the testis and the epididymis
   ___ WR / WR / S

10. disease of the male
    ___ WR / CV / S

Disease and Disorder Terms
NOT BUILT FROM WORD PARTS

Word parts may be present in the following terms; however, their full meanings cannot be translated using definitions of word parts alone.

TERM	DEFINITION
1. **erectile dysfunction (ED)** (e-REK-tīl) (dis-FUNK-shun)	inability to attain or maintain an erection sufficient to perform sexual intercourse (formerly called **impotence**)
ERECTILE DYSFUNCTION (ED) Oral therapies, such as sildenafil, vardenafil, tadalafil, and avanafil are currently first-line treatment for erectile dysfunction and work by increasing the flow of blood in the genital area. Second-line treatment includes penile self-injectable drugs and vacuum devices. Surgical implantation of a penile prosthesis may be considered when other treatments are not effective.	
2. **hydrocele** (HĪ-drō-sēl)	fluid-filled sac around the testicle; causes scrotal swelling

Disease and Disorder Terms—cont'd
NOT BUILT FROM WORD PARTS

TERM	DEFINITION
3. **infertility** (*in*-fer-TIL-i-tē)	reduced or absent ability to achieve pregnancy; generally defined after one year of frequent, unprotected sexual intercourse; may relate to male or female
4. **phimosis** (fī-MŌ-sis)	tightness of the prepuce (foreskin of the penis) that prevents its retraction over the glans penis; it may be congenital or a result of balanitis. Circumcision is the usual treatment.
5. **priapism** (PRĪ-a-*piz*-m)	persistent abnormal erection of the penis accompanied by pain and tenderness
6. **prostate cancer** (PROS-tāt) (KAN-cer)	cancer of the prostate gland, usually occurring in men middle-aged and older (Table 7.1)
7. **spermatocele** (SPER-ma-tō-sēl)	distension of the epididymis containing an abnormal cyst-like collection of fluid and sperm cells; may cause scrotal swelling
8. **testicular cancer** (tes-TIK-ū-ler) (KAN-cer)	cancer of the testicle, usually occurring in men 15 to 35 years of age

TABLE 7.1 Prostate Cancer

Prostate cancer is the most commonly diagnosed cancer in men and the second most common cause of cancer death among men in the United States. Approximately 95% of all cancers of the prostate are adenocarcinomas, arising from epithelial cells.

DIAGNOSTIC AND STAGING PROCEDURES
1. Digital rectal examination (DRE)
2. Prostate-specific antigen (PSA)
3. Transrectal ultrasound (TRUS)
4. Transrectal ultrasonically guided biopsy
5. MRI ultrasound fusion biopsy
6. MRI with endorectal surface coil (used for staging, not diagnosis)
7. Multiparametric MRI (used for staging, not diagnosis)

TREATMENT
Treatment depends on the stage of the prostate cancer, the age of the patient, and the choices of therapy by the patient and his physician. Options include the following:

1. Active surveillance, with the intent to pursue active therapy if the disease progresses. Used in the earliest stages of cancer, or for men who are much older or have other serious health problems.
2. Radiation therapy, which may be performed with an external beam or with radioactive seeds (brachytherapy). It may be used in all stages of prostate cancer and is often combined with other therapies, especially in more advanced stages.
3. Radical prostatectomy, which may be performed as an open surgery, laparoscopically, or with the use of robotic-assisted devices. Used in all stages of prostate cancer; in later stages, removal of the pelvic lymph nodes is also performed.
4. Hormonal therapy, to reduce the production of testosterone, which fuels the growth of prostate cancer. May be accomplished with medications or with surgical orchiectomy (castration). Used mainly in later stages.
5. Chemotherapy, treating cancer with drugs. Used mainly in later stages.
6. Treatments used for prostate cancer that returns (recurrence) or doesn't respond to other therapies include **cryotherapy**, the use of very cold temperatures to freeze and kill prostate cells, and **immunotherapy**, which helps boost the body's response to the cancer cells.

TABLE 7.1 Prostate Cancer—cont'd

PROGRESSION OF PROSTATE CANCER

TERM	DEFINITION
9. **testicular torsion** (tes-TIK-ū-ler) (TOR-shun)	twisting of the spermatic cord causing decreased blood flow to the testis; occurs most often during puberty and often presents with a sudden onset of severe testicular or scrotal pain. Because of lack of blood flow to the testis, it is considered a surgical emergency.
10. **varicocele** (VAR-i-kō-sēl)	enlarged veins of the spermatic cord; may cause scrotal swelling

EXERCISE 8 ■ Pronounce and Spell

Practice pronunciation and spelling on paper and online.

1. **Practice on Paper**
   a. **Pronounce:** Read the phonetic spelling and say aloud the terms listed in the previous table. Refer to Table 2.2 Pronunciation Key as needed.
   b. **Spell:** Have a study partner read the terms aloud. Write the spelling of the terms on a separate sheet of paper.
2. **Practice Online**
   a. **Access** online learning resources. Go to evolve.elsevier.com > Evolve Resources > Student Resources.
   b. **Pronounce:** Select Audio Glossary > Chapter 7 > Exercise 8. Select a term to hear its pronunciation and repeat aloud.
   c. **Spell:** Select Activities > Chapter 7 > Spell Terms > Exercise 8. Select the audio icon and type the correct spelling of the term.
❑ Check the box when complete.

EXERCISE 9 ■ Fill In

A Identify

Fill in the blanks with the correct terms.

1. Another way of referring to cancer of the testicle is _____.
2. Inability to attain or maintain an erection is called _____.
3. Persistent abnormal erection is called _____.
4. _____ is the twisting of the spermatic cord, causing decreased blood flow.
5. Distension of the epididymis containing an abnormal cyst-like collection of fluid and sperm cells is called a(n) _____.
6. _____ is the reduced or absent ability to achieve pregnancy, generally after one year of unprotected sexual intercourse.

B Label

Write the medical terms pictured and defined.

1. _____
cancer of the prostate gland

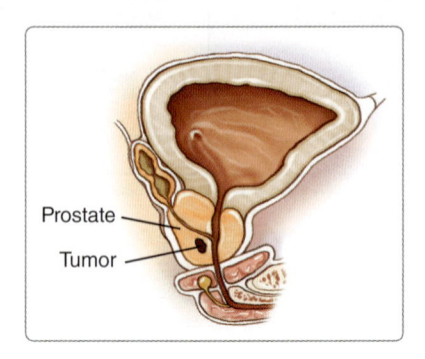

2. _____
tightness of the prepuce (foreskin of the penis) that prevents its retraction over the glans penis

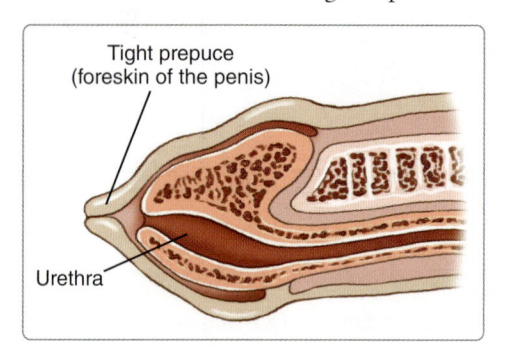

3. _____
fluid-filled sac around the testicle; causes scrotal swelling

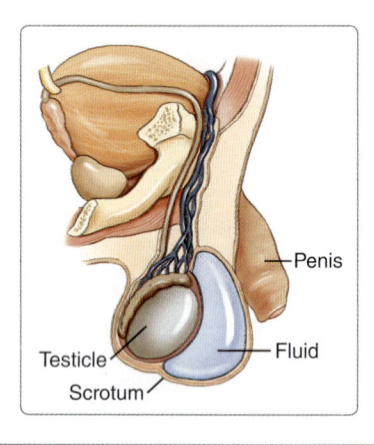

4. _____
enlarged veins of the spermatic cord

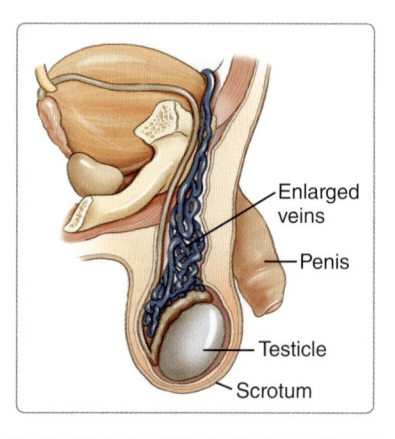

EXERCISE 10 ■ Match

Match the terms in the first column with the correct definitions in the second column.

_____ 1. varicocele
_____ 2. phimosis
_____ 3. testicular cancer
_____ 4. erectile dysfunction
_____ 5. hydrocele
_____ 6. prostate cancer
_____ 7. testicular torsion
_____ 8. priapism
_____ 9. spermatocele
_____ 10. infertility

a. reduced or absent ability to achieve pregnancy
b. inability to attain or maintain an erection
c. tightness of the prepuce
d. enlarged veins of the spermatic cord; may cause scrotal swelling
e. cancer of the testicle
f. cancer of the prostate gland
g. distension of the epididymis containing an abnormal cyst-like collection of fluid and sperm cells
h. persistent abnormal erection
i. twisting of the spermatic cord causing decreased blood flow
j. fluid-filled sac around the testicle; causes scrotal swelling

Chapter 7 Male Reproductive System 243

EXERCISE 11 ■ Review of Disease and Disorder Terms

Can you define, pronounce, and spell the following terms?

andropathy	erectile dysfunction (ED)	priapism	spermatocele
anorchism		prostate cancer	testicular cancer
balanitis	hydrocele	prostatitis	testicular torsion
benign prostatic hyperplasia (BPH)	infertility	prostatocystitis	varicocele
	orchiepididymitis	prostatolith	
cryptorchidism	orchitis	prostatorrhea	
epididymitis	phimosis	prostatovesiculitis	

Surgical Terms
BUILT FROM WORD PARTS

The following terms can be translated using definitions of word parts. Further explanation is provided within parentheses as needed.

TERM	DEFINITION	TERM	DEFINITION
1. **balanoplasty** (BAL-a-nō-*plas*-tē)	surgical repair of the glans penis	5. **orchioplasty** (OR-kē-ō-*plas*-tē)	surgical repair of the testis
2. **epididymectomy** (ep-i-*did*-i-MEK-to-mē)	excision of the epididymis	6. **orchiotomy** (*or*-kē-OT-o-mē)	incision into the testis (also called **orchidotomy**)
3. **orchiectomy** (*or*-kē-EK-to-mē)	excision of the testis (bilateral orchiectomy is called **castration**) (also called **orchidectomy**)	7. **prostatectomy** (*pros*-ta-TEK-to-mē)	excision of the prostate gland (Tables 7.1, 7.2, and 7.3)
4. **orchiopexy** (OR-kē-ō-pek-sē)	surgical fixation of the testicle (performed to bring undescended testicle[s] into the scrotum) (also called **orchidopexy**)	8. **prostatocystotomy** (*pros*-tat-ō-sis-TOT-o-mē)	incision into the prostate gland and the (urinary) bladder
		9. **prostatolithotomy** (*pros*-tat-ō-li-THOT-o-mē)	incision into the prostate gland to remove stone(s)

TABLE 7.2 Types of Prostatectomies

	SIMPLE PROSTATECTOMY	RADICAL PROSTATECTOMY (RP)
Used to treat	benign prostatic hyperplasia (BPH) and its lower urinary tract symptoms (LUTS)	prostate cancer, especially in its early stages
Procedure	excision of the inside portion of the prostate gland, often through an abdominal incision made above the pubic bone	excision of the prostate gland with its capsule, seminal vesicles, vas deferens, and sometimes pelvic lymph nodes
Technique	open (OSP), laparoscopic (LSP), or robot-assisted (RASP)	open (ORP), laparoscopic (LRP), or robot-assisted (RARP)
Alternatives	transurethral incision of the prostate (TUIP), transurethral resection of the prostate gland (TURP), laser therapies (HoLEP and PVP), prostate artery embolization (PAE), minimally invasive surgical treatments (MISTs)	active surveillance (watchful waiting), radiation therapy, hormone therapy, chemotherapy (one or more of these methods may be combined with radical prostatectomy)

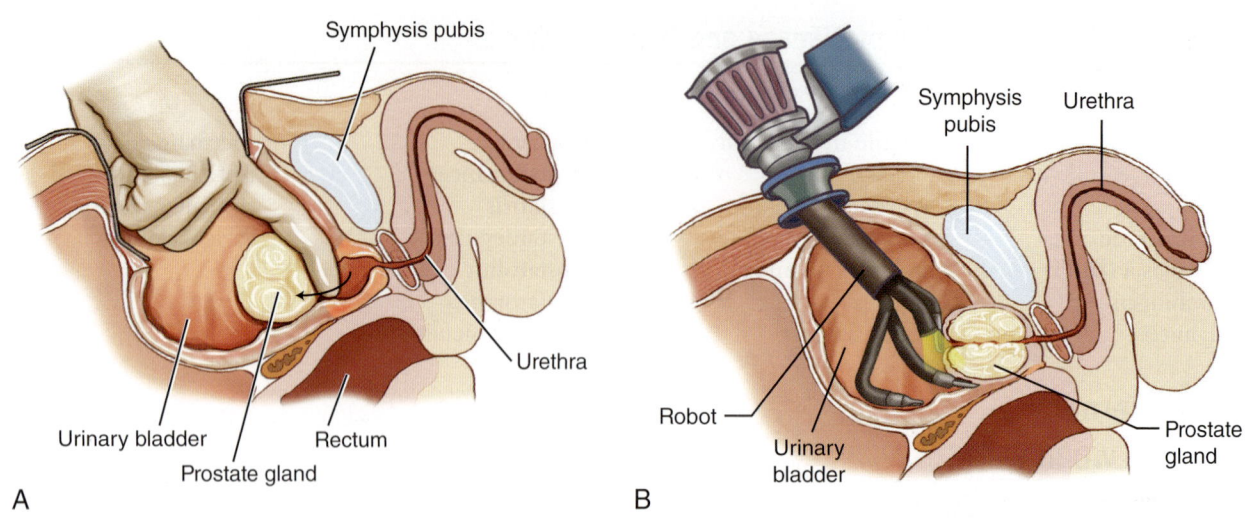

FIG. 7.5 Prostatectomy techniques. Both simple and radical prostatectomies may be performed using open incision, laparoscopic, or robot-assisted methods. The procedures may be performed by various approaches, including retropubic, perineal, and suprapubic. Open procedures tend to have more blood loss and longer recovery periods. Robot-assisted methods are more costly and require advanced training by the surgeon. **A,** Open prostatectomy with a suprapubic approach. **B,** Single port (opening) robot-assisted prostatectomy.

Surgical Terms—cont'd
BUILT FROM WORD PARTS

TERM	DEFINITION	TERM	DEFINITION
10. prostatovesiculectomy (*pros*-tat-ō-ves-*ik*-ū-LEK-to-mē)	excision of the prostate gland and the seminal vesicles	12. vasovasostomy (*vas*-ō-vā-ZOS-to-mē)	creation of artificial openings between ducts (the severed ends of the vas deferens are reconnected in an attempt to restore fertility in men who have had a vasectomy)
11. vasectomy (va-SEK-to-mē)	excision of a duct (partial excision of the vas deferens bilaterally, resulting in male sterilization)		
		13. vesiculectomy (ve-*sik*-ū-LEK-to-mē)	excision of the seminal vesicle(s)

EXERCISE 12 ■ Pronounce and Spell

Practice pronunciation and spelling on paper and online.

1. **Practice on Paper**
    a. **Pronounce:** Read the phonetic spelling and say aloud the terms listed in the previous table. Refer to Table 2.2 Pronunciation Key as needed.
    b. **Spell:** Have a study partner read the terms aloud. Write the spelling of the terms on a separate sheet of paper.

Chapter 7   Male Reproductive System   245

2. **Practice Online**
   a. **Access** online learning resources. Go to evolve.elsevier.com > Evolve Resources > Student Resources.
   b. **Pronounce:** Select Audio Glossary > Chapter 7 > Exercise 12. Select a term to hear its pronunciation and repeat aloud.
   c. **Spell:** Select Activities > Chapter 7 > Spell Terms > Exercise 12. Select the audio icon and type the correct spelling of the term.

❏ Check the box when complete.

EXERCISE 13 ■ Analyze and Define

Analyze and define the following terms by drawing slashes between word parts, writing word part abbreviations above the term, underlining combining forms, and writing combining form abbreviations below the term.

EXAMPLE:
```
              WR   CV  WR  CV   S
   prostat / o / lith / o / tomy
            CF        CF
   incision into the prostate gland to remove stone(s)
```

1. vasectomy

2. prostatocystotomy

3. orchiotomy

4. epididymectomy

5. orchiopexy

6. prostatovesiculectomy

7. orchioplasty

8. vesiculectomy

9. prostatectomy

10. balanoplasty

11. vasovasostomy

12. orchiectomy

EXERCISE 14 ■ Build

A Label

Build the surgical terms pictured by writing word parts above definitions.

1.
_____ / _____
   duct   excision

1. incision is made into the covering of the vas deferens
2. vas deferens is exposed and ligated (tied off)
3. segment of vas deferens is excised
4. vas deferens is repositioned and skin is sutured

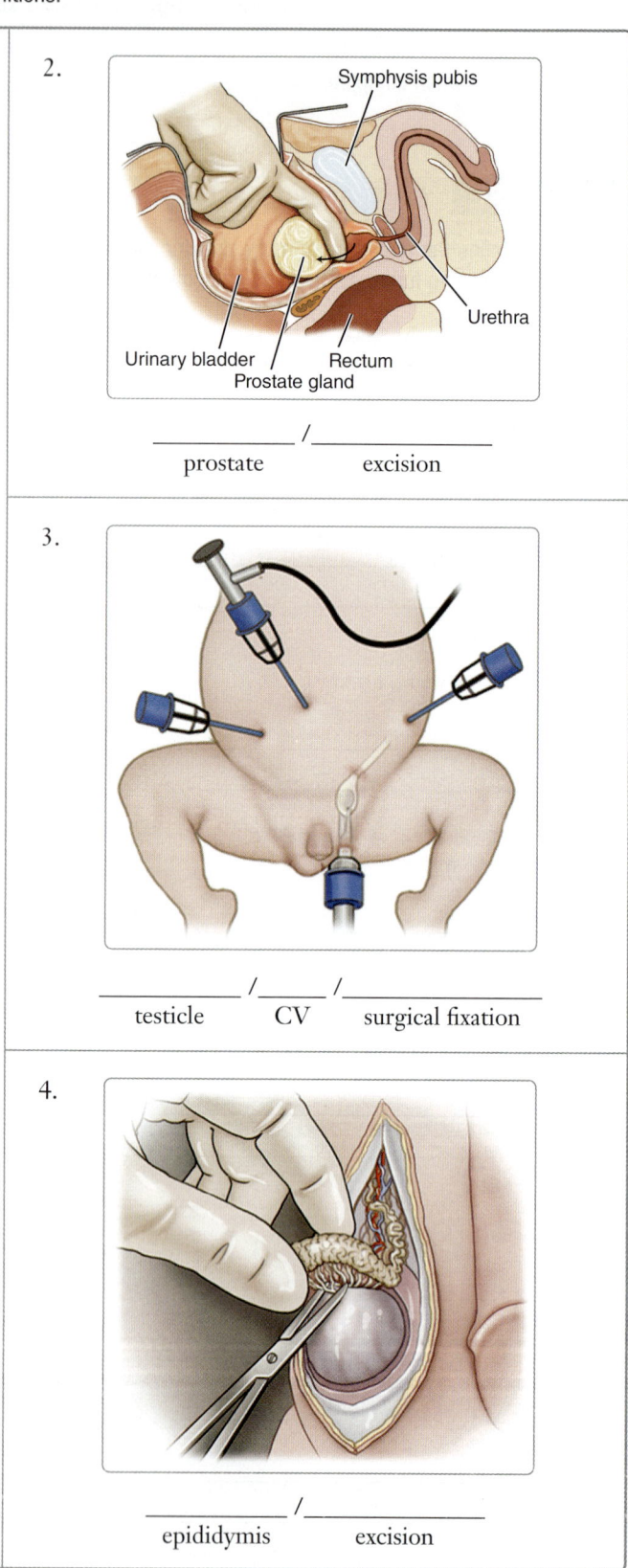

2.
_____ / _____
  prostate   excision

3.
_____ / _____ / _____
  testicle   CV   surgical fixation

4.
_____ / _____
 epididymis   excision

B Fill In

Build surgical terms for the following definitions by using the word parts you have learned.

EXAMPLE: excision of the prostate gland   prostat / ectomy
                                               WR   /   S

1. excision of the testis _____ WR / S

2. surgical repair of the glans penis _____ WR / CV / S

3. incision into the prostate gland and the (urinary) bladder _____ WR / CV / WR / CV / S

4. excision of the seminal vesicle(s) _____ WR / S

5. incision into the prostate gland to remove stone(s) _____ WR / CV / WR / CV / S

6. incision into the testis _____ WR / CV / S

7. excision of the prostate gland and the seminal vesicles _____ WR / CV / WR / S

8. surgical repair of the testis _____ WR / CV / S

9. creation of artificial openings between ducts _____ WR / CV / WR / CV / S

Surgical Terms
NOT BUILT FROM WORD PARTS

Word parts may be present in the following terms; however, their full meanings cannot be translated using definitions of word parts alone.

TERM	DEFINITION
1. ablation (ab-LĀ-shun)	destruction of abnormal or excessive tissue by melting, vaporizing, or eroding
2. circumcision (ser-kum-SI-zhun)	surgical removal of the prepuce (foreskin); all or part of the foreskin may be removed
3. enucleation (ē-nū-klē-Ā-shun)	excision of a whole organ or mass without cutting into it
4. hydrocelectomy (hī-drō-sē-LEK-to-mē)	surgical removal of a fluid-filled sac around the testicle causing scrotal swelling (hydrocele)
5. laser surgery (LĀ-ser) (SUR-jer-ē)	use of a focused beam of light to excise or vaporize abnormal tissue and to control bleeding; uses a variety of noninvasive and minimally invasive procedures. Two common types of laser surgery used to treat BPH are **holmium laser enucleation of the prostate gland (HoLEP)** and **photoselective vaporization of the prostate gland (PVP)**. (Table 7.3, Fig 7.6)

Surgical Terms—cont'd
NOT BUILT FROM WORD PARTS

TERM	DEFINITION
6. minimally invasive surgical treatments (MISTs) (MIN-e-*mel*-ē) (in-VĀS-iv) (SIR-ji-kel) (TRĒT-mentz)	procedures for benign prostatic hyperplasia that are characterized by fewer side effects, outpatient (office-based) locations, and shorter recovery times. Examples include prostatic urethral lift (PUL) and water vapor thermal therapy (WVTT). Limited data exists regarding the long-term success rate and the need for retreatment. (Table 7.3, Fig 7.9)
7. morcellation (*mor*-se-LĀ-shun)	cutting or grinding solid tissue into smaller pieces for removal
8. robotic surgery (rō-BOT-ik) (SUR-jer-ē)	use of small surgical instruments attached to a computer and operated by the surgeon from a console several feet from the operating table (Table 7.2, Fig. 7.7)
9. sterilization (*star*-i-li-ZĀ-shun)	surgical procedure that prevents pregnancy, either the ability of the female to conceive or of the male to induce conception
10. transurethral incision of the prostate gland (TUIP) (*trans*-ū-RĒ-thral) (in-SIZH-en) (of) (the) (PROS-tāt) (gland)	surgical procedure that widens the urethra by making a few small incisions in the bladder neck and the prostate gland. No prostate tissue is removed. TUIP may be used instead of TURP when the prostate gland is less enlarged. (Table 7.3)
11. transurethral resection of the prostate gland (TURP) (*trans*-ū-RĒ-thral) (rē-SEK-shun) (of) (the) (PROS-tāt) (gland)	surgical removal of pieces of prostate gland tissue by using an instrument inserted through the urethra. The capsule is left intact; usually performed when the enlarged prostate gland interferes with urination. (Table 7.3, Fig 7.8)

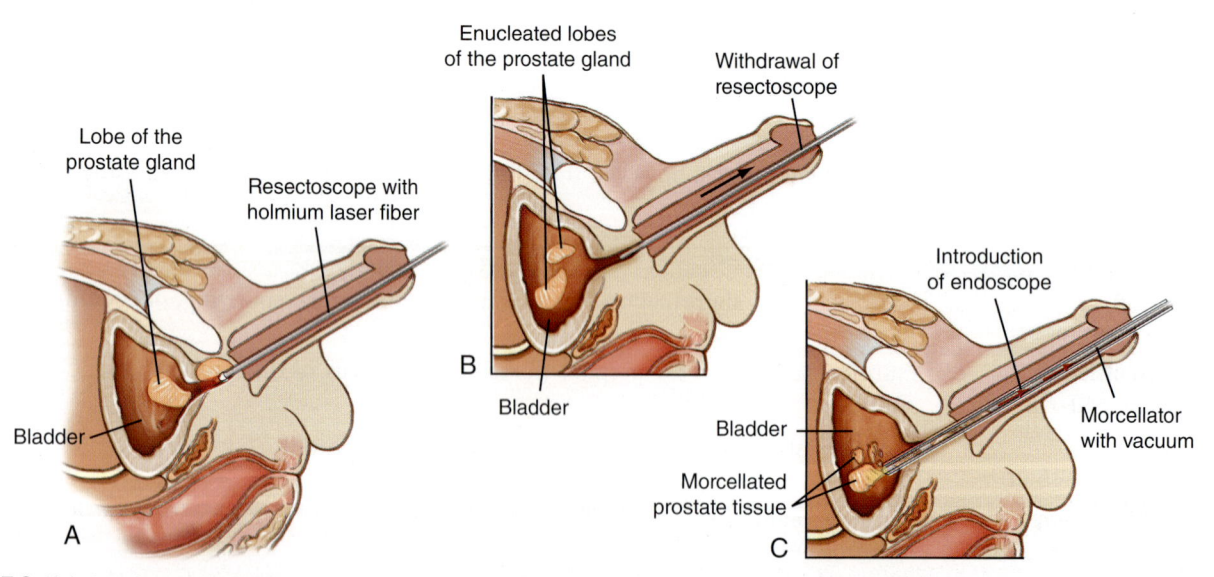

FIG. 7.6 Holmium laser enucleation of the prostate (HoLEP) is a minimally invasive laser surgery performed endoscopically to treat benign prostatic hyperplasia. **A,** The lobes of the prostate gland are removed intact from surrounding structures using a holmium laser. **B,** The enucleated lobes are temporarily placed in the urinary bladder. **C,** The lobes of the prostate are morcellated within the urinary bladder and removed through the endoscope using suction.

Chapter 7 Male Reproductive System   249

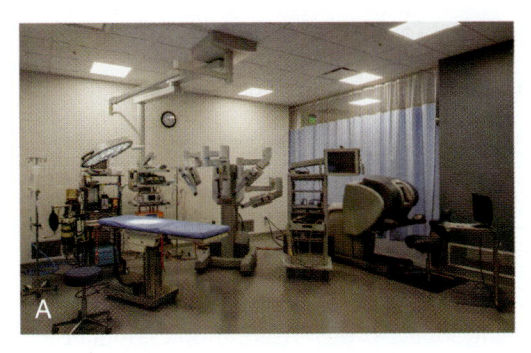

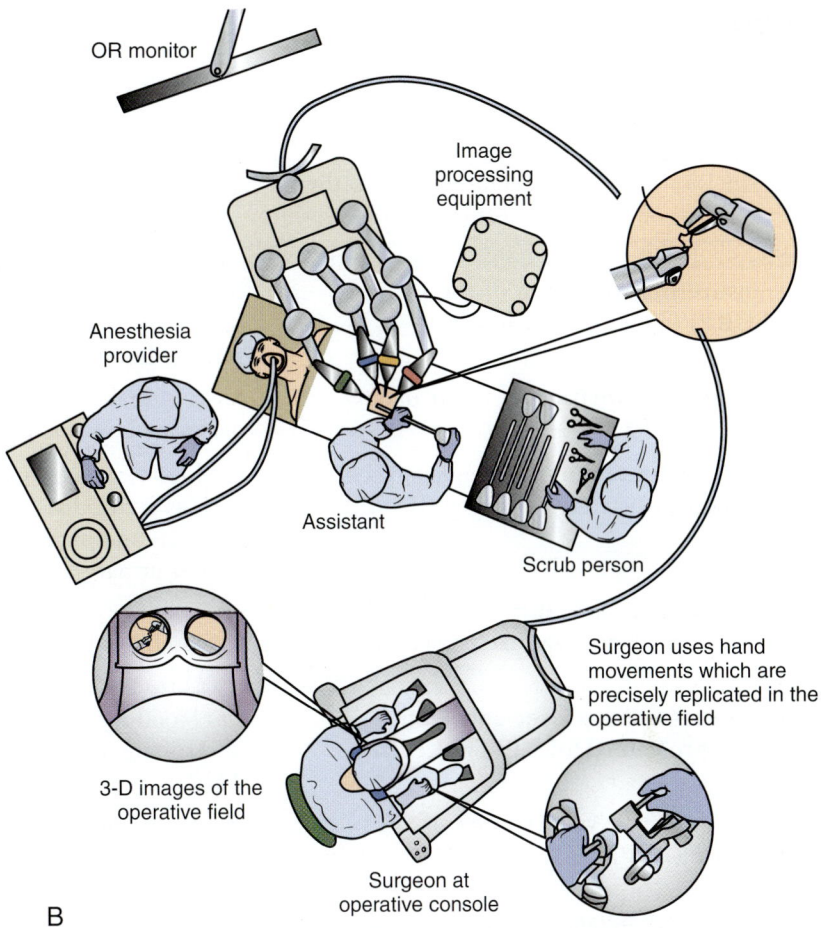

FIG. 7.7 Robotic surgery. **A,** Surgical suite. **B,** Operating room setup for robotic-assisted laparoscopic radical prostatectomy (RALRP) with a robotic system. Note that the surgeon performs the procedure at an operative console rather than hands-on surgery.

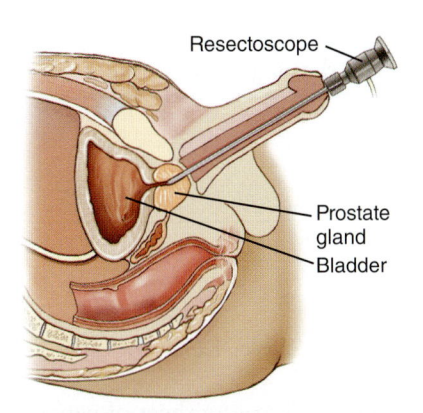

FIG. 7.8 Transurethral resection of the prostate gland (TURP) uses a resectoscope inserted through the urethra to the prostate gland. The end of the instrument is equipped to remove pieces of the enlarged gland.

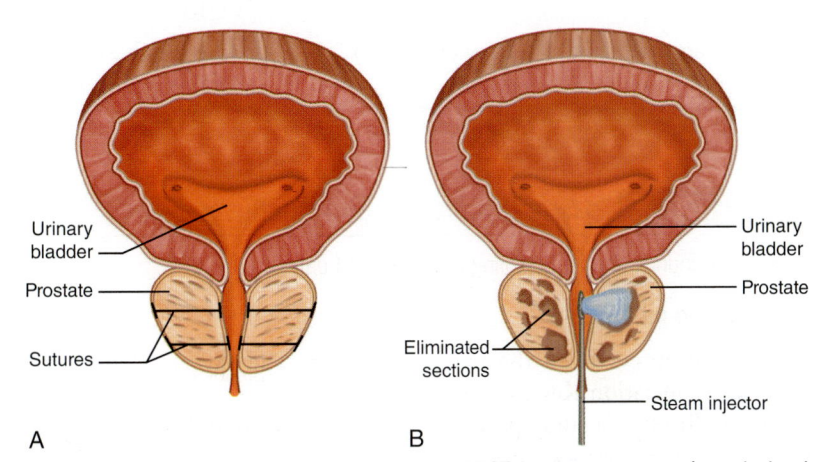

FIG. 7.9 Minimally invasive surgical therapies (MISTs) are newer procedures to treat benign prostatic hypertrophy. **A,** Prostatic urethral lift (PUL), in which sutures are used to lift and hold the prostate gland away from the urethra. **B,** Water vapor thermal therapy (WVTT), in which steam is injected into the gland to eliminate sections of the prostate.

TABLE 7.3 Surgical Treatments for Benign Prostatic Hyperplasia

Surgical treatments for benign prostatic hyperplasia can be grouped into three categories: incisional surgeries, laser surgeries, and minimally invasive surgeries.

1. INCISIONAL SURGERIES

Incisional surgeries require access to the prostate from outside the body (through the skin and subcutaneous tissues) or from within (through the urethra).

SURGICAL PROCEDURE	ADVANTAGES & DISADVANTAGES
transurethral resection of the prostate (TURP) (monopolar or bipolar)	most effective, most common procedure; disadvantages include sexual function impairment, longer catheterization times, higher rates of blood loss
transurethral incision of the prostate gland (TUIP)	fewer sexual side effects compared with TURP; can only be performed on smaller prostate glands
simple prostatectomy (open, laparoscopic, or robotic-assisted laparoscopic [RASP])	used for very large prostate glands or when other abnormalities, such as cystolithiasis, exist. Disadvantages include abdominal incisions and higher rates of blood loss (with open procedure), as well as urinary and sexual side effects.

2. LASER SURGERIES

Laser surgeries vaporize prostate tissue using a focused beam of light.

SURGICAL PROCEDURE	ADVANTAGES & DISADVANTAGES
holmium/thulium laser enucleation of the prostate (HoLEP/ThuLEP)	less blood loss, shorter hospitalizations, highly effective, no limits on prostate size. Risk of sexual function impairments similar to TURP. Not available in all communities.
photo-selective vaporization of the prostate (PVP)	shorter hospitalization and catheterization, lower bleeding risk, but less effective and therefore higher retreatment rates in larger prostate glands

3. MINIMALLY INVASIVE SURGICAL TREATMENTS (MISTs)

MISTs can be performed in the outpatient (office) setting or as a very short hospital stay; they are associated with minimal blood loss and faster recovery times.

SURGICAL PROCEDURE	ADVANTAGES & DISADVANTAGES
prostatic urethral lift (PUL)	local anesthesia, shorter catheterization time, preserved sexual function. Not for very large prostate glands, less effective than TURP, and thus more likely to require retreatment.
water vapor thermal therapy (WVTT)	local anesthesia, preserved sexual function, but longer catheterization time, less effective, and thus higher retreatment rates

EXERCISE 15 ■ Pronounce and Spell

Practice pronunciation and spelling on paper and online.

1. **Practice on Paper**
   a. **Pronounce:** Read the phonetic spelling and say aloud the terms listed in the term table. Refer to Table 2.2 Pronunciation Key as needed.
   b. **Spell:** Have a study partner read the terms aloud. Write the spelling of the terms on a separate sheet of paper.

2. **Practice Online**
   a. **Access** online learning resources. Go to evolve.elsevier.com > Evolve Resources > Student Resources.
   b. **Pronounce:** Select Audio Glossary > Chapter 7 > Exercise 15. Select a term to hear its pronunciation and repeat aloud.
   c. **Spell:** Select Activities > Chapter 7 > Spell Terms > Exercise 15. Select the audio icon and type the correct spelling of the term.

❏ Check the box when complete.

Chapter 7   Male Reproductive System   251

EXERCISE 16 ■ Fill In

A   Label

Write the surgical terms pictured and defined.

1. _____
   use of small surgical instruments attached to a computer and operated by the surgeon from a console several feet from the operating table

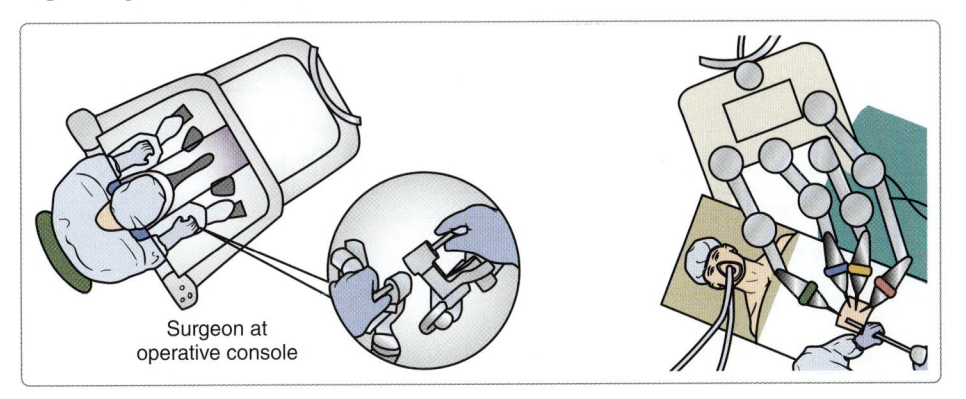

2. _____
   surgical removal of pieces of the prostate gland tissue by using an instrument inserted through the urethra

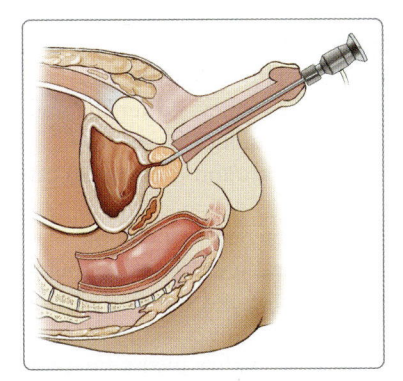

3. _____
   procedures for benign prostatic hyperplasia that are characterized by fewer side effects, outpatient locations, and shorter recovery times

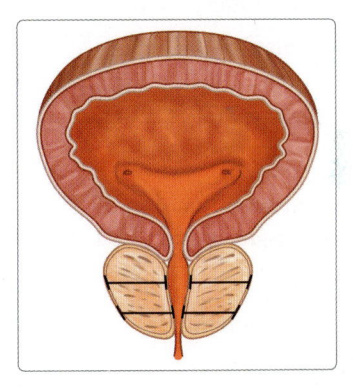

4. _____
   surgical removal of the prepuce (foreskin)

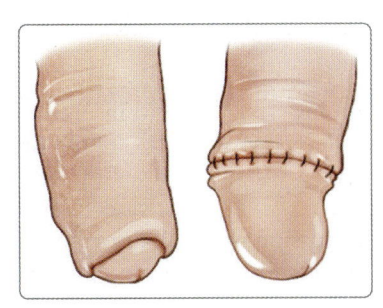

5. _____
   excision of a whole organ or mass without cutting into it

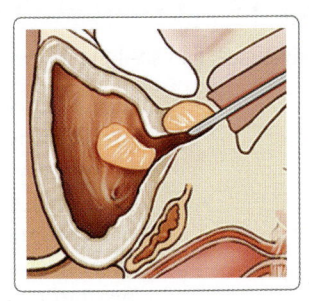

B Identify

Fill in the blanks with the correct term.

1. A surgical procedure that prevents pregnancy, either the ability of the female to conceive or of the male to induce conception is called _____.
2. Photoselective vaporization of the prostate (PVP) is one form of _____, the destruction of abnormal or excessive tissue by melting, vaporizing, or eroding.
3. Surgical removal of a fluid-filled sac around the testicle causing scrotal swelling is _____.
4. A surgical procedure for benign prostatic hyperplasia that widens the urethra by making small incisions is called _____.
5. One type of _____, in which a focused beam of light is used to excise or vaporize abnormal tissue and to control bleeding, is holmium laser enucleation of the prostate gland (HoLEP).
6. Endoscopic surgeries often involve _____, in which solid tissue is cut or ground into smaller pieces for removal.

EXERCISE 17 ■ Match

Match the terms in the first column with the correct definitions in the second column.

_____ 1. hydrocelectomy
_____ 2. transurethral resection of the prostate gland (TURP)
_____ 3. robotic surgery
_____ 4. morcellation
_____ 5. minimally invasive surgical treatments (MISTs)
_____ 6. sterilization
_____ 7. transurethral incision of the prostate gland (TUIP)
_____ 8. ablation
_____ 9. circumcision
_____ 10. laser surgery
_____ 11. enucleation

a. destruction of abnormal or excessive tissue by melting, vaporizing, or eroding
b. surgical procedure that widens the urethra by making a few small incisions in the bladder neck and the prostate gland
c. use of a focused beam of light to excise or vaporize abnormal tissue and to control bleeding
d. surgical removal of the prepuce (foreskin)
e. excision of a whole organ or mass without cutting into it
f. surgical procedure that prevents pregnancy, either the ability of the female to conceive or of the male to induce conception
g. surgical removal of a fluid-filled sac around the testicle causing scrotal swelling
h. use of small surgical instruments attached to a computer and operated by the surgeon from a console several feet from the operating table
i. examples include prostatic urethral lift and water vapor thermal therapy
j. cutting or grinding solid tissue into smaller pieces for removal
k. surgical removal of pieces of the prostate gland tissue by using an instrument inserted through the urethra

EXERCISE 18 ■ Review of Surgical Terms

Can you define, pronounce, and spell the following terms?

ablation
balanoplasty
circumcision
enucleation
epididymectomy
hydrocelectomy
laser surgery
minimally invasive surgical treatments (MISTs)
morcellation
orchiectomy
orchiopexy
orchioplasty
orchiotomy
prostatectomy
prostatocystotomy
prostatolithotomy
prostatovesiculectomy
robotic surgery
sterilization
transurethral incision of the prostate gland (TUIP)
transurethral resection of the prostate gland (TURP)
vasectomy
vasovasostomy
vesiculectomy

Diagnostic Terms
NOT BUILT FROM WORD PARTS

Word parts may be present in the following terms; however, their full meanings cannot be translated using definitions of word parts alone.

DIAGNOSTIC IMAGING

TERM	DEFINITION
1. **MRI ultrasound fusion biopsy** (M-R-I) (UL-tra-sound) (FŪ-shun) (BĪ-op-sē)	combination of magnetic resonance imaging with transrectal ultrasound (TRUS) to obtain tissue from a prostate lesion. Software merges an existing MR image with live ultrasound images. The combined, or fused, MRI-TRUS image is used to direct the biopsy needle into the area of the prostate that looks suspicious on MRI. (also called **MRI-TRUS fusion**, **MR-ultrasound fusion**, and **fusion guided biopsy**) (Table 7.1)
2. **multiparametric MRI** (MUL-ti-par-a-*met*-rik) (M-R-I)	magnetic resonance imaging procedure providing information of anatomic structure and physiology for the staging of prostate cancer. It uses a combination of different MRI modalities to better understand the size and extent of prostate tumors. (Table 7.1)
3. **transrectal ultrasound (TRUS)** (trans-REK-tal) (UL-tra-sound)	ultrasound procedure used to diagnose prostate cancer. Sound waves are sent and received by a transducer probe that is placed into the rectum. (Table 7.1)

LABORATORY

TERM	DEFINITION
4. **prostate-specific antigen (PSA)** (PROS-tāt) (spe-SIF-ik) (AN-ti-jen)	blood test that measures the level of prostate-specific antigen in the blood. Elevated test results may indicate the presence of prostate cancer, urinary or prostatic infection, or excess prostate tissue, as found in benign prostatic hyperplasia or prostatitis. (Table 7.1)
5. **semen analysis** (SĒ-men) (a-NAL-i-sis)	microscopic observation of ejaculated semen, revealing the size, structure, and movement of sperm; used to evaluate male infertility and to determine the effectiveness of a vasectomy (also called **sperm count** and **sperm test**)
6. **total testosterone** (TŌ-tal) (tes-TOS-ta-rōn)	blood test to measure the level of the hormone responsible for male physical characteristics (testosterone); used to detect multiple conditions in men and women, including infertility

OTHER

TERM	DEFINITION
7. **digital rectal examination (DRE)** (DIJ-i-tal) (REK-tal) (eg-*zam*-i-NĀ-shun)	physical examination in which the healthcare provider inserts a gloved finger into the rectum and palpates the prostate through the rectal wall to determine the size, shape, and consistency of the gland; used to screen for BPH and prostate cancer. BPH usually presents as a uniform, nontender enlargement, whereas cancer usually presents as a stony hard nodule. (Table 7.1)

EXERCISE 19 ■ Pronounce and Spell

Practice pronunciation and spelling on paper and online.

1. **Practice on Paper**

    a. **Pronounce:** Read the phonetic spelling and say aloud the terms listed in the previous table. Refer to Table 2.2 Pronunciation Key as needed.
    b. **Spell:** Have a study partner read the terms aloud. Write the spelling of the terms on a separate sheet of paper.

254 Chapter 7 Male Reproductive System

2. **Practice Online**
   a. **Access** online learning resources. Go to evolve.elsevier.com > Evolve Resources > Student Resources.
   b. **Pronounce:** Select Audio Glossary > Chapter 7 > Exercise 19. Select a term to hear its pronunciation and repeat aloud.
   c. **Spell:** Select Activities > Chapter 7 > Spell Terms > Exercise 19. Select the audio icon and type the correct spelling of the term.
   ❏ Check the box when complete.

EXERCISE 20 ■ Fill In

Fill in the blanks with the correct terms.

1. A physical examination in which the healthcare provider palpates the prostate through the rectal wall to determine the size, shape, and consistency of the gland is called _____.
2. A blood test that, when elevated, may indicate the presence of prostate cancer is called _____.
3. A diagnostic ultrasound procedure used to obtain images of the prostate gland is called _____.
4. A laboratory test for microscopic observation of ejaculated semen to evaluate male infertility is called _____.
5. A magnetic resonance imaging procedure that provides structural and physiological information for the staging of prostate cancer is called _____.
6. _____ is a blood test to measure the level of the hormone responsible for male physical characteristics and may be used to detect infertility.
7. A diagnostic imaging test that uses a combination of magnetic resonance imaging with transrectal ultrasound to obtain tissue from a prostate lesion is called _____.

EXERCISE 21 ■ Match

Match the terms in the first column with the correct definitions in the second column.

_____ 1. semen analysis
_____ 2. prostate-specific antigen (PSA)
_____ 3. transrectal ultrasound (TRUS)
_____ 4. total testosterone
_____ 5. MRI ultrasound fusion biopsy
_____ 6. digital rectal examination (DRE)
_____ 7. multiparametric MRI

a. test that uses a combination of different MRI modalities to better understand the size and extent of prostate tumors
b. a gloved finger palpates the prostate through the rectal wall to determine the size, shape, and consistency of the gland
c. blood test to measure the level of the hormone responsible for male physical characteristics
d. elevated results of this blood test may indicate the presence of prostate cancer, urinary or prostatic infection, or excess prostate tissue
e. microscopic observation of ejaculated semen, used to evaluate male infertility and to determine the effectiveness of a vasectomy
f. ultrasound procedure used to diagnose prostate cancer
g. combination of magnetic resonance imaging with transrectal ultrasound to obtain tissue from a prostate lesion

EXERCISE 22 ■ Review of Diagnostic Terms

Can you define, pronounce, and spell the following terms?

digital rectal examination (DRE)
MRI ultrasound fusion biopsy
multiparametric MRI
prostate-specific antigen (PSA)
semen analysis
total testosterone
transrectal ultrasound (TRUS)

Chapter 7 Male Reproductive System

Complementary Terms

Included in this section of the chapter are a few terms, including sexually transmitted infections, that apply to all genders. These infections can cause damage to reproductive organs and other potentially serious health consequences if left untreated. Any sexual behavior involving contact with the body fluids of another person puts an individual at risk for infection.

BUILT FROM WORD PARTS AND *NOT* BUILT FROM WORD PARTS

The first portion of the table contains Male Reproductive System Terms that can be translated using definitions of word parts. The second portion of the table contains terms that cannot be fully understood using the definitions of word parts.

■ Built from Word Parts

SIGNS AND SYMPTOMS

TERM	DEFINITION	TERM	DEFINITION
1. aspermia (a-SPER-mē-a)	condition of without sperm (characterized by absence of semen or ejaculation)	3. oligospermia (ol-i-gō-SPER-mē-a)	condition of scanty sperm (in the semen; may contribute to infertility); (also called **low sperm count**)
ASPERMIA may indicate the lack of production of spermatozoa, the lack of production of semen, or the lack of ejaculation of semen.		4. orchialgia (ōr-kē-AL-ja)	pain in the testis (also called **testalgia**)
2. balanorrhea (*bal*-a-nō-RĒ-a)	discharge from the glans penis		

■ *NOT* Built from Word Parts

INFECTIONS

TERM	DEFINITION
1. chlamydia (kla-MID-ē-a)	sexually transmitted infection caused by the bacterium *C. trachomatis*; sometimes referred to as a **silent STI** because many people are not aware they have the disease. Symptoms that occur when the disease becomes serious are painful urination and discharge from the penis in men and genital itching, vaginal discharge, and bleeding between menstrual periods in women.
2. genital herpes (JEN-i-tal) (HER-pēz)	sexually transmitted infection caused by herpes simplex virus type 2
3. gonorrhea (gon-ō-RĒ-a)	sexually transmitted infection caused by a bacterial organism that inflames the mucous membranes of the genitourinary tract
4. human immunodeficiency virus (HIV) (HŪ-man) (*im*-ū-nō-de-FISH-en-sē) (VĪ-rus)	sexually transmitted infection caused by a retrovirus that infects T-helper cells of the immune system; may also be acquired in utero or transmitted through infected blood via needle sharing. Advanced HIV infection progresses to AIDS (acquired immunodeficiency syndrome).
5. human papillomavirus (HPV) (HŪ-man) (*pap*-i-LŌ-ma-*vī*-rus)	sexually transmitted infection caused by viral infection; there are more than 40 types of HPV that cause benign or cancerous growths in male and female genitals (also called **genital warts**)
HUMAN PAPILLOMAVIRUS is the cause of most cervical cancers. Some penile, vulvar, vaginal, throat, and anal cancers are also linked to HPV infection. HPV is the most prevalent sexually transmitted disease, and vaccines are available to protect men and women from HPV infection.	
6. sexually transmitted infection (STI) (SEK-shū-al-ē) (TRANS-mi-ted) (in-FEK-shun)	infection spread through sexual contact; STIs affect males and females, causing damage to reproductive organs and potentially serious health consequences if left untreated (also called **sexually transmitted disease [STD]**)
SEXUALLY TRANSMITTED INFECTION (STI) VS. SEXUALLY TRANSMITTED DISEASE (STD): WHAT'S THE DIFFERENCE? Usually, a "disease" refers to a clear medical problem, often with signs or symptoms. But patients with an infection may have no signs or symptoms and still have the problem. While **STI** is medically more accurate, you will also frequently hear the term **STD**. Sexual behaviors that involve contact with body fluids put individuals at risk for infection.	

256 Chapter 7 Male Reproductive System

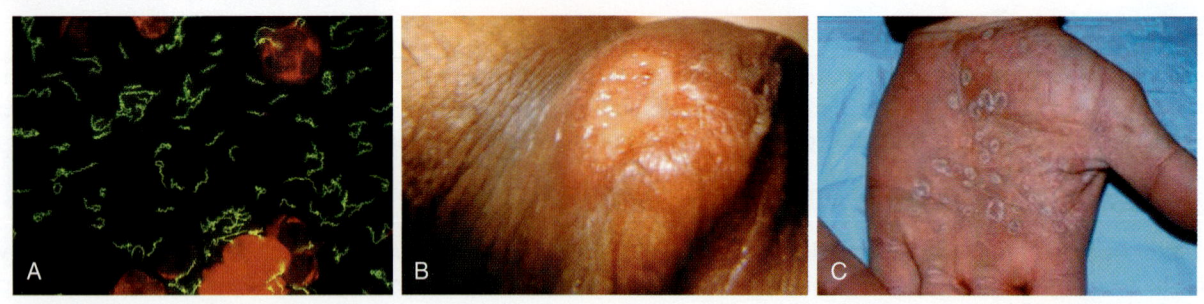

FIG. 7.10 Syphilis. **A,** *Treponema pallidum*, organism responsible for syphilis viewed microscopically. **B,** Primary syphilis, depicting a syphilitic chancre. **C,** Secondary syphilis, depicting rash on palms of hands.

Complementary Terms—cont'd
■ **NOT Built from Word Parts**

INFECTIONS	
TERM	**DEFINITION**
7. syphilis (SIF-i-lis)	infection caused by the bacterium *Treponema pallidum*. Rapidly spreads throughout the body, and if untreated becomes systemic and can progress through three stages separated by latent periods. Usually sexually transmitted, but may be acquired in utero and by direct contact with infected skin. (Fig. 7.10)
8. trichomoniasis (trik-ō-mō-NĪ-a-sis)	sexually transmitted infection caused by a one-celled organism *Trichomonas*. It infects the genitourinary tract. Men may be asymptomatic or may develop urethritis, an enlarged prostate gland, or epididymitis. Women may have vaginal itching, dysuria, and vaginal or urethral discharge.

TREATMENTS	
TERM	**DEFINITION**
9. artificial insemination (ar-ti-FISH-al) (in-*sem*-i-NĀ-shun)	introduction of washed and concentrated sperm into the female reproductive tract; used as a treatment for infertility
10. condom (KON-dum)	cover for the penis worn to prevent conception and the spread of sexually transmitted infections
11. spermicide (SPUR-mi-sīd)	an agent that destroys spermatozoa; used to prevent conception

Refer to **Appendix E** for pharmacology terms.

OTHER	
TERM	**DEFINITION**
12. azoospermia (ā-zō-a-SPUR-mē-a)	lack of live sperm in the semen (characterized by absence of semen or ejaculation)

AZOOSPERMIA may be:
- obstructive, caused by blocked vessels or ducts
- nonobstructive, caused by infection, lack of production of spermatozoa, or retrograde ejaculation (in which semen travels into the urinary bladder rather than exiting through the urethra)

13. ejaculation (ē-*jak*-ū-LĀ-shun)	ejection of semen from the male urethra
14. orgasm (ŌR-gazm)	climax of sexual stimulation
15. puberty (PŪ-ber-tē)	period when secondary sex characteristics (such as pubic and armpit hair, deepening of voice in men, breast development in women) develop and the ability to reproduce sexually begins

Chapter 7 Male Reproductive System 257

EXERCISE 23 ■ Pronounce and Spell

Practice pronunciation and spelling on paper and online.

1. **Practice on Paper**
   a. **Pronounce:** Read the phonetic spelling and say aloud the terms listed in the previous table. Refer to Table 2.2 Pronunciation Key as needed.
   b. **Spell:** Have a study partner read the terms aloud. Write the spelling of the terms on a separate sheet of paper.

2. **Practice Online**
   a. **Access** online learning resources. Go to evolve.elsevier.com > Evolve Resources > Student Resources.
   b. **Pronounce:** Select Audio Glossary > Chapter 7 > Exercise 23. Select a term to hear its pronunciation and repeat aloud.
   c. **Spell:** Select Activities > Chapter 7 > Spell Terms > Exercise 23. Select the audio icon and type the correct spelling of the term.

❏ Check the box when complete.

EXERCISE 24 ■ Complementary Terms Built from Word Parts

A Analyze and Define

Analyze and define the following terms by drawing slashes between word parts, writing word part abbreviations above the term, underlining combining forms, and writing combining form abbreviations below the term.

1. orchialgia

3. aspermia

2. oligospermia

4. balanorrhea

B Build

Build the complementary terms for the following definitions by using the word parts you have learned.

1. condition of without sperm (or semen or ejaculation)   _____ / _____ / _____
       P   WR   S

2. condition of scanty sperm (in the semen)   _____ / _____ / _____ / _____
      WR   CV   WR   S

3. pain in the testis   _____ / _____
      WR   S

4. discharge from the glans penis   _____ / _____ / _____
      WR   CV   S

Chapter 7 Male Reproductive System

EXERCISE 25 ■ Complementary Terms NOT Built from Word Parts

A Match

Match the terms in the first column with their correct definitions in the second column.

_____ 1. ejaculation
_____ 2. human papillomavirus
_____ 3. genital herpes
_____ 4. gonorrhea
_____ 5. orgasm
_____ 6. condom
_____ 7. azoospermia

a. climax of sexual stimulation
b. STI caused by herpes simplex virus type 2
c. ejection of semen
d. lack of live sperm in the semen
e. cover for the penis worn to prevent conception and the spread of sexually transmitted infections
f. also called genital warts
g. STI caused by a bacterium that inflames mucous membranes

B Match

Match the terms in the first column with their correct definitions in the second column.

_____ 1. sexually transmitted infection
_____ 2. spermicide
_____ 3. syphilis
_____ 4. puberty
_____ 5. human immunodeficiency virus
_____ 6. trichomoniasis
_____ 7. artificial insemination
_____ 8. chlamydia

a. infection spread through sexual contact
b. period when secondary sex characteristics develop and the ability to reproduce sexually begins
c. retrovirus that progresses to AIDS
d. infection caused by *Treponema pallidum*; if untreated, progresses through three stages
e. introduction of washed and concentrated sperm into the female reproductive tract
f. STI caused by a bacterium, *C. trachomatis* (silent STD)
g. an agent that destroys spermatozoa; used to prevent conception
h. STI caused by a one-celled organism, *Trichomonas*

EXERCISE 26 ■ Review of Complementary Terms

Can you define, pronounce, and spell the following terms?

artificial insemination
aspermia
azoospermia
balanorrhea
chlamydia
condom
ejaculation
genital herpes
gonorrhea
human immunodeficiency virus (HIV)
human papillomavirus (HPV)
oligospermia
orchialgia
orgasm
puberty
sexually transmitted infection (STI)
spermicide
syphilis
trichomoniasis

Abbreviations

SIGNS AND SYMPTOMS

ABBREVIATION	TERM	ABBREVIATION	TERM
BOO	bladder outlet obstruction	LUTS	lower urinary tract symptoms; spoken as a whole word (lutz)

DISEASE AND DISORDERS

ABBREVIATION	TERM	ABBREVIATION	TERM
BPH	benign prostatic hyperplasia	HPV	human papillomavirus
ED	erectile dysfunction	STD	sexually transmitted disease
HIV	human immunodeficiency virus	STI	sexually transmitted infection

Chapter 7 Male Reproductive System

DIAGNOSTIC

ABBREVIATION	TERM	ABBREVIATION	TERM
DRE	digital rectal examination	TRUS	transrectal ultrasound
PSA	prostate-specific antigen		

TREATMENT

ABBREVIATION	TERM	ABBREVIATION	TERM
HoLEP	holmium laser enucleation of the prostate gland; spoken as a whole word (HŌL-ep)	RARP	robot-assisted radical prostatectomy
		RASP	robot-assisted simple prostatectomy
MISTs	minimally invasive surgical treatments; spoken as a whole word (mistz)	TUIP	transurethral incision of the prostate gland; spoken as a whole word (twip)
PUL	prostatic urethral lift	TURP	transurethral resection of the prostate gland; spoken as a whole word (terp)
PVP	photoselective vaporization of the prostate gland	WVTT	water vapor thermal therapy
RP	radical prostatectomy		

Refer to **Appendix D** for a complete list of abbreviations.

EXERCISE 27 ■ Fill In

Write the terms abbreviated.

1. The patient experienced **LUTS** _____ caused by **BOO** _____.
2. The physician performed a **DRE** _____ on the patient to assist in diagnosing **BPH** _____.
3. Incisional surgeries for BPH include **TUIP** _____ of the prostate and **TURP** _____ of the prostate. Simple prostatectomy may be performed when the prostate gland is very large; two techniques for this are an open procedure and a **RASP** _____.
4. Laser surgeries for benign prostatic hyperplasia include **HoLEP** _____ and **PVP** _____.
5. **MISTs** _____ are relatively new procedures for BPH. Two examples are **PUL** _____ and **WVTT** _____.
6. **HIV** _____ is a type of retrovirus that infects T-helper cells of the immune system.
7. **HPV** _____ causes female and male genital warts and most cervical cancers.
8. **STI** _____ is the preferred term for **STD** _____.
9. **PSA** _____ is a laboratory test used to diagnose cancer of the prostate.
10. **RP** _____ is a surgical procedure to treat prostate cancer. It may be performed as an open procedure, laparoscopically, or by **RARP** _____.
11. **ED** _____ was formerly referred to as impotence.
12. **TRUS** _____, used in the diagnosis of prostate cancer, provides imaging of the prostate gland and is used as a guide for biopsy of the prostate.

Chapter 7 Male Reproductive System

PRACTICAL APPLICATION

EXERCISE 28 ■ Case Study: Translate Between Everyday Language and Medical Language

CASE STUDY: Jimmie Zeller

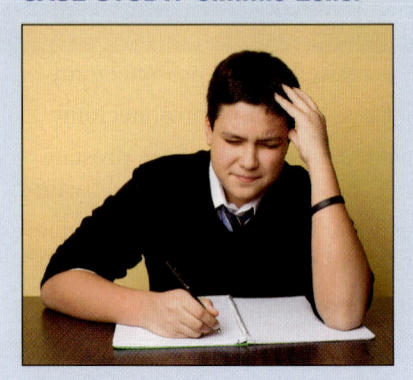

Jimmie, a 15-year-old male, is in the emergency department (ED) because of pain in his testicle that started about 6 hours ago. The pain started suddenly. He felt nauseated and vomited twice. The ED physician examined him and found that his scrotum was swollen, and the painful testicle was higher than the other. A Doppler ultrasound was performed and the findings suggested twisting of the spermatic cord with decreased blood flow to the testis. A surgeon was called immediately to examine Jimmie, since this condition requires immediate surgical fixation of the testis or even surgical removal of the testis. The surgeon examined him quickly and took him immediately to the operating room, since she knew that the risk of reduced or absent ability to achieve pregnancy increases when this condition is left untreated.

Now that you have worked through Chapter 7, on the male reproductive system, consider the medical terms that might be used to describe Jimmie's experience. See the Chapter at a Glance section at the end of the chapter for a list of terms that might apply.

A. Underline phrases in the case study that could be substituted with medical terms.

B. Write the medical term and its definition for three of the phrases you underlined.

MEDICAL TERM	DEFINITION
1. _____	_____
2. _____	_____
3. _____	_____

DOCUMENTATION: Excerpt From Operative Note

This 15-year-old male presented to the emergency department with orchialgia and a swollen scrotum of approximately 6 hours duration. A Doppler ultrasound was suspicious for testicular torsion and physical examination was also highly suggestive of this. He was brought to the operating room for surgical exploration. The patient and his mother received informed consent in which the possibilities of orchiectomy and future infertility were addressed. After appropriate anesthesia and sterile preparation of the surgical field were performed, a transscrotal approach was used to bring the affected testicle into the operative field. Testicular torsion was confirmed and the spermatic cord was detorsed until no twists were visible. Orchiopexy was then performed on both testes using permanent sutures.

C. Underline medical terms presented in Chapter 7 used in the previous excerpt from Jimmie's medical record. See the Chapter at a Glance section at the end of the chapter for a complete list.

D. Select and define three of the medical terms you underlined. To check your answers, go to Appendix A.

MEDICAL TERM	DEFINITION
1. _____	_____
2. _____	_____
3. _____	_____

Chapter 7 Male Reproductive System

EXERCISE 29 ■ Interact with Medical Documents

A

Read the report and complete it by writing medical terms on answer lines within the document. Definitions of terms to be written appear after the document.

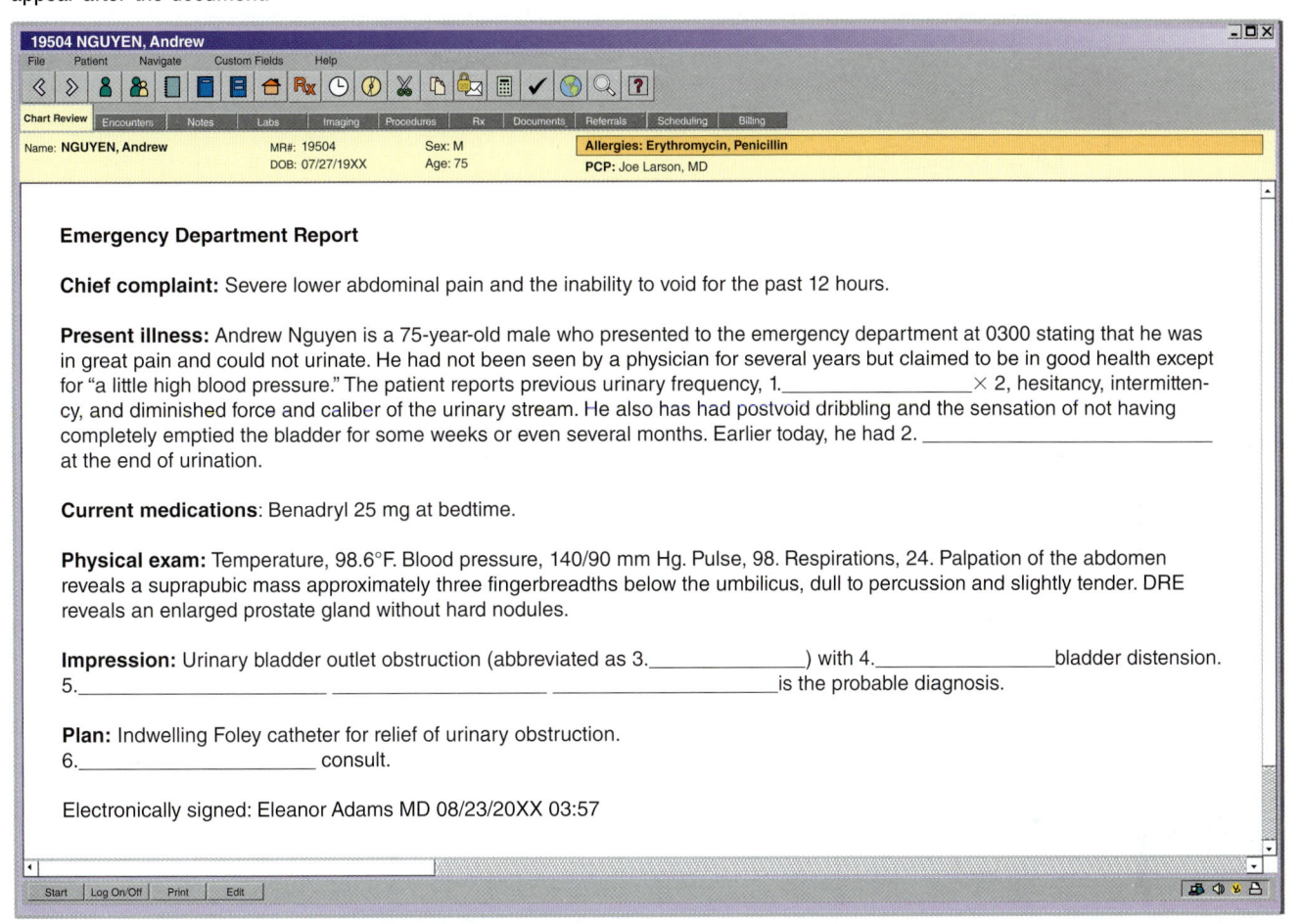

19504 NGUYEN, Andrew

File | Patient | Navigate | Custom Fields | Help

Chart Review | Encounters | Notes | Labs | Imaging | Procedures | Rx | Documents | Referrals | Scheduling | Billing

Name: **NGUYEN, Andrew** MR#: 19504 Sex: M **Allergies: Erythromycin, Penicillin**
DOB: 07/27/19XX Age: 75 PCP: Joe Larson, MD

Emergency Department Report

Chief complaint: Severe lower abdominal pain and the inability to void for the past 12 hours.

Present illness: Andrew Nguyen is a 75-year-old male who presented to the emergency department at 0300 stating that he was in great pain and could not urinate. He had not been seen by a physician for several years but claimed to be in good health except for "a little high blood pressure." The patient reports previous urinary frequency, 1._____ × 2, hesitancy, intermittency, and diminished force and caliber of the urinary stream. He also has had postvoid dribbling and the sensation of not having completely emptied the bladder for some weeks or even several months. Earlier today, he had 2._____ at the end of urination.

Current medications: Benadryl 25 mg at bedtime.

Physical exam: Temperature, 98.6°F. Blood pressure, 140/90 mm Hg. Pulse, 98. Respirations, 24. Palpation of the abdomen reveals a suprapubic mass approximately three fingerbreadths below the umbilicus, dull to percussion and slightly tender. DRE reveals an enlarged prostate gland without hard nodules.

Impression: Urinary bladder outlet obstruction (abbreviated as 3._____) with 4._____ bladder distension. 5._____ _____ _____ is the probable diagnosis.

Plan: Indwelling Foley catheter for relief of urinary obstruction.
6._____ consult.

Electronically signed: Eleanor Adams MD 08/23/20XX 03:57

Definitions of Medical Terms to Complete the Document

Write the medical terms defined on corresponding answer lines in the document.

1. night urination
2. blood in the urine
3. abbreviation for bladder outlet obstruction
4. pertaining to urine
5. nonmalignant excessive development pertaining to the prostate gland (enlargement of the prostate gland)
6. study of the urinary tract

Chapter 7 Male Reproductive System

EXERCISE 29 ■ Interact with Medical Documents—cont'd

B

Read the medical report and answer the questions below it.

Michigan Oncology Group   44976 East Lincoln   Detroit, MI 97654

January 23, 20XX

Kathryn S. Marcus, MD
Internal Medicine Services
2301 North Brinkley
Detroit, MI 97654

Re: Brindley, Javier
DOB: 08/24/19XX

Dear Dr. Marcus:

It is now 3 years since this patient had brachytherapy using radioactive seeds for his T2a, Gleason 5 prostate cancer. He continues to experience nocturia and some erectile dysfunction with a prostate obstruction score of 3.

His weight is stable at 209 pounds and blood pressure is 122/82 mm Hg. He has no adenopathy. DRE reveals a smooth prostate with no nodules. There is a slight asymmetry with greater prominence on the right side. The PSA remains 0.1 as of August 20, 20XX.

He is doing well and is likely cured of his cancer. I would like to continue seeing him on a yearly basis with a repeat PSA. He will continue seeing you as needed.

Joseph P. Potter, MD
JPP/bko

Use the medical report above to answer the questions.

1. In addition to erectile dysfunction, the patient's symptoms include:
   a. pus in the urine
   b. excessive urine
   c. night urination
   d. blood in the urine

2. Brachytherapy using radioactive seeds was used to treat:
   a. benign prostatic hyperplasia
   b. prostate cancer
   c. erectile dysfunction

3. Which diagnostic test revealed "a smooth prostate"?
   a. transrectal ultrasound
   b. prostate-specific antigen
   c. digital rectal examination

4. Three years after treatment, the patient:
   a. appears to be cancer free
   b. shows disease progression
   c. has been recommended for a radical prostatectomy

EXERCISE 30 ■ Use Medical Language in Online Electronic Health Records

Select the correct medical terms to complete three medical records in one patient's electronic file.

🌐 Access online resources at evolve.elsevier.com > Evolve Resources > Student Resources > Activities > Chapter 7 > Electronic Health Records

Topic: Prostate Cancer
Record 1, Encounters: Office Visit
Record 2, Lab: Pathology report
Record 3, Chart Review: Progress Note

❏ Check the box when complete.

EXERCISE 31 ■ Use Medical Terms in Clinical Statements

For each phrase printed in bold, circle the medical term or abbreviation defined. Answers are listed in Appendix A. For pronunciation practice read the answers aloud.

1. Mr. Potts had a high **blood test that measures the level of prostate-specific antigen in the blood** (PSA, PVP, HPV) level and was referred to a **physician who studies and treats diseases of the urinary tract** (nephrologist, proctologist, urologist). A **combination of magnetic resonance imaging with transrectal ultrasound to obtain tissue from a prostate lesion** (transrectal ultrasound, MRI ultrasound fusion biopsy, digital rectal examination) was performed. The results indicated prostate cancer.

2. A child born with **state of hidden testis** (orchitis, cryptorchidism, anorchism) is at higher risk for developing **cancer of the testicle** (testicular torsion, testicular cancer, prostate cancer). **Surgical fixation of the testicle** (orchiopexy, orchiectomy, orchioplasty) may be performed to help decrease this risk.

3. **Excessive development pertaining to the prostate gland** (prostate cancer, prostatitis, benign prostatic hyperplasia) is very common, and mainly affects men over the age of 50. It is usually diagnosed by digital rectal examination. Treatments include **surgical removal of pieces of prostate gland tissue by using an instrument inserted through the urethra** (TURP, TUIP, TRUS), **use of a focused beam of light to excise or vaporize abnormal tissue and to control bleeding** (hydrocelectomy, morcellation, laser surgery), and simple **excision of the prostate gland** (prostatectomy, prostatolithotomy, prostatovesiculectomy).

4. **Infection spread through sexual contact** (STI, PSA, MIST) may be caused by a virus, such as **a retrovirus that infects T-helper cells of the immune system** (syphilis, trichomoniasis, human immunodeficiency virus), a bacterium, such as *Treponema pallidum* (genital herpes, syphilis, chlamydia), or a protozoan, such as **a one-celled organism** (human papillomavirus, gonorrhea, trichomoniasis).

EXERCISE 32 ■ Pronounce Medical Terms in Use

Practice pronunciation of terms by reading aloud the following paragraph. Use the phonetic spellings to assist with pronunciation. The script also contains medical terms not presented in the chapter. If interested, research their meanings in a medical dictionary or a reliable online source.

A 62-year-old male was found to have an elevated **prostate-specific antigen** (PROS-tāt) (spe-SIF-ik) (AN-ti-jen) test during a routine physical examination. At the age of 42 years he underwent a **vasectomy** (va-SEK-to-mē). The patient denies having nocturia or any significant change in his urinary stream. **Digital rectal examination** (DIJ-i-tal) (REK-tal) (eg-zam-i-NĀ-shun) revealed a mildly enlarged prostate gland with a 1.0 cm stony hard nodule of the right lobe. The urologist performed a **transrectal ultrasound** (trans-REK-tal) (UL-tra-sound) and biopsy. A diagnosis of adenocarcinoma of the prostate was made. The patient elected to undergo a robot-assisted radical **prostatectomy** (pros-ta-TEK-to-mē). Urinary incontinence complicated his postoperative course but this lasted for only 3 months. No **erectile dysfunction** (e-REK-tīl) (dis-FUNK-shun) was reported. His prognosis for full recovery should be excellent.

CHAPTER REVIEW

EXERCISE 33 ■ Chapter Content Quiz

Test your understanding of terms and abbreviations introduced in this chapter. Circle the letter for the medical term or abbreviation related to the words in italics.

1. *Inflammation of the testis* is often caused by a bacterial or viral infection.
   a. orchitis
   b. epididymitis
   c. prostatitis

2. The medical term for *discharge from the glans penis* is:
   a. balanitis
   b. balanorrhea
   c. balanorrhaphy

3. Radical *excision of the prostate gland* is used to treat prostate cancer.
   a. prostatectomy
   b. orchiectomy
   c. epididymectomy

4. HoLEP and PVP are surgical procedures used to treat *nonmalignant enlargement of the prostate gland*.
   a. anorchism
   b. testicular cancer
   c. benign prostatic hyperplasia

5. An STI may be asymptomatic, or it may cause symptoms such as *pain in the testis*, dysuria, and *discharge from the glans penis*.
   a. orchialgia, balanorrhea
   b. aspermia, infertility
   c. phimosis, priapism

6. *Inflammation of the testis and the epididymis* may be caused by an STI.
   a. prostatocystitis
   b. prostatovesiculitis
   c. orchiepididymitis

7. *A fluid-filled sac around the testicle causing scrotal swelling* is common in newborns.
   a. spermatocele
   b. hydrocele
   c. varicocele

8. *Surgical repair of the glans penis* is performed to correct anterior hypospadias.
   a. balanoplasty
   b. orchioplasty
   c. prostatocystotomy

9. The surgical procedure circumcision is the removal of all or part of the *foreskin*.
   a. glans penis
   b. testes
   c. prepuce

10. A surgical procedure that *destroys abnormal or excessive tissue by melting, vaporizing, or eroding* utilizes:
    a. morcellation
    b. enucleation
    c. ablation

11. The abbreviation for the *ultrasound procedure used to diagnose prostate cancer* with use of a transducer probe placed in the rectum is:
    a. RASP
    b. TRUS
    c. PSA

12. Sudden onset of *pain in the testis* can be a symptom of *twisting of the spermatic cord*.
    a. orchialgia, testicular torsion
    b. aspermia, anorchism
    c. prostatolith, prostatolithotomy

13. A *microscopic observation of ejaculated semen* was ordered after the patient's *excision of a duct (vas deferens)* to evaluate the success of the procedure.
    a. prostate-specific antigen, prostatovesiculectomy
    b. digital rectal examination, vasovasostomy
    c. semen analysis, vasectomy

14. Upon diagnosis of an intratesticular mass, a radical inguinal *excision of the testis* was recommended as a diagnostic and therapeutic procedure.
    a. orchiectomy
    b. prostatectomy
    c. vasectomy

15. The term meaning *reduced or absent ability to achieve pregnancy* does not mean complete inability to create offspring.
    a. erectile dysfunction
    b. sterilization
    c. infertility

16. *Condition of scanty sperm* and *lack of live sperm in semen* are terms frequently used in discussions of male infertility.
    a. oligospermia, azoospermia
    b. puberty, ejaculation
    c. chlamydia, syphilis

17. *A procedure in which sound waves are sent and received by a transducer probe that is placed into the rectum* is used to assess the prostate and the surrounding tissues.
    a. multiparametric MRI
    b. transrectal ultrasound
    c. prostate-specific antigen (PSA)

18. *A blood test to measure the level of the hormone responsible for male physical characteristics* level may be sufficient for screening, but additional tests may be necessary for those with mild symptoms of deficiency.
    a. total testosterone
    b. prostate-specific antigen (PSA)
    c. semen analysis

19. A vaccine for *sexually transmitted infection caused by viral infection that causes benign or cancerous growths in male and female genitals* can help prevent the majority of infections that cause cervical cancer.
    a. chlamydia
    b. human immunodeficiency virus
    c. human papillomavirus

20. *A tightness of the prepuce (foreskin of the penis) that prevents its retraction over the glans penis* is normal in babies and toddlers, but may be caused by infection in older boys and adults.
    a. priapism
    b. phimosis
    c. balanitis

CHAPTER AT A GLANCE — Word Parts New to This Chapter

COMBINING FORMS

andr/o	orch/o	prostat/o	vas/o	
balan/o	orchi/o	sperm/o	vesicul/o	
epididym/o	orchid/o	spermat/o		

SUFFIXES

-algia
-ism

CHAPTER AT A GLANCE — Male Reproductive System Terms Built from Word Parts

DISEASE AND DISORDER
andropathy
anorchism
balanitis
benign prostatic hyperplasia (BPH)
cryptorchidism
epididymitis
orchiepididymitis
orchitis
prostatitis
prostatocystitis
prostatolith
prostatorrhea
prostatovesiculitis

SURGICAL
balanoplasty
epididymectomy
orchiectomy
orchiopexy
orchioplasty
orchiotomy
prostatectomy
prostatocystotomy
prostatolithotomy
prostatovesiculectomy
vasectomy
vasovasostomy
vesiculectomy

COMPLEMENTARY
aspermia
balanorrhea
oligospermia
orchialgia

CHAPTER AT A GLANCE — Male Reproductive System Terms NOT Built from Word Parts

DISEASE AND DISORDER
erectile dysfunction (ED)
hydrocele
infertility
phimosis
priapism
prostate cancer
spermatocele
testicular cancer
testicular torsion
varicocele

SURGICAL
ablation
circumcision
enucleation
hydrocelectomy
laser surgery
minimally invasive surgical treatments (MISTs)
morcellation
robotic surgery
sterilization
transurethral incision of the prostate gland (TUIP)
transurethral resection of the prostate gland (TURP)

DIAGNOSTIC
digital rectal examination (DRE)
MRI ultrasound fusion biopsy
multiparametric MRI
prostate-specific antigen (PSA)
semen analysis
total testosterone
transrectal ultrasound (TRUS)

COMPLEMENTARY
artificial insemination
azoospermia
chlamydia
condom
ejaculation
genital herpes
gonorrhea
human immunodeficiency virus (HIV)
human papillomavirus (HPV)
orgasm
puberty
sexually transmitted infection (STI)
spermicide
syphilis
trichomoniasis

PART 2 BODY SYSTEMS

8 Female Reproductive System

Objectives

Upon completion of this chapter, you will be able to:

1. Pronounce organs and anatomic structures of the female reproductive system.
2. Define and spell word parts related to the female reproductive system.
3. Define, pronounce, and spell disease and disorder terms related to the female reproductive system.
4. Define, pronounce, and spell surgical terms related to the female reproductive system.
5. Define, pronounce, and spell diagnostic terms related to the female reproductive system.
6. Define, pronounce, and spell complementary terms related to the female reproductive system.
7. Interpret the meaning of abbreviations related to the female reproductive system.
8. Apply medical language in clinical contexts.

TABLE 8.1 Types, Symptoms, and Causes of Vaginal Fistulas, 281
TABLE 8.2 Types of Hysterectomies, 285
TABLE 8.3 Types of Surgeries Performed to Treat Malignant Breast Tumors, 286
TABLE 8.4 Comparison of the Pap Test and the HPV Test, 295

Outline

ANATOMY, 267
Function, 267
Organs and Anatomic Structures of the Female Reproductive System, 268
Glands of the Female Reproductive System, 270

WORD PARTS, 270
Female Reproductive System Combining Forms, 270
Combining Forms Used with Female Reproductive System Terms, 271
Prefixes, 271
Suffixes, 271

MEDICAL TERMS, 275
Disease and Disorder Terms, 275
   Built from Word Parts, 275
   NOT Built from Word Parts, 279
Surgical Terms, 284
   Built from Word Parts, 284
   NOT Built from Word Parts, 288
Diagnostic Terms, 291
   Built from Word Parts and
      NOT Built from Word Parts, 291
Complementary Terms, 298
   Built from Word Parts and
      NOT Built from Word Parts, 298
Abbreviations, 303

PRACTICAL APPLICATION, 305
CASE STUDY Translate Between Everyday Language and Medical Language, 305
Interact with Medical Documents, 306
Use Medical Language in Online Electronic Health Records, 308
Use Medical Terms in Clinical Statements, 308
Pronounce Medical Terms in Use, 309

CHAPTER REVIEW, 310
Chapter Content Quiz, 310
Chapter at a Glance, 311

Answers to Chapter Exercises, Appendix A

266

Chapter 8 Female Reproductive System

ANATOMY

The female reproductive system is composed of internal and external structures (Fig. 8.1). Internal structures of the female reproductive system are the clitoral body and crura, clitoral bulbs, vagina, uterus, fallopian tubes, and ovaries. External structures include the vulva and mammary glands.

Function

The female reproductive system is responsible for supporting conception and pregnancy. As the female matures throughout her lifespan, this system develops and changes based on the influence of hormones produced by the ovaries. Estrogen and progesterone are female hormones essential for sexual maturation and the overall health of the female. These hormones affect the structure and function of the integumentary, urinary, cardiac, musculoskeletal, and neurologic systems.

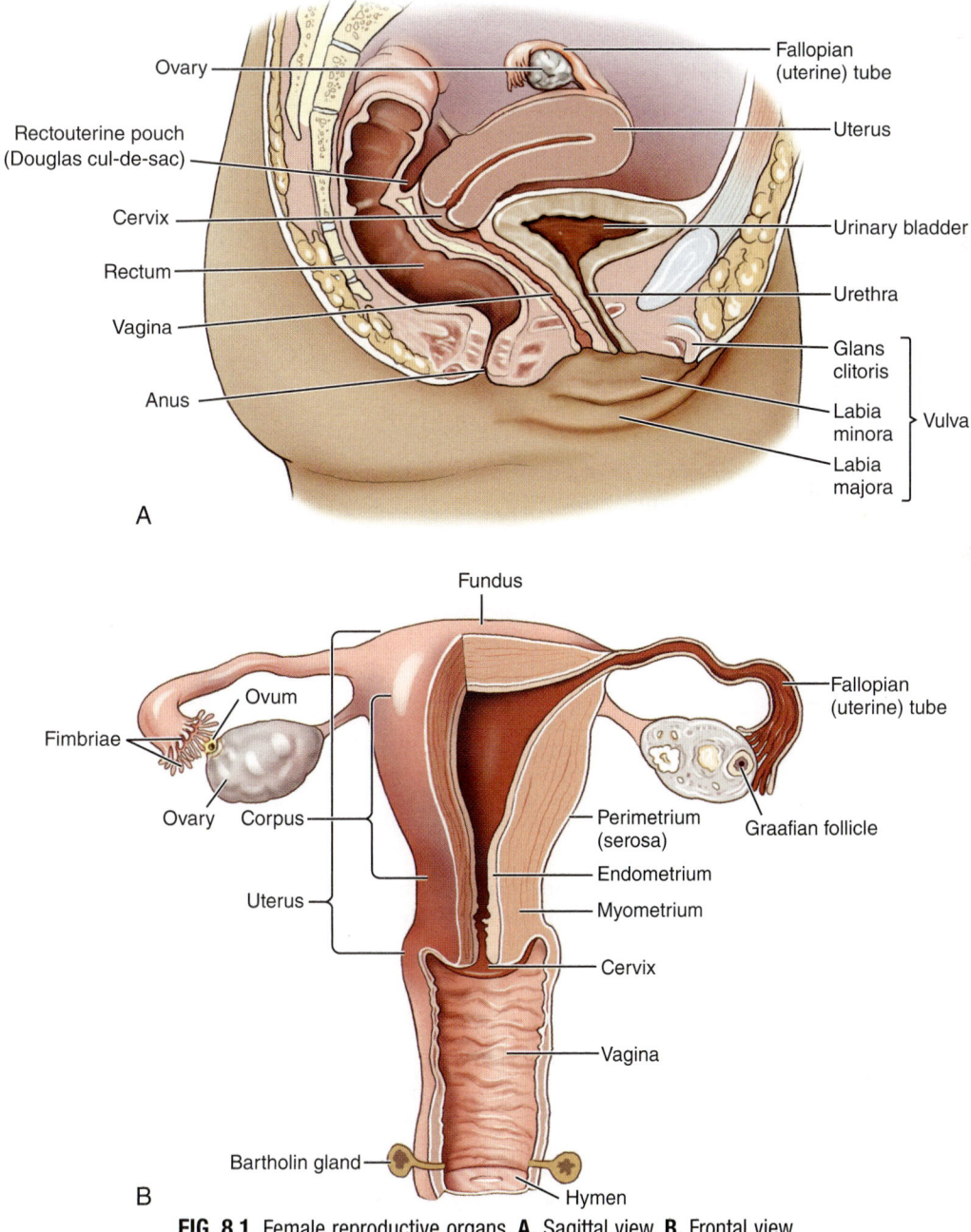

FIG. 8.1 Female reproductive organs. **A,** Sagittal view. **B,** Frontal view.

Organs and Anatomic Structures of the Female Reproductive System

TERM	DEFINITION
ovaries (Ō-var-ēs)	almond-shaped organs located in the pelvic cavity; form and store egg cells (ova) and produce the hormones estrogen and progesterone. **Ovulation** is the release of an egg from the ovaries, which can then travel through the fallopian tubes to the uterus.
ovum *(pl.* **ova)** (Ō-vum) (Ō-vah)	female egg cell
graafian follicles (GRA-fē-en) (FOL-i-kels)	100,000 microscopic sacs that make up a large portion of the ovaries. Each follicle contains an immature ovum. Normally one graafian follicle develops to maturity monthly between puberty and menopause. It moves to the surface of the ovary and releases the ovum, which passes into the fallopian tube.
🏛 **THE GRAAFIAN FOLLICLE** is named for Dutch anatomist Reinier de Graaf, who discovered the sac in 1672.	
fallopian tubes (fa-LŌ-pē-an) (toobz)	pair of tubes attached to the uterus that provide a passageway for the ovum to move from the ovary to the uterus (also called **uterine tubes**)
🏛 **THE FALLOPIAN TUBE** was named in honor of Gabriele Falloppio, 1523-1562, one of the most important anatomists and physicians of the sixteenth century. Falloppio also gave the **vagina** and the **placenta** their names. Fallopian, an eponym, has become so common in medical terminlogy that it is often not capitalized.	
fimbria *(pl.* **fimbriae)** (FIM-brē-a) (FIM-brē-ā)	finger-like projection at the free end of the fallopian tube
uterus (Ū-ter-us)	pear-sized and shaped muscular organ that lies in the pelvic cavity, except during pregnancy when it enlarges and extends up into the abdominal cavity. Its functions are menstruation, pregnancy, and labor.
endometrium (*en*-dō-MĒ-trē-um)	inner lining of the uterus
myometrium (*mī*-ō-MĒ-trē-um)	muscular middle layer of the uterus
perimetrium (*per*-i-MĒ-trē-um)	outer protective layer of the uterus that secretes watery serous fluid to reduce friction (also called **uterine serosa**)
corpus (KŌR-pus)	large central portion of the uterus (also called **uterine body**)
fundus (FUN-dus)	rounded upper portion of the uterus
cervix (Cx) (SER-vicks)	narrow lower portion of the uterus
vagina (va-JĪ-nah)	passageway between the uterus and the outside of the body
hymen (HĪ-men)	fold of membrane found near the opening of the vagina
clitoris (KLIT-a-ris)	network of erectile tissue and nerves with external and internal components: the majority of the structure is located inside the body and not visible to the eye (Fig. 8.2B)
glans clitoris (glanz) (KLIT-a-ris)	external portion of the clitoris protruding below the shelter formed where the labia majora meet in the anterior portion of the vulva (the shelter is called the clitoral hood)
body (BAH-dē)	internal erectile tissue posterior to the glans clitoris, extending distally and branching around the vagina (also called **shaft**)
crura (*s.* **crus**) (KRŪ-ra) (krus)	internal erectile tissue branching from the clitoral body posteriorly, forming long structures often called legs
clitoral bulbs (KLIT-ar-al) (buhlbz)	internal erectile tissue located between the crura and vaginal wall that increases in size during sexual stimulation

Chapter 8 Female Reproductive System   269

TERM	DEFINITION
vulva (VUL-va)	external genitals of the female reproductive system, including the mons pubis, labia majora, labia minora, glans clitoris, urinary meatus, and vaginal opening (Fig. 8.2)
perineum (*per*-i-NĒ-um)	pelvic floor in the male and female reproductive systems. In the female reproductive system it refers to the area between the vaginal opening and the anus.

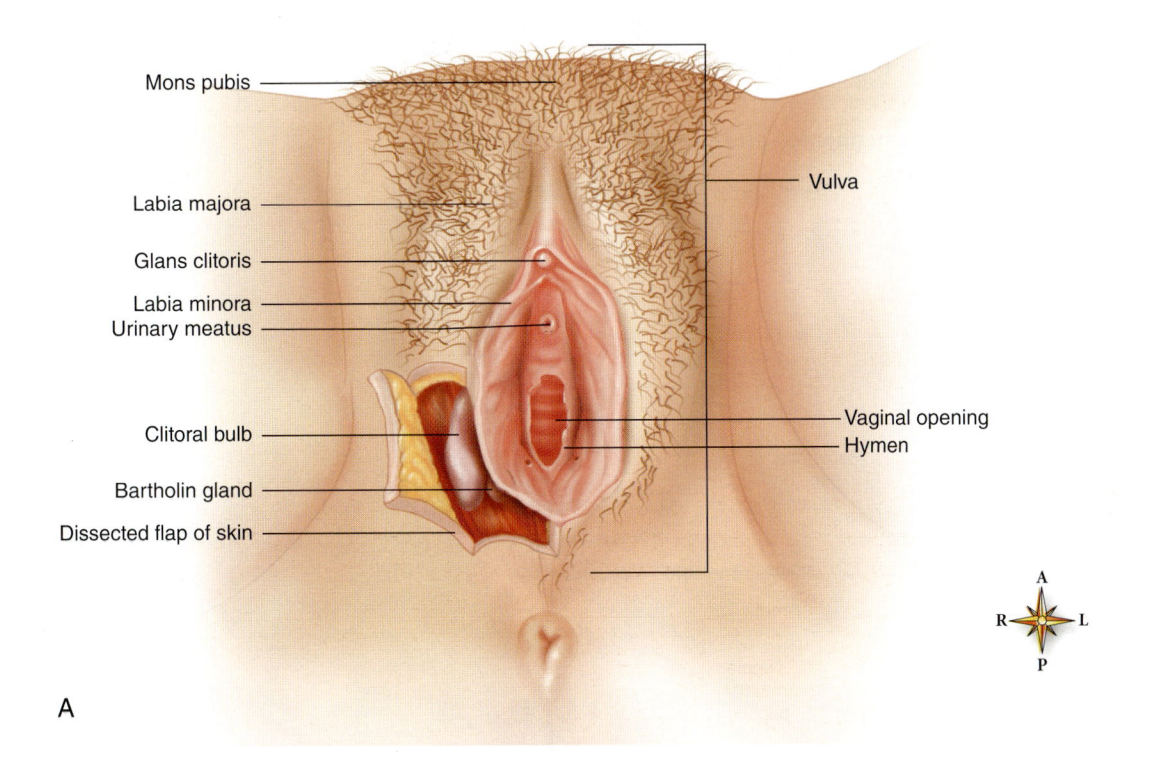

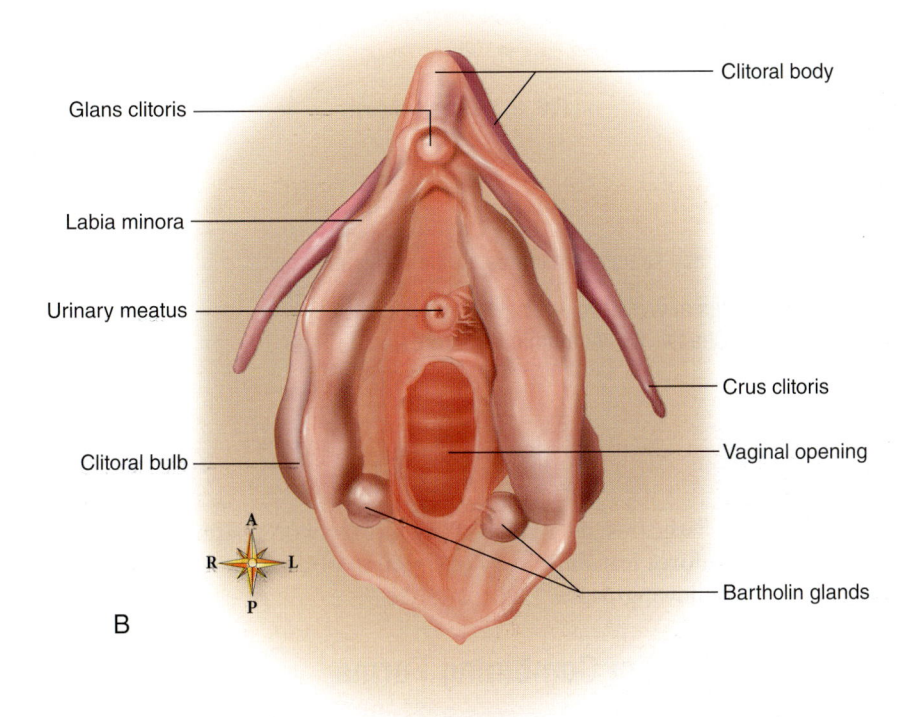

FIG. 8.2 Vulva. **A,** External reproductive structures, which together are called the vulva. **B,** The full structure of the clitoris, most of which is located internally.

Chapter 8 Female Reproductive System

Glands of the Female Reproductive System

TERM	DEFINITION
Bartholin glands (BAR-tō-lin) (glans)	pair of mucus-producing glands located on each side of the vagina, near the vaginal opening (also called **greater vestibular glands**); (Fig. 8.2)
🏛 **BARTHOLIN GLANDS** were described by Caspar Bartholin, a Danish anatomist, in 1675.	
breasts (brests)	milk-producing glands. Each breast consists of 15 to 20 divisions or lobules. (also called **mammary glands**); (Fig. 8.3)
mammary papilla (MAM-a-rē) (pa-PIL-a)	breast nipple
areola (a-RĒ-ō-la)	pigmented area around the breast nipple

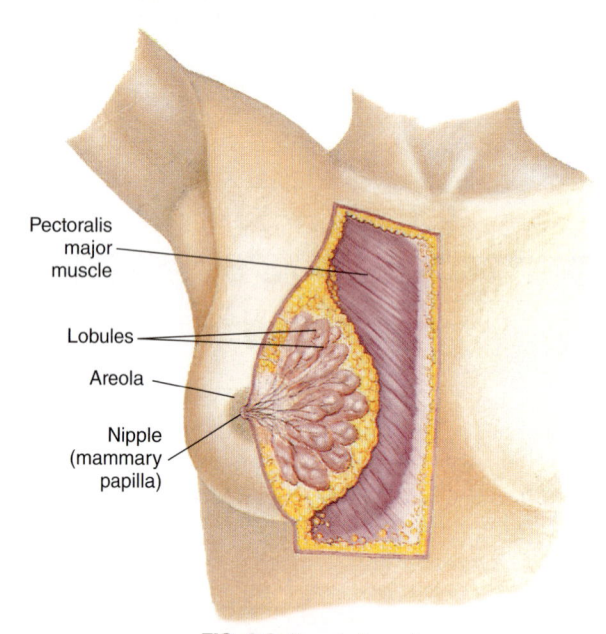

FIG. 8.3 Female breast.

PRONOUNCE ANATOMIC STRUCTURES

Practice saying aloud each of the organs and specific structures on the previous pages.

To hear the terms, go to Evolve Resources at www.evolve.elsevier.com and select:
Student Resources > Audio Glossary > Chapter 8 > **Anatomic Structures**.

❑ Check the box when complete.

🔗 WORD PARTS

Use paper flashcards or electronic flashcards on Evolve to memorize word parts used to analyze, define, and build medical terms in this chapter. To reinforce learning, study one section of the Word Parts Table at a time, then complete the corresponding exercise on the following pages.

1 ▪ Female Reproductive System Combining Forms

COMBINING FORM	DEFINITION	COMBINING FORM	DEFINITION
cervic/o	cervix	**endometri/o**	endometrium
colp/o	vagina	**episi/o**	vulva

COMBINING FORM	DEFINITION	COMBINING FORM	DEFINITION
gynec/o	woman, female reproductive organs	oophor/o	ovary
hymen/o	hymen	pelv/i	pelvis, pelvic cavity (Note: the combining vowel is an *i*)
hyster/o	uterus		
mamm/o	breast	perine/o	perineum
mast/o	breast	salping/o	fallopian tube (uterine tube) (Fig. 8.4)
men/o	menstruation	trachel/o	cervix
metr/o	uterus	vagin/o	vagina
		vulv/o	vulva

2 ■ Combining Forms Used with Female Reproductive System Terms

COMBINING FORM	DEFINITION	COMBINING FORM	DEFINITION
hemat/o	blood	my/o	muscle(s), muscle tissue
hydr/o	water	olig/o	scanty, few
leuk/o	white	py/o	pus

3 ■ Prefixes

PREFIX	DEFINITION	PREFIX	DEFINITION
a-	absence of, without	endo-	within
dys-	painful, abnormal, difficult, labored	peri-	surrounding (outer)

4 ■ Suffixes

SUFFIX	DEFINITION	SUFFIX	DEFINITION
-al	pertaining to	-osis	abnormal condition
-algia	pain	-pexy	surgical fixation
-cele	hernia, protrusion	-plasty	surgical repair
-cleisis	surgical closure	-rrhagia	excessive bleeding
-ectomy	excision, surgical removal	-rrhaphy	suturing, repairing
-gram	the record, radiographic image	-rrhea	flow, discharge
-graphy	process of recording, radiographic imaging	-salpinx	fallopian tube (uterine tube)
		-scope	instrument used for visual examination
-ic	pertaining to		
-itis	inflammation	-scopic	pertaining to visual examination
-logist	one who studies and treats (specialist, physician)	-scopy	visual examination
		-tomy	cut into, incision
-logy	study of		

Refer to **Appendix B** and **Appendix C** for alphabetized word parts and their meanings.

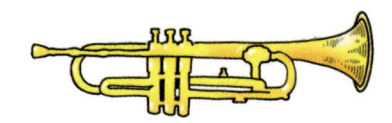

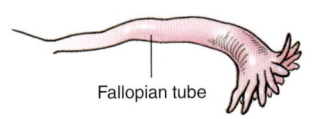

FIG. 8.4 Salpinx is derived from the Greek term for trumpet. The term was used for the fallopian tubes because of their trumpet-like shape.

272 Chapter 8 Female Reproductive System

EXERCISE 1 ■ Female Reproductive System Combining Forms

Refer to the first section of the word parts table.

A Label

Fill in the blanks with combining forms in this diagram of internal female reproductive organs and anatomic structures.
To check your answers, go to Appendix A at the back of the textbook.

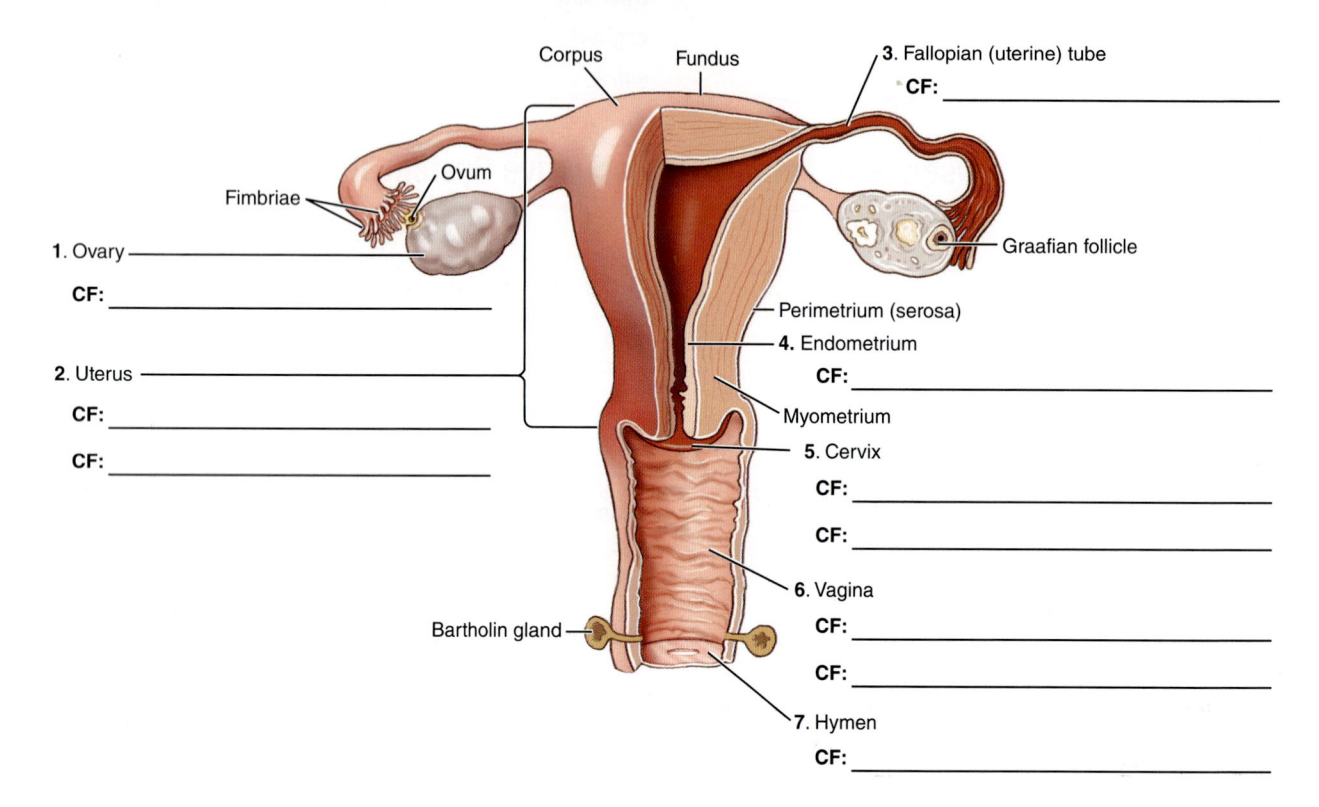

Corpus Fundus 3. Fallopian (uterine) tube
CF: _____

Ovum
Fimbriae
Graafian follicle
1. Ovary
CF: _____

Perimetrium (serosa)
4. Endometrium
CF: _____

2. Uterus
CF: _____
CF: _____

Myometrium
5. Cervix
CF: _____
CF: _____

6. Vagina
Bartholin gland
CF: _____
CF: _____

7. Hymen
CF: _____

B Label

Fill in the blanks with combining forms in this diagram of external female reproductive organs and anatomic structures.

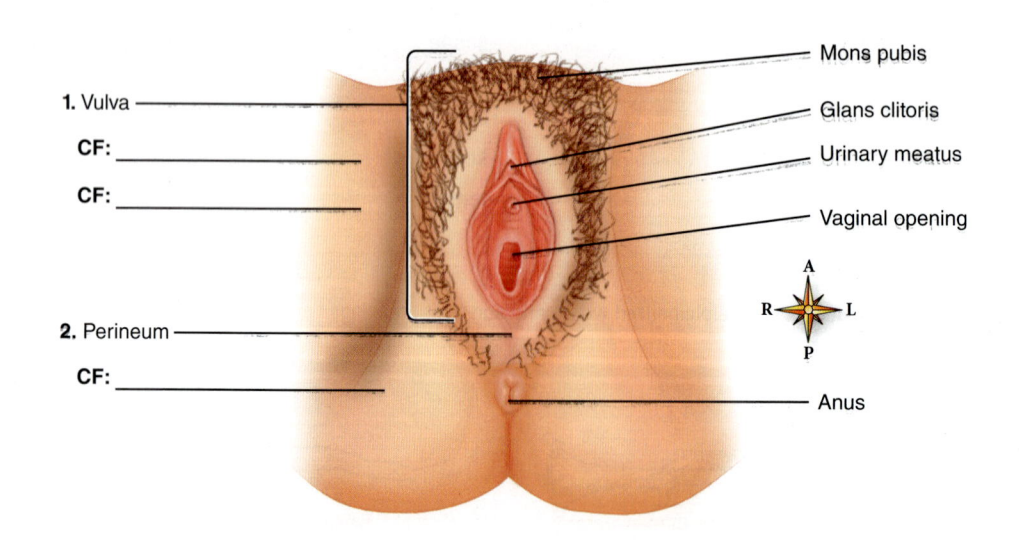

Mons pubis
1. Vulva
Glans clitoris
CF: _____
Urinary meatus
CF: _____
Vaginal opening

2. Perineum
CF: _____

Anus

Chapter 8   Female Reproductive System   273

C   Identify

Write the combining form for each of the following.

1. menstruation _____
2. woman, female reproductive organs _____
3. breast   a. _____ , b. _____
4. pelvis, pelvic cavity _____

D   Define and Match

Step 1: Write the definitions after the following combining forms.
Step 2: Match the descriptions on the right with the combining forms and definitions. Answers may be used more than once; no answer line appears for those not described in a lettered item.

_____ 1. salping/o, _____
_____ 2. metr/o, _____
_____ 3. perine/o, _____
_____ 4. cervic /o, _____
_____ 5. colp/o, _____
_____ 6. trachel/o, _____
_____ 7. mamm/o, _____
_____ 8. pelv/i, _____

a. pelvic floor in male and female anatomy
b. passageway between the uterus and the outside of the body
c. narrow lower portion of the uterus
d. milk-producing glands
e. pear-sized and shaped muscular organ
f. passageway for ovum to move from the ovary to the uterus

E   Define and Match

Step 1: Write the definitions after the following combining forms.
Step 2: Match the descriptions on the right with the combining forms and definitions. Answers may be used more than once; no answer line appears for those not described in a lettered item.

_____ 1. vagin/o, _____
_____ 2. hymen/o, _____
_____ 3. episi/o, _____
_____ 4. hyster/o, _____
_____ 5. mast/o, _____
_____ 6. oophor/o, _____
_____ 7. vulv/o, _____
_____ 8. endometri/o, _____
_____ 9. men/o, _____
_____ 10. gynec/o, _____

a. fold of membrane near the opening of the vagina
b. passageway between the uterus and the outside of the body
c. inner lining of the uterus
d. external genitals of the female reproductive system
e. milk-producing glands
f. pear-sized and shaped muscular organ
g. almond-shaped organs located in the pelvic cavity that produce and store female reproductive cells

EXERCISE 2 ■ Combining Forms Used with Female Reproductive System Terms

Refer to the second section of the word parts table.

A   Define

Write the definitions of the following combining forms.

1. olig/o _____
2. hemat/o _____
3. my/o _____
4. leuk/o _____
5. py/o _____
6. hydr/o _____

274 Chapter 8 Female Reproductive System

B Identify

Write the combining form for each of the following.

1. pus _____
2. water _____
3. blood _____
4. muscle(s), muscle tissue _____
5. scanty, few _____
6. white _____

EXERCISE 3 ■ Prefixes

Refer to the third section of the word parts table.

A Define

Write the definitions of the following prefixes.

1. endo- _____
2. a- _____
3. peri- _____
4. dys- _____

B Identify

Write the prefix for each of the following definitions.

1. painful, abnormal, difficult, labored _____
2. within _____
3. absence of, without _____
4. surrounding (outer) _____

EXERCISE 4 ■ Suffixes

Refer to the fourth section of the word parts table.

A Match

Match the suffixes in the first column with their correct definitions in the second column.

_____ 1. -graphy   a. pertaining to visual examination
_____ 2. -pexy   b. pertaining to
_____ 3. -cele   c. process of recording, radiographic imaging
_____ 4. -scopic   d. inflammation
_____ 5. -logy   e. study of
_____ 6. -itis   f. hernia, protrusion
_____ 7. -al   g. suturing, repairing
_____ 8. -rrhaphy   h. surgical fixation

B Define

Write the definitions of the following suffixes.

1. -gram _____
2. -osis _____
3. -algia _____
4. -rrhea _____
5. -scopy _____
6. -ic _____
7. -ectomy _____
8. -plasty _____
9. -rrhagia _____
10. -scope _____
11. -tomy _____
12. -logist _____

C Label

Write the suffixes pictured and defined.

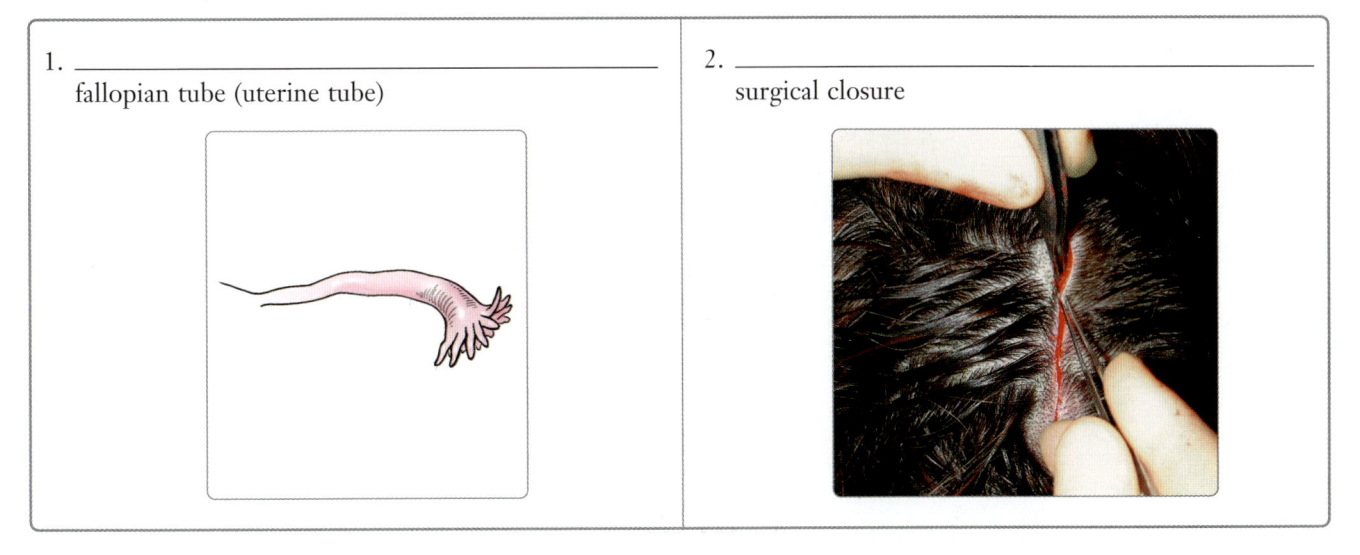

1. _____
fallopian tube (uterine tube)

2. _____
surgical closure

MEDICAL TERMS

Medical terms relevant to this chapter have been grouped by topics, such as Disease and Disorder, and are listed in tables designated as Built from Word Parts or *NOT* Built from Word Parts. The exercises following each table assist with learning term definitions, pronunciations, and spellings.

Disease and Disorder Terms
BUILT FROM WORD PARTS

The following terms can be translated using definitions of word parts. Further explanation is provided within parentheses as needed.

TERM	DEFINITION	TERM	DEFINITION
1. **cervicitis** (*ser*-vi-SĪ-tis)	inflammation of the cervix (Fig. 8.8)	6. **mastitis** (*mas*-TĪ-tis)	inflammation of the breast
2. **endometriosis** (*en*-dō-*mē*-trē-Ō-sis)	abnormal condition of the endometrium (endometrial tissue grows outside of the uterus in various areas in the pelvic cavity, including ovaries, fallopian tubes, intestines, and uterus) (Fig. 8.5)	7. **menometrorrhagia** (*men*-ō-*met*-rō-RĀ-jea)	excessive bleeding from the uterus at menstruation (and between menstrual cycles; heavy and irregular bleeding)
		8. **menorrhagia** (*men*-ō-RĀ-jea)	excessive bleeding at menstruation (heavy bleeding in regular, cyclical pattern); (also called **heavy menstrual bleeding**)
3. **endometritis** (*en*-dō-mē-TRĪ-tis)	inflammation of the endometrium (Fig. 8.8)		
4. **hematosalpinx** (*hem*-a-tō-SAL-pinks)	blood in the fallopian tube	9. **metrorrhagia** (*mē*-trō-RĀ-jea)	excessive bleeding from the uterus (irregular, out-of-cycle bleeding ranging from heavy to light, including spotting); (also called **intermenstrual bleeding**)
5. **hydrosalpinx** (*hī*-drō-SAL-pinks)	water in the fallopian tube (a clear, watery fluid collects in the tube, and can cause blockage)		

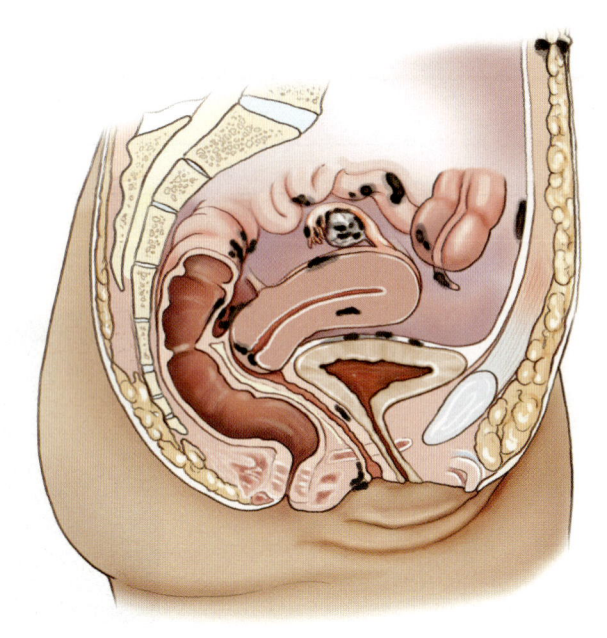

FIG. 8.5 Endometriosis. Spots indicate common sites of endometrial deposits.

Disease and Disorder Terms—cont'd
BUILT FROM WORD PARTS

TERM	DEFINITION	TERM	DEFINITION
10. **myometritis** (*mī*-o-me-TRĪ-tis)	inflammation of the uterine muscle (myometrium)	15. **salpingocele** (sal-PING-gō-sēl)	hernia of the fallopian tube
11. **oophoritis** (*ō*-of-o-RĪ-tis)	inflammation of the ovary	16. **vaginitis** (*vaj*-i-NĪ-tis)	inflammation of the vagina (Fig. 8.8)
12. **perimetritis** (*per*-i-me-TRĪ-tis)	inflammation surrounding the uterus (perimetrium)	17. **vaginosis** (*vaj*-i-NŌ-sis)	abnormal condition of the vagina (caused by a bacterial imbalance) (also called **bacterial vaginosis**)
13. **pyosalpinx** (*pī*-ō-SAL-pinks)	pus in the fallopian tube		
14. **salpingitis** (*sal*-pin-JĪ-tis)	inflammation of the fallopian tube (Fig. 8.8)	18. **vulvovaginitis** (*vul*-vō-*vaj*-i-NĪ-tis)	inflammation of the vulva and vagina

EXERCISE 5 ■ Pronounce and Spell

Practice pronunciation and spelling on paper and online.

1. **Practice on Paper**
    a. **Pronounce:** Read the phonetic spelling and say aloud the terms listed in the previous table. Refer to Table 2.2 Pronunciation Key as needed.
    b. **Spell:** Have a study partner read the terms aloud. Write the spelling of the terms on a separate sheet of paper.
2. **Practice Online**
    a. **Access** online learning resources. Go to evolve.elsevier.com > Evolve Resources > Student Resources.
    b. **Pronounce:** Select Audio Glossary > Chapter 8 > Exercise 5. Select a term to hear its pronunciation and repeat aloud.
    c. **Spell:** Select Activities > Chapter 8 > Spell Terms > Exercise 5. Select the audio icon and type the correct spelling of the term.

❏ Check the box when complete.

Chapter 8 Female Reproductive System 277

EXERCISE 6 ■ Analyze and Define

Analyze and define the following terms by drawing slashes between word parts, writing word part abbreviations above the term, underlining combining forms, and writing the combining form abbreviations below the term.

1. vaginosis

2. hematosalpinx

3. metrorrhagia

4. oophoritis

5. perimetritis

6. vulvovaginitis

7. salpingocele

8. menometrorrhagia

EXERCISE 7 ■ Build

A Label

Build terms pictured by writing word parts above definitions.

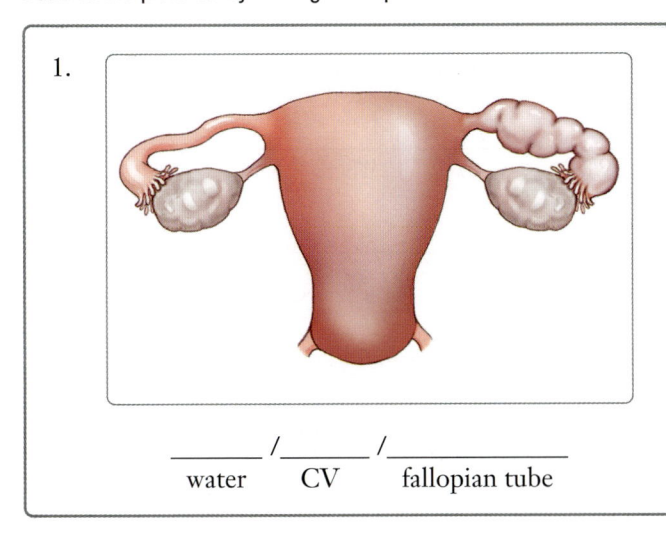

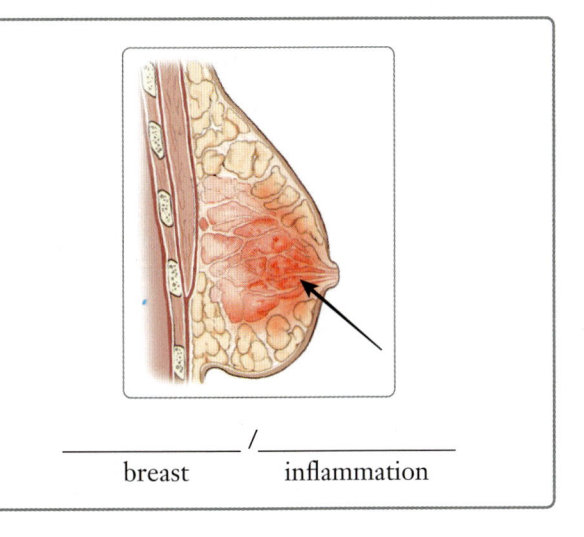

1.
_____ / _____ / _____
water   CV   fallopian tube

2.
_____ / _____
breast   inflammation

278 Chapter 8 Female Reproductive System

3.

_____ / _____
vagina   abnormal condition
(caused by a bacterial imbalance)

4.

_____ / _____
endometrium   abnormal condition

5.

_____ / _____
fallopian tube   inflammation

6.

_____ / _____
endometrium   inflammation

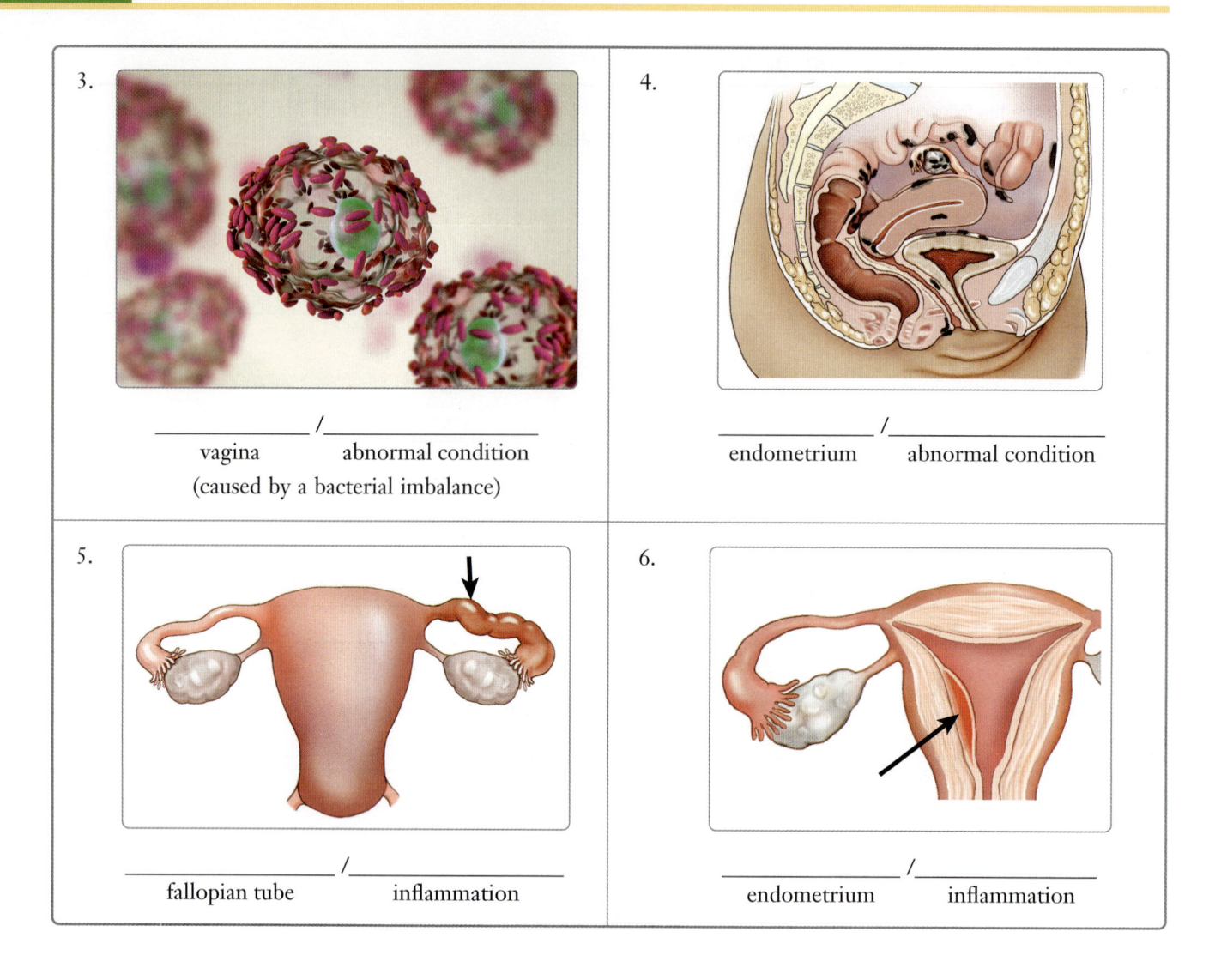

B Fill In

Build disease and disorder terms for the following definitions by using the word parts you have learned.

1. inflammation of the uterine muscle

   _____ / _____ / _____ / _____
   WR   CV   WR   S

2. excessive bleeding at menstruation (heavy bleeding in regular, cyclical pattern)

   _____ / _____ / _____
   WR   CV   S

3. pus in the fallopian tube

   _____ / _____ / _____
   WR   CV   S

4. inflammation of the cervix

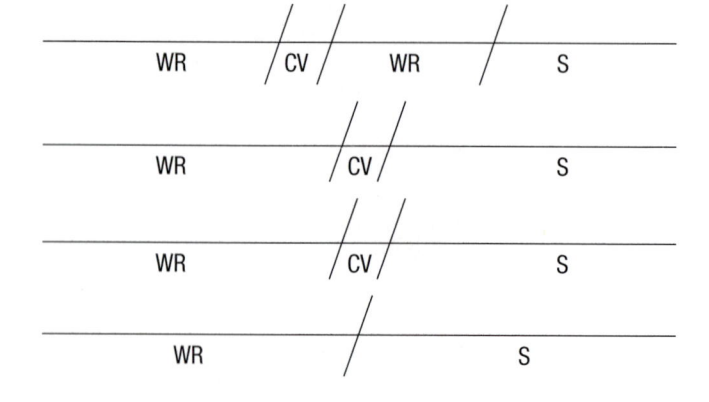

   _____ / _____
   WR   S

Disease and Disorder Terms
NOT BUILT FROM WORD PARTS

Word parts may be present in the following terms; however, their full meanings cannot be translated using definitions of word parts alone.

TERM	DEFINITION
1. **abnormal uterine bleeding (AUB)** (ab-NOR-mul) (Ū-ter-in) (BLĒD-ing)	irregular bleeding in the absence of pregnancy; menometrorrhagia, menorrhagia, and metrorrhagia are some types of AUB
2. **adenomyosis** (ad-e-nō-mī-Ō-sis)	growth of endometrium into the muscular portion of the uterus
3. **Bartholin cyst** (BAR-tō-lin) (sist)	blockage of one of the glands on either side of the vagina; usually causes a tender, swollen lump on the affected side, which may become infected, resulting in a Bartholin abscess
4. **breast cancer** (brest) (KAN-cer)	malignant tumor of the breast (Fig. 8.6)
5. **cervical cancer** (SER-vi-kal) (KAN-cer)	malignant tumor of the cervix, which progresses from cervical dysplasia to carcinoma. Its cause is linked to human papillomavirus (HPV) infection.

HPV VACCINE The Food and Drug Administration (FDA) approved a vaccine for human papillomavirus (HPV) in 2006, directly impacting the prevention of **cervical cancer**. The vaccine is highly effective in protecting against several forms of HPV as long as it is administered before a male or female becomes sexually active. Because vaccination does not combat all strains of HPV and is not 100% effective, periodic cervical cancer screening is strongly recommended.

6. **endometrial cancer** (en-dō-MĒ-trē-al) (KAN-cer)	malignant tumor of the endometrium (also called **uterine cancer**) (Fig. 8.7)

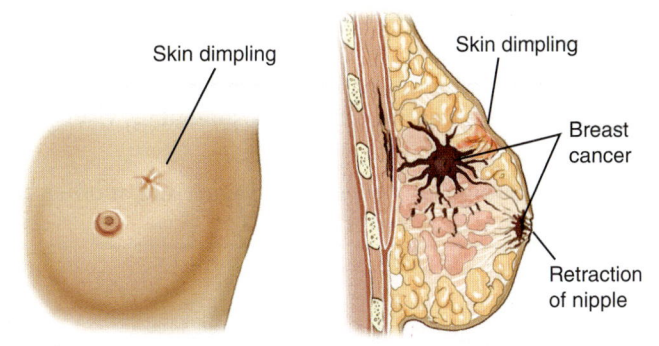

FIG. 8.6 Clinical signs of breast cancer.

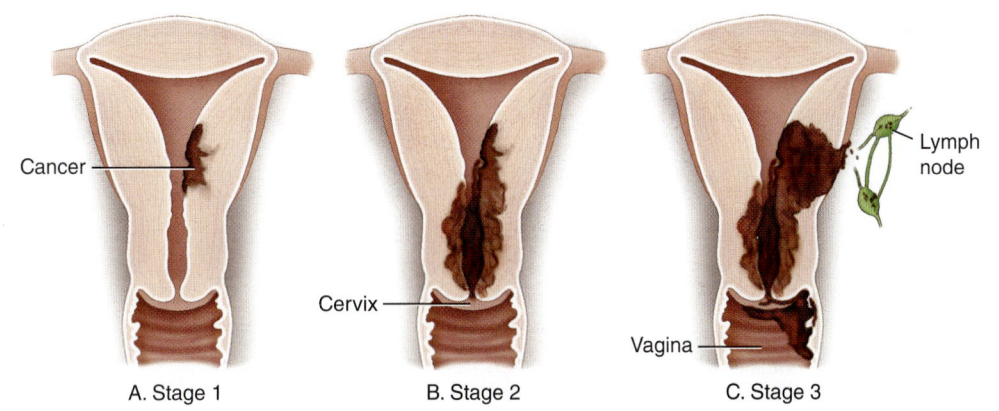

FIG. 8.7 Endometrial cancer. **A,** Stage 1: Confined to the endometrium. **B,** Stage 2: Spread into support structures of the cervix from the body of the uterus. **C,** Stage 3: Spreads to other organs such as the vagina.

Disease and Disorder Terms
NOT BUILT FROM WORD PARTS—cont'd

TERM	DEFINITION
7. **fibrocystic breast changes (FCC)** (fī-brō-SIS-tik) (brest) (CHĀN-jiz)	thickening of tissue (fibrosis), benign cysts, and pain or tenderness in one or both breasts; thought to be caused by monthly hormonal changes (also called **fibrocystic breasts**; formerly called **fibrocystic breast disease**)
8. **ovarian cancer** (ō-VAR-ē-an) (KAN-cer)	malignant tumor of the ovary
9. **pelvic inflammatory disease (PID)** (PEL-vik) (in-FLAM-a-tor-ē) (di-ZĒZ)	inflammation of some or all of the female pelvic organs; can be caused by many different pathogens. If untreated, the infection may spread upward from the vagina, involving the uterus, fallopian tubes, ovaries, and other pelvic organs. An ascending infection may result in infertility and, in acute cases, fatal septicemia (Fig. 8.8).
10. **polycystic ovary syndrome (PCOS)** (pol-ē-SIS-tik) (Ō-vah-rē) (SIN-drōm)	condition typically characterized by hormonal imbalances, ovulatory dysfunction, and multiple ovarian cysts; symptoms can include irregular menstruation, acne, excess facial and body hair, and infertility. People with this condition have increased risks of cardiovascular disease, obesity, and glucose intolerance.
11. **premenstrual syndrome (PMS)** (prē-MEN-stroo-al) (SIN-drōm)	condition involving physical and emotional symptoms occurring up to 10 days before menstruation. Symptoms include nervous tension, irritability, mastalgia (pain in the breast), edema, and headache.
12. **toxic shock syndrome (TSS)** (TOK-sik) (shok) (SIN-drōm)	severe illness characterized by high fever, rash, vomiting, diarrhea, and myalgia, followed by hypotension and, in severe cases, shock and death; usually affects menstruating women using tampons; caused by *Staphylococcus aureus* and *Streptococcus pyogenes*
13. **uterine fibroid** (Ū-ter-in) (FĪ-broyd)	benign tumor of the uterine muscle (also called **myoma of the uterus** or **leiomyoma**)
14. **uterovaginal prolapse** (ū-ter-ō-VAJ-i-nal) (prō-LAPS)	dropping of the uterus (and sometimes vagina) due to weakened pelvic muscles; the uterus moves downward into and is sometimes visible outside the vagina
15. **vaginal fistula** (VAJ-i-nal) (FIS-tū-la)	abnormal passageway between the vagina and another organ, such as the urinary bladder, colon, or rectum (Table 8.1)

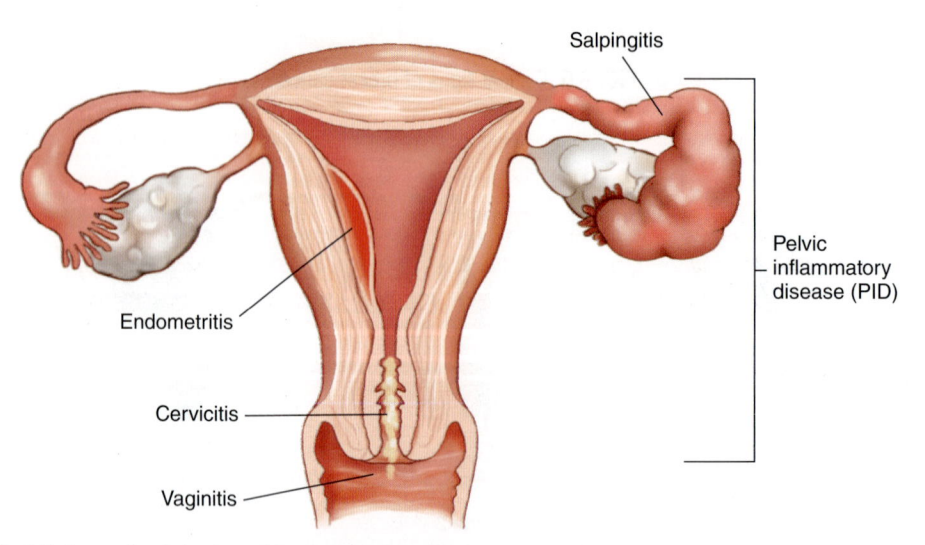

FIG. 8.8 Ascending infection of the female reproductive system as seen in pelvic inflammatory disease.

TABLE 8.1 Types, Symptoms, and Causes of Vaginal Fistulas

TYPES OF VAGINAL FISTULAS	SYMPTOMS	CAUSES OF VAGINAL FISTULAS
• **Vesicovaginal fistula,** abnormal passageway between the urinary bladder and the vagina • **Colovaginal fistula,** abnormal passageway between the colon (large intestine) and the vagina • **Rectovaginal fistula,** abnormal passageway between the rectum and the vagina	• **Vesicovaginal fistula,** urine may leak or flow out of the vagina, causing incontinence, bad smells, sores or discomfort • **Colovaginal and rectovaginal fistulas,** foul-smelling discharge (feces) or gas may come out of the vagina, which may be painful or cause infections	• **Gynecologic surgery,** including hysterectomy and cesarean section, and injuries during childbirth (occurs more frequently in developing countries where access to medical care may be limited) • **Gastrointestinal diseases** including inflammatory bowel disease (Crohn disease and ulcerative colitis) and diverticulitis • **Malignancies** in the pelvic region and radiation therapy for pelvic cancers

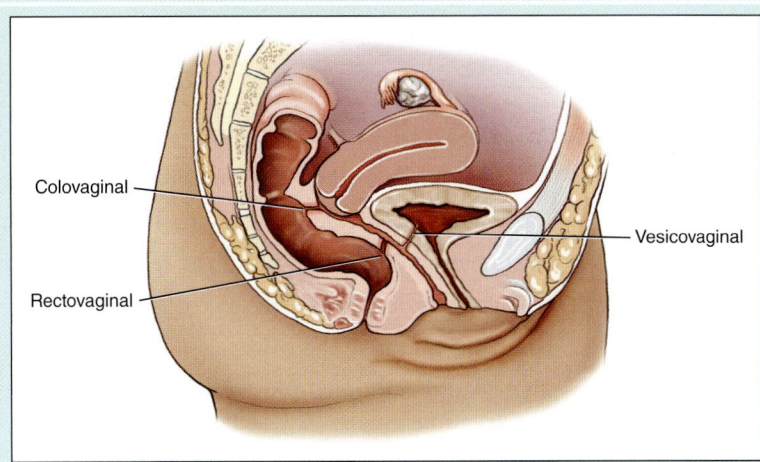

Vaginal fistulas: vesicovaginal, colovaginal, and rectovaginal.

EXERCISE 8 ■ Pronounce and Spell

Practice pronunciation and spelling on paper and online.

1. Practice on Paper
   a. **Pronounce:** Read the phonetic spelling and say aloud the terms listed in the term table. Refer to Table 2.2 Pronunciation Key as needed.
   b. **Spell:** Have a study partner read the terms aloud. Write the spelling of the terms on a separate sheet of paper.

2. Practice Online
   a. **Access** online learning resources. Go to evolve.elsevier.com > Evolve Resources > Student Resources.
   b. **Pronounce:** Select Audio Glossary > Chapter 8 > Exercise 8. Select a term to hear its pronunciation and repeat aloud.
   c. **Spell:** Select Activities > Chapter 8 > Spell Terms > Exercise 8. Select the audio icon and type the correct spelling of the term.

❏ Check the box when complete.

EXERCISE 9 ■ Match

Match the terms in the first column with their correct definitions in the second column.

_____ 1. vaginal fistula
_____ 2. uterovaginal prolapse
_____ 3. uterine fibroid
_____ 4. fibrocystic breast changes
_____ 5. endometrial cancer
_____ 6. breast cancer
_____ 7. adenomyosis

a. abnormal passageway between the vagina and another organ
b. also called myoma of the uterus or leiomyoma
c. also called uterine cancer
d. dropping of the uterus (and sometimes vagina) due to weakened pelvic muscles
e. growth of endometrium into the muscular portion of the uterus
f. malignant tumor of the breast
g. thickening of tissue (fibrosis), benign cysts, and pain or tenderness in one or both breasts

EXERCISE 10 ■ Match

Match the terms in the first column with their correct definitions in the second column.

_____ 1. toxic shock syndrome
_____ 2. premenstrual syndrome
_____ 3. polycystic ovary syndrome
_____ 4. pelvic inflammatory disease
_____ 5. ovarian cancer
_____ 6. cervical cancer
_____ 7. Bartholin cyst
_____ 8. abnormal uterine bleeding

a. blockage of one of the glands on either side of the vagina
b. hormonal imbalances, ovulatory dysfunction, and multiple ovarian cysts
c. inflammation of some or all of the female pelvic organs
d. irregular bleeding in the absence of pregnancy
e. malignant tumor of the ovary
f. physical and emotional symptoms occurring up to 10 days before menstruation
g. progresses from cervical dysplasia to carcinoma
h. severe illness characterized by high fever, rash, vomiting, diarrhea, and myalgia, followed by hypotension and, in severe cases, shock and death

EXERCISE 11 ■ Fill In

A Identify

Fill in the blanks with the correct terms.

1. A malignant tumor of the ovary is referred to as _____ _____.
2. _____ is growth of endometrium into the muscular portion of the uterus.
3. A severe illness characterized by high fever, rash, vomiting, diarrhea, and myalgia, followed by hypotension, which is associated with the use of tampons. is known as _____ _____ _____.
4. _____ _____ is a malignant tumor, which progresses from cervical dysplasia to carcinoma, and is linked to human papillomavirus (HPV) infection.
5. A condition involving physical and emotional symptoms occurring up to 10 days before menstruation is called _____.
6. Irregular bleeding in the absence of pregnancy is _____ _____ _____; menometrorrhagia, menorrhagia, and metrorrhagia are examples.
7. _____ _____ _____ refers to thickening of tissue (fibrosis), benign cysts, and pain or tenderness in one or both breasts.

B Label

Write the medical terms pictured and defined.

1. _____
dropping of the uterus (and sometimes vagina) due to weakened pelvic muscles

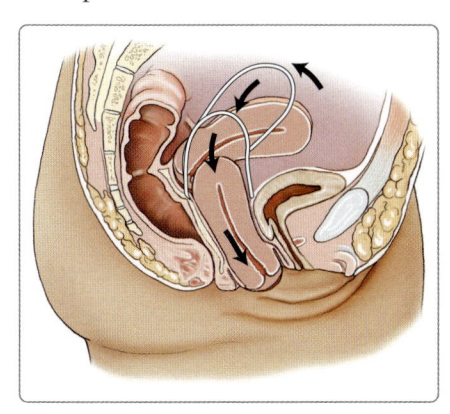

2. _____
benign tumor of the uterine muscle

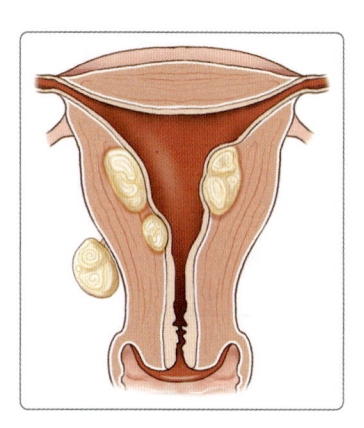

3. _____
malignant tumor of the endometrium

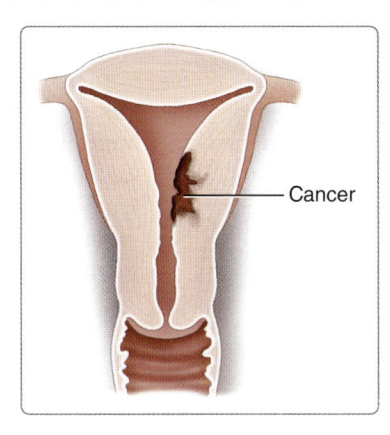

4. _____
malignant tumor of the breast

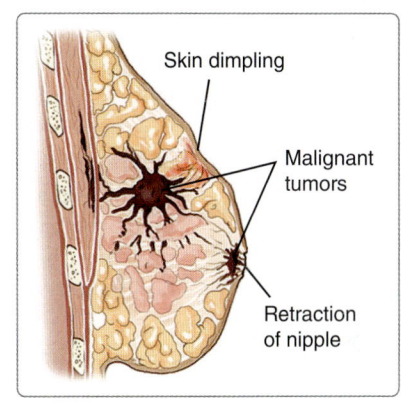

5. _____
inflammation of some or all of the female pelvic organs

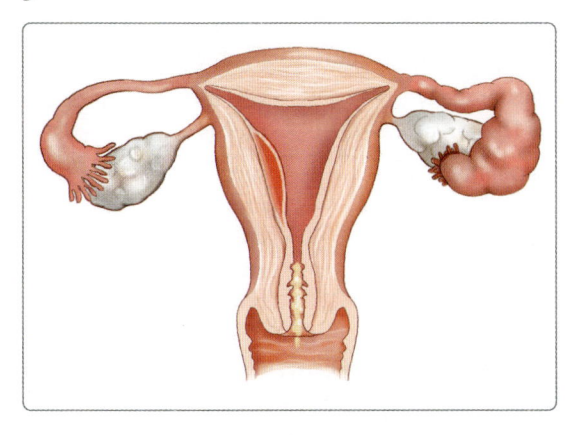

6. _____
abnormal passageway between the vagina and another organ, such as the urinary bladder, colon, or rectum

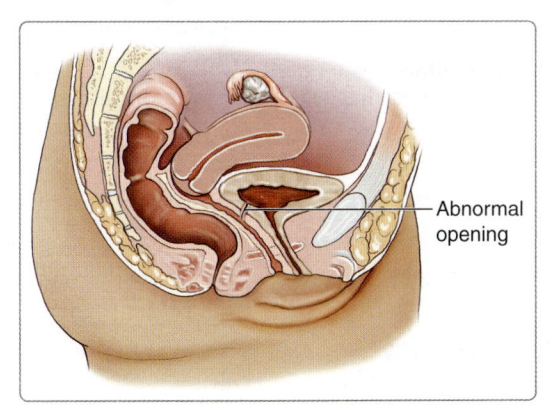

284　Chapter 8　Female Reproductive System

7. _____
condition typically characterized by hormonal imbalances, ovulatory dysfunction, and multiple ovarian cysts

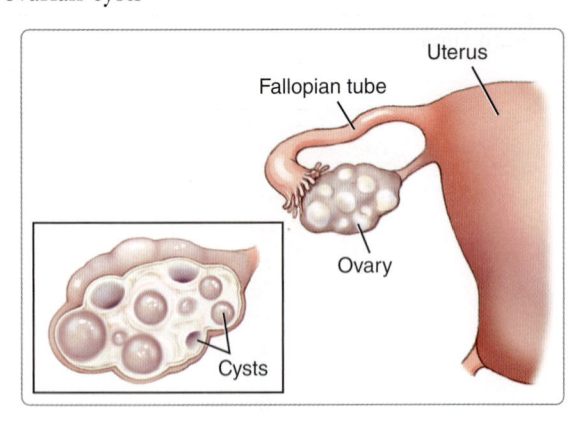

8. _____
blockage of one of the glands on either side of the vagina; usually causes a tender, swollen lump on the affected side

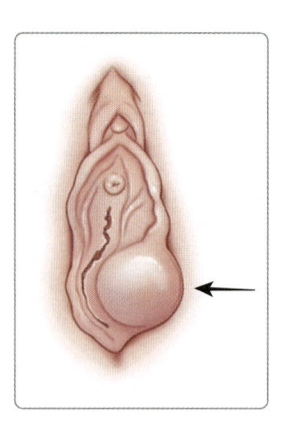

EXERCISE 12 ■ Review of Disease and Disorder Terms

Can you define, pronounce, and spell the following terms?

abnormal uterine bleeding (AUB)	fibrocystic breast changes (FCC)	ovarian cancer	salpingocele
adenomyosis	hematosalpinx	pelvic inflammatory disease (PID)	toxic shock syndrome (TSS)
Bartholin cyst	hydrosalpinx	perimetritis	uterine fibroid
breast cancer	mastitis	polycystic ovary syndrome (PCOS)	uterovaginal prolapse
cervical cancer	menometrorrhagia	premenstrual syndrome (PMS)	vaginal fistula
cervicitis	menorrhagia	pyosalpinx	vaginitis
endometrial cancer	metrorrhagia	salpingitis	vaginosis
endometriosis	myometritis		vulvovaginitis
endometritis	oophoritis		

Surgical Terms
BUILT FROM WORD PARTS

The following terms can be translated using definitions of word parts. Further explanation is provided within parentheses as needed.

TERM	DEFINITION	TERM	DEFINITION
1. colpocleisis (*kol*-pō-KLĪ-sis)	surgical closure of the vagina	7. hysterectomy (*his*-te-REK-to-mē)	excision of the uterus (Table 8.2, Fig. 8.9)
2. colpoperineorrhaphy (kol-pō-*per*-i-nē-OR-a-fē)	suturing of the vagina and the perineum (performed to mend perineal vaginal tears)	8. hysteropexy (HIS-ter-ō-*pek*-sē)	surgical fixation of the uterus
3. colpoplasty (KOL-pō-*plas*-tē)	surgical repair of the vagina	9. mammoplasty (MAM-ō-*plas*-tē)	surgical repair of the breast (performed to enlarge or reduce in size, and to reconstruct after removal of a tumor) (Fig. 8.10)
4. colporrhaphy (kol-POR-a-fē)	suturing of the vagina (wall of the vagina)		
5. episiorrhaphy (e-*piz*-ē-OR-a-fē)	suturing of (a tear in) the vulva		
6. hymenotomy (*hī*-men-OT-o-mē)	incision into the hymen		

TYPES OF MAMMOPLASTY include **implants**, which use a silicone or saline insert to create a breast, and **flap reconstruction**, which transfers the patient's muscle or fat and surrounding tissue from another area to the chest to create a breast mound.

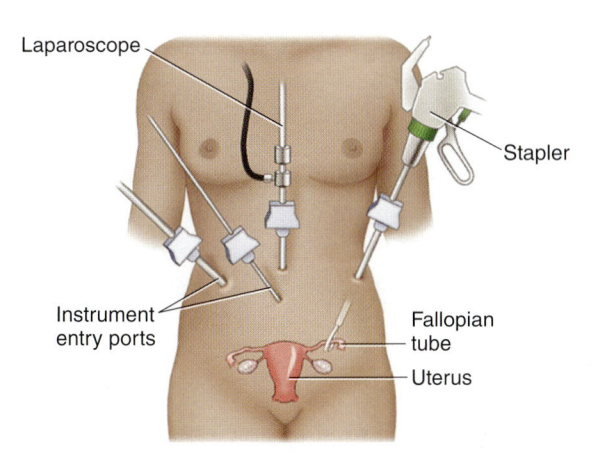

FIG. 8.9 Laparoscopically assisted vaginal hysterectomy (LAVH). The laparoscope, a type of endoscope, is inserted into the abdominopelvic cavity through a tiny incision near the umbilicus, allowing direct observation of the pelvic organs and structures. Three or four additional tiny incisions may be made to accommodate other instruments and devices. Numerous gynecological surgeries can be performed laparoscopically, including **hysterectomy, hysteropexy, myomectomy, oophorectomy, salpingectomy, salpingostomy,** and **tubal ligation.**

TABLE 8.2 Types of Hysterectomies

Total hysterectomy	Excision of the entire uterus, including the cervix; can be performed abdominally, vaginally, or laparoscopically
Subtotal hysterectomy	Excision of the upper part of the uterus leaving the cervix in place; can be performed abdominally or laparoscopically (also called **supracervical hysterectomy**)
Radical hysterectomy	Excision of the entire uterus, upper portion of the vagina, and surrounding tissues; performed abdominally

TERM	DEFINITION	TERM	DEFINITION
10. mastectomy (mas-TEK-to-mē)	excision of the breast (Table 8.3, Fig. 8.10)	15. salpingo-oophorectomy (sal-*ping*-gō-ō-*of*-o-REK-to-mē)	excision of the fallopian tube and the ovary
11. mastopexy (MAS-tō-pek-sē)	surgical fixation of the breast (performed to lift sagging breast tissue or to create symmetry) (Fig. 8.10)	16. salpingostomy (*sal*-ping-GOS-to-mē)	creation of an artificial opening in the fallopian tube (performed to restore patency)
12. oophorectomy (ō-of-o-REK-to-mē)	excision of the ovary	17. trachelectomy (trā-ke-LEK-to-mē)	excision of the cervix (also called **cervicectomy**)
13. perineorrhaphy (*per*-i-nē-OR-a-fē)	suturing of (a tear in) the perineum	18. vulvectomy (vul-VEK-to-mē)	excision of the vulva
14. salpingectomy (*sal*-pin-JEK-to-mē)	excision of the fallopian tube		

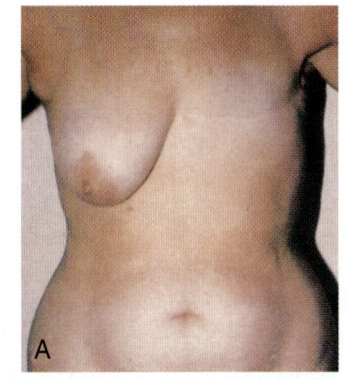

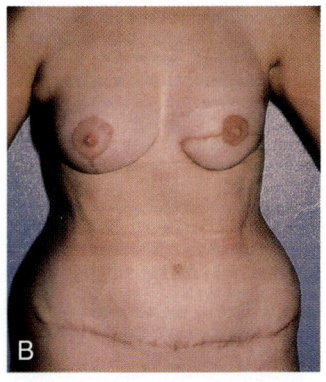

FIG. 8.10 Breast surgery and reconstruction. **A,** Left breast shows modified radical mastectomy scar. **B,** Left breast shows mammoplasty by TRAM (transverse rectus abdominis muscle) reconstruction (note the extensive lower abdominal scar, repositioned navel, and reconstructed nipple) and right mastopexy.

286 Chapter 8 Female Reproductive System

TABLE 8.3 Types of Surgeries Performed to Treat Malignant Breast Tumors

Surgeries to treat malignant breast tumors can be by grouped into three categories, Traditional Surgeries, Breast Conserving Surgeries, and Breast Reconstruction.

TRADITIONAL SURGERIES	Mastectomy was the main surgery for breast cancer until the mid-1980's. It is still used for patients with larger tumors, inflammatory breast cancers, and those who have a recurrence after a breast-conserving surgery.
Radical mastectomy	Removal of breast tissue, nipple, lymph nodes, and underlying chest wall muscle (rarely performed)
Modified radical mastectomy	Removal of breast tissue, nipple, and lymph nodes
Simple mastectomy	Removal of breast tissue, nipple, and skin (also called **total mastectomy**)
BREAST-CONSERVING SURGERIES	Less invasive procedures that preserve more of the breast are now an option for many people with breast cancer
Lumpectomy	Removal of the cancerous lesion along with a margin of surrounding healthy breast tissue. Radiation therapy may be needed as well.
Segmental mastectomy	Removal of a quadrant, or wedge, of breast tissue (also called **quadrantectomy**)
Skin-sparing mastectomy	Removal of the breast tissue, nipple, and areola, leaving most of the skin over the breast intact. Used only for smaller tumors that are not close to the skin.
Nipple-sparing mastectomy	Removal of breast tissue only, preserving the overlying skin, nipple and areola (also called **subcutaneous mastectomy**). Used mainly for small, early-stage cancers that are near the outer part of the breast.
BREAST RECONSTRUCTION	Type of surgery that can restore the original appearance of the breasts. It may be performed at the time of mastectomy or during a second surgery, 6 to 12 months later. Some people choose not to have reconstructive surgery.

EXERCISE 13 ■ Pronounce and Spell

Practice pronunciation and spelling on paper and online.

1. **Practice on Paper**

    a. **Pronounce:** Read the phonetic spelling and say aloud the terms listed in the term table. Refer to Table 2.2 Pronunciation Key as needed.
    b. **Spell:** Have a study partner read the terms aloud. Write the spelling of the terms on a separate sheet of paper.

2. **Practice Online**

    a. **Access** online learning resources. Go to evolve.elsevier.com > Evolve Resources > Student Resources.
    b. **Pronounce:** Select Audio Glossary > Chapter 8 > Exercise 13. Select a term to hear its pronunciation and repeat aloud.
    c. **Spell:** Select Activities > Chapter 8 > Spell Terms > Exercise 13. Select the audio icon and type the correct spelling of the term.

❏ Check the box when complete.

EXERCISE 14 ■ Analyze and Define

Analyze and define the following terms by drawing slashes between word parts, writing word part abbreviations above the term, underlining combining forms, and writing the combining form abbreviations below the term.

1. colpoplasty

2. hymenotomy

3. vulvectomy

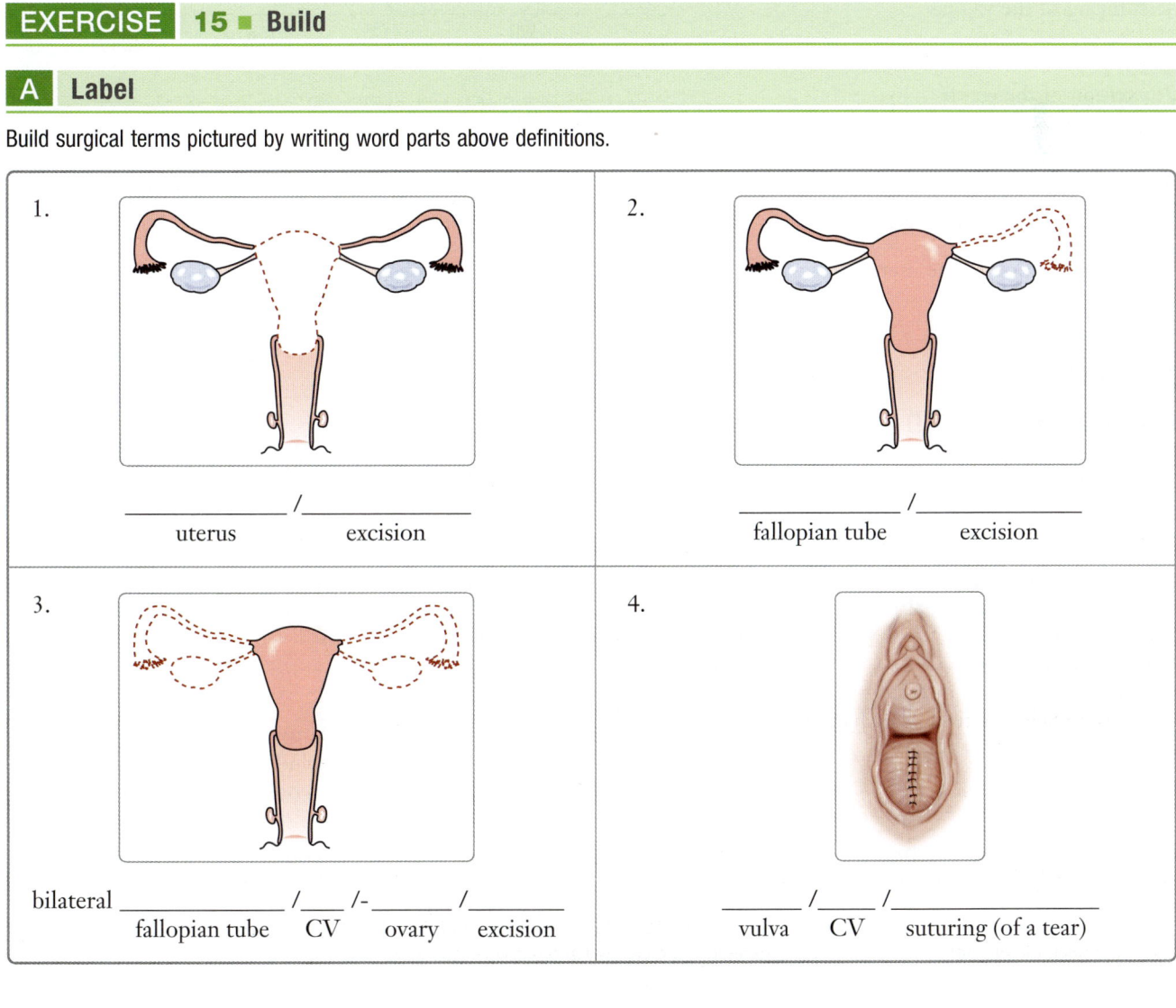

_____

_____

4. perineorrhaphy

_____

_____

5. salpingostomy

_____

_____

6. oophorectomy

_____

_____

7. mastopexy

_____

_____

8. colpoperineorrhaphy

_____

_____

EXERCISE 15 ■ Build

A Label

Build surgical terms pictured by writing word parts above definitions.

1. _____ / _____
   uterus   excision

2. _____ / _____
   fallopian tube   excision

3. bilateral _____ / ___ /- _____ / _____
              fallopian tube   CV   ovary   excision

4. _____ / ___ / _____
   vulva   CV   suturing (of a tear)

288 Chapter 8 Female Reproductive System

5.

_____ / _____
breast   excision

6.

_____ / ____ / _____
breast   CV   surgical repair

B Fill In

Build surgical terms for the following definitions by using the word parts you have learned.

1. suturing of the vagina

   _____ / ____ / _____
   WR   CV   S

2. excision of the cervix

   _____ / _____
   WR   S

3. surgical closure of the vagina

   _____ / ____ / _____
   WR   CV   S

4. surgical fixation of the uterus

   _____ / ____ / _____
   WR   CV   S

Surgical Terms
NOT BUILT FROM WORD PARTS

Word parts may be present in the following terms; however, their full meanings cannot be translated using definitions of word parts alone.

TERM	DEFINITION
1. anterior and posterior colporrhaphy (A&P repair) (an-TĒR-ē-or) (pos-TĒR-ē-or) (kol-POR-a-fē)	surgical repair of a weakened vaginal wall to correct a cystocele (protrusion of the bladder against the anterior wall of the vagina) and a rectocele (protrusion of the rectum against the posterior wall of the vagina)
2. conization (kon-i-ZĀ-shun)	surgical removal of a cone-shaped area of the cervix; used in the diagnosis and treatment of cervical cancer. Types of conization include loop electrosurgical excision procedure (LEEP), cryosurgery (cold-knife conization), and laser. (also called **cone biopsy**)
3. dilation and curettage (D&C) (dī-LĀ-shun) (kū-re-TAHZH)	surgical procedure to widen the cervix and remove contents from the uterus using a curette, an instrument for scraping or suctioning; the procedure can be diagnostic or therapeutic (Fig. 8.11)
4. endometrial ablation (en-dō-MĒ-trē-al) (ab-LĀ-shun)	procedure to destroy or remove the endometrium by use of laser, electrical, or thermal energy; used to treat abnormal uterine bleeding (Fig. 8.12)

🏛 **ABLATION** is from the Latin **ablatum**, meaning **to carry away**. In surgery, **ablation** means **excision or eradication**, especially by cutting with laser or electrical energy.

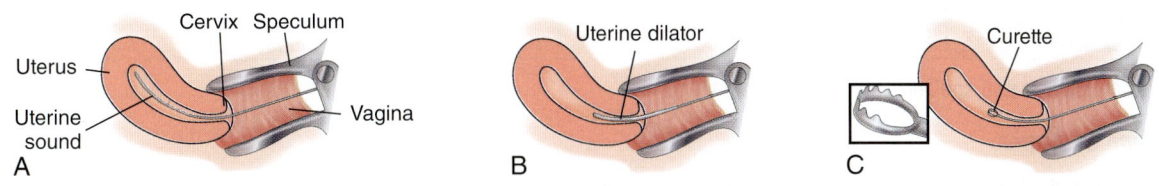

FIG. 8.11 Dilation and curettage (D&C). **A,** Uterine sound is a device used to measure the size of the uterus, to help determine how far to insert the instruments. **B,** Uterine dilator helps to open the cervix to allow easier access. **C,** Curette scrapes the endometrium and removes contents.

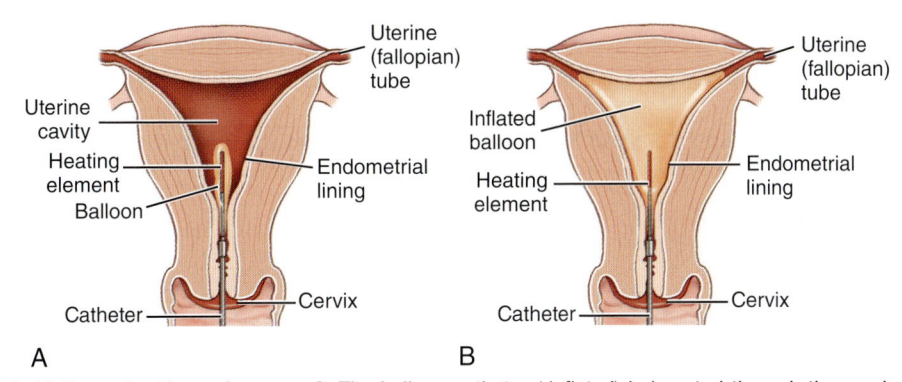

FIG. 8.12 Endometrial ablation using thermal energy. **A,** The balloon catheter (deflated) is inserted through the cervix into the uterine cavity. **B,** The balloon is inflated with a solution of 5% dextrose and water and heated to 87°C for 8 minutes, ablating the endometrial lining.

TERM	DEFINITION
5. myomectomy (mī-ō-MEK-to-mē)	excision of a uterine fibroid (myoma)
6. tubal ligation (TOO-bul) (lī-GĀ-shun)	surgical closure of the fallopian tubes for sterilization; tubes may be cut and tied (ligated), cut and cauterized, or closed off with a clip, clamp, ring, or band (also called **tubal sterilization** and **female surgical sterilization**) (Fig. 8.13)
7. uterine artery embolization (UAE) (Ū-ter-in) (AR-ter-ē) (em-be-li-ZĀ-shun)	placement of metal coils or small gelatin beads into uterine arteries to stop blood flow supplying uterine fibroids or to stop severe hemorrhage after childbirth; performed by an interventional radiologist (also called **uterine fibroid embolization** when used to treat uterine fibroids)

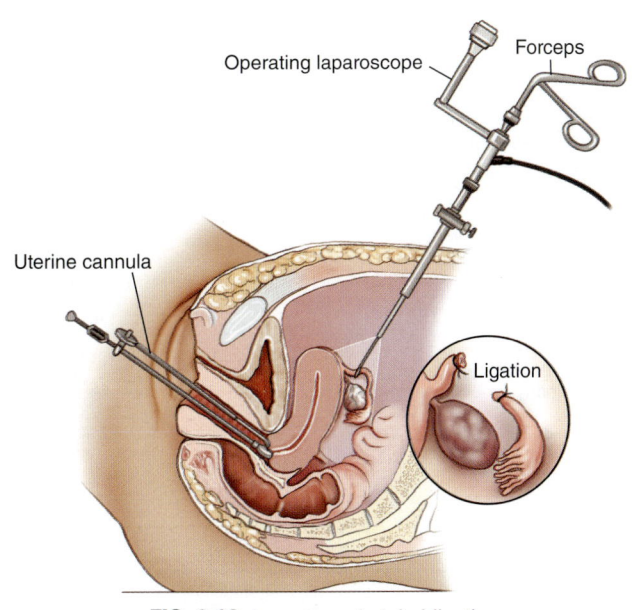

FIG. 8.13 Laparoscopic tubal ligation.

Chapter 8 Female Reproductive System

EXERCISE 16 ■ Pronounce and Spell

Practice pronunciation and spelling on paper and online.

1. **Practice on Paper**
   a. **Pronounce:** Read the phonetic spelling and say aloud the terms listed in the term table. Refer to Table 2.2 Pronunciation Key as needed.
   b. **Spell:** Have a study partner read the terms aloud. Write the spelling of the terms on a separate sheet of paper.

2. **Practice Online**
   a. **Access** online learning resources. Go to evolve.elsevier.com > Evolve Resources > Student Resources.
   b. **Pronounce:** Select Audio Glossary > Chapter 8 > Exercise 16. Select a term to hear its pronunciation and repeat aloud.
   c. **Spell:** Select Activities > Chapter 8 > Spell Terms > Exercise 16. Select the audio icon and type the correct spelling of the term.

❏ Check the box when complete.

EXERCISE 17 ■ Fill In

A Label

Write the surgical terms pictured and defined.

1. _____
   surgical closure of the fallopian tubes for sterilization

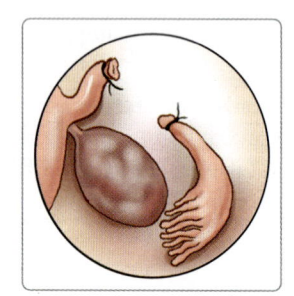

2. _____
   surgical procedure to widen the cervix and remove contents from the uterus using an instrument for scraping or suctioning

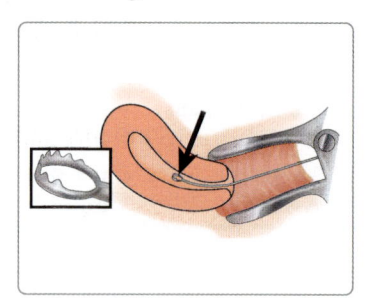

3. _____
   procedure to destroy or remove the endometrium by use of laser, electrical, or thermal energy

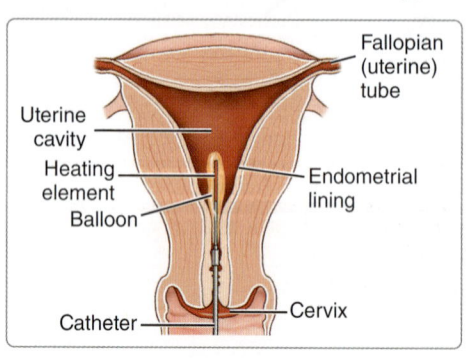

4. _____
   excision of a uterine fibroid

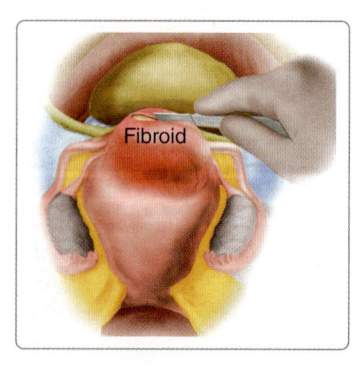

B Identify

Fill in the blanks with the correct terms.

1. The surgery used to repair a cystocele and rectocele is a(n) _____ and _____.

2. A procedure used to treat uterine fibroids by blocking the blood supply is called _____.

3. Surgical removal of a cone-shaped area of the cervix is called _____.

C Match

Match the surgical procedures in the first column with their corresponding organs in the second column. You may use the answers in the second column more than once.

_____ 1. dilation and curettage   a. fallopian tubes
_____ 2. tubal ligation   b. vagina
_____ 3. anterior and posterior colporrhaphy   c. uterus
_____ 4. myomectomy   d. ovaries
_____ 5. conization   e. vulva
_____ 6. endometrial ablation   f. lymph nodes
_____ 7. uterine artery embolization   g. cervix

EXERCISE 18 ■ Review of Surgical Terms

Can you define, pronounce, and spell the following terms?

anterior and posterior colporrhaphy (A&P repair)	dilation and curettage (D&C)	mastectomy	trachelectomy
colpocleisis	endometrial ablation	mastopexy	tubal ligation
colpoperineorrhaphy	episiorrhaphy	myomectomy	uterine artery embolization (UAE)
colpoplasty	hymenotomy	oophorectomy	vulvectomy
colporrhaphy	hysterectomy	perineorrhaphy	
conization	hysteropexy	salpingectomy	
	mammoplasty	salpingo-oophorectomy	
		salpingostomy	

Diagnostic Terms

BUILT FROM WORD PARTS AND *NOT* BUILT FROM WORD PARTS

The first portion of the table contains Female Reproductive System Terms that can be translated using definitions of word parts. The second portion of the table contains Female Reproductive System Terms that cannot be fully understood using the definitions of word parts.

■ Built from Word Parts

DIAGNOSTIC IMAGING			
TERM	**DEFINITION**	**TERM**	**DEFINITION**
1. **hysterosalpingogram (HSG)** (*his*-ter-ō-*sal*-PING-gō-gram)	radiographic image of the uterus and fallopian tubes (after an injection of contrast materials)	2. **mammogram** (MAM-ō-gram)	radiographic image of the breast

Complementary Terms—cont'd
BUILT FROM WORD PARTS AND *NOT* BUILT FROM WORD PARTS

Built from Word Parts—cont'd

DIAGNOSTIC IMAGING—CONT'D

TERM	DEFINITION	TERM	DEFINITION
3. mammography (ma-MOG-ra-fē)	radiographic imaging of the breast (also called **digital mammography** when images are obtained electronically and viewed on a computer)	4. sonohysterography (SHG) (*son*-ō-*his*-ter-OG-ra-fē)	process of recording the uterus by use of sound (Saline solution is injected into the uterine cavity during transvaginal sonography. Used to diagnose abnormalities inside the uterus, including polyps, fibroids, adhesions.) (also called **hysterosonography**)

ENDOSCOPY

TERM	DEFINITION	TERM	DEFINITION
5. colposcope (KOL-pō-skōp)	instrument used for visual examination of the vagina (and cervix)	9. pelviscopic (pel-vi-SKOP-ik)	pertaining to visual examination of the pelvic cavity (female reproductive organs)
6. colposcopy (kol-POS-ko-pē)	visual examination (with a magnified view) of the vagina (and cervix)	10. pelviscopy (pel-VIS-ku-pē)	visual examination of the pelvic cavity (female reproductive organs) (also called **gynecologic laparoscopy**)
7. hysteroscope (HIS-ter-ō-skōp)	instrument used for visual examination of the uterus (uterine cavity)		
8. hysteroscopy (*his*-ter-OS-ko-pē)	visual examination of the uterus (uterine cavity)		

NOT Built from Word Parts

DIAGNOSTIC IMAGING

TERM	DEFINITION
1. sentinel lymph node biopsy (SEN-tin-el) (limf) (nōd) (BĪ-op-sē)	injection of blue dye and/or radioactive isotope used to identify the sentinel lymph node(s), the first in the axillary chain and most likely to contain metastasis of breast cancer. The nodes are removed and microscopically examined. If the nodes closest to the cancer (called "sentinel nodes") are negative, additional nodes are not removed. (Fig. 8.14)
2. stereotactic breast biopsy (*ster*-ē-ō-TAK-tik) (brest) (BĪ-op-sē)	technique that combines mammography and computer-assisted biopsy to obtain tissue from a breast lesion (Fig. 8.15)
TYPES OF BREAST BIOPSY	
• **Image-guided breast biopsy** uses mammography, sonography, or magnetic resonance (MR) images to guide a biopsy needle.	
• **Surgical breast biopsy** involves making an incision to remove a palpable breast lesion (also called **open** or **incisional biopsy**).	
• **Wire localization biopsy** uses image guidance to place a thin, flexible wire directly into a breast lesion. The lesion is removed surgically with the wire intact.	
3. transvaginal sonography (TVS) (trans-VAJ-i-nal) (so-NOG-ra-fē)	ultrasound procedure that uses a transducer placed in the vagina to obtain images of the ovaries, uterus, cervix, fallopian tubes, and surrounding structures; used to diagnose masses such as ovarian cysts or tumors, to monitor pregnancy, and to evaluate ovulation for the treatment of infertility (Fig. 8.16)

Chapter 8 Female Reproductive System 293

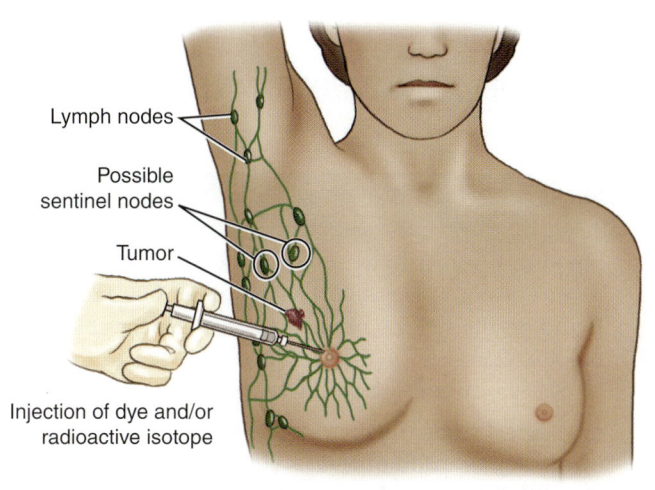

FIG. 8.14 Preparation for sentinel lymph node biopsy. The process of identifying the sentinel node(s) is performed in the nuclear medicine department of radiology. The biopsy is performed in surgery. The sentinel lymph node biopsy procedure was first developed for patients with melanoma. It is now also used to determine metastasis of breast cancer to the lymph nodes. Previously, surgeons would remove 10 to 20 lymph nodes to determine the spread of cancer, which often caused lymphedema and painful swelling of the affected arm.

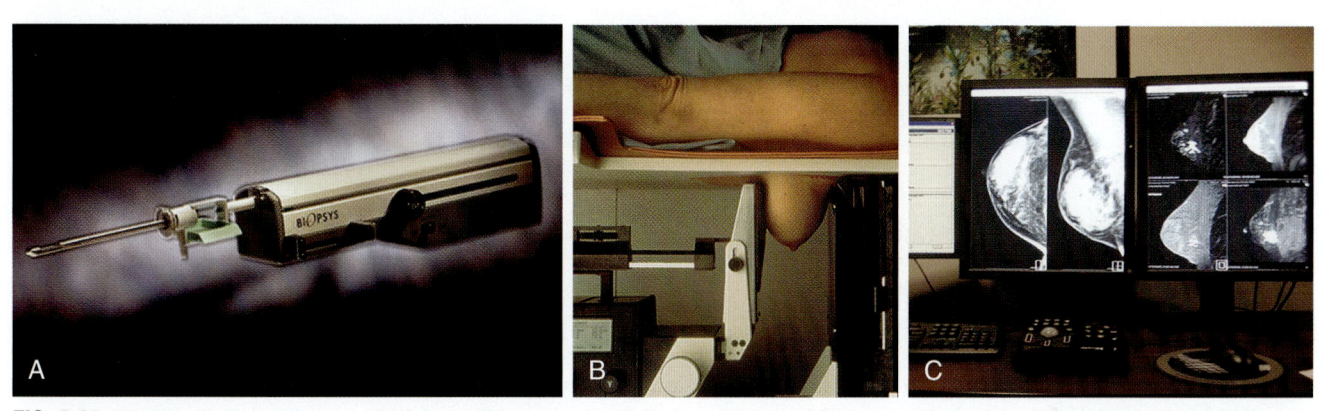

FIG. 8.15 Stereotactic breast biopsy, which is used for nonpalpable lesions that are visible on mammography. The patient is placed prone on a special table with the breast suspended through an opening. The breast is placed in a mammography machine under the table, which produces a digital mammography image that identifies the exact location of the lesion. The biopsy instrument is guided by a radiologist or surgeon. **A,** The stereotactic needle is used to obtain the specimen for biopsy. **B,** The patient is positioned for stereotactic breast biopsy. **C,** The mammogram appears digitally and is used to determine the placement of the biopsy needle.

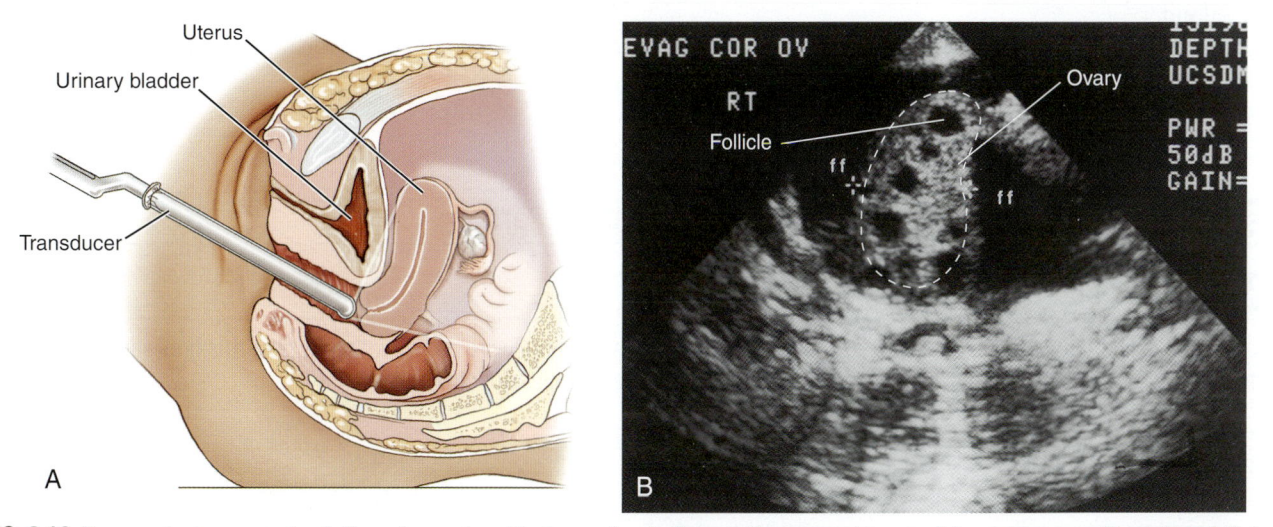

FIG. 8.16 Transvaginal sonography. **A,** Transducer placed in the vagina. **B,** Transvaginal coronal image of the right ovary with multiple follicles, showing free fluid surrounding the ovary.

Diagnostic Terms—cont'd
BUILT FROM WORD PARTS AND *NOT* BUILT FROM WORD PARTS
- *NOT* Built from Word Parts

LABORATORY

TERM	DEFINITION
4. **CA-125 test** (C-A-1-25) (test)	blood test primarily used to monitor treatment for ovarian cancer and to detect recurrence once treatment is complete. CA-125 (cancer antigen 125) is a protein found on the surface of most ovarian cancer cells and is released into the bloodstream. Elevated amounts of CA-125 in the blood may indicate the presence of ovarian cancer. (also called **CA-125** and **CA 125 tumor marker**)
5. **HPV test** (H-P-V) (test)	cytological study of cervical and vaginal secretions to detect high-risk forms of the human papillomavirus (HPV) that can cause abnormal cervical cells and cervical cancer; used for cervical cancer screening (Table 8.4)
6. **Pap test** (pap) (test)	cytological study of cervical and vaginal secretions to detect abnormal and cancerous cells; primarily used for cervical cancer screening (also called **Papanicolaou** [*pap*-a-NIK-kō-lā-oo] **test**; formerly called **Pap smear**) (Table 8.4)

🏛 **PAP TEST** is named after Dr. George N. Papanicolaou (1883-1962), a Greek physician practicing in the United States, who developed the cell smear method for the diagnosis of cancer in 1943. Though the smear method could be used to sample cells from any organ, it has been commonly used on cervical and vaginal secretions to detect cervical cancer. In 1966 the FDA approved a liquid-based screening system, which improved the detection of squamous intraepithelial lesions. With use of the liquid-based method surpassing use of the smear method, the procedure is more commonly called a Pap test, rather than a Pap smear.

EXERCISE 19 ■ Pronounce and Spell

Practice pronunciation and spelling on paper and online.

1. **Practice on Paper**
   a. **Pronounce:** Read the phonetic spelling and say aloud the terms listed in the term table. Refer to Table 2.2 Pronunciation Key as needed.
   b. **Spell:** Have a study partner read the terms aloud. Write the spelling of the terms on a separate sheet of paper.

2. **Practice Online** 🌐
   a. **Access** online learning resources. Go to evolve.elsevier.com > Evolve Resources > Student Resources.
   b. **Pronounce:** Select Audio Glossary > Chapter 8 > Exercise 19. Select a term to hear its pronunciation and repeat aloud.
   c. **Spell:** Select Activities > Chapter 8 > Spell Terms > Exercise 19. Select the audio icon and type the correct spelling of the term.

❑ Check the box when complete.

EXERCISE 20 ■ Diagnostic Terms Built from Word Parts

A Analyze and Define

Analyze and define the following diagnostic terms by drawing slashes between word parts, writing word part abbreviations above the term, underlining combining forms, and writing combining form abbreviations below the term.

1. colposcopy

2. mammogram

3. colposcope

_____

_____

4. hysteroscopy

_____

_____

5. hysterosalpingogram

_____

_____

6. pelviscopic

_____

_____

TABLE 8.4 Comparison of the Pap Test and the HPV Test

	PAP TEST	HPV TEST
Purpose of the test	Checks the cervix for any abnormal cells that could lead to cervical cancer	Looks for DNA from humanpapilloma virus in cells from the cervix
Who should have the test	Women between the ages of 21 and 65, every 3 to 5 years	Women age 30 to 65, every 5 years with or without a Pap test at the same time; performing the tests at the same time is called **co-testing**
How the tests are performed	The healthcare provider inserts a speculum (an instrument used to see the cervix) into the vagina and uses a flat stick and a soft brush to collect cells from the cervix (A). This sample of cells is then placed in a bottle with a liquid preservative (B) and sent to the lab for interpretation. 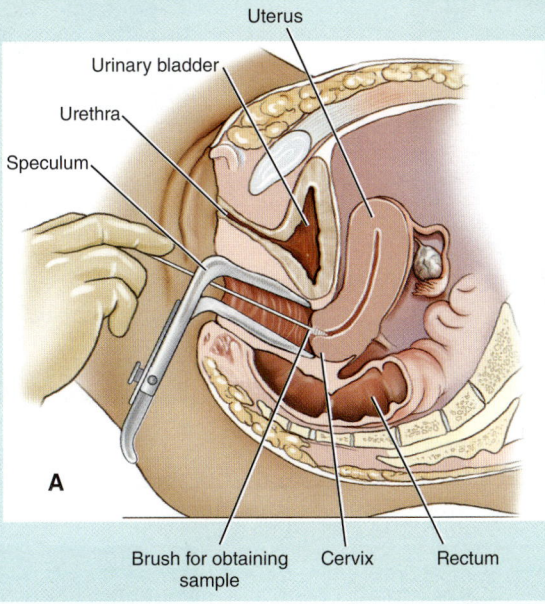	
Interpreting the results	• **Normal** • **ASC-US** (unclear, could be abnormal) • **Abnormal** (low grade or high grade)	• **Positive** (an HPV type is present that is associated with cervical cancer) • **Negative** (no HPV type associated with cervical cancer is present)
Next steps	• **Normal:** return to usual screening recommendations • **ASC-US:** perform HPV testing if not yet done, more frequent testing or colposcopy • **Abnormal:** more frequent testing, colposcopy and biopsy, or immediate treatment (depending on level of abnormality, age, and HPV test results)	• **Negative:** return to usual screening recommendations • **Positive:** Further testing may be done to determine the virus subtype (HPV 16 and 18 have the strongest association to cervical cancer). Options also include watchful waiting (many HPV infections will resolve on their own), colposcopy, biopsy, and possible treatment depending on results.

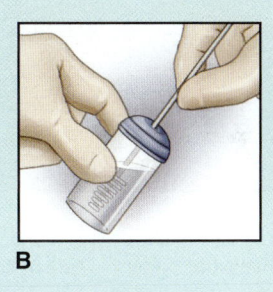

296 Chapter 8 Female Reproductive System

A Analyze and Define—cont'd

7. pelviscopy

_____

_____

8. mammography

_____

_____

9. hysteroscope

_____

_____

10. sonohysterography

_____

_____

B Build

Build diagnostic terms pictured by writing word parts above definitions.

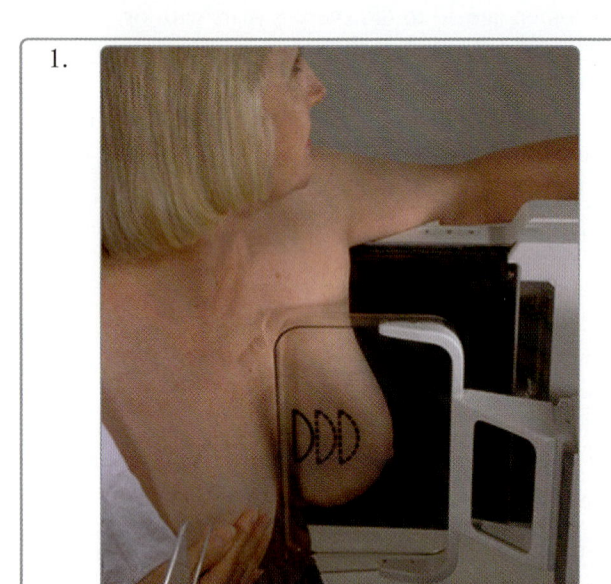

1.

_____ / ____ / _____
breast / CV / radiographic imaging

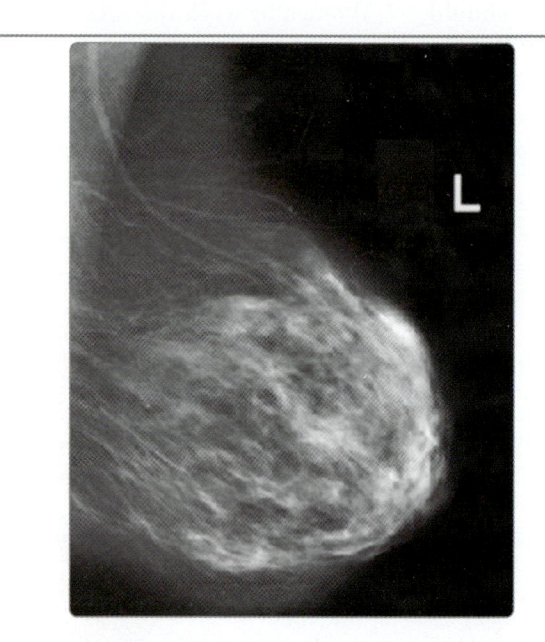

2.

_____ / ____ / _____
breast / CV / radiographic image

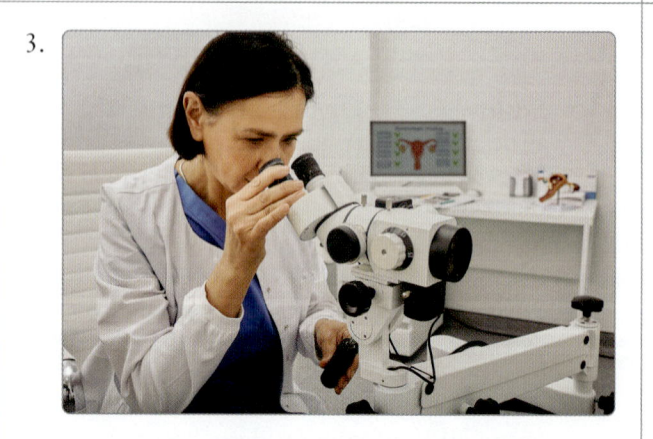

3.

_____ / ____ / _____
vagina / CV / instrument used for visual examination

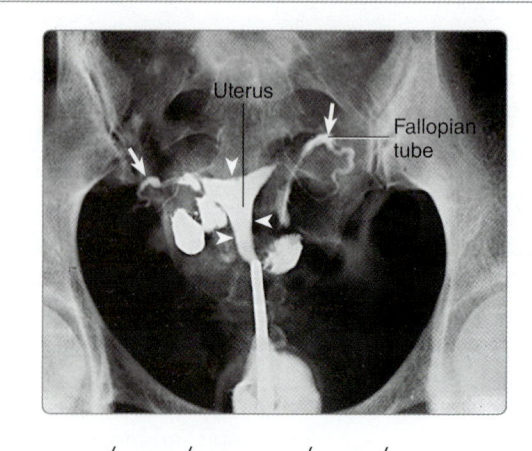

4.

_____ / ____ / _____ / ____ / _____
uterus / CV / fallopian tubes / CV / radiographic image

C Build

Build diagnostic terms for the following definitions by using the word parts you have learned.

1. visual examination of the vagina (and cervix)   _____ / _____ / _____
                                                                                  WR   CV   S

2. visual examination of the uterus   _____ / _____ / _____
                                                                      WR   CV   S

3. pertaining to visual examination of the pelvic cavity (female reproductive organs)   _____ / _____ / _____
                                             WR   CV   S

4. visual examination of the pelvic cavity (female reproductive organs)   _____ / _____ / _____
                                             WR   CV   S

5. instrument used for visual examination of the uterus   _____ / _____ / _____
                                             WR   CV   S

6. process of recording the uterus with sound   _____ / _____ / _____ / _____ / _____
                                             WR   CV   WR   CV   S

EXERCISE 21 ■ Diagnostic Terms NOT Built from Word Parts

A Label

Write the diagnostic terms pictured and defined.

1. _____
procedure that uses a transducer placed in the vagina to obtain images of the ovaries, uterus, cervix, fallopian tubes, and surrounding structures

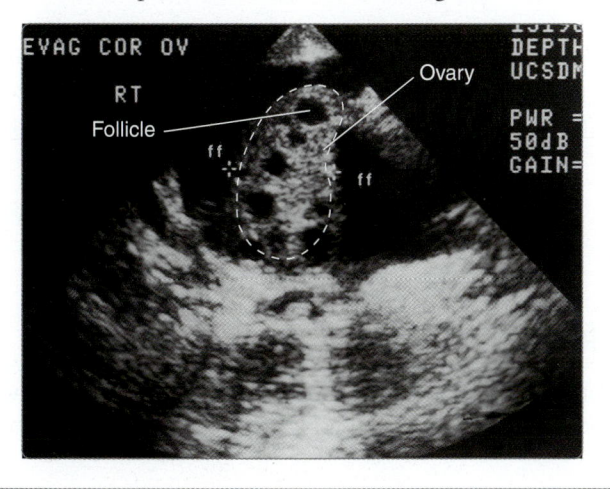

2. _____
cytological study of cervical and vaginal secretions; primarily used for cervical cancer screening

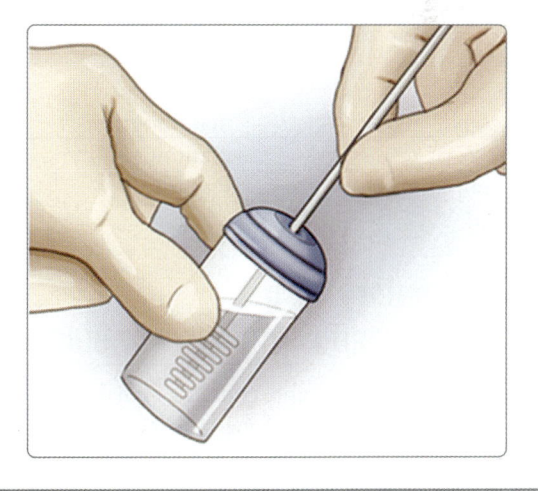

298 Chapter 8 Female Reproductive System

B Match

Match the terms in the first column with their correct definitions in the second column

_____ 1. Pap test
_____ 2. transvaginal sonography
_____ 3. sentinel lymph node biopsy
_____ 4. HPV test
_____ 5. CA-125 test
_____ 6. stereotactic breast biopsy

a. blood test used to monitor treatment for ovarian cancer and to detect recurrence
b. combines mammography and computer-assisted biopsy to obtain tissue from a breast lesion
c. cytological study of cervical and vaginal secretions to detect abnormal and cancerous cells
d. ultrasound procedure that uses a transducer placed in the vagina to obtain images of internal female reproductive structures
e. identification of the first lymph nodes in the axillary chain, using blue dye and/or radioactive isotope
f. cytological study of cervical and vaginal secretions to detect high-risk forms of the human papillomavirus

C Identify

Fill in the blanks with the correct terms.

1. _____ _____ _____ _____ uses a blue dye to identify lymph nodes most likely to contain metastasis of breast cancer.
2. A technique that combines mammography and computer-assisted biopsy of the breast is known as _____ _____.
3. _____ _____ is a blood test used to monitor treatment and detect recurrence of ovarian cancer.
4. A cytological study of cervical and vaginal secretions used to test for the virus that can cause cervical cancer is called _____ _____.

EXERCISE 22 ■ Review of Diagnostic Terms

Can you define, pronounce, and spell the following terms?

CA-125 test	hysteroscope	pelviscopic	sonohysterography (SHG)
colposcope	hysteroscopy	pelviscopy	stereotactic breast biopsy
colposcopy	mammogram	sentinel lymph node biopsy	transvaginal sonography (TVS)
HPV test	mammography		
hysterosalpingogram (HSG)	Pap test		

Complementary Terms
BUILT FROM WORD PARTS AND *NOT* BUILT FROM WORD PARTS

The first portion of the table contains Female Reproductive System Terms that can be translated using definitions of word parts. The second portion of the table contains terms that cannot be fully understood using the definitions of word parts.

■ Built from Word Parts

SIGNS AND SYMPTOMS			
TERM	**DEFINITION**	**TERM**	**DEFINITION**
1. amenorrhea (a-*men*-ō-RĒ-a)	absence of menstrual flow	2. dysmenorrhea (dis-*men*-ō-RĒ-a)	painful menstrual flow

TERM	DEFINITION	TERM	DEFINITION
3. leukorrhea (lū-kō-RĒ-a)	white discharge (from the vagina)	5. oligomenorrhea (ol-i-gō-men-ō-RĒ-a)	scanty menstrual flow (infrequent menstrual flow)
4. mastalgia (mas-TAL-ja)	pain in the breast		

MEDICAL SPECIALTIES

TERM	DEFINITION	TERM	DEFINITION
6. gynecologist (gīn-ek-OL-o-jist)	physician who studies and treats diseases of women (female reproductive system)	7. gynecology (GYN) (gīn-ek-OL-o-jē)	study of women (branch of medicine dealing with health and diseases of the female reproductive system)

DESCRIPTIVE TERMS

TERM	DEFINITION	TERM	DEFINITION
8. endocervical (en-dō-SER-vi-kal)	pertaining to within the cervix	11. vesicovaginal (ves-i-kō-VAJ-i-nal)	pertaining to the (urinary) bladder and the vagina
9. pelvic (PEL-vik)	pertaining to the pelvis	12. vulvovaginal (vul-vō-VAJ-i-nal)	pertaining to the vulva and vagina
10. vaginal (VAJ-i-nal)	pertaining to the vagina		

■ NOT Built from Word Parts

SIGNS AND SYMPTOMS

TERM	DEFINITION
1. anovulation (an-ov-ū-LĀ-shun)	failure of the ovary to release an egg
2. dyspareunia (dis-pa-RŪ-nē-a)	difficult or painful intercourse
3. fistula (FIS-tū-la)	abnormal passageway between two organs or between an internal organ and the body surface
4. oligoovulation (ol-i-gō-ov-ū-LĀ-shun)	infrequent release of an egg

TREATMENTS

TERM	DEFINITION
5. contraception (kon-tra-SEP-shen)	intentional prevention of conception (pregnancy) (also called **birth control** [**BC**]) (Fig. 8.17)
METHODS OF CONTRACEPTION include barrier (condoms), chemical (spermicides), oral pharmaceutical (birth control pills), and long-acting reversible contraception (LARC) such as an intrauterine device (IUD), intrauterine system (IUS), implant, and injection.	
6. hormone therapy (HŌR-mōn) (THER-a-pē)	use of hormones, estrogen and progesterone, to treat symptoms associated with menopause (also called **hormone replacement therapy** [**HRT**])

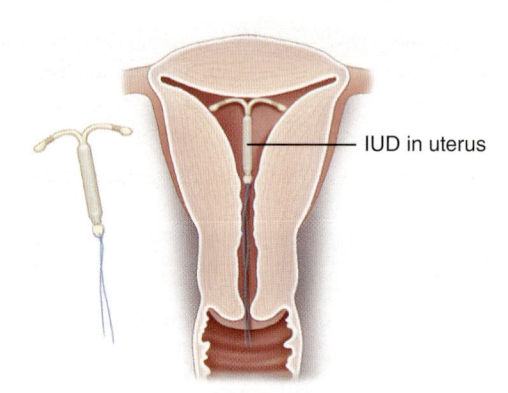

FIG. 8.17 Intrauterine device (IUD). Inserted through the cervix, this T-shaped device provides long-term contraception by changing the intrauterine environment.

Complementary Terms—cont'd
BUILT FROM WORD PARTS AND *NOT* BUILT FROM WORD PARTS

- *NOT* **Built from Word Parts**

EQUIPMENT	
TERM	**DEFINITION**
7. **speculum** (SPEK-ū-lum)	instrument for opening a body cavity to allow visual inspection

OTHERS	
TERM	**DEFINITION**
8. **menarche** (me-NAR-kē)	beginning of menstruation (specifically, onset of the first menstrual period)
9. **menopause** (MEN-o-pawz)	cessation of menstruation, usually around the ages of 48 to 53 years; may be induced at an earlier age surgically (bilateral oophorectomy) or medically (side effect of chemotherapy treatment)

Refer to **Appendix E** for pharmacology terms related to the female reproductive system.

EXERCISE 23 ■ Pronounce and Spell

Practice pronunciation and spelling on paper and online.

1. **Practice on Paper**
   a. **Pronounce:** Read the phonetic spelling and say aloud the terms listed in the previous table. Refer to Table 2.2 Pronunciation Key as needed.
   b. **Spell:** Have a study partner read the terms aloud. Write the spelling of the terms on a separate sheet of paper.

2. **Practice Online**
   a. **Access** online learning resources. Go to evolve.elsevier.com > Evolve Resources > Student Resources.
   b. **Pronounce:** Select Audio Glossary > Chapter 8 > Exercise 23. Select a term to hear its pronunciation and repeat aloud.
   c. **Spell:** Select Activities > Chapter 8 > Spell Terms > Exercise 23. Select the audio icon and type the correct spelling of the term.

❏ Check the box when complete.

Chapter 8 Female Reproductive System 301

EXERCISE 24 ■ Complementary Terms Built from Word Parts

A Analyze and Define

Analyze and define the following complementary terms by drawing slashes between word parts, writing word part abbreviations above the term, underlining combining forms, and writing combining form abbreviations below the term.

1. gynecologist

2. gynecology

3. vulvovaginal

4. mastalgia

5. pelvic

6. leukorrhea

7. vesicovaginal

8. vaginal

9. endocervical

10. oligomenorrhea

B Build

Build complementary terms for the following definitions by using the word parts you have learned.

1. white discharge (from the vagina) — WR / CV / S

2. pertaining to the pelvis — WR / S

3. pain in the breast — WR / S

4. pertaining to the vulva and vagina — WR / CV / WR / S

5. physician who studies and treats diseases of women — WR / CV / S

Chapter 8 Female Reproductive System

6. study of women (branch of medicine dealing with health and diseases of the female reproductive system) _____ WR / CV / S

7. pertaining to the (urinary) bladder and the vagina _____ WR / CV / WR / S

8. pertaining to the vagina _____ WR / S

9. pertaining to within the cervix _____ P / WR / S

10. absence of menstrual flow _____ P / WR / CV / S

11. painful menstrual flow _____ P / WR / CV / S

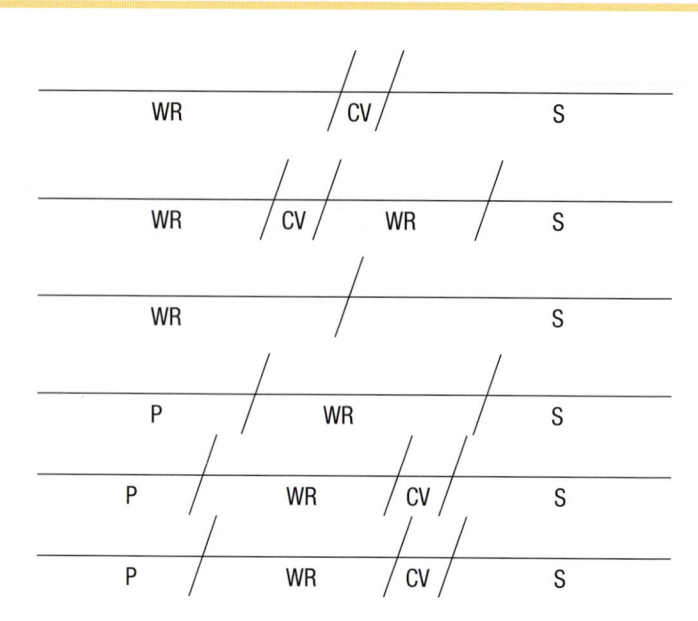

EXERCISE 25 ■ Complementary Terms NOT Built from Word Parts

A Match

Match the terms in the first column with their correct definitions in the second column.

_____ 1. dyspareunia   a. abnormal passageway between two organs
_____ 2. contraception   b. instrument for opening a body cavity to allow visual inspection
_____ 3. hormone therapy   c. failure of the ovary to release an egg
_____ 4. speculum   d. also called birth control
_____ 5. anovulation   e. onset of the first menstrual period
_____ 6. menarche   f. infrequent release of an egg
_____ 7. fistula   g. difficult or painful intercourse
_____ 8. menopause   h. cessation of menstruation
_____ 9. oligoovulation   i. use of hormones to treat symptoms associated with menopause

B Label

Write the medical terms pictured and defined.

1. _____
instrument for opening a body cavity to allow visual inspection

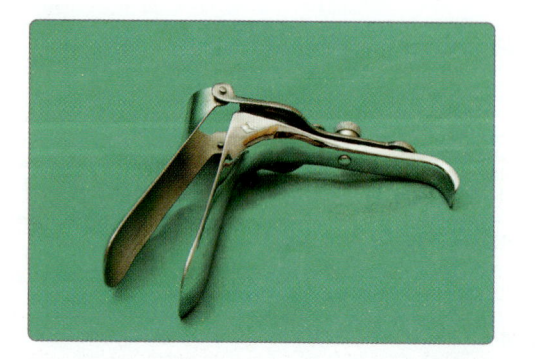

2. _____
intentional prevention of conception (pregnancy)

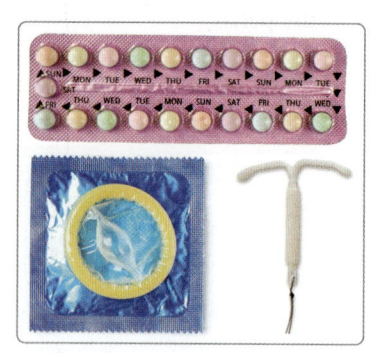

C Identify

Write the term for each of the following.

1. abnormal passageway _____
2. beginning of menstruation (specifically, onset of the first menstrual period) _____
3. painful intercourse _____
4. cessation of menstruation _____
5. use of hormones to treat symptoms associated with menopause _____
6. failure of the ovary to release an egg _____
7. infrequent release of an egg _____

EXERCISE 26 ■ Review of Complementary Terms

Can you define, pronounce, and spell the following terms?

amenorrhea	dyspareunia	gynecology	leukorrhea	oligomeno-	speculum
anovulation	endocervical	(GYN)	mastalgia	rrhea	vaginal
contraception	fistula	hormone	menarche	oligoovulation	vesicovaginal
dysmenorrhea	gynecologist	therapy	menopause	pelvic	vulvovaginal

Abbreviations

DISEASES AND DISORDERS

ABBREVIATION	TERM	ABBREVIATION	TERM
AUB	abnormal uterine bleeding	PID	pelvic inflammatory disease
FCC	fibrocystic breast changes	PMS	premenstrual syndrome
PCOS	polycystic ovary syndrome	TSS	toxic shock syndrome

DIAGNOSTIC

ABBREVIATION	TERM	ABBREVIATION	TERM
HSG	hysterosalpingogram	TVS	transvaginal sonography
SHG	sonohysterography		

TREATMENT

ABBREVIATION	TERM	ABBREVIATION	TERM
A&P repair	anterior and posterior colporrhaphy	LEEP	loop electrosurgical excision procedure; spoken as a whole word (lēp)
BC	birth control	TAH/BSO	total abdominal hysterectomy/bilateral salpingo-oophorectomy
D&C	dilation and curettage		
HRT	hormone replacement therapy	TLH	total laparoscopic hysterectomy
IUD	intrauterine device	UAE	uterine artery embolization
IUS	intrauterine system	VH	vaginal hysterectomy
LAVH	laparoscopically assisted vaginal hysterectomy		

MEDICAL SPECIALTIES

ABBREVIATION	TERM
GYN	gynecology

OTHER

ABBREVIATION	TERM	ABBREVIATION	TERM
Cx	cervix		Refer to **Appendix D** for a complete list of abbreviations.

304 Chapter 8 Female Reproductive System

EXERCISE 27 ■ Fill In

Write the terms abbreviated.

1. To repair a cystocele and rectocele the patient is scheduled in surgery for an **A&P repair** _____ and _____ _____.

2. Following a **TAH/BSO** _____ _____ _____ and _____ _____ _____ the gynecologist prescribed **HRT** _____ _____ _____ for the patient to take for 3 months after surgery.

3. **SHG** _____ and **TVS** _____ _____ are diagnostic ultrasound procedures used to assist in diagnosing diseases and disorders of the female reproductive organs.

4. When performing a **VH** _____ _____ the surgeon removes the uterus through the vagina without a surgical incision into the abdomen. During a(n) **LAVH** _____-_____ _____ _____ the surgeon uses a fiberoptic laparoscope inserted through a tiny incision near the umbilicus to visualize the uterus and guide removal through the vagina. In a **TLH** _____ _____ _____, morcellation is used to remove the uterus through the laparoscope.

5. **D&C** _____ and _____ is the dilation of the **Cx** _____ and scraping of the endometrium. **LEEP** _____ _____ _____ _____ is used for conization, the surgical removal of abnormal cervical tissue for the diagnosis and treatment of cervical cancer.

6. **FCC** _____ _____ _____ is the most common breast problem of women in their 20s.

7. A female patient with probable **PID** _____ _____ _____ was referred to the **GYN** _____ clinic for evaluation and care.

8. The medical management of **PMS** _____ _____ emphasizes the relief of symptoms.

9. **UAE** _____ _____ _____ offers a minimally invasive treatment option for some women with symptomatic uterine fibroids.

10. For long-acting reversible contraception, the patient considered an **IUD** _____ _____ and **IUS** _____ _____, either of which would be inserted by a gynecologist. While these methods of **BC** _____ _____ are effective in preventing pregnancy, they do not protect against sexually transmitted infections.

11. A diagnosis of **PCOS** _____ _____ _____ may be made if two of the following criteria are met: 1) chronic anovulation, 2) hyperandrogenism (excessive secretion of androgens with clinical or biological manifestations), and 3) polycystic ovaries.

12. When investigating the cause of **AUB** _____ _____ _____ in women over 50, endometrial cancer must be considered and ruled out.

Chapter 8 Female Reproductive System

PRACTICAL APPLICATION

EXERCISE 28 ■ Case Study: Translate Between Everyday Language and Medical Language

CASE STUDY: Cindy Collier and Rajive Modi

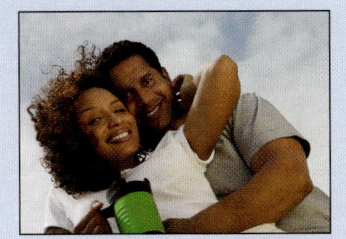

Cindy and Rajive want to have a baby. They have been trying for over a year to get pregnant, but it hasn't happened. Cindy worries something is wrong. Even though she has her period every month, menstruating is very painful, and she bleeds a lot. She often has pain low in her belly. She had sexual partners before Rajive, and she is worried that one may have given her a disease. Rajive is also concerned, and wonders if something might be wrong with him that is keeping Cindy from getting pregnant. When he was born, only one of his testicles was down, and they had to do surgery to fix the other one. He hasn't had any problems since then. He had partners before Cindy, and he is worried that he may have passed something on to her.

Now that you have worked through Chapters 7 and 8 on the reproductive systems, consider the medical terms that might be used to describe Cindy and Rajive's experience. See the Chapter at a Glance sections at the end of Chapters 7 and 8 for a list of terms that might apply.

A. Underline phrases in the case study that could be substituted with medical terms.

B. Write the medical term and its definition for three of the phrases you underlined.

MEDICAL TERM	DEFINITION
1. _____	_____
2. _____	_____
3. _____	_____

DOCUMENTATION: Excerpt from Infertility Clinic Consultation

Cindy, a 31-year-old female, and her husband Rajive, a 32-year-old male, present for workup and treatment for infertility. They have been trying to conceive for 14 months. Rajive: past medical history is significant for cryptorchidism at birth, which was repaired by orchidopexy at age 2. Cindy: menarche at 14, symptoms of dysmenorrhea and menorrhagia, both of which have worsened since discontinuing birth control pills. She had a normal Pap test approximately 1 year ago.

Diagnostic Studies: A complete blood count (CBC) was ordered, as well as serum tests for thyroid-stimulating hormone (TSH), follicle-stimulating hormone (FSH), and prolactin level (PRL). A urine pregnancy test was negative.
Impression: Primary infertility; cause undetermined. Possible cervicitis caused by chlamydia and possible pelvic inflammatory disease.
Recommendation: We will await culture results and treat both partners with antibiotics if necessary. If labs are normal, we will proceed with a semen analysis for Rajive. We should consider a hysterosalpingogram (HSG) for Cindy based on her history and physical exam findings.

C. Underline medical terms presented in Chapters 7 and 8 used in the previous excerpt from the infertility consultation. See the Chapter at a Glance sections at the end of the chapter for a complete list.

D. Select and define three of the medical terms you underlined. To check your answers, go to Appendix A.

MEDICAL TERM	DEFINITION
1. _____	_____
2. _____	_____
3. _____	_____

306   Chapter 8   Female Reproductive System

EXERCISE 29 ■ Interact with Medical Documents

A

Read the report and complete it by writing medical terms on answer lines within the document. Definitions of terms to be written appear after the document.

234-5678BR GARCIA, Evelina

File Patient Navigate Custom Fields Help

Chart Review | Encounters | Notes | Labs | Imaging | Procedures | Rx | Documents | Referrals | Scheduling | Billing

Name: GARCIA, Evelina   MR#: 234-5678BR   Sex: F   Allergies: Peanuts
                        DOB: 10/08/19XX   Age: 48   PCP: Emily Fowler MD

Surgical Progress Note: Evelina Garcia is a 48-year-old woman here for follow-up after a suspicious lesion in the left breast was discovered during routine 1._____. Her husband and sister are present for this visit.

Family history is positive for breast 2._____ in two maternal aunts, both under age 50 at diagnosis.

Past medical history includes 3._____ for 4._____ and 5._____. She has been on 6._____ for menopause since age 46 years.

The patient consented to a 7._____.

The pathology report is as follows:
Gross description: Received in formalin are four, pink-tan, cylindrical fragments of fibroadipose tissue, which range from 0.8 to 1.3 cm in length, each with a 0.1-cm diameter. The specimen is entirely submitted in one cassette.

Final diagnosis: Mammary parenchyma, left breast guided needle biopsy: Infiltrating, moderately differentiated ductal carcinoma with focal ductal carcinoma in situ, Grade 2, involving all four specimens. Lymphovascular invasion is identified.

Upon examination, the biopsy site reveals a 1-cm, healing surgical scar on the 8._____ aspect of the left breast. The patient reports mild tenderness, alleviated with ibuprofen, but denies any signs or symptoms of infection.

Extensive education provided to patient and family regarding diagnosis and surgical treatment options. Patient states that she is interested in 9._____ with immediate reconstruction. Due to presence of lymphovascular invasion, 10._____ will be scheduled at the time of definitive surgery.

Consultation appointments arranged through Breast Center with medical oncology and plastic surgery clinics within 1 week. Follow-up appointment scheduled for next week.

Electronically signed: Meredith Woolridge, MD 11/17/20XX 09:17

Start | Log On/Off | Print | Edit

Definitions of Medical Terms to Complete the Document

Write the medical terms defined on corresponding answer lines in the document.

1. radiographic imaging of the breast
2. cancerous tumor
3. excision of the uterus
4. growth of endometrium into the muscular portion of the uterus
5. abnormal condition in which endometrial tissue occurs in various areas of the pelvic cavity
6. use of estrogen and progesterone to treat symptoms associated with menopause
7. combines mammography and computer-assisted biopsy to obtain tissue from a breast lesion
8. pertaining to the middle and to (one) side
9. surgical removal of a breast
10. an injection of blue dye and/or radioactive isotope used to identify the first in the axillary chain and most likely to contain metastasis of breast cancer

B

Read the medical report and answer the questions below it.

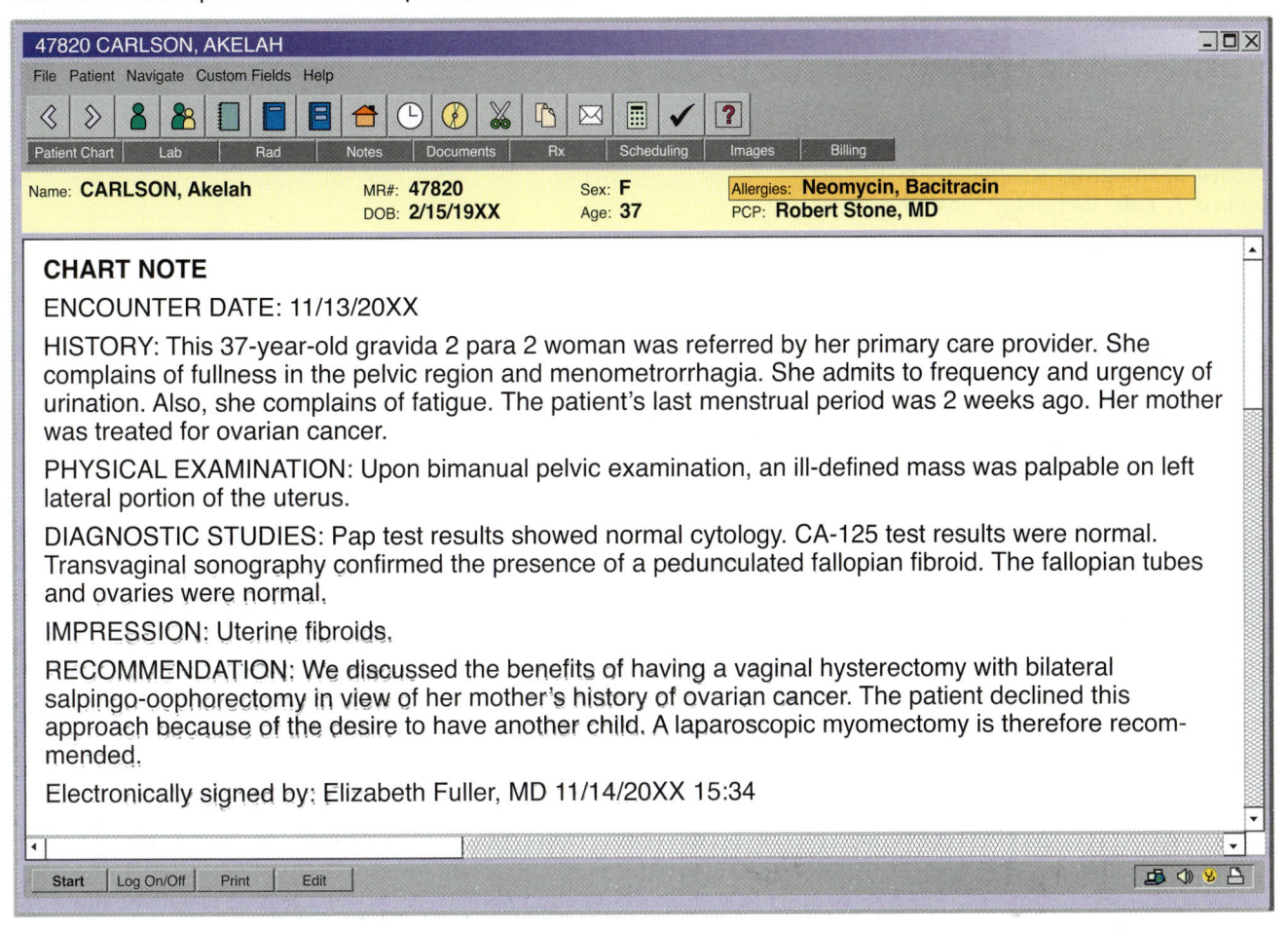

47820 CARLSON, AKELAH

File Patient Navigate Custom Fields Help

| Patient Chart | Lab | Rad | Notes | Documents | Rx | Scheduling | Images | Billing |

Name: **CARLSON, Akelah** MR#: **47820** Sex: **F** Allergies: **Neomycin, Bacitracin**
DOB: **2/15/19XX** Age: **37** PCP: **Robert Stone, MD**

CHART NOTE

ENCOUNTER DATE: 11/13/20XX

HISTORY: This 37-year-old gravida 2 para 2 woman was referred by her primary care provider. She complains of fullness in the pelvic region and menometrorrhagia. She admits to frequency and urgency of urination. Also, she complains of fatigue. The patient's last menstrual period was 2 weeks ago. Her mother was treated for ovarian cancer.

PHYSICAL EXAMINATION: Upon bimanual pelvic examination, an ill-defined mass was palpable on left lateral portion of the uterus.

DIAGNOSTIC STUDIES: Pap test results showed normal cytology. CA-125 test results were normal. Transvaginal sonography confirmed the presence of a pedunculated fallopian fibroid. The fallopian tubes and ovaries were normal.

IMPRESSION: Uterine fibroids.

RECOMMENDATION: We discussed the benefits of having a vaginal hysterectomy with bilateral salpingo-oophorectomy in view of her mother's history of ovarian cancer. The patient declined this approach because of the desire to have another child. A laparoscopic myomectomy is therefore recommended.

Electronically signed by: Elizabeth Fuller, MD 11/14/20XX 15:34

Start Log On/Off Print Edit

Use the medical report above to answer the questions.

1. The patient's symptoms include:
   a. absence of menstrual flow
   b. scanty menstrual flow
   c. increased amount of menstrual flow during menses and bleeding between periods
   d. painful menstruation

2. The CA-125 diagnostic study was used to detect the presence of:
   a. ovarian cancer
   b. cervical cancer
   c. endometrial cancer
   d. endometriosis

3. The recommended procedure, a myomectomy, will entail the surgical excision of:
   a. the breast
   b. the uterus
   c. ovarian cancer
   d. uterine fibroids

EXERCISE 30 ■ Use Medical Language in Online Electronic Health Records

Select the correct medical terms to complete three medical records in one patient's electronic file.

🌐 Access online resources at evolve.elsevier.com > Evolve Resources > Student Resources > Activities > Chapter 8 > Electronic Health Records

Topic: Invasive Ductal Carcinoma
Record 1, Encounters: Gynecology Clinic Visit
Record 2, Imaging: Radiology Final Report
Record 3, Lab: Pathology Final Diagnosis

❏ Check the box when complete.

EXERCISE 31 ■ Use Medical Terms in Clinical Statements

For each phrase printed in bold, circle the medical term or abbreviation defined. Answers are listed in Appendix A. For pronunciation practice read the answers aloud.

1. Mariana Esteban was experiencing **pertaining to the vagina** (endometrial, cervical, vaginal) itching, burning, and excessive **white discharge from the vagina** (leukorrhea, amenorrhea, dysmenorrhea). After a pelvic exam and testing of a sample of vaginal fluid, she was diagnosed with **inflammation of the vagina** (cervicitis, vaginitis, endometritis) caused by *Candida albicans*, a yeastlike fungus.

2. A **visual examination of the vagina** (hysterosalpingogram, colposcopy, colposcope) is used to further evaluate abnormal **cytologic study of the cervical and vaginal secretions to detect abnormal and cancerous cells** (Pap test, HPV test, CA-125 test) results and to identify suspicious lesions. **Surgical removal of a cone-shaped area of the cervix** (trachelectomy, colpoplasty, conization) may be performed to obtain a biopsy tissue sample for lab testing to rule out a **malignant tumor of the cervix** (cervical cancer, endometrial cancer, ovarian cancer).

3. After Lin Xiang's routine **process of radiographic imaging of the breast** (mammogram, mammography) exam, the radiologist discovered a breast lesion on the **radiographic image of the breast** (mammogram, mammography). A biopsy revealed a malignant tumor. A(n) **excision of the breast** (mastectomy, mammoplasty, mastopexy) was performed. The patient is scheduled, at a later date, for reconstructive **surgical repair of the breast** (mastectomy, mammoplasty, mastopexy) with an implant.

4. After 12 months of the **absence of menstrual flow** (dysmenorrhea, menorrhagia, amenorrhea), the 49-year-old patient was experiencing the **cessation of menstruation** (menarche, pregnancy, menopause). In consultation with her health provider, she was prescribed **use of estrogen and progesterone** (contraception, hormone therapy, uterine artery embolization) to treat symptoms such as **difficult or painful intercourse** (dyspareunia, dysmenorrhea, vaginosis), hot flashes, and night sweats. Physical therapy was also offered to strengthen her pelvic floor muscles to prevent **dropping of the uterus and vagina due to weakened pelvic muscles** (adenomyosis, uterovaginal prolapse, vaginal fistula).

EXERCISE 32 ■ Pronounce Medical Terms in Use

Practice pronunciation of terms by reading aloud the following paragraphs. Use the phonetic spellings to assist with pronunciation. The script also contains medical terms not presented in the chapter. If interested, research their meanings in a medical dictionary or a reliable online source.

CANCERS OF THE FEMALE REPRODUCTIVE SYSTEM

Breast Cancer
The breast is the most common site of cancer in women. More than 80% of **breast cancer** (brest) (KAN-cer) is infiltrating ductal cancer (IDC), which originates in the mammary ducts. The rate of growth depends on hormonal influences. As long as the cancer remains in the duct, it is considered noninvasive and is called *ductal carcinoma in situ (DCIS)*.

    Mammography (ma-MOG-ra-fē) is the most common method used for diagnosing cancer of the breast. Confirmation is done with a biopsy obtained by conventional surgery or guided breast biopsy, such as **stereotactic breast biopsy** (ster-ē-ō-TAK-tik) (brest) (BĪ-op-sē). Treatment may include lumpectomy, **mastectomy** (mas-TEK-to-mē), chemotherapy, radiation therapy, and hormonal therapy.

Cervical Cancer
In many regions of the world **cervical cancer** (SER-vi-kal) (KAN-cer) is the leading cause of death in women. Cervical cancer frequently results from a sexually transmitted infection, a feature that distinguishes it from other cancers. Abnormal **vaginal** (VAJ-i-nal) bleeding is the most common symptom. **Pap tests** (pap) (tests) and **HPV tests** (H-P-V) (tests), followed by **colposcopy** (kol-POS-ko-pē) with biopsy, are used to diagnose this disease. Surgical treatment options include **conization** (kon-i-ZĀ-shun), such as **LEEP**, and **hysterectomy** (his-te-REK-to-mē). Chemotherapy and radiation therapy may also be used. A vaccine for human papillomavirus is now available for both boys and girls and can be used for the prevention of cervical cancer.

Endometrial Cancer
Currently 75% of women diagnosed with **endometrial cancer** (en-dō-MĒ-trē-al) (KAN-cer) are postmenopausal. Inappropriate bleeding is a warning sign; hence early diagnosis is common. **Pelvic** (PEL-vik) examination, Pap test, and endometrial sampling are used to diagnose this disease. Treatment is **hysterosalpingo-oophorectomy** (his-ter-ō-sal-ping-gō-ō-of-o-REK-to-mē), which may be followed by chemotherapy and radiation therapy. Laparoscopically assisted vaginal hysterectomy may also be used.

Ovarian Cancer
Ovarian cancer (ō-VAR-ē-an) (KAN-cer) is the ninth most common form of cancer in women, yet it is the most challenging to diagnose and causes more deaths than any other cancer of the female reproductive system. Early symptoms are often absent or associated with other problems; thus early diagnosis is uncommon. Early symptoms include abdominal discomfort and bloating; later stages include abdominal or pelvic pain and urinary or menstrual irregularities. **CA-125 test** (C-A-1-25) (test) and **transvaginal sonography** (trans-VAJ-i-nal) (so-NOG-ra-fē) are used in diagnosing this disease. Treatment is total abdominal hysterectomy and bilateral **salpingo-oophorectomy** (sal-ping-gō-ō-of-o-REK-to-mē) and removal of as much additional involved tissue as possible, including lymph nodes in the pelvic area. Chemotherapy is usually prescribed following surgery.

Chapter 8 Female Reproductive System

CHAPTER REVIEW

EXERCISE 33 ■ Chapter Content Quiz

Test your understanding of terms and abbreviations introduced in this chapter. Circle the letter for the medical term or abbreviation related to the words in italics.

1. *A severe illness that may affect menstruating women after using tampons* is abbreviated as:
   a. TSS
   b. TVS
   c. TLH

2. *Blockage of one of the glands on either side of the vagina* can lead to infection, which may result in an abscess.
   a. cervicitis
   b. vulvovaginitis
   c. Bartholin cyst

3. *Inflammation of the breast*, is an infection characterized by *pain in the breast*, edema, warmth, and erythema and most commonly occurs with breastfeeding.
   a. mastitis, mastalgia
   b. myometritis, mastopexy
   c. perimetritis, mammoplasty

4. Bilateral *water in the fallopian tube* indicates both tubes are blocked by watery liquid and can be a cause of female infertility.
   a. salpingocele
   b. hematosalpinx
   c. hydrosalpinx

5. Symptoms of *growth of the endometrium into the muscular portion of the uterus* include dysmenorrhea, menorrhagia, and *difficult or painful intercourse*.
   a. endometriosis, mastalgia
   b. adenomyosis, dyspareunia
   c. myometritis, amenorrhea

6. Monthly hormonal changes may cause *thickening of tissue (fibrosis), benign cysts, and pain or tenderness in one or both breasts*.
   a. FCC
   b. PMS
   c. PID

7. Cryosurgery, laser, and LEEP are various surgical techniques performed to *remove a cone-shaped area of the cervix*.
   a. colporrhaphy
   b. conization
   c. myomectomy

8. The *surgical procedure to widen the cervix and remove contents from the uterus* can be used for both diagnosis and treatment.
   a. CX
   b. D&C
   c. SHG

9. A *surgical repair of the breast* to reduce size is called reduction:
   a. mammoplasty
   b. mammogram
   c. mastectomy

10. Partial *surgical closure of the vagina* may be used to treat vaginal prolapse for patients who are not candidates for more complex reconstructive surgeries and who are no longer sexually active.
    a. colpocleisis
    b. episiorrhaphy
    c. trachelectomy

11. In *total excision of the uterus performed laparoscopically*, the uterus, including the cervix, is morcellated and withdrawn through the laparoscope.
    a. TAH/BSO
    b. TLH
    c. TSS

12. The *instrument used for visual examination of the uterus* is a thin, lighted device inserted through the vagina that transmits images of the inside of the uterus to a computer screen.
    a. hysteroscope
    b. colposcope
    c. pelviscopy

13. The *cytological study of cervical and vaginal secretions to detect high-risk forms of the human papillomavirus* is a lab test conducted to screen for cervical cancer.
    a. CA-125 test
    b. Pap test
    c. HPV test

14. *Infrequent release of an ovum from a mature graafian follicle* generally refers to having eight or fewer menstrual cycles in 1 year.
    a. oligomenorrhea
    b. oligoovulation
    c. anovulation

15. A *vesicovaginal* fistula is an abnormal passageway between the vagina and the:
    a. rectum
    b. urinary bladder
    c. vulva

16. The *instrument used to open* the vagina to conduct a pelvic exam is called:
    a. speculum
    b. hysteroscope
    c. colposcope

17. *The beginning of menstruation*, when the first menstrual period occurs, is called
    a. menopause
    b. anovulation
    c. menarche

18. Symptoms of *dropping of the uterus (and sometimes vagina) due to weakened pelvic muscles* may include urine leaks, discomfort in the *pertaining to the pelvis* area, and lower back pain.
    a. vaginal fistula, endocervical
    b. uterovaginal prolapse, pelvic
    c. abnormal uterine bleeding, vulvovaginal

19. *Syndrome involving physical and emotional symptoms occurring up to 10 days before menstruation* may range from mild to severe, and affect up to 90% of women of reproductive age.
    a. Premenstrual syndrome
    b. Toxic shock syndrome
    c. Polycystic ovary syndrome

20. A *technique that combines mammography and computer-assisted biopsy to obtain tissue from a breast lesion* may be performed if the lesion can be seen on imaging but cannot be felt by the patient or medical care provider.
    a. transvaginal sonography
    b. sentinel lymph node biopsy
    c. stereotactic breast biopsy

CHAPTER AT A GLANCE — Word Parts New to This Chapter

COMBINING FORMS

cervic/o	hymen/o	metr/o	salping/o	
colp/o	hyster/o	oophor/o	trachel/o	
endometri/o	mamm/o	pelv/i	vagin/o	
episi/o	mast/o	perine/o	vulv/o	
gynec/o	men/o			

PREFIXES
peri-

SUFFIXES
-cleisis
-rrhaphy
-salpinx

CHAPTER AT A GLANCE — Female Reproductive System Terms Built from Word Parts

DISEASE AND DISORDER
cervicitis
endometriosis
endometritis
hematosalpinx
hydrosalpinx
mastitis
menometrorrhagia
menorrhagia
metrorrhagia
myometritis
oophoritis
perimetritis
pyosalpinx
salpingitis
salpingocele
vaginitis
vaginosis
vulvovaginitis

SURGICAL
colpocleisis
colpoperineorrhaphy
colpoplasty
colporrhaphy
episiorrhaphy
hymenotomy
hysterectomy
hysteropexy
mammoplasty
mastectomy
mastopexy
oophorectomy
perineorrhaphy
salpingectomy
salpingo-oophorectomy
salpingostomy
trachelectomy
vulvectomy

DIAGNOSTIC
colposcope
colposcopy
hysterosalpingogram (HSG)
hysteroscope
hysteroscopy
mammogram
mammography
pelviscopic
pelviscopy
sonohysterography (SHG)

COMPLEMENTARY
amenorrhea
dysmenorrhea
endocervical
gynecologist
leukorrhea
mastalgia
oligomenorrhea
pelvic
vaginal
vesicovaginal
vulvovaginal

CHAPTER AT A GLANCE — Female Reproductive System Terms *NOT* Built from Word Parts

DISEASE AND DISORDER
abnormal uterine bleeding (AUB)
adenomyosis
Bartholin cyst
breast cancer
cervical cancer
endometrial cancer
fibrocystic breast changes (FCC)
ovarian cancer
pelvic inflammatory disease (PID)
polycystic ovary syndrome (PCOS)
premenstrual syndrome (PMS)
toxic shock syndrome (TSS)
uterine fibroid
uterovaginal prolapse
vaginal fistula

SURGICAL
anterior and posterior colporrhaphy (A&P repair)
conization
dilation and curettage (D&C)
endometrial ablation
myomectomy
tubal ligation
uterine artery embolization (UAE)

DIAGNOSTIC
CA-125 test
HPV test
Pap test
sentinel lymph node biopsy
stereotactic breast biopsy
transvaginal sonography (TVS)

COMPLEMENTARY
anovulation
contraception
dyspareunia
fistula
hormone therapy
menarche
menopause
oligoovulation
speculum

PART 2 BODY SYSTEMS

Obstetrics and Neonatology

9

Outline

ANATOMY, 314
Terms Relating to Pregnancy, 314

WORD PARTS, 315
Obstetric and Neonatology Combining Forms, 315
Combining Forms Used with Obstetric and Neonatology Terms, 316
Prefixes, 316
Suffixes, 316

MEDICAL TERMS, 320
Obstetric Disease and Disorder Terms, 320
    Built from Word Parts and
      NOT Built from Word Parts, 320
Neonatology Disease and Disorder Terms, 326
    Built from Word Parts and
      NOT Built from Word Parts, 326
Obstetric Surgical Terms, 331
    Built from Word Parts and
      NOT Built from Word Parts, 331
Obstetric and Neonatology Diagnostic Terms, 334
    Built from Word Parts and
      NOT Built from Word Parts, 334
Obstetric Complementary Terms, 338
    Built from Word Parts and
      NOT Built from Word Parts, 338
Neonatalogy Complementary Terms, 344
    Built from Word Parts and
      NOT Built from Word Parts, 344
Abbreviations, 348

PRACTICAL APPLICATION, 350
CASE STUDY Translate Between Everyday Language and Medical Language, 350
Interact with Medical Documents, 351
Use Medical Terms in Clinical Statements, 352
Use Medical Language in Online Electronic Health Records, 353
Pronounce Medical Terms in Use, 353

CHAPTER REVIEW, 354
Chapter Content Quiz, 354
Chapter at a Glance, 355

Answers to Chapter Exercises, Appendix A

Objectives

Upon completion of this chapter, you will be able to:

1. Pronounce organs and anatomic structures relating to pregnancy.
2. Define and spell word parts related to obstetrics and neonatology.
3. Define, pronounce, and spell disease and disorder terms related to obstetrics and neonatology.
4. Define, pronounce, and spell surgical and diagnostic terms related to obstetrics and neonatology.
5. Define, pronounce, and spell complementary terms related to obstetrics and neonatology.
6. Interpret the meaning of abbreviations related to obstetrics and neonatology.
7. Apply medical language in clinical contexts.

TABLE 9.1 Comparing Terms: Gravid/o and Par/o, 338
TABLE 9.2 Terms Relating to Mother and Newborn, 345

Chapter 9 Obstetrics and Neonatology

ANATOMY

Obstetrics is the branch of medicine that deals with childbirth and the care of the mother before, during, and after birth. **Neonatology** is the branch of medicine that deals with the diagnosis and treatment of disorders of the newborn.

Terms Relating to Pregnancy

TERM	DEFINITION
gamete (GAM-ēt)	mature germ cell, either sperm (male) or ovum (female)
fertilization (fer-ti-li-ZĀ-shun)	beginning of pregnancy, when the sperm enters the ovum. Fertilization normally occurs in the fallopian tubes. (also called **conception**) (Fig. 9.1A)
zygote (ZĪ-gōt)	cell formed by the union of the sperm and the ovum
embryo (EM-brē-ō)	unborn offspring in the stage of development from implantation of the zygote to the end of the eighth week of pregnancy. This period is characterized by rapid growth of the embryo.
fetus (FĒ-tus)	unborn offspring from the beginning of the ninth week of pregnancy until birth (Fig. 9.1B)
gestation (jes-TĀ-shun)	development of a new individual from conception to birth (also called **pregnancy**)
gestation period (jes-TĀ-shun) (PĒR-ē-ed)	duration of pregnancy; normally 38 to 42 weeks (starting from the first day of the last menstrual period), which can be divided into three equal periods, called *trimesters*
implantation (*im*-plan-TĀ-shun)	embedding of the zygote in the uterine lining. The process normally begins about 7 days after fertilization and continues for several days. (Fig. 9.1A)
placenta (pla-SEN-ta)	temporary organ attached to the uterine wall that forms during pregnancy and provides oxygen and nutrients to the fetus. Typically, the placenta detaches from the endometrium after delivery and is commonly referred to as **afterbirth**. (Fig. 9.1B)
amniotic sac (*am*-nē-OT-ic) (sak)	membranous bag that surrounds the fetus before delivery (also called **amnionic sac**, **fetal membrane**, and commonly referred to as **bag of waters**) (Fig. 9.1B)
chorion (KOR-ē-on)	outermost layer of the amniotic sac

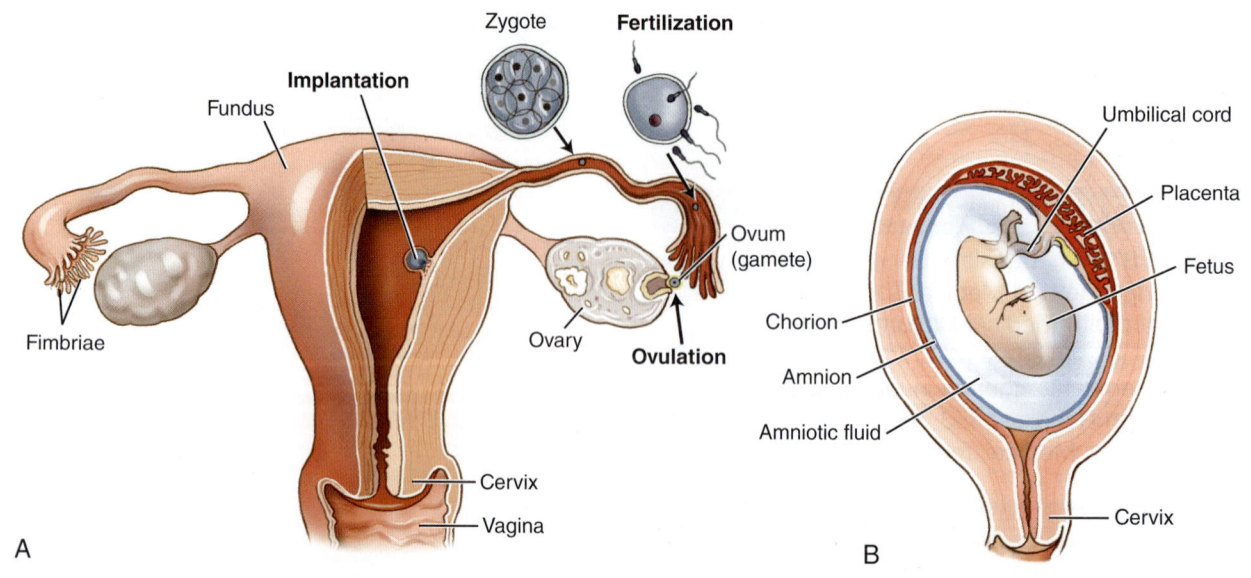

FIG. 9.1 A, Ovulation, fertilization, and implantation. **B,** Development of the fetus.

Chapter 9 Obstetrics and Neonatology

TERM	DEFINITION
amnion (*am*-nē-ON)	innermost layer of the amniotic sac
amniotic fluid (*am*-nē-OT-ic) (flu-id)	fluid within the amniotic sac, which surrounds the fetus (also called **amnionic fluid**)
umbilicus (um-BIL-i-cus)	navel (belly button); marks the site of attachment of the umbilical cord to the fetus

SKIN CHANGES THAT OCCUR THROUGHOUT PREGNANCY
- **striae gravidarum**: "stretch marks" occurring on the abdomen, breast, buttocks, and thighs from weakening of elastic tissues
- **linea nigra**: dark medial line extending from the pubis upward
- **chloasma**: hyperpigmentation of blotchy brown macules usually evenly distributed over the cheeks and forehead

PRONOUNCE ANATOMIC STRUCTURES

Practice saying aloud each of the organs and specific structures on the previous pages.

To hear the terms, go to Evolve Resources at www.evolve.elsevier.com and select:
Student Resources > Audio Glossary > Chapter 9 > **Anatomic Structures**.

❏ Check the box when complete.

🔗 WORD PARTS

Use paper flashcards or electronic flashcards on Evolve to memorize word parts used to analyze, define, and build medical terms in this chapter. To reinforce learning, study one section of the Word Parts Table at a time, and then complete the corresponding exercise on the following pages.

1 ▪ Obstetric and Neonatology Combining Forms

COMBINING FORM	DEFINITION	COMBINING FORM	DEFINITION
amni/o	amnion, amniotic fluid	omphal/o	umbilicus, navel
amnion/o	amnion, amniotic fluid	par/o	bear, give birth to, labor, childbirth
chori/o	chorion	part/o	bear, give birth to, labor, childbirth
fet/o	fetus, unborn offspring	puerper/o	childbirth
gravid/o	pregnancy	🏛 **PUERPER** is made up of two Latin word roots: **puer**, meaning **child**, and **per**, meaning **through**.	
lact/o	milk		
nat/o	birth		

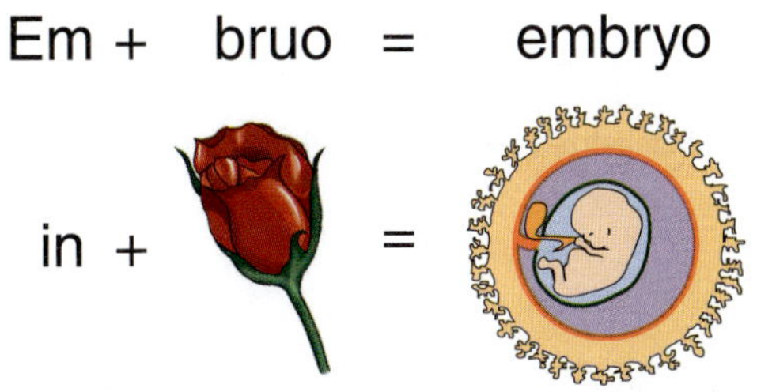

Em + bruo = embryo

in + 🌹 = 🥚

FIG. 9.2 *Embryo* comes from the Greek *em*, meaning "in," plus *bruo*, meaning "to bud" or "to shoot."

2 ■ Combining Forms Used with Obstetric and Neonatology Terms

COMBINING FORM	DEFINITION	COMBINING FORM	DEFINITION
carcin/o	cancer	pseud/o	false
cephal/o	head	pylor/o	pylorus, pyloric sphincter (see Fig. 11.4)
episi/o	vulva		
esophag/o	esophagus (tube leading from the throat to the stomach) (see Fig. 11.1)	**PYLORUS** refers to portion of the stomach that connects to the small intestine, and the **pyloric sphincter** is a ring of muscle between the two.	
		son/o	sound
hydr/o	water	terat/o	malformations
hyster/o	uterus	**TERAT/O** is translated literally as **monster**; however, in terms containing terat/o relating to obstetrics, terat/o refers to malformations or abnormal development.	
olig/o	scanty, few		
pelv/i	pelvis, pelvic cavity	trache/o	trachea
prim/i	first *(Note: the combining vowel is i.)*		

3 ■ Prefixes

PREFIX	DEFINITION	PREFIX	DEFINITION
ante-	before	neo-	new
dys-	painful, abnormal, difficult, labored	nulli-	none
intra-	within	poly-	many, much
micro-	small	post-	after
multi-	many	pre-	before

4 ■ Suffixes

SUFFIX	DEFINITION	SUFFIX	DEFINITION
-a	noun suffix, no meaning	-ic	pertaining to
-al	pertaining to	-itis	inflammation
-amnios	amnion, amniotic fluid	-logist	one who studies and treats (specialist, physician)
-cele	hernia, protrusion		
-centesis	surgical puncture to aspirate fluid (with a sterile needle)	-logy	study of
		-malacia	softening
-cyesis	pregnancy	-oma	tumor, swelling
-e	noun suffix, no meaning	-rrhea	flow, discharge
-gen	substance or agent that produces or causes	-rrhexis	rupture
		-tocia	birth, labor
-genic	producing, originating, causing	-tomy	cut into, incision
-graphy	process of recording, radiographic imaging	-um	noun suffix, no meaning
		-us	noun suffix, no meaning

Refer to **Appendix B** and **Appendix C** for alphabetized word parts and their meanings.

Chapter 9 Obstetrics and Neonatology

EXERCISE 1 ■ Obstetric and Neonatology Combining Forms

Refer to the first section of the word parts table.

A Label

Fill in the blanks with combining forms to label this diagram of fetal development. To check your answers, go to Appendix A at the back of the textbook.

1. Umbilicus
   CF: _____

2. Fetus
   CF: _____

3. Amnion, amniotic fluid
   CF: _____
   CF: _____

4. Chorion
   CF: _____

B Identify

Write the combining form for each of the following definitions.

1. childbirth _____
2. bear, give birth to, labor, childbirth
   a. _____
   b. _____
3. pregnancy _____
4. milk _____
5. birth _____

C Define and Match

Step 1: Write the definitions after the following combining forms.
Step 2: Match the descriptions on the right with the combining forms and definitions. Answers may be used more than once.

_____ 1. amni/o, _____
_____ 2. omphal/o, _____
_____ 3. amnion/o, _____
_____ 4. fet/o, _____
_____ 5. chori/o, _____

a. outermost layer of the amniotic sac
b. 9 weeks of pregnancy to birth
c. innermost layer of amniotic sac; fluid surrounding the fetus
d. site of the umbilical cord attachment to the fetus

D Define

Write the definitions of the following combining forms.

1. lact/o _____
2. par/o, part/o _____
3. puerper/o _____
4. gravid/o _____
5. nat/o _____

318 Chapter 9 Obstetrics and Neonatology

EXERCISE 2 ■ Combining Forms Used with Obstetric and Neonatology Terms

Refer to the second section of the word parts table.

A Define

Write the definitions of the following combining forms.

1. prim/i _____
2. olig/o _____
3. pylor/o _____
4. hydr/o _____
5. cephal/o _____
6. episi/o _____
7. hyster/o _____
8. esophag/o _____
9. carcin/o _____
10. pseud/o _____
11. terat/o _____
12. trache/o _____
13. son/o _____
14. pelv/i _____

B Identify

Write the combining form for each of the following definitions.

1. head _____
2. scanty, few _____
3. first _____
4. uterus _____
5. pylorus, pyloric sphincter _____
6. pelvis, pelvic cavity _____
7. false _____
8. vulva _____
9. malformations _____
10. esophagus _____
11. cancer _____
12. trachea _____
13. water _____
14. sound _____

EXERCISE 3 ■ Prefixes

Refer to the third section of the word parts table.

A Define

Write the definitions of the following prefixes.

1. pre- _____
2. micro- _____
3. neo- _____
4. multi- _____
5. post- _____
6. dys- _____
7. ante- _____
8. poly- _____
9. intra- _____
10. nulli- _____

B Identify

Write the prefix for each of the following definitions.

1. none _____
2. after _____
3. small _____
4. within _____
5. before a. _____
   b. _____
6. many, much _____
7. many _____
8. new _____
9. painful, abnormal, difficult, labored _____

Chapter 9   Obstetrics and Neonatology   319

EXERCISE 4 ■ Suffixes

Refer to the fourth section of the word parts table.

A Define

Write the definitions of the following suffixes.

1. -logy _____
2. -gen _____
3. -oma _____
4. -ic _____
5. -tomy _____
6. -logist _____

7. -cele _____
8. -genic _____
9. -malacia _____
10. -itis _____
11. -rrhea _____
12. -graphy _____

B Label

Write the suffixes pictured and defined.

1. _____
   birth, labor

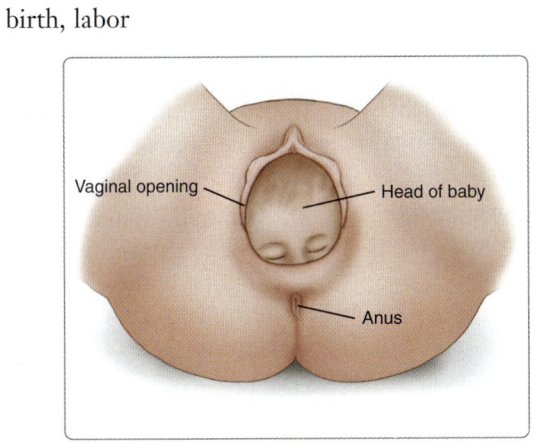

2. _____
   rupture

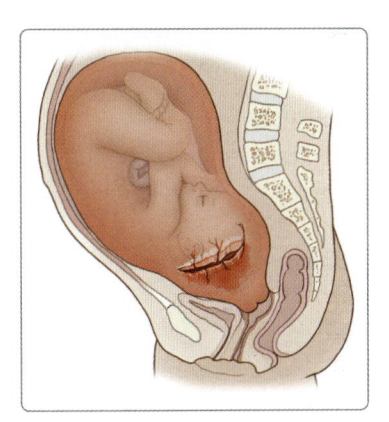

3. _____
   pregnancy

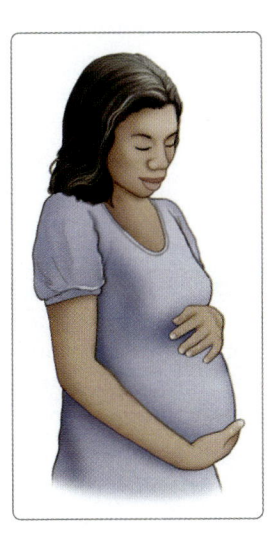

4. _____
   amnion, amniotic fluid

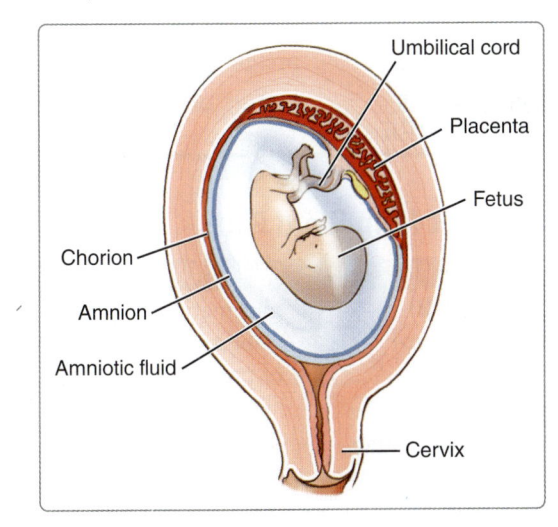

C Identify

Write the suffixes in this chapter that have no meaning. Place in alphabetical order.

1. _____   3. _____
2. _____   4. _____

MEDICAL TERMS

Medical terms relevant to this chapter have been grouped by topics, such as Disease and Disorder, and are listed in tables designated as Built from Word Parts or *NOT* Built from Word Parts. The exercises following each table assist with learning term definitions, pronunciations, and spellings.

Obstetric Disease and Disorder Terms
BUILT FROM WORD PARTS AND *NOT* BUILT FROM WORD PARTS

The first portion of the table contains Obstetric Disease and Disorder Terms that can be translated using definitions of word parts. The second portion of the table contains Obstetric Disease and Disorder Terms that cannot be fully understood using the definitions of word parts.

■ Built from Word Parts

TERM	DEFINITION	TERM	DEFINITION
1. amnionitis (am-nē-ō-NĪ-tis)	inflammation of the amnion	6. oligohydramnios (ol-i-gō-hī-DRAM-nē-os)	scanty amnion water (less than the normal amount of amniotic fluid; 500 mL or less)
2. chorioamnionitis (kor-ē-ō-am-nē-ō-NĪ-tis)	inflammation of the chorion and amnion	7. polyhydramnios (pol-ē-hī-DRAM-nē-os)	much amnion water (more than the normal amount of amniotic fluid; 2000 mL or more) (also called **hydramnios**)
3. choriocarcinoma (kor-ē-ō-kar-si-NŌ-ma)	cancerous tumor of the chorion		
4. dystocia (dis-TŌ-sha)	difficult labor (obstructed or prolonged; causes may be from maternal factors, such as ineffective uterine contractions and abnormal pelvic shape, or from fetal causes, such as large size and abnormal birth presentation)	8. pseudocyesis (sū-dō-sī-Ē-sis)	false pregnancy (belief one is pregnant, often with physical symptoms such as a swollen abdomen, though a fetus is not present; contributing factors may be psychological, hormonal, or related to underlying pathology, such as a uterine tumor)
5. hysterorrhexis (his-ter-ō-REK-sis)	rupture of the uterus		

■ *NOT* Built from Word Parts

TERM	DEFINITION
1. abortion (AB) (a-BŌR-shun)	termination of pregnancy by the expulsion from the uterus of an embryo or fetus before viability, usually before 20 weeks of gestation. Spontaneous abortion is the termination of pregnancy that occurs naturally and is commonly referred to as *miscarriage*. Induced abortion is the intentional termination of pregnancy by surgical or medical intervention.
2. abruptio placentae (ab-RUP-shē-ō) (pla-SEN-tē)	premature separation of the placenta from the uterine wall; can cause antepartum hemorrhage (severe bleeding before giving birth); (also called **placental abruption**) (Fig. 9.3A)

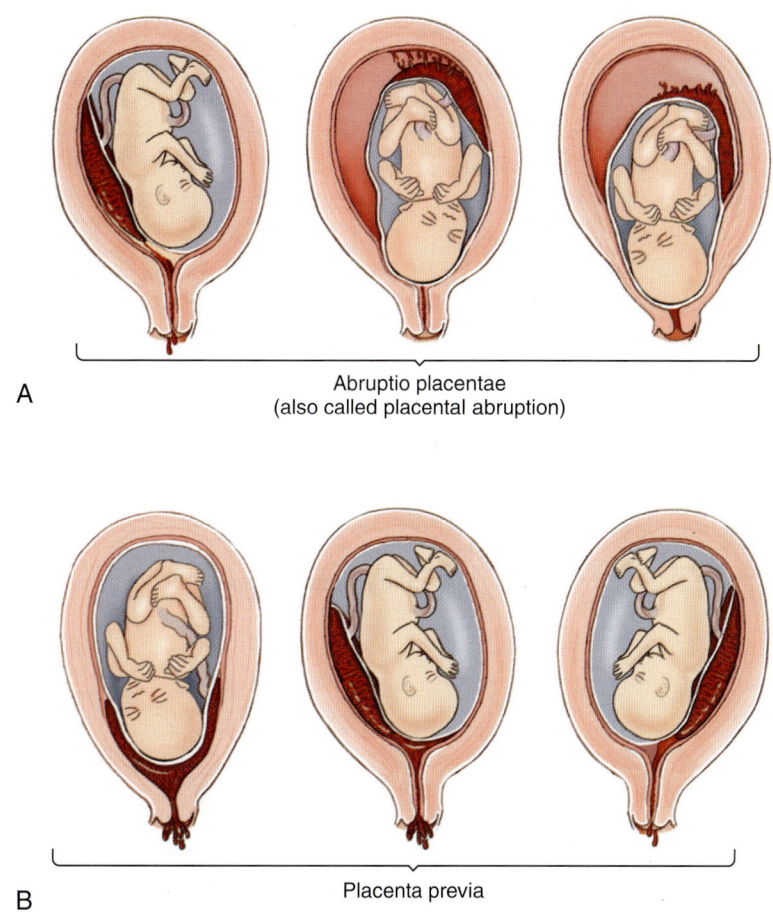

FIG. 9.3 Various presentations of abruptio placentae **(A)** and placenta previa **(B)**.

TERM	DEFINITION
3. eclampsia (e-KLAMP-sē-a)	severe complication and progression of preeclampsia characterized by convulsion (see *preeclampsia* later). Eclampsia is a potentially life-threatening disorder.
4. ectopic pregnancy (ek-TOP-ik) (PREG-nan-sē)	nonviable pregnancy occurring outside the uterus, commonly in the fallopian tubes; life-threatening if left untreated
5. placenta accreta spectrum (PAS) (pla-SEN-ta) (a-KRĒ-ta) (spek-trum)	growth of the placenta into the uterine wall, resulting in the inability to detach after delivery; types describing the severity of the abnormal attachment include accreta, increta, and percreta. Serious condition that increases the risk of postpartum hemorrhage (severe bleeding after giving birth). (Fig. 9.4)
6. placenta previa (pla-SEN-ta) (PRĒ-vē-a)	abnormally low implantation of the placenta on the uterine wall completely or partially covering the cervix. Dilation of the cervix can cause separation of the placenta from the uterine wall, resulting in bleeding. With severe hemorrhage, a cesarean section is necessary to save the mother and baby's life. (Fig. 9.3B)
7. preeclampsia (prē-ē-KLAMP-sē-a)	abnormal condition encountered during pregnancy or shortly after delivery characterized by high blood pressure and proteinuria, but with no convulsions. The cause is unknown; if not successfully treated, the condition can progress to eclampsia.

322 Chapter 9 Obstetrics and Neonatology

A **Placenta accreta**

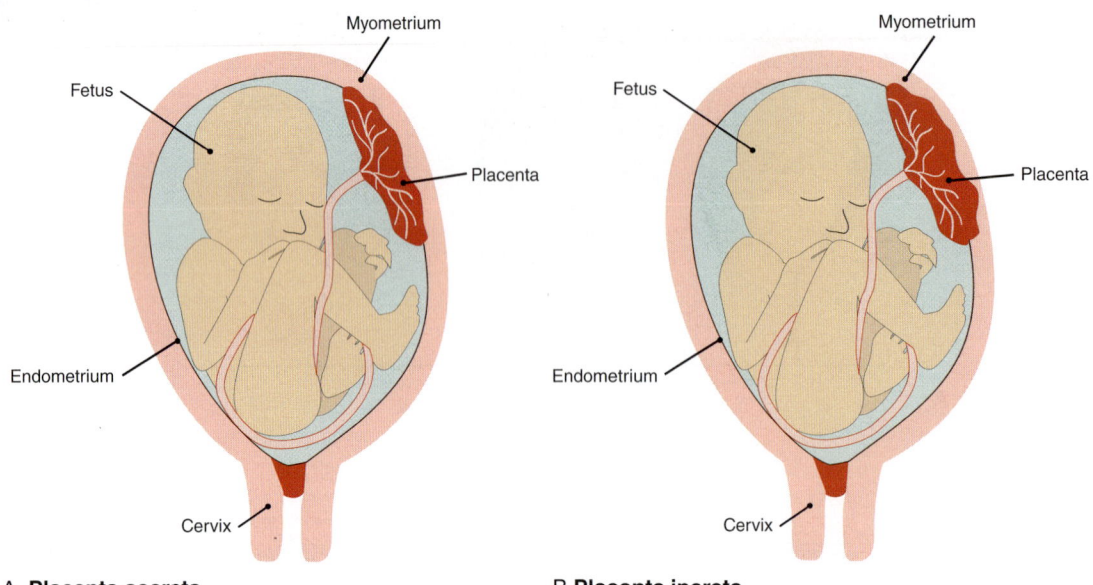

B **Placenta increta**

C **Placenta percreta**

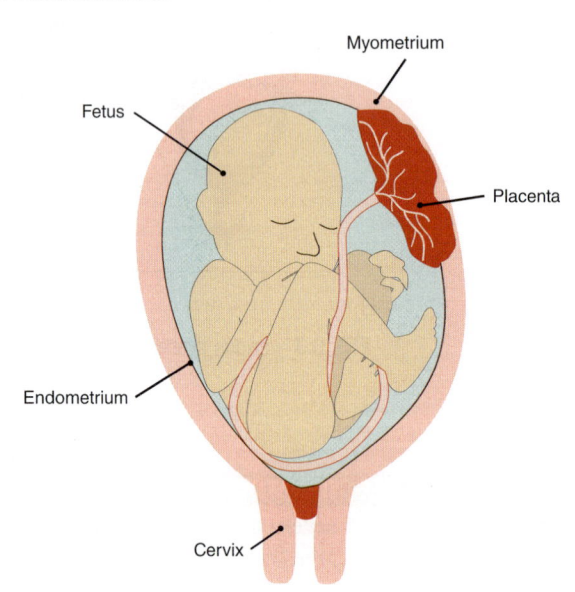

FIG. 9.4 Placenta accreta spectrum. Types describe the severity of the condition and the depth of the growth into the uterine wall. **A, Placenta accreta** occurs when the placenta attaches too firmly to the uterine wall but has not grown into the uterine muscle (myometrium). **B, Placenta increta** occurs when the placenta has grown into the uterine muscle. **C, Placenta percreta** occurs when the placenta grows through the uterine wall and potentially into surrounding organs.

EXERCISE 5 ■ Pronounce and Spell

Practice pronunciation and spelling on paper and online.

1. **Practice on Paper**
   a. **Pronounce:** Read the phonetic spelling and say aloud the terms listed in the previous table. Refer to Table 2.2 Pronunciation Key as needed.
   b. **Spell:** Have a study partner read the terms aloud. Write the spelling of the terms on a separate sheet of paper.

2. **Practice Online**
   a. **Access** online learning resources. Go to evolve.elsevier.com > Evolve Resources > Student Resources.
   b. **Pronounce:** Select Audio Glossary > Chapter 9 > Exercise 5. Select a term to hear its pronunciation and repeat aloud.
   c. **Spell:** Select Activities > Chapter 9 > Spell Terms > Exercise 5. Select the audio icon and type the correct spelling of the term.

☐ Check the box when complete.

Chapter 9 Obstetrics and Neonatology

EXERCISE 6 ■ Obstetric Disease and Disorder Terms Built from Word Parts

A Analyze and Define

Analyze and define the following disease and disorder terms.

1. chorioamnionitis

2. choriocarcinoma

3. pseudocyesis

4. amnionitis

5. hysterorrhexis

6. oligohydramnios

7. polyhydramnios

8. dystocia

B Label

Build terms pictured by writing word parts above definitions.

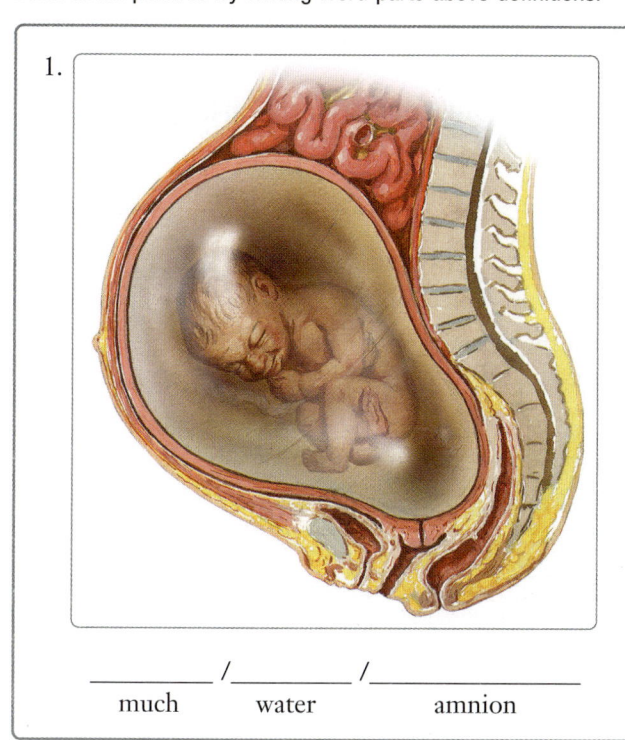

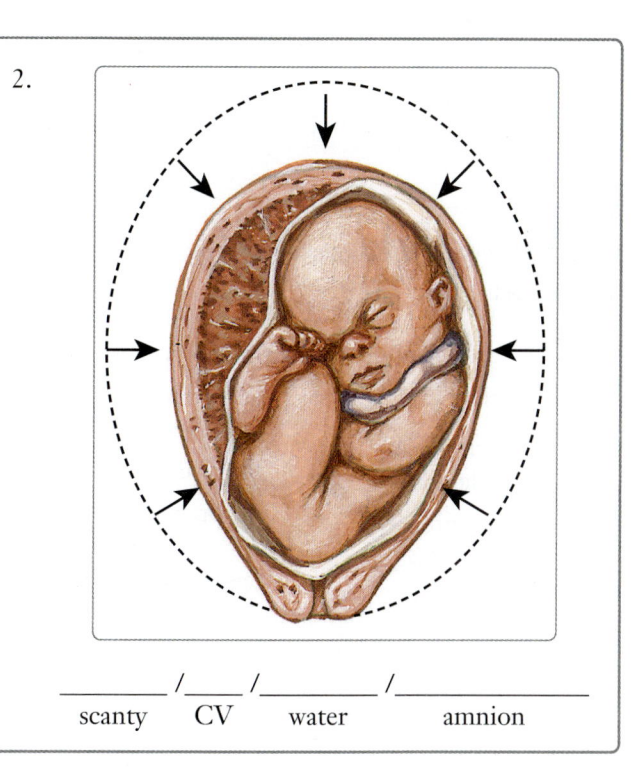

1.

_____ / _____ / _____
much   water   amnion

2.

_____ / ____ / _____ / _____
scanty   CV   water   amnion

324　Chapter 9　Obstetrics and Neonatology

3.

_____ / ___ / _____
uterus　　CV　　rupture

4.

_____ / _____
difficult　　　　　labor

C Fill In

Build disease and disorder terms for the following definitions by using the word parts you have learned.

1. cancerous tumor of the chorion   _____ / __ / _____ / __
　　　　　　　　　　　　　　　　　　WR　CV　WR　　S

2. inflammation of the amnion   _____ / __
　　　　　　　　　　　　　　　　WR　　S

3. inflammation of the chorion and amnion   _____ / __ / _____ / __
　　　　　　　　　　　　　　　　　　　　　　WR　CV　WR　　S

4. false pregnancy   _____ / __ / __
　　　　　　　　　　WR　CV　S

EXERCISE 7 ■ Obstetric Disease and Disorder Terms NOT Built from Word Parts

A Match

Match the terms in the first column with their correct definitions in the second column.

_____ 1. abruptio placentae
_____ 2. preeclampsia
_____ 3. ectopic pregnancy
_____ 4. placenta previa
_____ 5. eclampsia
_____ 6. abortion
_____ 7. placenta accreta spectrum

a. severe complication and progression of preeclampsia characterized by convulsion
b. abnormally low implantation of the placenta on the uterine wall
c. termination of pregnancy by the expulsion from the uterus of an embryo or fetus before viability
d. placenta grows into the uterine wall and is unable to detach after delivery
e. premature separation of the placenta from the uterine wall
f. nonviable pregnancy occurring outside the uterus
g. abnormal condition characterized by high blood pressure and proteinuria, but with no convulsions

Chapter 9   Obstetrics and Neonatology   325

B Label

Write the medical terms pictured and defined.

1. _____
   nonviable pregnancy occurring outside the uterus, commonly in the fallopian tubes; life-threatening if left untreated

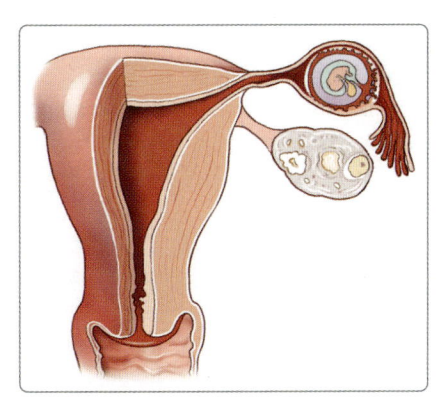

2. _____
   premature separation of the placenta from the uterine wall

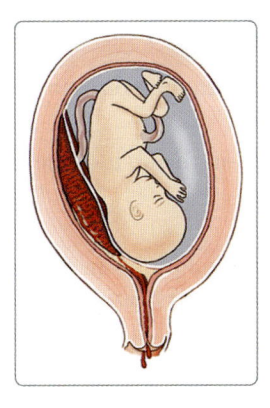

3. _____
   abnormally low implantation of the placenta on the uterine wall

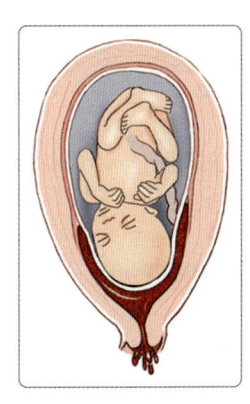

C Identify

Fill in the blanks with the correct terms.

1. serious condition in which the placenta grows into the uterine wall _____
2. severe complication and progression of preeclampsia _____
3. termination of pregnancy by the expulsion from the uterus of an embryo or fetus _____
4. characterized by high blood pressure and proteinuria, but with no convulsions _____

EXERCISE 8 ■ Review of Obstetric Disease and Disorder Terms

Can you define, pronounce, and spell the following terms?

abortion (AB)	choriocarcinoma	hysterorrhexis	placenta previa
abruptio placentae	dystocia	oligohydramnios	polyhydramnios
amnionitis	eclampsia	placenta accreta	preeclampsia
chorioamnionitis	ectopic pregnancy	spectrum (PAS)	pseudocyesis

Neonatalogy Disease and Disorder Terms
BUILT FROM WORD PARTS AND *NOT* BUILT FROM WORD PARTS

The first portion of the table contains Neonatology Disease and Disorder Terms that can be translated using definitions of word parts. The second portion of the table contains Neonatology Disease and Disorder Terms that cannot be fully understood using the definitions of word parts.

■ Built from Word Parts

TERM	DEFINITION	TERM	DEFINITION
1. **laryngomalacia** (la-*ring*-gō-ma-LĀ-sha)	softening of the larynx (causes inhalation stridor in infants)	5. **pyloric stenosis** (pī-LOR-ik) (ste-NŌ-sis)	narrowing pertaining to the pyloric sphincter (Congenital pyloric stenosis occurs in 1 of every 200 newborns.)
2. **microcephalus** (mī-krō-SEF-a-lus)	(fetus with a very) small head		
3. **omphalitis** (*om*-fa-LĪ-tis)	inflammation of the umbilicus	🏛 **STENOSIS** comes from the Greek word of the same spelling meaning *to narrow*. In medical language, it may appear as a suffix, -stenosis, or as a standalone word, as in pyloric stenosis.	
4. **omphalocele** (OM-fal-ō-*sēl*)	hernia at the umbilicus (a part of the intestine protrudes through the abdominal wall at birth)	6. **tracheoesophageal fistula** (trā-kē-ō-ē-*sof*-a-JĒ-al) (FIS-tū-la)	abnormal passageway pertaining to the trachea and esophagus (between the trachea and esophagus)

■ *NOT* Built from Word Parts

TERM	DEFINITION
1. **cleft lip or palate** (kleft) (lip) (or) (PAL-at)	congenital split of the lip or roof of the mouth; one or both deformities may be present (*cleft* indicates a fissure) (Fig. 9.5)
2. **coarctation of the aorta** (kō-ark-TĀ-shun) (of) (the) (ā-OR-ta)	congenital stenosis (narrowing) that occurs in the arch of the aorta
3. **congenital cytomegalovirus (CMV) infection** (kon-JEN-i-tal) (sī-to-MEG-a-lō-*vī*-rus) (in-FEK-shun)	herpes-type virus that crosses the placenta. Symptoms in newborns may include jaundice, microcephaly, developmental delay and hearing loss; some infants may have no symptoms.
4. **congenital heart disease** (kon-JEN-i-tal) (hart) (di-ZĒZ)	heart abnormality present at birth
5. **Down syndrome** (down) (SIN-drōm)	genetic condition caused by a chromosomal abnormality characterized by varying degrees of intellectual, developmental, and physical disorders or defects (there is an extra 21st chromosome; hence, it is also called **trisomy 21**) (Fig. 9.6)
6. **erythroblastosis fetalis** (e-*rith*-rō-blas-TŌ-sis) (fē-TAL-is)	condition of the fetus and newborn characterized by destruction of erythrocytes, usually caused by incompatibility of maternal and fetal blood Rh factors; may result in anemia, limiting the blood's ability to carry enough oxygen to tissues. (also called **hemolytic disease of the newborn**)
7. **esophageal atresia** (e-*sof*-a-JĒ-al) (a-TRĒ-zha)	congenital absence of part of the esophagus. Food cannot pass from the baby's mouth to the stomach.
8. **fetal alcohol syndrome (FAS)** (FĒ-tal) (AL-kō-hol) (SIN-drōm)	condition caused by excessive alcohol consumption during pregnancy. Various birth defects may be present, including central nervous system dysfunction and malformations of the skull and face.
9. **gastroschisis** (gas-TROS-ki-sis)	congenital fissure of the abdominal wall that is not at the umbilicus. Enterocele, protrusion of the intestine, is usually present.

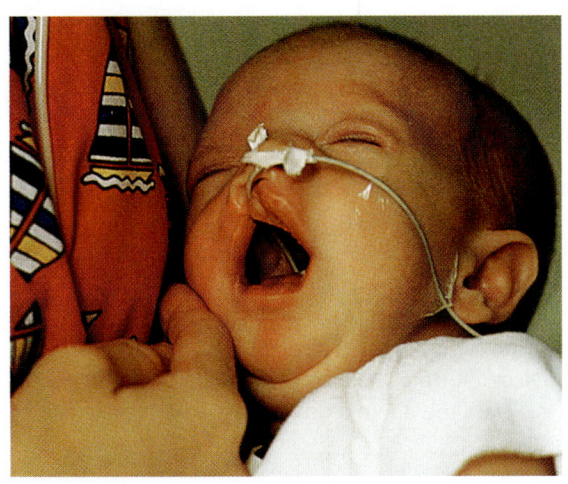

Chapter 9   Obstetrics and Neonatology   327

FIG. 9.5 Unilateral cleft lip. Note the nasogastric feeding tube in place. Neonates born with a cleft lip, palate, or both may require assistive feeding due to an impaired ability to suck.

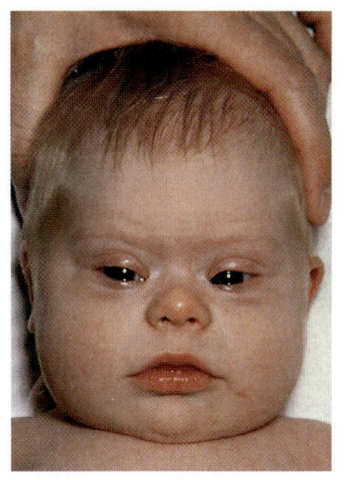

FIG. 9.6 Neonate with Down syndrome.

TERM	DEFINITION
10. **respiratory distress syndrome (RDS)** (RES-pi-ra-*tōr*-ē) (di-STRESS) (SIN-drōm)	respiratory complication in the newborn, especially in premature infants. In premature infants RDS is caused by normal immaturity of the respiratory system, resulting in compromised respiration. (formerly called **hyaline membrane disease**)
11. **spina bifida** (SPĪ-na) (BIF-i-da)	congenital defect in the vertebral column caused by the failure of the vertebral arch to close. If the meninges protrude through the opening, the condition is called meningocele. Protrusion of both the meninges and spinal cord is called myelomeningocele. (Fig. 9.7)

BIRTHMARKS are benign discolorations in the neonate's skin. Common birthmarks include **congenital dermal melanocytosis**, which appear as bluish-black areas of hyperpigmentation often found on the lower back or buttocks of darker-skinned neonates, and **hemangiomas**, which are various benign vascular tumors or stains that cause reddish discoloration and/or malformations of the skin surface. **Nevus flammeus**, also called port-wine stain, is common, often temporary, and is caused by the dilation of certain blood vessels.

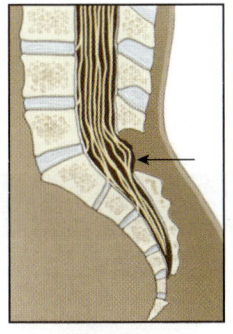

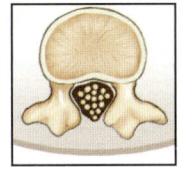

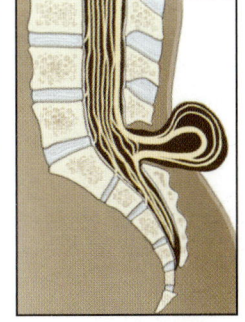

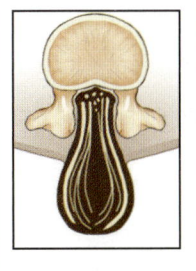

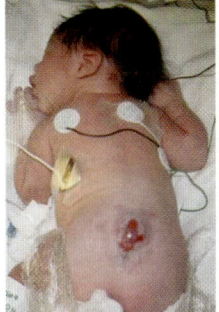

A   Spina bifida   Meningomyelocele   B

FIG. 9.7 A, Drawings of spina bifida and meningomyelocele. **B,** Photograph of meningomyelocele.

328 Chapter 9 Obstetrics and Neonatology

EXERCISE 9 ■ Pronounce and Spell

Practice pronunciation and spelling on paper and online.

1. **Practice on Paper**
   a. **Pronounce:** Read the phonetic spelling and say aloud the terms listed in the previous table. Refer to Table 2.2 Pronunciation Key as needed.
   b. **Spell:** Have a study partner read the terms aloud. Write the spelling of the terms on a separate sheet of paper.

2. **Practice Online**
   a. **Access** online learning resources. Go to evolve.elsevier.com > Evolve Resources > Student Resources.
   b. **Pronounce:** Select Audio Glossary > Chapter 9 > Exercise 9. Select a term to hear its pronunciation and repeat aloud.
   c. **Spell:** Select Activities > Chapter 9 > Spell Terms > Exercise 9. Select the audio icon and type the correct spelling of the term.

❏ Check the box when complete.

EXERCISE 10 ■ Neonatology Disease and Disorder Terms Built from Word Parts

A Analyze and Define

Analyze and define the following disease and disorder terms.

1. pyloric (stenosis)
   _____
   _____

2. omphalocele
   _____
   _____

3. omphalitis
   _____
   _____

4. microcephalus
   _____
   _____

5. tracheoesophageal (fistula)
   _____
   _____

6. laryngomalacia
   _____
   _____

B Label

Build terms pictured by writing word parts above definitions.

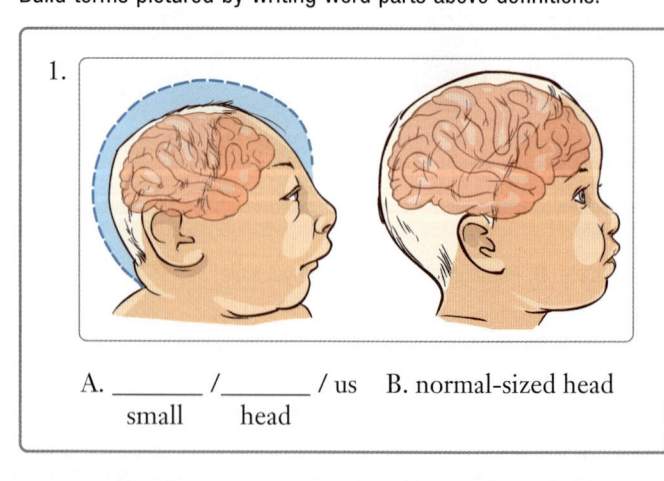

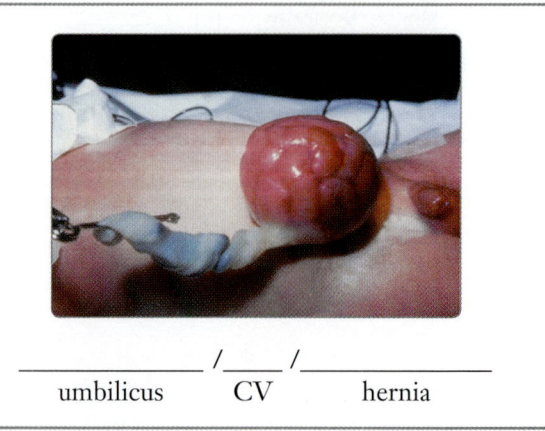

1. A. _____ / _____ / us   B. normal-sized head
       small   head

2. _____ / ____ / _____
   umbilicus   CV   hernia

Chapter 9   Obstetrics and Neonatology   329

C Fill In

Build disease and disorder terms for the following definitions by using the word parts you have learned.

1. softening of the larynx

   _____ / ___ / _____
   WR   CV   S

2. (narrowing) pertaining to the pyloric sphincter

   _____ / _____ stenosis
   WR   S

3. abnormal passageway pertaining to the trachea and the esophagus (between the trachea and esophagus)

   _____ / __ / _____ / _____ fistula
   WR   CV   WR   S

4. inflammation of the umbilicus

   _____ / _____
   WR   S

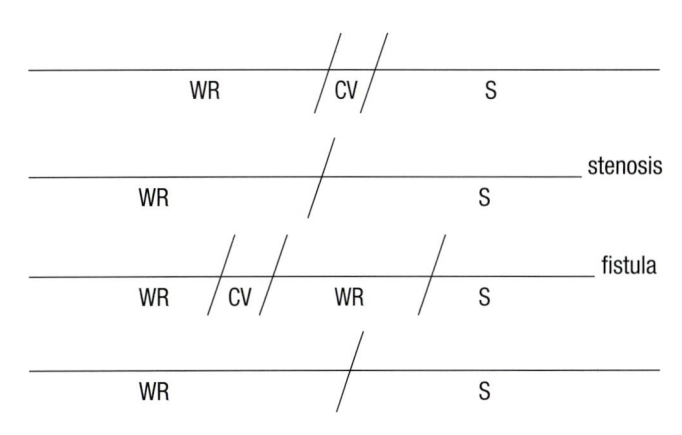

EXERCISE 11 ■ Neonatology Disease and Disorder Terms NOT Built from Word Parts

A Match

Match the terms in the first column with their correct definitions in the second column.

_____ 1. Down syndrome
_____ 2. cleft lip or palate
_____ 3. spina bifida
_____ 4. coarctation of the aorta
_____ 5. congenital cytomegalovirus infection
_____ 6. respiratory distress syndrome
_____ 7. esophageal atresia
_____ 8. gastroschisis
_____ 9. fetal alchohol syndrome
_____ 10. congenital heart disease
_____ 11. erythroblastosis fetalis

a. heart abnormality present at birth
b. respiratory complication of neonates
c. split of the lip or roof of the mouth
d. caused by incompatibility of maternal and fetal blood Rh factors
e. congenital fissure of the abdominal wall
f. congenital stenosis of the aorta
g. congenital absence of part of the esophagus
h. causes various birth defects, including central nervous system dysfunction
i. genetic condition caused by chromosomal abnormality
j. defect of the vertebral column
k. herpes-type virus that crosses the placenta

B Label

Write the medical terms pictured and defined.

1. _____
   congenital absence of part of the esophagus

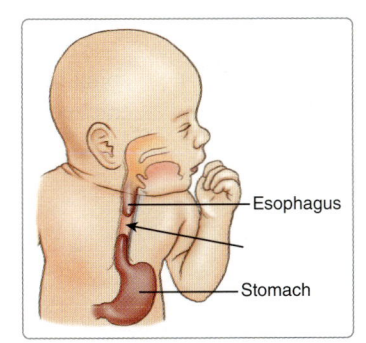

2. _____
   congenital stenosis (narrowing) that occurs in the arch of the aorta

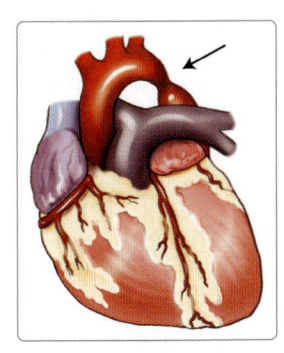

330 Chapter 9 Obstetrics and Neonatology

3. _____
congenital defect in the vertebral column caused by the failure of the vertebral arch to close.

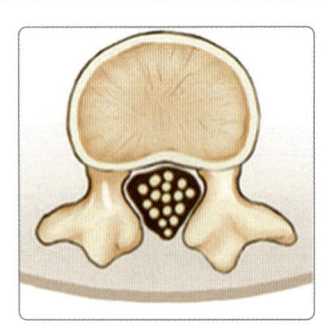

4. _____
congenital fissure of the abdominal wall that is not at the umbilicus.

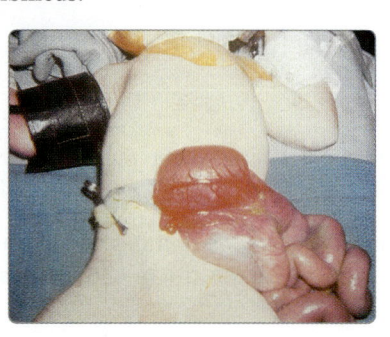

C Identify

Fill in the blanks with the correct terms.

1. A neonate affected by _____ _____, or the destruction of erythrocytes caused by fetal and maternal Rh factor incompatibility, may present with pallor, yellowing of skin and eyes, and enlargement of the liver and spleen.
2. Ventricular septal defect is an example of _____ _____ _____, a heart abnormality present at birth.
3. A respiratory complication that occurs more commonly in premature infants is _____ _____ _____.
4. While some infants have no symptoms, _____ _____ _____, a herpes-type virus, may cause jaundice, microcephaly, developmental delay, and hearing loss.
5. _____ _____ _____ is a condition caused by excessive alcohol consumption during pregnancy.
6. A congenital split of the lip or roof of the mouth is called _____ _____ or _____.
7. _____ _____, a genetic condition caused by a chromosomal abnormality, is also called trisomy 21.

EXERCISE 12 ■ Review of Neonatalogy Disease and Disorder Terms

Can you define, pronounce, and spell the following terms?

cleft lip or palate	Down syndrome	gastroschisis	pyloric stenosis
coarctation of the aorta	erythroblastosis fetalis	laryngomalacia	respiratory distress
congenital cytomegalovirus (CMV) infection	esophageal atresia	microcephalus	syndrome (RDS)
	fetal alcohol syndrome (FAS)	omphalitis	spina bifida
congenital heart disease		omphalocele	tracheoesophageal fistula

Chapter 9 Obstetrics and Neonatology   331

Obstetric Surgical Terms
BUILT FROM WORD PARTS AND *NOT* BUILT FROM WORD PARTS

The first portion of the table contains Obstetric Surgical Terms that can be translated using definitions of word parts. The second portion of the table contains Obstetric Surgical Terms that cannot be fully understood using the definitions of word parts.

■ Built from Word Parts

TERM	DEFINITION	TERM	DEFINITION
1. **amniotomy** (*am*-nē-OT-o-mē)	incision into the amnion (rupture of the amniotic sac to induce labor; a special hook is generally used to make the incision) (Fig. 9.8)	2. **episiotomy** (e-*piz*-ē-OT-o-mē)	incision into the vulva (perineum) (sometimes performed during delivery to prevent a traumatic tear of the vulva) (also called **perineotomy**) (Fig. 9.9)

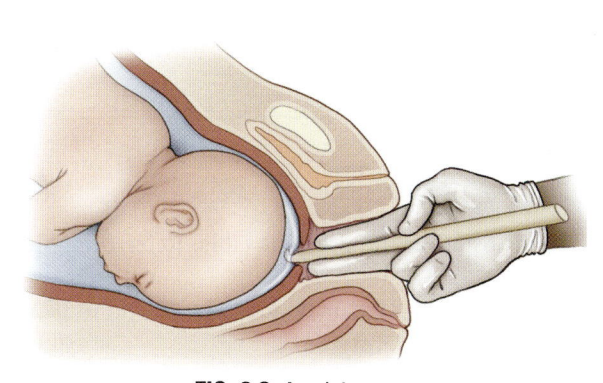

FIG. 9.8 Amniotomy.

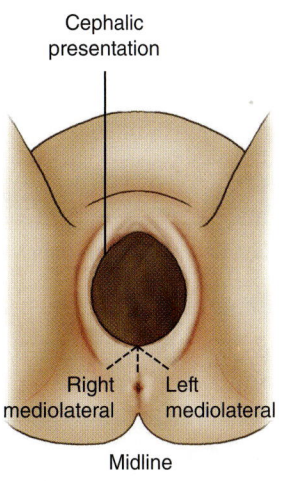

FIG. 9.9 Episiotomies.

■ *NOT* Built from Word Parts

TERM	DEFINITION
1. **cervical cerclage** (SER-vi-kal) (ser-KLAHZH)	suturing the cervix closed to prevent dilation and premature delivery
2. **cesarean section (CS, C-section)** (se-ZĀR-ē-an) (SEK-shun)	birth of a fetus through an incision in the mother's abdomen and uterus (may also be spelled **caesarean**)
🏛 **CESAREAN SECTION (C-SECTION)** The origin of this term has no relation to the birth of Julius Caesar, as is commonly believed. One suggested etymology is that, from 715 to 672 BC, it was Roman law that the operation be performed on dying women in the last few months of pregnancy in the hope of saving the child. At that time the operation was called a **caeso matris utero**, which means **the cutting of the mother's uterus**.	
3. **in vitro fertilization (IVF)** (in) (VĒ-trō) (*fer*-ti-li-ZĀ-shun)	method of fertilizing human ova outside the body and placing the zygote into the uterus; used when infertility is present. Infertility management techniques that artificially combine both the ova and the sperm are called **assisted reproductive technology (ART)**. (Fig. 9.10)

332   Chapter 9   Obstetrics and Neonatology

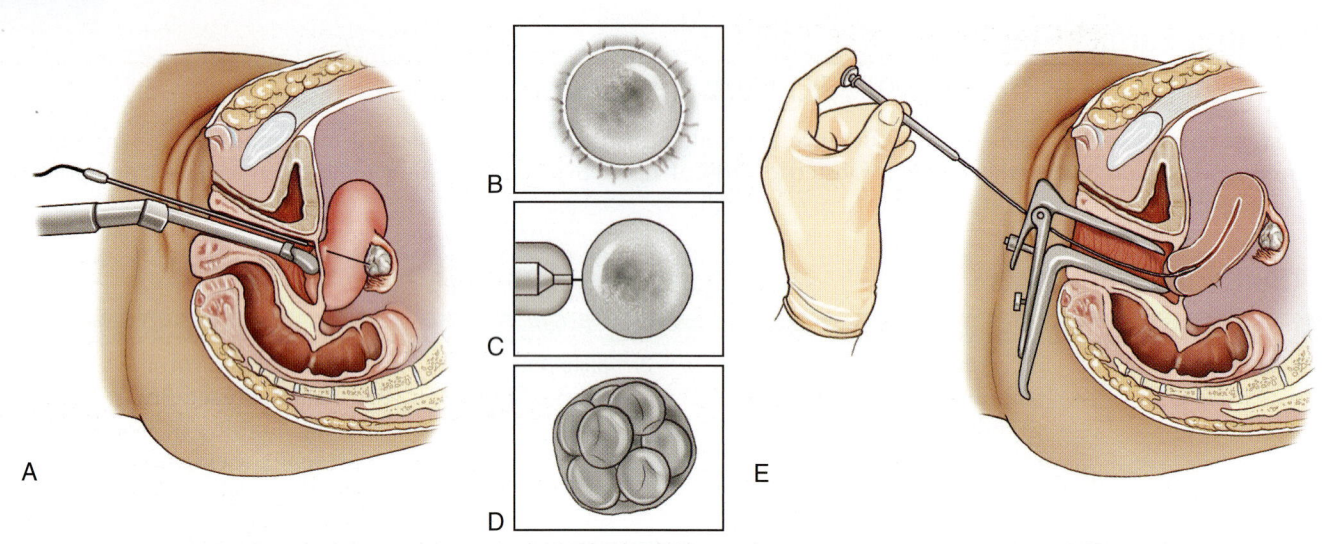

FIG. 9.10 In vitro fertilization (IVF). After ovarian stimulation, ova are retrieved from the ovary by ultrasound-guided transvaginal needle aspiration **(A)**. The ova are fertilized outside the body in a dish with spermatozoa obtained from semen **(B)**. A technique using a single sperm called intracytoplasmic sperm injection may also be used **(C)**. After 48 hours the fertilized ova (zygotes) **(D)** are injected into the uterus for implantation **(E)**. The first pregnancy after in vitro fertilization was reported more than 3 decades ago. Since then **assisted reproductive technology (ART)** has achieved millions of pregnancies worldwide.

EXERCISE 13 ■ Pronounce and Spell

Practice pronunciation and spelling on paper and online.

1. **Practice on Paper**
    a. **Pronounce:** Read the phonetic spelling and say aloud the terms listed in the previous table. Refer to Table 2.2 Pronunciation Key as needed.
    b. **Spell:** Have a study partner read the terms aloud. Write the spelling of the terms on a separate sheet of paper.

2. **Practice Online**
    a. **Access** online learning resources. Go to evolve.elsevier.com > Evolve Resources > Student Resources.
    b. **Pronounce:** Select Audio Glossary > Chapter 9 > Exercise 13. Select a term to hear its pronunciation and repeat aloud.
    c. **Spell:** Select Activities > Chapter 9 > Spell Terms > Exercise 13. Select the audio icon and type the correct spelling of the term.

❑ Check the box when complete.

EXERCISE 14 ■ Obstetric Surgical Terms Built from Word Parts

A Analyze and Define

Analyze and define the following surgical terms.

1. episiotomy

2. amniotomy

Chapter 9   Obstetrics and Neonatology   333

B Build

Build surgical terms for the following definitions by using the word parts you have learned.

1. incision into the amnion   _____ / ____ / _____
                                       WR   CV   S

2. incision into the vulva   _____ / ____ / _____
                                       WR   CV   S

EXERCISE 15 ■ Obstetric Surgical Terms NOT Built from Word Parts

A Label

Write the surgical terms pictured and defined.

1. _____
suturing the cervix closed to prevent premature delivery

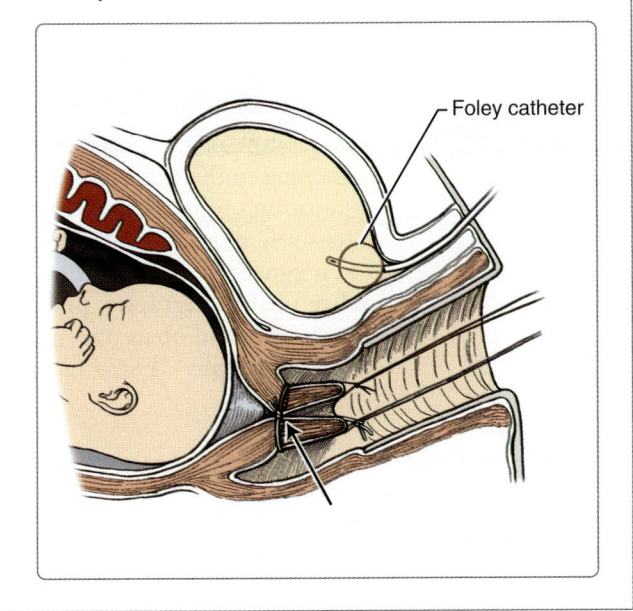

2. _____
method of fertilizing human ova outside the body and placing the zygote into the uterus

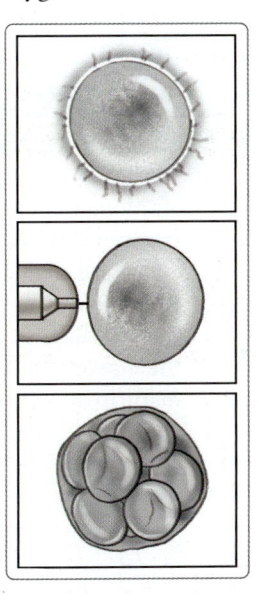

3. _____
birth of a fetus through an incision in the mother's abdomen and uterus

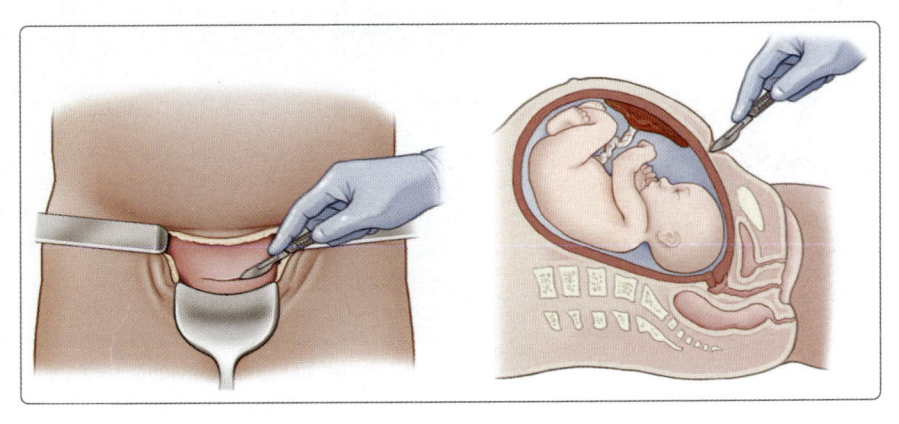

334 Chapter 9 Obstetrics and Neonatology

B Match

Match the terms in the first column with their correct definitions in the second column.

_____ 1. cesarean section
_____ 2. cervical cerclage
_____ 3. in vitro fertilization

a. method of fertilizing human ova outside the body
b. birth of a fetus through an incision in the mother's abdomen
c. suturing the cervix closed

EXERCISE 16 ■ Review of Obstetric Surgical Terms

Can you define, pronounce, and spell the following terms?

amniotomy	cesarean section	episiotomy	in vitro fertilization
cervical cerclage	(CS, C-section)		(IVF)

Obstetric and Neonatology Diagnostic Terms
BUILT FROM WORD PARTS AND *NOT* BUILT FROM WORD PARTS

The first portion of the table contains Obstetric and Neonatology Diagnostic Terms that can be translated using definitions of word parts. The second portion of the table contains Obstetric and Neonatology Diagnostic Terms that cannot be fully understood using the definitions of word parts.

■ Built from Word Parts

DIAGNOSTIC IMAGING

TERM	DEFINITION	TERM	DEFINITION
1. **amniocentesis** (am-nē-ō-sen-TĒ-sis)	surgical puncture to aspirate amniotic fluid (The needle is inserted through the abdominal and uterine walls, using ultrasound to guide the needle. It is a prenatal test in which the fluid is used for the assessment of fetal health and maturity to aid in diagnosing fetal abnormalities.) (Fig. 9.11)	2. **pelvic sonography** (PEL-vik) (so-NOG-ra-fē)	pertaining to the pelvis, process of recording sound; used extensively to evaluate the fetus and pregnancy (also called **pelvic ultrasonography, pelvic ultrasound,** and **obstetric ultrasonography**) (Fig. 9.12)

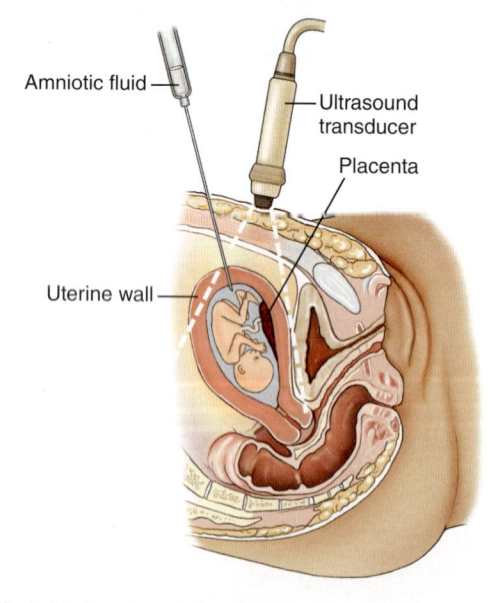

FIG. 9.11 Amniocentesis. Ultrasound is used to guide the needle through the abdominal and uterine walls.

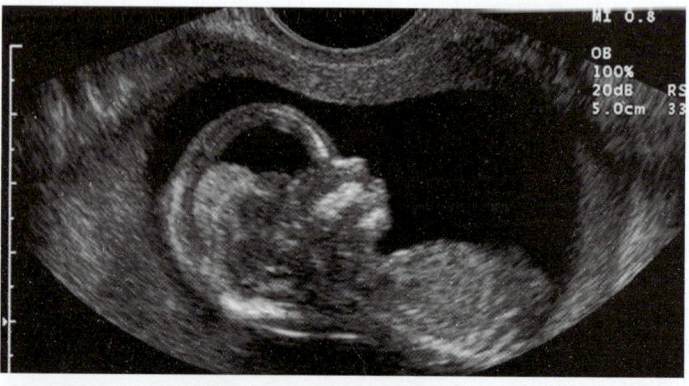

FIG. 9.12 Pelvic sonography image showing a fetal profile. Some specific uses are to: (1) diagnose early abnormal pregnancy, (2) determine the age of the fetus, (3) measure fetal growth, and (4) determine fetal position.

NOT Built from Word Parts

DIAGNOSTIC IMAGING

TERM	DEFINITION
1. nuchal translucency screening (NŪ-kal) (trans-LŪ-sen-sē) (SKRĒN-ing)	ultrasound test to check the back of the fetal neck for extra fluid or thickening. It is usually performed between 11 and 13 weeks of pregnancy and, when combined with first trimester screening blood tests, may reveal an increased risk for Down syndrome or other congenital disorders.

LABORATORY

TERM	DEFINITION
2. quad screen (kwod) (skrēn)	blood test performed during the second trimester measuring four hormone levels that can reveal an increased risk of certain disorders in the developing fetus. It measures the levels of alpha-fetoprotein, human chorionic gonadotropin, unconjugated estriol, and inhibin, and can indicate the possibility of Down syndrome (trisomy 21), trisomy 18, and neural tube defects such as spina bifida. An abnormal quad screen requires a confirming diagnostic test, such as ultrasound or amniocentesis, and genetic counseling is an important part of the workup.

OTHER

TERM	DEFINITION
3. Apgar score (AP-gar) (skor)	system for rapid neonatal assessment at 1 and 5 minutes after birth. Five vital criteria, including heart rate, respiration, muscle tone, response to stimulation, and color, are assessed and scored on a 0-2 scale, with 7-10 considered normal. (Fig. 9.13)

🏛 **APGAR SCORE** Developed in 1952 by Virginia Apgar, MD, the Apgar score provides a basic framework for rapid neonatal assessment by health care providers at 1 minute and 5 minutes after birth. Five vital criteria (**heart rate, respiration, muscle tone, response to stimulation,** and **color**) are assessed and scored on a 0-2 scale. The score is totaled, with a 5-minute Apgar score of 7 to 10 considered normal. The Apgar score is used only for quickly reporting a neonate's status and does not predict future health outcomes.

TERM	DEFINITION
4. chorionic villus sampling (CVS) (kor-ē-A-nik) (VIL-us) (SAM-pling)	prenatal test that takes a sample of the area of blood supply in the placenta either through the abdominal wall or the vagina. It is usually performed between 10 and 13 weeks of pregnancy and tests for chromosomal and other genetic problems. It has a small risk of miscarriage and is thus usually performed only in high-risk pregnancies or when a screening test is positive for an abnormality. (Fig. 9.14)

SIGN	SCORE 0	SCORE 1	SCORE 2
Heart rate	Absent	Below 100	Over 100
Respiratory effort	Absent	Slow, irregular	Good, crying
Muscle tone	Limp	Some flexion of extremities	Active motion
Response to catheter in nostril (tested after oropharynx is clear)	No response	Grimace	Cough or sneeze
Color	Blue, pale	Body pink, extremities blue	Completely pink

FIG. 9.13 Apgar Score

336 Chapter 9 Obstetrics and Neonatology

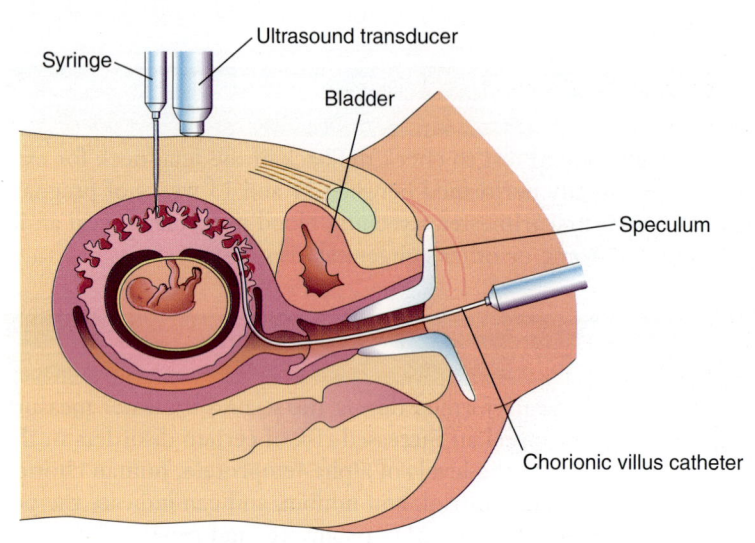

FIG. 9.14 Chorionic villus sampling.

EXERCISE 17 ■ Pronounce and Spell

Practice pronunciation and spelling on paper and online.

1. **Practice on Paper**
   a. **Pronounce:** Read the phonetic spelling and say aloud the terms listed in the previous table. Refer to Table 2.2 Pronunciation Key as needed.
   b. **Spell:** Have a study partner read the terms aloud. Write the spelling of the terms on a separate sheet of paper.

2. **Practice Online**
   a. **Access** online learning resources. Go to evolve.elsevier.com > Evolve Resources > Student Resources.
   b. **Pronounce:** Select Audio Glossary > Chapter 9 > Exercise 17. Select a term to hear its pronunciation and repeat aloud.
   c. **Spell:** Select Activities > Chapter 9 > Spell Terms > Exercise 17. Select the audio icon and type the correct spelling of the term.

❏ Check the box when complete.

EXERCISE 18 ■ Obstetric and Neonatalogy Diagnostic Terms Built from Word Parts

A Analyze and Define

Analyze and define the following obstetric and neonatology diagnostic terms.

1. amniocentesis

2. pelvic sonography

Chapter 9 Obstetrics and Neonatology   337

B Label

Build diagnostic terms pictured by writing word parts above definitions.

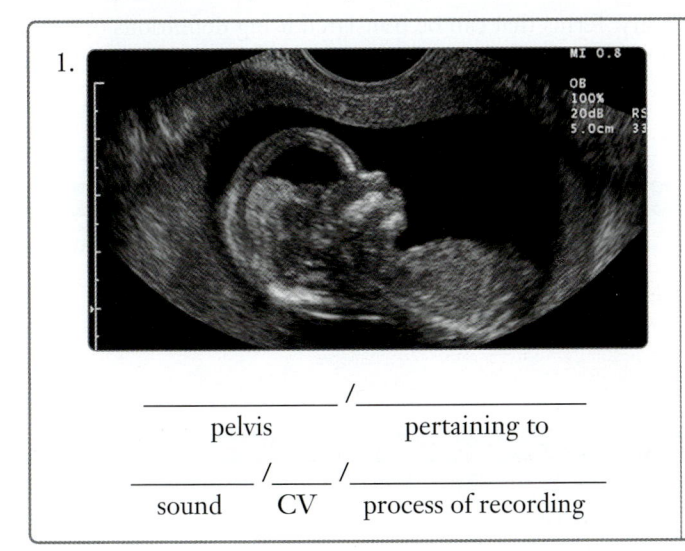

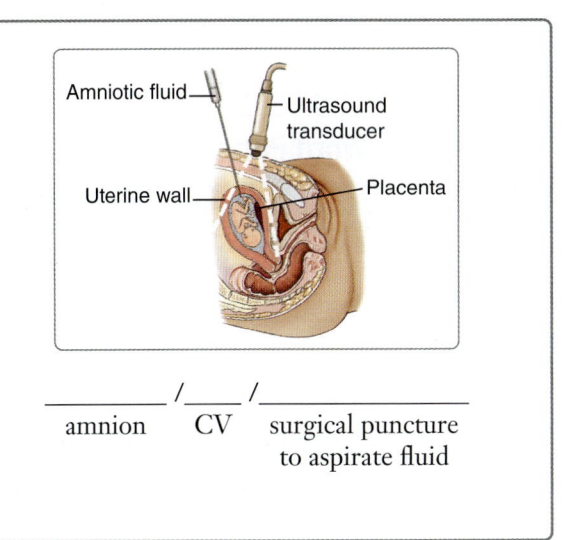

1.

_____ / _____
pelvis   pertaining to

_____ / ___ / _____
sound   CV   process of recording

2.

_____ / ___ / _____
amnion   CV   surgical puncture
                to aspirate fluid

EXERCISE 19 ■ Diagnostic Terms NOT Built from Word Parts

A Match

Match the terms in the first column with their correct definitions in the second column.

_____ 1. quad screen
_____ 2. Apgar score
_____ 3. nuchal translucency screening
_____ 4. chorionic villus sampling

a. system for rapid neonatal assessment at 1 and 5 minutes after birth
b. takes a sample of the the area of blood supply in the placenta
c. test that measures four hormone levels, can reveal increased risk
d. ultrasound test to check the back of the fetal neck for extra fluid or thickening

B Identify

Fill in the blanks with the correct terms.

1. A system for rapid neonatal assessment judging five vital criteria is called _____ _____.
2. _____ _____ _____ is usually performed between 10 and 13 weeks of pregnancy and tests for chromosomal and other genetic problems.
3. A blood test that measures levels of alpha-fetoprotein, human chorionic gonadotropin, unconjugated estriol, and inhibin is called a _____ _____.
4. _____ _____ _____ uses ultrasound to look for extra fluid or thickening, and when combined with first trimester screening blood tests, may reveal an increased risk for Down syndrome or other congenital disorders.

EXERCISE 20 ■ Review of Obstetric and Neonatology Diagnostic Terms

Can you define, pronounce, and spell the following terms?

amniocentesis	chorionic villus sampling	nuchal translucency	pelvic sonography
Apgar score	(CVS)	screening	quad screen

Obstetric Complementary Terms
BUILT FROM WORD PARTS AND *NOT* BUILT FROM WORD PARTS

The first portion of the table contains Obstetric Complementary Terms that can be translated using definitions of word parts. The second portion of the table contains Obstetric Complementary Terms that cannot be fully understood using the definitions of word parts.

■ Built from Word Parts

SIGNS AND SYMPTOMS

TERM	DEFINITION	TERM	DEFINITION
1. **amniorrhea** (*am*-nē-ō-RĒ-a)	discharge (escape) of amniotic fluid	3. **lactorrhea** (*lak*-tō-RĒ-a)	(spontaneous) discharge of milk (also called **galactorrhea**)
2. **amniorrhexis** (*am*-nē-ō-REK-sis)	rupture of the amnion		

DESCRIPTIVE TERMS

TERM	DEFINITION	TERM	DEFINITION
4. **antepartum** (*an*-tē-PAR-tum)	before childbirth (reference to the mother)	12. **nullipara** (nu-LIP-a-ra)	no births (has not given birth to a viable offspring)
5. **gravida** (GRAV-i-da)	pregnant (is or has been pregnant, regardless of pregnancy outcome)	13. **para** (PAR-a)	birth (has given birth to an offspring after the point of viability—20 weeks, whether the fetus is alive or stillborn)
6. **gravidopuerperal** (*grav*-i-dō-pū-ER-per-al)	pertaining to pregnancy and childbirth (from pregnancy until reproductive organs return to normal after delivery)	14. **postpartum** (pōst-PAR-tum)	after childbirth (reference to the mother)
		15. **primigravida** (*prī*-mi-GRAV-i-da)	first pregnancy (pregnant for the first time)
7. **intrapartum** (*in*-tra-PAR-tum)	within (during) labor and childbirth	16. **primipara (primip)** (*prī*-MIP-a-ra)	first birth (has given birth to an offspring after the point of viability—20 weeks)
8. **lactogenic** (*lak*-tō-JEN-ik)	producing milk (by stimulation)		
9. **multigravida** (*mul*-ti-GRAV-i-da)	many pregnancies (has been pregnant two or more times)	**VARIATION IN PRONUNCIATION** *Primigravida* and *primipara* are sometimes pronounced with a long **e** in the first syllable: (*prē*-mi-GRAV-i-da) and (*prē*-MIP-a-ra), respectively.	
10. **multipara (multip)** (mul-TIP-a-ra)	many births (has given birth to two or more viable offspring)	17. **puerperal** (pū-ER-per-al)	pertaining to childbirth (immediately after childbirth and the time until reproductive organs return to normal)
11. **nulligravida** (*nul*-li-GRAV-i-da)	no pregnancies (has never been pregnant)		

TABLE 9.1 Comparing Terms: Gravid/o and Par/o

GRAVID/O (PREGNANCY)	PAR/O (BIRTH)
nulli/gravid/a – no pregnancies	nulli/par/a – no births
primi/gravid/a – first pregnancy	primi/par/a – first birth
multi/gravid/a – many pregnancies	multi/par/a – many births

AN EXAMPLE OF USING GRAVIDA AND PARA IN MEDICAL SHORTHAND IN A CLINICAL SETTING
A 27 y/o G4P2113 has had **four** pregnancies, **two** term births, **one** preterm birth, **one** abortion, and has **three** living children.

NOT Built from Word Parts

SIGNS AND SYMPTOMS

TERM	DEFINITION
1. colostrum (ke-LOS-trem)	thin, milky fluid secreted by the breast during pregnancy and during the first days after birth before lactation begins
2. lochia (LŌ-kē-a)	vaginal discharge after childbirth
3. quickening (KWIK-en-ing)	first feeling of movement of the fetus in utero by the pregnant woman. It usually occurs between 16 and 20 weeks of gestation.

MEDICAL SPECIALTIES

TERM	DEFINITION
4. midwife (MID-wīf)	individual who practices midwifery
5. midwifery (MID-wif-rē)	practice of assisting in childbirth

COMPARE MIDWIFE AND DOULA Midwives practice midwifery and supervise pregnancy, labor, delivery, and puerperium. They assist with delivery independently, care for the newborn, and obtain medical assistance as necessary. A **midwife** may or may not be a registered nurse. Education, certification, and licensure vary by state and country. A **doula** (DOO-la) is a trained birth attendant who provides continual physical and emotional support to the laboring woman. **Doulas** provide a complementary role to the obstetric healthcare team.

TERM	DEFINITION
6. obstetrician (*ob*-ste-TRISH-an)	physician who specializes in obstetrics
7. obstetrics (OB) (ob-STET-riks)	medical specialty dealing with pregnancy, childbirth, and puerperium

DESCRIPTIVE TERMS

TERM	DEFINITION
8. breech presentation (brēch) (prē-zen-TĀ-shun)	birth position in which the buttocks, feet, or knees emerge first
9. cephalic presentation (se-FAL-ik) (prē-zen-TĀ-shun)	birth position in which any part of the head emerges first. It is the most common presentation.
10. in vitro (in) (VĒ-trō)	outside the body or in a lab setting
11. in vivo (in) (VĒ-vō)	within the living body

OTHER

TERM	DEFINITION
12. lactation (lak-TĀ-shun)	secretion of milk
13. parturition (*par*-tū-RISH-un)	act of giving birth
14. puerperium (*pū*-er-PĒ-rē-um)	period from delivery until the reproductive organs return to normal (approximately 6 weeks)

Refer to **Appendix E** for pharmacology terms related to obstetrics and neonatology.

340　Chapter 9　Obstetrics and Neonatology

EXERCISE 21 ■ Pronounce and Spell

Practice pronunciation and spelling on paper and online.

1. **Practice on Paper**
   a. **Pronounce:** Read the phonetic spelling and say aloud the terms listed in the previous table. Refer to Table 2.2 Pronunciation Key as needed.
   b. **Spell:** Have a study partner read the terms aloud. Write the spelling of the terms on a separate sheet of paper.

2. **Practice Online**
   a. **Access** online learning resources. Go to evolve.elsevier.com > Evolve Resources > Student Resources.
   b. **Pronounce:** Select Audio Glossary > Chapter 9 > Exercise 21. Select a term to hear its pronunciation and repeat aloud.
   c. **Spell:** Select Activities > Chapter 9 > Spell Terms > Exercise 21. Select the audio icon and type the correct spelling of the term.

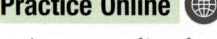

❑ Check the box when complete.

EXERCISE 22 ■ Obstetric Complementary Terms Built from Word Parts

A Analyze and Define

Analyze and define the following obstetric complementary terms.

1. multigravida

2. lactorrhea

3. puerperal

4. amniorrhea

5. nullipara

6. amniorrhexis

7. postpartum

8. primipara

9. gravida

B Label

Build terms pictured by writing word parts above definitions.

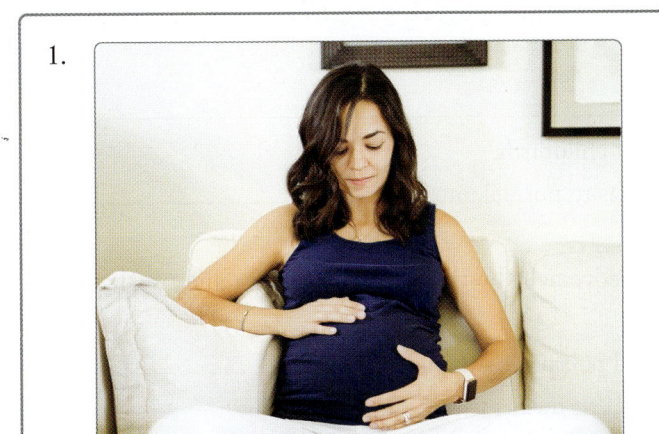

1. _____ / _____ / um
   before   childbirth
   (reference to the mother)

2. 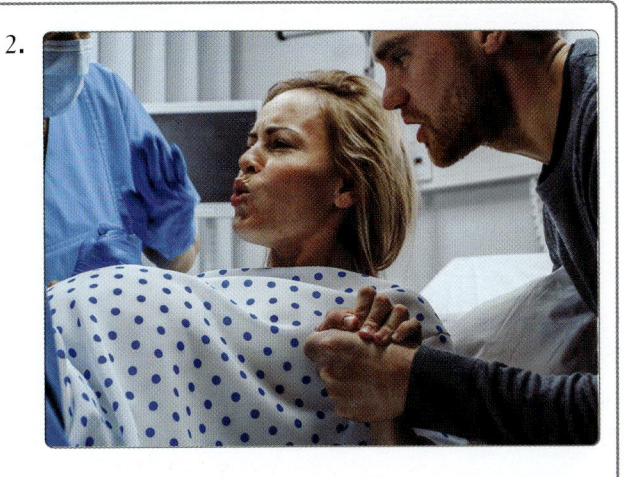 _____ / _____ / um
   within (during)   labor and childbirth

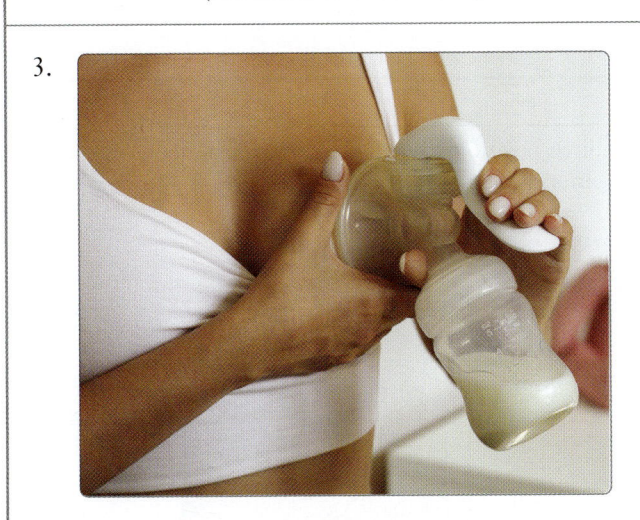

3. _____ / ___ / _____
   milk   CV   producing

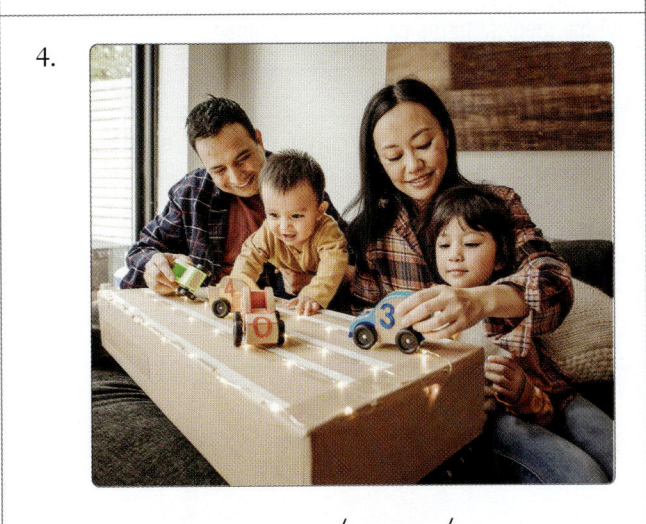

4. _____ / _____ / a
   many   births

C Fill In

Build obstetric complementary terms for the following definitions by using the word parts you have learned.

1. pertaining to pregnancy and childbirth (from pregnancy until reproductive organs return to normal after delivery)   _____ / WR / CV / WR / S

2. first pregnancy   _____ / WR / CV / WR / S

3. birth (has given birth to an offspring after the point of viability)   _____ / WR / S

4. no pregnancies (has never been pregnant)   _____ / P / WR / S

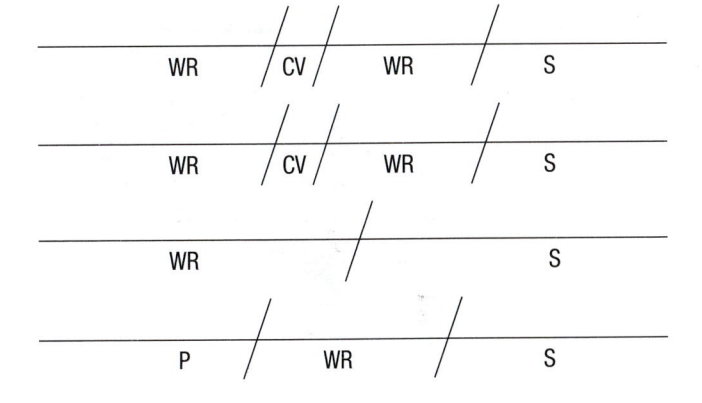

EXERCISE 23 ■ Obstetric Complementary Terms *NOT* Built from Word Parts

A Identify

Fill in the blanks with the correct terms.

1. The act of giving birth is called _____.
2. _____ is the practice of assisting in childbirth.
3. The period from delivery until the reproductive system returns to normal, or _____, lasts about 6 weeks.
4. _____ is the first feeling of fetal movement by the pregnant woman and usually occurs between 16 and 20 weeks of gestation.
5. The medical specialty dealing with pregnancy, childbirth, and puerperium is called _____.
6. _____ _____ means within the living body.
7. The thin, milky fluid secreted by the breast during pregnancy and shortly after birth is called _____.
8. _____ is vaginal discharge after childbirth.

B Label

Write the medical terms pictured and defined.

1. _____
   birth position in which any part of the head emerges first.

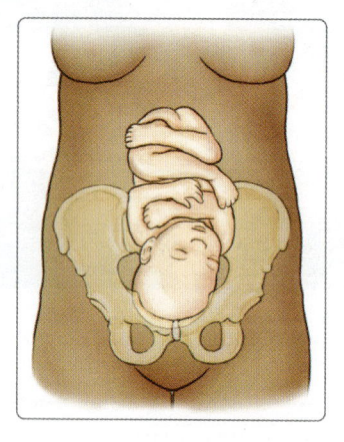

2. _____
   birth position in which the buttocks, feet, or knees emerge first

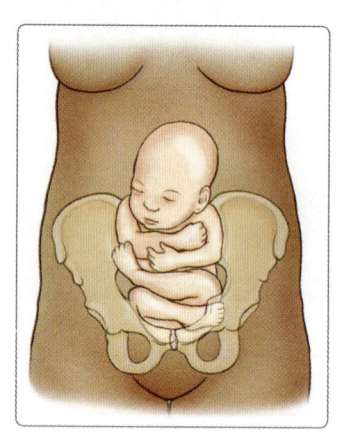

3. _____
   secretion of milk

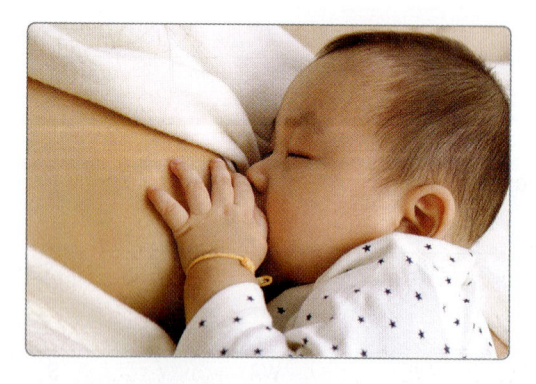

4. _____
   outside the body or in a lab setting

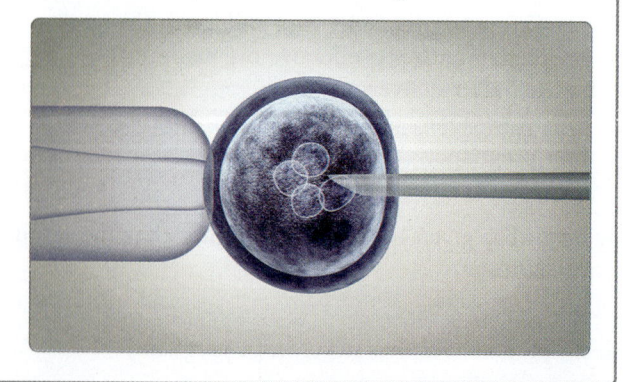

Chapter 9 Obstetrics and Neonatology 343

5. _____
individual who practices the assistance of childbirth

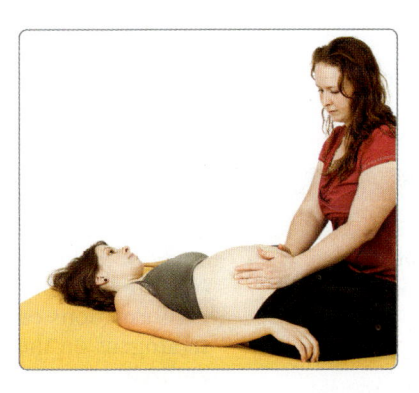

6. _____
physician who specializes in pregnancy, childbirth, and the puerperium

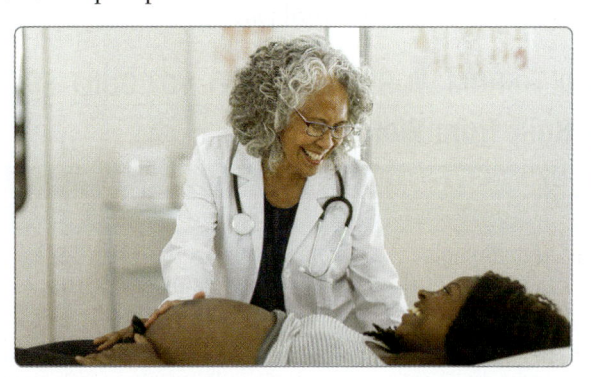

C Match

Match the terms in the first column with their correct definitions in the second column.

_____ 1. parturition
_____ 2. lochia
_____ 3. in vivo
_____ 4. lactation
_____ 5. midwifery
_____ 6. obstetrician
_____ 7. cephalic presentation

a. within the living body
b. secretion of milk
c. practice of assisting in childbirth
d. physician who specializes in pregnancy, childbirth, and the puerperium
e. act of giving birth
f. birth position in which any part of the head emerges first
g. vaginal discharge after childbirth

D Match

Match the terms in the first column with their correct definitions in the second column.

_____ 1. breech presentation
_____ 2. midwife
_____ 3. quickening
_____ 4. puerperium
_____ 5. colostrum
_____ 6. obstetrics
_____ 7. in vitro

a. period from delivery until the reproductive organs return to normal
b. thin, milky fluid secreted by the breast during pregnancy and in the first few days after
c. first feeling of movement of the fetus in utero by the pregnant woman
d. birth position in which the buttocks, feet, or knees emerge first
e. outside the body or in a lab setting
f. individual who practices assisting in childbirth
g. medical specialty dealing with pregnancy, childbirth, and the puerperium

EXERCISE 24 ■ Review of Obstetric Complementary Terms

Can you define, pronounce, and spell the following terms?

amniorrhea	intrapartum	midwifery	parturition
amniorrhexis	in vitro	multigravida	postpartum
antepartum	in vivo	multipara (multip)	primigravida
breech presentation	lactation	nulligravida	primipara (primip)
cephalic presentation	lactogenic	nullipara	puerperal
colostrum	lactorrhea	obstetrician	puerperium
gravida	lochia	obstetrics (OB)	quickening
gravidopuerperal	midwife	para	

Neonatalogy Complementary Terms

The first portion of the table contains Neonatalogy Complementary Terms that can be translated using definitions of word parts. The second portion of the table contains Neonatal Complementary Terms that cannot be fully understood using the definitions of word parts.

BUILT FROM WORD PARTS AND *NOT* BUILT FROM WORD PARTS

■ Built from Word Parts

MEDICAL SPECIALTIES

TERM	DEFINITION	TERM	DEFINITION
1. neonatologist (nē-ō-nā-TOL-o-jist)	physician who studies and treats disorders of the newborn	3. teratology (ter-a-TOL-o-jē)	study of malformations (usually in regard to malformations caused by teratogens on the developing embryo)
2. neonatology (nē-ō-nā-TOL-o-jē)	study of the newborn (branch of medicine that deals with diagnosis and treatment of disorders in newborns)		

DESCRIPTIVE TERMS

TERM	DEFINITION	TERM	DEFINITION
4. fetal (FĒ-tal)	pertaining to the fetus	8. prenatal (prē-NĀ-tal)	pertaining to before birth (reference to the newborn)
5. natal (NĀ-tal)	pertaining to birth	9. teratogen (ter-A-tō-jen)	(any agent) producing malformations (in the developing embryo)
6. neonate (NĒ-ō-nāt)	new birth (an infant from birth to 4 weeks of age) (synonymous with **newborn [NB]**)	**TERATOGENS** include drugs, alcohol, viruses, x-rays, and environmental factors.	
7. postnatal (pōst-NĀ-tal)	pertaining to after birth (reference to the newborn)	10. teratogenic (ter-a-tō-JEN-ik)	producing malformations (in the developing embryo)

■ *NOT* Built from Word Parts

SIGNS AND SYMPTOMS

TERM	DEFINITION
1. congenital anomaly (kon-JEN-i-tal) (a-NOM-a-lē)	abnormality present at birth; often discovered before birth by sonography or amniocentesis
2. meconium (me-KŌ-nē-um)	first stool of the newborn (greenish-black)

TREATMENTS

TERM	DEFINITION
3. gavage (ga-VOZH)	process of feeding through a tube; used for critically ill newborns and others who are unconscious, unable to swallow, or too weak to eat (also called **gastric gavage**)

DESCRIPTIVE TERMS

TERM	DEFINITION
4. premature infant (PRĒ-ma-tur) (IN-fent)	infant born before completing 37 weeks of gestation (also called **preterm infant**)
5. stillborn (STIL-born)	born dead (death of fetus after 20 weeks of pregnancy)

Chapter 9 Obstetrics and Neonatology 345

TABLE 9.2 Terms Relating to Mother and Newborn

	BEFORE BIRTH	AFTER BIRTH
Mother	antepartum	postpartum
Newborn	prenatal	postnatal

EXERCISE 25 ■ Pronounce and Spell

Practice pronunciation and spelling on paper and online.

1. **Practice on Paper**
   a. **Pronounce:** Read the phonetic spelling and say aloud the terms listed in the previous table. Refer to Table 2.2 Pronunciation Key as needed.
   b. **Spell:** Have a study partner read the terms aloud. Write the spelling of the terms on a separate sheet of paper.

2. **Practice Online**
   a. **Access** online learning resources. Go to evolve.elsevier.com > Evolve Resources > Student Resources.
   b. **Pronounce:** Select Audio Glossary > Chapter 9 > Exercise 25. Select a term to hear its pronunciation and repeat aloud.
   c. **Spell:** Select Activities > Chapter 9 > Spell Terms > Exercise 25. Select the audio icon and type the correct spelling of the term.

❏ Check the box when complete.

EXERCISE 26 ■ Neonatalogy Complementary Terms Built from Word Parts

A Analyze and Define

Analyze and define the following neonatology complementary terms.

1. teratogenic

2. neonatology

3. neonate

4. fetal

5. prenatal

6. teratology

7. natal

8. neonatologist

346 Chapter 9 Obstetrics and Neonatology

9. teratogen

10. postnatal

B Label

Build terms pictured by writing word parts above definitions.

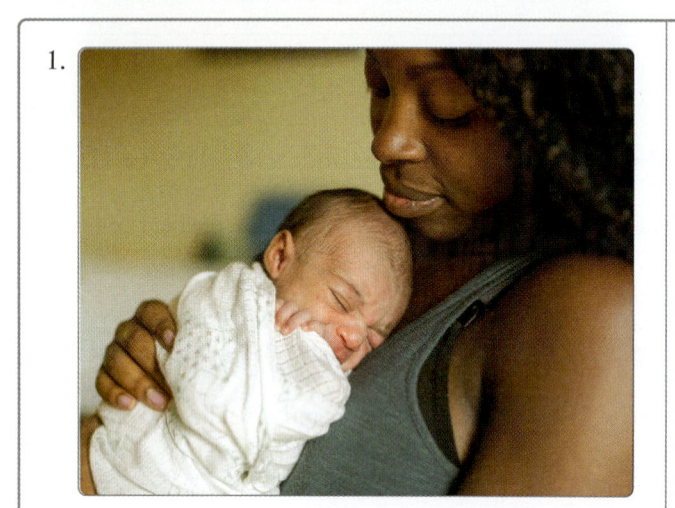

1. _____ / _____ / _____
   new   birth   noun suffix
                     (no meaning)

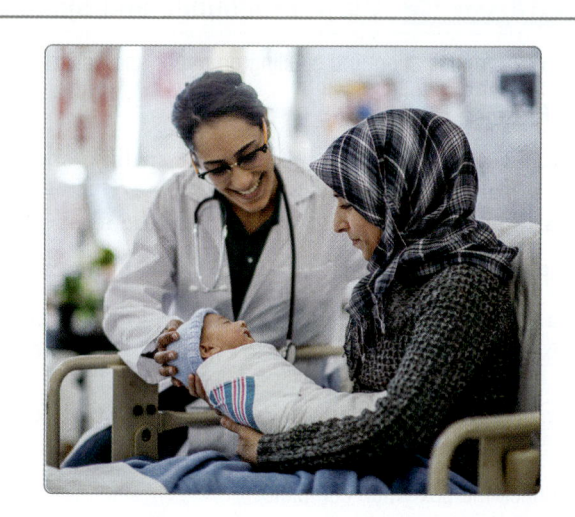

2. _____ / _____ / ____ / _____
   new   birth   CV   physician who studies
                         and treats

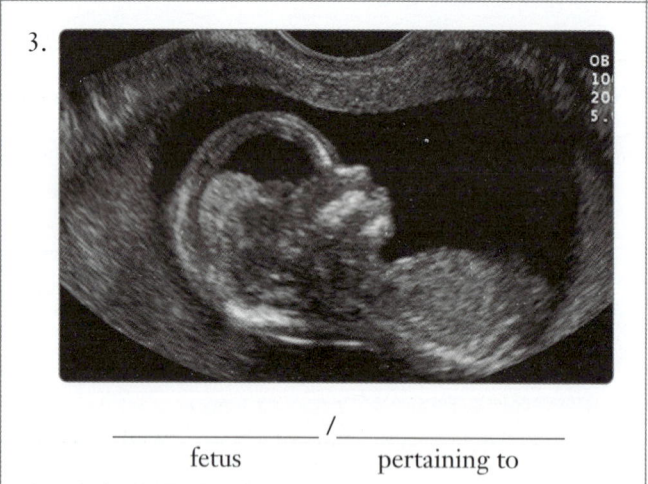

3. _____ / _____
   fetus   pertaining to

4. _____ / ____ / _____
   malformations   CV   agent that produces

C Fill In

Build neonatology complementary terms for the following definitions by using the word parts you have learned.

1. pertaining to after birth (reference to the newborn)   _____ / _____ / _____
                                                            P   WR   S

2. study of malformations   _____ / ____ / _____
                             WR   CV   S

Chapter 9   Obstetrics and Neonatology   347

3. study of the newborn

P / WR / CV / S

4. producing malformations

WR / CV / S

5. pertaining to birth

WR / S

6. pertaining to before birth (reference to the newborn)

P / WR / S

EXERCISE 27 ■ Neonatalogy Complementary Terms NOT Built from Word Parts

A Identify

Fill in the blanks with the correct terms.

1. An abnormality present at birth, _____ _____, may be discovered before birth by sonography or amniocentesis.
2. _____ is the term for the death of a fetus after 20 weeks of pregnancy.
3. The first stool of the newborn is called _____.

B Label

Write the medical terms pictured and defined.

1. _____
   process of feeding through a tube

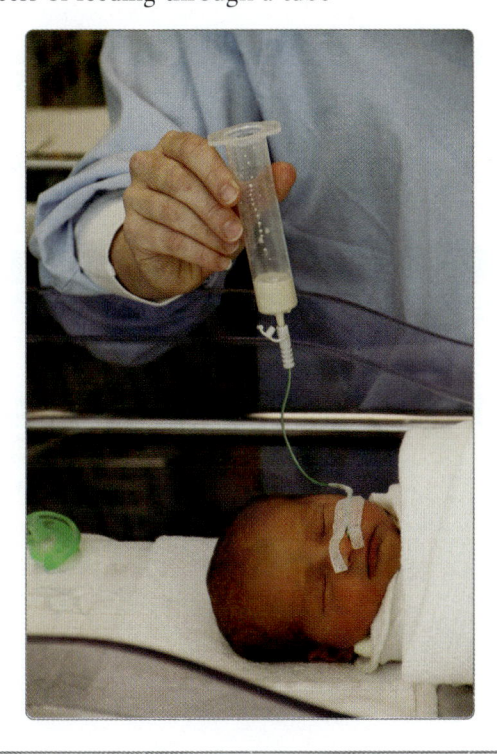

2. _____
   infant born before completing 37 weeks of gestation

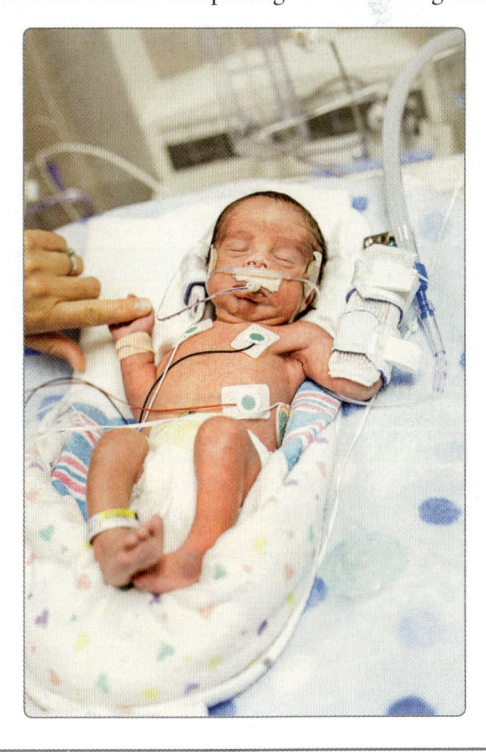

C Match

Match the terms in the first column with their correct definitions in the second column.

_____ 1. meconium   a. infant born before completing 37 weeks of gestation
_____ 2. stillborn   b. abnormality present at birth
_____ 3. gavage   c. process of feeding through a tube
_____ 4. premature infant   d. first stool of the newborn
_____ 5. congenital anomaly e. born dead (death of fetus after 20 weeks of pregnancy)

EXERCISE 28 ■ Review of Neonatalogy Complementary Terms

Can you define, pronounce, and spell the following terms?

congenital anomaly	natal	postnatal	teratogen
fetal	neonate	premature infant	teratogenic
gavage	neonatologist	prenatal	teratology
meconium	neonatology	stillborn	

Abbreviations

DISEASES AND DISORDERS

ABBREVIATION	TERM	ABBREVIATION	TERM
APH	antepartum hemorrhage	PAS	placenta accreta spectrum
CMV	cytomegalovirus	PPH	postpartum hemorrhage
FAS	fetal alcohol syndrome	RDS	respiratory distress syndrome

DIAGNOSTIC

ABBREVIATION	TERM
CVS	chorionic villus sampling

TREATMENT

ABBREVIATION	TERM	ABBREVIATION	TERM
AB	abortion	IVF	in vitro fertilization
CS, C-section	cesarean section	VBAC	vaginal birth after cesarean (section); spoken as (VĔ-bak)

MEDICAL SPECIALTIES

ABBREVIATION	TERM
OB	obstetrics

DESCRIPTIVE

ABBREVIATION	TERM	ABBREVIATION	TERM
multip	multipara; spoken as a whole word (MUL-tip)	primip	primipara; spoken as a whole word (PRĪ-mip)
NB	newborn		

Chapter 9 Obstetrics and Neonatology 349

OTHER			
ABBREVIATION	**TERM**	**ABBREVIATION**	**TERM**
DOB	date of birth	**LMP**	last menstrual period
EDD	expected (estimated) date of delivery		

Refer to **Appendix D** for a complete list of abbreviations.

EXERCISE 29 ■ Fill In

Write the terms abbreviated.

1. The **EDD** _____ _____ _____ for a pregnant woman is based on the date of the first day of her **LMP** _____ _____ _____; a first trimester ultrasound may help if this date is unclear. An infant's **DOB** _____ _____ _____ may occur before or after this date.

2. **OB** _____ pertains to the care of the mother during pregnancy, delivery, and the puerperium, while neonatology deals with care of the **NB** _____.

3. A **primip** _____ has given birth to only one offspring, but a **multip** _____ has given birth to two or more.

4. **CVS** _____ _____ _____ can be used earlier in pregnancy than amniocentesis to diagnose genetic disorders such as Down syndrome; however, it has a greater risk of spontaneous **AB** _____, and thus is usually only used when quad screens or other tests are abnormal, or in very high-risk pregnancies.

5. **FAS** _____ _____ _____ is caused by a known teratogen, and no amount of alcohol is considered safe during pregnancy.

6. Congenital **CMV** _____ infection can be acquired from the mother at any time during pregnancy, but it most often occurs in the third trimester (the last 13 weeks of pregnancy).

7. For women who are at risk of premature delivery, corticosteroids can be given to help reduce the symptoms of **RDS** _____ _____ _____.

8. **CS** _____ _____, also abbreviated as **C-section**, may be performed for a number of reasons, including nonreassuring fetal status, failure to progress during labor, or breech presentation.

9. On a later pregnancy, women who have had a previous C-section may choose to repeat this procedure, or they may consider **VBAC** _____ _____ _____ _____ (section), provided their risk for hysterorrhexis is low.

10. Since the first birth due to **IVF** _____ _____ _____ in 1978, more than 7 million pregnancies have been achieved by this and other assisted reproductive technologies.

11. Placental disorders include abruptio placentae, placenta previa, and **PAS** _____ _____ _____. Abruptio placentae and placenta previa can cause **APH** _____ _____ _____, while PAS can cause **PPH** _____ _____.

Chapter 9 Obstetrics and Neonatology

PRACTICAL APPLICATION

EXERCISE 30 ■ Case Study: Translate Between Everyday Language and Medical Language

CASE STUDY: Charlene Birch

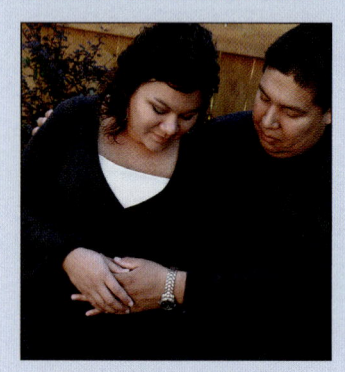

Charlene Birch is pregnant for the third time. She gave birth to one healthy baby about 4 years ago. The other baby was born dead when she was about 7 months into her pregnancy. Now she is about 3 months pregnant. She had an ultrasound test done when she first found out she was pregnant. This week she had some blood tests done, and the doctor told her that the results suggest that her developing baby may have a genetic condition that causes physical and mental problems. He is suggesting a test where they use a needle to take fluid out of her womb and look at it under a microscope. She and her husband are very concerned and are not sure what to do.

Now that you have worked through Chapter 9 on obstetrics and neonatology, consider the medical terms that might be used to describe Charlene's experience. See the Chapter at a Glance section at the end of the chapter for a list of terms that might apply.

A. Underline phrases in the case study that could be substituted with medical terms presented in Chapter 9 and previous chapters.

B. Write the medical term and its definition for three of the phrases you underlined.

MEDICAL TERM	DEFINITION
1. _____	_____
2. _____	_____
3. _____	_____

DOCUMENTATION: Excerpt from the Obstetrics Clinic Visit

Charlene is a 37-year-old gravida 3 para 2 female with an EDD of January 15, 20xx. Her prenatal history has been unremarkable up to this point. Recently, however, her prenatal screening tests came back suspicious for Down syndrome. I have recommended an amniocentesis to confirm this diagnosis. She is aware of the risks of the procedure, including the small possibility of spontaneous abortion. I have recommended that she have a very close follow-up. We will attempt to detect any conditions of concern, including cardiac congenital anomalies or gastrointestinal malformation such as tracheoesophageal fistula. We will plan to have a neonatologist present at the time of birth.

C. Underline medical terms presented in Chapter 9 used in the previous excerpt from Charlene's medical record. See the Chapter at a Glance section at the end of the chapter for a complete list.

D. Select and define three of the medical terms you underlined. To check your answers, go to Appendix A.

MEDICAL TERM	DEFINITION
1. _____	_____
2. _____	_____
3. _____	_____

Chapter 9   Obstetrics and Neonatology   351

EXERCISE 31 ■ Interact with Medical Documents

A

Read the report and complete it by writing medical terms on answer lines within the document. Definitions of terms to be written appear after the document.

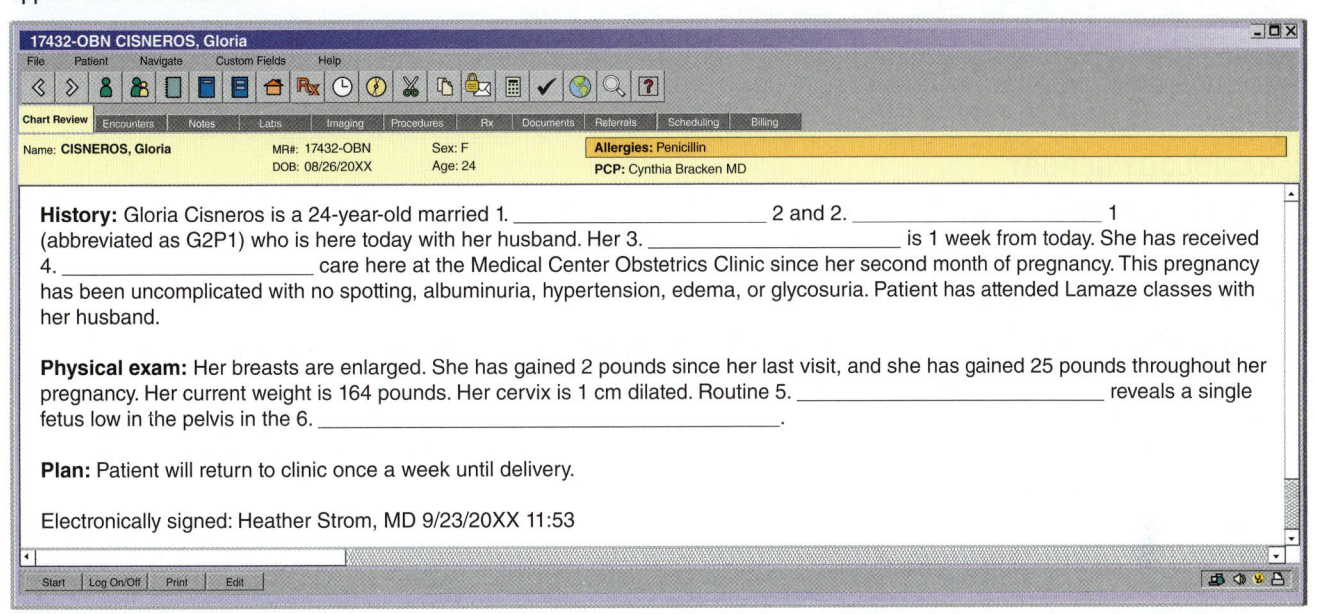

17432-OBN CISNEROS, Gloria

File   Patient   Navigate   Custom Fields   Help

Chart Review | Encounters | Notes | Labs | Imaging | Procedures | Rx | Documents | Referrals | Scheduling | Billing

Name: CISNEROS, Gloria   **MR#:** 17432-OBN   **Sex:** F   **Allergies:** Penicillin
                              DOB: 08/26/20XX   **Age:** 24   **PCP:** Cynthia Bracken MD

History: Gloria Cisneros is a 24-year-old married 1. _____ 2 and 2. _____ 1 (abbreviated as G2P1) who is here today with her husband. Her 3. _____ is 1 week from today. She has received 4. _____ care here at the Medical Center Obstetrics Clinic since her second month of pregnancy. This pregnancy has been uncomplicated with no spotting, albuminuria, hypertension, edema, or glycosuria. Patient has attended Lamaze classes with her husband.

Physical exam: Her breasts are enlarged. She has gained 2 pounds since her last visit, and she has gained 25 pounds throughout her pregnancy. Her current weight is 164 pounds. Her cervix is 1 cm dilated. Routine 5. _____ reveals a single fetus low in the pelvis in the 6. _____.

Plan: Patient will return to clinic once a week until delivery.

Electronically signed: Heather Strom, MD 9/23/20XX 11:53

Start | Log On/Off | Print | Edit

🏛 **LAMAZE** is a method of psychophysical preparation for childbirth started in the 1950s by a French obstetrician, Fernand Lamaze. The method requires classes and practice before and coaching during labor and delivery.

Definitions of Medical Terms to Complete the Document

Write the medical terms defined on corresponding answer lines in the document.

1. pregnant (is or has been pregnant, regardless of pregnancy outcome)
2. birth
3. abbreviation for expected delivery date
4. pertaining to before birth (reference to the newborn)
5. pertaining to the pelvis, process of recording sound
6. birth position in which any part of the head emerges first

352 Chapter 9 Obstetrics and Neonatology

B

Read the medical report and answer the questions below it.

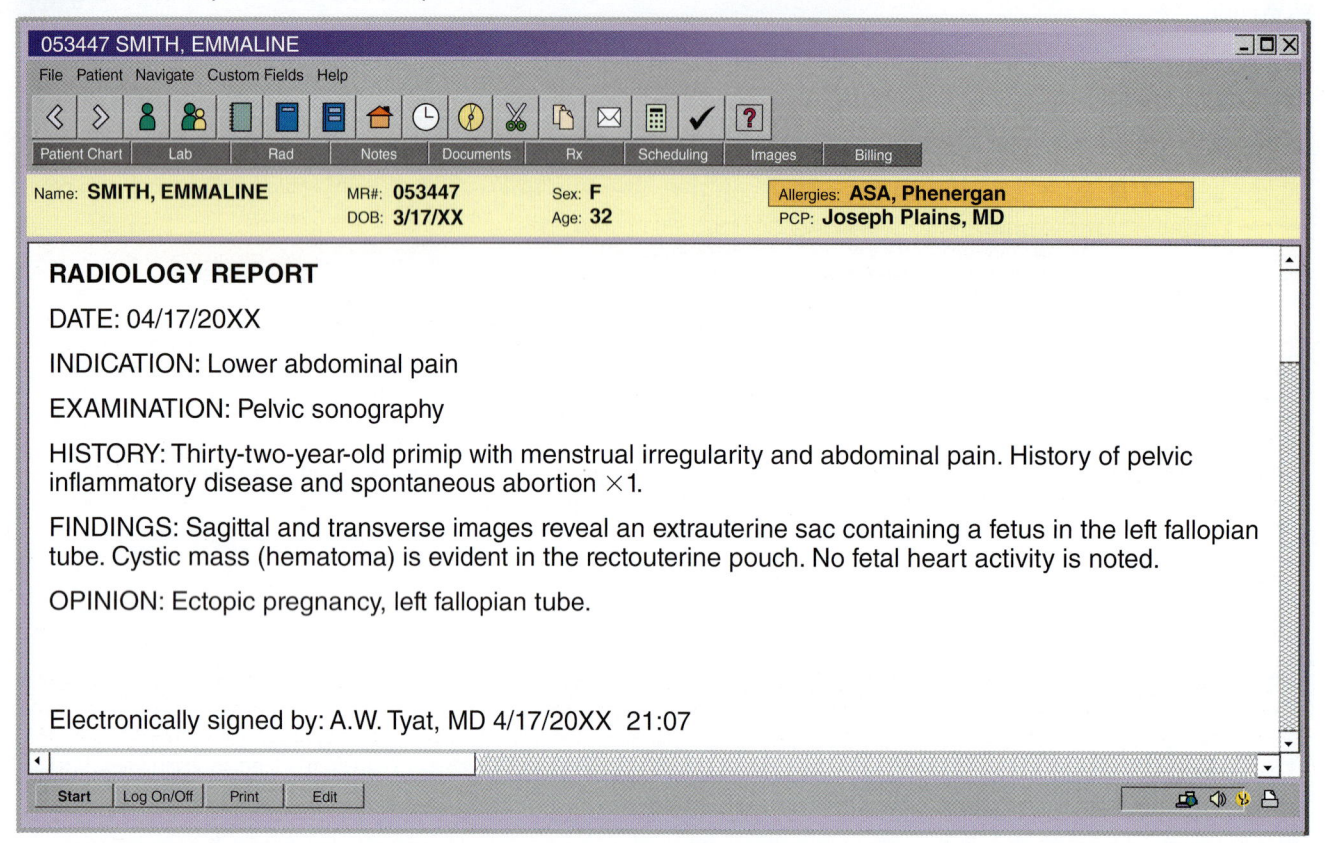

053447 SMITH, EMMALINE

File Patient Navigate Custom Fields Help

| Patient Chart | Lab | Rad | Notes | Documents | Rx | Scheduling | Images | Billing |

Name: **SMITH, EMMALINE**   MR#: **053447**   Sex: **F**   Allergies: **ASA, Phenergan**
                             DOB: **3/17/XX**   Age: **32**   PCP: **Joseph Plains, MD**

RADIOLOGY REPORT

DATE: 04/17/20XX

INDICATION: Lower abdominal pain

EXAMINATION: Pelvic sonography

HISTORY: Thirty-two-year-old primip with menstrual irregularity and abdominal pain. History of pelvic inflammatory disease and spontaneous abortion ×1.

FINDINGS: Sagittal and transverse images reveal an extrauterine sac containing a fetus in the left fallopian tube. Cystic mass (hematoma) is evident in the rectouterine pouch. No fetal heart activity is noted.

OPINION: Ectopic pregnancy, left fallopian tube.

Electronically signed by: A.W. Tyat, MD 4/17/20XX 21:07

Use the medical report above to answer the questions.

1. The patient has:
   a. never been pregnant
   b. given birth to two or more viable offspring
   c. borne one viable offspring

2. **True** or **False** The patient has experienced one abortion.

3. **True** or **False** Radiographic images were used to determine the findings.

EXERCISE 32 ■ Use Medical Terms in Clinical Statements

For each phrase printed in bold, circle the medical term or abbreviation defined. Answers are listed in Appendix A. For pronunciation practice read the answers aloud.

1. The patient who **had never been pregnant** was identified in the medical record as (nulligravida, nullipara, puerpera), whereas the patient who **had never given birth to a viable offspring** was identified as (nulligravida, nullipara, puerpera).

2. Antepartum hemorrhage may be caused by the **abnormally low implantation of the placenta on the uterine wall covering the cervix** (abruptio placentae, placenta accreta spectrum, placenta previa) or **the premature separation of the placenta from the uterine wall** (abruptio placentae, placenta accreta spectrum, placenta previa). Postpartum hemorrhage may be caused by the **growth of the placenta into the uterine wall, resulting in the inability to detach** (abruptio placentae, placenta accreta spectrum, placenta previa).

Chapter 9   Obstetrics and Neonatology   353

3. During the **period of time from delivery until the reproductive organs return to normal** (quickening, parturition, puerperium), the amount of **vaginal discharge after childbirth** (lochia, colostrum, lactation) decreases and changes to a watery consistency.

4. The neonate with **congenital absence of part of the esophagus** (erythroblastosis fetalis, esophageal atresia, CMV infection) required **process of feeding through a tube** (gavage, lactation, colostrum).

5. **After childbirth** (prenatal, intrapartum, postpartum) depression is a common but treatable condition.

EXERCISE 33 ■ Use Medical Language in Online Electronic Health Records

Select the correct medical terms to complete three medical records in one patient's electronic file.

Access online resources at evolve.elsevier.com > Evolve Resources > Student Resources > Activities > Chapter 9 > Electronic Health Records

Topic: Cesarean Section
Record 1, Procedures: Operative Report
Record 2, Imaging: Ultrasound Report
Record 3, Notes: Obstetrics Delivery Note

❏ Check the box when complete.

EXERCISE 34 ■ Pronounce Medical Terms in Use

Practice pronunciation of terms by reading aloud the following paragraph. Use the phonetic spellings to assist with pronunciation. The script also contains medical terms not presented in the chapter. If interested, research their meanings in a medical dictionary or a reliable online source.

> Josephine Alcotts is a 34-year-old **gravida** (GRAV-i-da) 2 **para** (PAR-a) 1 woman. Her LMP was April 20, 20XX. The EDD is January 25, 20XX. The **obstetrician** (ob-ste-TRISH-an) prescribed folic acid to prevent **spina bifida** (SPĪ-na) (BIF-i-da). The patient's first pregnancy was complicated by **preeclampsia** (prē-ē-KLAMP-sē-a) and a **breech presentation** (brēch) (prē-zen-TĀ-shun), which required a **cesarean section** (se-ZĀR-ē-an) (SEK-shun). **Pelvic sonography** (PEL-vik) (so-NOG-ra-fē) showed a single female fetus with normal development. She went on to deliver a healthy baby by VBAC 3 days before her expected delivery date.

CHAPTER REVIEW

EXERCISE 35 — Chapter Content Quiz

Test your understanding of terms and abbreviations introduced in this chapter. Circle the letter for the medical term, definition, or abbreviation related to the words in italics.

1. During the second trimester, the patient had a pelvic sonogram, which revealed *less than the normal amount of amniotic fluid*. Etiology may be related to disorders of the fetal urinary system.
   a. chorioamnionitis
   b. oligohydramnios
   c. polyhydramnios

2. Because of inadequate uterine contractions, the patient was experiencing *difficult labor*.
   a. dysphasia
   b. dystocia
   c. dysuria

3. Down syndrome can be diagnosed by two prenatal tests: chorionic villus sampling done at 10 to 13 weeks of pregnancy, or a *surgical puncture to aspirate amniotic fluid* after 15 weeks of pregnancy.
   a. amniocentesis
   b. CVS
   c. amniorrhea

4. Infection of the Zika virus during pregnancy is linked to an increase in premature births, blindness, neurological disorders, and *small head*s in newborns.
   a. microcephalus
   b. omphalocele
   c. gastroschisis

5. *Antepartum* hemorrhage is considered an emergency.
   a. during labor
   b. after childbirth
   c. before childbirth

6. In the EHR, the medical assistant recorded that the patient *has never been pregnant*.
   a. nullipara
   b. nulligravida
   c. prenatal

7. At 20 weeks of gestation, the patient was diagnosed with preeclampsia. The *disease progressed and she began having convulsions*. She was then diagnosed as having:
   a. eclampsia
   b. abruptio placentae
   c. placenta previa

8. The premature newborn with tachypnea and cyanosis of the skin and mucous membranes was diagnosed with *RDS*.
   a. respiratory distress symptom
   b. right dominant syndrome
   c. respiratory distress syndrome

9. The mother was experiencing *vaginal discharge* throughout her postpartum period.
   a. lactation
   b. lochia
   c. meconium

10. The drug thalidomide taken during pregnancy was a *producing malformation* risk for the fetus.
    a. lactogenic
    b. teratogenic
    c. embryogenic

11. After a complete infertility evaluation, the physician recommended *IVF* for the couple.
    a. in vivo fertilization
    b. in vitro fertilization
    c. in vitro fetus

12. The patient was *pregnant with her third child*. She was referred to as:
    a. multigravida
    b. multipara
    c. nullipara

13. The patient required a *cesarean section* when her labor failed to progress, and a low fetal heart rate was detected.
    a. CMV
    b. CVS
    c. CS

14. The premature infant was unable to nurse on her own; thus *process of feeding through a tube* was recommended.
    a. cesarean section
    b. gavage
    c. amniocentesis

15. *Congenital stenosis that occurs in the arch of the aorta* was discovered on the fetal ultrasound.
    a. coarctation of the aorta
    b. congenital cytomegalovirus infection
    c. Down syndrome

16. A woman with a previous history of premature labor and delivery underwent *suturing the cervix closed to prevent dilation and premature delivery* during her second trimester.
    a. cervicitis
    b. cervical cerclage
    c. cervicectomy

17. *Congenital fissure of the abdominal wall that is not at the umbilicus* is most commonly diagnosed by ultrasound around 18 to 20 weeks of pregnancy.
    a. omphalitis
    b. omphalocele
    c. gastroschisis

18. The physician ordered an amniocentesis after the patient had an abnormal *blood test performed during the second trimester measuring four hormone levels that can reveal an increased risk of certain disorders in the developing fetus*.
    a. quad screen
    b. Apgar score
    c. pelvic sonography

19. The obstetrician ordered a(n) *ultrasound test to check the back of the fetal neck for extra fluid or thickening*, along with blood tests, at the patient's first prenatal visit.
    a. chorionic villus sampling
    b. pelvic sonography
    c. nuchal translucency screening

20. Gamete intrafallopian transfer is another form of reproductive technology that is performed *outside the body or in a lab setting*.
    a. in vivo
    b. in vitro
    c. en vivo

CHAPTER AT A GLANCE — Word Parts New to This Chapter

COMBINING FORMS
amni/o
amnion/o
cephal/o
chori/o
esophag/o
fet/o
gravid/o
lact/o
nat/o
omphal/o
par/o
part/o

prim/i
pseud/o
puerper/o
pylor/o
terat/o

PREFIXES
ante-
multi-
nulli-
post-
pre-

SUFFIXES
-amnios
-cyesis
-e
-is
-rrhexis

-tocia
-um
-us

CHAPTER AT A GLANCE — Obstetric and Neonatology Terms Built from Word Parts

OBSTETRIC DISEASE AND DISORDER
amnionitis
chorioamnionitis
choriocarcinoma
dystocia
hysterorrhexis
oligohydramnios
polyhydramnios
pseudocyesis

NEONATAL DISEASE AND DISORDER
laryngomalacia
microcephalus
omphalitis

omphalocele
pyloric stenosis
tracheoesophageal fistula

OBSTETRIC SURGICAL
amniotomy
episiotomy

DIAGNOSTIC
amniocentesis
pelvic sonography

OBSTETRIC COMPLEMENTARY
amniorrhea

amniorrhexis
antepartum
gravida
gravidopuerperal
intrapartum
lactogenic
lactorrhea
multigravida
multipara (multip)
nulligravida
nullipara
para
postpartum
primigravida
primipara (primip)
puerperal

NEONATAL COMPLEMENTARY
fetal
natal
neonate
neonatologist
neonatology
postnatal
prenatal
teratogen
teratogenic
teratology

CHAPTER AT A GLANCE: Obstetric and Neonatal Terms NOT Built from Word Parts

OBSTETRIC DISEASE AND DISORDER
abortion (AB)
abruptio placentae
eclampsia
ectopic pregnancy
placenta accreta spectrum (PAS)
placenta previa
preeclampsia

NEONATAL DISEASE AND DISORDER
cleft lip or palate
coarctation of the aorta
congenital cytomegalovirus infection (CMV)
congenital heart disease
Down syndrome
erythroblastosis fetalis
esophageal atresia
fetal alcohol syndrome (FAS)
gastroschisis
respiratory distress syndrome (RDS)
spina bifida

OBSTETRIC SURGICAL
cervical cerclage
cesarean section (CS, C-section)
in vitro fertilization (IVF)

DIAGNOSTIC
Apgar score
chorionic villus sampling (CVS)
nuchal translucency screening
quad screen

OBSTETRIC COMPLEMENTARY
breech presentation
cephalic presentation
colostrum
in vitro
in vivo
lactation
lochia
midwife
midwifery
obstetrician
obstetrics (OB)
parturition
puerperium
quickening

NEONATAL COMPLEMENTARY
congenital anomaly
gavage
meconium
premature infant
stillborn

PART 2 BODY SYSTEMS

Cardiovascular, Lymphatic, Immune Systems and Blood

10

Outline

ANATOMY, 358
Cardiovascular System, 358
Blood, 360
Lymphatic System, 361
Immune System, 363

WORD PARTS, 364
Anatomic Structures Combining Forms, 364
Combining Forms Used with Cardiovascular, Blood, Lymphatic, and Immune System Terms, 364
Prefixes, 364
Suffixes, 364

MEDICAL TERMS, 369
Cardiovascular System Terms, 369
 Built from Word Parts, 369
 NOT Built from Word Parts, 376
Blood Terms, 390
 Built from Word Parts, 390
 NOT Built from Word Parts, 393
Lymphatic System Terms, 398
 Built from Word Parts and
  NOT Built from Word Parts, 398
Immune System Terms, 401
 Built from Word Parts and
  NOT Built from Word Parts, 401
Abbreviations, 405

PRACTICAL APPLICATION, 408
CASE STUDY Translate Between Everyday Language and Medical Language, 408
Interact with Medical Documents, 409
Use Medical Language in Online Electronic Health Records, 410
Use Medical Terms in Clinical Statements, 411
Pronounce Medical Terms in Use, 411

CHAPTER REVIEW, 412
Chapter Content Quiz, 412
Chapter at a Glance, 413

Answers to Chapter Exercises, Appendix A

Objectives

Upon completion of this chapter, you will be able to:

1. Pronounce organs and anatomic structures.
2. Define and spell word parts.
3. Define, pronounce, and spell cardiovascular system terms.
4. Define, pronounce, and spell blood terms.
5. Define, pronounce, and spell lymphatic system terms.
6. Define, pronounce, and spell immune system terms.
7. Interpret the meaning of abbreviations presented in the chapter.
8. Apply medical language in clinical contexts.

TABLE 10.1 Types of Angiography, 371
TABLE 10.2 Understanding a Lipid Profile, 382
TABLE 10.3 Common Types of Anemia, 393
TABLE 10.4 Leukemia, 393

ANATOMY

At first glance this may seem like an overabundance of material in one chapter. It is a lot to cover, but as you will see, **the systems have interactive functions**. The lymphatic and immune systems support each other by providing an immune response to invading microorganisms and foreign substances. The lymphatic system and blood share macrophages and lymphocytes. Lymph is drained into large veins of the cardiovascular system, and the cardiovascular system is responsible for circulating blood throughout the body.

Cardiovascular System

The cardiovascular system consists of the heart and a closed network of blood vessels composed of arteries, capillaries, and veins (Fig. 10.1).

FUNCTION

The heart functions as two pumps operating simultaneously. The right side of the heart pumps blood to the lungs while the left side pumps blood to the rest of the body. The exchange of gases, nutrients, and waste between the blood and body tissue takes place in the capillaries. The blood with carbon dioxide and waste is carried from the tissues through veins to organs of excretion. The cardiovascular system also serves a critical role in the body's ability to regulate temperature.

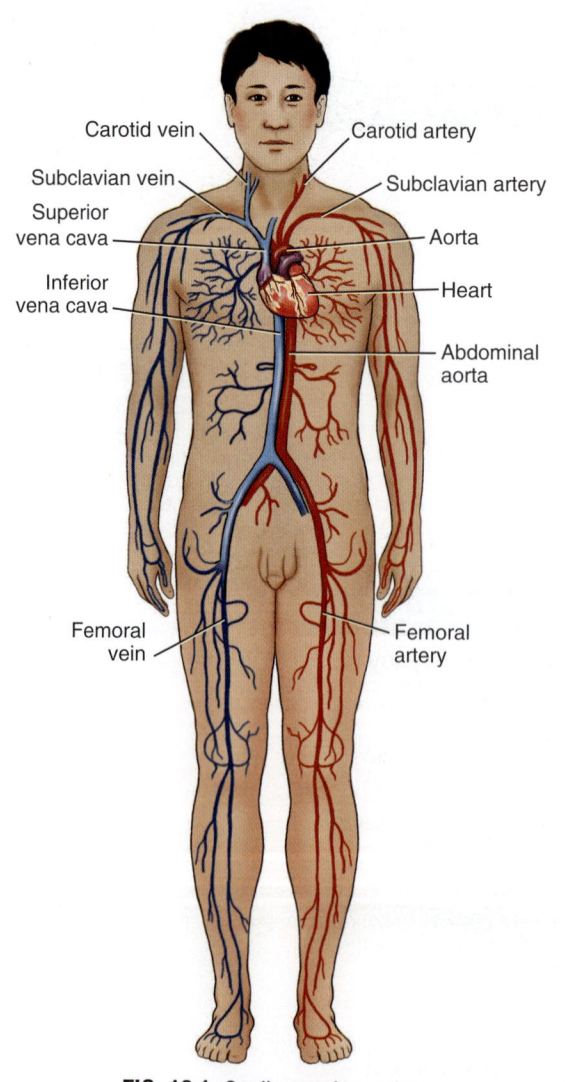

FIG. 10.1 Cardiovascular system.

Organs and Anatomic Structures of the Cardiovascular System

TERM	DEFINITION
heart (hart)	muscular cone-shaped organ the size of a fist, located behind and slightly to the left of the sternum (breastbone) and between the lungs. The pumping action of the heart circulates blood throughout the body. The heart consists of two smaller upper chambers, the **right atrium** and the **left atrium** (*pl.* **atria**), and two larger lower chambers, the **right ventricle** and the **left ventricle** (*pl.* **ventricles**). The right atrium receives blood returning from the body through the veins and contracts to fill the right ventricle, which then pumps blood to the lungs. The left atrium receives blood from the lungs and contracts to fill the left ventricle, which then contracts to pump blood from the heart through the arteries to body tissues. The **atrial septum** separates the atria and the **ventricular septum** separates the ventricles. (Fig. 10.2)
atrioventricular valves (*ā*-trē-ō-ven-TRIK-ū-ler) (valvz)	consist of the **tricuspid** and **mitral** valves, which lie between the right atrium and the right ventricle and the left atrium and left ventricle, respectively. Valves of the heart keep blood flowing in one direction.
semilunar valves (*sem*-ē-LOO-ner) (valvz)	**pulmonary** and **aortic** valves located between the right ventricle and the pulmonary artery and between the left ventricle and the aorta, respectively.
pericardium (*per*-i-KAR-dē-um)	two-layer sac surrounding the heart, consisting of an external fibrous and an internal serous layer. The internal serous layer is then divided into two parts: the outer layer, called the parietal pericardium, and the inner layer, called the epicardium. Between these is the pericardial space, which contains fluid produced by the serous layer that allows the heart to move without friction.
epicardium (*ep*-i-KAR-dē-um)	outer lining covering the heart (also called **visceral pericardium**)
myocardium (*my*-ō-KAR-dē-um)	middle, thick, muscular layer of the heart
endocardium (*en*-dō-KAR-dē-um)	inner lining of the heart
blood vessels (blud) (VES-els)	tubelike structures that carry blood throughout the body (Fig. 10.3)
arteries (AR-ter-ēz)	blood vessels that carry blood away from the heart. All arteries, with the exception of the pulmonary artery, carry oxygen and other nutrients from the heart to the body cells. The **pulmonary artery**, in contrast, carries carbon dioxide and other waste products from the heart to the lungs.
arterioles (ar-TĒR-ē-ōlz)	smallest arteries
aorta (ā-OR-ta)	largest artery in the body, which originates at the left ventricle, briefly ascends as the arch of the aorta, then descends through the thorax and abdomen
veins (vānz)	blood vessels that carry blood back to the heart. All veins, with the exception of the pulmonary veins, carry blood containing carbon dioxide and other waste products. The **pulmonary veins** carry oxygenated blood from the lungs to the heart.
venules (VEN-ūlz)	smallest veins
venae cavae (VĒ-nā) (KĀ-vā)	largest veins in the body. The **inferior vena cava** carries oxygen-poor blood to the right ventricle of the heart from body parts below the diaphragm, and the **superior vena cava** returns the blood to the right ventricle of the heart from the upper part of the body.
capillaries (KAP-i-*lār*-ēz)	microscopic blood vessels that connect arterioles with venules. Materials are passed between the blood and tissue through the capillary walls.

FIG. 10.2 Interior of the heart.

FIG. 10.3 Types of blood vessels.

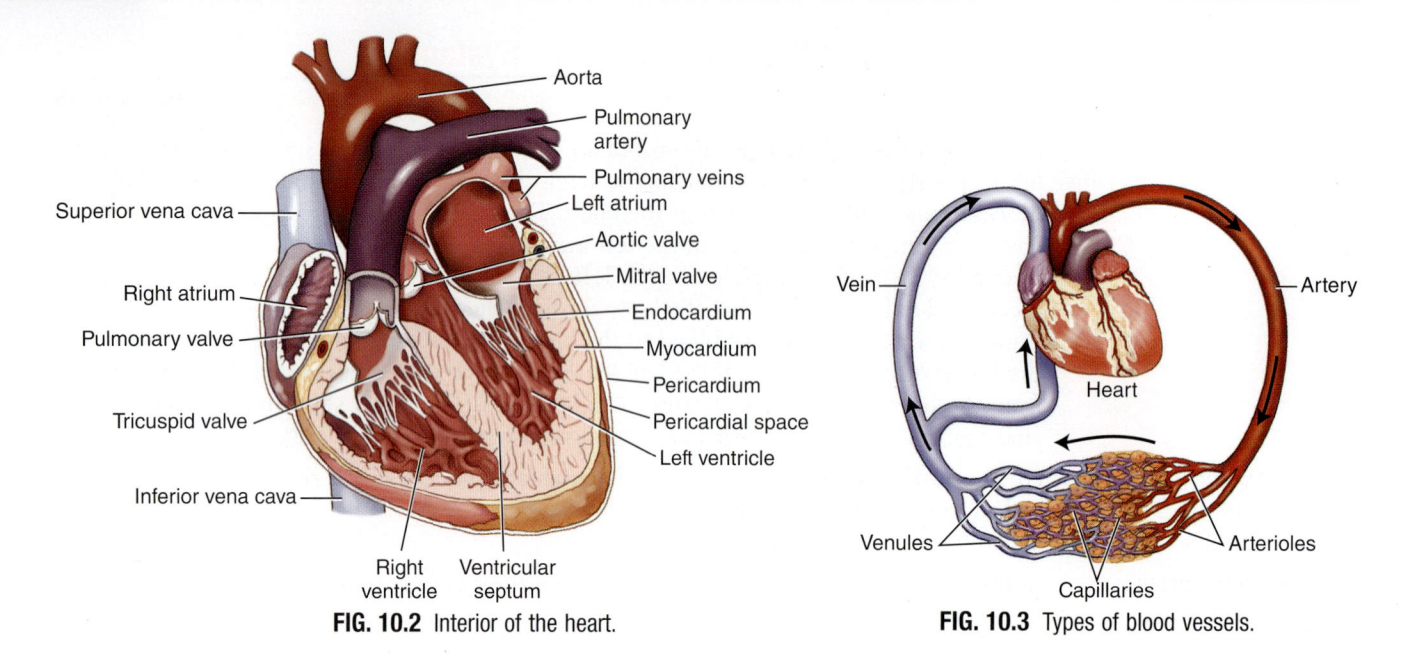

Blood

The adult body contains about 5 liters of blood. Blood cells, also known as formed elements, make up 45% of blood, while plasma accounts for 55% (Fig. 10.4). All blood cells originate from bone marrow, which is the soft inner tissue found in flat bones, such as the hip and shoulder blade, and also in the ends of long bones, such as the femur and humerus. Stem cells in the bone marrow develop into different types of blood cells in a process known as a **hematopoiesis**. These blood cells increase in number and mature, giving rise to specialized blood cells such as erythrocytes, leukocytes, and thrombocytes (platelets).

FUNCTION

Activities of the blood include transportation of nutrients, waste, oxygen, carbon dioxide, and hormones; protection of the body against microorganisms; regulation by controlling body temperature; and maintaining fluid and electrolyte balance.

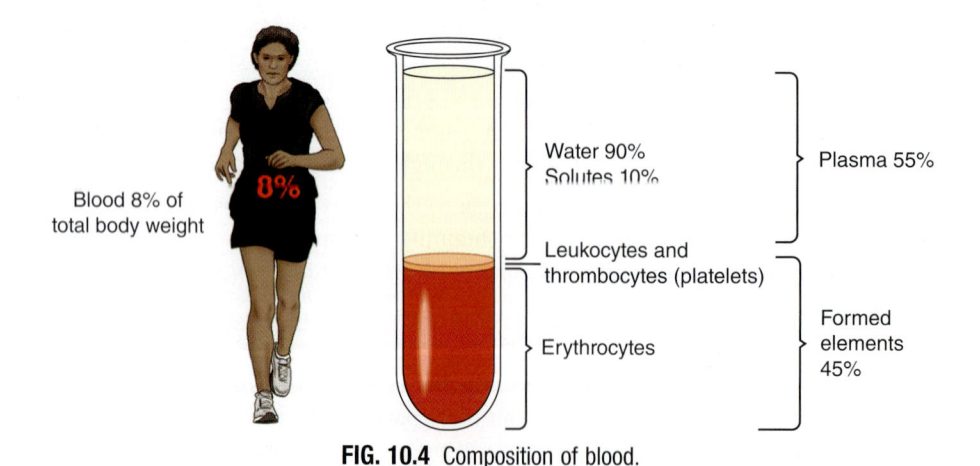

FIG. 10.4 Composition of blood.

Chapter 10 Cardiovascular, Lymphatic, Immune Systems and Blood

Composition of Blood

TERM	DEFINITION
blood (blud)	fluid circulated through the heart, arteries, capillaries, and veins; composed of **plasma** and **formed elements**, such as erythrocytes, leukocytes, and thrombocytes (platelets)
plasma (PLAZ-ma)	clear, straw-colored liquid portion of blood in which cells are suspended. Plasma is approximately 90% water. The other 10% is composed of solutes (dissolved substances), which include proteins, electrolytes, and vitamins. Plasma comprises approximately 55% of the total blood volume.
serum (SĒR-um)	clear, watery fluid portion of the blood that remains after a clot has formed
blood cells (formed elements)	production of new blood cells takes place in bone marrow, the spongy tissue inside some bones
erythrocytes (e-RITH-rō-sītes)	red blood cells that carry oxygen
leukocytes (LOO-kō-sītes)	white blood cells that combat infection and respond to inflammation. There are five types of white blood cells. (Fig. 10.5)
thrombocytes (THROM-bō-sītes)	one of the formed elements in the blood that is responsible for aiding in the clotting process (also called **platelets**)

> **STEM CELLS**
> **Hematopoietic stem cells** are immature cells found in the bone marrow and peripheral blood. They have the potential to develop into all types of blood cells, including erythrocytes, leukocytes, and thrombocytes.
> Stem cell transplantation is used to treat **leukemia** (cancer involving the white blood cells), **aplastic anemia** (disease in which there is inadequate production of blood cells), **multiple myeloma** (cancer that forms tumors in the bone marrow), **lymphoma** (cancer involving lymphoid cells), and **immune deficiency disorders**.
> Transplant cells may be obtained from the patient (**autologous**), from an identical twin (**synergetic**), or from a sibling or other individual (**allogenic**).

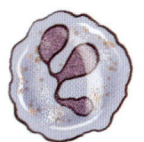

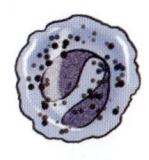

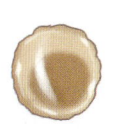

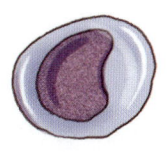

Neutrophil   Eosinophil   Basophil   Lymphocyte   Monocyte

FIG. 10.5 Types of leukocytes. Each leukocyte plays a different role in providing immune responses to pathogens, foreign agents, allergies, and abnormal body cells.

Lymphatic System

The lymphatic system consists of lymph, a transparent, colorless fluid mostly composed of white blood cells, which is transported through lymphatic vessels, lymph nodes, the spleen, and thymus gland (Fig. 10.6).

FUNCTION

Three functions of the lymphatic system are to return excessive tissue fluid to the blood, absorb fats and fat-soluble vitamins from the small intestine and transport them to the blood, and provide defense against infections and other diseases. Collected extracellular fluid called lymph travels away from body tissues toward the heart and is drained into the cardiovascular system through ducts in the upper chest. Breathing and muscular contractions help propel lymph through the vessels.

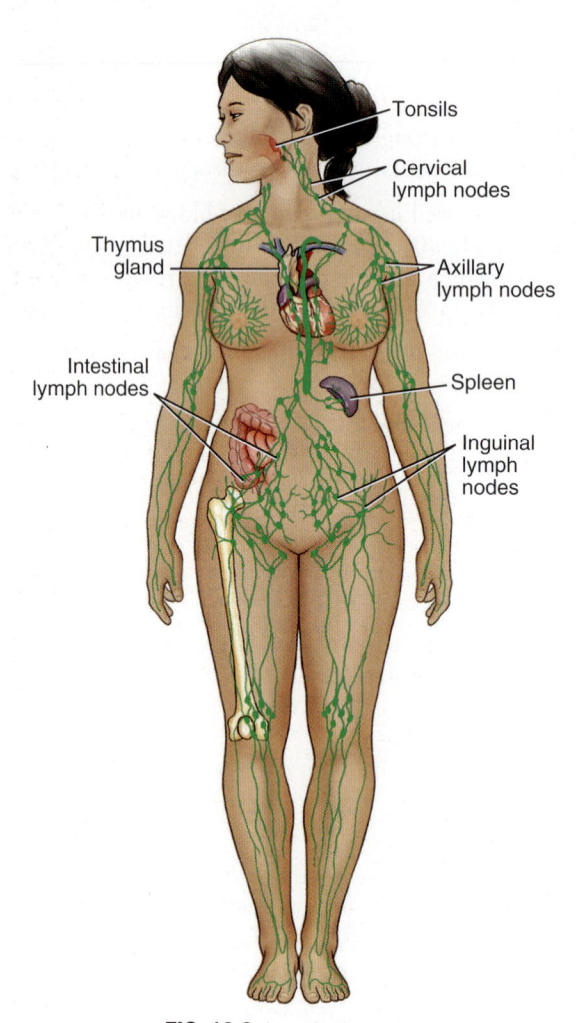

FIG. 10.6 Lymphatic system.

Organs and Anatomic Structures of the Lymphatic System

TERM	DEFINITION
lymph (limf)	transparent, colorless tissue fluid; contains **lymphocytes** and **monocytes** and flows in a one-way direction toward the heart
lymphatic vessels (lim-FAT-ik) (VES-els)	transport lymph from body tissues into the right and left subclavian veins, which then empty into the superior vena cava. The lymphatic vessels begin as capillaries spread throughout the body then merge into larger tubes that eventually become ducts in the chest. They provide a one-way flow for lymph, which enters through veins into the circulatory system.
lymph nodes (limf) (nōdz)	small, spherical bodies composed of lymphoid tissue. They may be singular or grouped together along the path of the lymph vessels. The nodes filter lymph to keep substances such as bacteria and other foreign agents from entering the blood. They also contain lymphocytes.
spleen (splēn)	located in the left side of the abdominal cavity between the stomach and the diaphragm. In adulthood, the spleen is the largest lymphatic organ in the body. Blood, rather than lymph, flows through the spleen. Blood is cleansed of microorganisms in the spleen. The spleen stores blood and destroys worn out red blood cells.
thymus gland (THĪ-mus) (gland)	one of the primary lymphatic organs, it is located anterior to the ascending aorta and posterior to the sternum between the lungs. It plays an important role in the development of the body's immune system, particularly from infancy to puberty. Around puberty the thymus gland shrinks so that most of the gland is connective tissue.

Chapter 10 Cardiovascular, Lymphatic, Immune Systems and Blood   363

Immune System

The immune system does not have its own organs and structures. Its function depends on organs and structures of other body systems, including the spleen, liver, intestinal tract, lymph nodes, and bone marrow.

FUNCTION

The immune system protects the body against pathogens (disease-causing organisms such as bacteria, fungi, and viruses), foreign agents that cause allergic reactions (e.g., peanuts), toxins (e.g., insect bites), and abnormal body cells (e.g., cancer). Immune function depends on three layers of protection, often referred to as lines of defense. (Fig. 10.7)

The first line of defense is the prevention of foreign substances from entering the body. Unbroken skin and mucous membranes act as physical barriers. Ear wax and saliva act as chemical barriers. If the first line of defense is penetrated by pathogens, a second line of defense continues to battle disease. Second-line defenses include inflammation and fever plus phagocytosis, a process in which some of the white blood cells destroy the invading microorganisms. Also activated are protective proteins such as interferons, which fight viruses, and natural killer (NK) cells, which are effective against microorganisms and cancer cells. Specific immunity, the third line of defense, provides protection against specific pathogens, such as the polio virus, by forming specific antibodies to fight against the infectious agent.

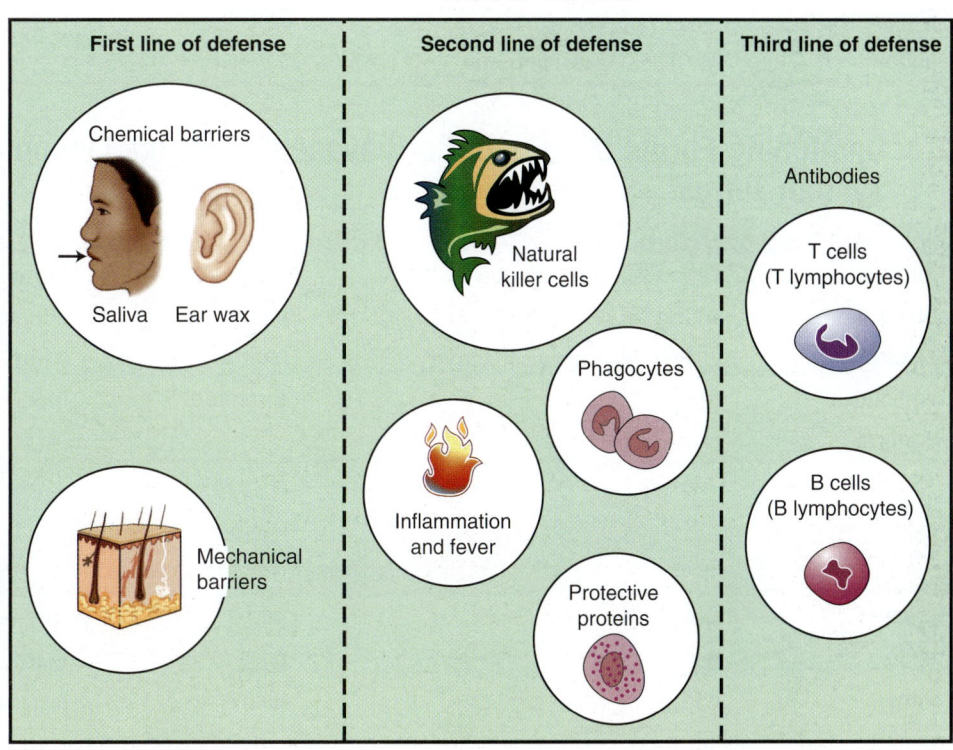

FIG. 10.7 Three lines of defense provided by the immune system to protect the body against pathogens, foreign agents, and cancer.

PRONOUNCE ANATOMIC STRUCTURES

Practice saying aloud each of the organs and specific structures on the previous pages.

To hear the terms, go to Evolve Resources at www.evolve.elsevier.com and select:
Student Resources > Audio Glossary > Chapter 10 > **Anatomic Structures**

❏ Check the box when complete.

Chapter 10 Cardiovascular, Lymphatic, Immune Systems and Blood

WORD PARTS

Use paper flashcards or electronic flashcards on Evolve to assist with memorization of word parts used to analyze, define, and build terms presented in this chapter. To reinforce learning, study one section of the Word Parts Table at a time, and then complete the corresponding exercise on the following pages.

1 ■ Anatomic Structures Combining Forms

COMBINING FORM	DEFINITION	COMBINING FORM	DEFINITION
angi/o	vessel(s); blood vessel(s)	myel/o	bone marrow
aort/o	aorta	**MYEL/O** also means spinal cord; see Chapter 15.	
arteri/o	artery (s.), arteries (pl.)	phleb/o	vein(s)
atri/o	atrium	plasm/o	plasma
cardi/o	heart	splen/o	spleen
cyt/o	cell(s)	**SPLEN/O** has only one "e" while its definition, spleen, has two.	
hem/o	blood	thym/o	thymus gland
hemat/o	blood	valvul/o	valve
lymph/o	lymph, lymph tissue	ven/o	vein(s)
lymphaden/o	lymph node	ventricul/o	ventricle
my/o	muscle(s), muscle tissue		

2 ■ Combining Forms Used with Cardiovascular, Blood, Lymphatic, and Immune System Terms

COMBINING FORM	DEFINITION	COMBINING FORM	DEFINITION
ather/o	yellowish, fatty plaque	immun/o	immune system
ech/o	sound	isch/o	deficiency, blockage
electr/o	electricity, electrical activity	leuk/o	white
embol/o	plug	thromb/o	blood clot
erythr/o	red		

3 ■ Prefixes

PREFIX	DEFINITION	PREFIX	DEFINITION
brady-	slow	peri-	surrounding (outer)
endo-	within	poly-	many, much
intra-	within	tachy-	fast, rapid
pan-	all, total		

4 ■ Suffixes

SUFFIX	DEFINITION	SUFFIX	DEFINITION
-apheresis	removal	-centesis	surgical puncture to aspirate fluid (with a sterile needle)
-ar	pertaining to	-ectomy	excision, surgical removal

Chapter 10 Cardiovascular, Lymphatic, Immune Systems and Blood

SUFFIX	DEFINITION
-emia	in the blood
-genic	producing, originating, causing
-gram	the record, radiographic image
-graphy	process of recording, radiographic imaging
-ia	diseased state, condition of
-ic	pertaining to
-ism	state of
-itis	inflammation
-logist	one who studies and treats (specialist, physician)
-logy	study of
-lysis	loosening, dissolution, separating
-megaly	enlargement
-oma	tumor, swelling

SUFFIX	DEFINITION
-osis	abnormal condition (means increase when used with blood cell word roots)
-ous	pertaining to
-pathy	disease
-penia	abnormal reduction in number
-plasty	surgical repair
-rrhage	excessive flow
-rrhaphy	suturing, repairing
-sclerosis	hardening
-scopy	visual examination
-stasis	control, stop, standing
-stenosis	constriction or narrowing
-us	noun suffix, no meaning

The suffixes **-RRHAGIA** and **-RRHAGE** come from the Greek word **rhegynai**, meaning to **burst forth**.

Refer to **Appendix B** and **Appendix C** for alphabetical lists of word parts and their meanings.

EXERCISE 1 ■ Anatomic Structures Combining Forms

Refer to the first section of the word parts table.

A Label

Fill in the blanks with combining forms to label this diagram of a cutaway section of the heart.
To check your answers, go to Appendix A.

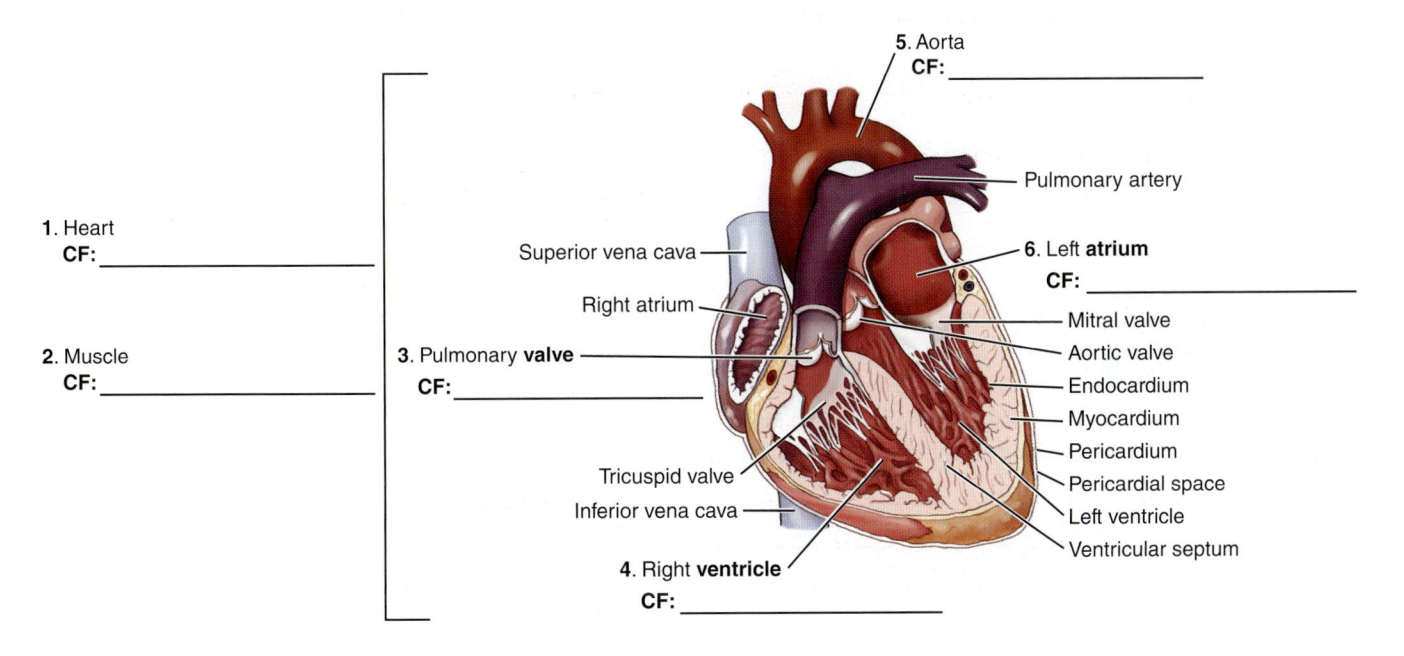

1. Heart
   CF: _____
2. Muscle
   CF: _____
3. Pulmonary **valve**
   CF: _____
4. Right **ventricle**
   CF: _____
5. Aorta
   CF: _____
6. Left **atrium**
   CF: _____

366 Chapter 10 Cardiovascular, Lymphatic, Immune Systems and Blood

B Define and Match

Step 1: Write the definitions after the following combining forms.
Step 2: Match the descriptions on the right with the combining forms and definitions.

_____ 1. cardi/o, _____   a. structures that keep blood flowing in one direction
_____ 2. atri/o, _____   b. larger lower chamber in the heart
_____ 3. valvul/o, _____   c. largest artery in the body
_____ 4. ventricul/o, _____   d. pumping action circulates blood throughout the body
_____ 5. aort/o, _____   e. small upper chamber in the heart
_____ 6. my/o, _____   f. tissue that produces movement

C Label

Fill in the blanks to label the illustrations of blood vessels and blood.

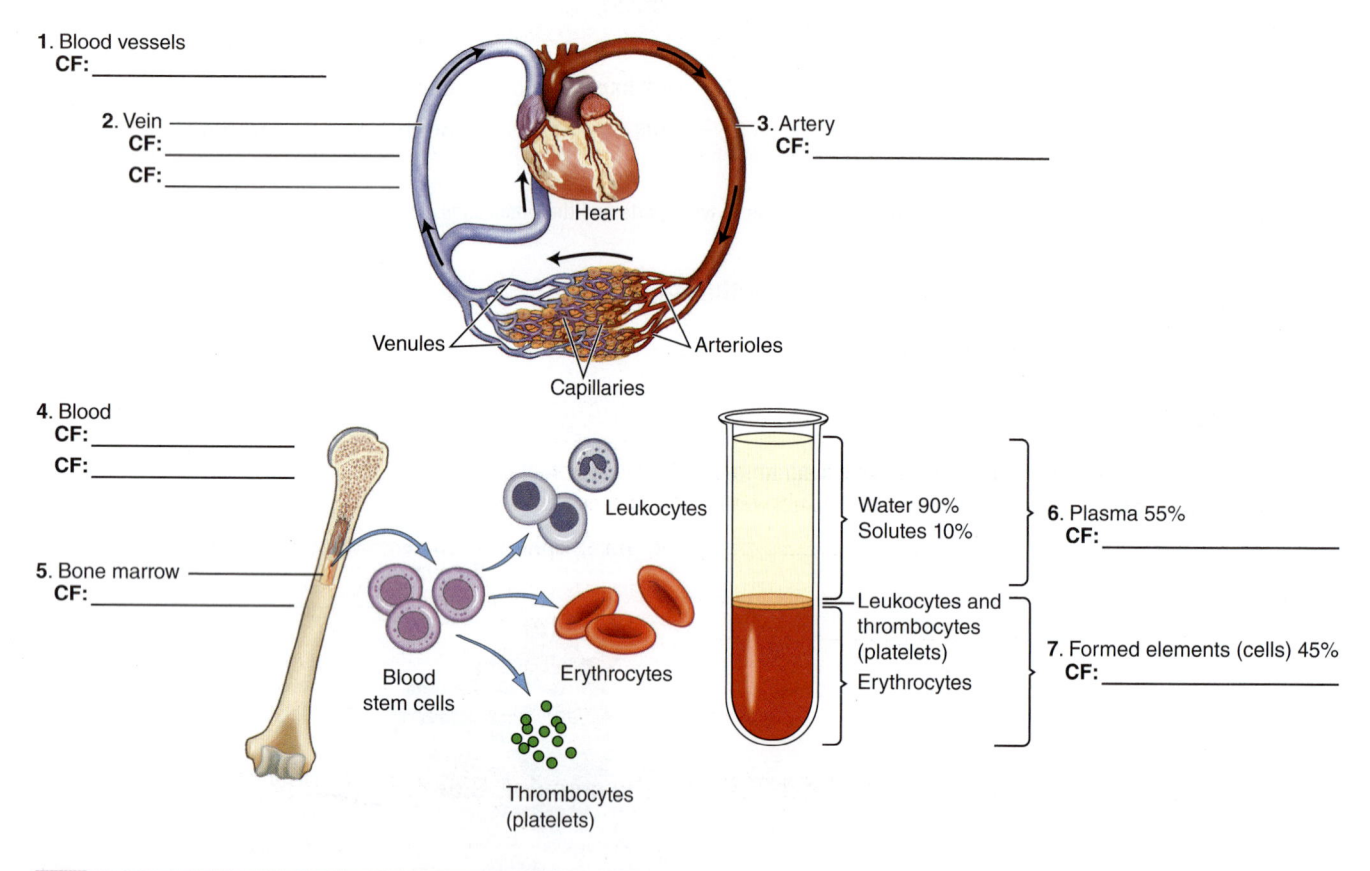

1. Blood vessels
   CF: _____

2. Vein
   CF: _____
   CF: _____

3. Artery
   CF: _____

4. Blood
   CF: _____
   CF: _____

5. Bone marrow
   CF: _____

6. Plasma 55%
   CF: _____

7. Formed elements (cells) 45%
   CF: _____

D Define and Match

Step 1: Write the definitions after the following combining forms.
Step 2: Match the descriptions on the right with the combining forms and definitions. Answers may be used more than once.

_____ 1. arteri/o, _____   a. fluid circulated through the heart, arteries, capillaries, and veins
_____ 2. myel/o, _____   b. clear, straw-colored liquid portion of blood
_____ 3. hemat/o, _____   c. blood vessels that carry blood away from the heart
_____ 4. phleb/o, _____   d. soft inner tissue of bones where blood cells are formed
_____ 5. angi/o, _____   e. blood vessels that carry blood back to the heart
_____ 6. ven/o, _____   f. tubelike structures that carry blood or other fluids
_____ 7. plasm/o, _____
_____ 8. hem/o, _____

Chapter 10   Cardiovascular, Lymphatic, Immune Systems and Blood   367

E Label

Fill in the blanks with combining forms to label the illustration of the lymphatic system.

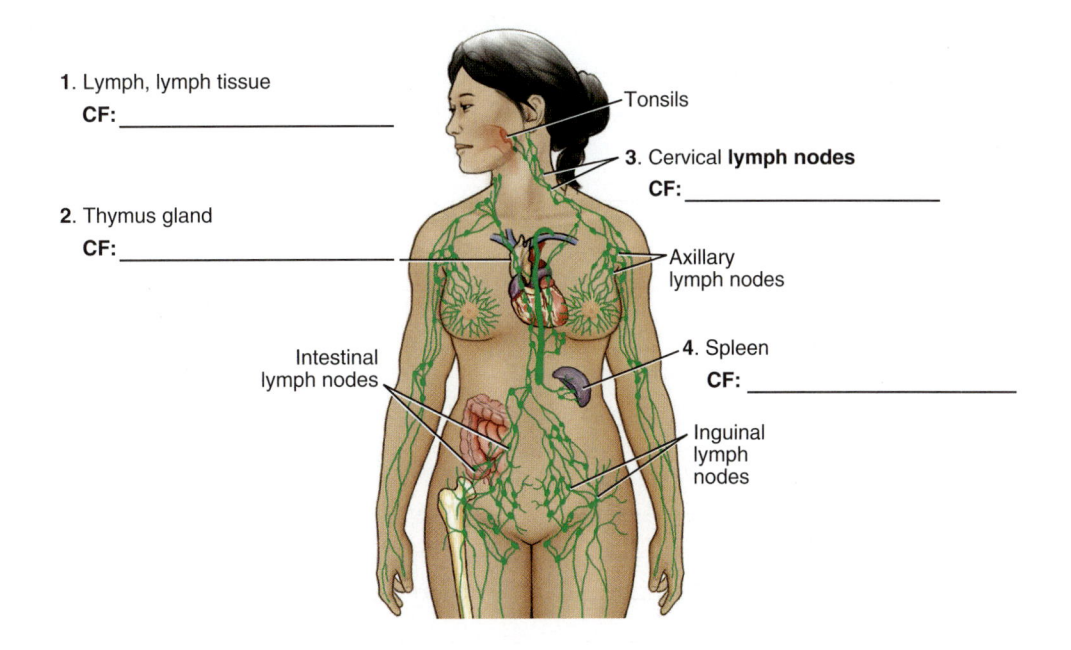

1. Lymph, lymph tissue
   CF: _____

2. Thymus gland
   CF: _____

3. Cervical **lymph nodes**
   CF: _____

4. Spleen
   CF: _____

> When used in reference to the lymphatic system, the combining form **lymphaden/o** refers to a collection of lymphatic tissue and is called a lymph **node** rather than the literal translation of lymph gland.

F Define and Match

Step 1: Write the definitions after the following combining forms.
Step 2: Match the descriptions on the right with the combining forms and definitions.

_____ 1. splen/o, _____
_____ 2. lymph/o, _____
_____ 3. thym/o, _____
_____ 4. lymphaden/o, _____

a. small, spherical bodies of tissue that filter lymph
b. lymphatic organ important in the development of immunity
c. largest lymphatic organ in adulthood that filters blood
d. transparent, colorless tissue fluid

EXERCISE 2 ■ Combining Forms Used with Cardiovascular, Blood, Lymphatic, and Immune System Terms

Refer to the second section of the word parts table.

A Define

Write the definitions of the following combining forms.

1. ech/o _____
2. thromb/o _____
3. isch/o _____
4. erythr/o _____
5. ather/o _____
6. electr/o _____
7. leuk/o _____
8. immun/o _____
9. embol/o _____

B Identify

Write the combining form for each of the following.

1. blood clot _____
2. sound _____
3. deficiency, blockage _____
4. yellowish, fatty plaque _____
5. immune system _____
6. electricity, electrical activity _____
7. plug _____
8. white _____
9. red _____

EXERCISE 3 ■ Prefixes

Refer to the third section of the word parts table.

A Define

Write the definitions of the following prefixes.

1. brady- _____
2. pan- _____
3. poly- _____
4. tachy- _____
5. intra- _____
6. peri- _____
7. endo- _____

B Identify

Write the prefix for each of the following.

1. fast _____
2. slow _____
3. many, much _____
4. surrounding (outer) _____
5. all, total _____
6. within _____ ; _____

EXERCISE 4 ■ Suffixes

Refer to the fourth section of the word parts table.

A Identify

Write the suffix for each of the following.

1. excessive flow _____
2. producing, originating, causing _____
3. hardening _____
4. loosening, dissolution, separating _____
5. abnormal reduction in number _____
6. control, stop, standing _____
7. removal _____
8. study of _____
9. one who studies and treats (specialist, physician) _____
10. noun suffix, no meaning _____
11. pertaining to _____ ; _____ ; _____

Chapter 10 Cardiovascular, Lymphatic, Immune Systems and Blood 369

B Match

Match the suffixes indicating disease or disorder in the first column with their correct definitions in the second column.

_____ 1. -stenosis   a. in the blood
_____ 2. -ia   b. inflammation
_____ 3. -rrhage   c. disease
_____ 4. -penia   d. state of
_____ 5. -pathy   e. hardening
_____ 6. -osis   f. constriction or narrowing
_____ 7. -oma   g. excessive flow
_____ 8. -itis   h. enlargement
_____ 9. -ism   i. abnormal reduction in number
_____ 10. -emia   j. tumor
_____ 11. -megaly   k. condition of (means increase when used with blood cell word roots)
_____ 12. -sclerosis   l. diseased or abnormal state, condition of

C Match

Match the suffixes indicating diagnostic or surgical procedures in the first column with their correct definitions in the second column.

_____ 1. -centesis   a. suturing, repairing
_____ 2. -ectomy   b. the record, radiographic image
_____ 3. -plasty   c. visual examination
_____ 4. -rrhaphy   d. surgical puncture to aspirate fluid (with a sterile needle)
_____ 5. -scopy   e. process of recording, radiographic imaging
_____ 6. -gram   f. excision, surgical removal
_____ 7. -graphy   g. surgical repair

-RRH SUFFIXES, of which there are five, have all now been introduced, including **-rrhage** and **-rrhaphy**. The other three are **-rrhea**, meaning flow or discharge; **-rrhagia**, meaning excessive bleeding; and **-rrhexis**, meaning rupture.

MEDICAL TERMS

Medical terms relevant to this chapter have been grouped by topics, such as Cardiovascular System Terms, and are listed in tables designated as Built from Word Parts or *NOT* Built from Word Parts. The exercises following each table assist with learning term definitions, pronunciations, and spellings.

Cardiovascular System Terms
BUILT FROM WORD PARTS

The following terms can be translated using definitions of word parts. Further explanation is provided within parentheses as needed.

DISEASE AND DISORDERS			
TERM	**DEFINITION**	**TERM**	**DEFINITION**
1. **angioma** (an-jē-Ō-ma)	tumor composed of blood vessels	4. **arteriosclerosis** (ar-tēr-ē-ō-skle-RŌ-sis)	hardening of the arteries
2. **angiostenosis** (an-jē-ō-ste-NŌ-sis)	narrowing of a blood vessel	5. **atherosclerosis** (ath-er-ō-skle-RŌ-sis)	hardening of fatty plaque (deposited on the arterial wall)
3. **aortic stenosis** (ā-OR-tik) (ste-NŌ-sis)	narrowing, pertaining to aorta (narrowing of the aortic valve) (Fig. 10.8)		

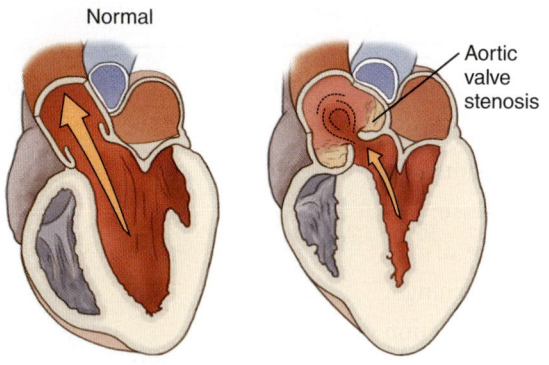

FIG. 10.8 Aortic stenosis.

Cardiovascular System Terms—cont'd
BUILT FROM WORD PARTS

TERM	DEFINITION	TERM	DEFINITION
6. **bradycardia** (*brad*-ē-KAR-dē-a)	condition of a slow heart (rate less than 60 beats per minute)	**MYOCARDIAL ISCHEMIA** is the deficient flow of blood to the heart muscle caused by vessel constriction commonly due to atherosclerosis and potentially leading to **myocardial infarction**.	
💡 The **i** from **cardi/o** is dropped when the suffix starts with an **i**. When analyzing several terms in this list, such as **bradycardia**, the last i in the term is considered to be a part of the suffix.		11. **myocarditis** (*mī*-ō-kar-DĪ-tis)	inflammation of the muscle of the heart
		12. **pericarditis** (*per*-i-kar-DĪ-tis)	inflammation (of the sac) surrounding the heart (Fig. 10.9)
7. **cardiomegaly** (*kar*-dē-ō-MEG-a-lē)	enlargement of the heart	13. **phlebitis** (fle-BĪ-tis)	inflammation of a vein
8. **cardiomyopathy** (*kar*-dē-ō-mī-OP-a-thē)	disease of the heart muscle	14. **polyarteritis** (*pol*-ē-*ar*-te-RĪ-tis)	inflammation of many (sites in the) arteries (Note: the i in arteri/o has been dropped)
9. **endocarditis** (*en*-dō-kar-DĪ-tis)	inflammation of the inner (lining) of the heart (particularly heart valves)	15. **tachycardia** (*tak*-i-KAR-dē-a)	condition of a rapid heart (rate of more than 100 beats per min)
10. **ischemia** (is-KĒ-mē-a)	deficiency in blood (flow); (caused by constriction or obstruction of a blood vessel)	16. **thrombophlebitis** (throm-bō-fle-BĪ-tis)	inflammation of a vein associated with a blood clot
		17. **valvulitis** (*val*-vū-LĪ-tis)	inflammation of a valve (of the heart)

SURGICAL TERMS

TERM	DEFINITION	TERM	DEFINITION
18. **angioplasty** (AN-jē-ō-*plas*-tē)	surgical repair of a blood vessel (also called **balloon angioplasty**)	21. **endarterectomy** (end-ar-ter-EK-to-mē)	excision within the artery (excision of plaque from the arterial wall). (Note: the o from endo- and the i from arteri/o have been dropped)
19. **atherectomy** (ath-er-EK-to-mē)	excision of fatty plaque (from a blocked artery using a specialized catheter and a rotary cutter)	**ENDARTERECTOMY** procedures are usually named for the artery to be cleaned out, such as **carotid endarterectomy**, which means removal of plaque from the wall of the carotid artery.	
20. **embolectomy** (*em*-bo-LEK-to-mē)	excision of a plug (embolus or clot, usually with a balloon catheter, inflating the balloon beyond the clot, then pulling the balloon back to the incision and bringing the plug with it)	22. **pericardiocentesis** (*per*-i-kar-dē-ō-sen-TĒ-sis)	surgical puncture to aspirate fluid from the sac surrounding the heart (usually to relieve cardiac tamponade and for diagnostic investigation) (Fig. 10.9)

Chapter 10   Cardiovascular, Lymphatic, Immune Systems and Blood   371

Pericarditis   Pericardiocentesis

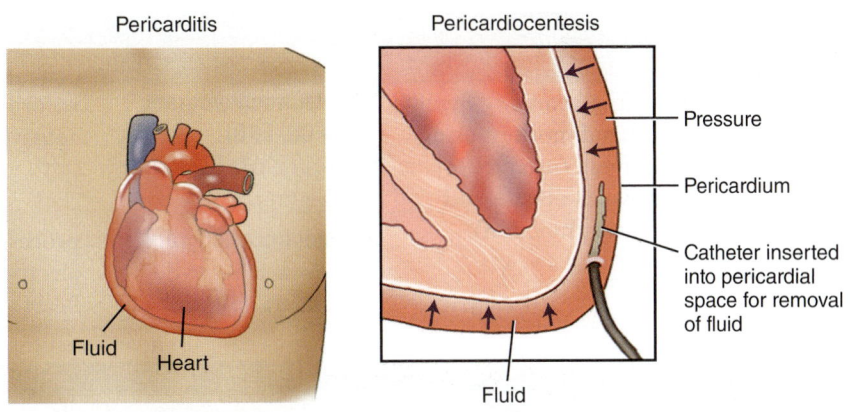

Pressure
Pericardium
Catheter inserted into pericardial space for removal of fluid

Fluid
Heart
Fluid

FIG. 10.9 Pericarditis may produce excess fluid in the pericardium. If the fluid seriously affects the heart's ability to pump blood, pericardiocentesis may be performed to remove the fluid.

TERM	DEFINITION	TERM	DEFINITION
23. phlebectomy (fle-BEK-to-mē)	excision of a vein	24. valvuloplasty (VAL-vū-lō-*plas*-tē)	surgical repair of a valve (cardiac or venous)

DIAGNOSTIC IMAGING TERMS

TERM	DEFINITION	TERM	DEFINITION
25. angiography (*an*-jē-OG-ra-fē)	radiographic imaging of blood vessels (the procedure is named for the vessel to be studied, e.g., **femoral angiography** or **coronary angiography**) (Table 10.1)	27. aortogram (ā-OR-to-gram)	radiographic image of the aorta (after an injection of contrast materials)
		28. arteriogram (ar-TĒR-ē-ō-gram)	radiographic image of an artery (after an injection of contrast materials)
26. angioscopy (*an*-jē-OS-ko-pē)	visual examination (of the inside) of a blood vessel	29. venogram (VĒ-nō-gram)	radiographic image of a vein (after an injection of contrast materials)

TABLE 10.1 Types of Angiography

CORONARY ARTERY VISUALIZATION
Coronary angiography is an **invasive procedure** in which a catheter is inserted into an artery in the groin, arm, or neck, and then advanced into the coronary vessels. Next, contrast materials are injected, and images are recorded. It is considered the best technique for determining the percentage of blockage in the coronary arteries.

OTHER VASCULAR VISUALIZATION
Magnetic resonance angiography (MRA) is a **noninvasive procedure** that does not require catheterization and uses specialized MR imaging to study vascular structures of the body. MRA may be chosen over computed tomography angiography because there is no exposure to ionizing radiation.

Computed tomography angiography (CTA) is a **noninvasive procedure** that uses a high-resolution CT system to study vascular structures of the body after the injection of intravenous contrast materials.

Digital subtraction angiography (DSA) is an **invasive procedure** in which an image is taken and stored in the computer, and then contrast material is injected. A second image is taken and stored in the computer. The computer compares the two images and subtracts the first image from the second, removing structures not being studied. DSA enables better visualization of the arteries than regular angiography.

DIAGNOSTIC PROCEDURES

TERM	DEFINITION	TERM	DEFINITION
30. echocardiogram (ECHO) (ek-ō-KAR-dē-ō-gram)	record of the heart (structure and motion) using sound (waves); (used to detect valvular disease and evaluate heart function)	31. electrocardiogram (ECG, EKG) (ē-*lek*-trō-KAR-dē-ō-gram)	record of the electrical activity of the heart
		32. electrocardiography (ē-*lek*-trō-*kar*-dē-OG-ra-fē)	process of recording the electrical activity of the heart

MEDICAL SPECIALTIES

TERM	DEFINITION	TERM	DEFINITION
33. cardiologist (*kar*-dē-OL-o-jist)	physician who studies and treats diseases of the heart	34. cardiology (*kar*-dē-OL-o-jē)	study of the heart (a branch of medicine that deals with diseases of the heart)

ELECTROPHYSIOLOGIST is a **cardiologist** who specializes in the diagnosis and treatment of patients with arrhythmias (electrical abnormalities in the heart's normal rhythmic pattern).

DESCRIPTIVE TERMS

TERM	DEFINITION	TERM	DEFINITION
35. atrioventricular (AV) (ā-trē-ō-ven-TRIK-ū-ler)	pertaining to the atrium and ventricle	37. intravenous (IV) (in-tra-VĒ-nus)	pertaining to within the vein
36. cardiogenic (kar-dē-ō-JEN-ik)	originating in the heart	**INTRAVENOUS (IV) THERAPY** is the infusion of a substance directly into a vein for therapeutic purposes. **IV therapy** is a very common and essential component of medical care, serving as a direct, efficient route for the administration of fluids, medications, and blood products.	

EXERCISE 5 ■ Pronounce and Spell

Practice pronunciation and spelling on paper and online.

1. **Practice on Paper**
   a. **Pronounce:** Read the phonetic spelling and say aloud the terms listed in the previous table. Refer to Table 2.2 Pronunciation Key as needed.
   b. **Spell:** Have a study partner read the terms aloud. Write the spelling of the terms on a separate sheet of paper.

2. **Practice Online**
   a. **Access** online learning resources. Go to evolve.elsevier.com > Evolve Resources > Student Resources.
   b. **Pronounce:** Select Audio Glossary > Chapter 10 > Exercise 5. Select a term to hear its pronunciation and repeat aloud.
   c. **Spell:** Select Activities > Chapter 10 > Spell Terms > Exercise 5. Select the audio icon and type the correct spelling of the term.

❏ Check the box when complete.

EXERCISE 6 ■ Analyze and Define

Analyze and define the following terms.

1. atrioventricular

2. electrocardiography

3. cardiologist

4. aortogram

5. valvulitis

6. phlebectomy

7. tachycardia

8. angioscopy

9. angiography

10. cardiogenic

11. ischemia

12. thrombophlebitis

13. atherectomy

14. valvuloplasty

15. angioma

16. myocarditis

Chapter 10 Cardiovascular, Lymphatic, Immune Systems and Blood

EXERCISE 7 ■ Build

A Label

Build terms pictured by writing word parts above definitions.

1.

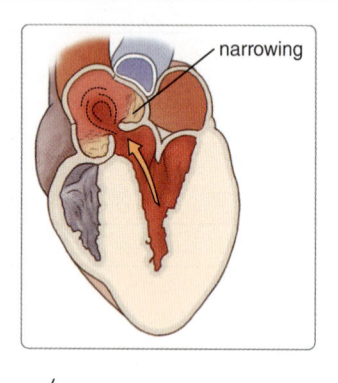

_____ / _____ _____
aorta   pertaining to   narrowing

2.

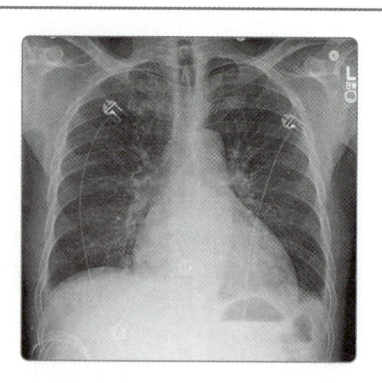

Chest radiography showing
_____ / ____ / _____
heart   CV   enlargement

3.

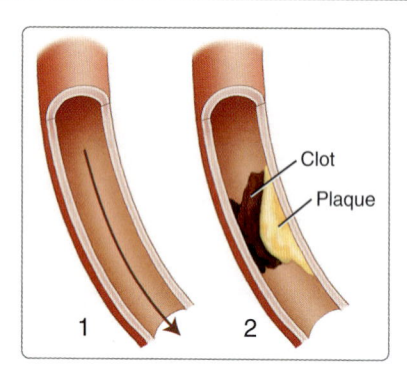

1. Healthy artery with smooth blood flow
2. Blocked artery due to blood clot and
_____ / _____ / _____
fatty plaque   CV   hardening

4.

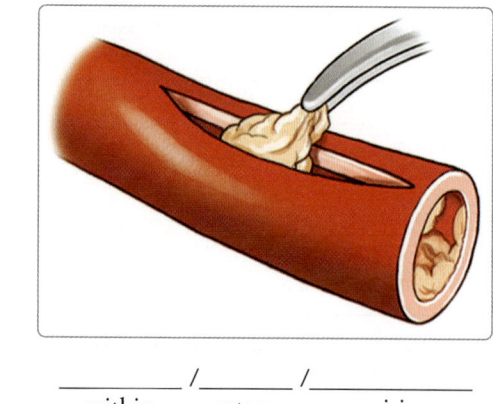

_____ / _____ / _____
within   artery   excision

5.

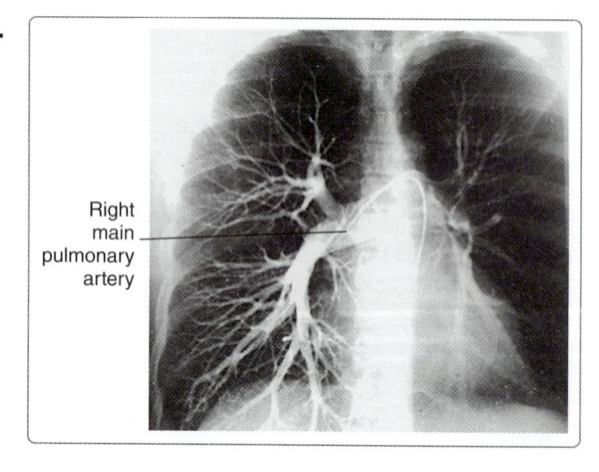

_____ / _____ / _____,
artery   CV   radiographic image
performed after injection of contrast materials

6.

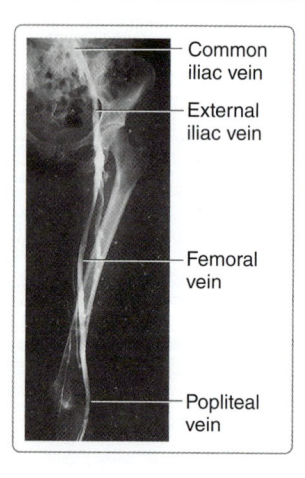

Normal _____ / ____ / _____, left lower limb
         vein   CV   radiographic
                         image

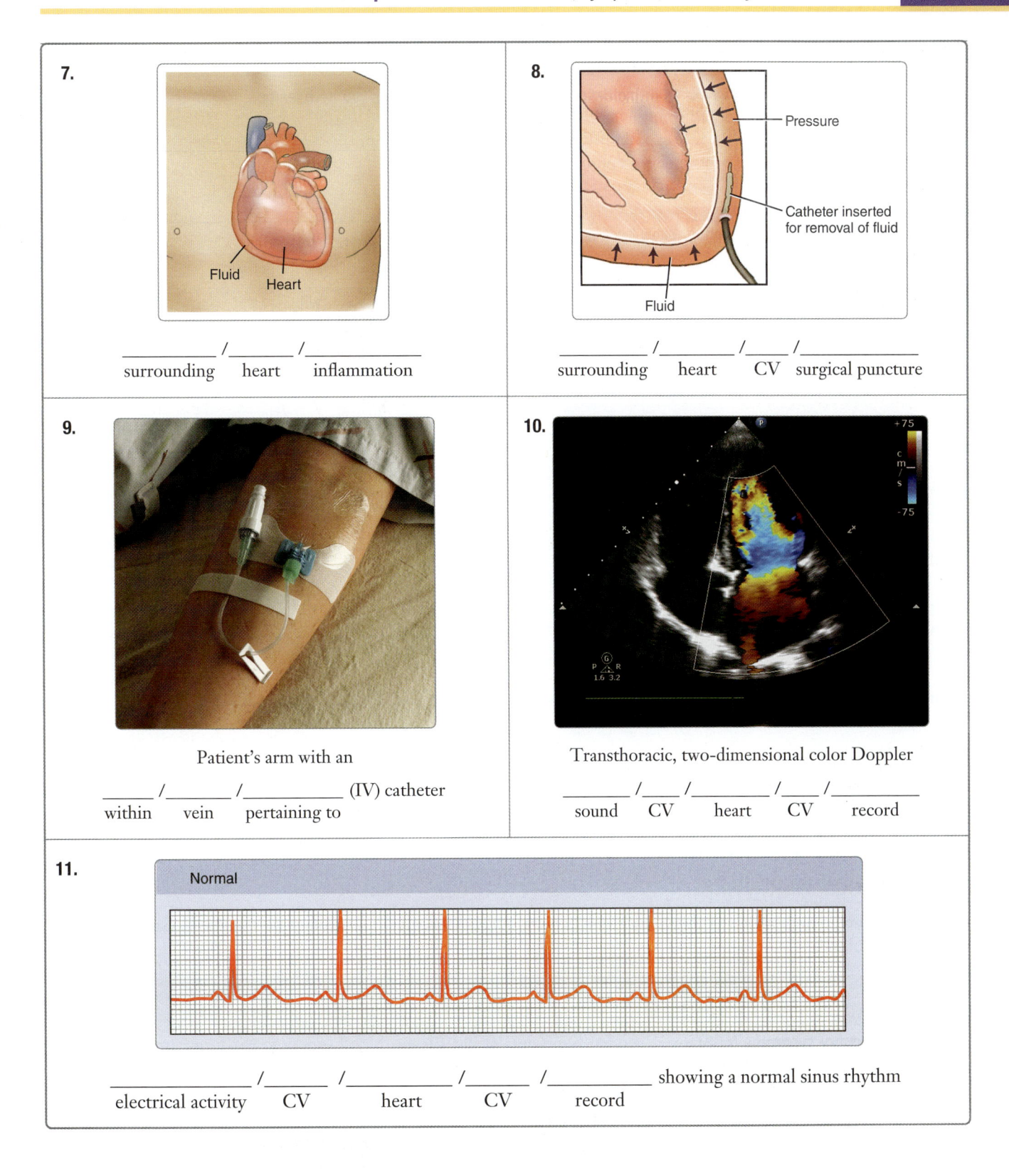

Chapter 10 Cardiovascular, Lymphatic, Immune Systems and Blood 375

7.

_____ / _____ / _____
surrounding   heart   inflammation

8.

_____ / _____ / ____ / _____
surrounding   heart   CV   surgical puncture

9. Patient's arm with an

_____ / _____ / _____ (IV) catheter
within   vein   pertaining to

10. Transthoracic, two-dimensional color Doppler

_____ / ____ / _____ / ____ / _____
sound   CV   heart   CV   record

11.

_____ / _____ / _____ / _____ / _____ showing a normal sinus rhythm
electrical activity   CV   heart   CV   record

B Fill In

Build cardiovascular system terms for the following definitions by using the word parts you have learned.

1. inflammation of a vein

   _____ / _____
   WR   S

2. surgical repair of a blood vessel

   _____ / ____ / _____
   WR   CV   S

3. inflammation of the inner (layer) of the heart

   ____ / _____ / _____
   P   WR   S

4. condition of slow heart rate

   ____ / _____ / _____
   P   WR   S

5. hardening of the arteries

   _____ / ____ / _____
   WR   CV   S

6. excision of a plug

   _____ / _____
   WR   S

7. disease of the heart muscle

   _____ / ____ / _____ / ____ / _____
   WR   CV   WR   CV   S

8. narrowing of a blood vessel

   _____ / ____ / _____
   WR   CV   S

9. inflammation of many (sites in the) arteries

   ____ / _____ / _____
   P   WR   S

10. study of the heart

    _____ / ____ / _____
    WR   CV   S

Cardiovascular System Terms
NOT BUILT FROM WORD PARTS

Word parts may be present in the following terms; however, their full meanings cannot be translated using definitions of word parts alone.

DISEASE AND DISORDERS	
TERM	**DEFINITION**
1. **acute coronary syndrome (ACS)** (a-KŪT) (KOR-o-nar-ē) (SIN-drōm)	sudden symptoms of insufficient blood supply to the heart, indicating unstable angina or acute myocardial infarction. Rapid assessment is necessary to determine the diagnosis and treatment and to minimize heart damage.
2. **aneurysm** (AN-ū-riz-em)	ballooning of a weakened portion of an arterial wall (Fig. 10.10)
3. **angina pectoris** (an-JĪ-na) (PEK-to-ris)	chest pain, which may radiate to the left arm and jaw, that occurs when there is an insufficient supply of blood to the heart muscle
🏛 **ANGINA PECTORIS** was believed by the ancients to be a disorder of the breast. The Latin **angere**, meaning to throttle, was used to represent the sudden pain and was added to pectus, meaning breast.	

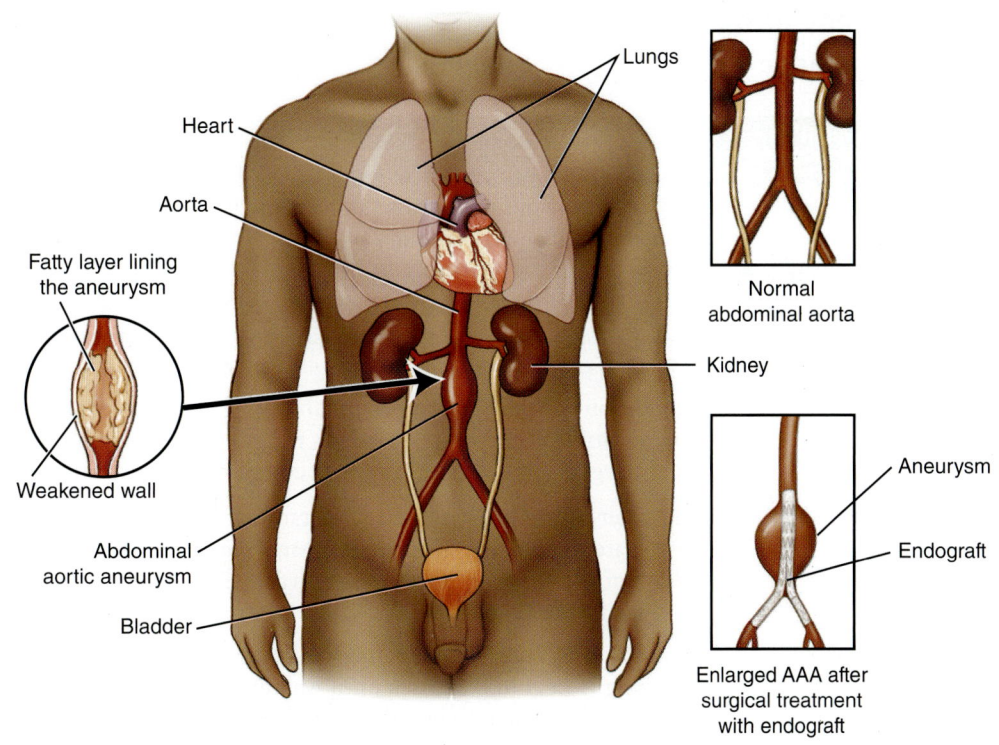

Chapter 10   Cardiovascular, Lymphatic, Immune Systems and Blood   377

FIG. 10.10 Abdominal aortic aneurysm. An abdominal aortic aneurysm (AAA) is located in the abdominal area of the aorta, the main blood vessel that transports blood away from the heart. Because the success rate of surgery is much lower once an aneurysm has ruptured, more emphasis is being placed on diagnosis. AAAs can be detected by physical examination but are more frequently detected by abdominal ultrasound or computerized tomography (CT). Smaller AAAs have a very low risk of rupture and are usually followed closely to make sure they don't enlarge. Larger AAAs are usually repaired surgically. The preferred surgical intervention, called **endovascular stenting,** is performed through a puncture in the femoral artery, using a radiographic procedure called fluoroscopy. With this technique, an **endograft** can be placed within an aneurysm.

TERM	DEFINITION
4. arrhythmia (ā-RITH-mē-a)	any disturbance or abnormality in the heart's normal rhythmic pattern
5. cardiac arrest (KAR-dē-ak) (a-REST)	sudden cessation of cardiac output and effective circulation, which requires cardiopulmonary resuscitation **(CPR)**
6. cardiac tamponade (KAR-dē-ak) (tam-po-NĀD)	acute compression of the heart caused by fluid accumulation in the pericardial cavity
7. coronary artery disease (CAD) (KOR-o-nar-ē) (AR-te-rē) (di-ZĒZ)	condition that reduces the flow of blood through the coronary arteries to the myocardium that may progress to depriving the heart tissue of sufficient oxygen and nutrients to function normally; most often caused by coronary atherosclerosis. CAD is a common cause of heart failure and myocardial infarction.
🏛 **CORONARY** is derived from the Latin coronalis, meaning crown or wreath. It describes the arteries encircling the heart.	
8. cor pulmonale (kor) (pul-mō-NAL-ē)	enlargement of the heart's right ventricle due to pulmonary disease
9. deep vein thrombosis (DVT) (dēp) (vān) (throm-BŌ-sis)	formation of a blood clot in a deep vein of the body. Most often occurs in the lower extremities. A clot, or part of a clot, can break off and travel to the lungs, causing a pulmonary embolism.

Cardiovascular System Terms—cont'd
NOT BUILT FROM WORD PARTS

DISEASE AND DISORDERS—cont'd	
TERM	**DEFINITION**
10. fibrillation (fi-bri-LĀ-shun)	rapid, quivering, uncoordinated contractions of the atria or ventricles, causing cardiac arrhythmia
TYPES OF FIBRILLATION In **atrial fibrillation (AF** or **AFib)**, the atria quiver instead of contracting, causing an irregular ventricular response. Not all of the blood is ejected with each contraction, and the remaining blood flow becomes turbulent. This increases the risk of clot formation. Two types of AFib are **paroxysmal atrial fibrillation (PAF)**, which is intermittent, and **chronic atrial fibrillation**, which is sustained (Fig. 10.11). In **ventricular fibrillation (VF** or **VFib)**, the heart does not contract and blood flow stops, causing a medical emergency that may result in sudden death.	
11. heart failure (HF) (hart) (fāl-ŪR)	condition in which there is an inability of the heart to pump enough blood through the body to supply the tissues and organs with nutrients and oxygen. One common type is **congestive heart failure (CHF)**.
12. hypertensive heart disease (HHD) (hī-per-TEN-siv) (hart) (di-ZĒZ)	disorder of the heart caused by persistent high blood pressure; it may be associated with hypertrophy (abnormal thickening of the heart muscle) or dilation of the chambers of the heart (due to thinning and stretching of the heart muscle)
13. intermittent claudication (in-ter-MIT-ent) (klaw-di-KĀ-shun)	condition of pain, tension, and weakness in a limb that starts when walking is begun, increases until walking is no longer possible, and then completely resolves when the patient is at rest. It is caused by reversible muscle ischemia that occurs with peripheral artery disease.
14. mitral valve stenosis (MĪ-tral) (valv) (ste-NŌ-sis)	narrowing of the mitral valve from scarring, usually caused by episodes of rheumatic fever
15. myocardial infarction (MI) (mī-ō-KAR-dē-al) (in-FARK-shun)	death (necrosis) of a portion of the myocardium caused by lack of oxygen resulting from an interrupted blood supply (also called **heart attack**)

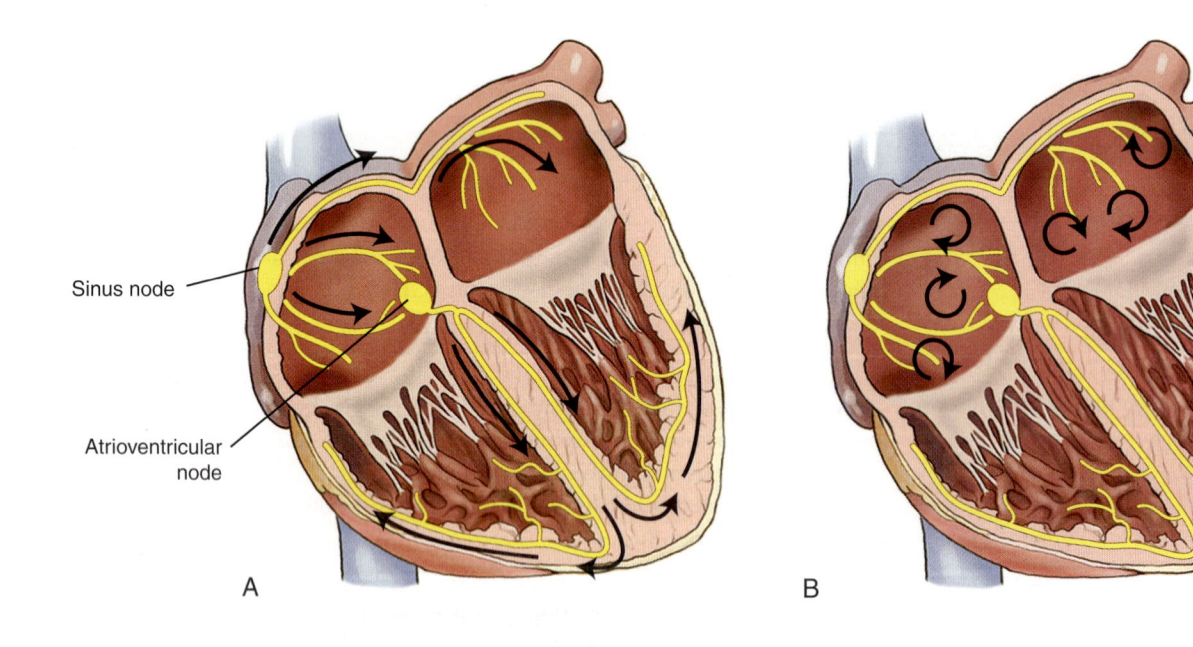

Normal heart rhythm (sinus rhythm)   **Atrial fibrillation**

FIG. 10.11 Atrial fibrillation (AFib). **A,** Normal heart rhythm. *Arrows* indicate the normal travel of electrical impulses though the heart, stimulating coordinated contraction of chambers. **B,** Atrial fibrillation, showing chaotic, rapid electrical impulses.

Chapter 10 Cardiovascular, Lymphatic, Immune Systems and Blood

TERM	DEFINITION
16. **peripheral artery disease (PAD)** (pe-RIF-er-al) (AR-ter-ē) (di-ZĒZ)	disease of the arteries in the arms and legs, resulting in narrowing or complete obstruction of the artery. This is caused most commonly by atherosclerosis, but occasionally by inflammatory diseases, emboli, or thrombus formation. The most common symptom of peripheral artery disease is intermittent claudication. (also called **peripheral vascular disease [PVD]**)

RAYNAUD (RĀ-NŌ) PHENOMENON is classified as a **peripheral artery disease (PAD)**. The condition was first described by Maurice Raynaud, a French physician, in 1862. Symptoms include intermittent, symmetric attacks of cyanosis and pallor of the distal ends of the fingers and toes, often caused by exposure to cold temperature.

17. **rheumatic heart disease** (rū-MAT-ik) (hart) (di-ZĒZ)	damage to the heart muscle or heart valves caused by one or more episodes of rheumatic fever

RHEUMATIC FEVER is an inflammatory disease, usually occurring in children and young adults after an upper respiratory tract streptococcal infection. One of the most serious symptoms is valvulitis (inflammation of a cardiac valve). While antibiotics have greatly decreased the incidence of this disease in developed nations, it is still a significant threat in developing nations.

18. **varicose veins** (VAR-i-kōs) (vānz)	distended or tortuous veins, usually found in the lower extremities (Fig. 10.12)

VARICOSE VEINS AND TREATMENT Varicose veins usually occur in the superficial veins of the legs. One-way valves in the veins help move the blood upward. When these valves fail, or the veins lose their elasticity, the blood flows backward, pools, and forms varicose veins. Causes are heredity, obesity, pregnancy, illness, or injury. Treatments include laser ablation, ambulatory phlebectomy, and sclerotherapy.

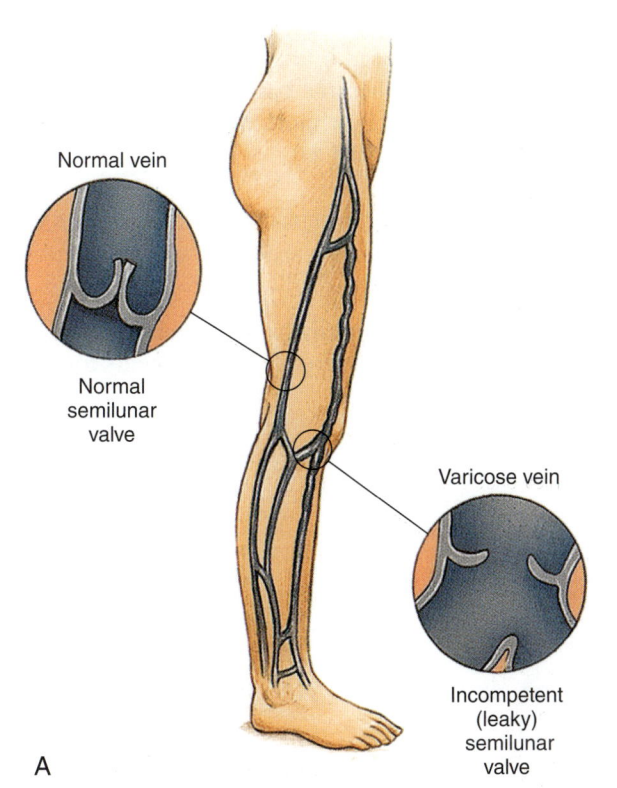

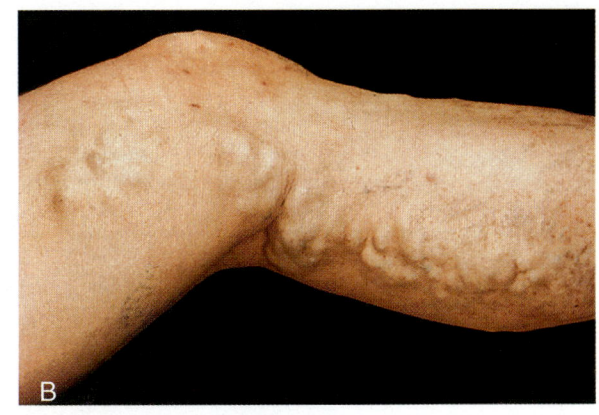

FIG. 10.12 A, Normal and varicose veins. **B,** Appearance of varicose veins.

Cardiovascular System Terms—cont'd
NOT BUILT FROM WORD PARTS

SURGICAL TERMS

TERM	DEFINITION
19. **artificial cardiac pacemaker** (ar-ti-FISH-el) (KAR-dē-ak) (PĀS-mā-kr)	battery-powered apparatus implanted under the skin, with leads placed on the heart or in the chamber of the heart; used to treat an abnormal heart rhythm, usually one that is too slow, due to an abnormal sinus node
SINUS NODE of the heart is the body's natural pacemaker. Also called the sinoatrial or SA node, it consists of specialized fibers that are responsible for initiating nerve impulses that tell the heart muscles when to contract. When the SA node is working properly, the pumping motion of the heart chambers is coordinated and well-timed. If the SA node (or other parts of the heart's conduction system) doesn't work properly, arrhythmias may occur.	
20. **automatic implantable cardiac defibrillator (AICD)** (aw-to-MAT-ik) (im-PLANT-a-bl) (KAR-dē-ak) (dē-FIB-ri-lā-tor)	device implanted in the body that continuously monitors the heart rhythm. If life-threatening arrhythmias occur, the device delivers an electric shock to convert the arrhythmia back to a normal rhythm.
21. **catheter ablation** (KATH-e-ter) (ab-LĀ-shun)	procedure in which abnormal cells that trigger abnormal heart rhythms (arrhythmias) are destroyed by using a device that heats or freezes the cells (Fig. 10.13)
22. **coronary artery bypass graft (CABG)** (KOR-o-nar-ē) (AR-te-rē) (BĪ-pas) (graft)	surgical technique to bring a new blood supply to heart muscle by detouring around blocked arteries
23. **coronary stent** (KOR-o-nar-ē) (stent)	supportive scaffold device placed in the coronary artery; used to prevent closure of the artery after angioplasty or atherectomy; used to treat an artery occluded by plaque
24. **femoropopliteal bypass** (fem-o-rō-pop-LIT-ē-al) (BĪ-pass)	surgery to establish an alternate route from femoral artery to popliteal artery to bypass an obstruction
25. **percutaneous transluminal coronary angioplasty (PTCA)** (per-kū-TĀ-nē-us) (trans-LŪ-min-al) (KOR-o-nar-ē) (AN-jē-ō-plas-tē)	procedure in which a balloon is advanced into a coronary artery to the area where plaque has formed. When the balloon is inflated, the vessel wall expands, allowing blood to flow more freely. (also called **percutaneous coronary intervention (PCI)**)
PERCUTANEOUS TRANSLUMINAL CORONARY ANGIOPLASTY (PTCA) VS. CORONARY ARTERY BYPASS GRAFTING (CABG): CABG is usually chosen when multiple vessels are diseased and when patients have blockage in the left main coronary artery. PTCA is used in patients with acute, unstable CAD and in patients who have only one or two vessels involved.	
26. **thrombolytic therapy** (throm-bō-LIT-ik) (THER-a-pē)	injection of a medication either intravenously or intraarterially to dissolve blood clots. It is often used in emergency departments for acute myocardial infarction.

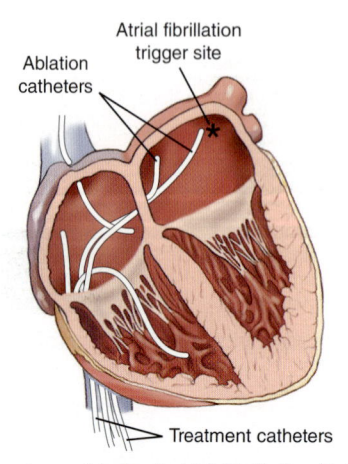

FIG. 10.13 Catheter ablation is used to treat atrial fibrillation if drug therapy is not effective.

DIAGNOSTIC IMAGING TERMS

TERM	DEFINITION
27. **digital subtraction angiography (DSA)** (DIJ-i-tal) (sub-TRAK-shun) (*an*-jē-OG-ra-fē)	process of digital radiographic imaging of the blood vessels that "subtracts" or removes structures not being studied (see Table 10.1)
28. **Doppler ultrasound** (DOP-ler) (UL-tra-sound)	study that uses high-frequency sound waves for detection of blood flow within the vessels; used to assess intermittent claudication, deep vein thrombosis, and other blood flow abnormalities
29. **sestamibi test** (*ses*-ta-MIB-ē) (test)	nuclear medicine test used to diagnose coronary artery disease and assess revascularization after coronary artery bypass surgery. Sestamibi, a radioactive isotope, is taken up by normal myocardial cells, but not in ischemia or infarction. These areas are identified as "cold" spots on the images produced.
30. **single-photon emission computed tomography (SPECT)** (SING-el) (FŌ-ton) (ē-MISH-on) (com-PŪ-ted) (tō-MOG-ra-fē)	nuclear medicine test that collects a series of images (projections) as a gamma camera rotates around the patient. These projections are then used by a computer to generate three-dimensional pictures; it also helps show the function of organs, such as coronary artery flow or active and inactive areas of the brain.
31. **transesophageal echocardiogram (TEE)** (*trans*-e-*sof*-a-JĒ-al) (ek-ō-KAR-dē-ō-*gram*)	ultrasound test that examines cardiac function and structure by using an ultrasound probe placed in the esophagus, which provides more direct views of the heart structures

DIAGNOSTIC PROCEDURES

TERM	DEFINITION
32. **cardiac catheterization** (KAR-dē-ak) (*kath*-e-ter-i-ZĀ-shun)	diagnostic procedure performed by passing a catheter into the heart from a blood vessel in the groin or arm to examine the condition of the heart and surrounding blood vessels; used to diagnose and treat cardiovascular conditions such as coronary artery disease
33. **exercise stress test** (EK-ser-sīz) (stres) (test)	study that evaluates cardiac function during physical stress by riding a bike or walking on a treadmill. **Electrocardiography** is the most common method, but **echocardiography** and **nuclear medicine scanning** (diagnostic imaging tests) can also be used to measure cardiac function while exercising.

CHEMICAL STRESS TESTING is the use of drugs to simulate the stress of physical exercise on the body. It is used to study cardiac function in patients who are unable to exercise.

OTHER DIAGNOSTIC MEASUREMENT TERMS

TERM	DEFINITION
34. **blood pressure (BP)** (blud) (PRES-ūr)	pressure exerted by the blood against the blood vessel walls. A blood pressure measurement written as **systolic** pressure (120) and **diastolic** pressure (80) is commonly recorded as 120/80 (blood pressure is measured in millimeters of mercury [mm Hg]).

SYSTOLE (SIS-tō-lē) is the cardiac-cycle phase in which the ventricles contract and eject blood. **Diastole** (dī-AS-tō-lē) is the phase in which the ventricles relax and fill with blood between contractions.

35. **pulse (P)** (puls)	contraction of the heart, which can be felt with a fingertip. The pulse is most commonly felt over the radial artery (in the wrist); however, the pulsations can be felt over a number of sites, including the femoral (groin) and carotid (neck) arteries.
36. **sphygmomanometer** (*sfig*-mō-ma-NOM-e-ter)	device used for measuring blood pressure

Cardiovascular System Terms—cont'd
NOT BUILT FROM WORD PARTS

LABORATORY TERMS

TERM	DEFINITION
37. **C-reactive protein (CRP)** (C)-(rē-AK-tiv) (PRŌ-tēn)	blood test to measure the amount of C-reactive protein in the blood, which when elevated, indicates inflammation in the body. It is sometimes used in assessing the risk of cardiovascular disease.
38. **creatine phosphokinase (CPK)** (KRĒ-a-tin) (fos-fō-KĪ-nās)	blood test used to measure the level of creatine phosphokinase, an enzyme of heart and skeletal muscle released into the blood after muscle injury or necrosis. The test is useful in evaluating patients with acute myocardial infarction.
39. **lipid profile** (LIP-id) (PRŌ-fīl)	blood test used to measure the amount and type of lipids (fat-like substances) in a sample of blood. This test is used to evaluate one of the risks of cardiovascular disease and to monitor therapy for patients taking lipid-lowering medications. (Table 10.2)
40. **troponin** (TRŌ-pō-nin)	blood test that measures troponin, a heart muscle enzyme. Troponins are released into the blood approximately 3 hours after necrosis of the heart muscle and may remain elevated from 7 to 10 days. The test is useful in the diagnosis of a myocardial infarction.

BIOMARKER is a naturally occurring substance of certain body cells that can be measured in the blood and used to aid in the diagnosis of various disorders. **Troponin, creatine phosphokinase**, and **C-reactive protein** are biomarkers, and elevated levels are used in diagnosing various disorders occurring in the body.

SIGNS AND SYMPTOMS

TERM	DEFINITION
41. **bruit** (broo-Ē)	sound heard over an artery during auscultation, resulting from vibration in the vessel wall caused by turbulent blood flow. Bruits are frequently caused by abnormal narrowing of an artery.

TABLE 10.2 Understanding a Lipid Profile

Cholesterol—a compound important in the production of sex hormones, steroids, cell membranes, and bile acids. Cholesterol is produced by the body and is also contained in foods such as animal fats. Cholesterol is transported by lipoproteins.

High-density lipoprotein (HDL)—a type of lipoprotein that removes cholesterol from the tissues and transports it to the liver to be excreted in the bile. Elevated levels of HDL are considered protective against development of atherosclerosis, which may lead to coronary artery disease. HDL is often referred to as the "good" cholesterol.

Low-density lipoprotein (LDL)—a type of lipoprotein that transports cholesterol to the tissue and deposits it on the walls of the arteries. High levels of LDL are associated with the presence of atherosclerosis, which may lead to coronary artery disease. LDL is often referred to as the "bad" cholesterol.

Total cholesterol—a measurement of the cholesterol components LDL, HDL, and VLDL (triglyceride carriers) in the blood.

Triglycerides (TGs)—a form of fat in the blood. Triglycerides are synthesized in the liver and used to store energy. Test results are used to assess the risk of coronary artery disease.

Very-low-density lipoprotein (VLDL)—a type of lipoprotein that transports most of the triglycerides in the blood. Elevated levels of VLDL, to a lesser degree than LDL, indicate a risk for developing coronary artery disease.

Chapter 10 Cardiovascular, Lymphatic, Immune Systems and Blood 383

TERM	DEFINITION
42. hypercholesterolemia (hī-per-k-*les*-ter-ol-Ē-mē-a)	excessive amount of cholesterol in the blood; associated with an increased risk of cardiovascular disease
43. hyperlipidemia (hī-per-*lip*-i-DĒ-mē-a)	excessive amount of any type of fats (lipoproteins, triglycerides, and cholesterol) in the blood; associated with an increased risk of cardiovascular disease
44. hypertension (HTN) (hī-per-TEN-shun)	blood pressure that is above normal (greater than 130/80 mm Hg in adults under the age of 60)
45. hypertriglyceridemia (hī-per-trī-*glis*-er-rī-DĒ-mē-a)	excessive amount of triglycerides in the blood; associated with an increased risk of cardiovascular disease
46. hypotension (hī-pō-TEN-shun)	blood pressure that is below normal (less than 90/60 mm Hg in adults under the age of 60)
47. murmur (MER-mer)	unusual sound heard during auscultation of the heart caused by turbulent blood flow. It may be "innocent" (not indicating disease), or it may reflect disease or malformation, such as an abnormal heart valve.
48. occlusion (a-KLOO-shun)	closing or blockage of a blood vessel or hollow organ

TREATMENTS

TERM	DEFINITION
49. cardiopulmonary resuscitation (CPR) (*kar*-dē-ō-PUL-mo-nar-ē) (rē-*sus*-i-TĀ-shun)	emergency procedure consisting of external cardiac compressions; may be accompanied by artificial ventilation
50. defibrillation (dē-*fib*-ri-LĀ-shun)	application of an electric shock to the myocardium through the chest wall to restore normal cardiac rhythm (Fig. 10.14)
51. vasoconstrictor (*vās*-ō-kon-STRIK-tor)	agent that narrows the diameter of the blood vessels
52. vasodilator (*vās*-ō-DĪ-lā-tor)	agent that expands the diameter of the blood vessels

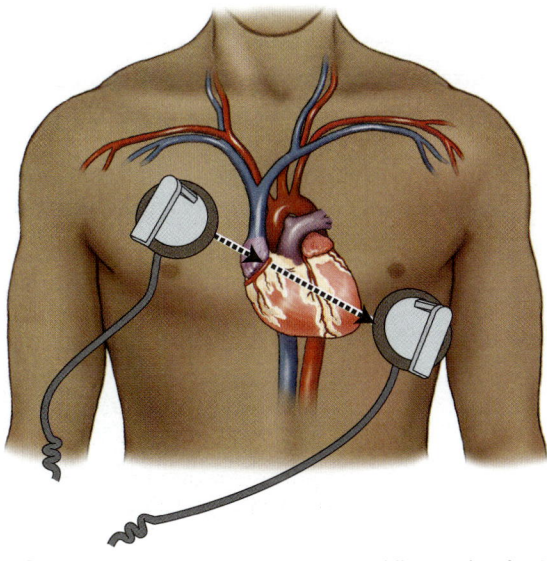

FIG. 10.14 Placement of defibrillator paddles on the chest.

384 Chapter 10 Cardiovascular, Lymphatic, Immune Systems and Blood

EXERCISE 8 ■ Pronounce and Spell

Practice pronunciation and spelling on paper and online.

1. **Practice on Paper**
   a. **Pronounce:** Read the phonetic spelling and say aloud the terms listed in the previous table. Refer to Table 2.2 Pronunciation Key as needed.
   b. **Spell:** Have a study partner read the terms aloud. Write the spelling of the terms on a separate sheet of paper.

2. **Practice Online**
   a. **Access** online learning resources. Go to evolve.elsevier.com > Evolve Resources > Student Resources.
   b. **Pronounce:** Select Audio Glossary > Chapter 10 > Exercise 8. Select a term to hear its pronunciation and repeat aloud.
   c. **Spell:** Select Activities > Chapter 10 > Spell Terms > Exercise 8. Select the audio icon and type the correct spelling of the term.

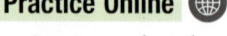

❏ Check the box when complete.

EXERCISE 9 ■ Fill In

A Disease and Disorder Terms

Fill in the blanks with the correct terms.

1. Sudden cessation of cardiac output and effective circulation is referred to as a(n) _____
   _____.
2. Veins that are distended or tortuous are called _____ _____.
3. _____ is the name given to the ballooning of a weakened portion of an artery wall.
4. _____ _____ _____ is a condition most often caused by coronary atherosclerosis, which deprives the heart tissue of sufficient oxygen and nutrients to function normally.
5. _____ _____ is a cardiac condition characterized by chest pain caused by an insufficient blood supply to the cardiac muscle.
6. Death of a portion of myocardial muscle caused by lack of oxygen resulting from an interrupted blood supply is called a(n) _____ _____.
7. Rapid, quivering, uncoordinated contractions of the atria or ventricles called _____ create a(n) _____, or a disturbance or abnormality in the heart's normal rhythmic pattern.
8. A disorder of the heart caused by a persistently high blood pressure is called _____ heart disease.
9. _____ _____ is the inability of the heart to pump enough blood through the body to supply tissues and organs.
10. _____ _____ _____ is a disease of the arteries in the arms and legs, resulting in narrowing or complete obstruction of an artery.
11. _____ _____ is a condition in which a patient has pain and discomfort in calf muscles while walking.
12. Acute compression of the heart caused by fluid accumulation in the pericardial cavity is known as _____
    _____.

Chapter 10   Cardiovascular, Lymphatic, Immune Systems and Blood   385

13. Episodes of rheumatic fever can cause _____ _____ _____ and _____ _____ _____ _____.

14. _____ _____ _____ is the formation of a blood clot, most often occurring in the lower extremities.

15. _____ _____ _____ is a sudden insufficient blood supply to the heart, indicating unstable angina or myocardial infarction.

16. Enlargement of the heart's right ventricle due to pulmonary disease is called _____ _____.

B Surgical Terms

Write the surgical terms pictured and defined.

1. _____

battery-powered apparatus implanted under the skin, with leads placed on the heart or in the chamber of the heart; used to treat an abnormal heart rhythm

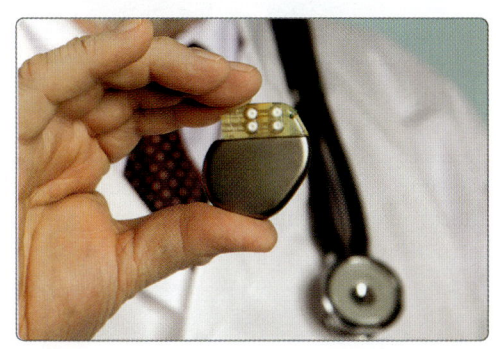

2. _____

injection of a medication either intravenously or intraarterially to dissolve blood clots

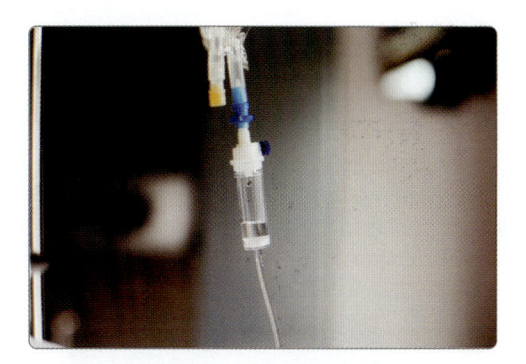

3. _____

surgical technique to bring a new blood supply to heart muscle by detouring around blocked arteries

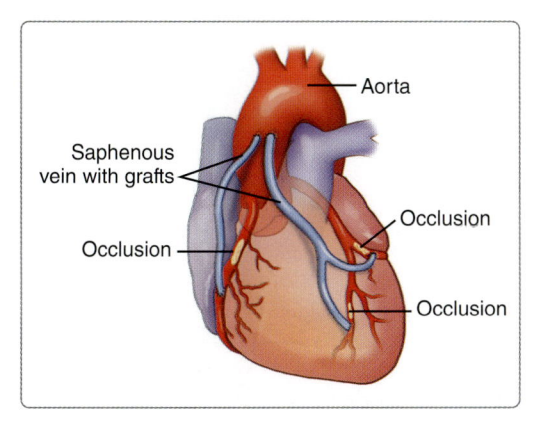

4. _____

procedure in which abnormal cells that trigger abnormal heart rhythms (arrhythmias) are destroyed by using a device that heats or freezes the cells

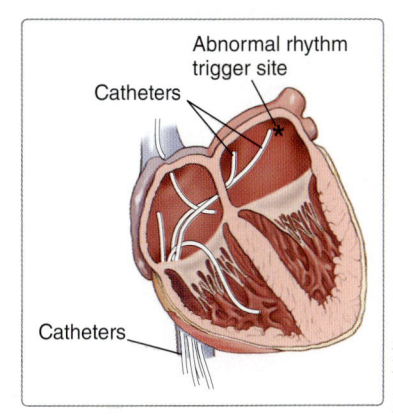

5. _____

supportive scaffold device placed in the coronary artery; used to prevent closure of the artery after angioplasty or atherectomy

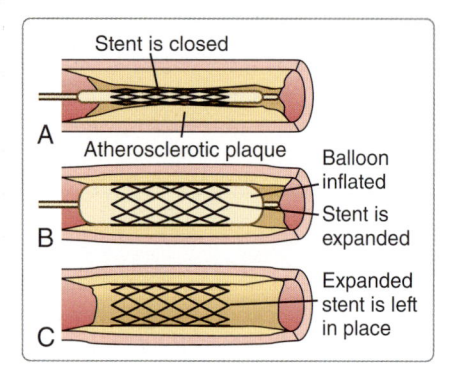

6. _____

procedure in which a balloon is advanced into the coronary artery to where plaque has formed. The balloon is inflated, and the vessel wall expands, allowing blood to flow more freely

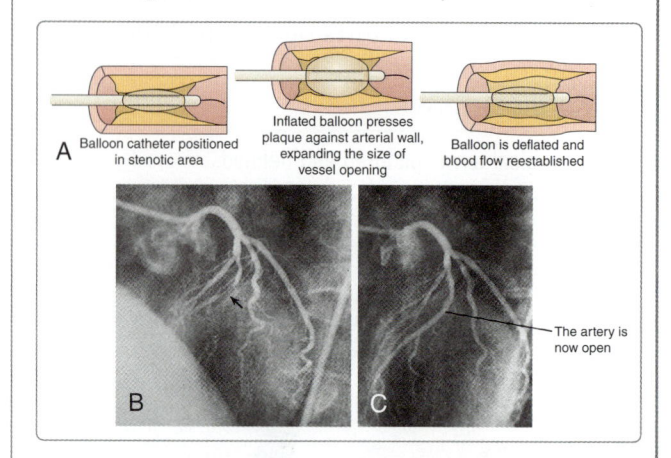

7. _____

device implanted in the body that can deliver an electric shock to convert arrhythmia back to a normal rhythm

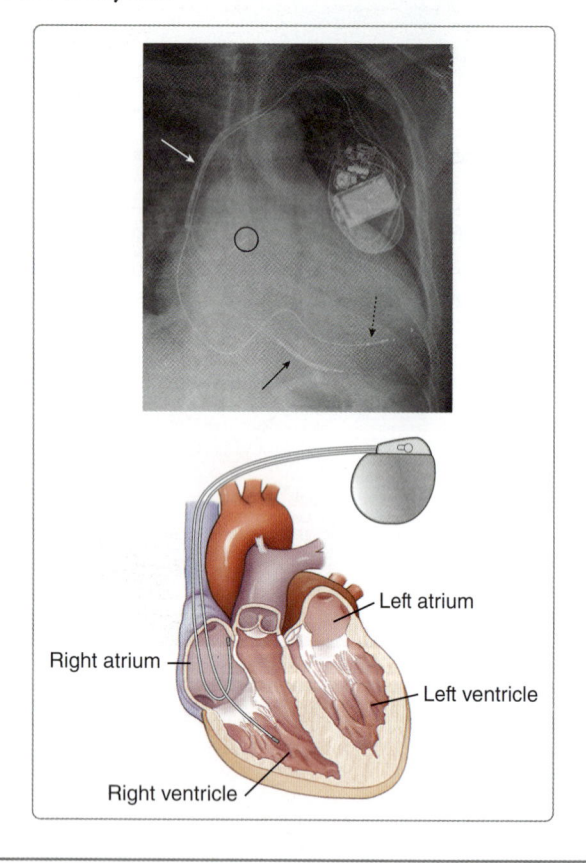

8. _____

surgery to establish an alternate route from the femoral artery to the popliteal artery to bypass an obstruction

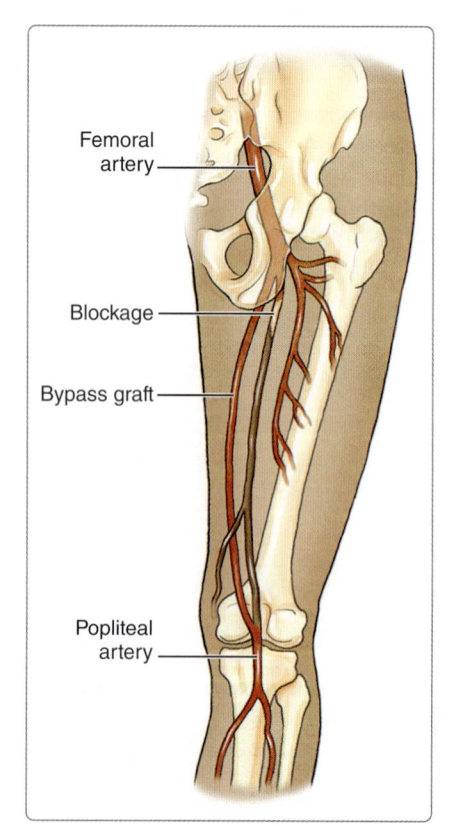

Chapter 10 Cardiovascular, Lymphatic, Immune Systems and Blood   387

EXERCISE 10 ■ Diagnostic Terms

A Label

Write the diagnostic terms pictured and defined.

1. _____
study that uses high-frequency sound waves for detection of blood flow within the vessels

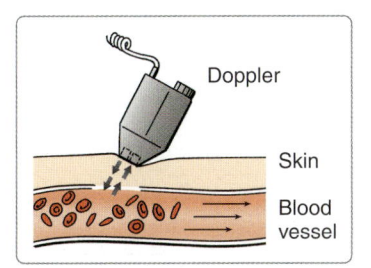

2. _____
blood test used to measure the amount and type of fat-like substances in a sample of blood

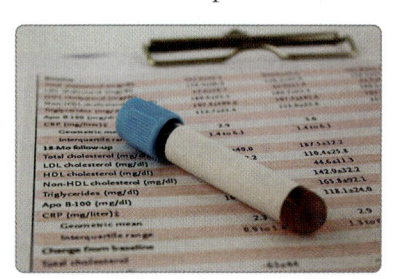

3. _____
study that elevates cardiac function during physical stress by riding a bike or walking on a treadmill

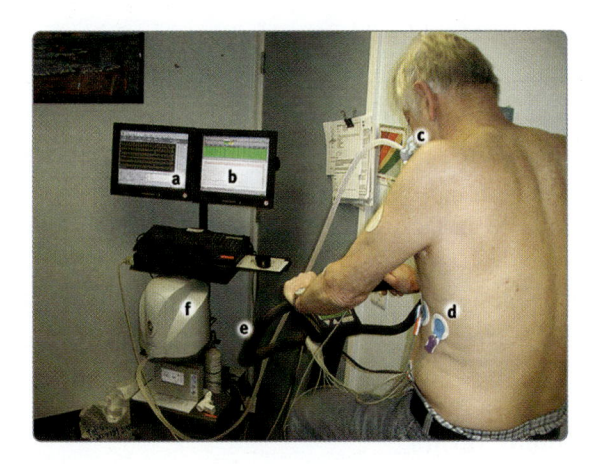

4. _____
nuclear medicine test used to diagnose coronary artery disease and assess revascularization after CABG surgery

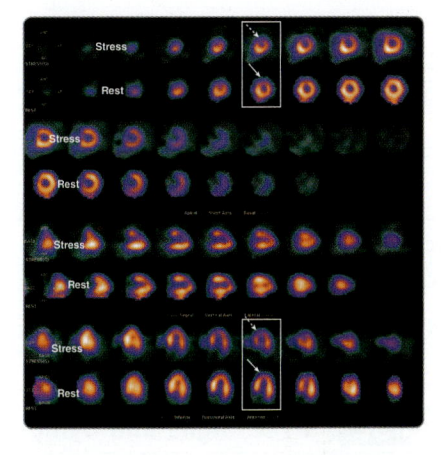

5. _____
process of digital radiographic imaging of the blood vessels that "subtracts" or removes structures not being studied

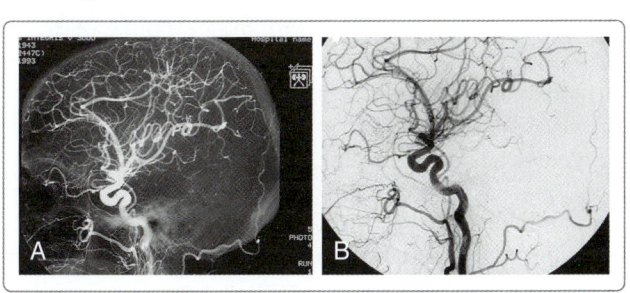

6. _____
device used to measure blood pressure

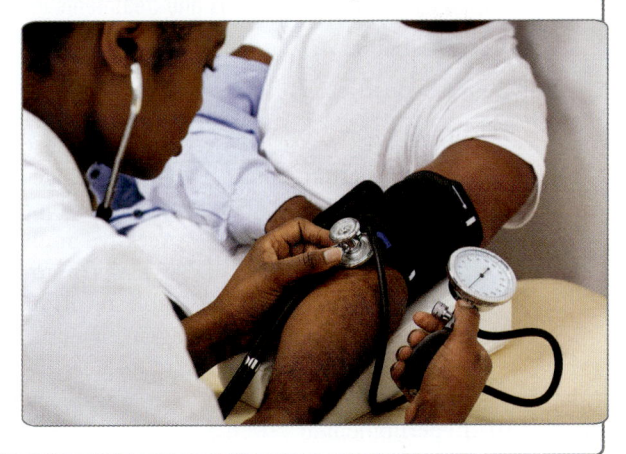

388 Chapter 10 Cardiovascular, Lymphatic, Immune Systems and Blood

7. _____
diagnostic procedure performed by passing a catheter into the heart from a vessel in the groin or arm to examine the condition of the heart and surrounding blood vessels

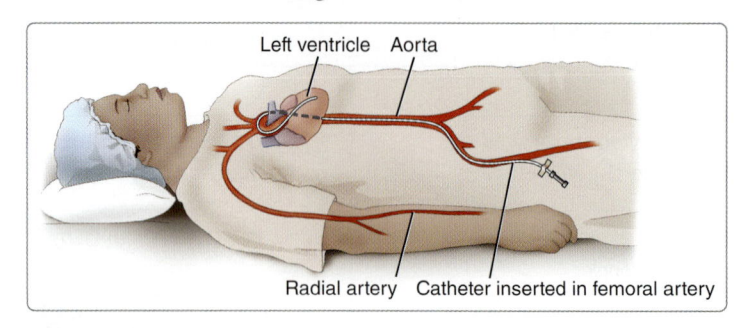

B Fill In

Fill in the blanks with the correct diagnostic terms.

1. _____ _____ is a test in which an ultrasound probe provides views of the heart structures from the esophagus.
2. A nuclear medicine test that visualizes the heart from several different angles, producing three-dimensional images, is called a(n) _____-_____ _____ _____ _____.
3. A blood test to measure an enzyme of the heart released into the bloodstream after muscle injury is called _____ _____.
4. An elevated _____ _____ indicates inflammation in the body.
5. _____ is the rhythmic expansion of an artery created by contraction of the heart that can be felt with a fingertip.
6. _____ is a heart muscle enzyme released into the bloodstream approximately 3 hours after heart muscle necrosis.
7. The vital sign measured with the use of a sphygmomanometer and stethoscope that is recorded in millimeters of mercury is _____ _____.

EXERCISE 11 ■ Signs and Symptoms and Treatment Terms

A Match

Match the terms for signs and symptoms and treatments in the first column with the correct definitions in the second column.

_____ 1. vasodilator
_____ 2. vasoconstrictor
_____ 3. bruit
_____ 4. hypercholesterolemia
_____ 5. occlusion
_____ 6. murmur
_____ 7. hypotension
_____ 8. hypertriglyceridemia
_____ 9. hypertension
_____ 10. hyperlipidemia

a. blood pressure that is below normal (less than 90/60 mm Hg in adults under the age of 60)
b. excessive amount of cholesterol in the blood
c. blood pressure that is above normal (greater than 130/80 mm Hg in adults under the age of 60)
d. closing or blockage of a blood vessel or hollow organ
e. excessive amount of triglycerides in the blood
f. excessive amount of any type of fats (lipoproteins, triglycerides, and cholesterol) in the blood
g. agent or nerve that narrows the diameter of the blood vessels
h. sound heard over an artery during auscultation, resulting from vibration in the vessel wall caused by turbulent blood flow
i. unusual sound heard during auscultation of the heart caused by turbulent blood flow
j. agent or nerve that expands the diameter of the blood vessels

B Label

Write the treatment terms pictured and defined.

1. _____
application of an electric shock to the myocardium through the chest wall to restore normal cardiac rhythm

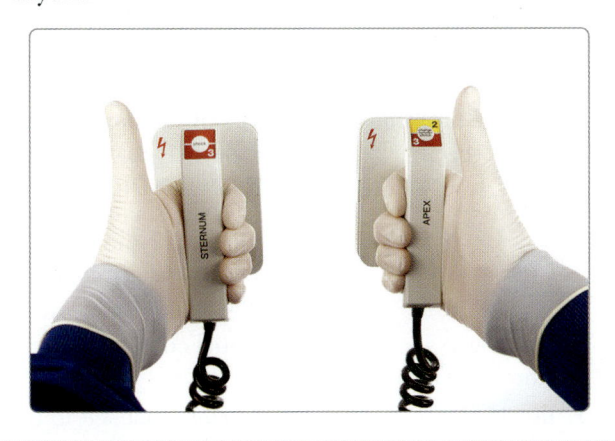

2. _____
emergency procedure consisting of external cardiac compressions; may be accompanied by artificial ventilation

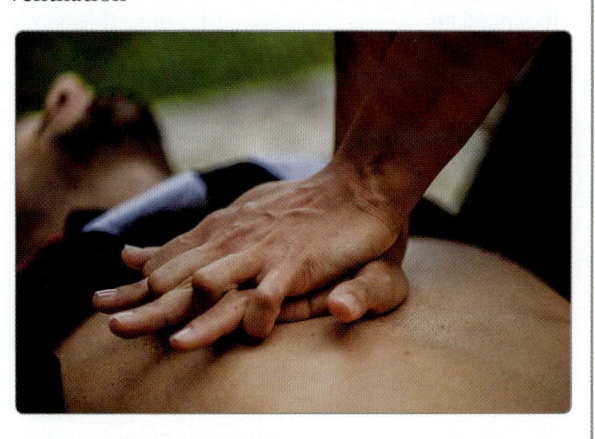

EXERCISE 12 ■ Review of Cardiovascular Terms

Can you define, pronounce, and spell the following cardiovascular system terms?

acute coronary syndrome (ACS)
aneurysm
angina pectoris
angiography
angioma
angioplasty
angioscopy
angiostenosis
aortic stenosis
aortogram
arrhythmia
arteriogram
arteriosclerosis
artificial cardiac pacemaker
atherectomy
atherosclerosis
atrioventricular (AV)
automatic implantable cardiac defibrillator (AICD)
blood pressure (BP)
bradycardia
bruit
cardiac arrest
cardiac catheterization
cardiac tamponade
cardiogenic
cardiologist
cardiology
cardiomegaly
cardiomyopathy
cardiopulmonary resuscitation (CPR)
catheter ablation
cor pulmonale
coronary artery bypass graft (CABG)
coronary artery disease (CAD)
coronary stent
C-reactive protein (CRP)
creatine phosphokinase (CPK)
deep vein thrombosis (DVT)
defibrillation
digital subtraction angiography (DSA)
Doppler ultrasound
echocardiogram (ECHO)
electrocardiogram (ECG, EKG)
electrocardiography
embolectomy
endarterectomy
endocarditis
exercise stress test
femoropopliteal bypass
fibrillation
heart failure (HF)
hypercholesterolemia
hyperlipidemia
hypertension (HTN)
hypertensive heart disease (HHD)
hypertriglyceridemia
hypotension
intermittent claudication
intravenous (IV)
ischemia
lipid profile
mitral valve stenosis
murmur
myocardial infarction (MI)
myocarditis
occlusion
percutaneous transluminal coronary angioplasty (PTCA)
pericardiocentesis
pericarditis
peripheral artery disease (PAD)
phlebectomy
phlebitis
polyarteritis
pulse
rheumatic heart disease
sestamibi test
single-photon emission computed tomography (SPECT)
sphygmomanometer
tachycardia
thrombolytic therapy
thrombophlebitis
transesophageal echocardiogram (TEE)
troponin
valvulitis
valvuloplasty
varicose veins
vasoconstrictor
vasodilator
venogram

Blood Terms
BUILT FROM WORD PARTS

The following terms can be translated using definitions of word parts. Further explanation is provided within parentheses as needed.

DISEASE AND DISORDERS

TERM	DEFINITION	TERM	DEFINITION
1. embolism (EM-bō-lizm)	state of a plug (blood clot or foreign material, such as air or fat, lodged inside a blood vessel)	4. hemorrhage (HEM-o-rij)	excessive flow of blood (bleeding internally or externally)
2. embolus (*pl.* emboli) (EM-bō-lus) (EM-bo-lī)	plug (blood clot or foreign material, such as air or fat, that enters the bloodstream and moves until it lodges at another point in the circulation)	5. multiple myeloma (MUL-te-pl) (mī-e-LŌ-ma)	tumors of the bone marrow (a blood malignancy that most often occurs after age 65. Signs and symptoms may include bone pain, infections, weight loss, anemia, and fatigue.)
3. hematoma (hē-ma-TŌ-ma)	tumor of blood (collection of blood that has leaked out of a broken vessel into the surrounding tissue)	6. thrombosis (throm-BŌ-sis)	abnormal condition of a blood clot
		7. thrombus (THROM-bus)	blood clot (attached to the interior wall of an artery or vein)

💡 **EMBOLUS/THROMBUS** An embolus circulates in the bloodstream until it becomes lodged in a vessel, whereas a thrombus is attached to the interior wall of a vessel. When any part of a thrombus breaks away and circulates in the bloodstream, it becomes known as an embolus.

SIGNS AND SYMPTOMS

TERM	DEFINITION	TERM	DEFINITION
8. erythrocytopenia (e-rith-rō-sī-tō-PĒ-nē-a)	abnormal reduction of red (blood) cells (a form of **anemia**); (lab finding)	10. lymphocytosis (lim-fō-sī-TŌ-sis)	increase in the number of lymphocytes; (lab finding)
9. leukocytopenia (lū-kō-sī-tō-PĒ-nē-a)	abnormal reduction of white (blood) cells (also called **leukopenia**); (lab finding)	11. pancytopenia (pan-sī-tō-PĒ-nē-a)	abnormal reduction of all (blood) cells; (lab finding)
		12. thrombocytopenia (throm-bō-sī-tō-PĒ-nē-a)	abnormal reduction of blood clotting cells (platelets); (lab finding)

OTHER TERMS

TERM	DEFINITION	TERM	DEFINITION
13. hematologist (hē-ma-TOL-o-jist)	physician who studies and treats diseases of the blood	16. plasmapheresis (plaz-ma-fe-RĒ-sis)	removal of plasma (from withdrawn blood; the cells, called formed elements, are then reinfused into the donor or into another patient who needs blood cells rather than whole blood)
14. hemolysis (hē-MOL-i-sis)	dissolution of (red) blood (cells)		
HEMOLYSIS refers to the breakdown of red blood cells at the end of their life cycles. Diseases, genetic defects, and medications can increase the rate of hemolysis, causing red blood cells to be destroyed too soon. The resulting shortage of healthy red blood cells leads to a form of anemia called **hemolytic anemia**.			
		17. phlebotomy (fle-BOT-o-mē)	incision into a vein (with a needle to remove blood for testing)
15. hemostasis (hē-mō-STĀ-sis)	stoppage of bleeding	18. thrombolysis (throm-BOL-i-sis)	dissolution of a blood clot

Chapter 10 Cardiovascular, Lymphatic, Immune Systems and Blood   391

EXERCISE 13 ■ Pronounce and Spell

Practice pronunciation and spelling on paper and online.

1. **Practice on Paper**
   a. **Pronounce:** Read the phonetic spelling and say aloud the terms listed in the previous table. Refer to Table 2.2 Pronunciation Key as needed.
   b. **Spell:** Have a study partner read the terms aloud. Write the spelling of the terms on a separate sheet of paper.

2. **Practice Online**
   a. **Access** online learning resources. Go to evolve.elsevier.com > Evolve Resources > Student Resources.
   b. **Pronounce:** Select Audio Glossary > Chapter 10 > Exercise 13. Select a term to hear its pronunciation and repeat aloud.
   c. **Spell:** Select Activities > Chapter 10 > Spell Terms > Exercise 13. Select the audio icon and type the correct spelling of the term.

❏ Check the box when complete.

EXERCISE 14 ■ Analyze and Define

Analyze and define the following blood terms.

1. hemostasis

2. hematologist

3. hemolysis

4. lymphocytosis

5. pancytopenia

6. erythrocytopenia

7. embolism

8. thrombus

EXERCISE 15 ■ Build

A Fill In

Build blood terms for the following definitions by using the word parts you have learned.

1. abnormal reduction of white (blood) cells   ___ / ___ / ___ / ___ / ___
                                                  WR   CV   WR   CV   S

392 Chapter 10 Cardiovascular, Lymphatic, Immune Systems and Blood

2. excessive flow of blood

_____ / _____ / _____
WR   CV   S

3. dissolution of a blood clot

_____ / _____ / _____
WR   CV   S

4. abnormal reduction of blood clotting cells (platelets)

_____ / ___ / _____ / ___ / _____
WR   CV   WR   CV   S

5. plug

_____ / _____
WR   S

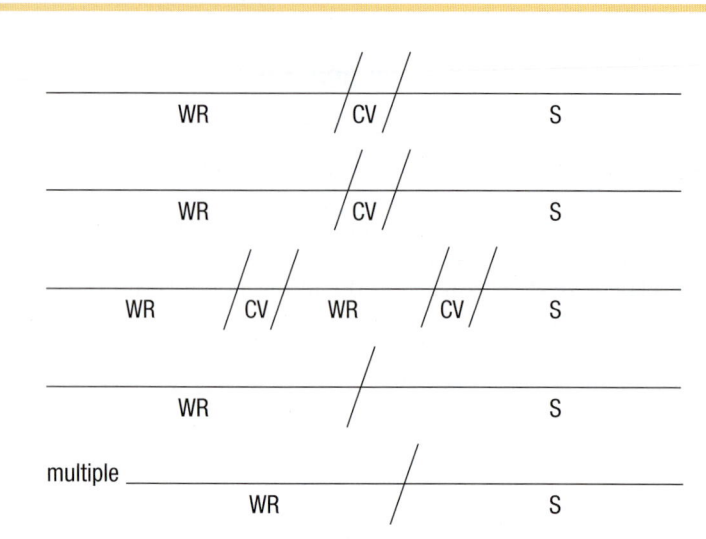

6. tumors of the bone marrow

multiple _____ / _____
           WR   S

B Label

Build terms pictured by writing word parts above definitions.

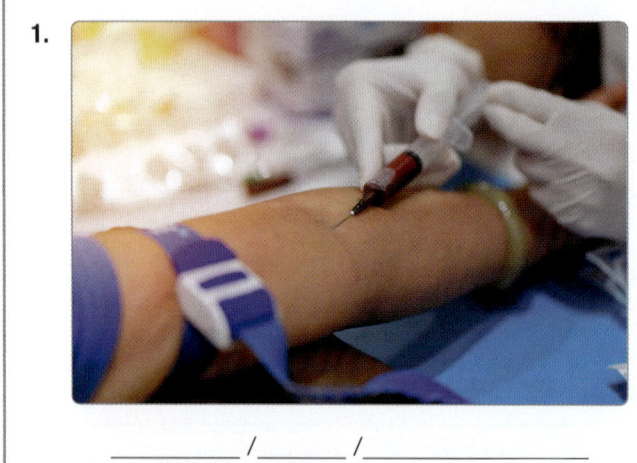

1.

_____ / _____ / _____
vein   CV   incision

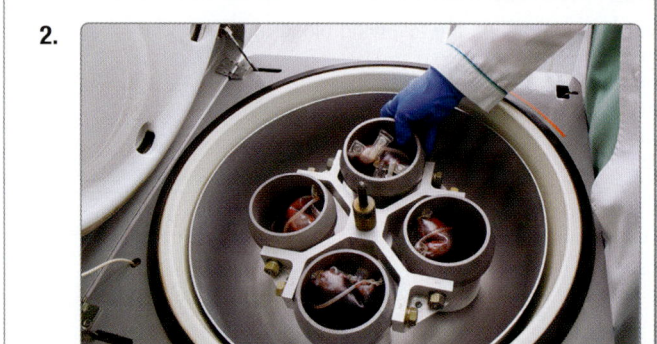

2.

_____ / _____
    plasma   removal

3.

Post-surgical site displaying swelling and formation of a _____ / _____
                                                             blood   tumor

4.

Blocked artery due to atherosclerosis and _____ / _____
                                          blood clot   abnormal
                                                       condition

Blood Terms
NOT BUILT FROM WORD PARTS

Word parts may be present in the following terms; however, their full meanings cannot be translated using definitions of word parts alone.

DISEASE AND DISORDERS

TERM	DEFINITION
1. **anemia** (a-NĒ-mē-a)	condition in which there is a reduction in the number of erythrocytes (RBCs). Anemia may be caused by blood loss, by decreased production of RBCs, or by increased destruction of RBCs. (Table 10.3)
2. **bleeding disorder** (BLĒD-ing) (dis-OR-der)	disease in which there is an inability to form proper blood clots; examples include hemophilia, von Willebrand disease, and clotting factor deficiencies
3. **hemophilia** (hē-mō-FIL-ē-a)	inherited bleeding disorder most commonly caused by a deficiency of the coagulation factor VIII
4. **leukemia** (lū-KĒ-mē-a)	malignant disease characterized by excessive increase in abnormal leukocytes (white blood cells) formed in the bone marrow (Table 10.4)

TABLE 10.3 Common Types of Anemia

TYPE	DESCRIPTION
Anemia due to blood loss	• acute blood loss anemia as a result of hemorrhage
Anemia due to decreased production of red blood cells	• iron deficiency anemia: not enough iron in the body to produce hemoglobin • pernicious anemia: ineffective production of red blood cells due to vitamin B_{12} deficiency • aplastic anemia: resulting from bone marrow failure
Anemia due to increased destruction of red blood cells	• hemolytic anemia: reduced life of blood cells (such as in sickle cell disease)

TABLE 10.4 Leukemia

Leukemia is differentiated by the type of leukocyte that is affected and how quickly the disease develops and progresses.

Acute leukemia develops quickly with rapid progression of the disease. Both adults and children may develop acute leukemia. Acute leukemia is the most common form of cancer in children and adolescents.

Chronic leukemia develops slowly with gradual disease progression and most often occurs in adults.

Lymphocytic leukemia affects the lymphoid cells (lymphocytes), which form lymph tissue (part of the immune system).

Myelogenous leukemia affects the myeloid cells, which form red blood cells, white blood cells, and platelets.

MAJOR TYPES OF LEUKEMIA
- **acute lymphocytic leukemia (ALL):** the most common type in young children; can affect adults (also called acute lymphoblastic leukemia)
- **acute myelogenous leukemia (AML):** most common acute leukemia in adults; can also affect children
- **chronic lymphocytic leukemia (CLL):** most common chronic adult leukemia; patient may feel well for years without needing treatment
- **chronic myelogenous leukemia (CML):** occurs mostly in older adults

Rare types of leukemia include hairy cell leukemia (**HCL**), myelodysplastic syndromes, and myeloproliferative disorders

Blood Terms—cont'd
NOT BUILT FROM WORD PARTS

DISEASE AND DISORDERS—CONT'D

TERM	DEFINITION
5. sepsis (SEP-sis)	systemic inflammatory response caused by pathogenic microorganisms, usually bacteria, entering the bloodstream and multiplying; life-threatening condition, which may lead to tissue damage, organ failure, and death. The overwhelming presence of pathogens in the blood is called septicemia.
6. sickle cell disease (SI-kl) (sel) (di-ZĒZ)	group of inherited red blood cell disorders (anemias) in which hemoglobin is abnormally shaped and has a shorter life cycle
7. thalassemia (*thal*-a-SĒ-mē-ah)	inherited bleeding disorder causing reduced production of healthy blood cells and hemoglobin

DIAGNOSTIC PROCEDURES

TERM	DEFINITION
8. bone marrow aspiration (bōn) (MAR-ō) (*as*-pi-RĀ-shun)	procedure to obtain a sample of the **liquid** portion of the bone marrow, usually from the ilium (upper hip bone) for study; used to diagnose leukemia, infections, some types of anemia, and other blood disorders
9. bone marrow biopsy (bōn) (MAR-ō) (BĪ-op-sē)	procedure to obtain a sample of the **solid** portion of bone marrow, usually from the ilium, for study; used to diagnose leukemia, infections, some types of anemia, and other blood disorders. May be performed at the same time as bone marrow aspiration.

BONE MARROW is contained within spongy bone, which is located primarily at the ends of long bones and in the center of other bones. Stem cells within the bone marrow turn into thrombocytes (platelets), red blood cells, and white blood cells.

LABORATORY

TERM	DEFINITION
10. activated partial thromboplastin time (aPTT) (AK-ti-*vāt*-ed) (PAR-shel) (*throm*-bō-PLAS-tin) (tīm)	blood test that measures the ability of the blood to clot by assessing intrinsic blood factors. Used to evaluate bleeding disorders, such as hemophilia A and B, and to monitor some types of anticoagulation therapy, such as heparin. Frequently ordered in conjunction with prothrombin time (PT/INR).
11. bleeding profile (BLĒD-ing) (PRŌ-fīl)	series of tests that measure the ability of various factors in the blood to form a clot. Usually includes PT/INR, aPTT, thrombin time, and tests for platelets and fibrinogen.

COAGULATION ABNORMALITIES Blood coagulation is the process that causes blood to clot and helps prevent excessive blood loss through a cut, puncture, or other trauma to blood vessels. The coagulation cascade involves a series of components called **blood clotting factors**, which act together in a step-wise manner to stop the flow of blood. These factors may be **intrinsic** (originating in the blood) or **extrinsic** (originating from tissues outside the blood). An abnormality in any of these factors, or in the ways in which they come together to form a clot, may result in either an inability to form a clot, such as **hemophilia**, or a tendency for the blood to form clots too easily, such as **deep vein thrombosis**. There are a number of laboratory tests in use to determine whether coagulation is functioning appropriately or to find the source of the abnormality if a patient is bleeding too much or clotting too easily.

TERM	DEFINITION
12. complete blood count with differential (CBC with diff) (com-PLĒT) (blud) (kownt) (with) (*dif*-er-EN-shal)	laboratory test for basic blood screening that measures various aspects of erythrocytes, leukocytes, and thrombocytes (platelets); this automated test quickly provides a tremendous amount of information about the blood
13. hematocrit (Hct) (hē-MAT-o-crit)	percentage of a blood sample that is composed of erythrocytes. It is used in the diagnosis and evaluation of anemic patients.

TERM	DEFINITION
14. hemoglobin (Hgb) (HĒ-mō-*glō*-bin)	blood test that measures the amount of hemoglobin (the protein in red blood cells that carries oxygen) in the blood
15. prothrombin time (PT/INR) (prō-THROM-bin) (tīm)	blood test that measures the ability of the blood to clot by assessing extrinsic blood factors. Used to evaluate bleeding disorders such as those caused by liver disease or vitamin K deficiency, or to monitor anticoagulation therapy such as warfarin. Frequently ordered in conjunction with activated partial thromboplastin time (aPTT).

PT/INR stands for **prothrombin time/international normalized ratio**. Most institutions, on the recommendation of the World Health Organization, report both absolute numbers and INR numbers, which provide uniform PT results to physicians worldwide.

TREATMENTS

TERM	DEFINITION
16. bone marrow transplant (BMT) (bōn) (MAR-ō) (TRANS-plant)	infusion of healthy bone marrow cells from a matched donor into a patient with severely diseased or damaged bone marrow; the donor cells may establish a new colony of healthy tissue in the recipient's bone marrow
17. peripheral blood stem cell transplant (PBSCT) (pe-RIF-er-al)(blud) (stem) (sel) (TRANS-plant)	infusion of blood-forming cells (stem cells) to replace blood cells damaged by disease or treatments, such as chemotherapy; stem cells are collected by apheresis, a process in which blood is removed from the patient or a matched donor and spun through a machine to harvest stem cells

INFUSION is the introduction of fluid into the bloodstream through a vein.

MEDICAL SPECIALTIES

TERM	DEFINITION
18. perfusionist (per-FŪ-shun-ist)	person who operates the heart-lung machine during surgeries in which the patient's blood must be oxygenated outside of the body; perfusionists monitor and are responsible for the circulatory and respiratory function of the patient during cardiothoracic surgery
19. phlebotomist (fle-BOT-ō-mist)	person who performs venipuncture for the purpose of drawing blood

OTHER TERMS

TERM	DEFINITION
20. anticoagulant (*an*-tī-kō-AG-ū-lant)	agent that slows the blood clotting process
21. blood dyscrasia (blud) (dis-KRĀ-zha)	any abnormal or pathologic condition of the blood

DYSCRASIA is made up of the Greek word parts **dys-**, meaning difficult, painful or abnormal, and **-crasia**, meaning mixture. Blood disease in ancient Greek times was thought to be an abnormal mixture of the four humors: blood, black bile, yellow bile, and phlegm. Today the term remains, but its full meaning can no longer be directly translated from its word parts.

TERM	DEFINITION
22. extravasation (ek-*strav*-a-SĀ-shun)	escape of blood or other fluid from a vessel into the tissue
23. venipuncture (VEN-i-*punk*-chur)	procedure used to puncture a vein with a needle to remove blood, instill a medication, or start an intravenous infusion

Chapter 10 Cardiovascular, Lymphatic, Immune Systems and Blood

EXERCISE 16 ■ Pronounce and Spell

Practice pronunciation and spelling on paper and online.

1. **Practice on Paper**
   a. **Pronounce:** Read the phonetic spelling and say aloud the terms listed in the previous table. Refer to Table 2.2 Pronunciation Key as needed.
   b. **Spell:** Have a study partner read the terms aloud. Write the spelling of the terms on a separate sheet of paper.
2. **Practice Online**
   a. **Access** online learning resources. Go to evolve.elsevier.com > Evolve Resources > Student Resources.
   b. **Pronounce:** Select Audio Glossary > Chapter 10 > Exercise 16. Select a term to hear its pronunciation and repeat aloud.
   c. **Spell:** Select Activities > Chapter 10 > Spell Terms > Exercise 16. Select the audio icon and type the correct spelling of the term.

❑ Check the box when complete.

EXERCISE 17 ■ Match

Match the disease and disorder terms in the first column with their correct definitions in the second column.

_____ 1. anemia
_____ 2. thalassemia
_____ 3. leukemia
_____ 4. sepsis
_____ 5. sickle cell disease
_____ 6. hemophilia
_____ 7. bleeding disorder

a. disease in which there is an inability to form proper blood clots (general term)
b. systemic inflammatory response caused by pathogenic microorganisms, usually bacteria, entering the bloodstream and multiplying
c. inherited bleeding disorder most commonly caused by a deficiency of the coagulation factor VIII
d. group of inherited red blood disorders in which hemoglobin is abnormally shaped and has a shorter life cycle
e. condition in which there is a reduction in the number of erythrocytes
f. malignant disease characterized by excessive increase in abnormal leukocytes
g. inherited blood disorder causing reduced production of healthy blood cells and hemoglobin

EXERCISE 18 ■ Label

Write the medical term pictured and defined.

1. _____

procedure to obtain a sample of the **liquid** portion of the bone marrow

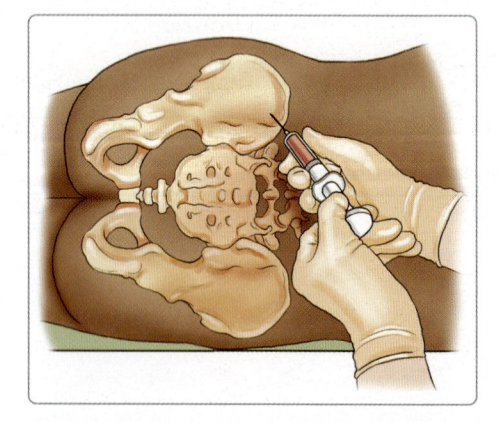

2. _____

procedure to obtain a sample of the **solid** portion of bone marrow

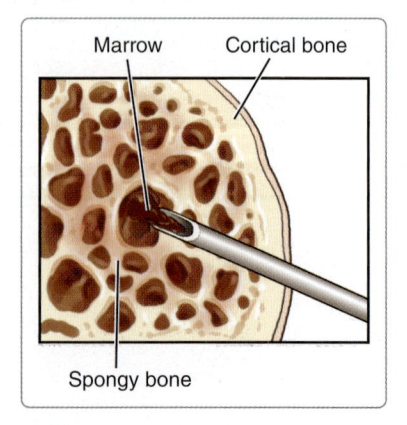

Chapter 10 Cardiovascular, Lymphatic, Immune Systems and Blood   397

3. _____
person who performs venipuncture for the purpose of drawing blood

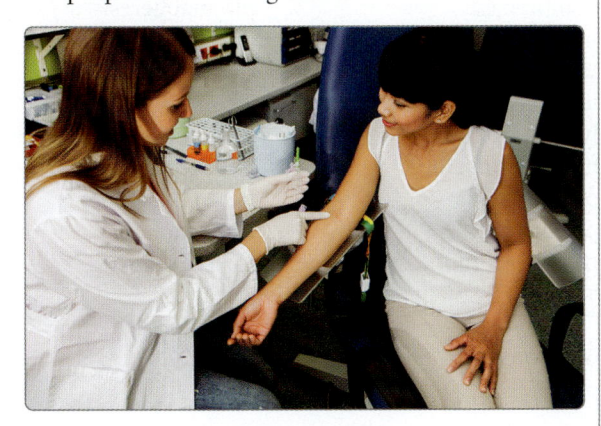

4. _____
person who operates the heart-lung machine during surgeries in which the patient's blood must be oxygenated outside of the body

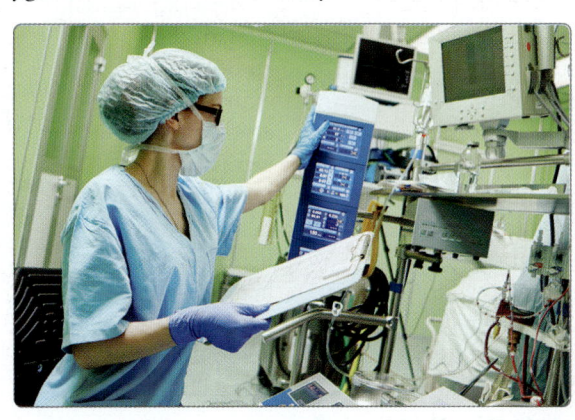

EXERCISE 19 ■ Fill In

Fill in the blanks with the correct terms.

1. Sickle cell disease, thalassemia, and leukemia are examples of _____ (plural form of the term), any abnormal or pathologic conditions of the blood.

2. A(n) _____, or agent that slows the blood clotting process, would be prescribed to prevent clots forming in blood vessels in patients diagnosed with atrial fibrillation, in patients with mechanical heart valves, and following certain surgeries.

3. A phlebotomist performs _____, the procedure used to puncture a vein with a needle to remove blood, instill a medication, or start an intravenous infusion. The escape of blood or fluid from a vessel, or _____, may occur at a venipuncture site. Tissue damage may occur if infused medicine leaks into surrounding tissue.

4. The infusion of healthy bone marrow cells, called a _____, and the infusion of blood-forming cells, called a _____, are used to treat multiple myeloma and some forms of leukemia, anemia, and lymphoma. Both treatments introduce stem cells into the bloodstream, where they can migrate to bone marrow and begin to make new blood cells.

5. This automated laboratory test for blood screening, or _____, measures various aspects of erythrocytes, leukocytes, and thrombocytes (platelets) and quickly gives a tremendous amount of information about the blood.

6. Two laboratory tests used in the diagnosis of anemia are _____, which reports the percentage of erythrocytes in a blood sample, and _____, which measures the amount of oxygen-carrying protein in erythrocytes.

7. A _____ measures the ability of various factors in the blood to form a clot using a series of tests, including _____, which assesses extrinsic blood factors, and _____, which assesses intrinsic blood factors.

EXERCISE 20 ■ Review of Blood Terms

Can you define, pronounce, and spell the following blood terms?

activated partial thromboplastin time (aPTT)	complete blood count with differential (CBC with diff)	hemorrhage	plasmapheresis
anemia	embolism	hemostasis	prothrombin time (PT/INR)
anticoagulant	embolus (*pl.* emboli)	leukemia	sepsis
bleeding disorder	erythrocytopenia	leukocytopenia	sickle cell disease
bleeding profile	extravasation	lymphocytosis	thalassemia
blood dyscrasia	hematocrit (Hct)	multiple myeloma	thrombocytopenia
bone marrow aspiration	hematologist	pancytopenia	thrombolysis
bone marrow biopsy	hematoma	perfusionist	thrombosis
bone marrow transplant (BMT)	hemoglobin (Hgb)	peripheral blood stem cell transplant (PBSCT)	thrombus
	hemolysis	phlebotomist	venipuncture
	hemophilia	phlebotomy	

Lymphatic System Terms
BUILT FROM WORD PARTS AND *NOT* BUILT FROM WORD PARTS

The first portion of the table contains Lymphatic System Terms that can be translated using definitions of word parts. The second portion of the table contains Lymphatic System Terms that cannot be fully understood through translation of word parts.

■ Built from Word Parts

DISEASE AND DISORDERS

TERM	DEFINITION	TERM	DEFINITION
1. **lymphadenitis** (*lim*-fad-e-NĪ-tis)	inflammation of lymph nodes	4. **lymphoma** (lim-FŌ-ma)	tumor of lymphatic tissue (malignant)
2. **lymphadenopathy** (lim-*fad*-e-NOP-a-thē)	disease of lymph nodes (characterized by abnormal enlargement of the lymph nodes associated with an infection or malignancy)	**LYMPHOMAS** are grouped into two general categories called **Hodgkin lymphoma** and **non-Hodgkin lymphoma**. While both forms are malignant and may involve painless swelling of lymph nodes, the diseases vary in pathology and progress differently.	
		5. **splenomegaly** (*sple*-nō-MEG-a-lē)	enlargement of the spleen
3. **lymphangitis** (lim-fan-JĪ-tis)	inflammation of lymph vessels	6. **thymoma** (thī-MŌ-ma)	tumor of the thymus gland

SURGICAL TERMS

TERM	DEFINITION	TERM	DEFINITION
7. **splenectomy** (sple-NEK-to-mē)	excision of the spleen	9. **thymectomy** (thī-MEK-to-mē)	excision of the thymus gland
8. **splenorrhaphy** (sple-NOR-a-fē)	suturing, repairing of the spleen		

DIAGNOSTIC IMAGING

TERM	DEFINITION
10. **lymphangiography** (*lim*-fan-jē-OG-ra-fē)	radiographic imaging of lymph vessels

NOT Built from Word Parts

DISEASE AND DISORDERS

TERM	DEFINITION
1. **infectious mononucleosis** (in-FEK-shus) (mon-ō-nū-klē-Ō-sis)	acute infection caused by the Epstein-Barr virus; characterized by swollen lymph nodes, sore throat, fatigue, and fever. The disease affects mostly young people and is often transmitted by saliva.
2. **lymphedema** (lim-fi-DĒ-ma)	swelling of tissue, usually of one arm or leg, caused by faulty lymphatic drainage

EXERCISE 21 ■ Pronounce and Spell

Practice pronunciation and spelling on paper and online.

1. **Practice on Paper**
   a. **Pronounce:** Read the phonetic spelling and say aloud the terms listed in the previous table. Refer to Table 2.2 Pronunciation Key as needed.
   b. **Spell:** Have a study partner read the terms aloud. Write the spelling of the terms on a separate sheet of paper.

2. **Practice Online**
   a. **Access** online learning resources. Go to evolve.elsevier.com > Evolve Resources > Student Resources.
   b. **Pronounce:** Select Audio Glossary > Chapter 10 > Exercise 21. Select a term to hear its pronunciation and repeat aloud.
   c. **Spell:** Select Activities > Chapter 10 > Spell Terms > Exercise 21. Select the audio icon and type the correct spelling of the term.

❏ Check the box when complete.

EXERCISE 22 ■ Lymphatic System Terms Built from Word Parts

A Analyze and Define

Analyze and define the following lymphatic system terms.

1. lymphangiography

2. thymectomy

3. splenorrhaphy

4. splenomegaly

5. lymphoma

6. lymphadenitis

B Build

Build lymphatic system terms for the following definitions by using the word parts you have learned.

1. inflammation of lymph vessels   _____ / _____ / _____
                                                 WR   WR   S

2. disease of lymph nodes   _____ / _____ / _____
                                                    WR   CV   S

3. tumor of the thymus gland   _____ / _____
                                                   WR   S

4. excision of the spleen   _____ / _____
                                                WR   S

EXERCISE 23 ■ Lymphatic System Terms NOT Built from Word Parts

A Label

Write the medical terms pictured and defined.

1. _____
   acute infection caused by the Epstein-Barr virus characterized by swollen lymph nodes, sore throat, fatigue, and fever

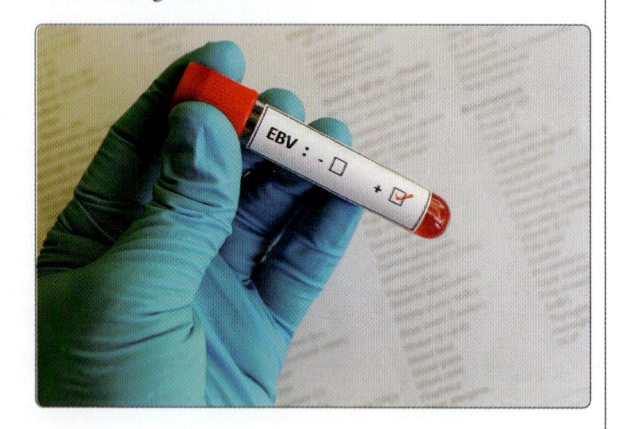

2. _____
   swelling of tissue, usually of one arm or leg, caused faulty lymphatic drainage

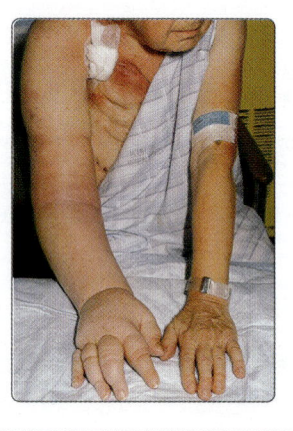

B Fill In

Fill in the blanks with the correct terms.

1. Hematologists and oncologists are medical specialists who treat _____, or tumor of lymphatic tissue. Treatment depends on the specific type, Hodgkin or non-Hodgkin, and subtype of the disease.

2. Radiographic imaging of lymph vessels, or _____, is a fluoroscopic procedure performed by an interventional radiologist; it can be used to assess the spread of cancer, determine the cause of lymphedema, and guide treatment.

3. Tumor of the thymus gland, or _____, is associated with myasthenia gravis and other autoimmune diseases. Excision of the thymus gland, or _____, is used as treatment for this type of tumor, which may be benign or malignant.

4. Excision of the spleen, or _____, may be performed to ease symptoms of pain or feelings of fullness caused by an enlarged spleen, or _____.

5. While a splenectomy would be used to treat a ruptured spleen, suturing of the spleen, or _____, would be used to repair a traumatic splenic injury.

6. Disease of the lymph nodes, or _____, is a palpable enlargement of lymph nodes commonly caused by upper respiratory infections.

7. Inflammation of lymph nodes, or _____, is the term used when lymphadenopathy is present along with redness and tenderness; it usually results from an infection.

8. Inflammation of lymph vessels, or _____, is an infection of the lymphatic channels, often resulting from an acute streptococcal infection, and can appear as red streaks on the skin. If untreated, it can lead to cellulitis.

EXERCISE 24 ■ Review of Lymphatic System Terms

Can you define, pronounce, and spell the following lymphatic system terms?

infectious mononucleosis	lymphangiography	lymphoma	splenorrhaphy
lymphadenitis	lymphangitis	splenectomy	thymectomy
lymphadenopathy	lymphedema	splenomegaly	thymoma

Immune System Terms
BUILT FROM WORD PARTS AND *NOT* BUILT FROM WORD PARTS

The first portion of the table contains Immune System Terms that can be translated using definitions of word parts. The second portion of the table contains Immune System Terms that cannot be fully understood through translation of word parts.

■ Built from Word Parts

MEDICAL SPECIALTIES

TERM	DEFINITION	TERM	DEFINITION
1. **immunologist** (im-ū-NOL-o-jist)	physician who studies and treats immune system disorders	2. **immunology** (im-ū-NOL-o-jē)	study of the immune system (branch of medicine dealing with immune system disorders)

OTHER TERMS

TERM	DEFINITION
3. **lymphocyte** (lim-fa-SĪT)	lymph cell (type of leukocyte found in lymph tissue that is a part of the immune system and fights infection)

Immune System Terms—cont'd
BUILT FROM WORD PARTS AND *NOT* BUILT FROM WORD PARTS

■ *NOT* Built from Word Parts

DISEASE AND DISORDERS

TERM	DEFINITION
1. acquired immunodeficiency syndrome (AIDS) (a-KWĪRD) (*im*-ū-nō-de-FISH-en-sē) (SIN-drōm)	advanced, chronic immune system suppression caused by human immunodeficiency virus (HIV) infection; manifested by opportunistic infections (such as candidiasis and tuberculosis), neurologic disease (peripheral neuropathy and cognitive motor impairment), and secondary neoplasms (Kaposi sarcoma)
2. allergy (AL-er-jē)	hypersensitivity to a substance, resulting in an inflammatory immune response
3. anaphylaxis (*an*-a-fe-LAK-sis)	exaggerated reaction to a previously encountered antigen such as bee venom, peanuts, or latex. While symptoms may initially be mild, such as hives or sneezing, anaphylaxis can quickly become severe. When it leads to a drop in blood pressure and blockage of the airway (which can lead to death within minutes), it is called **anaphylactic shock**.
4. autoimmune disease (*aw*-tō-i-MŪN) (di-ZĒZ)	disease caused by the body's inability to distinguish its own cells from foreign bodies, thus producing antibodies that attack its own tissue. **Rheumatoid arthritis** and **systemic lupus erythematosus** are examples of autoimmune diseases.
5. immunodeficiency (*im*-ū-nō-de-FISH-en-sē)	inability of the immune system to respond effectively to pathogens due to a lack of functioning antibodies, lymphocytes, or both. May be inherited, acquired by an infection, or caused by treatments, such as chemotherapy (also called **immunocompromised**)
6. opportunistic infections (*op*-ar-too-NIS-tik) (in-FEK-shuns)	illnesses caused by microorganisms that are not usually pathogenic but result in disease because of a weakened immune system
7. sarcoidosis (*sar*-koi-DŌ-sis)	disease in which clumps of inflammatory cells form in one or more organs of the body, frequently the lungs and lymph nodes. Thought to be caused by an overreaction of the immune system to an unknown substance.

DIAGNOSTIC LABORATORY

TERM	DEFINITION
8. erythrocyte sedimentation rate (ESR) (e-RITH-rō-sīt) (*sed*-a-men-TĀ-shun) (rāt)	blood test that determines the amount of time it takes for red blood cells to settle at the bottom of a tube of blood. A faster than normal rate may indicate inflammation, part of the immune response. Because the test cannot identify a specific disease, it is usually combined with other, more specific tests. (also called **sed rate**)

MEDICAL SPECIALTY

TERM	DEFINITION
9. allergist (AL-er-jist)	physician who studies and treats allergic conditions

OTHER TERMS

TERM	DEFINITION
10. allergen (AL-er-jen)	environmental substance capable of producing a hypersensitivity reaction (allergy) in the body. Common allergens are house dust, pollen, animal dander, and various foods.

Chapter 10 Cardiovascular, Lymphatic, Immune Systems and Blood   403

TERM	DEFINITION
HYPERSENSITIVITY refers to a condition in which the body "overreacts" to something that it perceives to be a foreign substance, such as an allergen.	
11. antibody (AN-ti-*bod*-ē)	protective protein produced by the immune system in response to the presence of a foreign substance (antigen)
12. antigen (AN-ti-jen)	substance that triggers an immune response when introduced into the body. Examples of antigens are transplant tissue, toxins, and infectious organisms.
13. immunity (i-MŪ-ni-tē)	being resistant to specific invading pathogens
TYPES OF IMMUNITY Inherited immunity develops before birth and is also called innate immunity. **Acquired immunity** develops after birth *naturally*, when antigen exposure is not deliberate, or *artificially*, when antigen exposure is deliberate.	
14. immunosuppression (*im*-ū-nō-su-PRESH-un)	state in which the body's ability to fight infections or disease is reduced; may be caused by a disease process, be a treatment side effect, or be induced with pharmaceuticals to prevent transplant rejection or treat autoimmune diseases
15. vaccine (vak-SĒN)	substance that is used to stimulate the body's immune response against infectious disease; may be administered by injection, mouth, or nasal spray

EXERCISE 25 ■ Pronounce and Spell

Practice pronunciation and spelling on paper and online.

1. **Practice on Paper**
    a. **Pronounce:** Read the phonetic spelling and say aloud the terms listed in the previous table. Refer to Table 2.2 Pronunciation Key as needed.
    b. **Spell:** Have a study partner read the terms aloud. Write the spelling of the terms on a separate sheet of paper.

2. **Practice Online**
    a. **Access** online learning resources. Go to evolve.elsevier.com > Evolve Resources > Student Resources.
    b. **Pronounce:** Select Audio Glossary > Chapter 10 > Exercise 25. Select a term to hear its pronunciation and repeat aloud.
    c. **Spell:** Select Activities > Chapter 10 > Spell Terms > Exercise 25. Select the audio icon and type the correct spelling of the term.

❏ Check the box when complete.

EXERCISE 26 ■ Immune System Terms Built from Word Parts

Analyze and define the following immune system terms.

1. lymphocyte

   _____

   _____

2. immunology

   _____

   _____

3. immunologist

   _____

   _____

Chapter 10 Cardiovascular, Lymphatic, Immune Systems and Blood

EXERCISE 27 ■ Immune System Terms NOT Built from Word Parts

A Match

Match the immune system terms in the first column with their definitions in the second column.

_____ 1. allergen
_____ 2. autoimmune disease
_____ 3. opportunistic infections
_____ 4. antigen
_____ 5. immunity
_____ 6. allergist
_____ 7. antibodies
_____ 8. immunodeficiency

a. inability of the immune system to respond effectively to pathogens due to a lack of functioning antibodies, lymphocytes, or both
b. illnesses caused by microorganisms that are not usually pathogenic but result in disease because of a weakened immune system
c. resistant to specific invading pathogens
d. protective protein produced by the immune system in response to the presence of a foreign substance
e. house dust, pollen, and animal dander are examples
f. transplant tissue, toxins, and infectious organisms are examples
g. physician who treats allergic conditions
h. rheumatoid arthritis is an example

B Match

Match the immune system terms in the first column with their definitions in the second column.

_____ 1. sarcoidosis
_____ 2. vaccine
_____ 3. allergy
_____ 4. acquired immunodeficiency syndrome
_____ 5. anaphylaxis
_____ 6. erythrocyte sedimentation rate
_____ 7. immunosuppression

a. hypersensitivity to a substance
b. advanced, chronic immune system suppression caused by HIV infection
c. administered by injection, nasal spray, or orally to prevent an infectious disease
d. the body's ability to fight infections or disease is reduced
e. blood test that determines the amount of time it takes for red blood cells to settle at the bottom of a tube of blood
f. exaggerated reaction to a previously encountered antigen
g. disease in which clumps of inflammatory cells form in one or more organs of the body, frequently the lungs and lymph nodes

EXERCISE 28 ■ Fill In

Fill in the blanks with the correct terms.

1. A(n) _____, an environmental substance capable of producing a hypersensitivity reaction, is a specific type of _____, a substance that triggers an immune response when introduced into the body. A(n) _____ is a protective protein produced by the immune system in response to the presence of an antigen.

2. An exaggerated reaction to a previously encountered antigen such as bee venom, peanuts, or latex is called _____. While symptoms may initially be mild, such as hives or sneezing, they can quickly become severe. When the reaction leads to a drop in blood pressure and blockage of the airway (which can lead to death within minutes), it is called anaphylactic shock.

3. _____ is a disease in which clumps of inflammatory cells form in one or more organs of the body, frequently the lungs and lymph nodes. It is thought to be caused by an overreaction of the immune system to an unknown substance.

4. A blood test that determines the amount of time it takes for red blood cells to settle at the bottom of a tube of blood, a test that may indicate inflammation, is called _____ and is abbreviated as _____.

Chapter 10   Cardiovascular, Lymphatic, Immune Systems and Blood   405

5. A lymph cell or _____ is a type of leukocyte found in lymph tissue that is a part of the immune system and fights infection.
6. A substance administered by injection, mouth, or nasal spray, or a(n) _____, aims to prevent infectious disease by causing _____, or being resistant to specific invading pathogens.
7. Patients with _____, abbreviated as _____, or advanced, chronic immune system suppression caused by human immunodeficiency virus, are particularly at risk for _____, or illnesses caused by microorganisms that are not usually pathogenic but result in disease because of a weakened immune system.
8. A state in which the body's ability to fight infections or disease is reduced, or _____, may be caused by a disease process, be a treatment side effect, or be induced with pharmaceuticals to prevent transplant rejection or treat autoimmune diseases.
9. Study of the immune system, or _____, is the branch of medicine concerned with how the body protects itself from pathogens. It is a medical specialty that treats disorders of the immune system, including its underperformance, such as an inability to respond effectively to pathogens, or _____, and overperformance, such as hypersensitivity to a substance resulting in an inflammatory response, or _____.
10. A clinical _____, or physician who studies and treats immune system disorders, treats patients with _____, or disease caused by the body's inability to distinguish its own cells from foreign bodies; physicians with this specialty may also be involved in the care of those receiving transplants or immunotherapy. A(n) _____, or physician who studies and treats allergic conditions, is a board-certified physician sometimes referred to as an allergist/immunologist, which indicates the ability to diagnose and treat allergies, asthma, and immune deficiency disorders.

EXERCISE 29 ■ Review of Immune System Terms

Can you define, pronounce, and spell the following immune system terms?

acquired immunodeficiency syndrome (AIDS)	anaphylaxis	immunity	lymphocyte
	antibody	immunodeficiency	opportunistic infections
	antigen	immunologist	sarcoidosis
allergen	autoimmune disease	immunology	vaccine
allergist	erythrocyte sedimentation rate (ESR)	immunosuppression	
allergy			

Abbreviations

DISEASE AND DISORDERS			
ABBREVIATION	TERM	ABBREVIATION	TERM
ACS	acute coronary syndrome	HHD	hypertensive heart disease
AF	atrial fibrillation	MI	myocardial infarction
AFib	atrial fibrillation; spoken as (Ā-fib)	PAD	peripheral artery disease
CAD	coronary artery disease	VF	ventricular fibrillation
DVT	deep vein thrombosis	VFib	ventricular fibrillation; spoken as (VĒ-fib)
HF	heart failure		

SIGNS AND SYMPTOMS	
ABBREVIATION	TERM
HTN	hypertension

Abbreviations—cont'd

DIAGNOSTIC

ABBREVIATION	TERM	ABBREVIATION	TERM
aPTT	activated partial thromboplastin time	ESR	erythrocyte sedimentation rate
BP	blood pressure	Hct	hematocrit
CBC with diff	complete blood count with differential	Hgb	hemoglobin
CPK	creatine phosphokinase	P	pulse
CRP	C-reactive protein	PT	prothrombin time
DSA	digital subtraction angiography	SPECT	single-photon emission computed tomography; spoken as a whole word (spekt)
ECG, EKG	electrocardiogram		
ECHO	echocardiogram; spoken as a whole word (EK-ō)	TEE	transesophageal echocardiogram

TREATMENTS

ABBREVIATION	TERM	ABBREVIATION	TERM
AICD	automatic implantable cardiac defibrillator	CPR	cardiopulmonary resuscitation
		PBSCT	peripheral blood stem cell transplant
BMT	bone marrow transplant	PCI	percutaneous coronary intervention
CABG	coronary artery bypass graft; spoken as a whole word (KA-bij)	PTCA	percutaneous transluminal coronary angioplasty

DESCRIPTIVE

ABBREVIATION	TERM	ABBREVIATION	TERM
AV	atrioventricular	IV	intravenous

OTHER

ABBREVIATION	TERM	ABBREVIATION	TERM
CCU	coronary care unit	WBC	white blood cell (leukocyte)
RBC	red blood cell (erythrocyte)		

Refer to **Appendix D** for a complete list of abbreviations.

EXERCISE 30 ■ Abbreviations

Write the terms abbreviated.

1. **CAD** _____ _____ _____ has received growing interest over the past several years. Diagnostic procedures for new patients usually begin with an exercise **ECG** _____. Patients whose stress tests are borderline usually proceed to noninvasive imaging such as **SPECT** _____-_____ _____ _____ _____ and stress **ECHO** _____.

2. **DVT** _____ _____ _____ is common in hospitalized patients. Early detection is important because DVT can result in death from a pulmonary embolism. Doppler ultrasound is a noninvasive diagnostic procedure used to diagnose DVT. MRI and venography may be used as well.

3. The **CBC** _____ _____ _____ **with diff** _____ is a series of automated laboratory tests of the peripheral blood that provide a great deal of information about the blood and

Chapter 10   Cardiovascular, Lymphatic, Immune Systems and Blood   407

other body organs. Tests performed as part of the CBC are **RBC** _____ _____ _____ count, **WBC** _____ _____ _____ count and differential, **Hgb** _____, and **Hct** _____.

4. Standard surgical treatment for CAD includes **CABG** _____ _____ _____ _____. There is a growth in the use of minimally invasive techniques to treat CAD, which include transmyocardial laser revascularization and **PTCA** _____ _____ _____ _____ (also called **PCI** _____ _____ _____), atherectomy, and coronary stent placement.

5. Hospitalized patients diagnosed with **MI** _____ _____ are cared for in the **CCU** _____ _____ _____.

6. A sphygmomanometer is used to measure **BP** _____ _____, while **P** _____ is measured using the fingertips.

7. Diagnosis used to indicate that a patient's heart is unable to pump enough blood through the body to supply tissues is **HF** _____ _____.

8. If the patient's heart and/or lungs have ceased to function, the medical team must begin **CPR** _____ _____.

9. A patient with persistently elevated blood pressure is likely to be diagnosed with **HHD** _____ _____ _____.

10. When scheduling blood tests for a patient on oral anticoagulant medication, the doctor is likely to include a **PT** _____ _____.

11. Any interruption of the conduction of electrical impulses from the atria to the ventricles is called **AV** _____ block.

12. The treatment of **ACS** _____ _____ _____ is aimed at preventing thrombus formation and restoring blood flow to the occluded coronary artery.

13. Stopping smoking, exercising, and proper diet are important in the medical management of **PAD** _____ _____ _____.

14. **DSA** _____ _____ _____ is especially valuable in cardiac diagnostic applications.

15. The physician ordered a **TEE** _____ _____ to examine the patient's heart structure and function.

16. Two blood tests used in assessing and evaluating cardiovascular diseases are **CRP** _____ _____ and **CPK** _____ _____.

17. A patient experiencing **AFib** _____ _____, also abbreviated as **AF**, may be referred to an electrophysiologist, a cardiology subspecialist.

18. An **AICD** _____ _____ _____ _____ delivers an electric shock to convert an arrhythmia, such as **VF** _____ _____, also known as **VFib**, back to normal rhythm.

19. The patient with dehydration was ordered **IV** _____ fluids by her physician.

20. **HTN** _____ is usually diagnosed when a patient has elevated blood pressure on two separate occasions.

21. The primary difference between **PBSCT** _____ _____ _____ _____ and **BMT** _____ _____ _____ is whether stem cells are collected from blood or bone marrow.

22. **ESR** _____ _____ _____, or sed rate, indirectly measures the degree of inflammation in the body and is used to help detect inflammation associated with infections, cancers, and autoimmune diseases.

Chapter 10 Cardiovascular, Lymphatic, Immune Systems and Blood

PRACTICAL APPLICATION

EXERCISE 31 ■ Case Study: Translate Between Everyday Language and Medical Language

CASE STUDY: Natalia Krouse

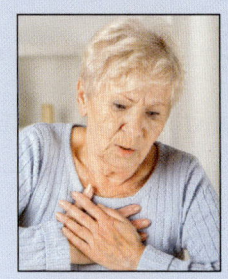

Natalia has not been feeling well lately. She seems to feel "wiped out" most of the time. She wonders if maybe her medicine for high blood pressure isn't working as well as it used to. Tonight she went for her usual walk after dinner with her dogs. She had barely made it down the driveway when she started feeling pain in her chest. It felt like something pushing down on her and squeezing her. She noticed pain in her left arm and even in her jaw. She noticed her heart was racing, and she was breathing faster than usual. She was also feeling dizzy at the same time and was afraid she might pass out. She stopped to sit down and after about 5 minutes she started feeling a little better. Her neighbor saw her and called 911. An ambulance came and took her to the emergency department.

Now that you have worked through Chapter 10 on the cardiovascular system, consider the medical terms that might be used to describe Natalia's experience. See the Chapter at a Glance section at the end of the chapter for a list of terms that might apply.

A. Underline phrases in the case study that could be substituted with medical terms.

B. Write the medical term and its definition for three of the phrases you underlined.

MEDICAL TERM	DEFINITION
1. _____	_____
2. _____	_____
3. _____	_____

DOCUMENTATION: Excerpt from Hospital Admission Report

Natalia was brought to the emergency department and was admitted to the cardiology floor of the hospital. A portion of her history from the electronic medical record is noted below.

The patient has an extensive history of chronic cardiovascular issues. Coronary artery disease risk factors include hypertension and hypercholesterolemia. She also has extensive varicose veins of the lower extremities bilaterally. Her family physician referred her to a cardiologist in 2003 for medical management of these complications. She smokes one pack of cigarettes a day and has previously declined participation in a smoking cessation program. She is not diabetic. Family history reveals a brother who had coronary artery bypass grafts and a mother deceased from abdominal aortic aneurysm rupture.

C. Underline medical terms presented in Chapter 10 in the previous excerpt from Natalia's medical record. See the Chapter at a Glance section at the end of the chapter for a complete list.

D. Select and define three of the medical terms you underlined. To check your answers, go to Appendix A.

MEDICAL TERM	DEFINITION
1. _____	_____
2. _____	_____
3. _____	_____

Chapter 10   Cardiovascular, Lymphatic, Immune Systems and Blood   409

EXERCISE 32 ■ Interact With Medical Documents

A

Read the report and complete it by writing medical terms on answer lines within the document. Definitions of terms to be written appear after the document.

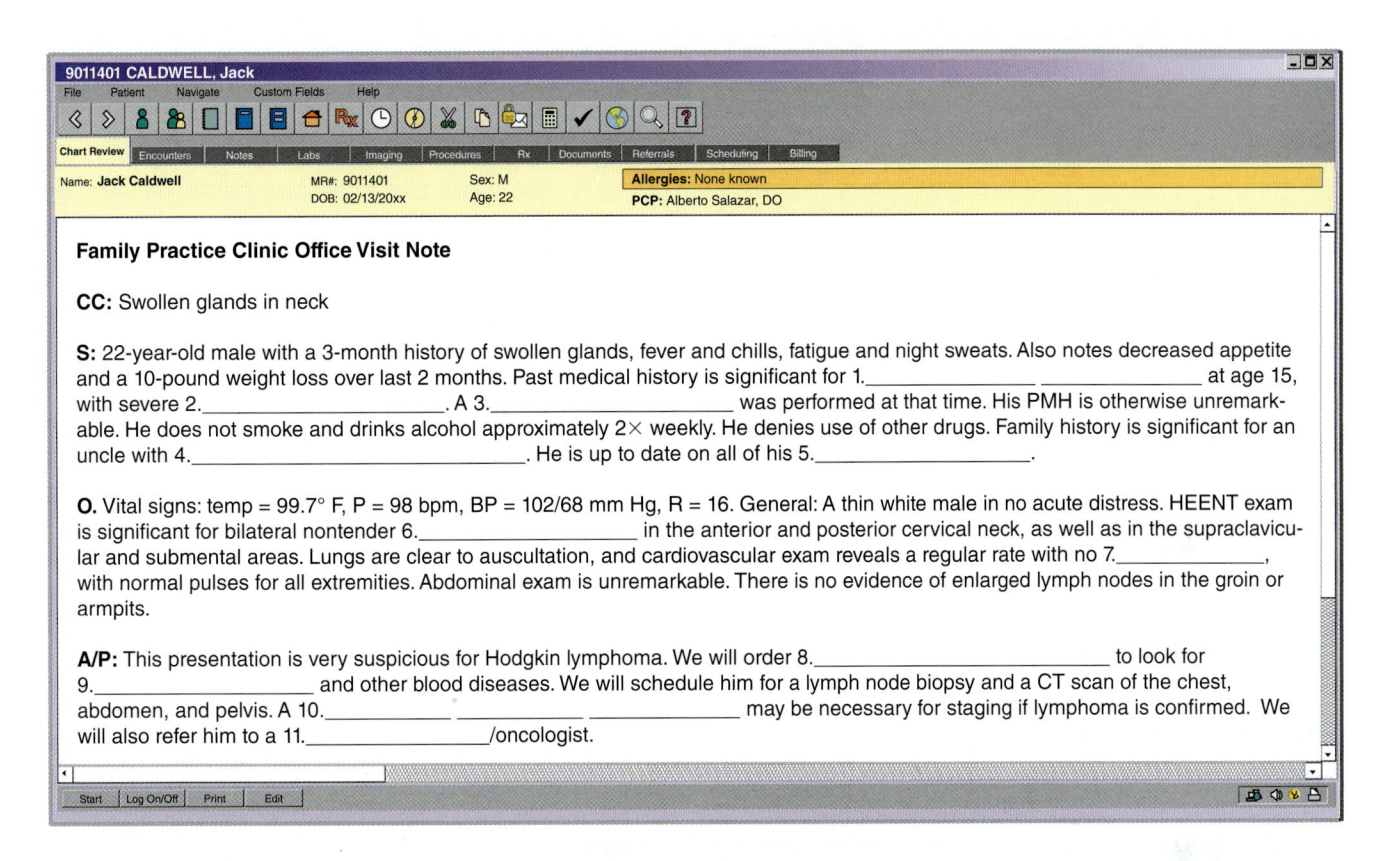

9011401 CALDWELL, Jack

Name: **Jack Caldwell**   MR#: 9011401   Sex: M   Allergies: None known
                          DOB: 02/13/20xx   Age: 22   PCP: Alberto Salazar, DO

Family Practice Clinic Office Visit Note

CC: Swollen glands in neck

S: 22-year-old male with a 3-month history of swollen glands, fever and chills, fatigue and night sweats. Also notes decreased appetite and a 10-pound weight loss over last 2 months. Past medical history is significant for 1._____ _____ at age 15, with severe 2._____. A 3._____ was performed at that time. His PMH is otherwise unremarkable. He does not smoke and drinks alcohol approximately 2× weekly. He denies use of other drugs. Family history is significant for an uncle with 4._____. He is up to date on all of his 5._____.

O. Vital signs: temp = 99.7° F, P = 98 bpm, BP = 102/68 mm Hg, R = 16. General: A thin white male in no acute distress. HEENT exam is significant for bilateral nontender 6._____ in the anterior and posterior cervical neck, as well as in the supraclavicular and submental areas. Lungs are clear to auscultation, and cardiovascular exam reveals a regular rate with no 7._____, with normal pulses for all extremities. Abdominal exam is unremarkable. There is no evidence of enlarged lymph nodes in the groin or armpits.

A/P: This presentation is very suspicious for Hodgkin lymphoma. We will order 8._____ to look for 9._____ and other blood diseases. We will schedule him for a lymph node biopsy and a CT scan of the chest, abdomen, and pelvis. A 10._____ _____ _____ may be necessary for staging if lymphoma is confirmed. We will also refer him to a 11._____/oncologist.

Definitions of Medical Terms to Complete the Document

Write the medical terms defined on corresponding answer lines in the document.

1. acute infection caused by the Epstein-Barr virus characterized by swollen lymph nodes, sore throat, fatigue, and fever
2. enlargement of the spleen
3. excision of the spleen
4. tumor of lymphatic tissue (malignant)
5. suspension of weakened or killed microorganisms administered by injection, mouth, or nasal spray (plural form of the term)
6. disease of lymph nodes
7. any disturbance or abnormality in the heart's normal rhythmic pattern
8. abbreviation for laboratory test for basic blood screening that measures various aspects of erythrocytes, leukocytes, and platelets
9. malignant disease characterized by excessive increase in abnormal leukocytes formed in the bone marrow
10. procedure to obtain a sample of the solid portion of bone marrow, usually from the ilium, for study
11. physician who studies and treats diseases of the blood

EXERCISE 32 — Interact With Medical Documents—cont'd

B

Read the medical report and answer the questions below it.

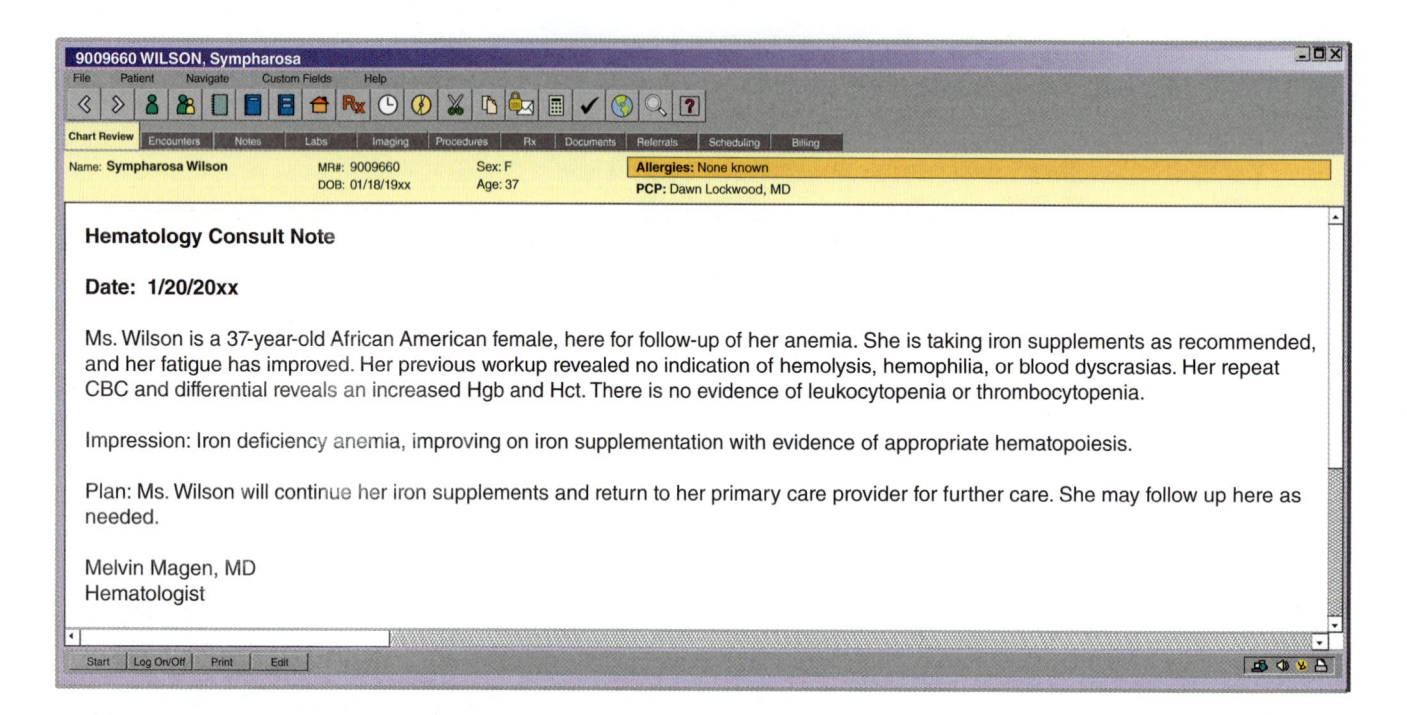

9009660 WILSON, Sympharosa

Name: **Sympharosa Wilson** MR#: 9009660 Sex: F Allergies: None known
DOB: 01/18/19xx Age: 37 PCP: Dawn Lockwood, MD

Hematology Consult Note

Date: 1/20/20xx

Ms. Wilson is a 37-year-old African American female, here for follow-up of her anemia. She is taking iron supplements as recommended, and her fatigue has improved. Her previous workup revealed no indication of hemolysis, hemophilia, or blood dyscrasias. Her repeat CBC and differential reveals an increased Hgb and Hct. There is no evidence of leukocytopenia or thrombocytopenia.

Impression: Iron deficiency anemia, improving on iron supplementation with evidence of appropriate hematopoiesis.

Plan: Ms. Wilson will continue her iron supplements and return to her primary care provider for further care. She may follow up here as needed.

Melvin Magen, MD
Hematologist

Use the medical report above to answer the questions.

1. Ms. Wilson was seen in the hematology clinic for:
   a. a low platelet count
   b. a low erythrocyte count
   c. a low white blood cell count

2. Her repeat CBC and differential revealed an improved:
   a. hemoglobin and C-reactive protein
   b. hematocrit and troponin
   c. hemoglobin and hematocrit

3. The consulting doctor was a physician who studies and treats:
   a. immune system disorders
   b. diseases of the blood
   c. diseases of the heart

4. **True** or **False**: the patient had evidence of dissolution of red blood cells.

5. **True** or **False**: the reason for the hematology consult was erythrocytopenia.

EXERCISE 33 — Use Medical Language in Online Electronic Health Records

Select the correct medical terms to complete three medical records in one patient's electronic file.

Access online resources at evolve.elsevier.com > Evolve Resources > Student Resources > Activities > Chapter 10 > Electronic Health Records

Topic: CAD
Record 1, Imaging: Echocardiogram Report
Record 2, Procedures: Cardiovascular Operative Report
Record 3, Discharge: Discharge Summary

❏ Check the box when complete.

Chapter 10   Cardiovascular, Lymphatic, Immune Systems and Blood   411

EXERCISE 34 ■ Use Medical Terms in Clinical Statements

For each phrase printed in bold, circle the medical term or abbreviation defined. Answers are listed in Appendix A. For pronunciation practice, read the answers aloud.

1. **Condition that reduces the flow of blood through the coronary arteries to the heart muscle** (thrombosis, arteriosclerosis, coronary artery disease) may eventually lead to an MI. Treatment includes restoring blood supply to the heart. **Surgical repair of the blood vessel** (angiography, arteriogram, angioplasty) is used in some cases, and for more severe blockage, the cardiac surgeon will perform a **surgical technique to bring a new blood supply to the myocardium by detouring around blocked arteries** (coronary artery bypass graft, cardiac catheterization, cardiopulmonary resuscitation).

2. **Rapid heart rate** (tachypnea, hypertension, tachycardia) may be noted by measuring the **contraction of the heart, which can be felt with a fingertip** (blood pressure, hemostasis, pulse) and may also be accompanied **by blood pressure that is below normal** (hypertension, heart failure, hypotension).

3. Utilizing a **basic blood screening that measures aspects of erythrocytes, leukocytes, and thrombocytes** (Hgb, PBSCT, CBC with diff) and a bone marrow biopsy, it was determined that Sophia Tompkins had **malignant disease characterized by excessive increase in abnormal leukocytes formed in the bone marrow** (lymphoma, leukemia, hematoma). She was referred to a **physician who studies and treats diseases of the blood** (hematologist, cardiologist, phlebotomist) for consultation and treatment.

4. **Abnormal reduction of blood clotting cells** (leukocytopenia, leukemia, thrombocytopenia) can contribute to **excessive flow of blood** (hemorrhage, aneurysm, thrombosis). If **stopping the flow of blood** (hematoma, hemostasis, hematology) can be achieved quickly, **condition in which there is a reduction in the number of erythrocytes** (anemia, leukemia, hypotension) may be avoided.

5. Sjögren syndrome, myasthenia gravis, and Hashimoto thyroiditis are examples of **disease caused by the body's inability to distinguish its own cells from foreign bodies, thus producing antibodies that attack its own tissue** (anaphylaxis, opportunistic infection, autoimmune disease). People with **tumor of the thymus gland** (lymphoma, thymoma, lymphedema) are at higher risk of these disorders. These patients may seek treatment from a(n) **physician who studies and treats immune system disorders** (immunologist, allergist, hematologist).

EXERCISE 35 ■ Pronounce Medical Terms in Use

Practice pronunciation of terms by reading aloud the following paragraph. Use the phonetic spellings to assist with pronunciation. The script also contains medical terms not presented in the chapter. If interested, research their meanings in a medical dictionary or a reliable online source.

A 55-year-old man presented to his doctor with pain in the calf and swelling in the left foot and ankle. Three days prior, the patient had completed trans-Pacific airline travel, spending several hours in a sitting position.
He has a history of **varicose veins** (VAR-i-kōs) (vānz). No previous history of **hypertension** (hī-per-TEN-shun) or **thrombophlebitis** (throm-bō-fle-BĪ-tis) existed. Physical examination revealed an edematous left lower extremity and a tender calf. The pedal **pulse** (puls) was intact. A **Doppler ultrasound** (DOP-ler) (UL-tra-sound) was obtained, which revealed **deep vein thrombosis** (dēp) (vān) (throm-BŌ-sis). He was treated as an outpatient with apixaban and will continue this therapy for at least 3 months. Unlike warfarin, this oral **anticoagulant** (an-tī-kō-AG-ū-lant) therapy does not require routine monitoring of the **prothrombin time** (prō-THROM-bin) (tīm).

CHAPTER REVIEW

EXERCISE 36 ▪ Chapter Content Quiz

Test your understanding of terms and abbreviations introduced in this chapter. Circle the letter for the medical term or abbreviation related to the words in italics.

1. Ms. Tompkins was diagnosed with sickle cell disease and was sent to a *physician who studies and treats diseases of the blood* for further evaluation.
   a. cardiologist
   b. immunologist
   c. hematologist

2. Following a trans-Pacific flight, Kenji Makoto developed *inflammation of the vein associated with a blood clot*, which was probably due to sitting for a long period of time.
   a. thrombophlebitis
   b. lymphadenitis
   c. atherosclerosis

3. Ted Lauer had a *record of the electrical activity of the heart* to follow up on his atrial fibrillation.
   a. CPR
   b. ECG
   c. ECHO

4. Mr. Schonfeld was diagnosed with a 6-cm abdominal aortic *ballooning of a weakened portion of a vessel wall*, which required surgical repair with an endograft.
   a. embolism
   b. thrombosis
   c. aneurysm

5. On physical examination of the neck, Samantha Winslow was noted to have *disease of lymph nodes (abnormal enlargement of the lymph nodes)*.
   a. lymphoma
   b. lymphadenopathy
   c. lymphadenitis

6. After finishing a course of immunosuppressive medication for cancer treatment, a CBC revealed that the patient had *abnormal reduction of white blood cells*.
   a. leukocytopenia
   b. anemia
   c. thrombocytopenia

7. Mr. Matthews has an allergy to peanuts; he carries an EpiPen to prevent *episodes of exaggerated reaction to a previously encountered antigen, which can lead to death within minutes*.
   a. immunodeficiency
   b. anaphylaxis
   c. autoimmune disease

8. Mrs. Patel was experiencing episodes of *chest pain that occur when there is an insufficient amount of blood to the heart muscle* and was scheduled for an exercise stress test.
   a. acute coronary syndrome
   b. atrial fibrillation
   c. angina pectoris

9. Because Mr. Jiang is taking warfarin, he needs to have his *blood test used to determine certain coagulation activity defects and to monitor anticoagulation therapy* tested regularly.
   a. prothrombin time
   b. hematocrit
   c. hemoglobin

10. Mr. MacDougal was brought to the emergency department after suffering chest trauma in a motor vehicle accident. His symptoms and chest x-ray were suspicious for aortic rupture, so a(n) *radiographic image of the aorta* was obtained.
    a. arteriogram
    b. aortogram
    c. venogram

11. After her myocardial infarction, Mrs. Alvarez was found to have 95% blockage in three sections of her coronary arteries. Thus, a *surgical technique to bring a new blood supply to heart muscle by detouring around blocked arteries* was performed.
    a. coronary stent
    b. angiography
    c. coronary artery bypass graft

12. Mr. Williams suffered from pancytopenia after his chemotherapy, so the hematologist ordered a(n) *infusion of healthy bone marrow cells from a matched donor into a patient with severely diseased or damaged bone marrow*.
    a. bone marrow aspiration
    b. bone marrow biopsy
    c. bone marrow transplant

13. Kelly Anastopoulis was recently diagnosed with rheumatoid arthritis, a(n) *disease caused by the body's inability to distinguish its own cells from foreign bodies*,

when she had symptoms of joint pain and swelling in her hands.
a. immunodeficiency
b. blood dyscrasia
c. autoimmune disease

14. Mrs. Rosenberg was admitted to the hospital to rule out a myocardial infarction. A phlebotomist performed a venipuncture to obtain labs, including a *blood test to measure the level of an enzyme of heart and skeletal muscle released into the blood after muscle injury or necrosis.*
a. CPK
b. CRP
c. CBC

15. Ryan Lee developed *inflammation of the sac surrounding the heart* after a viral upper respiratory infection.
a. myocarditis
b. pericarditis
c. endocarditis

16. Mr. O'Leary presented with symptoms of a stroke. *Process of digital radiographic imaging of the blood vessels that "subtracts" or removes structures not being studied* was performed to see if thrombolytic therapy was appropriate.
a. digital subtraction angiography
b. transesophageal echocardiogram
c. single-photon emission computed tomography

17. During his high school sports physical, Habib El-Amin was found to have a(n) *unusual sound heard during auscultation of the heart caused by turbulent blood flow.*
a. extravasation
b. murmur
c. bruit

18. The surgeon performed an emergency *suturing, repairing of the spleen* after Theresa Pangilinan ruptured it playing lacrosse.
a. splenectomy
b. thymectomy
c. splenorrhaphy

19. The cardiologist recommended a *battery-powered apparatus implanted under the skin to treat an abnormal heart rhythm* for Mr. Jones, who had episodes of severe bradycardia.
a. artificial cardiac pacemaker
b. automatic implantable cardiac defibrillator
c. percutaneous transluminal coronary angioplasty

20. Because she was over the age of 65, the physician recommended a pneumonia *substance that is used to stimulate the body's immune response against infectious disease* for Mrs. Kurtz.
a. venipuncture
b. vaccine
c. vasoconstrictor

CHAPTER AT A GLANCE — Word Parts New to This Chapter

COMBINING FORMS

angi/o	ech/o	lymphaden/o	thym/o	
aort/o	electr/o	myel/o	valvul/o	
arteri/o	embol/o	phleb/o	ven/o	
ather/o	immun/o	plasm/o	ventricul/o	
atri/o	isch/o	splen/o		
cardi/o	lymph/o	thromb/o		

PREFIXES
brady-
pan-

SUFFIXES
-apheresis
-penia
-rrhage
-sclerosis

CHAPTER AT A GLANCE — Terms Built from Word Parts

CARDIOVASCULAR
angiography
angioma
angioplasty
angioscopy
angiostenosis
aortic stenosis
aortogram
arteriogram
arteriosclerosis
atherectomy
atherosclerosis
atrioventricular (AV)
bradycardia
cardiogenic
cardiologist
cardiology
cardiomegaly
cardiomyopathy
echocardiogram (ECHO)
electrocardiogram (ECG, EKG)
electrocardiography
embolectomy
endarterectomy
endocarditis
intravenous (IV)
ischemia
myocarditis
pericardiocentesis
pericarditis
phlebectomy
phlebitis
polyarteritis
tachycardia
thrombophlebitis
valvulitis
valvuloplasty
venogram

Chapter 10 Cardiovascular, Lymphatic, Immune Systems and Blood

BLOOD
embolism
embolus (*pl.* emboli)
erythrocytopenia
hematologist
hematoma
hemolysis
hemorrhage
hemostasis
leukocytopenia
lymphocytosis
multiple myeloma
pancytopenia
phlebotomy
plasmapheresis
thrombocytopenia
thrombolysis
thrombosis
thrombus

LYMPHATIC
lymphadenitis
lymphadenopathy
lymphangiography
lymphangitis
lymphoma
splenectomy
splenomegaly
splenorrhaphy
thymectomy
thymoma

IMMUNE
immunologist
immunology
lymphocyte

CHAPTER AT A GLANCE — Terms *NOT* Built from Word Parts

CARDIOVASCULAR
acute coronary syndrome (ACS)
aneurysm
angina pectoris
arrhythmia
artificial cardiac pacemaker
automatic implantable cardiac defibrillator (AICD)
blood pressure (BP)
bruit
cardiac arrest
cardiac catheterization
cardiac tamponade
cardiopulmonary resuscitation (CPR)
catheter ablation
cor pulmonale
coronary artery bypass graft (CABG)
coronary artery disease (CAD)
coronary stent
C-reactive protein (CRP)
creatine phosphokinase (CPK)
deep vein thrombosis (DVT)
defibrillation
digital subtraction angiography (DSA)
Doppler ultrasound
exercise stress test
femoropopliteal bypass
fibrillation
heart failure (HF)
hypercholesterolemia
hyperlipidemia
hypertension (HTN)
hypertensive heart disease (HHD)
hypertriglyceridemia
hypotension
intermittent claudication
lipid profile
mitral valve stenosis
murmur
myocardial infarction (MI)
occlusion
percutaneous transluminal coronary angioplasty (PTCA)
peripheral artery disease (PAD)
pulse (P)
rheumatic heart disease
sestamibi test
single-photon emission computed tomography (SPECT)
sphygmomanometer
thrombolytic therapy
transesophageal echocardiogram (TEE)
troponin
varicose veins
vasoconstrictor
vasodilator

BLOOD
activated partial thromboplastin time (aPTT)
anemia
anticoagulant
bleeding disorder
bleeding profile
blood dyscrasia
bone marrow aspiration
bone marrow biopsy
bone marrow transplant (BMT)
complete blood count with differential (CBC with diff)
extravasation
hematocrit (Hct)
hemoglobin (Hgb)
hemophilia
leukemia
perfusionist
peripheral blood stem cell transplant (PBSCT)
phlebotomist
prothrombin time (PT/INR)
sepsis
sickle cell disease
thalassemia
venipuncture

LYMPHATIC
infectious mononucleosis
lymphedema

IMMUNE
acquired immunodeficiency syndrome (AIDS)
allergen
allergist
allergy
anaphylaxis
antibody
antigen
autoimmune disease
erythrocyte
immunodeficiency
opportunistic infections
sarcoidosis
sedimentation rate (ESR)
vaccine

PART 2 BODY SYSTEMS

Digestive System

11

Outline

ANATOMY, 416
Function, 417
Organs and Anatomic Structures of the Digestive System, 417

WORD PARTS, 420
Digestive System Combining Forms, 420
Accessory Organs and Combining Forms Used with Digestive System Terms, 420
Prefixes, 421
Suffixes, 421

MEDICAL TERMS, 426
Disease and Disorder Terms, 426
   Built from Word Parts, 426
   NOT Built from Word Parts, 430
Surgical Terms, 434
   Built from Word Parts, 434
   NOT Built from Word Parts, 439
Diagnostic Terms, 441
   Built from Word Parts, 441
   NOT Built from Word Parts, 445
Complementary Terms, 449
   Built from Word Parts, 449
   NOT Built from Word Parts, 451
Abbreviations, 455

PRACTICAL APPLICATION, 457
CASE STUDY Translate Between Everyday Language and Medical Language, 457
Interact with Medical Documents, 458
Use Medical Language in Online Electronic Health Records, 460
Use Medical Terms in Clinical Statements, 460
Pronounce Medical Terms in Use, 461

CHAPTER REVIEW, 462
Chapter Content Quiz, 462
Chapter at a Glance, 463

Answers to Chapter Exercises, Appendix A

Objectives

Upon completion of this chapter, you will be able to:

1. Pronounce organs and anatomic structures of the digestive system.
2. Define and spell word parts related to the digestive system.
3. Define, pronounce, and spell disease and disorder terms related to the digestive system.
4. Define, pronounce, and spell surgical terms related to the digestive system.
5. Define, pronounce, and spell diagnostic terms related to the digestive system.
6. Define, pronounce, and spell complementary terms related to the digestive system.
7. Interpret the meaning of abbreviations related to the digestive system.
8. Apply medical language in clinical contexts.

TABLE 11.1 Abdominal Sonography, 445

Chapter 11 Digestive System

ANATOMY

The digestive system, also known as the alimentary canal or the gastrointestinal tract and abbreviated as GI tract, is a long continuous tube comprising the mouth, pharynx, esophagus, stomach, small intestine, large intestine, rectum, and anus. Accessory organs of the digestive system are the salivary glands, liver, bile ducts, gallbladder, and pancreas. (Figs. 11.1 through 11.5)

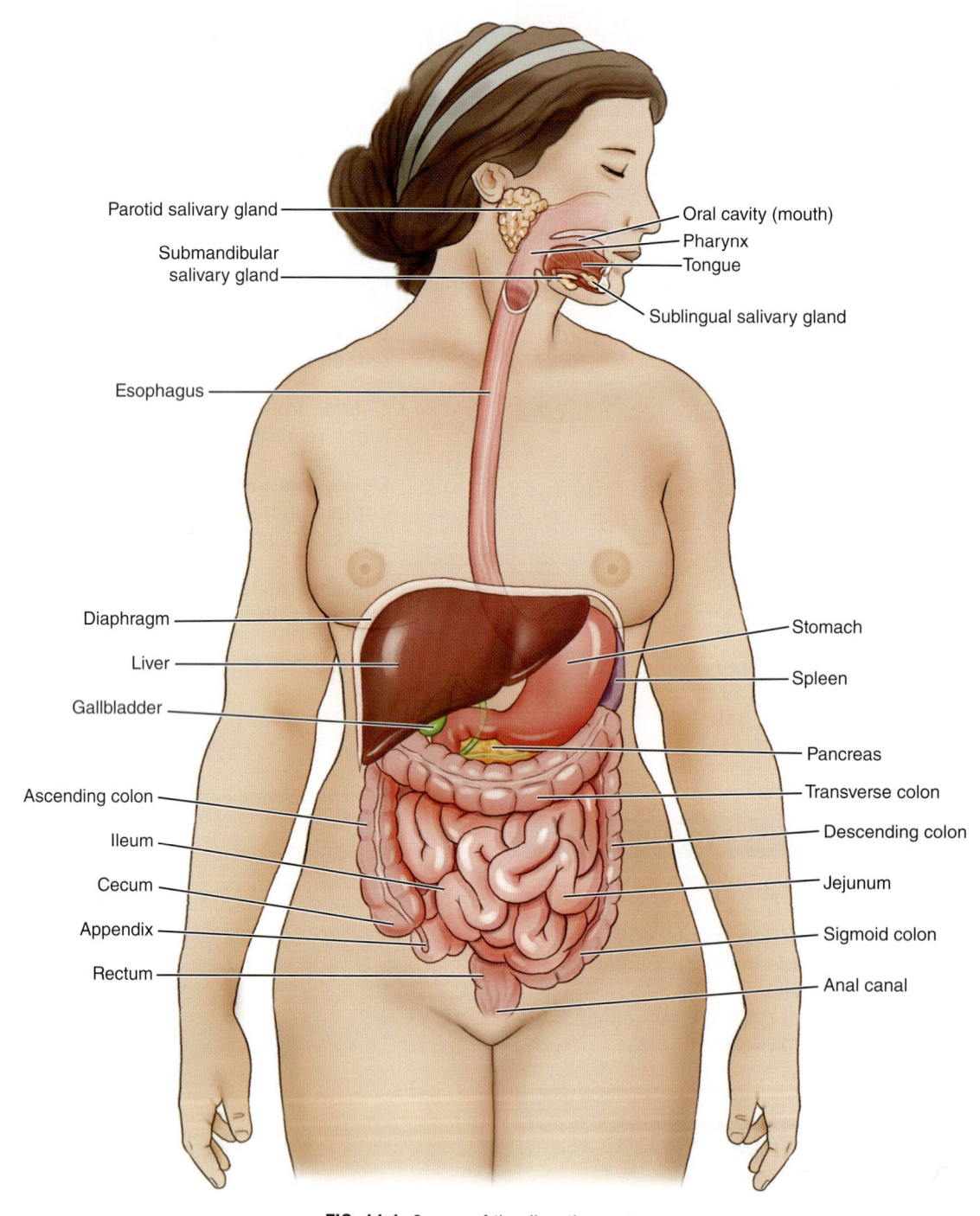

FIG. 11.1 Organs of the digestive system.

Chapter 11   Digestive System   417

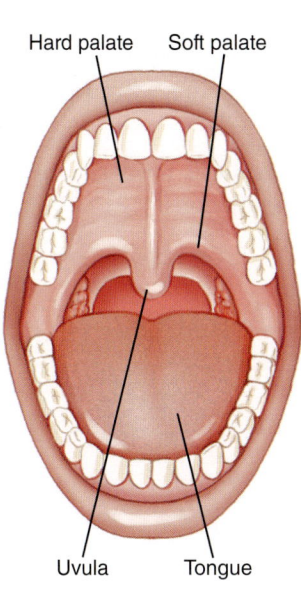

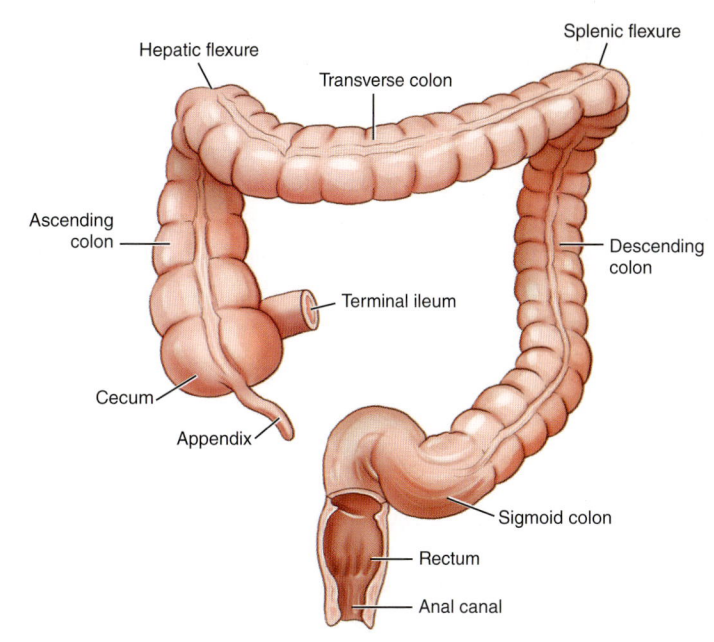

FIG. 11.2 The oral cavity.

FIG. 11.3 Anatomy of the large intestine.

Function

Functions of the digestive system are **ingestion**, the taking in of nutrients through the mouth; **digestion**, the mechanical and chemical breakdown of food for use by body cells; **absorption**, the transfer of digested food from the small intestine to the bloodstream; and **elimination**, the removal of solid waste from the body.

Organs and Anatomic Structures of the Digestive System

TERM	DEFINITION
mouth (mouth)	opening through which food passes into the body (ingestion); breaks food into small particles by mastication (chewing) and mixing with saliva (Fig. 11.2)
tongue (tung)	major organ for taste and speech; consists mostly of skeletal muscle and is attached in the posterior region of the mouth. The tongue moves food for mastication and directs it to the pharynx for swallowing.
palate (PAL-et)	roof of the mouth; separates the nasal cavity from the oral cavity
soft palate (sawft) (PAL-et)	posterior portion, not supported by bone
hard palate (hard) (PAL-et)	anterior portion, supported by bone
uvula (Ū-vū-la)	soft V-shaped structure that extends from the soft palate; directs food into the throat
pharynx (FAR-inks)	food and air passageway. Chewed food enters the pharynx from the mouth and is swallowed, directing it into the esophagus. Air enters the pharynx from the nasal cavities or mouth and passes into the larynx. (also called **throat**)

Organs and Anatomic Structures of the Digestive System—cont'd

TERM	DEFINITION
esophagus (e-SOF-a-gus)	10-inch (25-cm) tube that is a passageway for food extending from the pharynx to the stomach. **Peristalsis**, involuntary wavelike movements that propel food along the gastrointestinal tract, begins in the esophagus.
stomach (STUM-ek)	J-shaped sac that mixes and stores food. It secretes chemicals for digestion and hormones that act locally to control digestive system functions.
cardia (KAR-dē-a)	area around the opening of the esophagus
fundus (FUN-dus)	proximal domed portion of the stomach
body (BOD-ē)	central portion of the stomach, distal to the fundus
antrum (AN-trum)	distal portion of the stomach
pylorus (pī-LOR-us)	portion of the stomach that connects to the small intestine
pyloric sphincter (pī-LOR-ik) (SFINK-ter)	ring of smooth muscle that guards the opening between the stomach and the duodenum
small intestine (smal) (in-TES-tin)	20-foot (6-m) tube extending from the pyloric sphincter to the large intestine. **Digestion** is completed in the small intestine. **Absorption**, the passage of the nutrients (end products of digestion) from the small intestine to the bloodstream, takes place through the **villi**, tiny fingerlike projections that line the walls of the small intestine.
duodenum (dū-OD-e-num)	first 10 to 12 inches (25 cm) of the small intestine

🏛 **DUODENUM** is derived from the Latin **duodeni**, meaning **12 each**, a reference to its length. It was named in 240 BC by a Greek physician. **Jejunum** is derived from the Latin **jejunus**, meaning **empty**; it was so named because the early anatomists always found it empty. **Ileum** is derived from the Greek **eilein**, meaning to **roll**, a reference to the peristaltic waves that move food along the gastrointestinal tract. This term was first used in the early part of the 17th century.

jejunum (je-JŪ-num)	second portion of the small intestine, approximately 8 feet (2.4 m) long
ileum (IL-ē-um)	third portion of the small intestine, approximately 11 feet (3.3 m) long, which connects with the large intestine
large intestine (larj) (in-TES-tin)	approximately 5 feet (1.5 m) long tube that extends from the ileum to the anus (Fig. 11.3). **Absorption** of water and transit of the solid waste products of digestion take place in the large intestine.
cecum (SĒ-kum)	U-shaped pouch that is the first portion of the large intestine
colon (KŌ-lun)	main portion of the large intestine. The colon is divided into four parts: ascending colon, transverse colon, descending colon, and sigmoid colon.
rectum (REK-tum)	distal portion of the large intestine, approximately 8 to 10 inches (20 cm) long, extending from the sigmoid colon to the anus
anus (Ā-nus)	sphincter muscle (ringlike band of muscle fiber that keeps an opening tight) at the end of the gastrointestinal tract. Provides for voluntary **elimination** of solid waste products of digestion.

Chapter 11 Digestive System   419

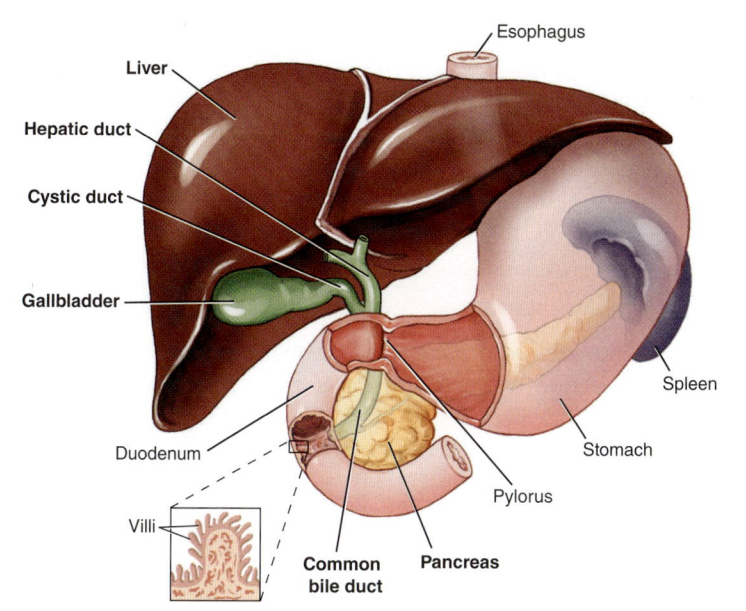

FIG. 11.4 Accessory organs: liver, hepatic duct, cystic duct, gallbladder, common bile duct, and pancreas. Salivary glands, also accessory organs, are shown in Fig. 11.1.

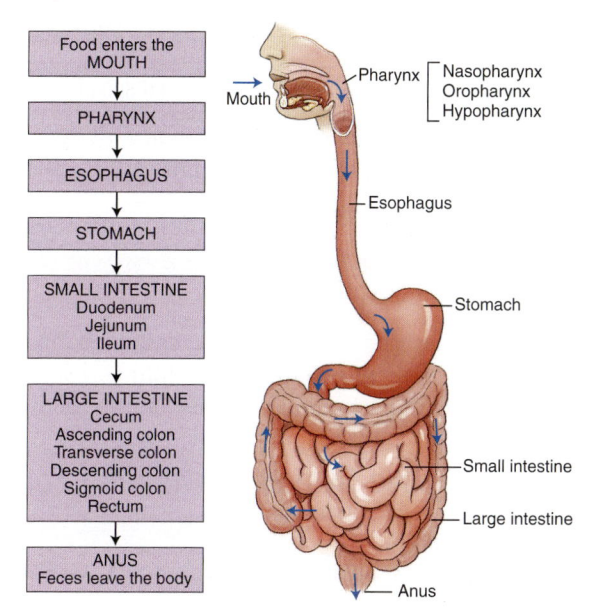

FIG. 11.5 Pathway of food.

TERM	DEFINITION
ACCESSORY ORGANS (Fig. 11.4)	
salivary glands (SAL-i-*ver*-ē) (glans)	produce saliva, which flows into the mouth (Fig. 11.1)
liver (LIV-er)	produces bile, which is necessary for the digestion of fats. The liver performs many other functions concerned with digestion and metabolism.
biliary tract (BIL-ē-ar-ē) (trakt)	organs and ducts (passageways) that transport, store, and release bile (also called **biliary system**)
bile ducts (bīl) (dukts)	passageways that carry bile. The **hepatic duct** collects bile formed in the liver. The **cystic duct** transports bile to and from the gallbladder for storage.
common bile duct (ka-mon)(bīl) (dukt)	small, tubelike structure where the hepatic duct and cystic duct join; conveys bile to the duodenum to aid in the breakdown of fats
gallbladder (GAWL-blad-er)	small, saclike structure that stores bile produced by the liver
pancreas (PAN-krē-us)	glandular organ that produces pancreatic juice, which helps digest all types of food; secretes insulin and glucagon to regulate blood sugar
🏛 **PANCREAS** is derived from the Greek **pan**, meaning **all**, and **krea**, meaning **flesh**. The pancreas was first described in 300 BC. It was so named because of its fleshy appearance.	
OTHER STRUCTURES	
peritoneum (*per*-i-tō-NĒ-um)	serous saclike lining of the abdominal and pelvic cavities
appendix (a-PEN-diks)	small pouch attached to the cecum. While its function is not fully understood, the appendix may play a role in supporting the immune system and maintaining beneficial microbes in the intestines. (also called **vermiform appendix**)
abdomen (AB-duh-men)	portion of the body between the thorax and the pelvis

PRONOUNCE ANATOMIC STRUCTURES

Practice saying aloud each of the organs and specific structures on the previous pages.

To hear the terms, go to Evolve Resources at www.evolve.elsevier.com and select:
Student Resources > Audio Glossary > Chapter 11 > Anatomic Structures

❏ Check the box when complete.

WORD PARTS

Use paper flashcards or electronic flashcards on Evolve to memorize word parts used to analyze, define, and build medical terms in this chapter. To reinforce learning, study one section of the Word Parts Table at a time, and then complete the corresponding exercise on the following pages.

1 ■ Digestive System Combining Forms

COMBINING FORM	DEFINITION	COMBINING FORM	DEFINITION
an/o	anus	gastr/o	stomach
antr/o	antrum	ile/o	ileum
cec/o	cecum	jejun/o	jejunum
col/o	colon (large intestine)	or/o	mouth
colon/o	colon (large intestine)	proct/o	rectum
duoden/o	duodenum	rect/o	rectum
enter/o	intestines (usually the small intestine)	sigmoid/o	sigmoid colon
esophag/o	esophagus	stomat/o	mouth

2 ■ Accessory Organs and Combining Forms Used with Digestive System Terms

COMBINING FORM	DEFINITION	COMBINING FORM	DEFINITION
abdomin/o	abdomen, abdominal cavity	**HERNIA** Types in the digestive system include abdominal, hiatal or diaphragmatic, inguinal, and umbilical hernias. (Fig. 11.7)	
append/o	appendix		
appendic/o	appendix	lapar/o	abdomen, abdominal cavity
celi/o	abdomen, abdominal cavity	lith/o	stone(s), calculus (*pl.* calculi)
cheil/o	lip(s)	lingu/o	tongue
cholangi/o	bile duct(s)	nas/o	nose
chol/e	gall, bile (Note: the combining vowel is e.)	palat/o	palate
choledoch/o	common bile duct	pancreat/o	pancreas
cyst/o	bladder, sac	peritone/o	peritoneum
diverticul/o	diverticulum, *pl.* diverticula (pouch extending from a hollow organ) (Fig. 11.6)	phag/o	eating, swallowing
		pharyng/o	pharynx
		polyp/o	polyp, small growth
gingiv/o	gum(s)	pylor/o	pylorus, pyloric sphincter
gloss/o	tongue	sial/o	saliva, salivary gland
hepat/o	liver	steat/o	fat
herni/o	hernia (protrusion of an organ through a membrane or cavity wall)	uvul/o	uvula

Chapter 11 Digestive System 421

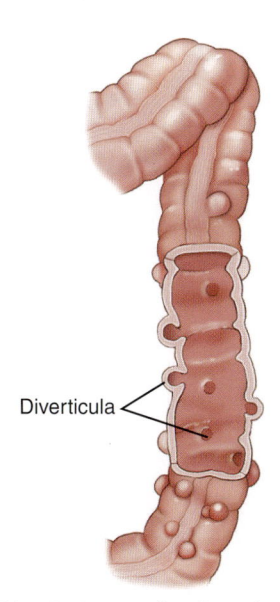

FIG. 11.6 Diverticula extending from the large intestine.

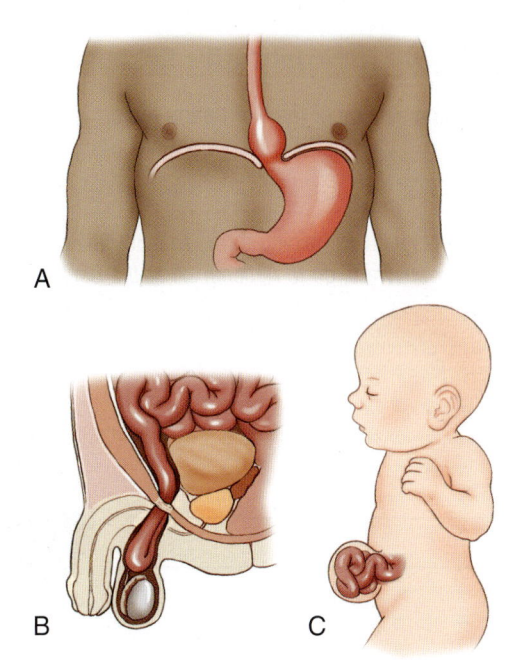

FIG. 11.7 Digestive hernias. **A**, Hiatal. **B**, Inguinal. **C**, Umbilical.

3 ■ Prefixes

PREFIX	DEFINITION	PREFIX	DEFINITION
a-	absence of, without	hemi-	half
dys-	painful, abnormal, difficult, labored		

4 ■ Suffixes

SUFFIX	DEFINITION	SUFFIX	DEFINITION
-ac	pertaining to	-logy	study of
-al	pertaining to	-megaly	enlargement
-cele	hernia, protrusion	-oma	tumor, swelling
-centesis	surgical puncture to aspirate fluid (with a sterile needle)	-osis	abnormal condition (means increase when used with blood cell word roots)
-eal	pertaining to	-pathy	disease
-ectomy	excision, surgical removal	-pepsia	digestion
-gram	the record, radiographic image	-plasty	surgical repair
-graphy	process of recording, radiographic imaging	-rrhaphy	suturing, repairing
		-rrhea	flow, discharge
-iasis	condition	-scope	instrument used for visual examination
-ia	diseased state, condition of	-scopy	visual examination
-ic	pertaining to	-stomy	creation of an artificial opening
-itis	inflammation	-tomy	cut into, incision
-lith	stone(s), calculus (*pl.* calculi)	-y	noun suffix, no meaning
-logist	one who studies and treats (specialist, physician)		

Refer to **Appendix B** and **Appendix C** for a complete listing of word parts.

422 Chapter 11 Digestive System

EXERCISE 1 ■ Digestive System Combining Forms

Refer to the first section of the word parts table.

A Label

Fill in the blanks with combining forms to label this diagram of the digestive system.
To check your answers, go to Appendix A at the back of the textbook.

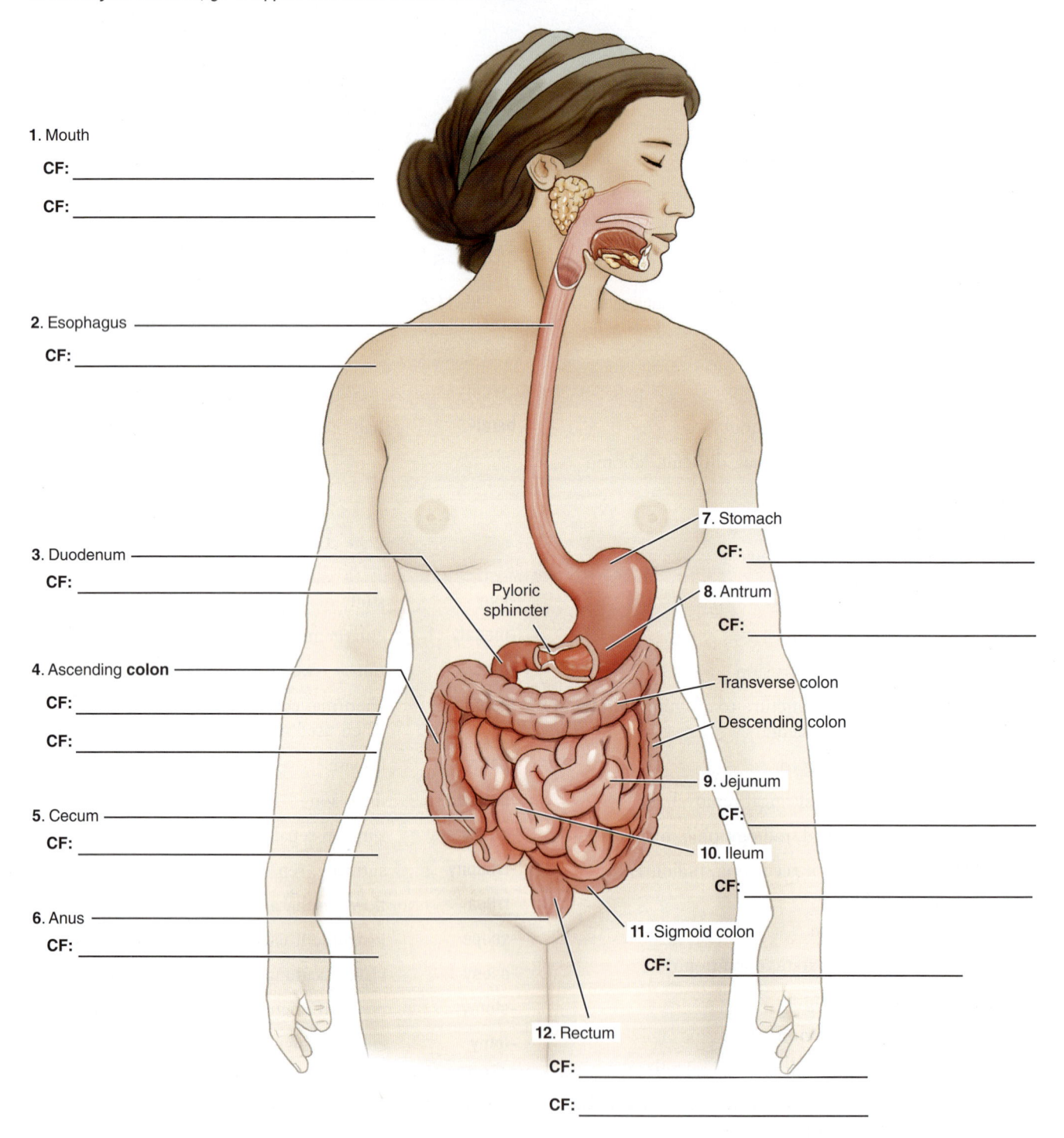

1. Mouth
   CF: _____
   CF: _____

2. Esophagus
   CF: _____

3. Duodenum
   CF: _____

4. Ascending **colon**
   CF: _____
   CF: _____

5. Cecum
   CF: _____

6. Anus
   CF: _____

7. Stomach
   CF: _____

8. Antrum
   CF: _____

Pyloric sphincter

Transverse colon
Descending colon

9. Jejunum
   CF: _____

10. Ileum
    CF: _____

11. Sigmoid colon
    CF: _____

12. Rectum
    CF: _____
    CF: _____

Chapter 11   Digestive System   423

B   Define and Match

Step 1: Write the definitions after the following combining forms.
Step 2: Match the descriptions on the right with the combining forms and definitions.

_____ 1. jejun/o, _____
_____ 2. an/o, _____
_____ 3. gastr/o, _____
_____ 4. rect/o, _____
_____ 5. or/o, _____
_____ 6. col/o, _____
_____ 7. sigmoid/o, _____
_____ 8. enter/o, _____

a. opening through which food passes into the body
b. distal portion of the large intestine
c. main portion of the large intestine
d. 20-foot (6-m) tube extending from the pyloric sphincter to the large intestine
e. second portion of the small intestine
f. portion of large intestine between descending colon and rectum
g. sphincter muscle at the end of the gastrointestinal tract
h. J-shaped sac that mixes and stores food

C   Define and Match

Step 1: Write the definitions after the following combining forms.
Step 2: Match the descriptions on the right with the combining forms and definitions.

_____ 1. ile/o, _____
_____ 2. stomat/o, _____
_____ 3. proct/o, _____
_____ 4. esophag/o, _____
_____ 5. antr/o, _____
_____ 6. colon/o, _____
_____ 7. duoden/o, _____
_____ 8. cec/o, _____

a. distal portion of the stomach
b. first 10 to 12 inches (25 cm) of the small intestine
c. U-shaped pouch that is the first portion of the large intestine
d. third portion of the small intestine, approximately 11 feet (3.3 m) long
e. 10-inch (25-cm) tube that is a passageway for food extending from the pharynx to the stomach
f. main portion of the large intestine
g. opening through which food passes into the body
h. distal portion of the large intestine

EXERCISE 2 ■ Accessory Organs and Combining Forms Used with Digestive System Terms

Refer to the second section of the word parts table.

A   Identify

Write the combining form for each of the following.

1. peritoneum _____
2. gall, bile _____
3. hernia _____
4. diverticulum _____
5. polyp, small growth _____
6. fat _____

B   Define

Write the definitions of the following combining forms.

1. herni/o _____
2. abdomin/o _____
3. sial/o _____
4. chol/e _____
5. diverticul/o _____
6. gingiv/o _____
7. appendic/o _____
8. gloss/o _____

424 Chapter 11 Digestive System

9. hepat/o _____
10. cheil/o _____
11. peritone/o _____
12. palat/o _____
13. pancreat/o _____
14. lapar/o _____
15. lingu/o _____
16. choledoch/o _____
17. pylor/o _____
18. uvul/o _____
19. cholangi/o _____
20. polyp/o _____
21. celi/o _____
22. steat/o _____
23. append/o _____
24. pharyng/o _____
25. cyst/o _____
26. phag/o _____

C Label

Fill in the blanks with combining forms to label this diagram of the digestive system and associated structures.

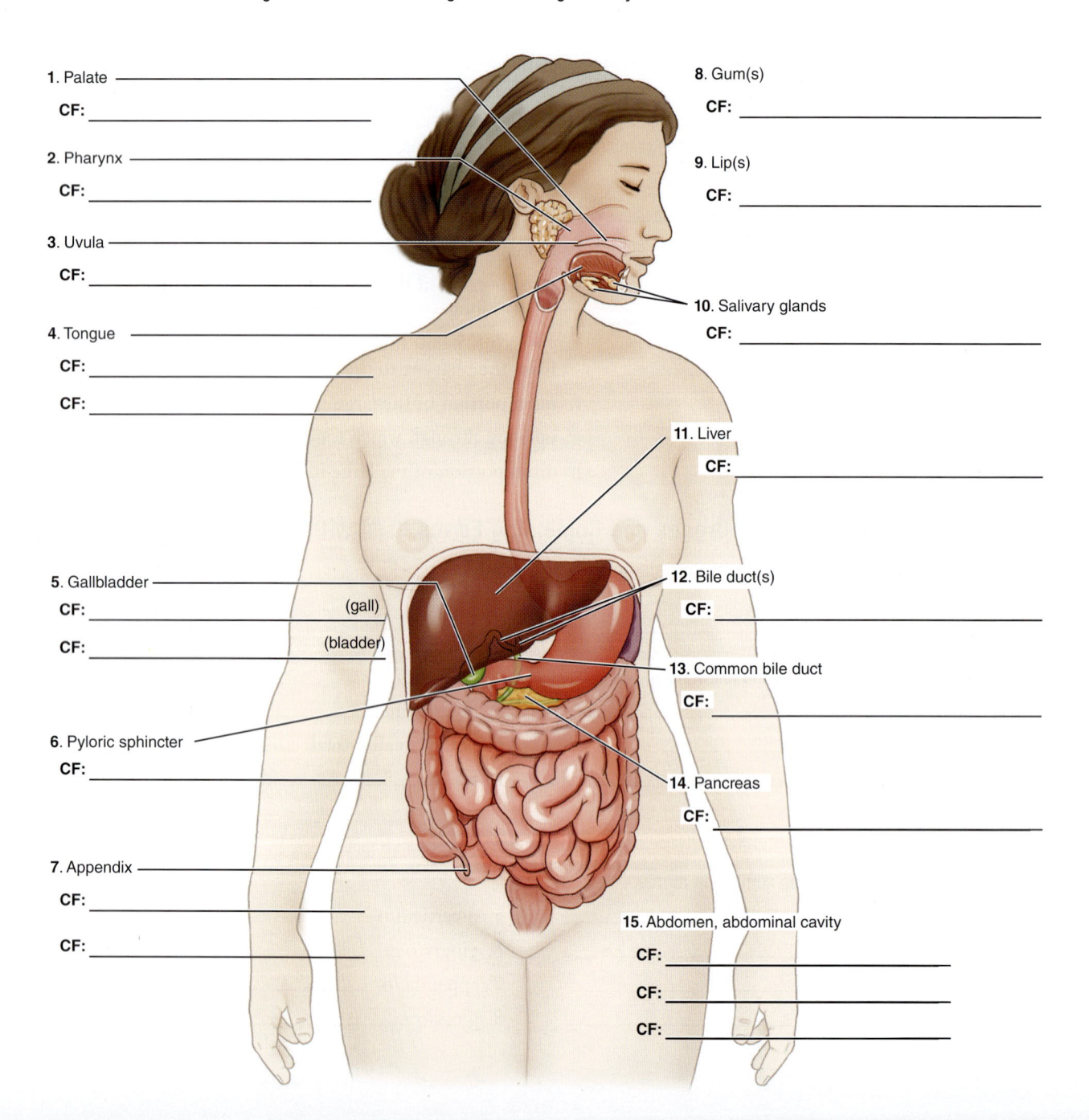

1. Palate
   CF: _____

2. Pharynx
   CF: _____

3. Uvula
   CF: _____

4. Tongue
   CF: _____
   CF: _____

5. Gallbladder
   CF: _____ (gall)
   CF: _____ (bladder)

6. Pyloric sphincter
   CF: _____

7. Appendix
   CF: _____
   CF: _____

8. Gum(s)
   CF: _____

9. Lip(s)
   CF: _____

10. Salivary glands
    CF: _____

11. Liver
    CF: _____

12. Bile duct(s)
    CF: _____

13. Common bile duct
    CF: _____

14. Pancreas
    CF: _____

15. Abdomen, abdominal cavity
    CF: _____
    CF: _____
    CF: _____

EXERCISE 3 ■ Prefixes

Refer to the third section of the word parts table.

A Define

Write the definitions of the following prefixes.

1. dys- _____
2. hemi- _____
3. a- _____

B Identify

Write the prefixes for the following definitions.

1. absence of, without _____
2. half _____
3. painful, abnormal, difficult, labored _____

EXERCISE 4 ■ Suffixes

Refer to the fourth section of the word parts table.

A Define

Write the definitions of the following suffixes.

1. -pepsia _____
2. -ac, -al, -ic _____
3. -y _____
4. -osis _____
5. -iasis _____
6. -ia _____

B Identify

Write the suffixes for the following definitions.

1. instrument used for visual examination _____
2. process of recording, radiographic imaging _____
3. one who studies and treats (specialist, physician) _____
4. study of _____
5. the record, radiographic image _____
6. visual examination _____

C Match

Match the suffixes in the first column with their correct definitions in the second column.

_____ 1. -rrhea   a. disease
_____ 2. -pathy   b. enlargement
_____ 3. -oma   c. flow, discharge
_____ 4. -megaly   d. hernia, protrusion
_____ 5. -lith   e. inflammation
_____ 6. -itis   f. tumor, swelling
_____ 7. -cele   g. stone(s), calculus (*pl.* calculi)

D Match

Match the suffixes in the first column with their correct definitions in the second column.

_____ 1. -centesis   a. creation of an artificial opening
_____ 2. -ectomy   b. cut into, incision
_____ 3. -plasty   c. excision, surgical removal
_____ 4. -rrhaphy   d. surgical puncture to aspirate fluid (with a sterile needle)
_____ 5. -stomy   e. pertaining to
_____ 6. -tomy   f. suturing, repairing
_____ 7. -eal   g. surgical repair

MEDICAL TERMS

Medical terms relevant to this chapter have been grouped by topics, such as Disease and Disorder, and are listed in tables designated as Built from Word Parts or *NOT* Built from Word Parts. The exercises following each table assist with learning term definitions, pronunciations, and spellings.

Disease and Disorder Terms

BUILT FROM WORD PARTS

The following terms can be translated using definitions of word parts. Further explanation is provided within parentheses as needed.

TERM	DEFINITION	TERM	DEFINITION
1. **appendicitis** (a-*pen*-di-SĪ-tis)	inflammation of the appendix	10. **dysentery** (DIS-en-ter-ē)	painful intestines (disorder that involves inflammation of the intestines, usually the large intestine, associated with abdominal pain and diarrhea that is often bloody)
2. **cheilitis** (kī-LĪ-tis)	inflammation of the lips		
3. **cholangioma** (kō-*lan*-jē-Ō-ma)	tumor of the bile duct		
4. **cholecystitis** (kō-lē-sis-TĪ-tis)	inflammation of the gallbladder	11. **enteritis** (*en*-ter-Ī-tis)	inflammation of the intestines
5. **choledocholithiasis** (kō-*led*-o-kō-li-THĪ-a-sis)	condition of stones in the common bile duct	12. **enteropathy** (en-ter-OP-a-thē)	disease of the intestines
		13. **esophagitis** (e-*sof*-a-JĪ-tis)	inflammation of the esophagus
6. **cholelithiasis** (kō-le-li-THĪ-a-sis)	condition of gallstones	14. **gastritis** (gas-TRĪ-tis)	inflammation of the stomach
7. **colitis** (ko-LĪ-tis)	inflammation of the colon	15. **gastroenteritis** (*gas*-trō-*en*-te-RĪ-tis)	inflammation of the stomach and intestines
ANTIBIOTIC-ASSOCIATED COLITIS is caused by a bacterium called **Clostridium difficile** (**C. difficile**). Though usually occurring in hospitalized patients, it is also now occurring more frequently in the general community. Symptoms include diarrhea and abdominal pain. Treatments include stopping the antibiotic and frequent hand washing to limit the spread of disease between patients. Oral vancomycin and other antibiotics work directly in the colon to kill *C. difficile* bacteria.		16. **gingivitis** (*jin*-ji-VĪ-tis)	inflammation of the gums
		17. **glossitis** (glos-Ī-tis)	inflammation of the tongue
		18. **hepatitis** (*hep*-a-TĪ-tis)	inflammation of the liver
8. **diverticulitis** (dī-ver-*tik*-ū-LĪ-tis)	inflammation of a diverticulum	19. **hepatoma** (*hep*-a-TŌ-ma)	tumor of the liver
9. **diverticulosis** (dī-ver-*tik*-ū-LŌ-sis)	abnormal condition of having diverticula (Figs. 11.6 and 11.15B)		

Chapter 11 Digestive System 427

TERM	DEFINITION	TERM	DEFINITION
20. pancreatitis (pan-krē-a-TĪ-tis)	inflammation of the pancreas	24. rectocele (REK-tō-sēl)	hernia of the rectum
21. peritonitis (per-i-tō-NĪ-tis)	inflammation of the peritoneum	25. sialolith (sī-AL-ō-lith)	stone in the salivary gland
💡 In the term **peritonitis**, the final **e** is dropped from the combining form **peritone/o**.		26. steatohepatitis (stē-a-tō-hep-a-TĪ-tis)	inflammation of the liver associated with (excess) fat; (often caused by alcohol abuse and obesity; over time may lead to cirrhosis)
22. polyposis (pol-i-PŌ-sis)	abnormal condition of (multiple) polyps (in the mucous membrane of the intestine, especially the colon.)	27. stomatitis (stō-ma-TĪ-tis)	inflammation of the mouth (mucous membrane)
FAMILIAL POLYPOSIS is an inherited syndrome with a high potential for malignancy if polyps are not removed when they are small.		28. uvulitis (ū-vū-LĪ-tis)	inflammation of the uvula
23. proctitis (prok-TĪ-tis)	inflammation of the rectum		

EXERCISE 5 ■ Pronounce and Spell

Practice pronunciation and spelling on paper and online.

1. **Practice on Paper**
    a. **Pronounce:** Read the phonetic spelling and say aloud the terms listed in the previous table. Refer to Table 2.2 Pronunciation Key as needed.
    b. **Spell:** Have a study partner read the terms aloud. Write the spelling of the terms on a separate sheet of paper.

2. **Practice Online** 🌐
    a. **Access** online learning resources. Go to evolve.elsevier.com > Evolve Resources > Student Resources.
    b. **Pronounce:** Select Audio Glossary > Chapter 11 > Exercise 5. Select a term to hear its pronunciation and repeat aloud.
    c. **Spell:** Select Activities > Chapter 11 > Spell Terms > Exercise 5. Select the audio icon and type the correct spelling of the term.

❏ Check the box when complete.

EXERCISE 6 ■ Analyze and Define

Analyze and define the following terms.

1. steatohepatitis

    _____

    _____

2. diverticulosis

    _____

    _____

3. cholangioma

    _____

    _____

4. hepatoma

    _____

    _____

428 Chapter 11 Digestive System

EXERCISE 6 ■ Analyze and Define—cont'd

5. uvulitis

6. pancreatitis

7. proctitis

8. cheilitis

9. gastritis

10. rectocele

11. enteropathy

12. peritonitis

13. enteritis

14. glossitis

EXERCISE 7 ■ Build

A Label

Build terms pictured by writing word parts above definitions.

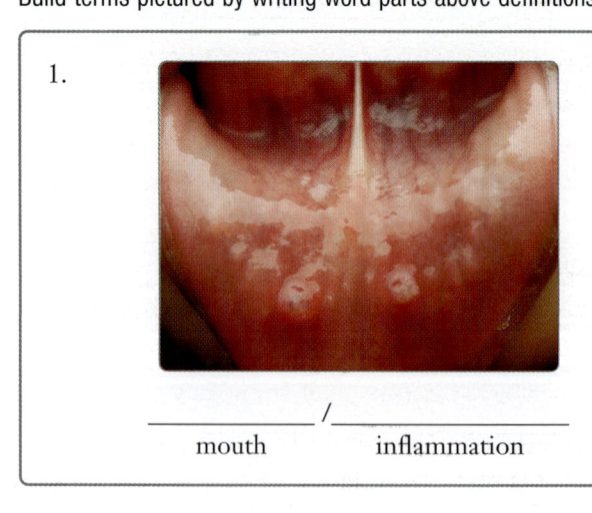

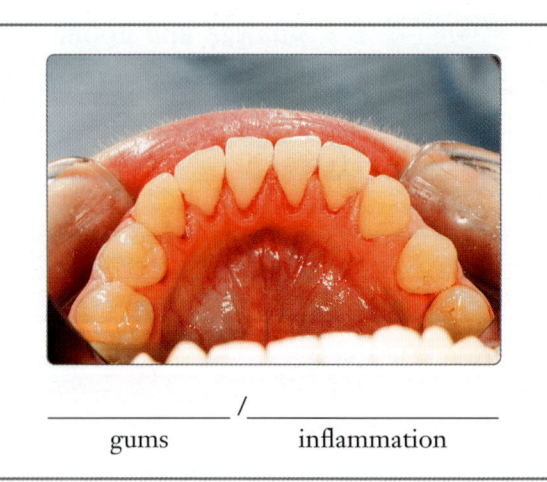

1. _____ / _____
   mouth   inflammation

2. _____ / _____
   gums   inflammation

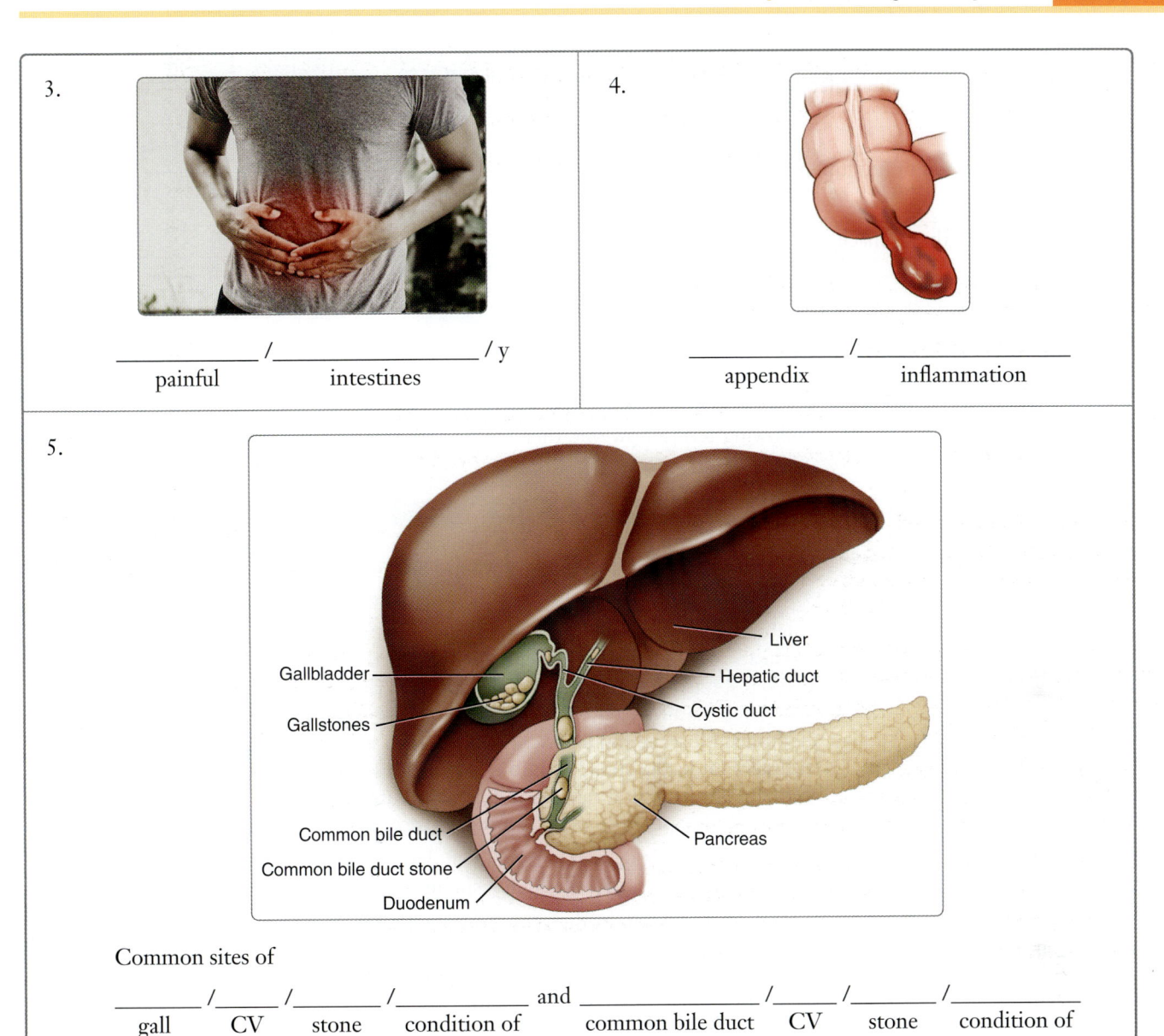

Chapter 11   Digestive System   429

3.

_____ / _____ / y
  painful   intestines

4.

_____ / _____
   appendix   inflammation

5.

Common sites of
_____ / _____ / _____ / _____ and _____ / _____ / _____ / _____
 gall   CV   stone   condition of   common bile duct   CV   stone   condition of

B Fill In

Build disease and disorder terms for the following definitions by using the word parts you have learned.

1. inflammation of the liver   _____ / _____
                                         WR   S

2. inflammation of the colon   _____ / _____
                                         WR   S

3. stone in the salivary gland   _____ / ____ / _____
                                         WR   CV   S

4. inflammation of the esophagus   _____ / _____
                                         WR   S

5. inflammation of a diverticulum   _____ / _____
                                         WR   S

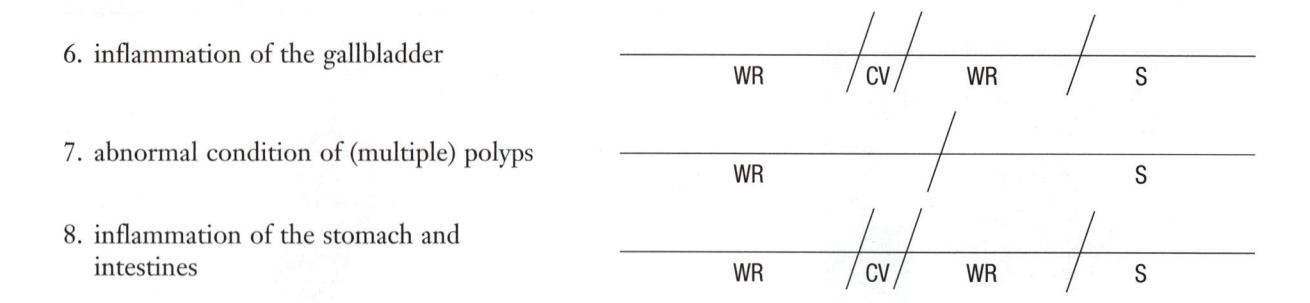

6. inflammation of the gallbladder _____ / _____ / _____ / _____
   WR / CV / WR / S

7. abnormal condition of (multiple) polyps _____ / _____
   WR / S

8. inflammation of the stomach and intestines _____ / _____ / _____ / _____
   WR / CV / WR / S

Disease and Disorder Terms
NOT BUILT FROM WORD PARTS

Word parts may be present in the following terms; however, their full meanings cannot be translated using definitions of word parts alone.

TERM	DEFINITION
1. **adhesion** (ad-HĒ-zhun)	abnormal growing together of two peritoneal surfaces that normally are separated. This may occur after abdominal surgery. Surgical treatment is called **adhesiolysis** or **adhesiotomy**.
2. **celiac disease** (SĒ-lē-ak) (di-ZĒZ)	malabsorption syndrome caused by an immune reaction to gluten (a protein in wheat, rye, and barley), which may damage the lining of the small intestine that is responsible for absorption of food into the bloodstream. Celiac disease is considered a multisystem disorder with varying signs and symptoms, including abdominal bloating and pain, chronic diarrhea or constipation, steatorrhea (excessive fat in the stool), vomiting, weight loss, fatigue, and iron deficiency anemia. A pruritic skin rash known as dermatitis herpetiformis may be associated with celiac disease. (also called **gluten enteropathy**)
3. **cirrhosis** (sir-RŌ-sis)	chronic disease of the liver with gradual destruction of cells and formation of scar tissue; commonly caused by alcoholism and certain types of viral hepatitis
4. **Crohn disease** (krōn) (di-ZĒZ)	chronic inflammation of the gastrointestinal tract, usually affecting the ileum and colon (but can occur anywhere between the mouth and anus); characterized by cobblestone ulcerations and the formation of scar tissue that may lead to intestinal obstruction (also called **regional ileitis** or **regional enteritis**)
5. **gastroesophageal reflux disease (GERD)** (gas-trō-e-sof-a-JĒ-al) (RĒ-fluks) (di-ZĒZ)	abnormal backward flow of the gastrointestinal contents into the esophagus, causing heartburn and the gradual breakdown of the mucous barrier of the esophagus

GASTROESOPHAGEAL REFLUX DISEASE (GERD) is a common gastrointestinal disorder. The acidity of the regurgitated stomach contents causes inflammation of the esophagus (reflux esophagitis). In addition to heartburn, GERD may also cause chronic cough and excessive throat clearing. **Chronic GERD** may cause cellular changes in the lower esophagus called **Barrett esophagus**, which increases the risk of cancer.

6. **hemochromatosis** (hē-mō-krō-ma-TŌ-sis)	iron metabolism disorder that occurs when too much iron is absorbed from food, resulting in excessive deposits of iron in the tissue; can cause heart failure, diabetes, cirrhosis, or cancer of the liver
7. **hemorrhoids** (HEM-o-roydz)	swollen or distended veins in the rectum or anus, which are called internal or external, respectively, and can be a source of rectal bleeding and pain
8. **ileus** (IL-ē-us)	nonmechanical obstruction of the intestine, caused by a lack of effective peristalsis (involuntary wavelike movements that propel food along the gastrointestinal tract)
9. **intussusception** (in-tu-sus-SEP-shun)	prolapse of one part of the intestine inside the part next to it. It is most common in infants; symptoms may include intestinal blockage, abdominal pain with cramping, or a lump that can be felt from the outside.

Chapter 11 Digestive System

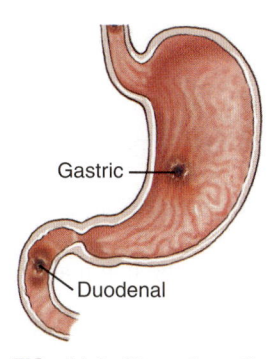

FIG. 11.8 Sites of peptic ulcers.

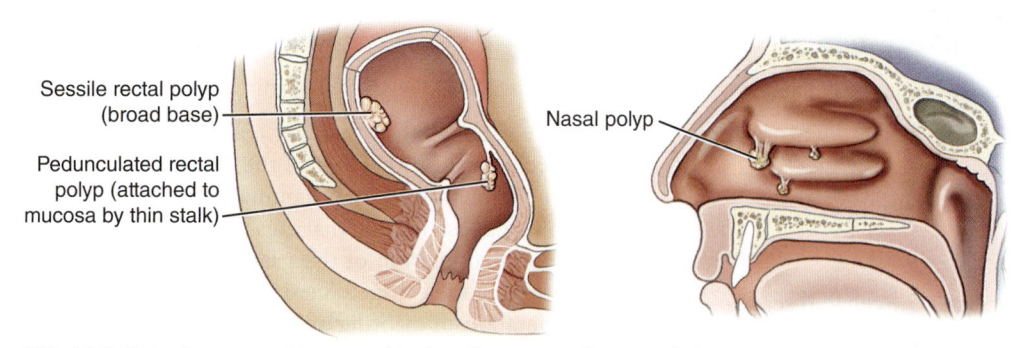

FIG. 11.9 Polyp is a general term used to describe a protruding growth from a mucous membrane. Polyps are commonly found in the nose, throat, intestines, uterus, and urinary bladder.

TERM	DEFINITION
10. **irritable bowel syndrome (IBS)** (IR-i-ta-bl) (BOW-el) (SIN-drōm)	periodic disturbances of bowel function, such as diarrhea and/or constipation, usually associated with abdominal pain
11. **nonalcoholic fatty liver disease (NAFLD)** (non-al-ka-HOL-ik) (FAT-ē) (LIV-er) (di-ZĒZ)	buildup of extra fat in the liver cells that is not due to alcohol consumption; strongly associated with obesity, type 2 diabetes mellitus, and lipid abnormalities. A more severe form, nonalcoholic steatohepatitis (NASH) is one of the leading causes of cirrhosis in the United States.
12. **peptic ulcer** (PEP-tik) (UL-ser)	erosion of the mucous membrane of the stomach or duodenum associated with increased secretion of acid from the stomach, bacterial infection (*H. pylori*), or medications such as nonsteroidal antiinflammatory drugs (often referred to as **gastric** or **duodenal ulcer**, depending on its location) (Fig. 11.8)
13. **polyp** (POL-ip)	tumorlike growth extending outward from a mucous membrane; usually benign; common sites are in the nose, throat, and intestines (Figs. 11.9 and 11.11)
14. **ulcerative colitis (UC)** (UL-ser-a-tiv) (kō-LĪ-tis)	disease characterized by inflammation of the colon with the formation of ulcers, which can cause bloody diarrhea. A proctocolectomy with permanent ileostomy may become necessary if the patient doesn't respond to medical therapy.
15. **volvulus** (VOL-vū-lus)	twisting or kinking of the intestine, causing intestinal obstruction

EXERCISE 8 ■ Pronounce and Spell

Practice pronunciation and spelling on paper and online.

1. **Practice on Paper**

    a. **Pronounce:** Read the phonetic spelling and say aloud the terms listed in the previous table. Refer to Table 2.2 Pronunciation Key as needed.
    b. **Spell:** Have a study partner read the terms aloud. Write the spelling of the terms on a separate sheet of paper.

2. **Practice Online**

    a. **Access** online learning resources. Go to evolve.elsevier.com > Evolve Resources > Student Resources.
    b. **Pronounce:** Select Audio Glossary > Chapter 11 > Exercise 8. Select a term to hear its pronunciation and repeat aloud.
    c. **Spell:** Select Activities > Chapter 11 > Spell Terms > Exercise 8. Select the audio icon and type the correct spelling of the term.

❏ Check the box when complete.

432 Chapter 11 Digestive System

EXERCISE 9 ■ Match

Match the terms in the first column with their definitions in the second column.

_____ 1. hemochromatosis
_____ 2. cirrhosis
_____ 3. ulcerative colitis
_____ 4. ileus
_____ 5. celiac disease
_____ 6. irritable bowel syndrome
_____ 7. Crohn disease
_____ 8. nonalcoholic fatty liver disease

a. buildup of extra fat in the liver cells that is not due to alcohol consumption
b. nonmechanical obstruction of the intestine
c. disease characterized by inflammation of the colon with the formation of ulcers, which can cause bloody diarrhea
d. chronic inflammation of the gastrointestinal tract usually affecting the ileum and colon with cobblestone ulcerations
e. iron metabolism disorder resulting in excessive deposits of iron in the tissue; can cause cirrhosis or liver cancer
f. malabsorption syndrome caused by an immune reaction to gluten
g. chronic disease of the liver with gradual destruction of cells and formation of scar tissue
h. periodic disturbances of bowel function, such as diarrhea and/or constipation, usually associated with abdominal pain

EXERCISE 10 ■ Label

Write the medical terms pictured and defined.

1. _____
erosion of the mucous membrane of the stomach or duodenum associated with increased secretion of acid from the stomach

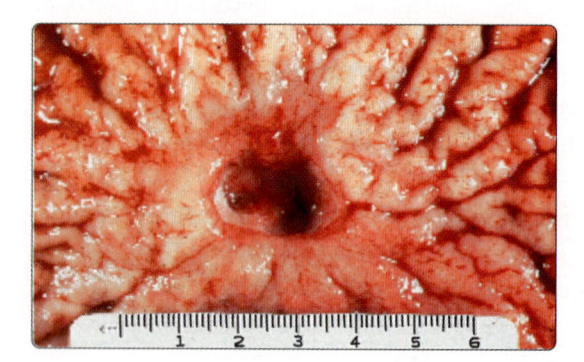

2. _____
twisting or kinking of the intestine, causing intestinal obstruction

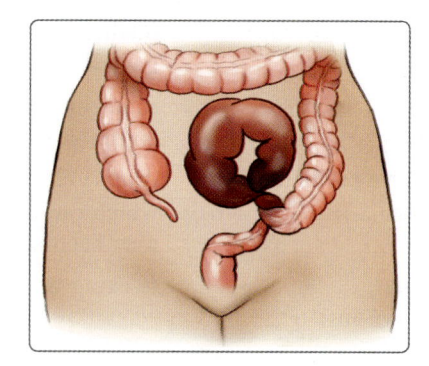

3. _____
tumorlike growth extending outward from a mucous membrane; usually benign

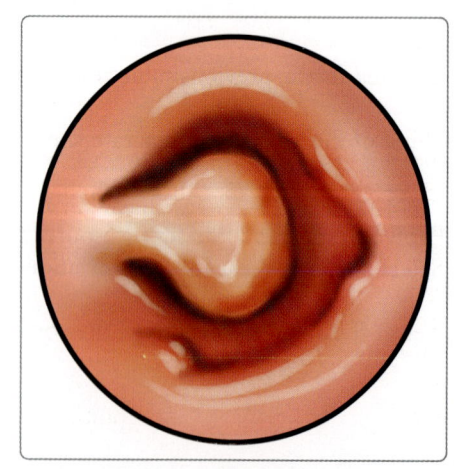

4. _____
abnormal backward flow of the gastrointestinal contents into the esophagus

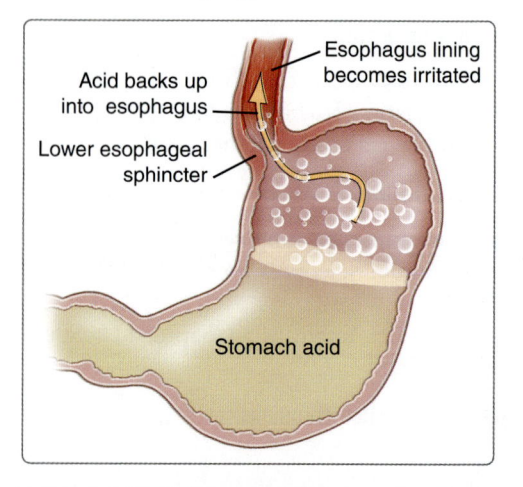

Chapter 11   Digestive System   433

5. _____
abnormal growing together of two peritoneal surfaces that normally are separated

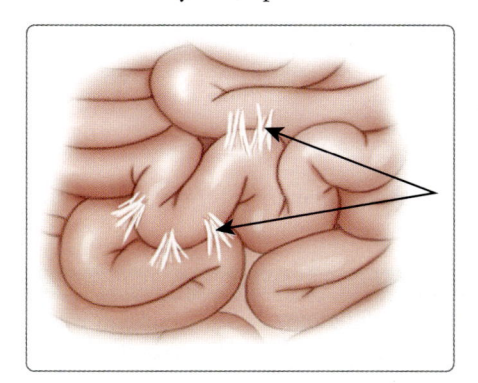

6. _____
prolapse of one part of the intestine inside the part next to it

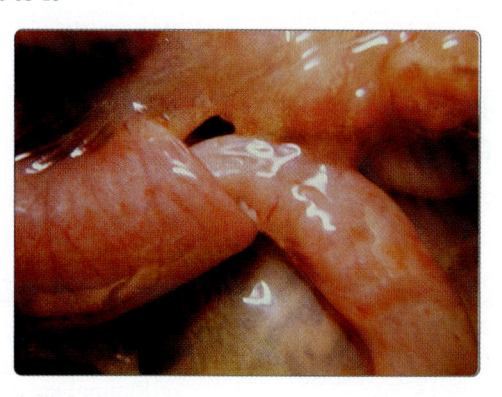

7. _____
swollen or distended veins in the rectum or anus, which can be a source of rectal bleeding and pain

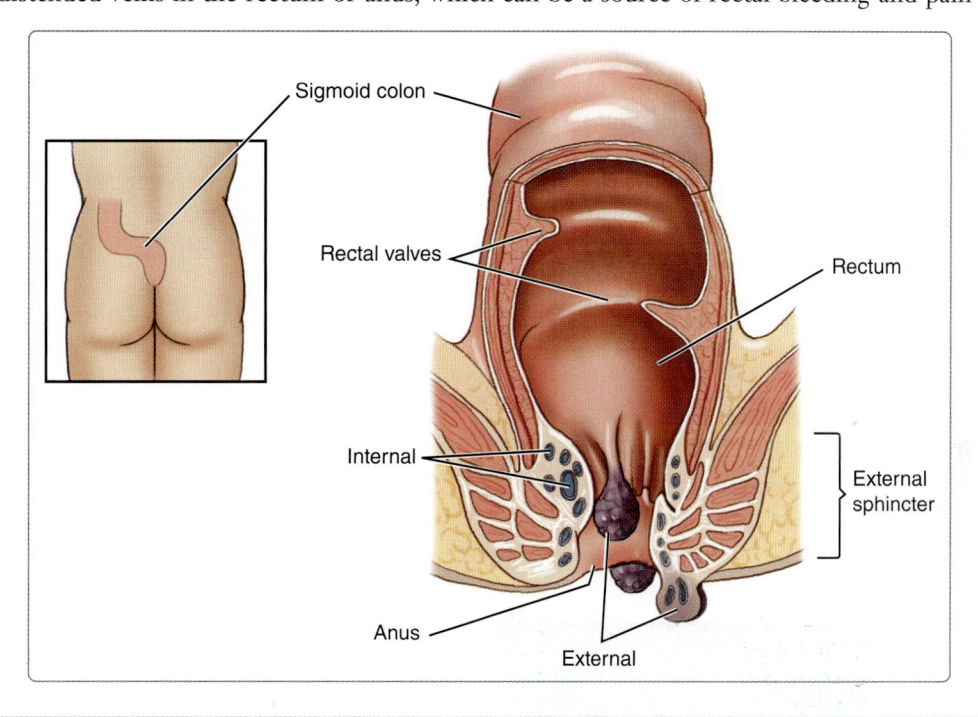

EXERCISE 11 ■ Review of Disease and Disorder Terms

Can you define, pronounce, and spell the following terms?

adhesion	colitis	gastroenteritis	ileus
appendicitis	Crohn disease	gastroesophageal reflux	intussusception
celiac disease	diverticulitis	disease (GERD)	irritable bowel syndrome
cheilitis	diverticulosis	gingivitis	(IBS)
cholangioma	dysentery	glossitis	nonalcoholic fatty liver
cholecystitis	enteritis	hemochromatosis	disease (NAFLD)
choledocholithiasis	enteropathy	hemorrhoids	pancreatitis
cholelithiasis	esophagitis	hepatitis	peptic ulcer
cirrhosis	gastritis	hepatoma	peritonitis

434 Chapter 11 Digestive System

> **EXERCISE 11** ■ **Review of Disease and Disorder Terms—cont'd**

polyp	rectocele	stomatitis	volvulus
polyposis	sialolith	ulcerative colitis (UC)	
proctitis	steatohepatitis	uvulitis	

Surgical Terms

BUILT FROM WORD PARTS

The following terms can be translated using definitions of word parts. Further explanation is provided within parentheses as needed.

TERM	DEFINITION	TERM	DEFINITION
1. **abdominocentesis** (ab-*dom*-i-nō-sen-TĒ-sis)	surgical puncture to aspirate fluid from the abdominal cavity (also called **paracentesis**)	8. **choledocholithotomy** (kō-*led*-o-kō-li-THOT-o-mē)	incision into the common bile duct to remove a stone
2. **abdominoplasty** (ab-DOM-i-nō-*plas*-tē)	surgical repair of the abdomen	9. **colectomy** (kō-LEK-to-mē)	excision of the colon
3. **anoplasty** (Ā-nō-*plas*-tē)	surgical repair of the anus	10. **colostomy** (ko-LOS-to-mē)	creation of an artificial opening into the colon (through the abdominal wall; used for the passage of stool)
4. **antrectomy** (an-TREK-to-mē)	excision of the antrum (of the stomach)		
5. **appendectomy** (*ap*-en-DEK-to-mē)	excision of the appendix	**COLOSTOMY** is a surgical procedure that creates a mouthlike opening called a **stoma** and may be permanent or temporary. It is performed as a treatment for bowel obstruction, cancer, or diverticulitis.	
6. **cheiloplasty** (KĪ-lō-*plas*-tē)	surgical repair of the lip	11. **diverticulectomy** (dī-ver-*tik*-ū-LEK-to-mē)	excision of a diverticulum
7. **cholecystectomy** (*kō*-le-sis-TEK-to-mē)	excision of the gallbladder (Fig. 11.10)	12. **enterorrhaphy** (*en*-ter-OR-a-fē)	suturing of the (small) intestine
🏛 **CHOLECYSTECTOMY** was first performed in 1882 by a German surgeon. **Laparoscopic cholecystectomy** was first performed in 1985.			

FIG. 11.10 In **laparoscopic cholecystectomy**, a type of endoscopic surgery, carbon dioxide (CO_2) is introduced into the abdominal cavity for better visualization. A tiny camera and surgical instruments, including a laparoscope, are passed through small incisions. **A,** External view. **B,** Internal view.

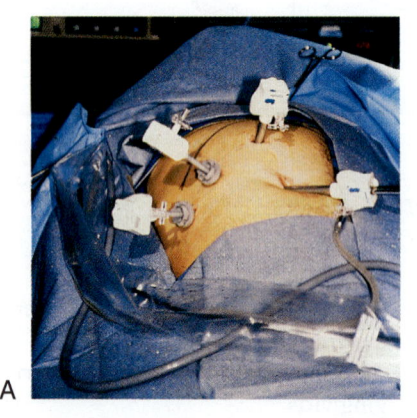

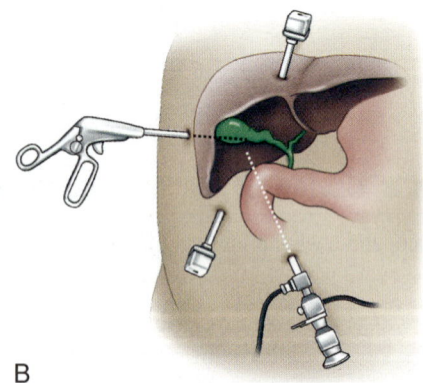

TERM	DEFINITION	TERM	DEFINITION
13. esophagogastroplasty (e-*sof*-a-gō-GAS-trō-*plas*-tē)	surgical repair of the esophagus and the stomach	22. ileostomy (*il*-ē-OS-to-mē)	creation of an artificial opening into the ileum (through the abdominal wall; used for passage of stool)
14. gastrectomy (gas-TREK-to-mē)	excision of the stomach (or part of the stomach)		
15. gastrojejunostomy (*gas*-trō-je-jū-NOS-to-mē)	creation of an artificial opening between the stomach and jejunum	**ILEOSTOMY** is a surgical procedure that creates a mouthlike opening called a **stoma**. It is performed following total proctocolectomy for ulcerative colitis, Crohn disease, or cancer.	
16. gastroplasty (GAS-trō-*plas*-tē)	surgical repair of the stomach	23. laparotomy (*lap*-a-ROT-o-mē)	incision into the abdominal cavity (also called **celiotomy**)
17. gastrostomy (gas-TROS-to-mē)	creation of an artificial opening into the stomach (through the abdominal wall)	24. palatoplasty (PAL-a-tō-*plas*-tē)	surgical repair of the palate
		25. pancreatectomy (pan-crē-a-TEK-ta-mē)	excision of the pancreas
GASTROSTOMY is a surgical procedure used to insert a tube, often referred to as a "G-tube," through the abdomen and into the stomach. This provides a route for long-term tube feeding if swallowing is impossible and to vent the stomach for air or drainage.		26. polypectomy (*pol*-i-PEK-to-mē)	excision of a polyp (Fig. 11.11)
		27. pyloroplasty (pī-LOR-ō-*plas*-tē)	surgical repair of the pylorus
18. gingivectomy (*jin*-ji-VEK-to-mē)	surgical removal of gum (tissue)	28. uvulectomy (ū-vū-LEK-to-mē)	excision of the uvula
19. glossorrhaphy (glo-SOR-a-fē)	suturing of the tongue	29. uvulopalatopharyngoplasty (UPPP) (ū-vū-lō-*pal*-a-tō-fa-RING-gō-*plas*-tē)	surgical repair of the uvula, palate, and pharynx (performed to correct obstructive sleep apnea) (see Fig. 5.6)
20. hemicolectomy (*hem*-ē-kō-LEK-to-mē)	excision of half of the colon		
21. herniorrhaphy (*her*-nē-OR-a-fē)	suturing of a hernia (for repair)		

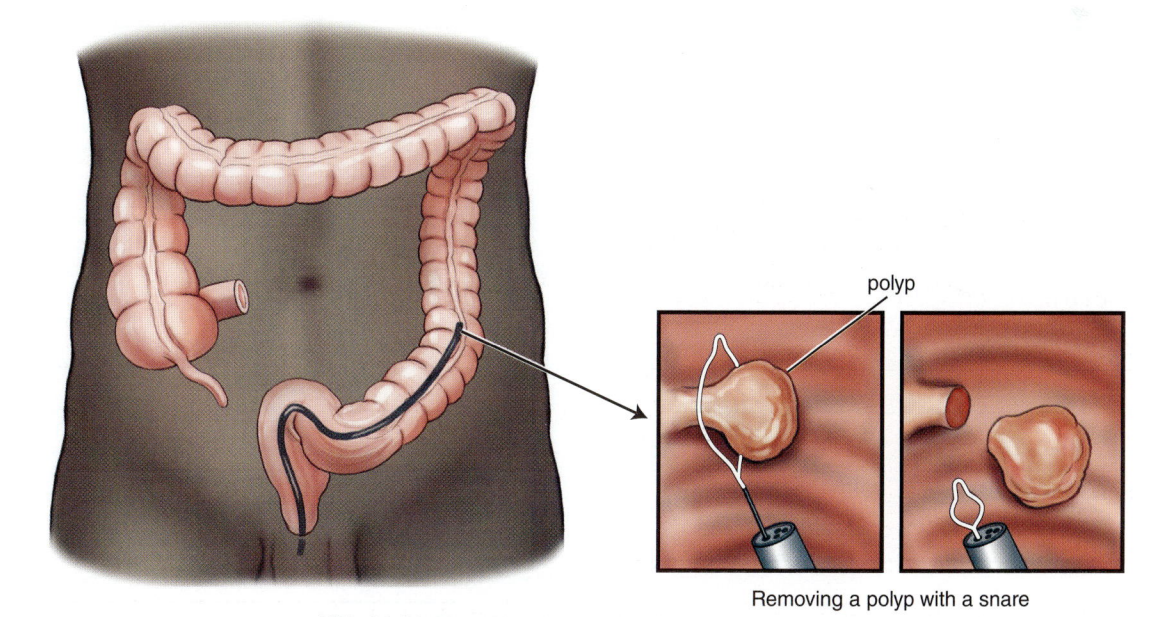

FIG. 11.11 Polypectomy performed using a colonoscope.

Removing a polyp with a snare

Chapter 11 Digestive System

EXERCISE 12 ■ Pronounce and Spell

Practice pronunciation and spelling on paper and online.

1. **Practice on Paper**
   a. **Pronounce:** Read the phonetic spelling and say aloud the terms listed in the previous table. Refer to Table 2.2 Pronunciation Key as needed.
   b. **Spell:** Have a study partner read the terms aloud. Write the spelling of the terms on a separate sheet of paper.

2. **Practice Online**
   a. **Access** online learning resources. Go to evolve.elsevier.com > Evolve Resources > Student Resources.
   b. **Pronounce:** Select Audio Glossary > Chapter 11 > Exercise 12. Select a term to hear its pronunciation and repeat aloud.
   c. **Spell:** Select Activities > Chapter 11 > Spell Terms > Exercise 12. Select the audio icon and type the correct spelling of the term.

❏ Check the box when complete.

EXERCISE 13 ■ Analyze and Define

Analyze and define the following terms.

1. herniorrhaphy

2. gastroplasty

3. hemicolectomy

4. antrectomy

5. enterorrhaphy

6. uvulectomy

7. gastrojejunostomy

8. cholecystectomy

9. abdominoplasty

10. pancreatectomy

Chapter 11   Digestive System   437

11. pyloroplasty

_____

_____

12. choledocholithotomy

_____

_____

13. uvulopalatopharyngoplasty

_____

_____

14. abdominocentesis

_____

_____

EXERCISE 14 ■ Build

A Label

Build terms pictured by writing word parts above definitions.

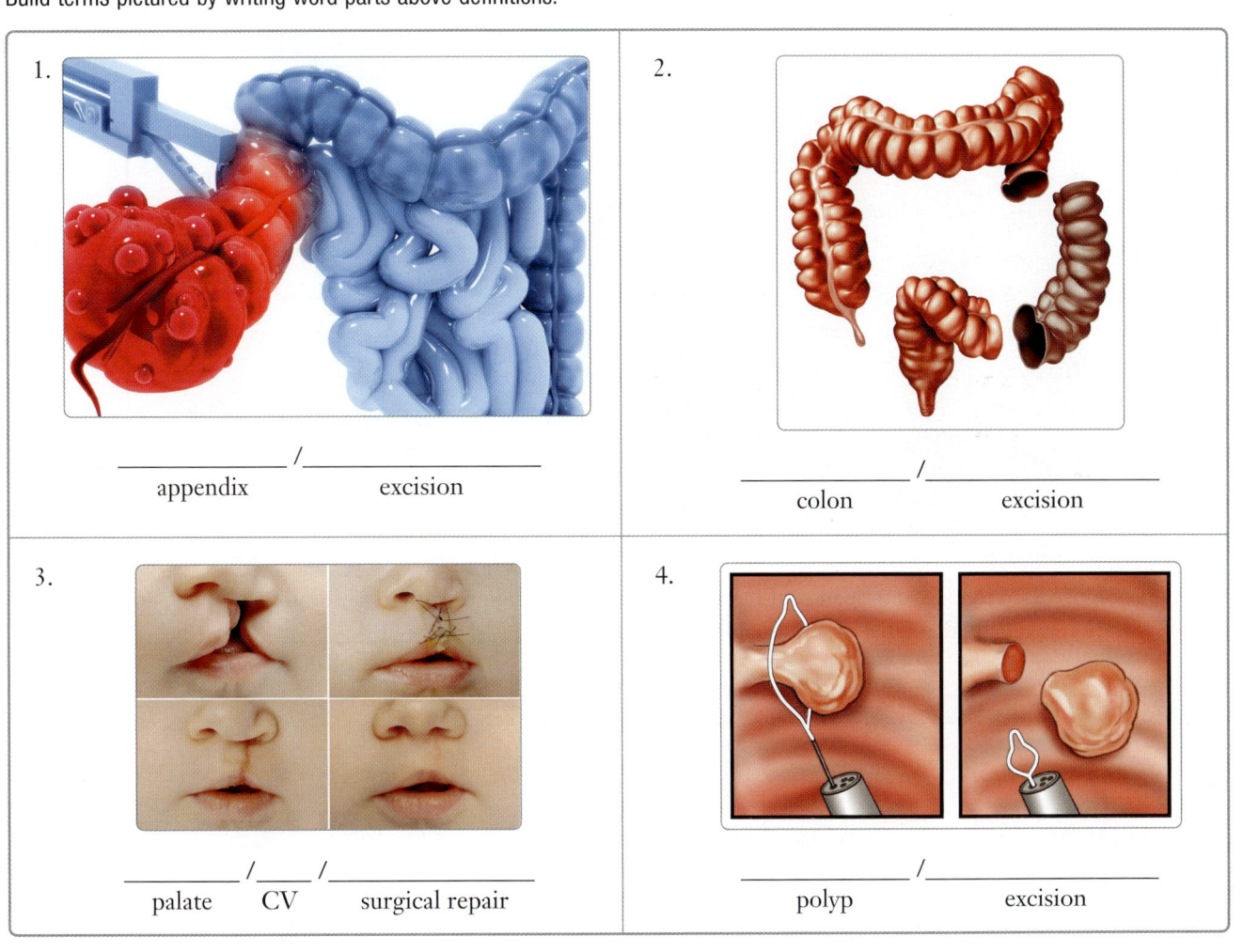

1.

_____/_____
appendix   excision

2.

_____/_____
colon   excision

3.

_____/___/_____
palate   CV   surgical repair

4.

_____/_____
polyp   excision

438　Chapter 11　Digestive System

5.

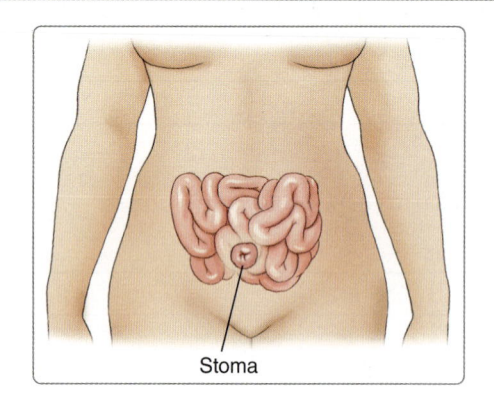

_____ / ____ / _____
ileum   CV   creation of an
                      artificial opening

after a total colectomy.

6.

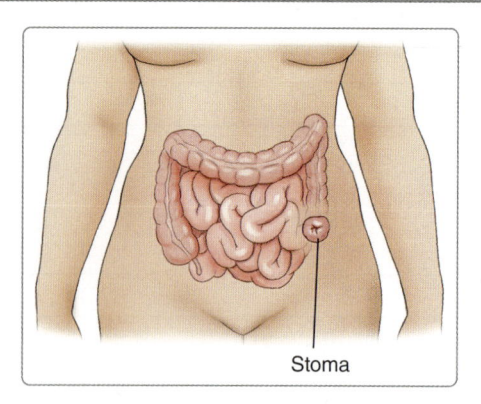

_____ / ____ / _____
colon   CV   creation of an
                      artificial opening

after an abdominoperineal resection.

7.

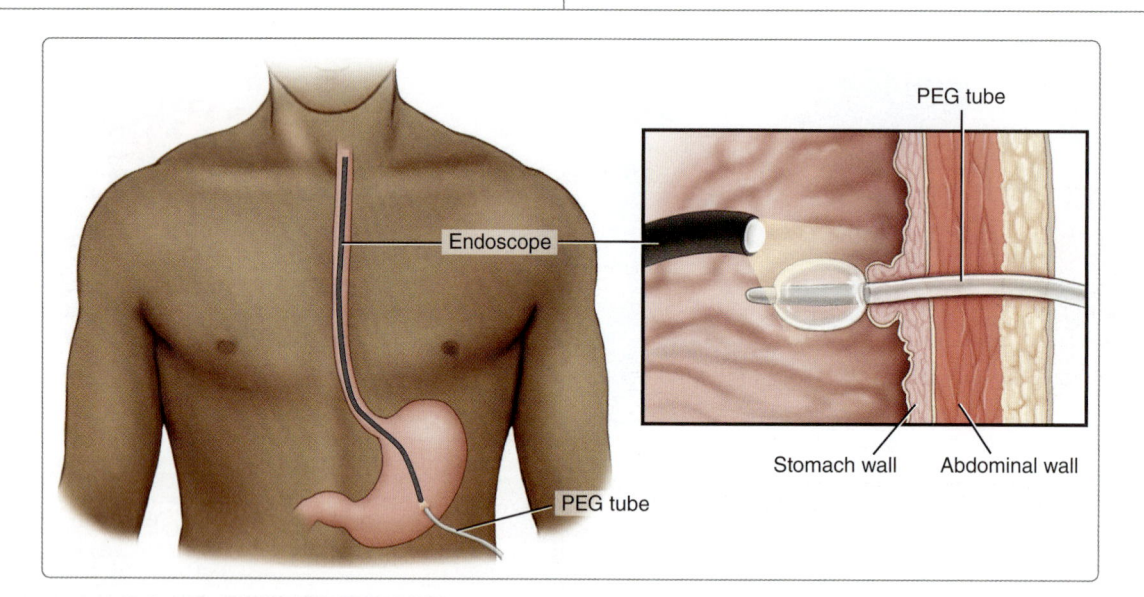

The procedure used to place a tube into the stomach through the abdominal wall to administer liquids for nutrition and hydration is called percutaneous endoscopic _____ / _____ / _____.
                                                                                                      stomach   CV   creation of an artificial opening

8.

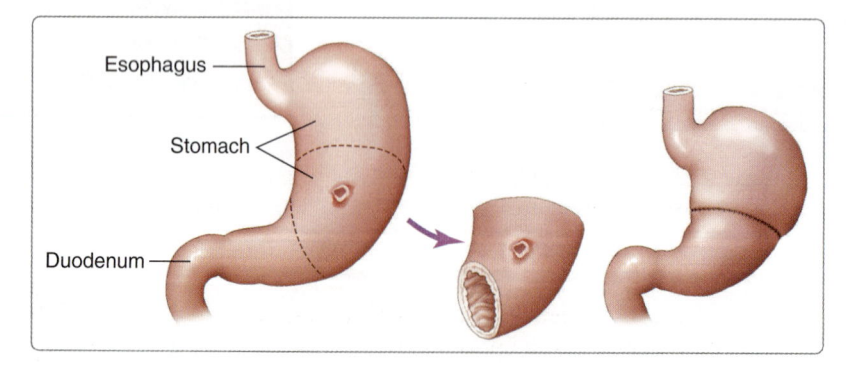

Partial _____ / _____ may be performed to treat chronic gastric ulcers.
         stomach   surgical removal

Chapter 11   Digestive System   439

B Fill In

Build surgical terms for the following definitions by using the word parts you have learned.

1. suturing of the tongue   ___WR___/CV/___S___

2. surgical repair of the esophagus and stomach   ___WR___/CV/___WR___/CV/___S___

3. excision of a diverticulum   ___WR___/___S___

4. surgical removal of gum (tissue)   ___WR___/___S___

5. incision into the abdominal cavity ___WR___/CV/___S___

6. surgical repair of the anus   ___WR___/CV/___S___

7. excision of the gallbladder   ___WR___/CV/___WR___/___S___

Surgical Terms
NOT BUILT FROM WORD PARTS

Word parts may be present in the following terms; however, their full meanings cannot be translated using definitions of word parts alone.

TERM	DEFINITION
1. **abdominoperineal resection (APR)** (ab-*dom*-i-nō-per-i-NĒ-el) (rē-SEK-shun)	removal of the distal colon, rectum, and anal sphincter through both abdominal and perineal approaches; performed to treat some colorectal cancers and inflammatory diseases of the lower large intestine. The patient will have a colostomy.
2. **anastomosis** (*pl.* **anastomoses**) (a-*nas*-to-MŌ-sis) (a-*nas*-to-MŌ-sēz)	connection created by surgically joining two structures, such as blood vessels or bowel segments (Fig. 11.12)
3. **bariatric surgery** (*bar*-ē-AT-rik) (SUR-jer-ē)	surgical reduction of gastric capacity to treat obesity (excess of body fat, which increases body weight), a condition that can cause serious illness
BARIATRIC SURGERY may be used to treat obesity for patients with a BMI (body mass index) greater than 35 or those with a BMI between 30 and 35 who also have type 2 diabetes. There are many types of bariatric surgery that are performed on the stomach, small intestine, or both. During surgery, the GI tract is reconstructed. A portion may be removed or bypassed in order to restrict the overall amount of food consumption and nutrient absorption.	
4. **hemorrhoidectomy** (*hem*-o-royd-EK-to-mē)	excision of hemorrhoids, the swollen or distended veins in the lower rectum and anus
5. **vagotomy** (vā-GOT-o-mē)	cutting of certain branches of the vagus nerve, performed with gastric surgery to reduce the amount of gastric acid produced and thus reduce the recurrence of ulcers

End to end   End to side   Side to side

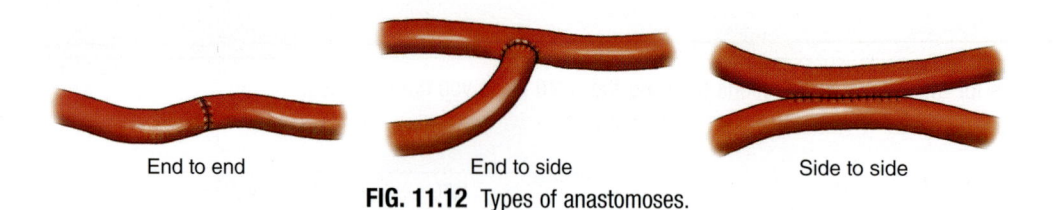

FIG. 11.12 Types of anastomoses.

EXERCISE 15 ■ Pronounce and Spell

Practice pronunciation and spelling on paper and online.

1. **Practice on Paper**
   a. **Pronounce:** Read the phonetic spelling and say aloud the terms listed in the previous table. Refer to Table 2.2 Pronunciation Key as needed.
   b. **Spell:** Have a study partner read the terms aloud. Write the spelling of the terms on a separate sheet of paper.

2. **Practice Online**
   a. **Access** online learning resources. Go to evolve.elsevier.com > Evolve Resources > Student Resources.
   b. **Pronounce:** Select Audio Glossary > Chapter 11 > Exercise 15. Select a term to hear its pronunciation and repeat aloud.
   c. **Spell:** Select Activities > Chapter 11 > Spell Terms > Exercise 15. Select the audio icon and type the correct spelling of the term.

❏ Check the box when complete.

EXERCISE 16 ■ Identify

Write the term for each of the following definitions.

1. cutting certain branches of the vagus nerve _____
2. connection created by surgically joining two structures _____
3. removal of the distal colon, rectum, and anal sphincter _____
4. surgical reduction of gastric capacity to treat obesity _____
5. excision of swollen or distended veins in the lower rectum and anus _____

EXERCISE 17 ■ Review of Surgical Terms

Can you define, pronounce, and spell the following terms?

abdominocentesis	cheiloplasty	gastroplasty	pancreatectomy
abdominoperineal resection (APR)	cholecystectomy	gastrostomy	polypectomy
	choledocholithotomy	gingivectomy	pyloroplasty
abdominoplasty	colectomy	glossorrhaphy	uvulectomy
anastomosis	colostomy	hemicolectomy	uvulopalatopharyngo-
(*pl.* anastomoses)	diverticulectomy	hemorrhoidectomy	plasty (UPPP)
anoplasty	enterorrhaphy	herniorrhaphy	vagotomy
antrectomy	esophagogastroplasty	ileostomy	
appendectomy	gastrectomy	laparotomy	
bariatric surgery	gastrojejunostomy	palatoplasty	

Diagnostic Terms
BUILT FROM WORD PARTS

The following terms can be translated using definitions of word parts. Further explanation is provided within parentheses as needed.

DIAGNOSTIC IMAGING

TERM	DEFINITION	TERM	DEFINITION
1. cholangiogram (kō-LAN-jē-ō-gram)	radiographic image of the bile ducts	4. esophagram (e-SOF-a-gram)	radiographic image of the esophagus (and pharynx); (also called **esophagogram** and **barium swallow**) *Note: the combining vowel "o" and the "g" in esophag/o are dropped in the term esophagram.*
2. cholangiography (kō-*lan*-jē-OG-ra-fē)	radiographic imaging of the bile ducts (after administration of contrast materials to outline the ducts)		

OPERATIVE CHOLANGIOGRAPHY is performed during surgery to check for residual stones after the removal of the gallbladder. **Postoperative cholangiography**, also called T-tube cholangiography, is performed in the radiology department after a cholecystectomy to check for residual stones. Both use the injection of contrast materials into the common bile duct.

ESOPHAGRAM During an **esophagram**, a contrast material, such as barium, is used to study the function and structure of the pharynx and esophagus as they relate to swallowing.

3. CT colonography (C-T) (*kō*-lon-OG-ra-fē)	radiographic imaging of the colon (using computed tomography); (also called **virtual colonoscopy**)		

ENDOSCOPY

TERM	DEFINITION	TERM	DEFINITION
5. capsule endoscopy (KAP-sel) (en-DOS-ko-pē)	(capsule) visual examination within (a hollow organ); (also called **camera endoscopy**) (Fig. 11.13)	**CAPSULE ENDOSCOPY** records pictures of the gastrointestinal tract and is especially helpful in visualizing the small intestine, which is not easily accessed. The procedure is used to find obscure causes of gastrointestinal bleeding and to help diagnose Crohn disease, celiac disease, and cancer.	

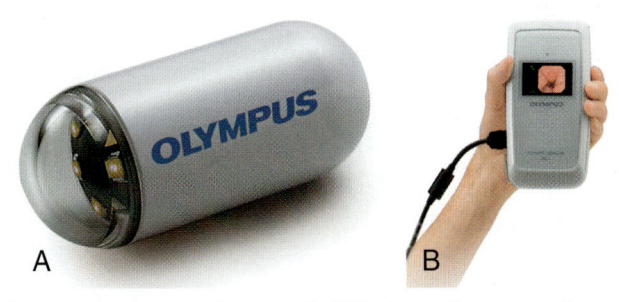

FIG. 11.13 Capsule endoscopy, also known as **camera endoscopy**. **A,** Patients swallow a capsule containing a camera, about the size of a pill. The camera takes pictures as it moves naturally through the gastrointestinal tract, and records thousands of images on a small device worn around the patient's waist. **B,** The recording device is then returned to the physician and the images are transferred to a computer for examination. The video capsule is expelled during a bowel movement and not retrieved.

Chapter 11 Digestive System

FIG. 11.14 Sigmoidoscopy, colonoscopy.

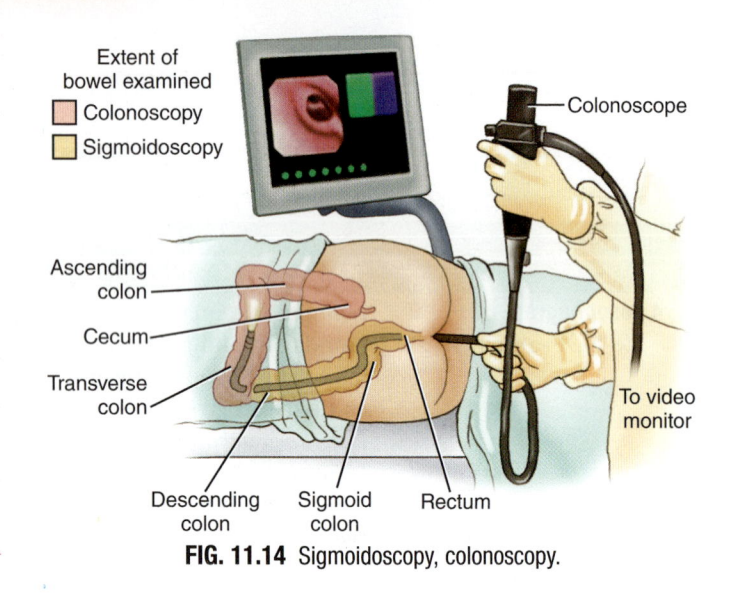

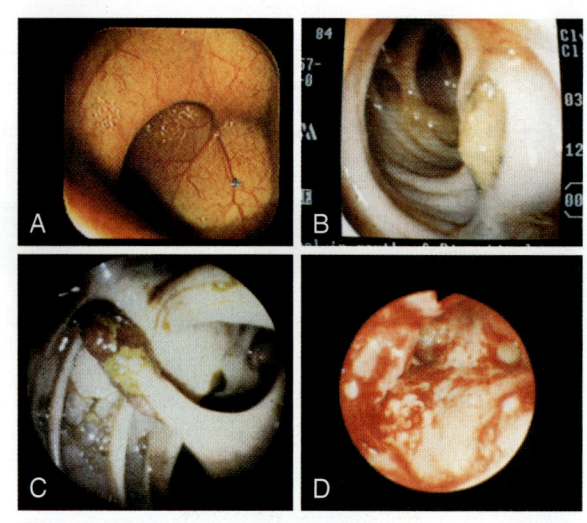

FIG. 11.15 Images obtained during colonoscopy reveal a normal colon **(A)**, diverticulosis **(B)**, a colon polyp **(C)**, and colon cancer **(D)**.

Diagnostic Terms—cont'd
BUILT FROM WORD PARTS

TERM	DEFINITION	TERM	DEFINITION
6. colonoscope (kō-LON-ō-skōp)	instrument used for visual examination of the colon	12. laparoscope (LAP-a-rō-skōp)	instrument used for visual examination of the abdominal cavity
7. colonoscopy (kō-lon-OS-ko-pē)	visual examination of the colon (Figs. 11.14 and 11.15)	**LAPAROSCOPES** are also used to perform laparoscopic surgery, which is less invasive than open abdominal surgery.	
8. esophagogastroduodenoscopy (EGD) (e-sof-a-gō-gas-trō-dū-od-e-NOS-ko-pē)	visual examination of the esophagus, stomach, and duodenum	13. laparoscopy (lap-a-ROS-ko-pē)	visual examination of the abdominal cavity
9. esophagoscopy (e-sof-a-GOS-ko-pē)	visual examination of the esophagus	14. proctoscope (PROK-tō-skōp)	instrument used for visual examination of the rectum
10. gastroscope (GAS-trō-skōp)	instrument used for visual examination of the stomach	15. proctoscopy (prok-TOS-ko-pē)	visual examination of the rectum
11. gastroscopy (gas-TROS-ko-pē)	visual examination of the stomach	16. sigmoidoscopy (sig-moy-DOS-ko-pē)	visual examination of the sigmoid colon (Fig. 11.14)

EXERCISE 18 ■ Pronounce and Spell

Practice pronunciation and spelling on paper and online.

1. **Practice on Paper**
   a. **Pronounce:** Read the phonetic spelling and say aloud the terms listed in the previous table. Refer to Table 2.2 Pronunciation Key as needed.
   b. **Spell:** Have a study partner read the terms aloud. Write the spelling of the terms on a separate sheet of paper.

Chapter 11 Digestive System 443

2. **Practice Online**

   a. **Access** online learning resources. Go to evolve.elsevier.com > Evolve Resources > Student Resources.
   b. **Pronounce:** Select Audio Glossary > Chapter 11 > Exercise 18. Select a term to hear its pronunciation and repeat aloud.
   c. **Spell:** Select Activities > Chapter 11 > Spell Terms > Exercise 18. Select the audio icon and type the correct spelling of the term.

   ❏ Check the box when complete.

EXERCISE 19 ■ Analyze and Define

Analyze and define the following terms.

1. proctoscope

2. proctoscopy

3. sigmoidoscopy

4. cholangiography

5. colonoscope

6. laparoscope

7. laparoscopy

8. esophagram

EXERCISE 20 ■ Build

A Fill In

Build diagnostic terms for the following definitions by using the word parts you have learned.

1. visual examination of the esophagus

   _____ / _____ / _____
        WR   CV   S

2. radiographic image of the bile ducts

   _____ / _____ / _____
        WR   CV   S

3. visual examination of the esophagus, stomach, and duodenum

   _____ / ___ / _____ / ___ / _____ / ___ / ___
    WR   CV   WR   CV   WR   CV   S

444 Chapter 11 Digestive System

B Label

Build terms pictured by writing word parts above definitions.

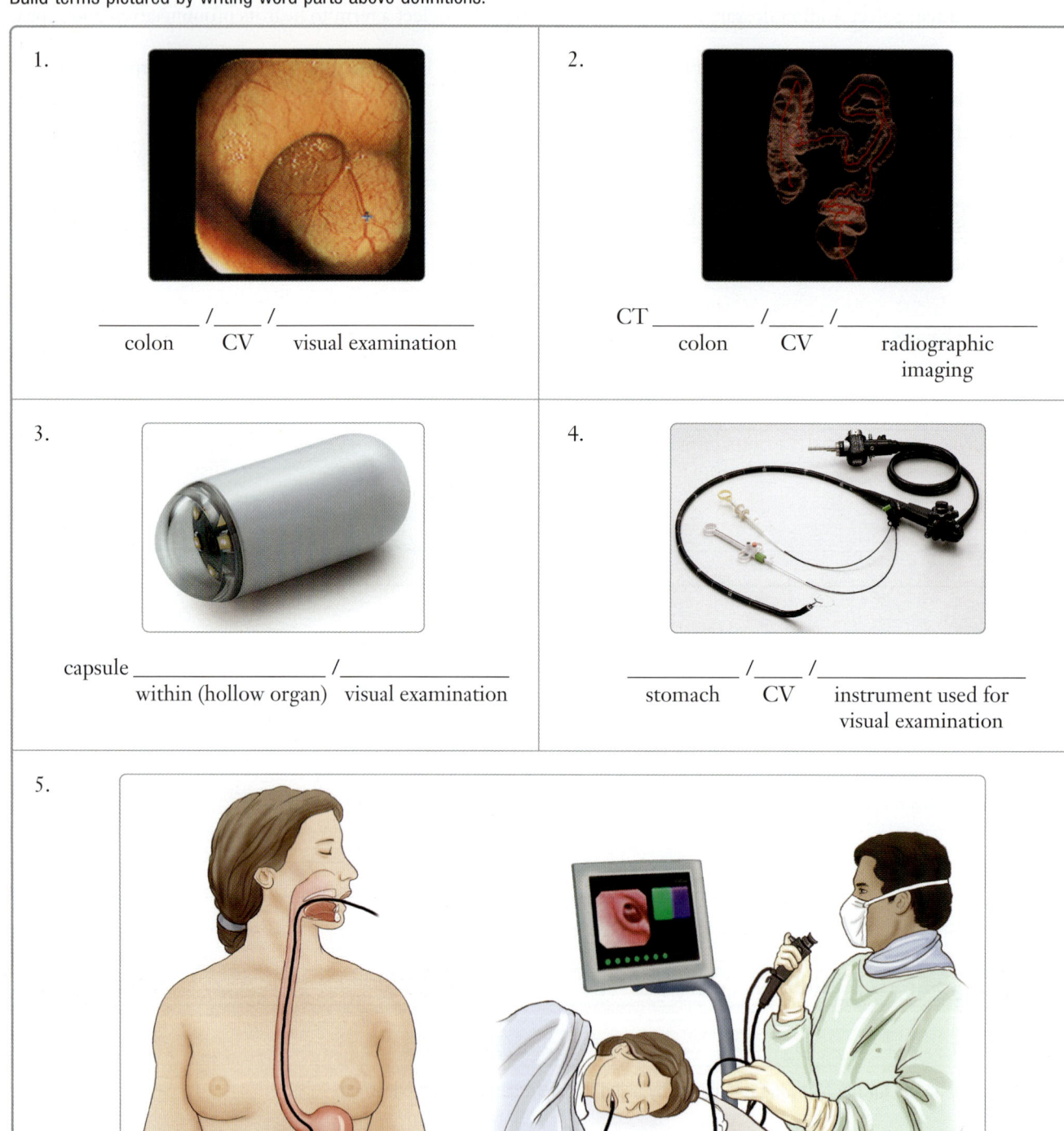

1.

_____ / ____ / _____
colon   CV   visual examination

2.

CT _____ / ____ / _____
    colon   CV   radiographic
                       imaging

3.

capsule _____ / _____
        within (hollow organ)   visual examination

4.

_____ / ____ / _____
stomach   CV   instrument used for
                   visual examination

5.

_____ / ____ / _____
stomach   CV   visual examination

Diagnostic Terms
NOT BUILT FROM WORD PARTS

Word parts may be present in the following terms; however, their full meanings cannot be translated using definitions of word parts alone.

DIAGNOSTIC IMAGING

TERM	DEFINITION
1. **abdominal sonography** (ab-DOM-i-nal) (so-NOG-ra-fē)	ultrasound scanning of the abdominal cavity in which the size and structure of organs such as the aorta, liver, gallbladder, bile ducts, and pancreas can be visualized (Table 11.1)
2. **barium enema (BE)** (BAR-ē-um) (EN-e-ma)	series of radiographic images taken of the large intestine after the contrast material barium has been administered rectally (Fig. 11.16)
3. **endoscopic retrograde cholangiopancreatography (ERCP)** (en-dō-SKOP-ic) (RET-rō-grād) (kō-lan-jē-ō-pan-krē-a-TOG-rah-fē)	procedure using an endoscope to visualize the biliary and pancreatic ducts, introduce contrast materials, and record x-ray images (fluoroscopy); used to evaluate obstructions, strictures, and some diseases of the liver and pancreas. Stone removal, biopsy, and stenting may be performed during the procedure for treatment.
4. **endoscopic ultrasound (EUS)** (en-dō-SKOP-ic) (UL-tra-sound)	procedure using an endoscope fitted with an ultrasound probe that provides images of the esophageal and gastric linings, as well as the walls of the small and large intestines; used to detect tumors and cystic growths and for staging of malignant tumors
5. **modified barium swallow (MBS)** (MOD-i-fīd) (BAR-ē-um) (SWAHL-ō)	radiographic procedure using fluoroscopy to evaluate swallowing function. Usually performed in the presence of a speech-language pathologist. May be performed in patients with difficulty swallowing or those who are at risk for aspiration pneumonia (lung infection caused by fluid or foreign material entering the respiratory tract).

TABLE 11.1 Abdominal Sonography

AREAS VISUALIZED AND POSSIBLE FINDINGS
- **Liver**—cysts, abscess, tumors, hepatitis, fatty infiltration, cirrhosis, hepatomegaly
- **Gallbladder and bile ducts**—cholelithiasis, choledocholithiasis, inflammation, obstruction, tumors (including polyps)
- **Pancreas**—inflammation, tumors, abscess, pseudocysts, obstruction
- **Kidney**—calculi, cysts, tumors, hydronephrosis, malformations, abscess, inflammation, scarring, atrophy
- **Aorta**—aneurysm, dissection, atherosclerosis

IMAGE
Abdominal ultrasound showing cholelithiasis.
GB, Gallbladder; *St*, stone

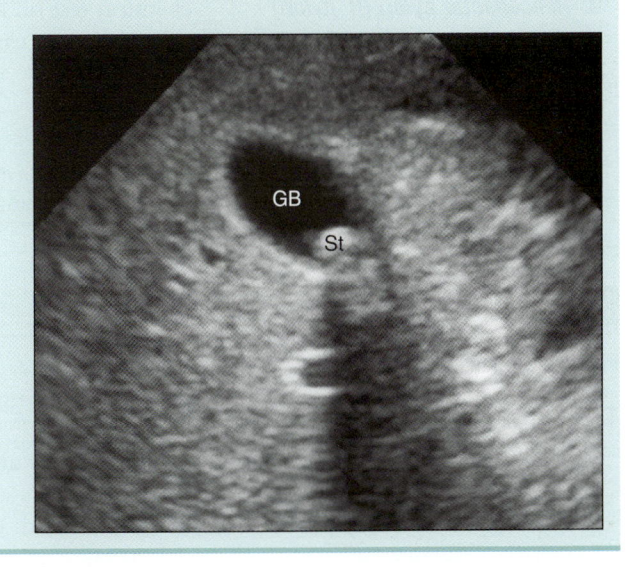

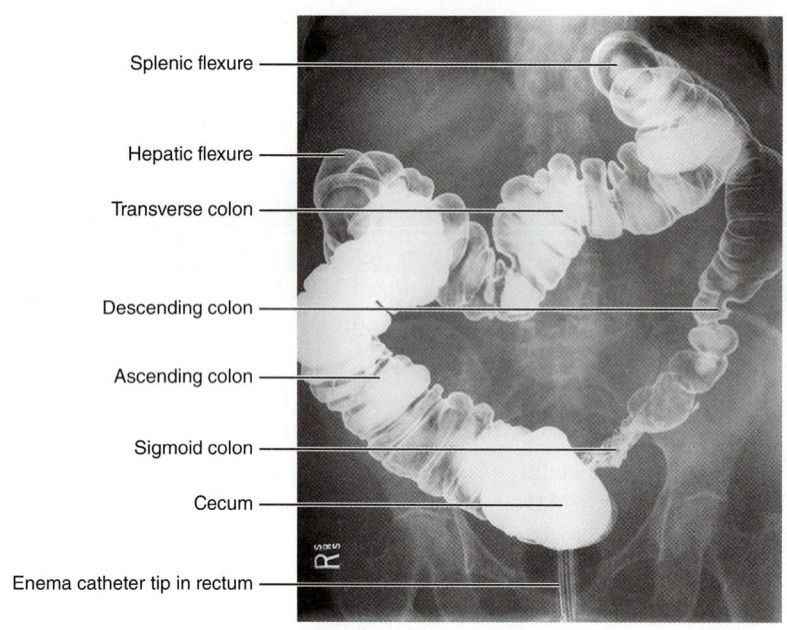

FIG. 11.16 Barium enema (BE).

Diagnostic Terms—cont'd
NOT BUILT FROM WORD PARTS

DIAGNOSTIC IMAGING—CONT'D	
TERM	**DEFINITION**
6. **upper GI series** (UP-per) (G-Ī) (SE-rēz)	series of radiographic images taken of the esophagus, stomach, and duodenum after the contrast material barium has been administered orally

LABORATORY	
TERM	**DEFINITION**
7. **fecal immunochemical test (FIT)** (FĒ-kl) (im-ū-nō-KEM-i-kl) (test)	examination of a stool sample using antibodies to detect hidden blood in the stool. Used to screen for colon cancer or polyps. (Fig. 11.17)
8. **guaiac-based fecal occult blood test (gFOBT)** (GWĪ-ak) (bāsd) (FĒ-kl) (o-KULT) (blud) (test)	examination of three stool samples using a chemical (guaiac) to detect blood not directly visible. An older test that requires dietary restrictions and medication adjustments prior to obtaining the sample.
9. *Helicobacter pylori* **(*H. pylori*) stool antigen** (*hel*-i-kō-BAK-ter) (pī-LŌ-rē) (stul) (AN-ti-jen)	chemical test on a fecal sample to determine the presence of the bacteria (*H. pylori*) that can cause peptic ulcers

HELICOBACTER PYLORI TESTING refers to various tests used to determine the presence of *Helicobacter pylori* (*H. pylori*) bacteria, which can cause peptic ulcers, increasing the risk of stomach cancer. Testing may be performed on a biopsy specimen during endoscopy (such as esophagogastroduodenoscopy), or via noninvasive testing, such as stool antigen or urea breath tests.

EXERCISE 21 ■ Pronounce and Spell

Practice pronunciation and spelling on paper and online.

1. **Practice on Paper**
   a. **Pronounce:** Read the phonetic spelling and say aloud the terms listed in the previous table. Refer to Table 2.2 Pronunciation Key as needed.
   b. **Spell:** Have a study partner read the terms aloud. Write the spelling of the terms on a separate sheet of paper.

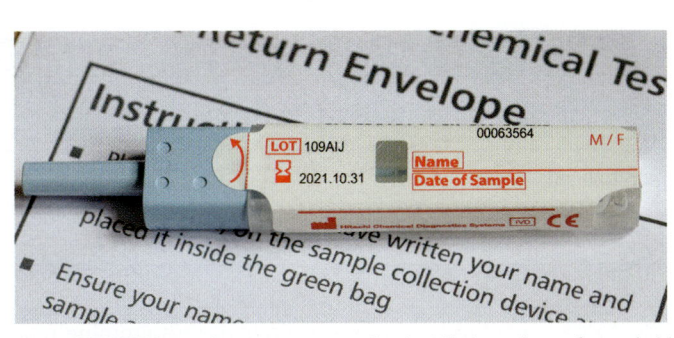

FIG. 11.17 Fecal immunochemical test (FIT). FIT is a colon cancer screening test that can be performed at home and does not require a prescription. If blood is detected in the stool a colonoscopy will be needed.

2. **Practice Online**
   a. **Access** online learning resources. Go to evolve.elsevier.com > Evolve Resources > Student Resources.
   b. **Pronounce:** Select Audio Glossary > Chapter 11 > Exercise 21. Select a term to hear its pronunciation and repeat aloud.
   c. **Spell:** Select Activities > Chapter 11 > Spell Terms > Exercise 21. Select the audio icon and type the correct spelling of the term.

❑ Check the box when complete.

EXERCISE 22 ■ Match

Match the diagnostic terms in the first column with their correct definitions in the second column.

_____ 1. guaiac-based fecal occult blood test
_____ 2. barium enema
_____ 3. *Helicobacter pylori* stool antigen
_____ 4. upper GI series
_____ 5. endoscopic retrograde cholangiopancreatography
_____ 6. abdominal sonography
_____ 7. endoscopic ultrasound
_____ 8. fecal immunochemical test
_____ 9. modified barium swallow

a. antibody test to detect hidden blood in a stool sample
b. radiographic images of the esophagus, stomach, and duodenum
c. provides images of esophageal and gastric linings, and also walls of the intestines
d. chemically detects blood in a series of three stool samples
e. radiographic imaging of biliary and pancreatic ducts
f. radiographic images of the large intestine
g. ultrasound to visualize a portion of the aorta, liver, gallbladder, bile ducts, and pancreas
h. procedure using fluoroscopy to evaluate swallowing function
i. used to identify bacteria that can cause peptic ulcers

448 Chapter 11 Digestive System

EXERCISE 23 ■ Fill In

A Label

Write the diagnostic terms pictured and defined.

1. _____

procedure using an endoscope to visualize the biliary and pancreatic ducts, introduce contrast materials, and record x-ray images

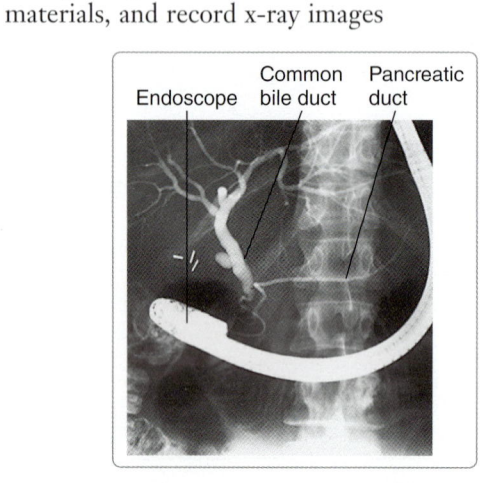

2. _____

series of radiographic images taken of the large intestine afer the contrast material barium has been administered rectally

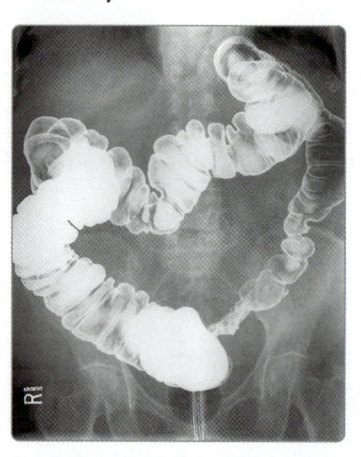

B Identify

Write the term for each of the following definitions.

1. chemical test on a fecal sample to determine the presence of the bacteria that can be found in the lining of the stomach and can cause peptic ulcers _____
2. antibody test of a stool sample to detect blood not directly visible _____
3. ultrasound scanning of the abdominal cavity to visualize the organs within _____
4. procedure using an endoscope fitted with an ultrasound probe that provides images of the esophageal and gastric linings, as well as the walls of the small and large intestines _____
5. series of radiographic images taken of the esophagus, stomach, and duodenum after the contrast material barium has been administered orally _____
6. radiographic procedure performed in patients with difficulty swallowing, or those who are at risk for aspiration pneumonia _____
7. older test using three stool samples and a chemical to detect blood that is not visible _____

EXERCISE 24 ■ Review of Diagnostic Terms

Can you define, pronounce, and spell the following terms?

abdominal sonography
abdominocentesis
barium enema (BE)
capsule endoscopy
cholangiography

colonoscope
colonoscopy
CT colonography

endoscopic retrograde cholangiopancreatography (ERCP)
endoscopic ultrasound (EUS)

esophagogastroduodenoscopy (EGD)
esophagram
esophagoscopy

Chapter 11   Digestive System   449

fecal immunochemical test (FIT)
gastroscope
gastroscopy
guaiac-based fecal occult blood test (gFOBT)
Helicobacter pylori stool antigen
laparoscope
laparoscopy
modified barium swallow (MBS)
proctoscope
proctoscopy
sigmoidoscopy
upper GI series

Complementary Terms
BUILT FROM WORD PARTS

The following terms can be translated using definitions of word parts. Further explanation is provided within parentheses as needed.

SIGNS AND SYMPTOMS

TERM	DEFINITION	TERM	DEFINITION
1. **aphagia** (a-FĀ-ja)	condition of without swallowing (the inability to)	5. **steatorrhea** (stē-a-tō-RĒ-a)	discharge of fat (excessive amount of fat in the stool, causing frothy, foul-smelling fecal matter usually associated with the malabsorption of fat in conditions such as chronic pancreatitis and celiac disease)
2. **dyspepsia** (dis-PEP-sē-a)	difficult digestion (often used to describe GI symptoms, such as abdominal pain and bloating)		
3. **dysphagia** (dis-FĀ-ja)	condition of difficult swallowing		
4. **hepatomegaly** (hep-a-tō-MEG-a-lē)	enlargement of the liver	6. **steatosis** (stē-a-TŌ-sis)	abnormal condition of fat (increased fat at the cellular level often affecting the liver); (lab finding)

MEDICAL SPECIALTIES

TERM	DEFINITION	TERM	DEFINITION
7. **gastroenterologist** (gas-trō-en-ter-OL-o-jist)	physician who studies and treats diseases of the stomach and intestines (GI tract and accessory organs)	8. **gastroenterology** (gas-trō-en-ter-OL-o-jē)	study of the stomach and intestines (branch of medicine that deals with treating diseases of the GI tract and accessory organs)

DESCRIPTIVE TERMS

TERM	DEFINITION	TERM	DEFINITION
9. **anal** (Ā-nal)	pertaining to the anus	15. **nasogastric** (nā-zō-GAS-trik)	pertaining to the nose and stomach
10. **celiac** (SĒ-lē-ak)	pertaining to the abdomen	16. **oral** (OR-al)	pertaining to the mouth
11. **colorectal** (kō-lō-REK-tal)	pertaining to the colon and rectum	17. **palatal** (PAL-a-tal)	pertaining to the palate
12. **duodenal** (dū-OD-e-nal)	pertaining to the duodenum	18. **pancreatic** (pan-krē-AT-ik)	pertaining to the pancreas
13. **esophageal** (e-sof-a-JĒ-al)	pertaining to the esophagus	19. **peritoneal** (per-i-tō-NĒ-al)	pertaining to the peritoneum
14. **ileocecal** (il-ē-ō-SĒ-kal)	pertaining to the ileum and cecum	20. **rectal** (REK-tal)	pertaining to the rectum
		21. **sublingual** (sub-LING-gwal)	pertaining to under the tongue

450 Chapter 11 Digestive System

EXERCISE 25 ■ Pronounce and Spell

Practice pronunciation and spelling on paper and online.

1. **Practice on Paper**
   a. **Pronounce:** Read the phonetic spelling and say aloud the terms listed in the previous table. Refer to Table 2.2 Pronunciation Key as needed.
   b. **Spell:** Have a study partner read the terms aloud. Write the spelling of the terms on a separate sheet of paper.

2. **Practice Online**
   a. **Access** online learning resources. Go to evolve.elsevier.com > Evolve Resources > Student Resources.
   b. **Pronounce:** Select Audio Glossary > Chapter 11 > Exercise 25. Select a term to hear its pronunciation and repeat aloud.
   c. **Spell:** Select Activities > Chapter 11 > Spell Terms > Exercise 25. Select the audio icon and type the correct spelling of the term.

❏ Check the box when complete.

EXERCISE 26 ■ Analyze and Define

Analyze and define the following complementary terms.

1. rectal

2. dyspepsia

3. palatal

4. esophageal

5. steatorrhea

6. duodenal

7. oral

8. gastroenterologist

9. steatosis

10. pancreatic

Chapter 11 Digestive System   451

EXERCISE 27 ■ Build

Build complementary terms for the following definitions by using the word parts you have learned.

1. enlargement of the liver
   _____ / _____ / _____
        WR   CV   S

2. condition of without swallowing (the inability to)
   _____ / _____ / _____
      P   WR   S

3. pertaining to under the tongue
   _____ / _____ / _____
      P   WR   S

4. pertaining to the nose and the stomach
   _____ / _____ / _____ / _____
      WR   CV   WR   S

5. pertaining to the mouth and the stomach
   _____ / _____ / _____ / _____
      WR   CV   WR   S

6. pertaining to the anus
   _____ / _____
          WR   S

7. pertaining to the peritoneum
   _____ / _____
          WR   S

8. pertaining to the abdomen
   _____ / _____
          WR   S

9. condition of difficult swallowing
   _____ / _____ / _____
      P   WR   S

10. pertaining to the ileum and cecum
    _____ / _____ / _____ / _____
       WR   CV   WR   S

11. pertaining to the colon and rectum
    _____ / _____ / _____ / _____
       WR   CV   WR   S

Complementary Terms
NOT BUILT FROM WORD PARTS

Word parts may be present in the following terms; however, their full meanings cannot be translated using definitions of word parts alone.

SIGNS AND SYMPTOMS	
TERM	**DEFINITION**
1. **ascites** (a-SĪ-tēz)	abnormal collection of fluid in the peritoneal cavity
2. **diarrhea** (dī-a-RĒ-a)	frequent discharge of liquid stool
DIARRHEA contains the prefix **dia-**, meaning **through**, and the suffix **-rrhea**, meaning **flow**.	
3. **emesis** (EM-e-sis)	expelling matter from the stomach through the mouth (also called **vomiting**)
4. **flatus** (FLĀ-tus)	gas in the gastrointestinal tract or expelled through the anus

Complementary Terms—cont'd
NOT BUILT FROM WORD PARTS

SIGNS AND SYMPTOMS	
TERM	**DEFINITION**
5. **hematemesis** (hē-ma-TEM-e-sis)	vomiting of blood
6. **hematochezia** (hē-ma-tō-KĒ-zha)	passage of visibly bloody feces
7. **malabsorption** (mal-ab-SORP-shun)	impaired digestion or intestinal absorption of nutrients
8. **melena** (me-LĒ-na)	black, tarry stool that contains digested blood; usually a result of bleeding in the upper GI tract
9. **nausea** (NAW-zē-a)	urge to vomit
10. **reflux** (RĒ-fluks)	abnormal backward flow. In esophageal reflux, the stomach contents flow back into the esophagus.

OTHER TERMS	
TERM	**DEFINITION**
11. **feces** (FĒ-sēz)	waste from the gastrointestinal tract expelled through the anus (also called **stool** or **fecal matter**)
12. **palpate** (PAL-pāt)	to examine by hand; to feel
13. **stoma** (STŌ-ma)	surgical opening between an organ and the surface of the body, such as the opening established in the abdominal wall by colostomy, ileostomy, or a similar operation. Stoma may also refer to an opening created between body structures or between portions of the intestines.

Refer to **Appendix E** for pharmacology terms related to the digestive system.

EXERCISE 28 ■ Pronounce and Spell

Practice pronunciation and spelling on paper and online.

1. **Practice on Paper**
   a. **Pronounce:** Read the phonetic spelling and say aloud the terms listed in the previous table. Refer to Table 2.2 Pronunciation Key as needed.
   b. **Spell:** Have a study partner read the terms aloud. Write the spelling of the terms on a separate sheet of paper.

2. **Practice Online**
   a. **Access** online learning resources. Go to evolve.elsevier.com > Evolve Resources > Student Resources.
   b. **Pronounce:** Select Audio Glossary > Chapter 11 > Exercise 28. Select a term to hear its pronunciation and repeat aloud.
   c. **Spell:** Select Activities > Chapter 11 > Spell Terms > Exercise 28. Select the audio icon and type the correct spelling of the term.

❏ Check the box when complete.

EXERCISE 29 ■ Match

Match the definitions in the first column with their correct terms in the second column.

_____ 1. abnormal collection of fluid in the peritoneal cavity
_____ 2. expelling matter from the stomach
_____ 3. to examine by hand
_____ 4. surgical opening between an organ and the surface of the body
_____ 5. urge to vomit
_____ 6. frequent discharge of liquid stool
_____ 7. waste expelled through the anus
_____ 8. vomiting of blood
_____ 9. abnormal backward flow
_____ 10. impaired digestion or intestinal absorption
_____ 11. gas expelled through the anus
_____ 12. passage of visibly bloody feces
_____ 13. black, tarry stools

a. hematemesis
b. flatus
c. hematochezia
d. reflux
e. emesis
f. stoma
g. melena
h. palpate
i. diarrhea
j. malabsorption
k. feces
l. nausea
m. ascites

EXERCISE 30 ■ Fill In

A Label

Write the medical terms pictured and defined.

1. _____
surgical opening between an organ and the surface of the body

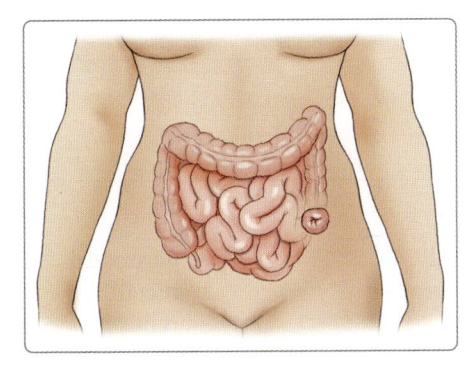

2. _____
to examine by hand; to feel

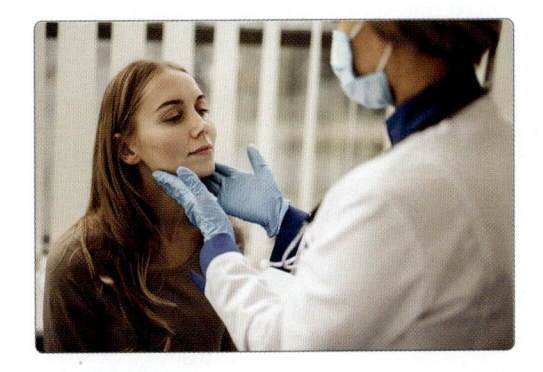

454　Chapter 11　Digestive System

3. _____
abnormal backward flow

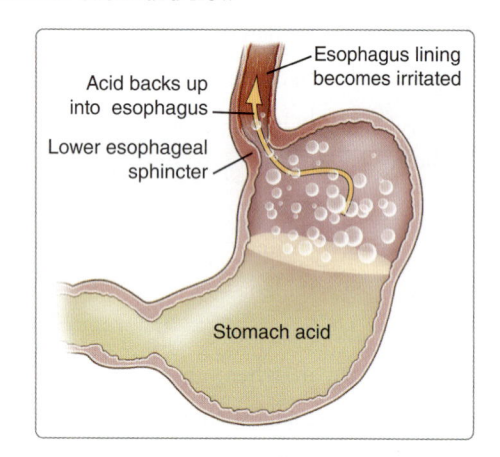

4. _____
abnormal collection of fluid in the peritoneal cavity

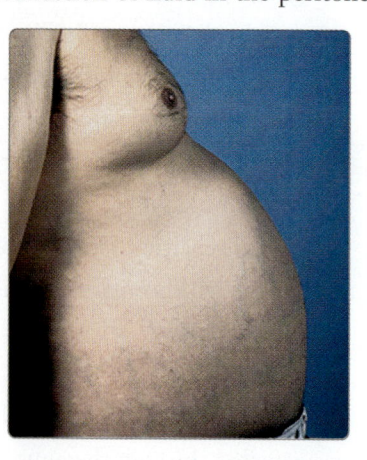

B Identify

Write the term for each of the following definitions.

1. also called stool _____
2. frequent discharge of liquid stool _____
3. gas in the gastrointestinal tract or expelled through the anus _____
4. also called vomiting _____
5. passage of visibly bloody feces _____
6. black, tarry stool that contains digested blood _____
7. urge to vomit _____
8. impaired digestion or intestinal absorption of nutrients _____
9. vomiting of blood _____

EXERCISE 31 ■ Review of Complementary Terms

Can you define, pronounce, and spell the following terms?

anal	emesis	ileocecal	peritoneal
aphagia	esophageal	malabsorption	rectal
ascites	feces	melena	reflux
celiac	flatus	nasogastric	steatorrhea
colorectal	gastroenterologist	nausea	steatosis
diarrhea	gastroenterology	oral	stoma
duodenal	hematemesis	palatal	sublingual
dyspepsia	hematochezia	palpate	
dysphagia	hepatomegaly	pancreatic	

Abbreviations

DISEASE AND DISORDER

ABBREVIATION	TERM	ABBREVIATION	TERM
IBS	irritable bowel syndrome	NASH	nonalcoholic steatohepatitis; spoken as a whole word (nash)
GERD	gastroesophageal reflux disease; spoken as a whole word (gurd)	UC	ulcerative colitis
NAFLD	nonalcoholic fatty liver disease; spoken as a whole word (NA-fuld)		

DIAGNOSTIC

ABBREVIATION	TERM	ABBREVIATION	TERM
BE	barium enema	FIT	fecal immunochemical test; spoken as a whole word (fit)
EGD	esophagogastroduodenoscopy	gFOBT	guaiac-based fecal occult blood test
ERCP	endoscopic retrograde cholangiopancreatography	MBS	modified barium swallow
EUS	endoscopic ultrasound		

TREATMENT

ABBREVIATION	TERM	ABBREVIATION	TERM
APR	abdominoperineal resection	UPPP	uvulopalatopharyngoplasty
PEG	percutaneous endoscopic gastrostomy; spoken as a whole word (peg)		

DESCRIPTIVE

ABBREVIATION	TERM	ABBREVIATION	TERM
GI	gastrointestinal	UGI	upper gastrointestinal

OTHER

ABBREVIATION	TERM	ABBREVIATION	TERM
H. pylori	*Helicobacter pylori* (bacteria that can cause peptic ulcers)	N&V	nausea and vomiting

Refer to **Appendix D** for a complete list of abbreviations.

EXERCISE 32 ■ Abbreviations

Write the terms abbreviated.

1. **MBS** _____ is a diagnostic imaging test that focuses on the pharynx and upper esophagus to evaluate swallowing function. An esophagram evaluates the pharynx and the entire esophagus, while a **UGI** _____ series visualizes the esophagus, stomach, and the beginning of the small intestine.

2. Laboratory tests that can be performed on stool samples include **H. pylori** _____ stool antigen, which detects the presence of a bacteria associated with **GERD** _____; **FIT** _____, which uses antibodies to detect blood in the stool and can screen for colon cancer and polyps; and **gFOBT** _____, an older test that requires dietary and medication restrictions prior to obtaining the sample.

3. **EGD** _____ may be performed by a gastroenterologist to diagnose numerous conditions; it can also be used for placement of a **PEG** _____ tube.

4. **ERCP** _____ and **EUS** _____ are procedures that can evaluate the biliary system and pancreas.

5. **BE** _____ is a diagnostic imaging test that can be used to diagnose **UC** _____ and Crohn disease. It may also be used in patients with **IBS** _____ to help rule out other causes of **GI** _____ symptoms.

6. **N&V** _____, ascites, and jaundice may be symptoms and signs of **NASH** _____, which may progress from **NAFLD** _____.

7. **APR** _____ is most commonly performed by general surgeons in patients with rectal cancer, while **UPPP** _____ is often performed by ENT surgeons for the treatment of obstructive sleep apnea.

Chapter 11 Digestive System 457

PRACTICAL APPLICATION

EXERCISE 33 ■ Case Study: Translate Between Everyday Language and Medical Language

CASE STUDY: Ruth Clifton

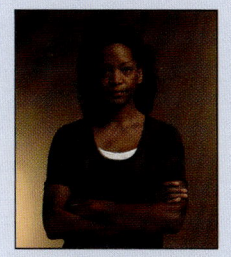

Ruth is worried about her stomach. She has been having pain on and off for about 3 months. At first it was just once in a while, but now it seems to be every day. Her pain seems to be worse when she hasn't eaten for a while, and after she eats something bland, it usually gets a bit better. She bought some antacids at the pharmacy, and chewing those also seems to help. Lately the pain in her stomach has been waking her up at night. A glass of milk usually helps with that. The last few days, however, she has felt sick to her stomach, has been throwing up, and is finding it difficult to eat. Her friend recommends that she see a stomach doctor, who helped her when she had similar problems.

Now that you have worked through Chapter 11 on the digestive system, consider the medical terms that might be used to describe Ruth Clifton's experience. See the Chapter at a Glance section at the end of this chapter for a list of terms that might apply.

A. Underline phrases in the case study that could be substituted with medical terms.

B. Write the medical term and its definition for three of the phrases you underlined.

MEDICAL TERM	DEFINITION
1. _____	_____
2. _____	_____
3. _____	_____

DOCUMENTATION: Excerpt from Endoscopic Procedure Report

Ms. Clifton made an appointment with a gastroenterologist. He recommended an endoscopic procedure; a portion of the report is documented below.

ENDOSCOPY REPORT: Procedure: Esophagogastroduodenoscopy

The patient was given 2 mg of intravenous midazolam along with lidocaine spray to the pharynx. After she was placed in the left lateral decubitus position, the gastroscope was passed into the pharynx without difficulty. No abnormalities were noted in the esophagus or in the cardia and the body of the stomach. A biopsy of the gastric mucosa was obtained for *Helicobacter pylori* testing. In the distal antrum, some mild erythematous changes were noted. The pylorus appeared normal, but a single 1-cm ulceration of the proximal duodenum, a peptic ulcer, was observed.

C. Underline medical terms presented in Chapter 11 in the previous excerpt from Ms. Clifton's medical record. See the Chapter at a Glance section at the end of the chapter for a complete list.

D. Select and define three of the medical terms you underlined. To check your answers, go to Appendix A.

MEDICAL TERM	DEFINITION
1. _____	_____
2. _____	_____
3. _____	_____

458 Chapter 11 Digestive System

EXERCISE 34 ■ Interact with Medical Documents

A

Read the report and complete it by writing medical terms on answer lines within the document. Definitions of terms to be written appear after the document.

01182003 JOHNSON, Sylvia

Name: Sylvia Johnson   MR#: 01182003   Sex: F   Allergies: None known
DOB: 11/03/19xx   Age: 63   PCP: Chambers, Jacqueline DO

Gastroenterology Consultation Note

Sylvia Johnson is a 63-year-old female who was referred by her PCP for evaluation of 1. _____.
She reports this has been occurring for the last 3 weeks. She also reports a change in bowel habits with alternating constipation and 2. _____ over the last 3 months. She denies 3. _____ or 4. _____. She has a history of 5. _____ and was tested for 6. _____ approximately 8 years ago. She denies any history of 7. _____, 8. _____, or 9. _____. Her family history is significant for 10. _____ cancer in her father, who died at age 70, and 11. _____ in her mother, who died of other causes at age 88.

On exam, she is a thin African American female, pleasant and in no acute distress. Vital signs are normal. Abdominal exam reveals normal bowel sounds, nontender to palpation with no 12. _____ or 13. _____.
Rectal exam reveals normal tone, external 14. _____, and no stool.

Impression and Plan: Hematochezia in a 63-year-old female with several risk factors for colon cancer. We will schedule her for a 15. _____ as soon as possible.

Abdul Ismail, MD
Gastroenterologist

Definitions of Medical Terms to Complete the Document

Write the medical terms defined on corresponding answer lines in the document.

1. discharge of visibly bloody feces
2. frequent discharge of liquid stool
3. urge to vomit
4. expelling matter from the stomach through the mouth
5. abnormal backward flow of the gastrointestinal contents into the esophagus
6. test on a fecal sample to determine the presence of a bacteria found in the lining of the stomach that can cause peptic ulcers
7. erosion of the mucous membrane of the stomach or duodenum
8. chronic inflammation of the gastrointestinal tract characterized by cobblestone ulcerations and the formation of scar tissue that may lead to intestinal obstruction
9. disease characterized by inflammation of the colon with the formation of ulcers, which can cause bloody diarrhea
10. pertaining to the colon and rectum
11. inflammation of the esophagus
12. abnormal collection of fluid in the peritoneal cavity
13. enlargement of the liver
14. swollen or distended veins in the rectum or anus
15. visual examination of the colon

B

Read the medical report and answer the questions below it.

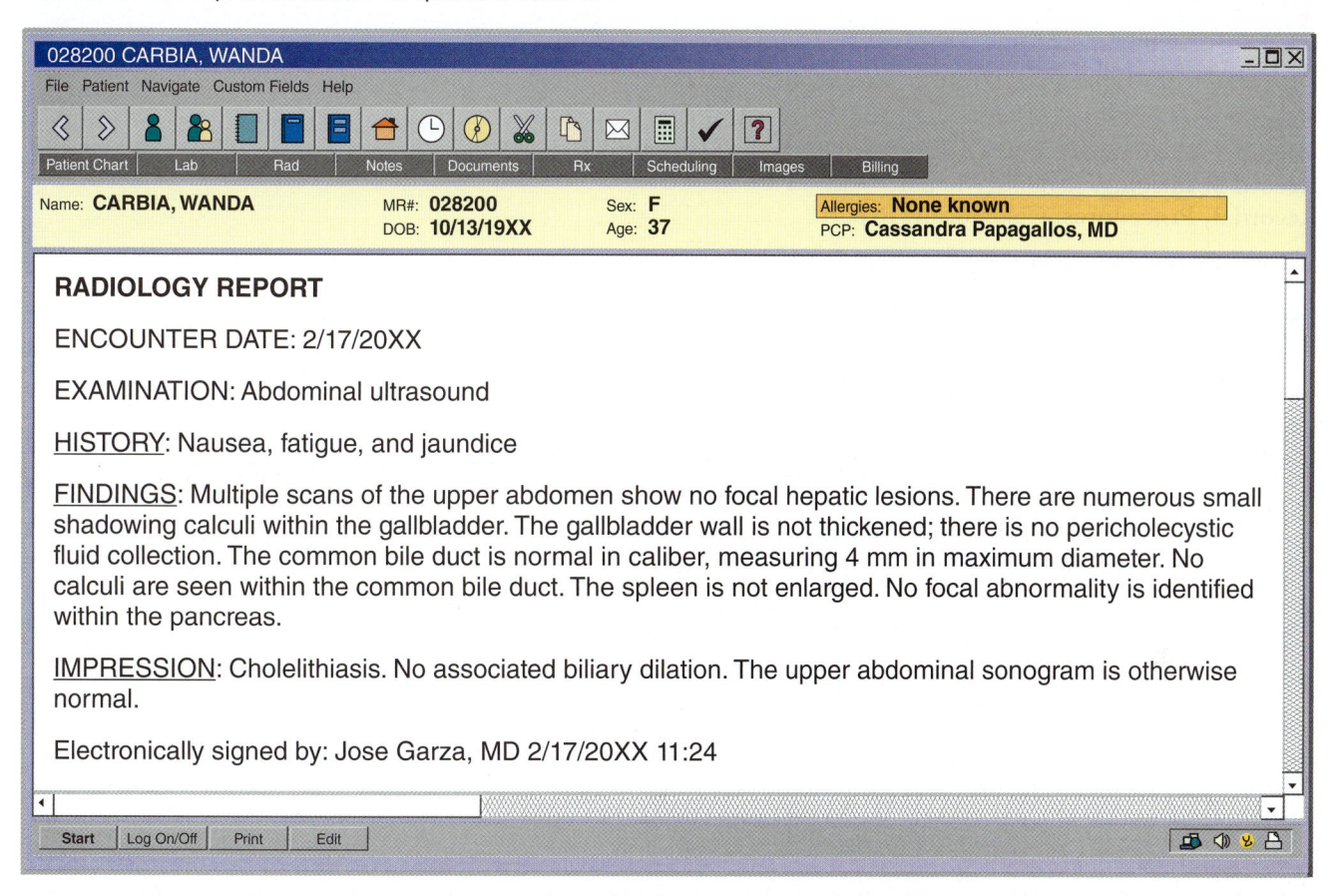

028200 CARBIA, WANDA

File Patient Navigate Custom Fields Help

| Patient Chart | Lab | Rad | Notes | Documents | Rx | Scheduling | Images | Billing |

Name: **CARBIA, WANDA** MR#: **028200** Sex: **F** Allergies: **None known**
DOB: **10/13/19XX** Age: **37** PCP: **Cassandra Papagallos, MD**

RADIOLOGY REPORT

ENCOUNTER DATE: 2/17/20XX

EXAMINATION: Abdominal ultrasound

HISTORY: Nausea, fatigue, and jaundice

FINDINGS: Multiple scans of the upper abdomen show no focal hepatic lesions. There are numerous small shadowing calculi within the gallbladder. The gallbladder wall is not thickened; there is no pericholecystic fluid collection. The common bile duct is normal in caliber, measuring 4 mm in maximum diameter. No calculi are seen within the common bile duct. The spleen is not enlarged. No focal abnormality is identified within the pancreas.

IMPRESSION: Cholelithiasis. No associated biliary dilation. The upper abdominal sonogram is otherwise normal.

Electronically signed by: Jose Garza, MD 2/17/20XX 11:24

Use the medical report above to answer the questions.

1. The exam included which diagnostic procedure:
   a. radiographic imaging of the colon with computerized tomography
   b. radiographic imaging of the bile ducts after administration of contrast materials
   c. use of an endoscope fitted with an ultrasound probe to obtain images of layers of the intestinal wall
   d. recording images of organs with sound waves produced by a transducer placed directly on the skin

2. The patient's symptoms included:
   a. expelling matter from the stomach through the mouth
   b. urge to vomit
   c. passage of visibly bloody feces
   d. vomiting of blood

3. The examination revealed the presence of:
   a. stones within the gallbladder
   b. stones within the common bile duct
   c. lesions in the liver
   d. inflammation of the pancreas

4. "Biliary dilation" would most likely refer to:
   a. inflammation of the pancreas
   b. the presence of fluid in the upper abdomen
   c. choledocholithiasis
   d. widening of the bile ducts or gallbladder

460 Chapter 11 Digestive System

EXERCISE 35 ■ Use Medical Language in Online Electronic Health Records

Select the correct medical terms to complete three medical records in one patient's electronic file.

🌐 Access online resources at evolve.elsevier.com > Evolve Resources > Student Resources > Activities > Chapter 11 > Electronic Health Records

Topic: Bowel Obstruction
Record 1, Encounters: Office Visit
Record 2, Imaging: Radiology Report
Record 3, Procedures: Colonoscopy Report

❏ Check the box when complete.

EXERCISE 36 ■ Use Medical Terms in Clinical Statements

For each phrase printed in bold, circle the medical term or abbreviation defined. Answers are listed in Appendix A. For pronunciation practice, read the answers aloud.

1. A **visual examination of the esophagus, stomach, and duodenum** (endoscopic retrograde cholangiopancreatography, esophagogastroduodenoscopy, abdominal ultrasonography) is performed by a **physician who studies and treats diseases of the stomach and intestines** (gastroenterologist, hepatologist, urologist) to diagnose **erosion of the mucous membrane of the stomach or duodenum** (ulcerative colitis, dysentery, peptic ulcer).

2. Dentists and dental hygienists treat disorders related to the **pertaining to the mouth** (oral, rectal, anal) cavity. They check for **inflammation of the gums** (gingivitis, glossitis, stomatitis) and **inflammation of the tongue** (gingivitis, glossitis, gastroenteritis), and examine the **pertaining to under the tongue** (subcostal, sublingual, subcutaneous) surface, looking for oral cancer or other abnormalities.

3. Three surgical procedures that may be performed on a patient with peptic ulcers are (1) partial **excision of the stomach** (gastrotomy, gastrostomy, gastrectomy), (2) **surgical repair of the pylorus** (pyloroplasty, enterorrhaphy, gastrojejunostomy, and (3) **cutting of certain branches of the vagus nerve** (colostomy, vagotomy, gingivectomy).

4. **Enlarged liver** (hepatitis, hepatomegaly, hepatoma) may be associated with **inflammation of the liver** (hepatitis, hepatomegaly, hepatoma), **tumor of the liver** (hepatitis, hepatomegaly, hepatoma), **chronic disease of the liver with gradual destruction of cells and formation of scar tissue** (celiac disease, cirrhosis, Crohn disease), fatty liver, or even normal pregnancy.

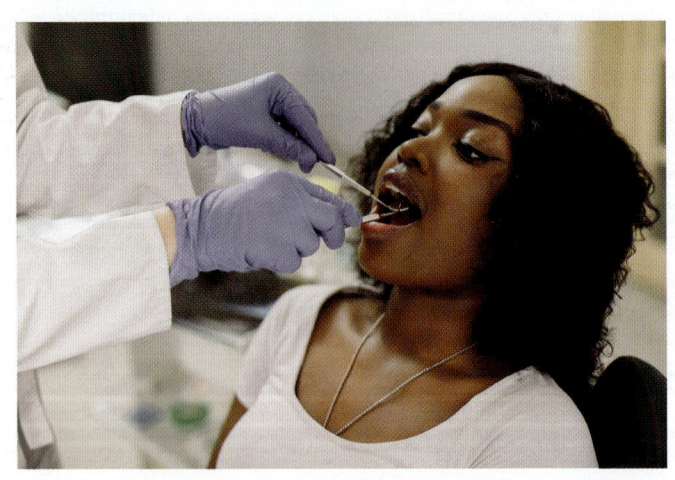

FIG. 11.18 Oral cancer screening is commonly performed by dentists as a part of routine exams.

EXERCISE 37 ■ Pronounce Medical Terms in Use

Practice pronunciation of terms by reading aloud the following paragraphs. Use the phonetic spellings following medical terms from the chapter to assist with pronunciation. The script also contains medical terms not presented in the chapter. If interested, research their meanings in a medical dictionary or a reliable online source.

COLORECTAL CANCER

Colorectal (kō-lō-REK-tal) cancer begins in the colon or rectum and is the second leading cause of cancer deaths in the United States. Most are adenocarcinomas that originate as a benign, adenomatous **polyp** (POL-ip).

Many people have no symptoms until the cancer is quite advanced, and symptoms may vary based on the location of the tumor. Typical symptoms and signs associated with colorectal cancer include **hematochezia** (hē-ma-tō-KĒ-zha) or **melena** (me-LĒ-na), abdominal pain, anemia, and/or a change in bowel habits.

Screening tests for colorectal cancer include stool-based tests such as the **fecal immunochemical test** (FĒ-kl) (im-ū-nō-KEM-i-kul) (test), multitarget stool DNA testing, and the **guaiac-based fecal occult blood test** (GWĪ-ak) (bāsd) (FĒ-kl) (o-KULT) (blud) (test). A patient with an abnormal stool test must have a follow-up colonoscopy (kō-lon-OS-ko-pē).

Colonoscopy is the most commonly used colorectal cancer screening test in the United States. It can also be used for biopsy and **polypectomy** (pol-i-PEK-to-mē). Disadvantages include the need for thorough bowel preparation and the use of conscious sedation. **Sigmoidoscopy** (sig-moy-DOS-ko-pē) can be performed without sedation, but it only visualizes the distal portion of the colon and must be done more frequently. **CT colonography** (C-T) (kō-lon-OG-ra-fē) might be suitable for older patients with multiple diseases that put them at higher risk for complications from colonoscopy; however, an abnormal result still requires endoscopic follow-up. **Barium enema** (BAR-ē-um) (EN-e-ma) is no longer routinely used for colorectal cancer screening.

Treatment for colorectal cancer depends on the location of the tumor and stage of the disease. **Colectomy** (kō-LEK-to-mē) with **anastomosis** (a-nas-to-MŌ-sis) may be used in patients with localized (limited to the colon) disease. In patients with complicated disease, a **colostomy** (ko-LOS-to-mē) may be necessary. Chemotherapy, immunotherapy, and/or radiotherapy may be used in these patients.

CHAPTER REVIEW

EXERCISE 38 ■ Chapter Content Quiz

Test your understanding of terms and abbreviations introduced in this chapter. Circle the letter for the medical term or abbreviation related to the words in italics.

1. Mr. Gomez complained of right upper quadrant pain after eating fatty foods, and was tentatively diagnosed with *inflammation of the gallbladder*.
   a. cholelithiasis
   b. cholecystitis
   c. choledocholithiasis

2. An abdominal ultrasound confirmed the diagnosis, and Mr. Gomez is now scheduled for a laparoscopic *excision of the gallbladder*.
   a. cholecystostomy
   b. cholecystectomy
   c. colectomy

3. After prior surgeries to remove portions of his intestines due to Crohn disease, Mr. Kipling was able to have *connections created by surgically joining two structures* when his disease went into remission. (Hint: plural form)
   a. anastomoses
   b. anastomosis
   c. anastomosices

4. Mrs. Marshall was having symptoms of bloody diarrhea, abdominal pain and cramping, and fatigue. She was eventually diagnosed with *disease characterized by inflammation of the colon with the formation of ulcers, which can cause bloody diarrhea*.
   a. UC
   b. UPPP
   c. UGI

5. As an infant, Cameron Liu had an episode of *prolapse of one part of the intestine inside the part next to it*, which was diagnosed and treated by a barium enema.
   a. irritable bowel syndrome
   b. ileum
   c. intussusception

6. Because of her frequent heartburn, Mrs. Patel had a(n) *series of radiographic images taken of the esophagus, stomach, and duodenum after the contrast material barium has been administered orally*.
   a. upper GI series
   b. endoscopic ultrasound
   c. barium enema

7. After years of taking medication for peptic ulcers with no relief, it was recommended that Mr. Ezaki have *cutting of certain branches of the vagus nerve* to help treat his symptoms.
   a. gastrectomy
   b. pyloroplasty
   c. vagotomy

8. Mrs. Schwartz found that she *experienced difficult digestion, such as abdominal pain and bloating*, shortly after taking her osteoporosis medication.
   a. dyspepsia
   b. diarrhea
   c. dysphagia

9. During the colonoscopy, Dr. Mostafa found it difficult to visualize the colon all the way to the *pertaining to the ileum and cecum* valve.
   a. esophageal
   b. ileocecal
   c. peritoneal

10. After multiple surgeries for various gynecologic and gastrointestinal problems, Ms. Harding developed *abnormal growing together of two peritoneal surfaces that normally are separated*.
    a. hemorrhoids
    b. celiac disease
    c. adhesions

11. Mrs. Palmeri complained of *discharge of fat (excessive amount of fat in the stool)*; lab tests and abdominal sonography suggested the diagnosis of *buildup of extra fat in the liver cells that is not due to alcohol consumption (abbreviation)*.
    a. steatosis, NASH
    b. hepatomegaly, GERD
    c. steatorrhea, NAFLD

12. A percutaneous endoscopic *creation of an artificial opening into the stomach (PEG)* tube was used for Mrs. McKee after her stroke.
    a. gastrostomy
    b. gastrectomy
    c. gastrotomy

13. John Begay saw his doctor because of right upper quadrant pain after eating fatty foods. An abdominal ultrasound revealed a stone in the common bile duct. A(n) *procedure using an endoscope to visualize the biliary and pancreatic ducts, introduce contrast materials, and record x-ray images* was performed and the stone was removed.
    a. ERCP
    b. EUS
    c. EGD

14. Mrs. Martinez, who had obesity, was diagnosed with diabetes and hypertension. Her physician referred her for *a surgical reduction of gastric capacity to treat obesity*, a condition which can cause serious illness.
    a. abdominocentesis
    b. bariatric surgery
    c. abdominoperineal resection

15. After his last episode of diverticulitis, Mr. Small developed *inflammation of the peritoneum*.
    a. cholecystitis
    b. pancreatitis
    c. peritonitis

16. As a result of her Parkinson disease, Mrs. Borders developed *difficult swallowing*.
    a. dysphagia
    b. aphagia
    c. dysentery

17. Laura Schmidt complained of *discharge of fat (excessive amount of fat in the stool, causing frothy, foul-smelling fecal matter)* which later led to her diagnosis of celiac disease.
    a. steatohepatitis
    b. steatosis
    c. steatorrhea

18. Many years ago, Jaime Garza had *excision of the uvula* for treatment of his sleep apnea.
    a. gingivectomy
    b. uvulectomy
    c. uvulopalatopharyngoplasty

19. Indu Deshmukh was born with cleft palate and cleft lip. She had palatoplasty and *surgical repair of the lip* during her childhood.
    a. pyloroplasty
    b. cheiloplasty
    c. gastroplasty

20. After eating very spicy Vietnamese food, Mr. Johanssen developed *inflammation of the tongue*.
    a. gingivitis
    b. cheilitis
    c. glossitis

CHAPTER AT A GLANCE — Word Parts New to This Chapter

COMBINING FORMS

abdomin/o	choledoch/o	hepat/o	peritone/o	
an/o	col/o	herni/o	polyp/o	
antr/o	colon/o	ile/o	proct/o	
append/o	cyst/o	jejun/o	rect/o	
appendic/o	diverticul/o	lapar/o	sial/o	
cec/o	duoden/o	lingu/o	sigmoid/o	
celi/o	enter/o	or/o	steat/o	
cheil/o	gastr/o	palat/o	stomat/o	
chol/e	gingiv/o	pancreat/o	uvul/o	
cholangi/o	gloss/o			

PREFIX
hemi-

SUFFIXES
-ac
-pepsia
-y

CHAPTER AT A GLANCE — Digestive System Terms Built from Word Parts

DISEASE AND DISORDER
appendicitis
cheilitis
cholangioma
cholecystitis
choledocholithiasis
cholelithiasis
colitis
dysentery
diverticulitis
diverticulosis
enteritis
enteropathy
esophagitis
gastritis
gastroenteritis
gingivitis
glossitis
hepatitis
hepatoma
pancreatitis
peritonitis
polyposis
proctitis
rectocele
sialolith
steatohepatitis
stomatitis
uvulitis

SURGICAL
abdominocentesis
abdominoplasty
anoplasty
antrectomy
appendectomy
cheiloplasty
cholecystectomy
choledocholithotomy
colectomy
colostomy
diverticulectomy
enterorrhaphy
esophagogastroplasty
gastrectomy
gastrojejunostomy
gastroplasty
gastrostomy
gingivectomy
glossorrhaphy
hemicolectomy
herniorrhaphy
ileostomy
laparotomy
palatoplasty
pancreatectomy
polypectomy
pyloroplasty
uvulectomy
uvulopalatopharyngoplasty (UPPP)

DIAGNOSTIC

capsule endoscopy
cholangiogram
cholangiography
colonoscope
colonoscopy
CT colonography
esophagogastroduodenoscopy (EGD)
esophagram
esophagoscopy
gastroscope
gastroscopy
laparoscope
laparoscopy
proctoscope
proctoscopy
sigmoidoscopy

COMPLEMENTARY

anal
aphagia
celiac
colorectal
duodenal
dyspepsia
dysphagia
esophageal
gastroenterologist
gastroenterology
hepatomegaly
ileocecal
nasogastric
oral
palatal
pancreatic
peritoneal
rectal
steatorrhea
steatosis
sublingual

CHAPTER AT A GLANCE — Digestive System Terms *NOT* Built from Word Parts

DISEASE AND DISORDER

adhesion
celiac disease
cirrhosis
Crohn disease
gastroesophageal reflux disease (GERD)
hemochromatosis
hemorrhoids
ileus
intussusception
irritable bowel syndrome (IBS)
nonalcoholic fatty liver disease (NAFLD)
peptic ulcer
polyp
ulcerative colitis (UC)
volvulus

SURGICAL

abdominoperineal resection (APR)
anastomosis (*pl.* anastomoses)
bariatric surgery
hemorrhoidectomy
vagotomy

DIAGNOSTIC

abdominal sonography
barium enema (BE)
endoscopic retrograde cholangiopancreatography (ERCP)
endoscopic ultrasound (EUS)
fecal immunochemical test (FIT)
guaiac-based fecal occult blood test (gFOBT)
Helicobacter pylori stool antigen
modified barium swallow (MBS)
upper GI series

COMPLEMENTARY

ascites
diarrhea
emesis
feces
flatus
hematemesis
hematochezia
malabsorption
melena
nausea
palpate
reflux
stoma

PART 2 BODY SYSTEMS

Eye 12

Outline

ANATOMY, 466
Function, 466
Organs and Anatomic Structures of the Eye, 466

WORD PARTS, 468
Combining Forms of the Eye, 468
Combining Forms Used with Eye Terms, 469
Prefixes, 469
Suffixes, 469

MEDICAL TERMS, 474
Disease and Disorder Terms, 474
  Built from Word Parts, 474
  NOT Built from Word Parts, 477
Surgical Terms, 483
  Built from Word Parts and
    NOT Built from Word Parts, 483
Diagnostic Terms, 487
  Built from Word Parts and
    NOT Built from Word Parts, 487
Complementary Terms, 492
  Built from Word Parts and
    NOT Built from Word Parts, 492
Abbreviations, 498

PRACTICAL APPLICATION, 499
CASE STUDY Translate Between Everyday Language and Medical Language, 499
Interact with Medical Documents, 500
Use Medical Language in Online Electronic Health Records, 501
Use Medical Terms in Clinical Statements, 502
Pronounce Medical Terms in Use, 502

CHAPTER REVIEW, 503
Chapter Content Quiz, 503
Chapter at a Glance, 504

Answers to Chapter Exercises, Appendix A

Objectives

Upon completion of this chapter, you will be able to:

1. Pronounce organs and anatomic structures of the eye.
2. Define and spell word parts related to the eye.
3. Define, pronounce, and spell disease and disorder terms related to the eye.
4. Define, pronounce, and spell surgical terms related to the eye.
5. Define, pronounce, and spell diagnostic terms related to the eye.
6. Define, pronounce, and spell complementary terms related to the eye.
7. Interpret the meaning of abbreviations related to the eye.
8. Apply medical language in clinical contexts.

ANATOMY

Function

The eyes are organs of vision and are located in a bony protective cavity of the skull called the orbit. Only a small portion of the eye is visible from the exterior (Figs. 12.1 and 12.2).

Organs and Anatomic Structures of the Eye

TERM	DEFINITION
eye (ī)	organ of vision
eyelids (ī) (lidz)	folds of skin, soft tissue, and a thin layer of muscle located above and below the eye; protect the front of the eye and keep its surface moist by distributing tear film (mixture of tears and oil)
meibomian glands (mī-BŌ-mē-an) (glans)	oil glands found in the upper and lower edges of the eyelids that help lubricate the eye (also called **tarsal glands**)
lacrimal apparatus (LAK-ri-mal) (*ap*-ah-RAT-us)	network of glands, ducts, canals, and sacs that produce and drain tears; the lacrimal gland produces tears, which then flow through the lacrimal ducts to cover the surface of the eye. Tears drain into lacrimal canals, flow into the lacrimal sac (tear sac) and then into the nasolacrimal duct, which opens into the nasal cavity. (Fig. 12.1C)
conjunctiva (kon-JUNK-ti-vah)	mucous membrane lining the eyelids and covering the anterior portion of the sclera
sclera (SKLER-ah)	outer protective layer of the eye; the portion seen on the anterior portion of the eyeball is referred to as the **white of the eye**
cornea (KŌR-nē-a)	transparent anterior part of the sclera, which is anterior to the aqueous humor and lies over the iris. It allows the light rays to enter the eye.
uvea (Ū-vē-a)	layer of tissue beneath the sclera and cornea; contains the choroid, iris, and ciliary body
choroid (KŌR-oid)	middle layer of the eye, which is interlaced with many blood vessels that supply nutrients to the eye
iris (Ī-ris)	pigmented muscular structure that regulates the amount of light entering the eye by controlling the size of the pupil
🏛 **IRIS** was the special messenger of the Queen of Heaven according to Greek mythology. In this role she passed from heaven to earth over the rainbow while dressed in rainbow hues. Her name was applied to the **circular eye muscle** because of its varied colors.	
ciliary body (SIL-ē-*ar*-ē) (BOD-ē)	connects the choroid to the iris; produces aqueous humor and helps change the shape of the lens for focusing
pupil (PŪ-pil)	opening in the center of the iris
lens (lenz)	lies directly behind the pupil; its function is to focus and bend light
retina (RET-i-nah)	innermost layer of the eye, which contains the vision receptors (Fig. 12.3)
macula (MAC-ū-la)	small portion of the retina at the back of the eye; responsible for detailed central vision
optic nerve (OP-tik) (nurv)	cranial nerve that carries visual impulses from the retina to the brain
aqueous humor (Ā-kwē-us) (HŪ-mor)	watery liquid found in the anterior cavity of the eye. It provides nourishment to nearby structures and maintains shape in the anterior part of the eye.
vitreous humor (VIT-rē-us) (HŪ-mor)	jellylike substance found behind the lens in the posterior cavity of the eye that maintains its shape

Chapter 12 Eye   467

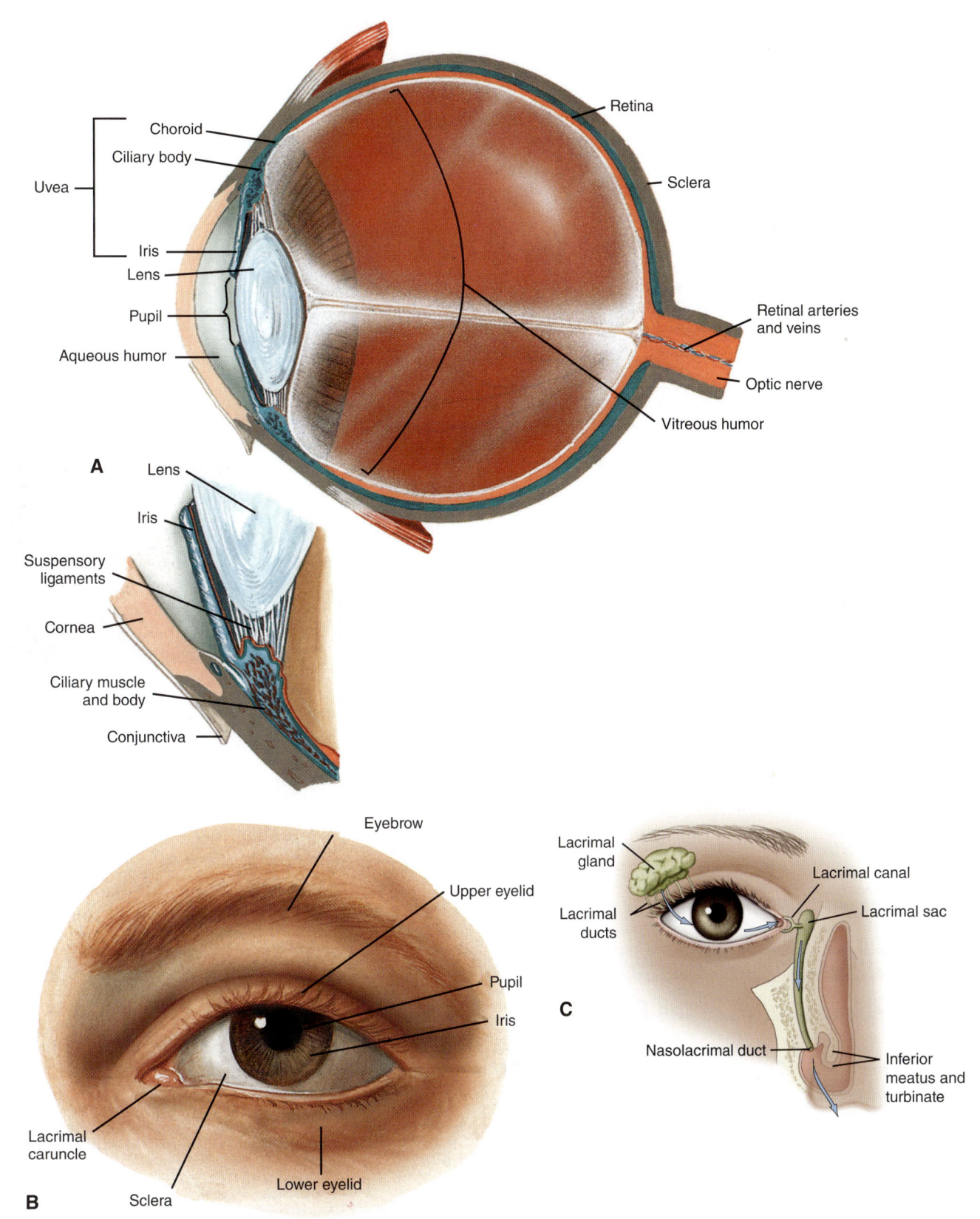

FIG. 12.1 **A,** Anatomy of the eye. **B,** Visible surface of the eye. **C,** Lacrimal apparatus.

468 Chapter 12 Eye

FIG. 12.2 Pathway of light.

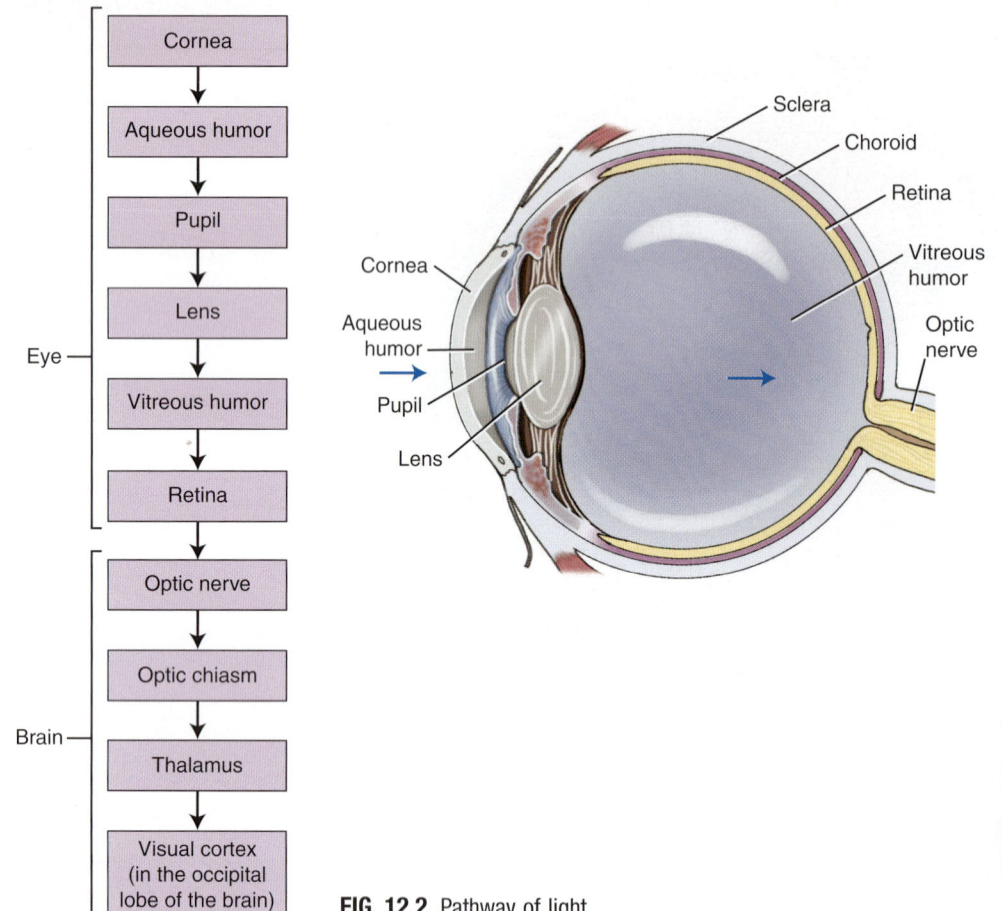

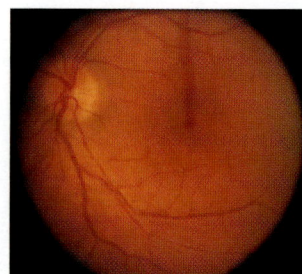

FIG. 12.3 Ophthalmoscopic view of the retina.

PRONOUNCE ANATOMIC STRUCTURES

Practice saying aloud each of the organs and specific structures on the previous pages.

To hear the terms, go to Evolve Resources at www.evolve.elsevier.com and select:
Student Resources > Audio Glossary > Chapter 12 > Anatomic Structures.

❏ Check the box when complete.

WORD PARTS

1 ■ Combining Forms of the Eye

Use paper flashcards or electronic flashcards on Evolve to memorize word parts used to analyze, define, and build medical terms in this chapter. To reinforce learning, study one section of the Word Parts Table at a time, and then complete the corresponding exercises on the following pages.

COMBINING FORM	DEFINITION	COMBINING FORM	DEFINITION
blephar/o	eyelid	irid/o	iris
conjunctiv/o	conjunctiva	kerat/o	cornea
cor/o	pupil	**KERAT/O** refers to hornlike tissue (keratin) or hard texture when used with dermatology terms.	
corne/o	cornea		
dacry/o	tear(s)	lacrim/o	tear(s)
ir/o	iris	ocul/o	eye

COMBINING FORM	DEFINITION
ophthalm/o	eye
💡 **SPELLING *OPHTHALM*** Look closely at the spelling of the word root **ophthalm**. Medical terms containing **ophthalm** are often misspelled by omitting the first h; **ph** gives the **f** sound followed by the sound of **thal**. Think pronunciation when spelling terms that contain **ophthalm**, as in ophthalmology (of[ph]-thal-MOL-o-jē).	
opt/o	vision
phac/o	lens

COMBINING FORM	DEFINITION
phak/o	lens
pupill/o	pupil *(Note: pupil has one l; the combining form has two ls.)*
retin/o	retina (Fig. 12.3)
scler/o	sclera
uve/o	uvea

2 ■ Combining Forms Used with Eye Terms

COMBINING FORM	DEFINITION	COMBINING FORM	DEFINITION
angi/o	vessel(s); blood vessel(s)	is/o	equal
blast/o	developing cell, germ cell	leuk/o	white
cry/o	cold	myc/o	fungus
cyst/o	bladder, sac *(Note: In terms describing the eye, the definition "sac" is used.)*	nas/o	nose
		phot/o	light
DACRY/O + CYST/O When the combining forms **dacry/o** and **cyst/o** appear together, the medical term refers to the lacrimal sac (directly translated as the "tear sac").		pseud/o	false
		rhin/o	nose
dipl/o	two, double	ton/o	tension, pressure
		xer/o	dry, dryness

3 ■ Prefixes

PREFIXES	DEFINITION	PREFIXES	DEFINITION
a-, an-	absence of, without	endo-	within
bin-	two	intra-	within

4 ■ Suffixes

SUFFIXES	DEFINITION	SUFFIXES	DEFINITION
-al	pertaining to	-metry	measurement
-algia	pain	-oma	tumor, swelling
-ar	pertaining to	-opia	vision
-ary	pertaining to	-osis	abnormal condition
-eal	pertaining to	-pathy	disease
-ectomy	excision, surgical removal	-pexy	surgical fixation
-graphy	process of recording, radiographic imaging	-phobia	abnormal fear or aversion
		-plasty	surgical repair
-ia	diseased state, condition of	-plegia	paralysis
-ic	pertaining to	-ptosis	drooping, sagging, prolapse
-itis	inflammation	-scope	instrument used for visual examination
-logist	one who studies and treats (specialist, physician)	-scopy	visual examination
-logy	study of	-stomy	creation of an artificial opening
-malacia	softening	-tomy	cut into, incision
-meter	instrument used to measure		

🔍 Refer to **Appendix B** and **Appendix C** for a complete listing of word parts.

Chapter 12 Eye

EXERCISE 1 ■ Combining Forms of the Eye

Refer to the first section of the word parts table.

A Label

Fill in the blanks with combining forms to label this diagram of the eye. *To check your answers, go to Appendix A at the back of the textbook.*

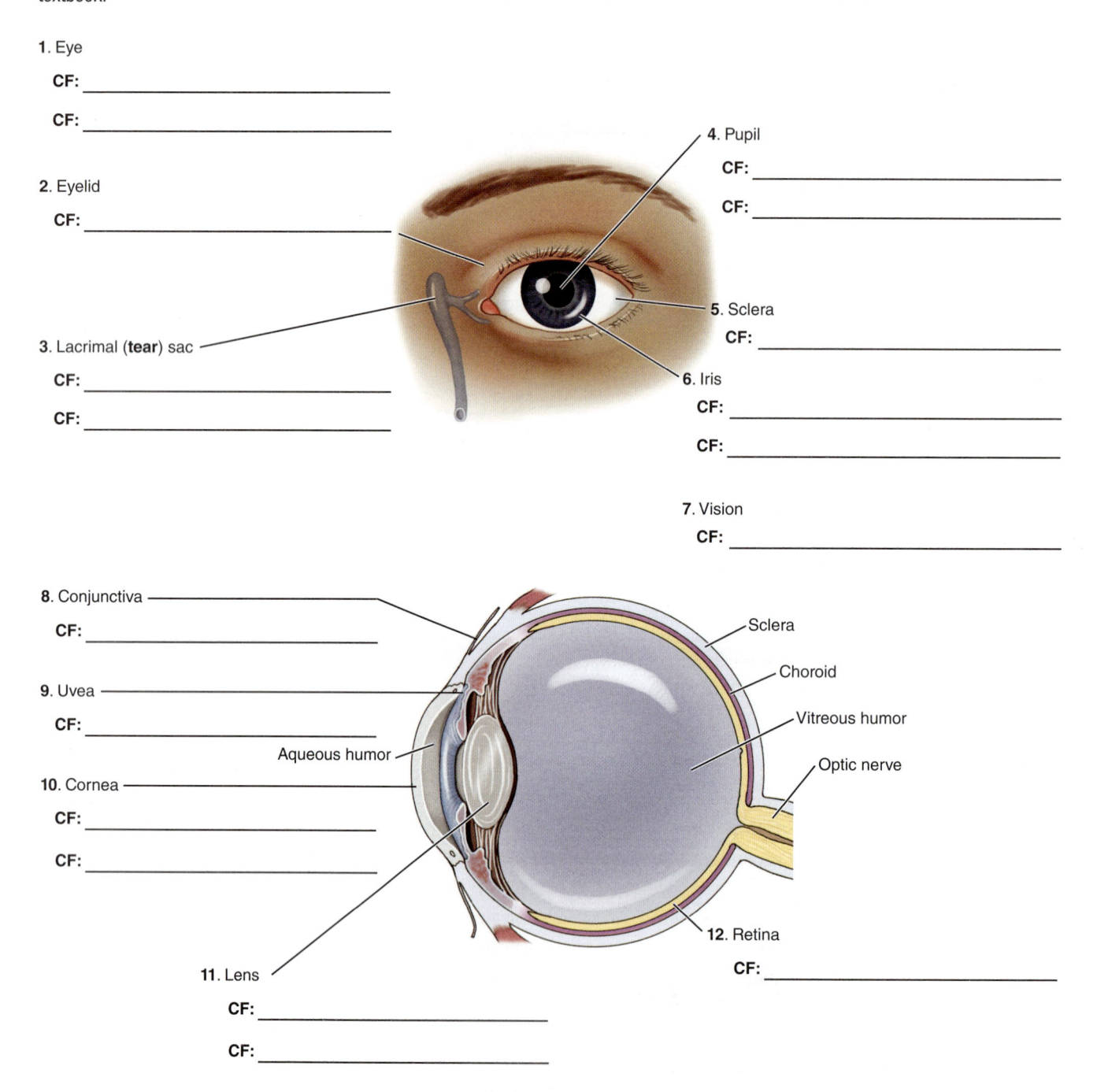

1. Eye
   CF: _____
   CF: _____

2. Eyelid
   CF: _____

3. Lacrimal (**tear**) sac
   CF: _____
   CF: _____

4. Pupil
   CF: _____
   CF: _____

5. Sclera
   CF: _____

6. Iris
   CF: _____
   CF: _____

7. Vision
   CF: _____

8. Conjunctiva
   CF: _____

9. Uvea
   CF: _____

10. Cornea
    CF: _____
    CF: _____

11. Lens
    CF: _____
    CF: _____

12. Retina
    CF: _____

B Define and Match

Step 1: Write the definitions after the following combining forms.
Step 2: Match the descriptions on the right with the combining forms and definitions. Answers may be used more than once; no answer line appears for those not described in a lettered item.

_____ 1. scler/o, _____
_____ 2. cor/o, _____
_____ 3. corne/o, _____
_____ 4. conjunctiv/o, _____
_____ 5. lacrim/o, _____
_____ 6. uve/o, _____
_____ 7. phac/o, phak/o, _____
_____ 8. ocul/o, _____
_____ 9. ir/o, irid/o, _____
_____ 10. pupill/o, _____
_____ 11. kerat/o, _____
_____ 12. ophthalm/o, _____
_____ 13. dacry/o, _____
_____ 14. retin/o, _____
_____ 15. blephar/o, _____
_____ 16. opt/o, _____

a. opening in the center of the iris
b. lies directly behind the pupil; focuses and bends light
c. organ of vision
d. pigmented muscular structure regulating the amount of light entering the eye
e. outer protective layer of the eye
f. produced by and drained by the lacrimal apparatus
g. innermost layer of the eye containing vision receptors
h. mucous membrane lining the eyelids and the anterior portion of the sclera
i. folds of skin, soft tissue, and a thin layer of muscle located above and below the eye
j. transparent anterior part of the sclera
k. layer that contains the choroid, iris, and ciliary body

EXERCISE 2 ■ Combining Forms Used with Eye Terms

Refer to the second section of the word parts table.

A Define

Write the definitions of the following combining forms.

1. ton/o _____
2. phot/o _____
3. cry/o _____
4. dipl/o _____
5. is/o _____
6. cyst/o _____
7. xer/o _____
8. angi/o _____
9. rhin/o _____
10. myc/o _____
11. blast/o _____
12. leuk/o _____
13. pseud/o _____
14. nas/o _____

B Identify

Write the combining form for each of the following definitions.

1. cold _____
2. tension, pressure _____
3. bladder, sac _____
4. two, double _____
5. light _____
6. equal _____
7. white _____
8. false _____
9. developing cell, germ cell _____
10. fungus _____
11. dry, dryness _____
12. vessel(s), blood vessel(s) _____
13. nose a. _____
   b. _____

EXERCISE 3 ■ Prefixes

Refer to the third section of the word parts table.

A Define

Write the definitions of the following prefixes.

1. intra- _____
2. an- _____
3. endo- _____
4. a- _____
5. bin- _____

B Identify

Write the prefixes for the following definitions.

1. two _____
2. without a. _____
   b. _____
3. within a. _____
   b. _____

EXERCISE 4 ■ Suffixes

Refer to the fourth section of the word parts table.

A Identify

Write the suffixes that mean "pertaining to."

1. _____
2. _____
3. _____
4. _____
5. _____

B Match

Match the suffixes in the first column with their correct definitions in the second column.

_____ 1. -stomy   a. disease
_____ 2. -graphy   b. instrument used to measure
_____ 3. -osis   c. drooping, sagging, prolapse
_____ 4. -scope   d. one who studies and treats (specialist, physician)
_____ 5. -algia   e. excision, surgical removal
_____ 6. -logist   f. abnormal condition
_____ 7. -ectomy   g. creation of an artificial opening
_____ 8. -meter   h. process of recording, radiographic imaging
_____ 9. -ptosis   i. instrument used for visual examination
_____ 10. -pathy   j. pain

C Label

Write the suffixes pictured and defined.

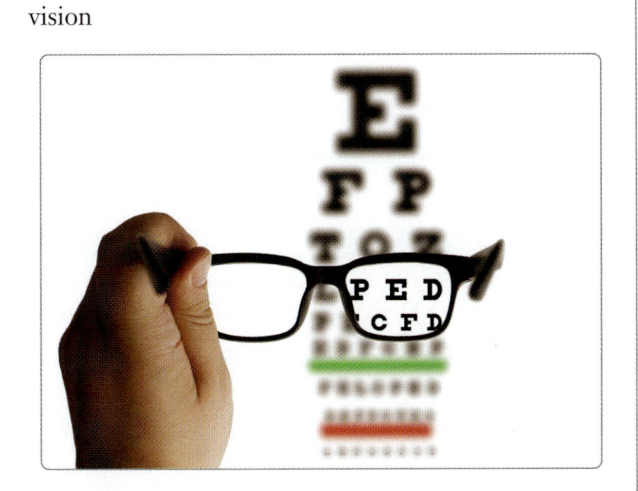

1. _____
   vision

2. _____
   abnormal fear or aversion

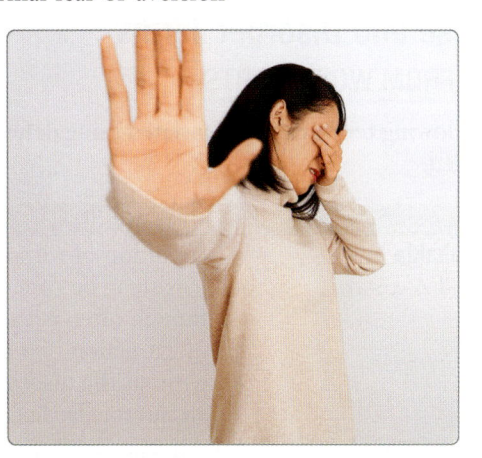

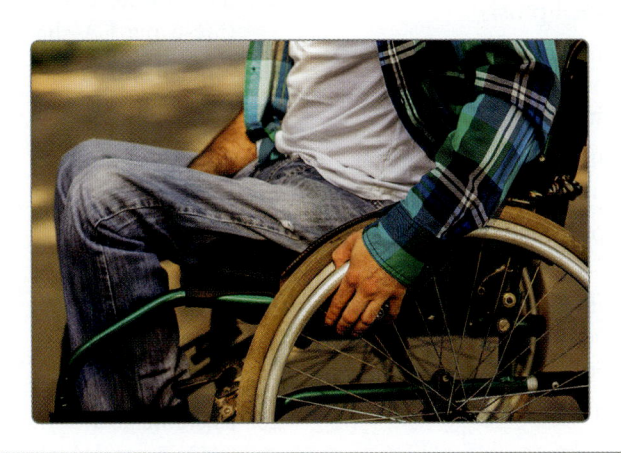

3. _____
   paralysis

D Define

Write the definitions of the following suffixes.

1. -scopy _____
2. -itis _____
3. -malacia _____
4. -plasty _____

E Identify

Write the suffix for each of the following definitions.

1. study of _____
2. measurement _____
3. cut into, incision _____
4. tumor, swelling _____
5. surgical fixation _____
6. diseased state, condition of _____

MEDICAL TERMS

Medical terms relevant to this chapter have been grouped by topics, such as Disease and Disorder, and are listed in tables designated as Built from Word Parts or *NOT* Built from Word Parts. The exercises following each table assist with learning term definitions, pronunciations, and spellings.

Disease and Disorder Terms

BUILT FROM WORD PARTS

The following terms can be translated using definitions of word parts. Further explanation is provided within parentheses as needed.

TERM	DEFINITION	TERM	DEFINITION
1. aphakia (a-FĀ-kē-a)	condition of without a lens (may be congenital, though often is the result of extraction of a cataract without the placement of an intraocular lens)	12. oculomycosis (ok-ū-lō-mī-KŌ-sis)	abnormal condition of the eye caused by a fungus
		13. ophthalmalgia (of-thal-MAL-ja)	pain in the eye
		14. ophthalmopathy (of-thal-MOP-a-thē)	(any) disease of the eye
2. blepharitis (blef-a-RĪ-tis)	inflammation of the eyelid	15. ophthalmoplegia (of-thal-mō-PLĒ-ja)	paralysis of the eye (muscle)
3. blepharoptosis (blef-ar-op-TŌ-sis)	drooping of the eyelid (also called **ptosis**)	16. phacomalacia (fāk-ō-ma-LĀ-sha)	softening of the lens
4. conjunctivitis (kon-junk-ti-VĪ-tis)	inflammation of the conjunctiva (also called **pink eye**)	17. retinoblastoma (ret-i-nō-blas-TŌ-ma)	tumor arising from a developing retinal cell (malignant, may be congenital; occurs mainly in children)
5. dacryocystitis (dak-rē-ō-sis-TĪ-tis)	inflammation of the tear (lacrimal) sac		
6. diplopia (di-PLŌ-pē-a)	double vision	18. retinopathy (ret-i-NOP-a-thē)	(any noninflammatory) disease of the retina (such as **diabetic retinopathy**)
7. endophthalmitis (en-dof-thal-MĪ-tis)	inflammation within the eye *(Note: the o in the prefix endo- is dropped.)*		
		19. scleritis (skle-RĪ-tis)	inflammation of the sclera
8. iridoplegia (īr-i-dō-PLĒ-ja)	paralysis of the iris	20. scleromalacia (sklēr-ō-ma-LĀ-sha)	softening of the sclera
9. iritis (ī-RĪ-tis)	inflammation of the iris	21. uveitis (ū-vē-Ī-tis)	inflammation of the uvea
10. keratitis (ker-a-TĪ-tis)	inflammation of the cornea	22. uveoscleritis (ū-vē-ō-sklē-RĪ-tis)	inflammation of the uvea and sclera
11. keratomalacia (ker-a-tō-ma-LĀ-sha)	softening of the cornea (usually a bilateral condition associated with vitamin A deficiency)	23. xerophthalmia (zēr-of-THAL-mē-a)	condition of dry eye (conjunctiva and cornea)

EXERCISE 5 ■ Pronounce and Spell

Practice pronunciation and spelling on paper and online.

1. **Practice on Paper**
   a. **Pronounce:** Read the phonetic spelling and say aloud the terms listed in the previous table. Refer to Table 2.2 Pronunciation Key as needed.
   b. **Spell:** Have a study partner read the terms aloud. Write the spelling of the terms on a separate sheet of paper.

2. **Practice Online**
   a. **Access** online learning resources. Go to evolve.elsevier.com > Evolve Resources > Student Resources.
   b. **Pronounce:** Select Audio Glossary > Chapter 12 > Exercise 5. Select a term to hear its pronunciation and repeat aloud.
   c. **Spell:** Select Activities > Chapter 12 > Spell Terms > Exercise 5. Select the audio icon and type the correct spelling of the term.

❏ Check the box when complete.

EXERCISE 6 ■ Analyze and Define

Analyze and define the following terms.

1. scleritis

2. ophthalmoplegia

3. retinopathy

4. endophthalmitis

5. xerophthalmia

6. aphakia

7. ophthalmopathy

8. scleromalacia

9. uveitis

10. keratomalacia

476   Chapter 12   Eye

EXERCISE 7 ■ Build

A Label

Build terms pictured by writing word parts above definitions.

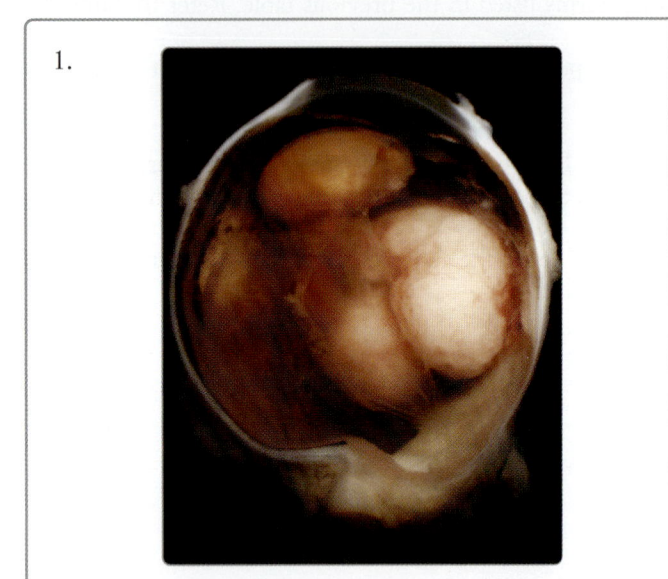

1.

_____ / ____ / _____ / _____
retina   CV   developing   tumor
                  cell

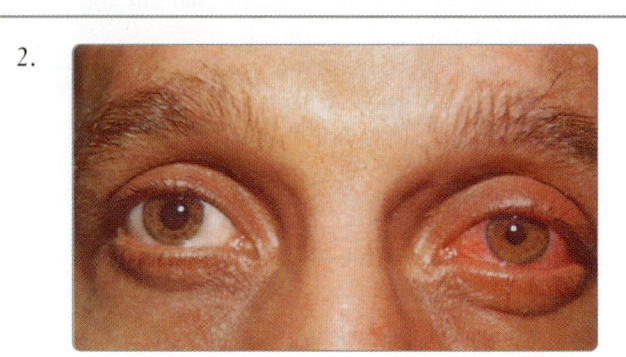

2.

_____ / _____
   sclera   inflammation

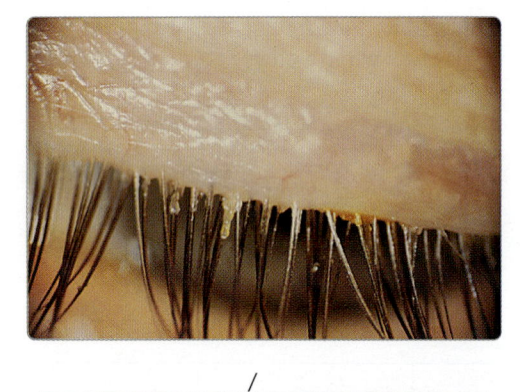

3.

_____ / _____
   eyelid   inflammation

4.

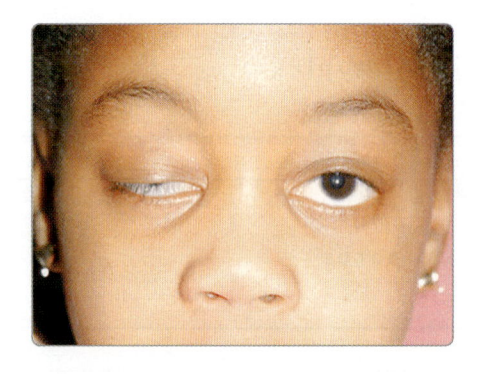

_____ / ____ / _____
  eyelid   CV   drooping

5.

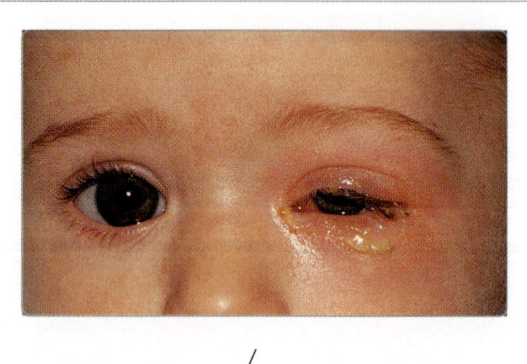

_____ / _____
 conjunctiva   inflammation

6.

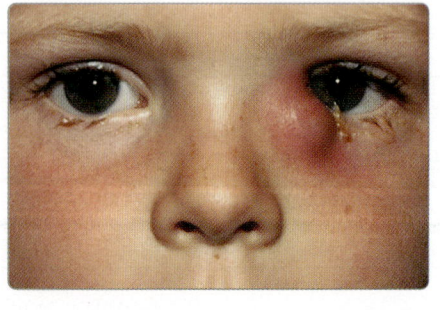

_____ / ____ / _____ / _____
  tear   CV   sac   inflammation

B Fill In

Build disease and disorder terms for the following definitions by using the word parts you have learned.

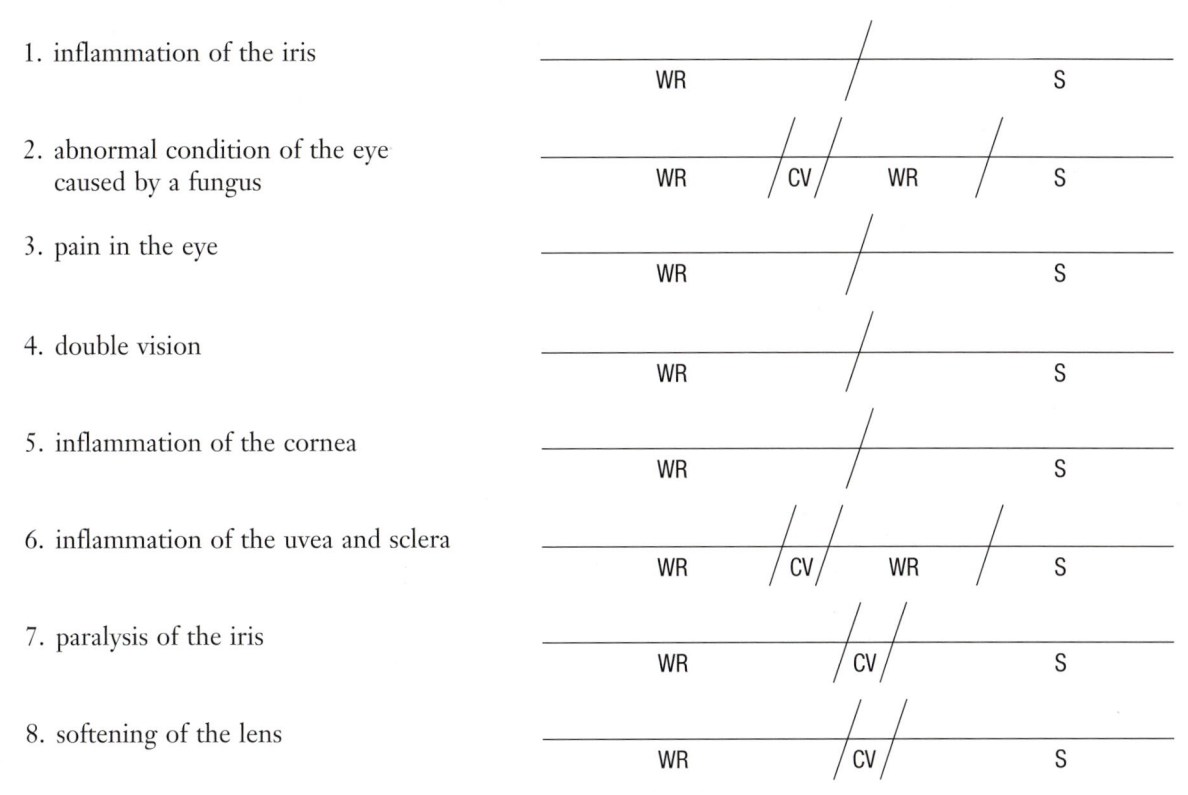

1. inflammation of the iris _____ / _____
   WR   S

2. abnormal condition of the eye caused by a fungus _____ / ___ / _____ / _____
   WR   CV   WR   S

3. pain in the eye _____ / _____
   WR   S

4. double vision _____ / _____
   WR   S

5. inflammation of the cornea _____ / _____
   WR   S

6. inflammation of the uvea and sclera _____ / ___ / _____ / _____
   WR   CV   WR   S

7. paralysis of the iris _____ / ___ / _____
   WR   CV   S

8. softening of the lens _____ / ___ / _____
   WR   CV   S

Disease and Disorder Terms
NOT BUILT FROM WORD PARTS

Word parts may be present in the following terms; however, their full meanings cannot be translated using definitions of word parts alone.

TERM	DEFINITION
1. amblyopia (am-blē-Ō-pē-a)	reduced vision in one eye caused by disuse or misuse associated with strabismus, unequal refractive errors, or otherwise impaired vision. The brain suppresses images from the impaired eye to avoid double vision. (also called **lazy eye**)
2. anisometropia (an-i-sō-ma-TRŌ-pē-a)	significant unequal refractive error between two eyes
3. astigmatism (Ast) (a-STIG-ma-tizm)	blurred vision caused by irregular curvature of the cornea or lens. Light refracts improperly, resulting in diffused, rather than points of light focusing on the retina. (Fig. 12.4C)
4. cataract (KAT-a-rakt)	clouding of the lens of the eye
CATARACT is derived from the Greek **kato**, meaning **down**, and **raktos**, meaning **precipice**. Together, the words were interpreted as **waterfall**. The individual with a cataract sees things as through a watery veil of mist or waterfall.	
5. chalazion (ka-LĀ-zē-on)	noninfected obstruction of an oil gland of the eyelid (also called **meibomian cyst**)
6. drusen (DRŪ-zen)	yellowish deposits located under the retina; commonly associated with aging and macular degeneration

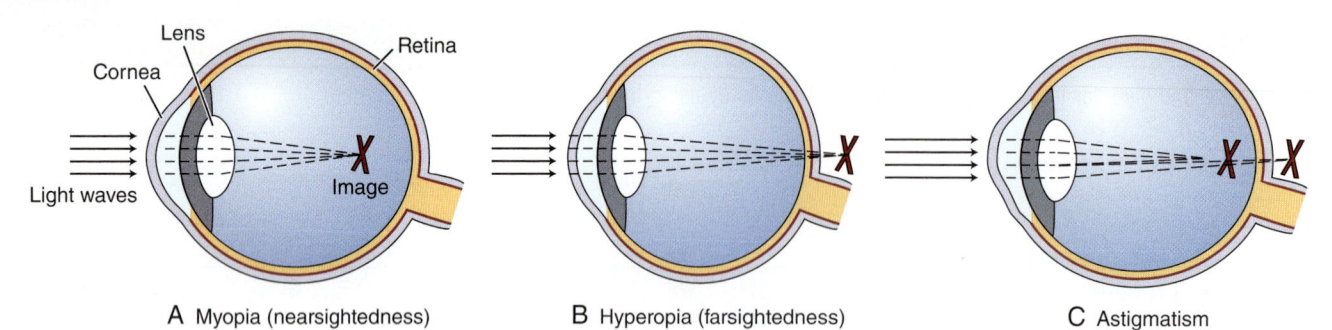

FIG. 12.4 Types of refractive errors. Refractive errors occur when light does not focus correctly on the retina because of the shape of the eye, cornea, or lens. **A,** Myopia, nearsightedness. **B,** Hyperopia, farsightedness. **C,** Astigmatism.

Disease and Disorder Terms—cont'd

NOT BUILT FROM WORD PARTS

TERM	DEFINITION
7. glaucoma (glaw-KŌ-ma)	eye disorder characterized by increase of intraocular pressure (IOP). If left untreated may progress to optic nerve damage and visual impairment or loss.
	GLAUCOMA is composed of the Greek **glaukos**, meaning **blue-gray** or **sea green**, and **oma**, meaning a morbid condition. The term was given to any condition in which gray or green replaced the black in the pupil.
8. hyperopia (hī-per-Ō-pē-a)	farsightedness (Fig. 12.4B)
9. hyphema (hī-FĒ-ma)	hemorrhage within the anterior chamber of the eye; most often caused by blunt trauma (also called **hyphemia**)
10. keratoconus (ker-a-tō-KŌ-nus)	progressive thinning of the cornea causing its normally rounded surface to bulge outward into a conelike shape and leading to vision impairment and, in some cases, vision loss; early symptoms, usually starting in the late teens and early twenties, include blurry vision and light sensitivity
11. macular degeneration (MAC-ū-lar) (dē-gen-e-RĀ-shun)	progressive deterioration of the portion of the retina called the **macula**, resulting in loss of central vision (Fig. 12.5). Age-related macular degeneration (AMD) is the leading cause of legal blindness in persons older than 65 years; onset occurs between the ages of 50 and 60.
12. myopia (mī-Ō-pē-a)	nearsightedness (Fig. 12.4A)
13. nyctalopia (nik-ta-LŌ-pē-a)	poor vision at night or in faint light (also called **night blindness**)
14. nystagmus (nis-TAG-mus)	involuntary, jerking movements of the eyes
15. pinguecula (ping-GWEH-kū-la)	yellowish mass on the conjunctiva that may be related to long-term exposure to ultraviolet light, dry climates, and dust. A pinguecula that spreads onto the cornea becomes a **pterygium**.
16. presbyopia (pres-bē-Ō-pē-a)	impaired vision as a result of aging
17. pterygium (te-RIJ-ē-um)	thin tissue growing onto the cornea from the conjunctiva, usually caused by sun exposure
18. retinal detachment (RET-in-al) (dē-TACH-ment)	separation of the retina from the choroid in the posterior portion of the eye resulting in a disruption of vision that may be permanent if treatment is delayed; onset may be gradual or sudden and is not painful (Fig. 12.6)

TERM	DEFINITION
19. retinitis pigmentosa (RP) (*ret*-i-NĪ-tis) (*pig*-men-TŌ-sa)	group of hereditary diseases marked by the destruction of retinal cells that causes low vision and blindness; usually the first symptom is impairment of night vision, followed by loss of peripheral vision, and then loss of central vision
20. strabismus (stra-BIZ-mus)	condition in which the eyes look in different directions; caused by dysfunction of the external eye muscles or an uncorrected refractive error (called **cross-eyed** when one eye turns in)
21. sty (stī)	infection of an oil gland of the eyelid (also spelled **stye** and also called **hordeolum**)

EXERCISE 8 ■ Pronounce and Spell

Practice pronunciation and spelling on paper and online.

1. **Practice on Paper**
   a. **Pronounce:** Read the phonetic spelling and say aloud the terms listed in the previous table. Refer to Table 2.2 Pronunciation Key as needed.
   b. **Spell:** Have a study partner read the terms aloud. Write the spelling of the terms on a separate sheet of paper.

2. **Practice Online**
   a. **Access** online learning resources. Go to evolve.elsevier.com > Evolve Resources > Student Resources.
   b. **Pronounce:** Select Audio Glossary > Chapter 12 > Exercise 8. Select a term to hear its pronunciation and repeat aloud.
   c. **Spell:** Select Activities > Chapter 12 > Spell Terms > Exercise 8. Select the audio icon and type the correct spelling of the term.

❏ Check the box when complete.

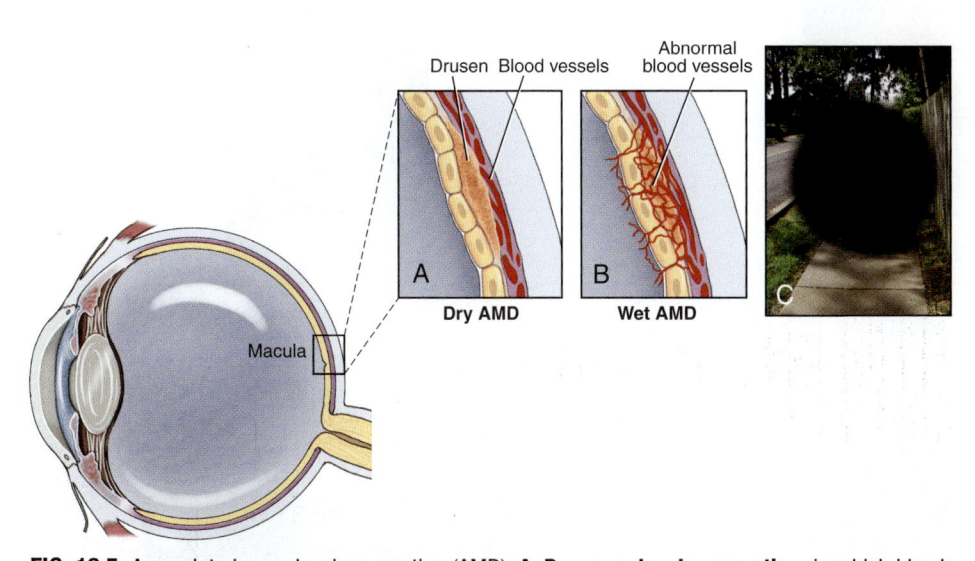

FIG. 12.5 Age-related macular degeneration (AMD). **A, Dry macular degeneration,** in which blood vessels under the macula become brittle and yellow deposits called drusen form, is the most common form of age-related macular degeneration (AMD). **B, Wet macular degeneration,** in which new abnormal blood vessels form under the macula, is less common though more likely to cause legal blindness. **C, Central vision loss** as may be experienced in AMD.

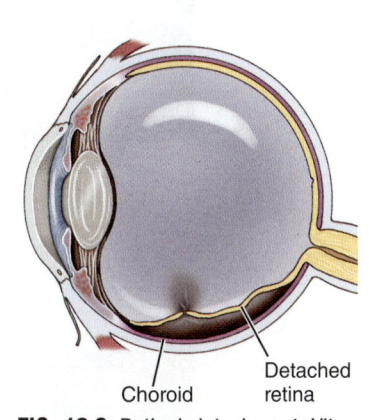

FIG. 12.6 Retinal detachment. Vitreous fluid has seeped through a tear in the retina, causing the retina to separate from the choroid.

EXERCISE 9 ■ Fill In

A Identify

Fill in the blanks with the correct terms.

1. Another name for nearsightedness is _____.
2. Impaired vision as a result of aging is _____.
3. Significant unequal refractive error between two eyes is _____.
4. Irregular curvature of the cornea or lens causes a condition known as _____.
5. _____ is the name given to involuntary, jerking movements of the eye.
6. Eye disorder characterized by the increase of intraocular pressure is _____.
7. Another name for farsightedness is _____.
8. _____ refers to a group of hereditary diseases marked by the destruction of retinal cells that causes low vision and blindness.
9. Another name for night blindness is _____.
10. Another name for lazy eye is _____.

B Label

Write the medical terms pictured and defined.

1. _____
   yellowish deposits located under the retina

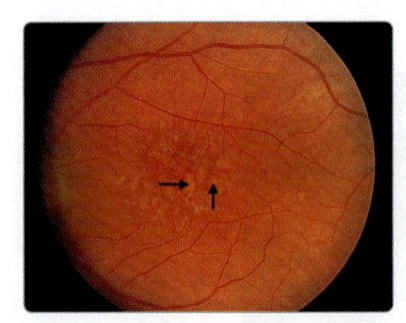

2. _____
   progressive deterioration of the portion of the retina called the macula, resulting in loss of central vision

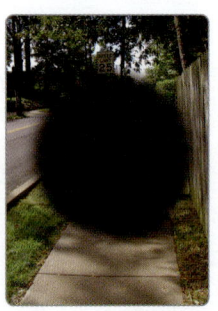

3. _____
   thin tissue growing onto the cornea from the conjunctiva, usually caused by sun exposure

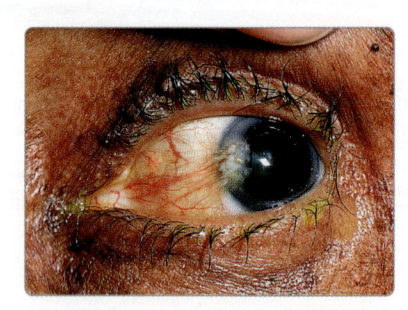

4. _____
   yellowish mass on the conjunctiva that may be related to long-term exposure to ultraviolet light, dry climates, and dust

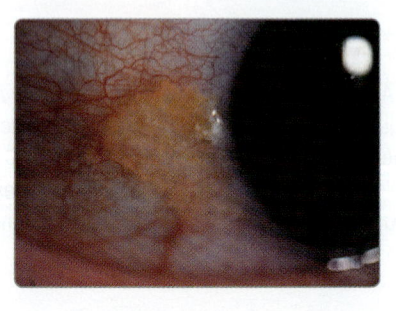

5. _____
noninfected obstruction of an oil gland of the eyelid

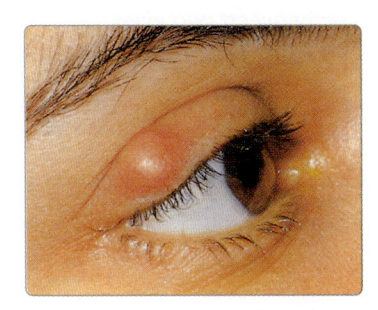

6. _____
infection of an oil gland of the eyelid

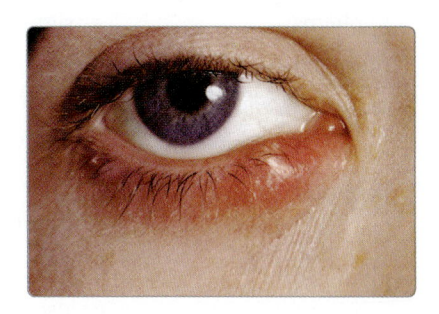

7. _____
clouding of the lens of the eye

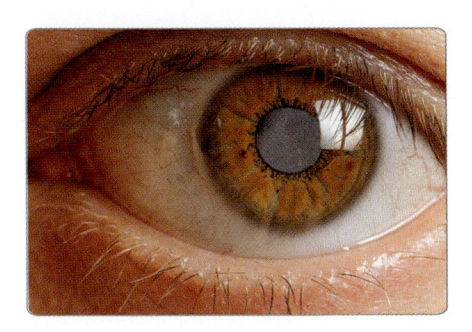

8. _____
hemorrhage within the anterior chamber of the eye; most often caused by blunt trauma

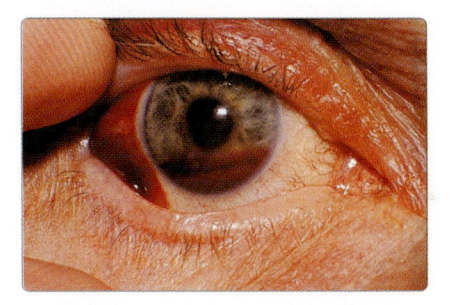

9. _____
condition in which the eyes look in different directions

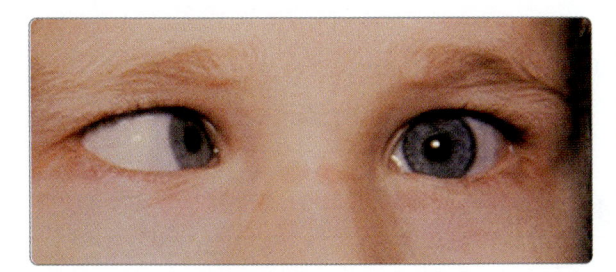

10. _____
separation of the retina from the choroid in the posterior portion of the eye

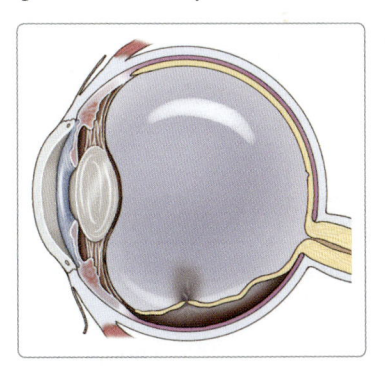

11. _____
eye disorder characterized by increase of intraocular pressure

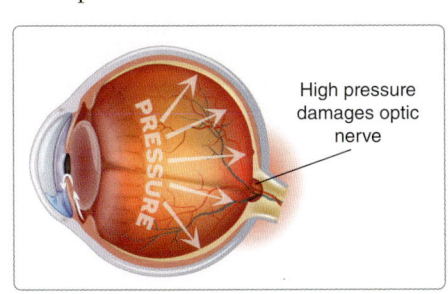

High pressure damages optic nerve

12. _____
progressive thinning of the cornea, causing it to bulge outward into a conelike shape

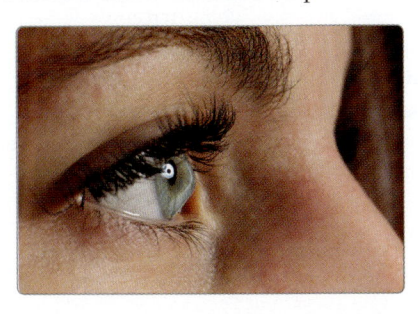

C Match

Match the terms in the first column with their correct definitions in the second column.

_____ 1. hyphema
_____ 2. pterygium
_____ 3. anisometropia
_____ 4. sty
_____ 5. keratoconus
_____ 6. chalazion
_____ 7. myopia
_____ 8. retinitis pigmentosa
_____ 9. astigmatism
_____ 10. pinguecula

a. significant unequal refractive error between two eyes
b. thinning of the cornea, causing a conelike bulge and leading to vision impairment
c. also called meibomian cyst
d. disease in which the first symptom is usually impaired night vision
e. thin tissue growing onto the cornea from the conjunctiva
f. irregular curvature of the cornea or lens
g. also called hordeolum
h. hemorrhage within the anterior chamber of the eye
i. yellowish mass on the conjunctiva
j. nearsightedness

D Match

Match the terms in the first column with their correct definitions in the second column.

_____ 1. nyctalopia
_____ 2. drusen
_____ 3. retinal detachment
_____ 4. amblyopia
_____ 5. strabismus
_____ 6. presbyopia
_____ 7. macular degeneration
_____ 8. hyperopia
_____ 9. nystagmus
_____ 10. cataract

a. called cross-eyed when one eye turns in
b. yellowish deposits located under the retina
c. impaired vision as a result of aging
d. results in loss of central vision
e. involuntary, jerking movements of the eyes
f. disruption of vision caused by separation of the retina from the choroid
g. clouding of the lens of the eye
h. also called lazy eye
i. also called night blindness
j. farsightedness

EXERCISE 10 ■ Review of Disease and Disorder Terms

Can you define, pronounce, and spell the following terms?

amblyopia	drusen	myopia	retinal detachment
anisometropia	endophthalmitis	nyctalopia	retinitis pigmentosa (RP)
aphakia	glaucoma	nystagmus	retinoblastoma
astigmatism (Ast)	hyperopia	oculomycosis	retinopathy
blepharitis	hyphema	ophthalmalgia	scleritis
blepharoptosis	iridoplegia	ophthalmopathy	scleromalacia
cataract	iritis	ophthalmoplegia	strabismus
chalazion	keratitis	phacomalacia	sty
conjunctivitis	keratoconus	pinguecula	uveitis
dacryocystitis	keratomalacia	presbyopia	uveoscleritis
diplopia	macular degeneration	pterygium	xerophthalmia

Chapter 12 Eye

Surgical Terms
BUILT FROM WORD PARTS AND *NOT* BUILT FROM WORD PARTS

The first portion of the table contains Surgical Terms that can be translated using definitions of word parts. The second portion of the table contains Surgical Terms that cannot be fully understood using the definitions of word parts.

■ Built from Word Parts

TERM	DEFINITION	TERM	DEFINITION
1. blepharoplasty (BLEF-a-rō-*plas*-tē)	surgical repair of the eyelid	4. iridectomy (*ir*-i-DEK-to-mē)	excision (of part) of the iris
2. cryoretinopexy (*krī*-ō-RE-tin-ō-*pek*-sē)	surgical fixation of the retina by using extreme cold (carbon dioxide)	5. iridotomy (*ir*-i-DOT-o-mē)	incision into the iris
		6. keratoplasty (KER-a-tō-*plas*-tē)	surgical repair of the cornea (corneal transplant)
3. dacryocystorhinostomy (*dak*-rē-ō-sis-tō-rī-NOS-to-mē)	creation of an artificial opening between the tear (lacrimal) sac and the nose (to restore drainage into the nose when the nasolacrimal duct is obstructed or obliterated)	7. sclerotomy (skle-ROT-o-mē)	incision into the sclera

■ *NOT* Built from Word Parts

TERM	DEFINITION
1. enucleation (ē-*nū*-klē-Ā-shun)	surgical removal of the eyeball (also, excision of a whole organ or mass without cutting into it)
2. LASIK (laser-assisted in situ keratomileusis) (LĀ-sik) (*ker*-a-tō-mi-LOO-sis)	laser procedure that reshapes the corneal tissue beneath the surface of the cornea to correct astigmatism, hyperopia, and myopia. It differs from photorefractive keratectomy (PRK) in that it reshapes corneal tissue beneath the surface rather than on the surface (Fig. 12.7B).
3. phacoemulsification (PHACO) (*fā*-kō-ē-*mul*-si-fi-KĀ-shun)	method to remove cataracts in which an ultrasonic needle probe breaks up the lens, which is then aspirated
4. photorefractive keratectomy (PRK) (*fō*-tō-rē-FRAK-tiv) (*ker*-a-TEK-to-mē)	procedure for the treatment of astigmatism, hyperopia, and myopia in which a laser is used to reshape (flatten) the corneal surface by removing a portion of the cornea (Fig. 12.7A)
5. posterior capsulotomy (pos-TĒR-ē-or) (*kap*-su-LOT-ō-mē)	laser procedure used to create an opening in the back center of the membrane holding an intraocular lens in place; performed to relieve vision impairment after cataract surgery (also called **YAG laser capsulotomy**)
6. retinal photocoagulation (RET-in-al) (*fō*-tō-kō-*ag*-ū-LĀ-shun)	intense beam of light from a laser condenses retinal tissue to seal leaking blood vessels, to destroy abnormal tissue or lesions, or to bond the retina to the back of the eye. Used to treat retinal tears, diabetic retinopathy, wet macular degeneration, glaucoma, and intraocular tumors.
7. scleral buckling (SKLER-al) (BUK-ling)	procedure to repair retinal detachment in which a piece of silicone is applied to the abnormal part of the sclera. This pushes in, or "buckles," the sclera toward the middle of the eye, decreasing the traction on the retina. For larger detachments, an entire band may encircle the eyeball. Cryoretinopexy is often used to repair the hole in the retina prior to the buckling procedure.
8. trabeculectomy (tra-*bek*-ū-LEK-to-mē)	surgical creation of an opening that allows aqueous humor to drain out of the eye to underneath the conjunctiva, where it is absorbed; used to treat glaucoma by reducing intraocular pressure. (Laser trabeculoplasty may also be used.)
9. vitrectomy (vi-TREK-to-mē)	surgical removal of all or part of the vitreous humor (to provide access to interior structures of the eye; used to treat diabetic retinopathy, retinal detachment, or a hole in the macula)

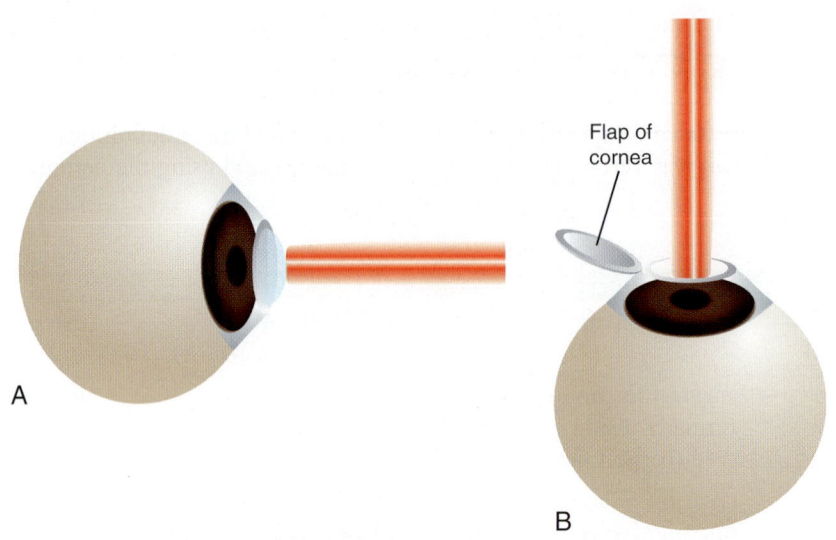

FIG. 12.7 Laser treatments for near-sightedness. **A, Photorefractive keratectomy** (PRK) removes tissue from the surface of the cornea. **B, LASIK** (laser-assisted in situ keratomileusis) reshapes corneal tissue below the surface of the cornea. The excimer laser was invented in the early 1980s. It is a computer-controlled ultraviolet beam of light that reshapes the cornea. It has replaced **RK** (radial keratotomy), a surgery in which spokelike incisions are made to reshape the cornea.

EXERCISE 11 ■ Pronounce and Spell

Practice pronunciation and spelling on paper and online.

1. **Practice on Paper**
    a. **Pronounce:** Read the phonetic spelling and say aloud the terms listed in the previous table. Refer to Table 2.2 Pronunciation Key as needed.
    b. **Spell:** Have a study partner read the terms aloud. Write the spelling of the terms on a separate sheet of paper.

2. **Practice Online**
    a. **Access** online learning resources. Go to evolve.elsevier.com > Evolve Resources > Student Resources.
    b. **Pronounce:** Select Audio Glossary > Chapter 12 > Exercise 11. Select a term to hear its pronunciation and repeat aloud.
    c. **Spell:** Select Activities > Chapter 12 > Spell Terms > Exercise 11. Select the audio icon and type the correct spelling of the term.

❏ Check the box when complete.

EXERCISE 12 ■ Surgical Terms Built from Word Parts

A Analyze and Define

Analyze and define the following surgical terms.

1. keratoplasty

3. cryoretinopexy

2. sclerotomy

4. blepharoplasty

Chapter 12 Eye 485

5. iridectomy

_____

_____

7. iridotomy

_____

_____

6. dacryocystorhinostomy

_____

_____

B Label

Build terms pictured by writing word parts above definitions.

1.

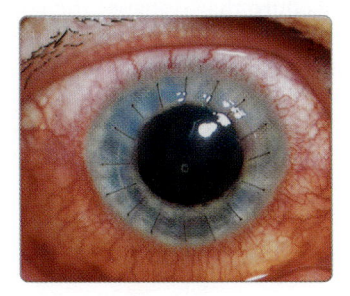

Appearance of the eye after
_____ / ____ / _____
cornea   CV   surgical repair

2.

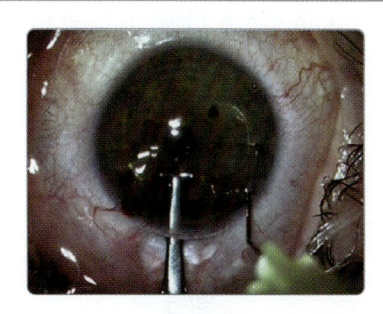

_____ / _____ / _____
iris   CV   incision

3.

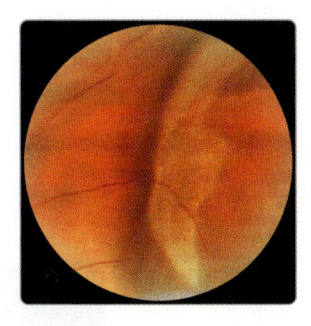

Retina after _____ / _____ / _____ / _____ / _____
              cold   CV   retina   CV   surgical
                                           fixation

C Fill In

Build surgical terms for the following definitions by using the word parts you have learned.

1. creation of an artificial opening between the tear (lacrimal) sac and the nose

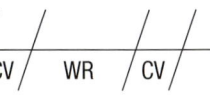

_____ / ___ / _____ / ___ / _____ / ___ / ___
 WR   CV   WR   CV   WR   CV   S

2. excision (of part) of the iris

_____ / _____
      WR   S

486   Chapter 12   Eye

3. incision into the sclera   _____ / ____ / _____
                                        WR   CV   S

4. surgical repair of the eyelid   _____ / ____ / _____
                                        WR   CV   S

EXERCISE 13 ■ Surgical Terms NOT Built from Word Parts

A Label

Write the surgical terms pictured and defined.

1. _____
procedure in which a laser is used to reshape (flatten) the corneal surface by removing a portion of the cornea

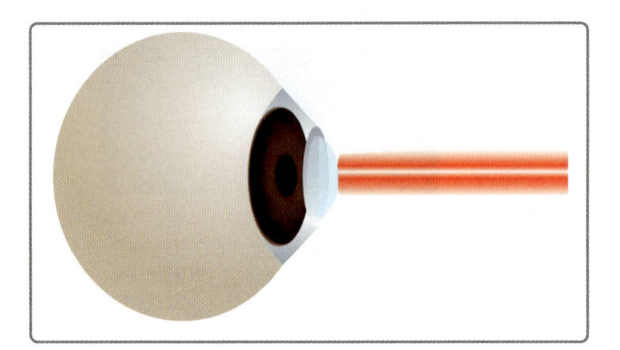

2. _____
laser procedure that reshapes the corneal tissue beneath the surface of the cornea to correct astigmatism, hyperopia, and myopia

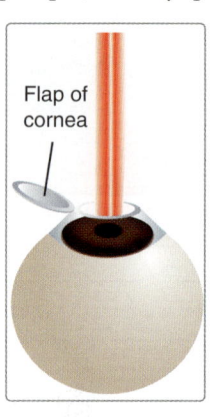

Flap of cornea

3. _____
procedure to repair retinal detachment in which a piece of silicone is applied to the abnormal part of the sclera

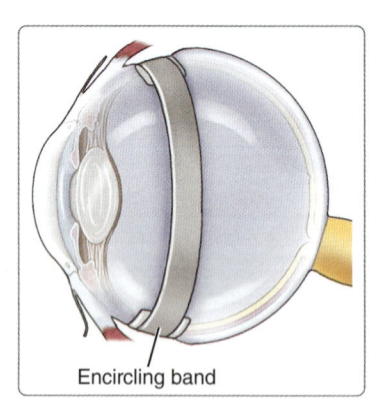

Encircling band

4. _____
method to remove cataracts in which an ultrasonic needle probe breaks up the lens, which is then aspirated

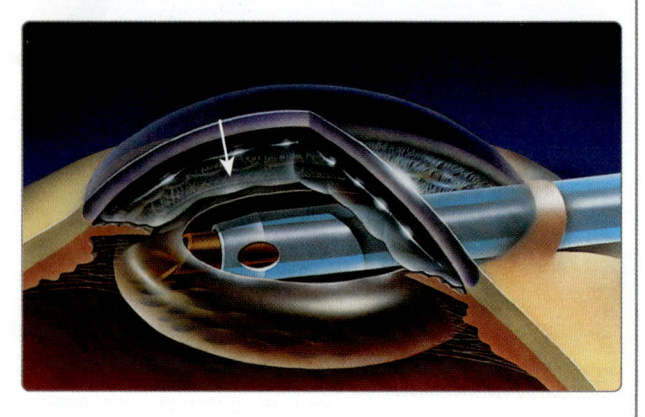

B Identify

Fill in the blanks with the correct terms.

1. _____ _____ is the use of a laser beam to condense retinal tissue to seal leaking blood vessels, destroy abnormal tissue, or bond the retina to the back of the eye.

2. Cloudiness affecting vision after cataract surgery can be treated with _____,
   a laser procedure that creates an opening in the back center of the lens membrane, allowing more light to pass through.
3. Surgical removal of an eyeball is called a(n) _____.
4. _____ is the surgical creation of an opening that allows aqueous humor to drain out of the eye to reduce intraocular pressure.
5. Surgery to remove vitreous humor from the eye is called _____.

C Match

Match the terms in the first column with their correct definitions in the second column.

_____ 1. LASIK
_____ 2. enucleation
_____ 3. trabeculectomy
_____ 4. retinal photocoagulation
_____ 5. phacoemulsification
_____ 6. scleral buckling
_____ 7. vitrectomy
_____ 8. photorefractive keratectomy
_____ 9. posterior capsulotomy

a. use of a laser beam to repair retinal tears and detachment, as well as other retinopathies
b. surgical creation of an opening to reduce intraocular pressure
c. procedure for the treatment of astigmatism, hyperopia, and myopia in which a laser is used to reshape the corneal surface by removing the outermost layer of the cornea
d. procedure in which the lens is broken up by ultrasound and aspirated
e. procedure used to correct astigmatism, nearsightedness, and farsightedness by reshaping tissue beneath the corneal surface
f. laser procedure used to create an opening in the back center of the membrane holding an intraocular lens in place
g. surgical removal of an eyeball
h. surgical removal of vitreous humor
i. procedure to repair retinal detachment in which a piece of silicone is applied to the abnormal part of the sclera

EXERCISE 14 ■ Review of Surgical Terms

Can you define, pronounce, and spell the following terms?

blepharoplasty	iridotomy	phacoemulsification (PHACO)	retinal photocoagulation
cryoretinopexy	keratoplasty	photorefractive keratectomy (PRK)	scleral buckling
dacryocystorhinostomy	LASIK (laser-assisted in situ keratomileusis)	posterior capsulotomy	sclerotomy
enucleation			trabeculectomy
iridectomy			vitrectomy

Diagnostic Terms
BUILT FROM WORD PARTS AND *NOT* BUILT FROM WORD PARTS

The first portion of the table contains Diagnostic Terms that can be translated using definitions of word parts. The second portion of the table contains Diagnostic Terms that cannot be fully understood using the definitions of word parts.

■ Built From Word Parts

DIAGNOSTIC IMAGING

TERM	DEFINITION
1. fluorescein angiography (FA) (flō-RES-ēn) (an-jē-OG-ra-fē)	radiographic imaging of blood vessels (of the eye with fluorescing dye)

OPHTHALMIC EVALUATION

TERM	DEFINITION
2. keratometer (ker-a-TOM-e-ter)	instrument used to measure (the curvature of) the cornea (used for fitting contact lenses)

TERM	DEFINITION
3. ophthalmoscope (of-THAL-mō-skōp)	instrument used for visual examination (of the interior) of the eye
4. ophthalmoscopy (of-thal-MOS-ko-pē)	visual examination of the eye
5. optometry (op-TOM-e-trē)	measurement of vision (also measurement of the eye and visual processing system)
6. pupillometer (pū-pil-OM-e-ter)	instrument used to measure (the diameter of) the pupil
7. pupilloscope (pū-PIL-ō-skōp)	instrument used for visual examination of the pupil
8. retinoscopy (ret-i-NOS-ko-pē)	visual examination of the retina
9. tonometer (tō-NOM-e-ter)	instrument used to measure pressure (within the eye, used to diagnose glaucoma)
10. tonometry (tō-NOM-e-trē)	measurement of pressure (within the eye)

■ **NOT Built from Word Parts**

DIAGNOSTIC IMAGING

TERM	DEFINITION
1. optical coherence tomography (OCT) (OP-ti-kul)(kō-HĒR-entz) (tō-MOG-rah-fē)	noninvasive test that uses light waves to take cross-sectional images of the retina; used to detect many eye conditions, including macular degeneration, glaucoma, retinopathy, and optic nerve damage.

OPHTHALMIC EVALUATION

TERM	DEFINITION
2. fundus examination (FUN-das) (eg-zam-i-NĀ-shun)	use of an ophthalmoscope to view the back of the eye, including the choroid, retina, macula, retinal blood vessels, and the optic disc (where the retina connects to the optic nerve); (also called **fundoscopy**)
3. slit lamp (slit) (lamp)	horizontally mounted binocular microscope that uses a very narrow vertical beam of light (slit) to examine the eye in great detail. It is especially useful for viewing the conjunctiva, cornea, lens, and vitreous humor.

OPTOMETRIC EXAMINATION

TERM	DEFINITION
4. phoropter (fōr-OP-tor)	instrument with many dials used to evaluate refractive errors and determine the lens curve and shape needed to correct vision. The patient reports which trial lens supports clearer vision in each eye, and then readings from the instrument are used to prescribe lenses.

EXERCISE 15 ■ Pronounce and Spell

Practice pronunciation and spelling on paper and online.

1. **Practice on Paper**
   a. **Pronounce:** Read the phonetic spelling and say aloud the terms listed in the previous table. Refer to Table 2.2 Pronunciation Key as needed.
   b. **Spell:** Have a study partner read the terms aloud. Write the spelling of the terms on a separate sheet of paper.

Chapter 12   Eye   489

2. **Practice Online**
   a. **Access** online learning resources. Go to evolve.elsevier.com > Evolve Resources > Student Resources.
   b. **Pronounce:** Select Audio Glossary > Chapter 12 > Exercise 15. Select a term to hear its pronunciation and repeat aloud.
   c. **Spell:** Select Activities > Chapter 12 > Spell Terms > Exercise 15. Select the audio icon and type the correct spelling of the term.
   ❑ Check the box when complete.

EXERCISE 16 ■ Diagnostic Terms Built from Word Parts

A Fill In

Build diagnostic terms for the following definitions by using the word parts you have learned.

1. measurement of pressure (within the eye)   _____ / ____ / _____
                                                                          WR   CV   S

2. instrument used to measure (the curvature of) the cornea   _____ / ____ / _____
                                                                           WR   CV   S

3. measurement of vision   _____ / ____ / _____
                                       WR   CV   S

4. instrument used to measure pressure (within the eye)   _____ / ____ / _____
                                                         WR   CV   S

5. instrument used for visual examination of the pupil   _____ / ____ / _____
                                                WR   CV   S

6. visual examination of the retina   _____ / ____ / _____
                                          WR   CV   S

B Label

Build terms pictured by writing word parts above definitions.

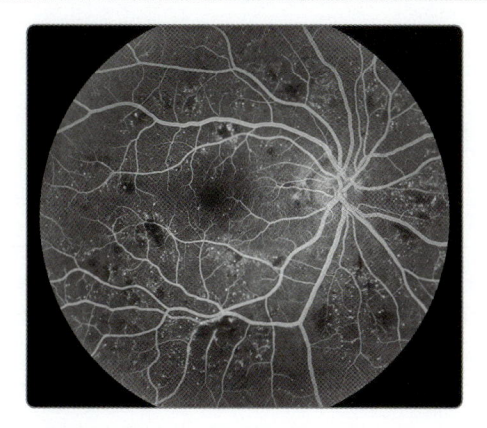

1. fluorescein _____ / ____ / _____
               blood vessel   CV radiographic imaging

2. _____ / ____ / _____
      pupil CV instrument used to measure

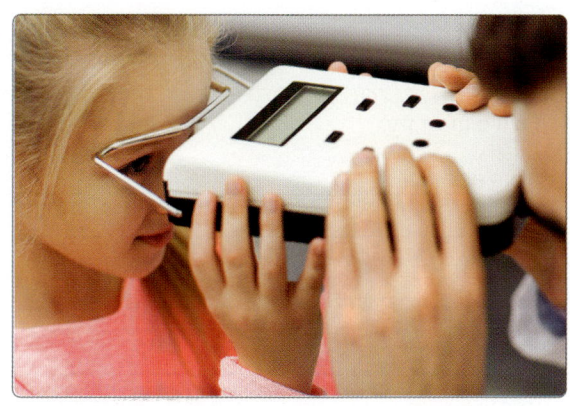

490　Chapter 12　Eye

3.

_____ / ___ / _____
　eye　　　CV　　visual examination

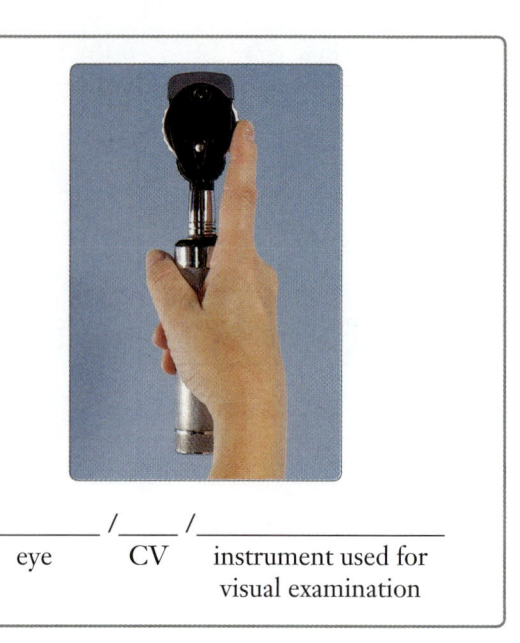

4.

_____ / ___ / _____
　eye　　　CV　　instrument used for
　　　　　　　　　visual examination

C　Analyze and Define

Analyze and define the following diagnostic terms.

1. pupilloscope
   _____
   _____

2. optometry
   _____
   _____

3. ophthalmoscope
   _____
   _____

4. tonometry
   _____
   _____

5. pupillometer
   _____
   _____

6. tonometer
   _____
   _____

7. keratometer
   _____
   _____

8. ophthalmoscopy
   _____
   _____

9. (fluorescein) angiography
   _____
   _____

10. retinoscopy
    _____
    _____

Chapter 12 Eye 491

EXERCISE 17 ■ Diagnostic Terms NOT Built from Word Parts

A Label

Write the diagnostic terms pictured and defined.

1. _____
horizontally mounted binocular microscope that uses a very narrow vertical beam of light to examine the eye in great detail

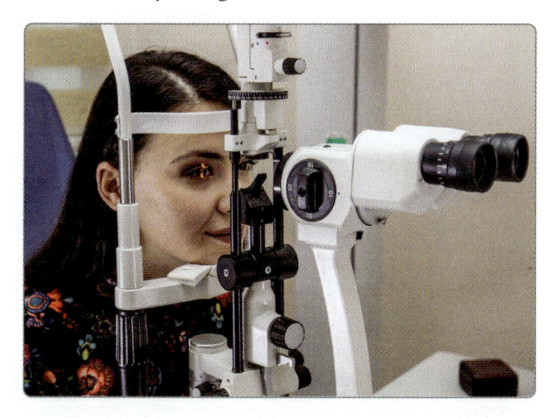

2. _____
noninvasive test that uses light waves to take cross-sectional images of the retina.

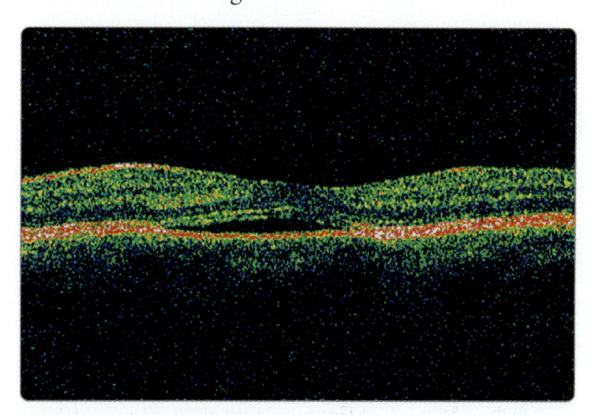

3. _____
use of an ophthalmoscope to view the back of the eye, including the choroid, retina, macula, retinal blood vessels, and the optic disc

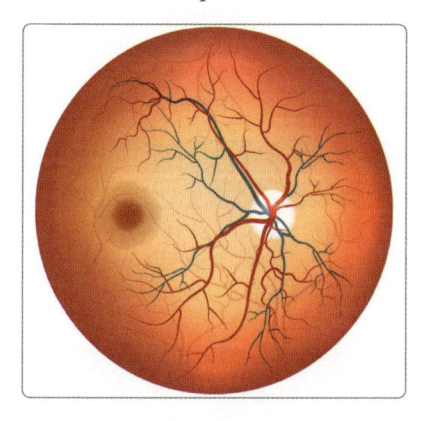

4. _____
instrument with many dials used to evaluate refractive errors and determine the lens curve and shape needed to correct vision

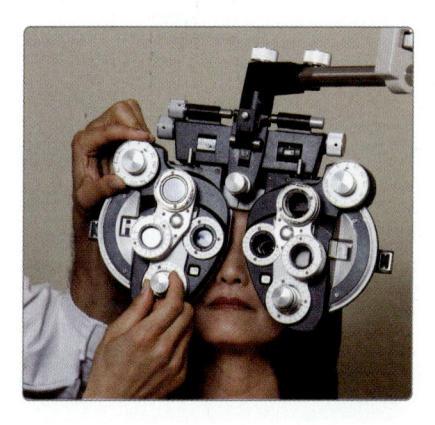

B Identify

Fill in the blanks with the correct terms.

1. _____ _____ _____ is used to detect many eye conditions, including retinopathy and optic nerve damage.

2. A binocular microscope, mounted horizontally, that uses a vertical beam of light, or _____ _____, is especially useful for viewing structures in the front of the eye, including the conjunctiva, cornea, and lens.

3. The _____, an instrument with many dials, is used by an optometrist to evaluate refractive errors and determine the lens curve and shape needed to correct vision.

4. The use of an ophthalmoscope to examine the back of the eye, or _____, is a routine part of examining the eye and can be done with or without dilation of the pupils.

EXERCISE 18 ■ Review of Diagnostic Terms

Can you define, pronounce, and spell the following terms?

fluorescein angiography (FA)	ophthalmoscope	optometry	retinoscopy
	ophthalmoscopy	phoropter	slit lamp
fundus examination	optical coherence tomography (OCT)	pupillometer	tonometer
keratometer		pupilloscope	tonometry

Complementary Terms
BUILT FROM WORD PARTS AND *NOT* BUILT FROM WORD PARTS

The first portion of the table contains Eye Complementary Terms that can be translated using definitions of word parts. The second portion of the table contains Eye Complementary Terms that cannot be fully understood using the definitions of word parts.

■ Built from Word Parts

SIGNS AND SYMPTOMS

TERM	DEFINITION	TERM	DEFINITION
1. anisocoria (an-ī-sō-KŌR-ē-a)	condition of absence of equal pupil (size) (unequal size of pupils)	4. photophobia (fō-tō-FŌ-bē-a)	abnormal fear of (sensitivity to) light
2. isocoria (ī-sō-KŌR-ē-a)	condition of equal pupil (size)	5. pseudophakia (soo-dō-FĀ-ke-a)	condition of false lens (placement of an intraocular lens during surgery to treat cataracts)
3. leukocoria (lū-kō-KŌ-rē-a)	condition of white pupil		

MEDICAL SPECIALTIES

TERM	DEFINITION	TERM	DEFINITION
6. ophthalmologist (of-thal-MOL-o-jist)	physician (surgeon) who studies and treats diseases of the eye	7. ophthalmology (Ophth) (of-thal-MOL-o-jē)	study of the eye (branch of medicine that treats diseases of the eye)

DESCRIPTIVE TERMS

TERM	DEFINITION	TERM	DEFINITION
8. binocular (bin-OK-ū-lar)	pertaining to two or both eyes	13. ophthalmic (of-THAL-mik)	pertaining to the eye
9. corneal (KOR-nē-al)	pertaining to the cornea	14. optic (OP-tik)	pertaining to vision
10. intraocular (in-tra-OK-ū-lar)	pertaining to within the eye	15. pupillary (PŪ-pi-lar-ē)	pertaining to the pupil
11. lacrimal (LAK-ri-mal)	pertaining to tear(s)	16. retinal (RET-i-nal)	pertaining to the retina
12. nasolacrimal (nā-zō-LAK-ri-mal)	pertaining to the nose and tear (ducts)		

■ *NOT* Built from Word Parts

SIGNS AND SYMPTOMS

TERM	DEFINITION
1. **emmetropia (Em)** (*em*-e-TRŌ-pē-a)	normal refractive condition of the eye
2. **visual acuity (VA)** (VIZH-ū-al) (a-KŪ-i-tē)	sharpness of vision measured from a distance using a standardized chart

MEDICAL SPECIALTIES

TERM	DEFINITION
3. **optician** (op-TISH-in)	specialist who fills prescriptions for lenses (cannot prescribe lenses)
4. **optometrist** (op-TOM-e-trist)	health professional who diagnoses, treats, and manages diseases and disorders of the eyes and visual processing system; doctor of optometry (OD)

🏛 **OPTOMETRIST** is derived from the Greek **optikos**, meaning **sight**, and **metron**, meaning **measure**. Literally, an optometrist is a person who measures sight.

TREATMENTS

TERM	DEFINITION
5. **intraocular lens (IOL)** (*in*-tra-OK-ū-lar) (lenz)	artificial lens implanted within the eye during cataract surgery
6. **miotic** (mī-OT-ik)	agent that contracts the pupil
7. **mydriatic** (*mid*-rē-AT-ik)	agent that dilates the pupil

🔍 Refer to **Appendix E** for pharmacology terms related to the eye.

EXERCISE 19 ■ Pronounce and Spell

Practice pronunciation and spelling on paper and online.

1. **Practice on Paper**
   a. **Pronounce:** Read the phonetic spelling and say aloud the terms listed in the previous table. Refer to Table 2.2 Pronunciation Key as needed.
   b. **Spell:** Have a study partner read the terms aloud. Write the spelling of the terms on a separate sheet of paper.

2. **Practice Online** 🌐
   a. **Access** online learning resources. Go to evolve.elsevier.com > Evolve Resources > Student Resources.
   b. **Pronounce:** Select Audio Glossary > Chapter 12 > Exercise 19. Select a term to hear its pronunciation and repeat aloud.
   c. **Spell:** Select Activities > Chapter 12 > Spell Terms > Exercise 19. Select the audio icon and type the correct spelling of the term.

❑ Check the box when complete.

EXERCISE 20 ■ Complementary Terms Built from Word Parts

A Analyze and Define

Analyze and define the following complementary terms.

1. ophthalmology

2. binocular

3. lacrimal

4. pupillary

5. ophthalmologist

6. corneal

7. ophthalmic

8. nasolacrimal

9. optic

10. intraocular

11. retinal

12. photophobia

13. isocoria

14. anisocoria

15. pseudophakia

16. leukocoria

B Label

Build terms pictured by writing word parts above definitions.

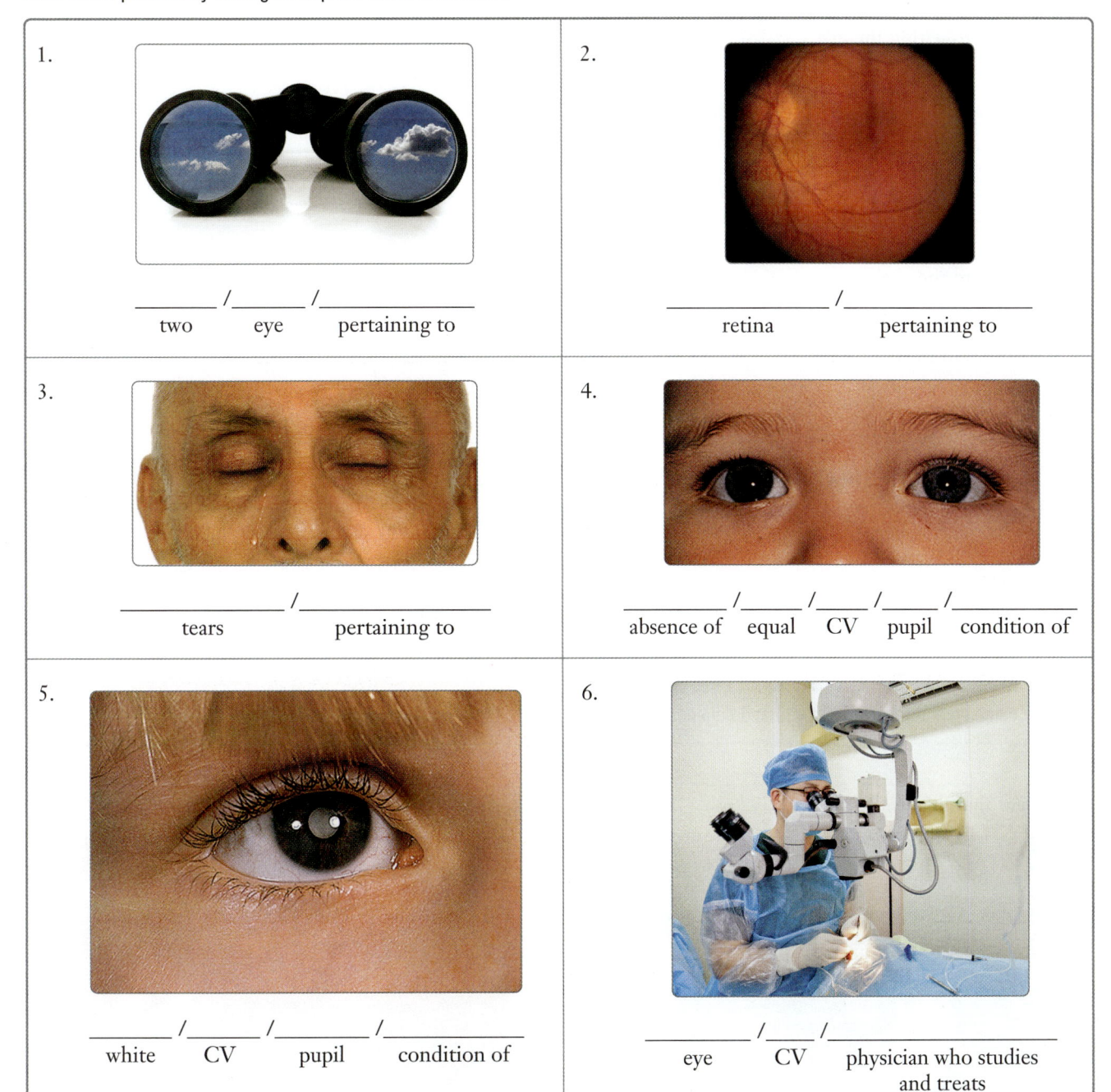

1. _____ / _____ / _____
   two   eye   pertaining to

2. _____ / _____
   retina   pertaining to

3. _____ / _____
   tears   pertaining to

4. _____ / _____ / ____ / _____ / _____
   absence of equal   CV   pupil   condition of

5. _____ / _____ / _____ / _____
   white   CV   pupil   condition of

6. _____ / ____ / _____
   eye   CV   physician who studies
                       and treats

C Fill In

Build complementary terms for the following definitions by using the word parts you have learned.

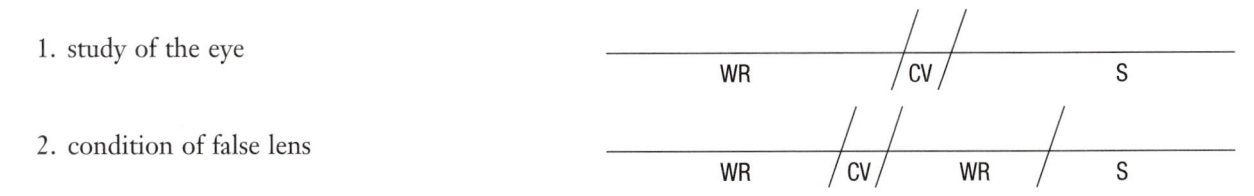

1. study of the eye   _____ / ____ / _____
                              WR   CV   S

2. condition of false lens _____ / ____ / _____ / _____
                              WR   CV   WR   S

3. condition of equal pupil (size) _____ / ____ / _____ / ____
   WR   CV   WR   S

4. pertaining to within the eye _____ / _____ / ____
   P   WR   S

5. abnormal fear of (sensitivity to) light _____ / ____ / ____
   WR   CV   S

6. pertaining to the pupil _____ / ____
   WR   S

7. pertaining to the eye _____ / ____
   WR   S

8. pertaining to the cornea _____ / ____
   WR   S

9. pertaining to the nose and tear (ducts) _____ / ____ / _____ / ____
   WR   CV   WR   S

10. pertaining to vision _____ / ____
    WR   S

EXERCISE 21 ■ Complementary Terms NOT Built from Word Parts

A Label

Write the complementary terms pictured and defined.

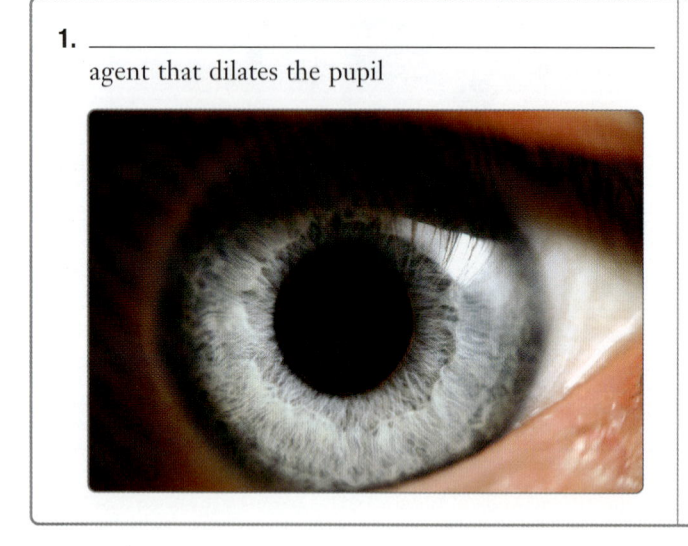

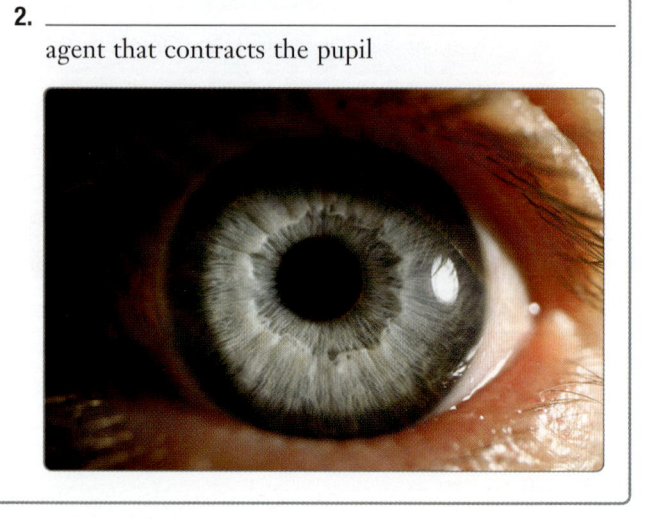

1. _____
   agent that dilates the pupil

2. _____
   agent that contracts the pupil

3. _____
artificial lens implanted within the eye during cataract surgery

4. _____
sharpness of vision measured from a distance using a standardized chart

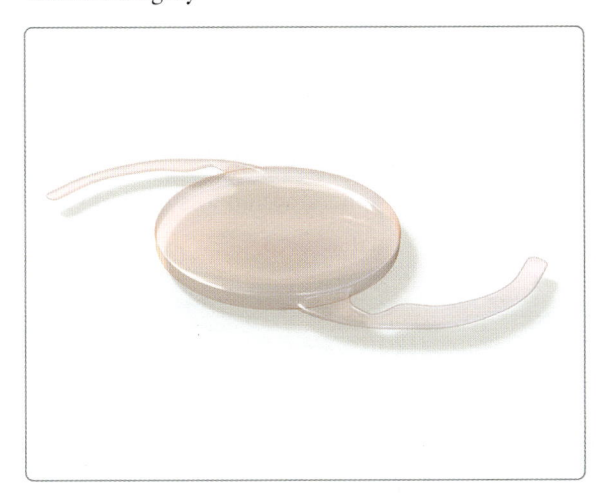

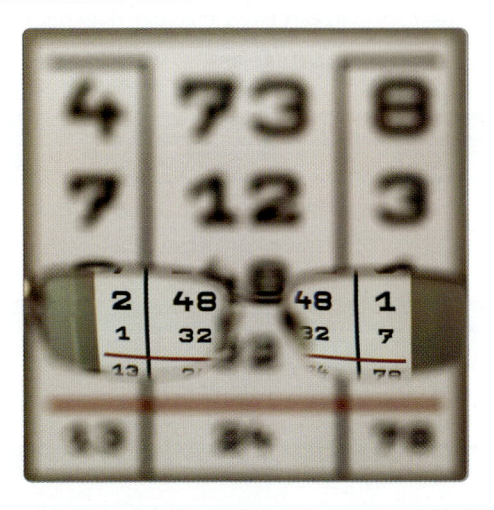

B Identify

Fill in the blanks with the correct terms.

1. Health professional who diagnoses, treats, and manages diseases and disorders of the eyes and visual processing system is a(n) _____.
2. Specialist who fills prescriptions for lenses but who cannot prescribe lenses is a(n) _____.
3. Normal refractive condition of the eye is called _____.

C Match

Match the terms in the first column with their correct definitions in the second column.

_____ 1. optician
_____ 2. intraocular lens
_____ 3. visual acuity
_____ 4. mydriatic
_____ 5. emmetropia
_____ 6. optometrist
_____ 7. miotic

a. sharpness of vision measured from a distance using a standardized chart
b. health professional who diagnoses, treats, and manages diseases and disorders of the eyes and visual processing system
c. agent that contracts the pupil
d. specialist who fills prescriptions for lenses (cannot prescribe lenses)
e. artificial lens implanted within the eye during cataract surgery
f. agent that dilates the pupil
g. normal refractive condition of the eye

EXERCISE 22 ■ Review of Complementary Terms

Can you define, pronounce, and spell the following terms?

anisocoria	isocoria	ophthalmic	photophobia
binocular	lacrimal	optic	pseudophakia
corneal	leukocoria	optician	pupillary
emmetropia (Em)	miotic	ophthalmologist	retinal
intraocular	mydriatic	ophthalmology (Ophth)	visual acuity (VA)
intraocular lens (IOL)	nasolacrimal	optometrist	

Abbreviations

DISEASE AND DISORDER

ABBREVIATION	TERM	ABBREVIATION	TERM
AMD	age-related macular degeneration	RP	retinitis pigmentosa
Ast	astigmatism		

SIGNS AND SYMPTOMS

ABBREVIATION	TERM	ABBREVIATION	TERM
Em	emmetropia	PVL	peripheral vision loss (tunnel vision)
IOP	intraocular pressure	VA	visual acuity

DIAGNOSTIC

ABBREVIATION	TERM	ABBREVIATION	TERM
FA	fluorescein angiography	OCT	optical coherence tomography

TREATMENTS

ABBREVIATION	TERM	ABBREVIATION	TERM
LASIK	laser-assisted in situ keratomileusis; spoken as a whole word (LĀ-sik)	PRK	photorefractive keratectomy
		IOL	intraocular lens
PHACO	phacoemulsification; spoken as a whole word (fā-kō)		

MEDICAL SPECIALTY

ABBREVIATION	TERM	ABBREVIATION	TERM
Ophth	ophthalmology	OD	doctor of optometry

DESCRIPTIVE

ABBREVIATION	TERM
OD	right eye
OS	left eye
OU	both eyes

ERROR-PRONE ABBREVIATIONS The Institute for Safe Medical Practices (ISMP) maintains a list of abbreviations that are frequently misinterpreted and can lead to medical errors. **OD**, **OS**, and **OU** appear on the list and are considered to be error-prone abbreviations.

EXERCISE 23 ■ Abbreviations

Write the terms abbreviated.

1. Diagnostic tests related to the eye include **FA** _____ _____ and **OCT** _____ _____ _____. Both tests can be used to assess the severity of **AMD** _____-_____ _____ _____.
2. Cataracts, if left untreated, can lead to a decrease in **VA** _____ _____. **PHACO** _____ is one type of treatment for this condition; an **IOL** _____ _____ is inserted during the same procedure.
3. **PRK** _____ _____ and **LASIK** _____-_____ _____ _____ _____ are both used to correct **Ast** _____, hyperopia, and myopia, with the goal of establishing **Em** _____.
4. Patients with glaucoma have increased **IOP** _____ _____. Treatment involves medications and/or surgery. Frequent **Ophth** _____ follow-up is required.
5. Symptoms of **RP** _____ include nyctalopia and **PVL** _____ _____ _____.
6. An optometrist is a healthcare professional who has received an **OD** _____ _____ and provides primary vision care.

7. Though considered error-prone, the following abbreviations are commonly used in eye exam documentation:

OD _____ _____, originating from the Latin meaning of *oculus dexter*

OS _____ _____, originating from the Latin meaning of *oculus sinister*

OU _____ _____, originating from the Latin meaning of *oculus uterque*

PRACTICAL APPLICATION

EXERCISE 24 ■ Case Study: Translate Between Everyday Language and Medical Language

CASE STUDY: Anjit Singh

Anjit Singh, a 2-year-old boy, was brought by his parents to the pediatrician for his well-child examination. His mother noted that lately he seemed to be having trouble seeing things that he could identify previously and that one of his eyes seemed to move more slowly and to look in a different direction. Also, the white part of the same eye seemed to be irritated and looked red and inflamed. She also noticed that on a recent flash photograph that she took of her son, one pupil had a typical "red eye" look, but the other pupil looked white. The pediatrician agreed that there was a problem and sent Anjit to an eye physician for further workup.

Now that you have worked through Chapter 12, consider the medical terms that might be used to describe Anjit's experience. See the Chapter at a Glance section at the end of the chapter for a list of terms that might apply.

A. Underline phrases in the case study that could be substituted with medical terms.

B. Write the medical term and its definition for three of the phrases you underlined.

MEDICAL TERM	DEFINITION
1. _____	_____
2. _____	_____
3. _____	_____

DOCUMENTATION: Excerpt From Ophthalmology Visit

Anjit was examined by an ophthalmologist; an excerpt from the medical record is documented below.

Anjit Singh is a 2-year-old male referred by his pediatrician for issues related to his left eye. He is accompanied by his mother and father. History is significant for leukocoria, strabismus with resultant amblyopia, and scleritis. There is no family history of eye disease. Ophthalmoscopy reveals the absence of a red reflex on the left, with confirmation of leukocoria in that eye. The left eye also deviates outward on extraocular motor testing, and visual acuity is markedly decreased on the left. Retinal exam reveals a normal right eye and a mass suspicious for retinoblastoma in the left.

C. Underline medical terms presented in Chapter 12 used in the previous excerpt from Anjit's medical record. See the Chapter at a Glance section at the end of the chapter for a complete list.

D. Select and define three of the medical terms you underlined. To check your answers, go to Appendix A.

MEDICAL TERM	DEFINITION
1. _____	_____
2. _____	_____
3. _____	_____

500 Chapter 12 Eye

EXERCISE 25 ■ Interact With Medical Documents

A

Read the report and complete it by writing medical terms on answer lines within the document. Definitions of terms to be written appear after the document.

763217 GRAVES, William

Name: GRAVES, William   MR#: 763217   Sex: M   Allergies: None known
DOB: 6/27/19XX   Age: 66   PCP: Murphy, Clara MD

Ophthalmology Clinic Visit
Date: 03 April 20XX 10:15

Subjective: Mr. Graves is a 66-year-old male here today for his annual 1._____ exam. He has no current complaint. He has a family history of 2._____ in his brother. He has a history of hypertension and type 2 diabetes mellitus. A 3._____ was removed from his right eye 5 years ago.

Medications: Glyburide 5 mg bid and metoprolol 50 mg bid.

Objective:
Visual Acuities: Aided: OD = 20/25, OS = 20/30-1, OU = 20/25
                Unaided: OD = 20/100, OS = 20/80-1, OU = 20/80

Externals: 2 mm 4._____, right eye.
    PERLA (pupils equal and reactive to light and accommodation).
    EOMI (extraocular movements intact).

Ophthalmoscopic:
    Lens: left eye showed early cortical spokes
    Disk: margins normal
    Cup-to-disk ratio: 0.2 both eyes
    Fundus: scattered microaneurysms bilaterally, with dot and blot hemorrhages noted in all four quadrants of both eyes
    Refraction: OD = 1.00-0.50 × 90 20/20, OS = 1.25-0.25 × 90 20/20
    Tonometry: OD = 14 mm Hg, OS = 13 mm Hg

Visual Field: Full

Assessment: Patient has compound myopic 5._____ and 6._____ with diabetic 7._____ and grade 2 hypertension. He also shows an early 8._____ in the left eye.

Plan: Provide prescription for corrective lenses. See patient for follow-up visit in 6 months to reevaluate diabetic retinopathy and cataract. Counseled patient to report any sudden changes in vision.

Electronically signed: Rwabunihi, Anella MD on 05 April 20XX 14:00

Definitions of Medical Terms to Complete the Document
Write the medical terms defined on corresponding answer lines in the document.

1. study of the eye
2. eye disorder characterized by the increase of intraocular pressure
3. thin tissue growing into the cornea from the conjunctiva
4. drooping of the eyelid
5. irregular curvature of the cornea or lens
6. impaired vision as a result of aging
7. (any noninflammatory) disease of the retina
8. clouding of the lens of the eye

B

Read the patient profile and answer the questions below it.

> **Patient Profile**
>
> This 70-year-old woman was admitted for surgical treatment of chronic, poorly controlled glaucoma and for cataract extraction.
>
> **Subjective:** The patient reported a progressive loss of **visual acuity** in her right eye; she complained of headaches and problems with glare (particularly at night) and said she perceives halos around lights.
>
> **Objective:** Vision testing and physical examination (i.e., **ophthalmoscopy, slit lamp** microscopy, and **tonometry**) revealed acuity (unaided) of 20/100 for the right eye and 20/60 for the left eye. Opacification of right lens was evident, as was moderate **corneal** edema. **Intraocular** pressure measurements were 28 mm Hg in the right eye and 21 mm Hg in the left eye.
>
> **Therapeutic Management:** After a **mydriatic** agent was applied to the right pupil, a combined procedure, **phacoemulsification** of the cataract and **trabeculectomy** with releasable sutures (to minimize **IOP**), was performed with the patient under local anesthesia. The patient tolerated the procedure well and returned to her room wearing a 12-hour collagen shield on the treated eye.

Use the patient profile above to answer the questions.

1. Vision testing and physical examination of the patient revealed opacification of the right lens, confirming the need for:
   a. PRK
   b. phacoemulsification
   c. scleral buckling
   d. enucleation

2. Application of a mydriatic agent would:
   a. reduce tears
   b. produce tears
   c. contract the pupil
   d. dilate the pupil

3. A trabeculectomy was performed because the patient had a history of:
   a. condition of crossed eyes
   b. disorder characterized by increased intraocular pressure
   c. nearsightedness
   d. progressive deterioration of a portion of the retina

4. The abbreviation IOP stands for:
   a. both eyes
   b. normal vision
   c. intraocular pressure
   d. iris outer pupil

EXERCISE 26 ■ Use Medical Language in Online Electronic Health Records

Select the correct medical terms to complete three medical records in one patient's electronic file.

🌐 Access online resources at evolve.elsevier.com > Evolve Resources > Student Resources > Activities > Chapter 12 > Electronic Health Records

Topic: Glaucoma
Record 1, Chart Review: New Patient Evaluation
Record 2, Referrals: Consultation
Record 3, Procedures: Operative Report

❏ Check the box when complete.

EXERCISE 27 — Use Medical Terms in Clinical Statements

For each phrase printed in bold, circle the medical term or abbreviation defined. Answers are listed in Appendix A. For pronunciation practice, read the answers aloud.

1. The **physician who studies and treats diseases of the eye** (ophthalmologist, optometrist, optician) is trained in surgery and specializes in eye and vision care, including the diagnosis and treatment of diseases and disorders of the eye, performing eye surgery, and prescribing lenses.

2. **A procedure using a laser to reshape corneal tissue** (posterior capsulotomy, LASIK, blepharoplasty) was performed to correct **farsightedness** (astigmatism, hyperopia, myopia).

3. **Excision of a portion of the iris**, called an (iridotomy, iridectomy, iridoplegia), may be performed to treat some forms of an **eye disorder characterized by optic nerve damage, usually caused by an abnormal increase of intraocular pressure** (glaucoma, cataracts, macular degeneration).

4. The goal of **surgical repair of the eyelids** (blepharoptosis, blepharoplasty, blepharitis) is to correct impaired peripheral vision caused by **drooping eyelids** (blepharoptosis, blepharoplasty, blepharitis).

5. The optometrist used a(n) **instrument used to measure (the curvature) of the cornea** (phoropter, keratometer, slit lamp) to collect data for the fitting of the patient's contact lenses.

6. **Vision loss occurring with age** (nyctalopia, presbyopia, keratoconus) may be diagnosed and treated by a(n) **healthcare professional who performs eye exams, administers vision tests, and prescribes corrective lenses** (ophthalmologist, optometrist, optician).

7. The patient presented with a painful redness in both eyes, photophobia, and diminished vision, which suggested the diagnosis of **inflammation of the pigmented muscular structure of the eye** (retinitis, scleritis, iritis).

8. Diabetic **disease of the retina** (retinopathy, retinitis pigmentosa, ophthalmalgia), which may involve swelling and leaking of blood vessels or development of new abnormal blood vessels on the surface of the retina, may be surgically treated by **removal of all or part of the vitreous humor** (trabeculectomy, vitrectomy, iridectomy) and **intense beam of light from a laser to condense, destroy, or bond tissue** (retinal photocoagulation, photorefractive keratectomy, phacoemulsification).

EXERCISE 28 — Pronounce Medical Terms in Use

Practice pronunciation of terms by reading aloud the following paragraphs. Use the phonetic spellings to assist with pronunciation. The script also contains medical terms not presented in the chapter. If interested, research their meanings in a medical dictionary or a reliable online source.

> An elderly gentleman visited his **ophthalmologist** (of-thal-MOL-o-jist) because of decreased vision. A **tonometry** (tō-NOM-e-trē) examination showed borderline readings. **Visual acuity** (VIZH-ū-al) (a-KŪ-i-tē) measurement indicated a mild degree of **myopia** (mī-Ō-pē–a) and **presbyopia** (pres-bē-Ō-pē-a). A diagnosis of **glaucoma** (glaw-KŌ-ma) was suspected in this case and timolol eye drops were prescribed, one drop daily.
>
> A **cataract** (KAT-a-rakt) of the right eye was found. Lens implant surgery, which places an **intraocular lens** (in-tra-OK-ū-lar) (lenz), will be performed when the cataract matures sufficiently. Approximately 5 years ago the patient had a **retinal detachment** (RET-in-al) (dē-TACH-ment) of the left eye. A **scleral buckling** (SKLER-al) (BUK-ling) procedure was performed and was successful in halting the progression of retinal detachment.

CHAPTER REVIEW

EXERCISE 29 ■ Chapter Content Quiz

Test your understanding of terms and abbreviations introduced in this chapter. Circle the letter for the medical term or abbreviation related to the words in italics.

1. Before the exam, a medication to *dilate the pupils* was placed in the patient's eyes using a dropper.
   a. miotic
   b. mydriatic
   c. myopia

2. A person with an *irregular curvature of the cornea or lens* of the eye has:
   a. astigmatism
   b. glaucoma
   c. strabismus

3. To *measure the pressure within the patient's eye*, the optometrist used a:
   a. pupillometer
   b. tonometer
   c. keratometer

4. A patient with an *involuntary jerking movement of the eyes* has a condition known as:
   a. astigmatism
   b. anisometropia
   c. nystagmus

5. The ophthalmologist ordered a *radiographic imaging of the blood vessels of the eye with a dye* to assess the progression of the patient's diabetic retinopathy.
   a. fluorescein angiography
   b. tonometry
   c. ophthalmoscopy

6. A person who is *farsighted* has:
   a. hyperopia
   b. myopia
   c. diplopia

7. *Health professionals who diagnose, treat, and manage diseases and disorders of the eyes and visual processing system* are licensed by the state and have earned doctorate degrees abbreviated as OD.
   a. optician
   b. optometrist
   c. ophthalmologist

8. *Inflammation of the white of the eye* can be very painful and may be associated with an underlying autoimmune disorder, such as rheumatoid arthritis and systemic lupus erythematosus.
   a. scleritis
   b. scleromalacia
   c. conjunctivitis

9. The surgery schedule indicated the patient being treated for cataracts would undergo right eye *PHACO* with IOL.
   a. photorefractive keratectomy
   b. photocoagulation
   c. phacoemulsification

10. During cataract surgery, an intraocular lens was placed in the patient's right eye, which would now be described as having *condition of false lens*.
    a. anisocoria
    b. aphakia
    c. pseudophakia

11. *Progressive deterioration of the retina, resulting in loss of central vision* may be described as dry, in which the blood vessels become thin and brittle, or wet, in which new abnormal vessels develop under the macula.
    a. retinitis pigmentosa
    b. macular degeneration
    c. presbyopia

12. The patient explained that she experienced an *abnormal sensitivity to light* before her migraine.
    a. photophobia
    b. nyctalopia
    c. isocoria

13. In hopes of giving up her glasses, the patient elected to have *a laser procedure to reshape her corneal tissue beneath the surface of the cornea* to treat nearsightedness.
    a. PRK
    b. LASIK
    c. IOP

14. In a surgical procedure, *retinal tissue was condensed using an intense beam of light* to repair retinal tears in the patient's left eye and prevent retinal detachment.
    a. retinal photocoagulation
    b. phacoemulsification
    c. scleral buckling

15. *Inflammation of the tear sac* is an infection of the lacrimal sac, which may be acute or chronic.
    a. blepharitis
    b. endophthalmitis
    c. dacryocystitis

504 Chapter 12 Eye

16. The *instrument used to measure the diameter of the pupil* may be used as a part of a neurological examination to provide an objective measure of pupillary response.
    a. tonometer
    b. pupillometer
    c. keratometer

17. Macular degeneration may be detected by *noninvasive test that uses light waves to take cross-sectional images of the retina.*
    a. fluorescein angiography
    b. tonometry
    c. optical coherence tomography

18. A corneal abrasion might be diagnosed using a *horizontally mounted binocular microscope that uses a very narrow vertical beam of light to examine the eye in great detail.*
    a. slit lamp
    b. keratometer
    c. pupilloscope

19. Autoimmune disorders such as rheumatoid arthritis and lupus may cause *inflammation of the uvea and sclera.*
    a. uveitis
    b. uveoscleritis
    c. scleritis

20. A patient with retinal detachment might require *surgical removal of all or part of the vitreous humor.*
    a. retinal photocoagulation
    b. scleral buckling
    c. vitrectomy

CHAPTER AT A GLANCE — Word Parts New to This Chapter

COMBINING FORMS

blephar/o	dipl/o	ocul/o	pupill/o	
conjunctiv/o	ir/o	ophthalm/o	retin/o	
cor/o	irid/o	opt/o	scler/o	
corne/o	is/o	phac/o	ton/o	
cry/o	kerat/o	phak/o	uve/o	
dacry/o	lacrim/o	phot/o		

PREFIX
bin-

SUFFIXES
-opia
-phobia
-plegia

CHAPTER AT A GLANCE — Eye Terms Built from Word Parts

DISEASE AND DISORDER
aphakia
blepharitis
blepharoptosis
conjunctivitis
dacryocystitis
diplopia
endophthalmitis
iridoplegia
iritis
keratitis
keratomalacia
oculomycosis
ophthalmalgia
ophthalmopathy
ophthalmoplegia
phacomalacia
retinoblastoma
retinopathy
scleritis
scleromalacia
uveitis
uveoscleritis
xerophthalmia

SURGICAL
blepharoplasty
cryoretinopexy
dacryocystorhinostomy
iridectomy
iridotomy
keratoplasty
sclerotomy

DIAGNOSTIC
fluorescein angiography (FA)
keratometer
ophthalmoscope
ophthalmoscopy
optometry
pupillometer
pupilloscope
retinoscopy
tonometer
tonometry

COMPLEMENTARY
anisocoria
binocular
corneal
intraocular
isocoria
lacrimal
leukocoria
nasolacrimal
ophthalmic
ophthalmologist
ophthalmology (Ophth)
optic
photophobia
pseudophakia
pupillary
retinal

CHAPTER AT A GLANCE: Eye Terms *NOT* Built from Word Parts

DISEASE AND DISORDER
amblyopia
anisometropia
astigmatism (Ast)
cataract
chalazion
drusen
glaucoma
hyperopia
hyphema
keratoconus
macular degeneration
myopia
nyctalopia
nystagmus
pinguecula
presbyopia
pterygium
retinal detachment
retinitis pigmentosa (RP)
strabismus
sty

SURGICAL
enucleation
LASIK (laser-assisted in situ keratomileusis)
phacoemulsification (PHACO)
photorefractive keratectomy (PRK)
posterior capsulotomy
retinal photocoagulation
scleral buckling
trabeculectomy
vitrectomy

DIAGNOSTIC
fundus examination
optical coherence tomography (OCT)
phoropter
slit lamp

COMPLEMENTARY
emmetropia (Em)
intraocular lens (IOL)
miotic
mydriatic
optician
optometrist
visual acuity (VA)

PART 2 BODY SYSTEMS

13 Ear

Objectives

Upon completion of this chapter, you will be able to:

1. Pronounce organs and anatomic structures of the ear.
2. Define and spell word parts related to the ear.
3. Define, pronounce, and spell disease and disorder terms related to the ear.
4. Define, pronounce, and spell surgical terms related to the ear.
5. Define, pronounce, and spell diagnostic terms related to the ear.
6. Define, pronounce, and spell complementary terms related to the ear.
7. Interpret the meaning of abbreviations related to the ear.
8. Apply medical language in clinical contexts.

Outline

ANATOMY, 507
Function, 507
Organs and Anatomic Structures of the Ear, 508

WORD PARTS, 509
Combining Forms of the Ear, 509
Combining Forms Used with Ear Terms, 509
Suffixes, 510

MEDICAL TERMS, 513
Disease and Disorder Terms, 513
   Built from Word Parts, 513
   NOT Built from Word Parts, 515
Surgical Terms, 518
   Built from Word Parts, 518
Diagnostic Terms, 521
   Built from Word Parts, 521
Complementary Terms, 523
   Built from Word Parts, 523
Abbreviations, 526

PRACTICAL APPLICATION, 527
CASE STUDY Translate Between Everyday Language and Medical Language, 527
Interact with Medical Documents, 528
Use Medical Language in Online Electronic Health Records, 530
Use Medical Terms in Clinical Statements, 530
Pronounce Medical Terms in Use, 530

CHAPTER REVIEW, 531
Chapter Content Quiz, 531
Chapter at a Glance, 532

Answers to Chapter Exercises, Appendix A

ANATOMY

Function

The two functions of the ear are to hear and to provide the sense of balance. The ear is made up of three parts: the **external ear**, the **middle ear**, and the **inner ear** (Figs. 13.1 and 13.2). The process of hearing begins with the **auricles** directing sound waves into the **external auditory canal.** As the sound waves ripple through the external ear, the **tympanic membrane** vibrates. The **ossicles,** three tiny bones in the middle ear, carry the vibration to the inner ear, where the stimulus is transmitted by the cochlear nerve to the brain and is interpreted as sound.

Balance is a function of the **inner ear** and is maintained through a series of complex processes. The vestibular nerve transmits information about motion and body position from the semicircular canals and the vestibule to the brain for interpretation.

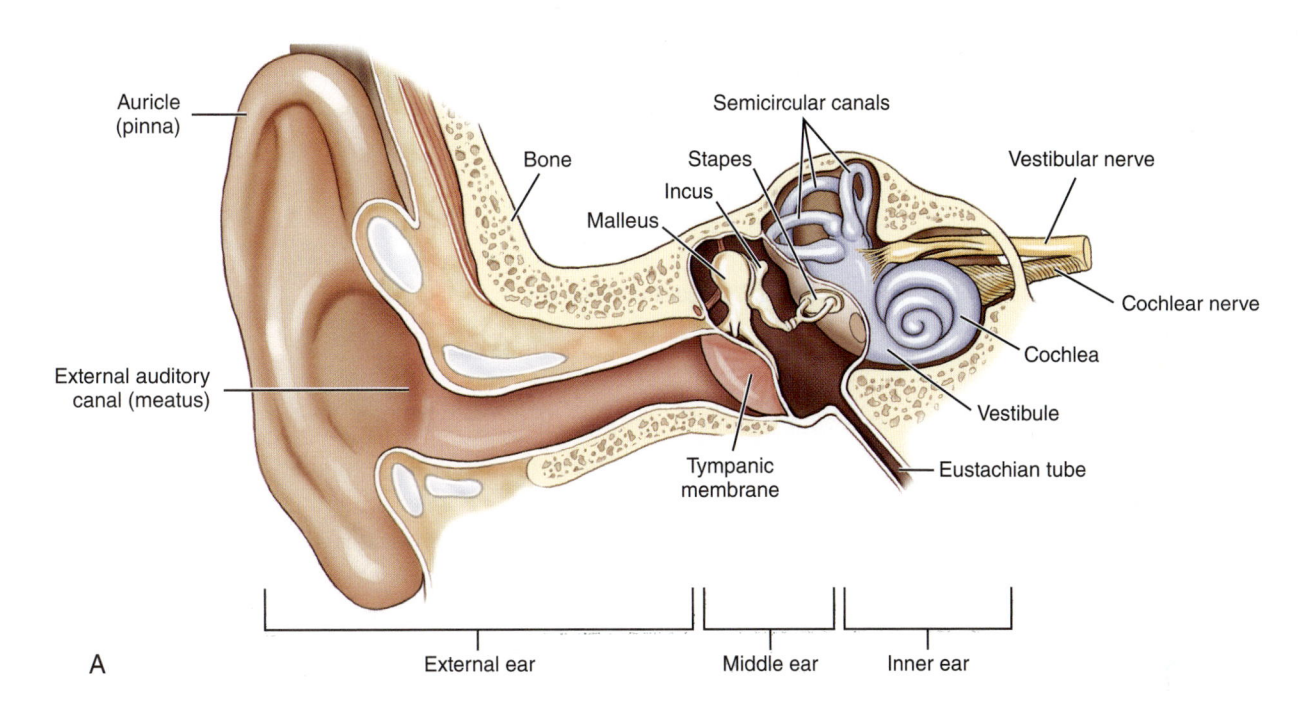

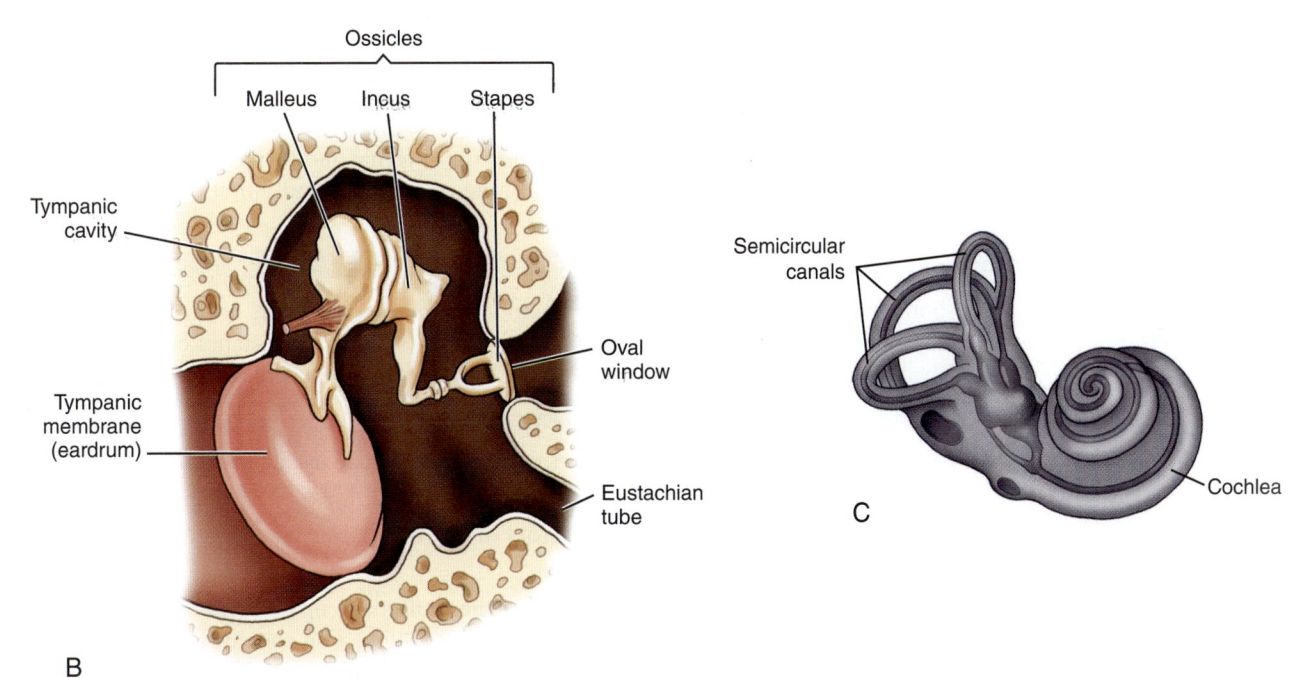

FIG. 13.1 A, Gross anatomy of the ear. **B,** The middle ear. **C,** Labyrinth.

508 Chapter 13 Ear

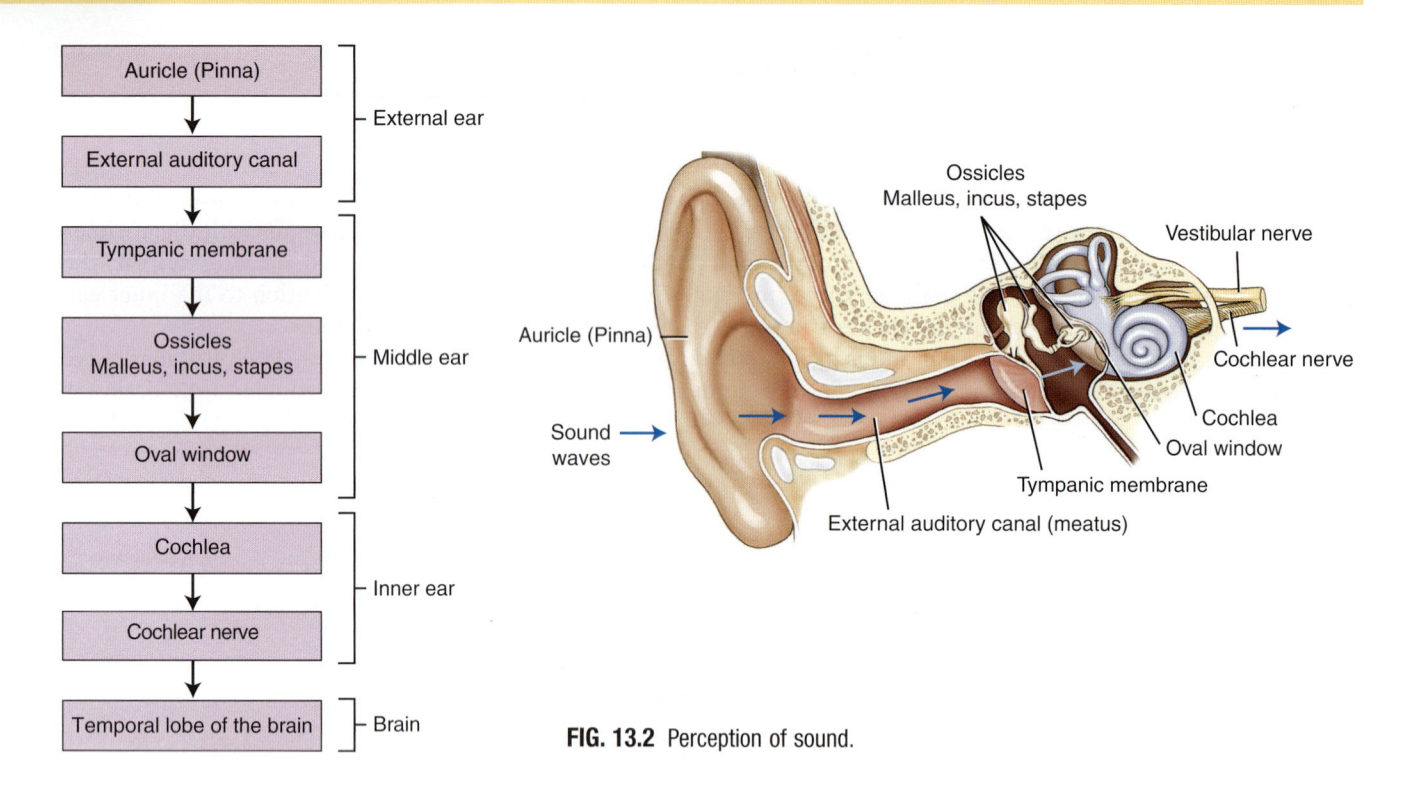

FIG. 13.2 Perception of sound.

Organs and Anatomic Structures of the Ear

TERM	DEFINITION
ear (ēr)	organ of hearing and balance; includes the external ear, middle ear, and labyrinth or inner ear
external ear (ek-STER-nal) (ēr)	consists of the auricle and external auditory canal (meatus)
auricle (AW-ri-kl)	external, visible part of the ear located on both sides of the head; directs sound waves into the external auditory canal (also called **pinna**)
external auditory canal (ek-STER-nal) (AW-di-tor-ē) (kah-NAL)	short tube that ends at the tympanic membrane. The inner part lies within the temporal bone of the skull and contains the glands that secrete earwax (cerumen). (also called **external auditory meatus**)
middle ear (MID-l) (ēr)	consists of the tympanic membrane and the tympanic cavity containing the ossicles
tympanic membrane (tim-PAN-ik) (MEM-brān)	semitransparent membrane that separates the external auditory canal and the middle ear cavity. The tympanic membrane transmits sound vibrations to the ossicles. (also called **eardrum**)
🏛 **TYMPANIC MEMBRANE** is derived from the Greek **tympanon**, meaning **drum**, because of its resemblance to a drum or tambourine.	
ossicles (OS-i-kalz)	bones of the middle ear that carry sound vibrations. The ossicles are composed of the **malleus** (hammer), **incus** (anvil), and **stapes** (stirrup). The stapes connects to the **oval window**, which transmits the sound vibrations to the cochlea of the inner ear.
🏛 **STAPES** is Latin for **stirrup**. The anatomic stapes was so named for its stirrup-like shape.	
eustachian tube (yū-STĀ-shan) (toob)	passage between the middle ear and the pharynx; equalizes air pressure on both sides of the tympanic membrane
inner ear (IN-ar) (ēr)	consists of the labyrinth and connectors of the vestibular and the cochlear nerves
labyrinth (LAB-e-rinth)	bony spaces within the temporal bone of the skull made up of three distinct parts: the cochlea, the semicircular canals, and the vestibule. The cochlea facilitates hearing. The semicircular canals and the vestibule facilitate equilibrium and balance.

TERM	DEFINITION
cochlea (KŌK-lē-ah)	coiled portion of the inner ear containing the sensory organ for hearing; connects to the oval window in the middle ear
semicircular canals and vestibule (sem-ī-SUR-kū-lar) (kah-NALS), (VES-ti-būl)	sensory organs of balance; contain receptors and endolymph that provide sensory information about the body's position to maintain equilibrium
vestibulocochlear nerve (ves-tib-ū-lō-KOK-lē-ar) (nurv)	cranial nerve responsible for hearing and balance; composed of vestibular fibers and cochlear fibers (also called **acoustic nerve** or **auditory nerve**)
vestibular nerve (ves-TIB-ū-lar) (nurv)	cranial nerve branch that conveys information about position and balance from the semicircular canals and vestibule to the brain
cochlear nerve (KOK-lē-ar) (nurv)	cranial nerve branch that conveys information about sound, including volume and frequency, from the cochlea to the brain
mastoid bone (MAS-toid) (bōn)	portion of the temporal bone of the skull posterior and inferior to each auditory canal; contains mastoid air cells that drain into the middle ear cavity behind the external auditory canal (also called **mastoid process**)

PRONOUNCE ANATOMIC STRUCTURES

Practice saying aloud each of the organs and specific structures on the previous pages.

To hear the terms, go to Evolve Resources at www.evolve.elsevier.com and select:

Student Resources > Audio Glossary > Chapter 13 > Anatomic Structures.

❏ Check the box when complete.

WORD PARTS

Use paper flashcards or electronic flashcards on Evolve to memorize word parts used to analyze, define, and build medical terms in this chapter. To reinforce learning, study one section of the Word Parts Table at a time, and then complete the corresponding exercise on the following pages.

1 ▪ Combining Forms of the Ear

COMBINING FORM	DEFINITION	COMBINING FORM	DEFINITION
audi/o	hearing	myring/o	tympanic membrane (eardrum)
aur/i	ear	ot/o	ear
cochle/o	cochlea	staped/o	stapes
labyrinth/o	labyrinth	tympan/o	middle ear
mastoid/o	mastoid bone	vestibul/o	vestibule

2 ▪ Combining Forms Used with Ear Terms

COMBINING FORM	DEFINITION	COMBINING FORM	DEFINITION
electr/o	electricity, electrical activity	py/o	pus
myc/o	fungus		

3 ■ Suffixes

SUFFIX	DEFINITION	SUFFIX	DEFINITION
-al	pertaining to	-metry	measurement
-algia	pain	-osis	abnormal condition (means increase when used with blood cell word roots)
-ar	pertaining to		
-ectomy	excision, surgical removal		
-gram	the record, radiographic image	-plasty	surgical repair
-graphy	process of recording, radiographic imaging	-rrhea	flow, discharge
		-sclerosis	hardening
-itis	inflammation	-scope	instrument used for visual examination
-logist	one who studies and treats (specialist, physician)	-scopy	visual examination
-logy	study of	-stomy	creation of an artificial opening
-meter	instrument used to measure	-tomy	cut into, incision

Refer to **Appendix B** and **Appendix C** for a complete list of word parts.

EXERCISE 1 ■ Combining Forms of the Ear

Refer to the first section of the word parts table.

A Label

Fill in the blanks with combining forms to label this diagram of the ear. *To check your answers, go to Appendix A at the the back of the textbook.*

1. Ear
   CF: _____
   CF: _____

2. Hearing
   CF: _____

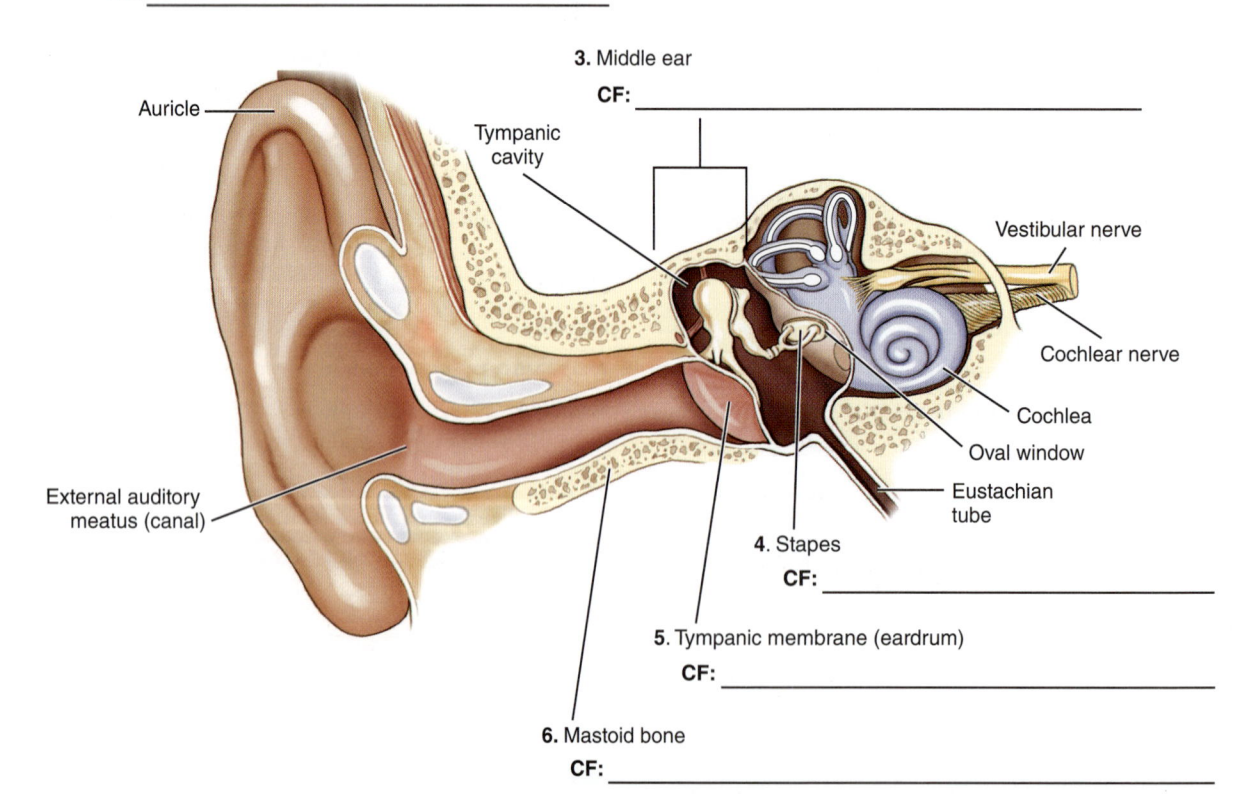

3. Middle ear
   CF: _____

4. Stapes
   CF: _____

5. Tympanic membrane (eardrum)
   CF: _____

6. Mastoid bone
   CF: _____

B Label

Fill in the blanks with combining forms of the ear.

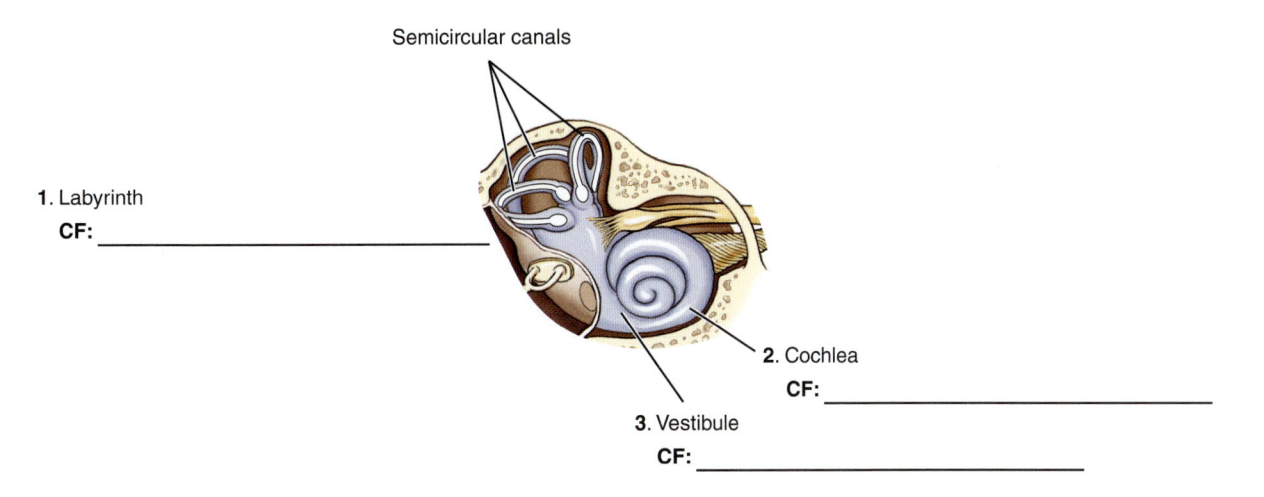

Semicircular canals

1. Labyrinth
   CF: _____

2. Cochlea
   CF: _____

3. Vestibule
   CF: _____

C Define and Match

Step 1: Write the definitions after the following combining forms.
Step 2: Match the descriptions on the right with the combining forms and definitions. Answers may be used more than once; no answer line appears for those not described in a lettered item.

_____ 1. staped/o, _____
_____ 2. vestibul/o, _____
_____ 3. aur/i, _____
_____ 4. cochle/o, _____
_____ 5. labyrinth/o, _____
_____ 6. myring/o, _____
_____ 7. tympan/o, _____
_____ 8. ot/o, _____
_____ 9. mastoid/o, _____
_____ 10. audi/o, _____

a. organ of hearing and balance
b. semitransparent membrane that separates the external auditory canal and the middle ear cavity
c. portion of the temporal bone of the skull posterior and inferior to each auditory canal
d. sensory organ of balance containing receptors and endolymph
e. bony spaces within the temporal bone of the skull made up of three distinct parts: the cochlea, the semicircular canals, and the vestibule
f. coiled portion of the inner ear containing the sensory organ for hearing
g. one of three bones of the middle ear; shaped like a stirrup and connected to the oval window
h. portion of the ear containing the tympanic membrane and the tympanic cavity

EXERCISE 2 ■ Combining Forms Used with Ear Terms

Refer to the second section of the word parts table.

A Define

Write the definitions of the following combining forms.

1. myc/o _____
2. py/o _____
3. electr/o _____

512 Chapter 13 Ear

B Identify

Write the combining form for each of the following.

1. electricity, electrical activity _____
2. fungus _____
3. pus _____

EXERCISE 3 ■ Suffixes

Refer to the third section of the word parts table.

A Match

Match the suffixes in the first column with their definitions in the second column.

_____ 1. -plasty   a. excision, surgical removal
_____ 2. -meter   b. one who studies and treats
_____ 3. -ectomy   c. abnormal condition
_____ 4. -rrhea   d. surgical repair
_____ 5. -osis   e. flow, discharge
_____ 6. -tomy   f. pain
_____ 7. -algia   g. instrument used to measure
_____ 8. -logist   h. instrument used for visual examination
_____ 9. -scope   i. hardening
_____ 10. -sclerosis   j. cut into, incision

B Define

Write definitions for the following suffixes.

1. -stomy _____
2. -scopy _____
3. -metry _____
4. -logy _____

C Identify

Write the suffix for each of the following.

1. process of recording, radiographic imaging _____
2. inflammation _____
3. pertaining to a. _____
             b. _____
4. the record, radiographic image _____

MEDICAL TERMS

Medical terms relevant to this chapter have been grouped by topics, such as Disease and Disorder, and are listed in tables designated as Built from Word Parts or *NOT* Built from Word Parts. The exercises following each table assist with learning term definitions, pronunciations, and spellings.

Disease and Disorder Terms
BUILT FROM WORD PARTS

The following terms can be translated using definitions of word parts. Further explanation is provided within parentheses as needed.

TERM	DEFINITION	TERM	DEFINITION
1. **labyrinthitis** (*lab*-i-rin-THĪ-tis)	inflammation of the labyrinth	6. **otopyorrhea** (ō-tō-*pī*-ō-RĒ-a)	discharge of pus from the ear
2. **mastoiditis** (*mas*-toyd-Ī-tis)	inflammation of the mastoid bone	7. **otorrhea** (ō-tō-RĒ-a)	discharge from the ear (may be serous, bloody, consisting of pus, or containing cerebrospinal fluid)
3. **myringitis** (*mir*-in-JĪ-tis)	inflammation of the tympanic membrane (eardrum)		
4. **otalgia** (ō-TAL-ja)	pain in the ear	8. **otosclerosis** (ō-tō-skle-RŌ-sis)	hardening of the ear (stapes) (caused by irregular bone development and resulting in hearing loss)
5. **otomycosis** (ō-tō-mī-KŌ-sis)	abnormal condition of fungus in the ear (usually affects the external auditory canal)		

EXERCISE 4 ■ Pronounce and Spell

Practice pronunciation and spelling on paper and online.

1. **Practice on Paper**
   a. **Pronounce:** Read the phonetic spelling and say aloud the terms listed in the previous table. Refer to Table 2.2 Pronunciation Key as needed.
   b. **Spell:** Have a study partner read the terms aloud. Write the spelling of the terms on a separate sheet of paper.

2. **Practice Online**
   a. **Access** online learning resources. Go to evolve.elsevier.com > Evolve Resources > Student Resources.
   b. **Pronounce:** Select Audio Glossary > Chapter 13 > Exercise 4. Select a term to hear its pronunciation and repeat aloud.
   c. **Spell:** Select Activities > Chapter 13 > Spell Terms > Exercise 4. Select the audio icon and type the correct spelling of the term.

❏ Check the box when complete.

EXERCISE 5 ■ Analyze and Define

Analyze and define the following terms.

1. otomycosis

2. otalgia

_____

_____

514 Chapter 13 Ear

3. labyrinthitis

_____

_____

4. myringitis

_____

_____

5. otosclerosis

_____

_____

6. mastoiditis

_____

_____

7. otopyorrhea

_____

_____

8. otorrhea

_____

_____

EXERCISE 6 ■ Build

A Label

Build terms pictured by writing word parts above definitions.

1.

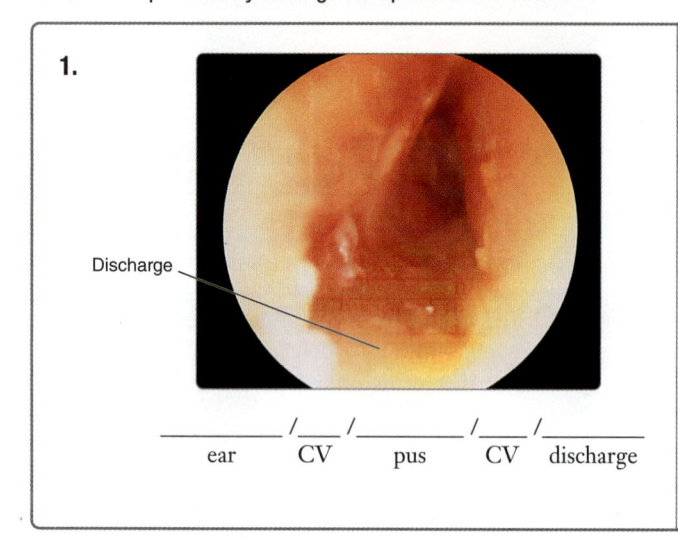

_____ / ___ / _____ / ___ / _____
  ear   CV   pus   CV   discharge

2.

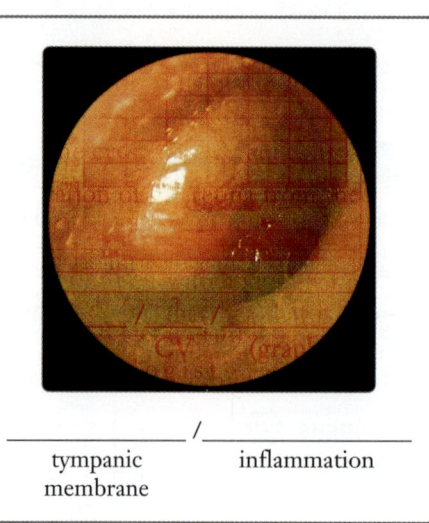

_____ / _____
 tympanic   inflammation
 membrane

B Fill In

Build disease and disorder terms for the following definitions by using the word parts you have learned.

1. inflammation of the mastoid bone

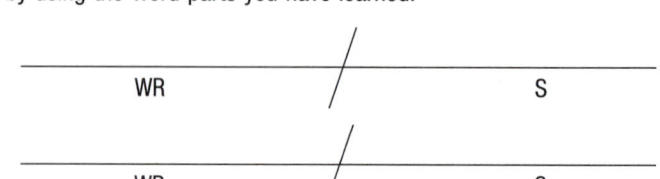

   _____ / _____
     WR   S

2. pain in the ear

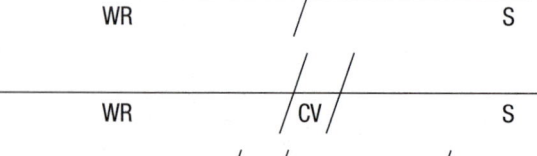

   _____ / _____
     WR   S

3. hardening of the ear (stapes)

   _____ / ___ / _____
     WR   CV   S

4. abnormal condition of fungus in the ear

   _____ / ___ / _____ / _____
     WR   CV   WR   S

5. inflammation of the labyrinth _____ / _____
                                        WR   S

6. discharge from the ear _____ / ___ / _____
                                WR   CV   S

Disease and Disorder Terms
NOT BUILT FROM WORD PARTS

Word parts may be present in the following terms; however, their full meanings cannot be translated using definitions of word parts alone.

TERM	DEFINITION
1. acoustic neuroma (a-KOOS-tik) (nū-RŌ-ma)	benign tumor within the inner ear that forms along the vestibulocochlear nerve; may cause hearing loss and damage structures of the cerebellum as it grows
2. cholesteatoma (ko-le-stē-a-TŌ-ma)	cystlike mass composed of epithelial cells and cholesterol occurring in the middle ear; may be associated with chronic otitis media
3. Ménière disease (me-NYĀR) (di-ZĒZ)	chronic disease of the inner ear characterized by a sensation of spinning motion (vertigo), ringing in the ear (tinnitus), aural fullness, and fluctuating hearing loss; symptoms are related to a change in volume or composition of fluid within the labyrinth
4. otitis externa (OE) (ō-TĪ-tis) (eks-TER-na)	inflammation of the outer ear, specifically the auditory canal
5. otitis media (OM) (ō-TĪ-tis) (MĒ-dē-a)	inflammation of the middle ear (Fig. 13.3A)
6. ototoxicity (ō-tō-tok-SIS-i-tē)	adverse pharmacologic reaction causing damage to the vestibulocochlear nerve; results in abnormalities of hearing and balance
7. presbycusis (prez-bi-KŪ-sis)	hearing impairment occurring with age
8. tinnitus (TIN-i-tus)	ringing in the ears (Note: the ending is **itus** and not **itis**, the usual ending for inflammation)
	The pronunciation of **tinnitus** varies. While healthcare professionals pronounce it as (TIN-i-tus), often the general population uses the alternate pronunciation (tin-NĪ-tus), as though the term ends with the suffix -itis.
9. vertigo (VER-ti-gō)	sense that either one's own body (subjective vertigo) or the environment (objective vertigo) is revolving; may indicate inner ear disease

BENIGN PAROXYSMAL POSITIONAL VERTIGO (BPPV) is characterized by brief episodes of vertigo associated with a change in the position of the head, such as turning over in bed or sitting up in the morning. In BPPV, normal calcium carbonate crystals called otoconia break loose and shift within the labyrinth, triggering an episode of vertigo.

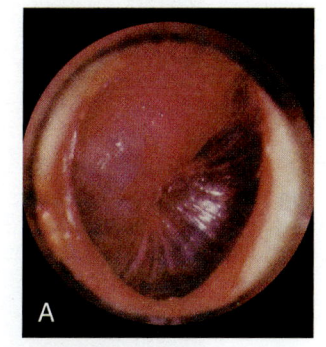

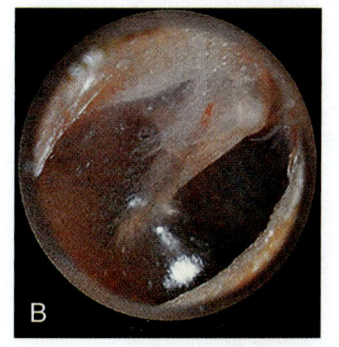

FIG. 13.3 Otitis media. Signs include bulging, perforated, reddened, or retracted tympanic membrane. **A,** Tympanic membrane demonstrating **acute otitis media (AOM)**. **B,** Normal tympanic membrane.

Chapter 13 Ear

EXERCISE 7 ■ Pronounce and Spell

Practice pronunciation and spelling on paper and online.

1. **Practice on Paper**
    a. **Pronounce:** Read the phonetic spelling and say aloud the terms listed in the previous table. Refer to Table 2.2 Pronunciation Key as needed.
    b. **Spell:** Have a study partner read the terms aloud. Write the spelling of the terms on a separate sheet of paper.

2. **Practice Online**
    a. **Access** online learning resources. Go to evolve.elsevier.com > Evolve Resources > Student Resources.
    b. **Pronounce:** Select Audio Glossary > Chapter 13 > Exercise 7. Select a term to hear its pronunciation and repeat aloud.
    c. **Spell:** Select Activities > Chapter 13 > Spell Terms > Exercise 7. Select the audio icon and type the correct spelling of the term.

❏ Check the box when complete.

EXERCISE 8 ■ Fill In

A Identify

Fill in the blanks with the correct terms.

1. The patient reported a sense that her body seemed to be revolving, or _____, and ringing in the ears, or _____.
2. A chronic ear disease characterized by vertigo, tinnitus, aural fullness, and fluctuating hearing loss is called _____ disease.
3. _____ is hearing impairment occurring with age.
4. An adverse reaction causing damage to the vestibulocochlear nerve that results in abnormalities of hearing and balance is _____.

B Label

Write the medical terms pictured and defined.

1. _____
inflammation of the outer ear, specifically the external auditory canal

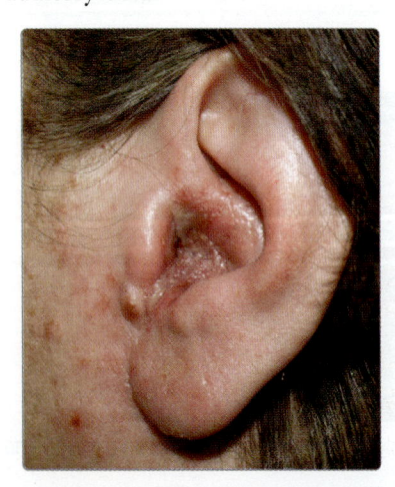

2. _____
inflammation of the middle ear

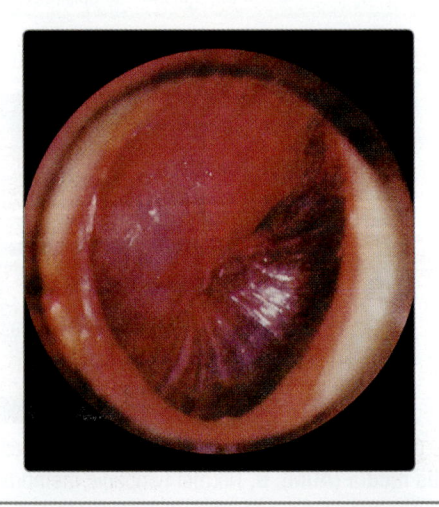

3. _____
cystlike mass composed of epithelial cells and cholesterol occurring in the middle ear

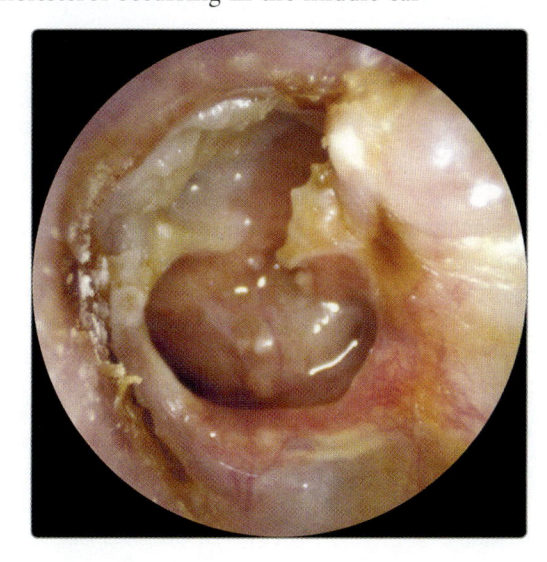

4. _____
benign tumor within the inner ear that forms along the vestibulocochlear nerve

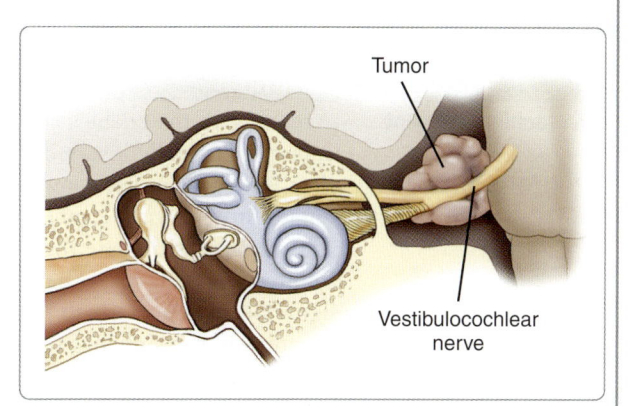

EXERCISE 9 ■ Match

Match the terms in the first column with their correct definitions in the second column.

_____ 1. vertigo
_____ 2. tinnitus
_____ 3. Ménière disease
_____ 4. otitis externa
_____ 5. acoustic neuroma
_____ 6. otitis media
_____ 7. presbycusis
_____ 8. cholesteatoma
_____ 9. ototoxicity

a. inflammation of the middle ear
b. adverse pharmacologic reaction causing damage to the vestibulocochlear nerve
c. benign tumor of the inner ear that forms along the vestibulocochlear nerve
d. sense of revolving of one's own body or the environment
e. ringing in the ears
f. inflammation of the outer ear, specifically the external auditory canal
g. hearing impairment occurring with age
h. mass composed of epithelial cells and cholesterol
i. chronic ear problem characterized by vertigo, tinnitus, and fluctuating hearing loss

EXERCISE 10 ■ Review of Disease and Disorder Terms

Can you define, pronounce, and spell the following terms?

acoustic neuroma	myringitis	otopyorrhea	tinnitus
cholesteatoma	otalgia	otorrhea	vertigo
labyrinthitis	otitis externa (OE)	otosclerosis	
mastoiditis	otitis media (OM)	ototoxicity	
Ménière disease	otomycosis	presbycusis	

Surgical Terms

BUILT FROM WORD PARTS

The following terms can be translated using definitions of word parts. Further explanation is provided within parentheses as needed.

TERM	DEFINITION	TERM	DEFINITION
1. **cochlear implant** (KŌK-lē-ar) (IM-plant)	pertaining to the cochlea implant (surgically inserted electronic device that converts sound into electrical impulses. The impulses stimulate the auditory nerve to carry the signal to the brain, which learns to interpret the signal as sound. The damaged part of the ear is bypassed.)	5. **myringoplasty** (mi-RING-gō-plas-tē)	surgical repair of the tympanic membrane
		6. **myringotomy** (mir-ing-GOT-o-mē)	incision into the tympanic membrane (performed to relieve pressure in the middle ear by releasing pus or fluid and for the placement of tubes)
		7. **otoplasty** (Ō-tō-plas-tē)	surgical repair of the (outer) ear
COCHLEAR IMPLANTS are fitted in adults and children who are deaf or severely hard of hearing.		8. **stapedectomy** (stā-pe-DEK-to-mē)	excision of the stapes (performed to restore hearing in cases of otosclerosis; the stapes is replaced by a prosthesis) (Fig. 13.4)
2. **labyrinthectomy** (lab-i-rin-THEK-to-mē)	excision of the labyrinth		
3. **mastoidectomy** (mas-toy-DEK-to-mē)	excision of the mastoid bone	9. **tympanoplasty** (TIM-pa-nō-plas-tē)	surgical repair (of the hearing mechanism) of the middle ear (including the tympanic membrane and the ossicles)
4. **mastoidotomy** (mas-toy-DOT-o-mē)	incision into the mastoid bone	10. **tympanostomy** (tim-pa-NOS-to-mē)	creation of an artificial opening into the middle ear

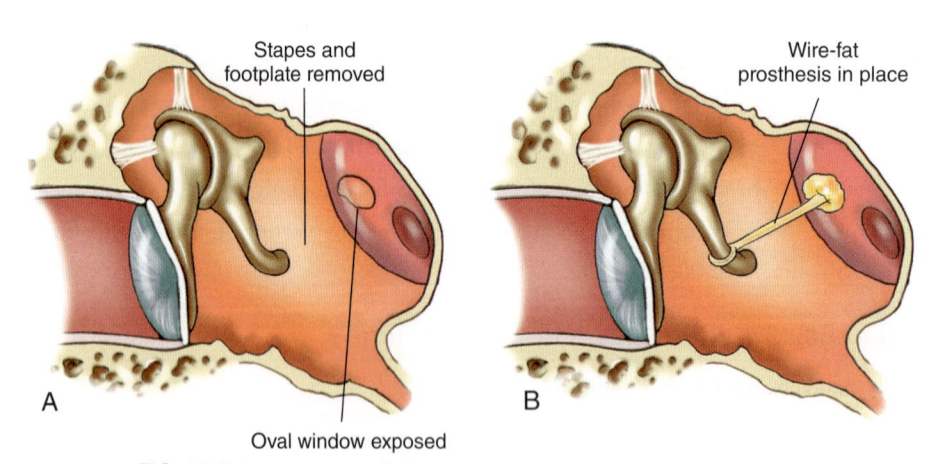

FIG. 13.4 Stapedectomy. **A,** Stapes is removed. **B,** Prosthesis is in place.

EXERCISE 11 ■ Pronounce and Spell

Practice pronunciation and spelling on paper and online.

1. **Practice on Paper**
   a. **Pronounce:** Read the phonetic spelling and say aloud the terms listed in the previous table. Refer to Table 2.2 Pronunciation Key as needed.
   b. **Spell:** Have a study partner read the terms aloud. Write the spelling of the terms on a separate sheet of paper.

2. Practice Online

a. **Access** online learning resources. Go to evolve.elsevier.com > Evolve Resources > Student Resources.
b. **Pronounce:** Select Audio Glossary > Chapter 13 > Exercise 11. Select a term to hear its pronunciation and repeat aloud.
c. **Spell:** Select Activities > Chapter 13 > Spell Terms > Exercise 11. Select the audio icon and type the correct spelling of the term.

❏ Check the box when complete.

EXERCISE 12 ■ Analyze and Define

Analyze and define the following surgical terms.

1. mastoidectomy

2. myringotomy

3. labyrinthectomy

4. mastoidotomy

5. tympanoplasty

6. myringoplasty

7. stapedectomy

8. cochlear (implant)

9. otoplasty

10. tympanostomy

EXERCISE 13 ■ Build

A Fill In

Build surgical terms for the following definitions by using the word parts you have learned.

1. incision into the mastoid bone _____ / _____ / _____
                                                                                  WR   CV   S

2. excision of the labyrinth _____ / _____
                                            WR   S

520 Chapter 13 Ear

3. surgical repair (of the hearing mechanism) of the middle ear

_____ / ____ / _____
WR   CV   S

4. excision of the mastoid bone

_____ / _____
WR   S

5. surgical repair of the (outer) ear

_____ / ____ / _____
WR   CV   S

6. surgical repair of the tympanic membrane

_____ / ____ / _____
WR   CV   S

B Label

Build terms pictured by writing word parts above definitions.

1.

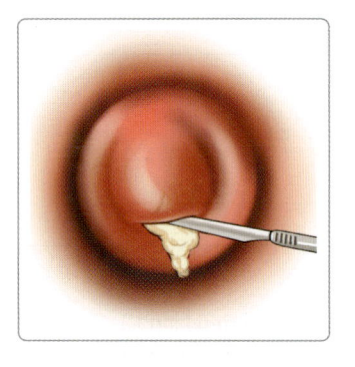

_____ / ____ / _____
tympanic   CV   incision
membrane

2.

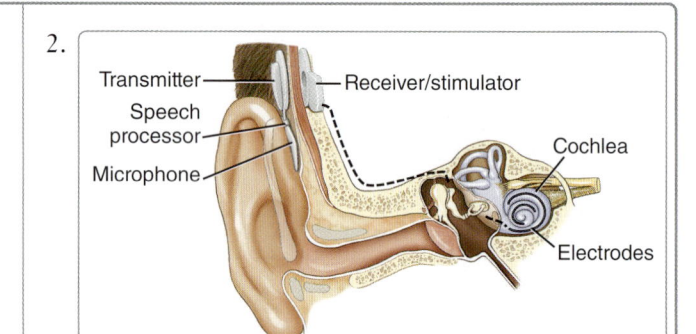

_____ / _____ implant
cochlea   pertaining to

3.

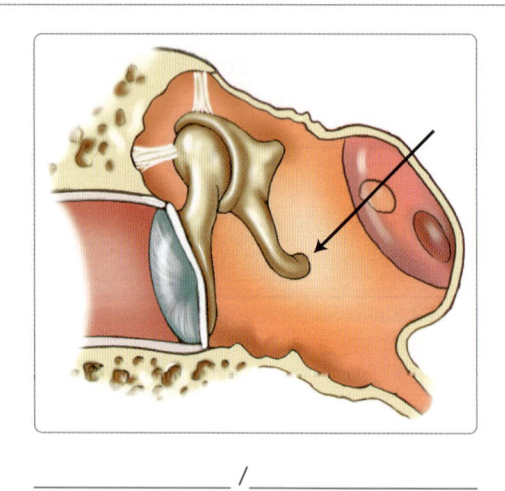

_____ / _____
stapes   excision

4.

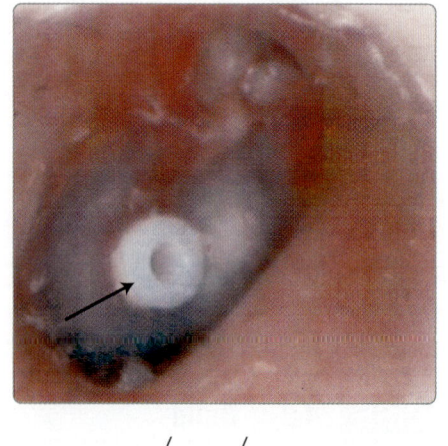

_____ / ____ / _____
middle ear   CV   creation of an
                    artificial opening

EXERCISE 14 ■ Review of Surgical Terms

Can you define, pronounce, and spell the following terms?

cochlear implant   mastoidotomy   otoplasty   tympanoplasty
labyrinthectomy   myringoplasty   stapedectomy   tympanostomy
mastoidectomy   myringotomy

Diagnostic Terms

BUILT FROM WORD PARTS

The following terms can be translated using definitions of word parts. Further explanation is provided within parentheses as needed.

TERM	DEFINITION	TERM	DEFINITION
1. **audiogram** (AW-dē-ō-*gram*)	(graphic) record of hearing	5. **otoscope** (Ō-tō-skōp)	instrument used for visual examination of the ear
2. **audiometer** (*aw*-dē-OM-e-ter)	instrument used to measure hearing	6. **otoscopy** (ō-TOS-ko-pē)	visual examination of the ear
3. **audiometry** (*aw*-dē-OM-e-trē)	measurement of hearing	7. **tympanometer** (*tim*-pa-NOM-e-ter)	instrument used to measure middle ear (function)
4. **electrocochleography** (ē-*lek*-trō-*kok*-lē-OG-ra-fē)	process of recording the electrical activity in the cochlea (in response to sound)	8. **tympanometry** (*tim*-pa-NOM-e-trē)	measurement of middle ear (function)

EXERCISE 15 ■ Pronounce and Spell

Practice pronunciation and spelling on paper and online.

1. **Practice on Paper**
   a. **Pronounce:** Read the phonetic spelling and say aloud the terms listed in the previous table. Refer to Table 2.2 Pronunciation Key as needed.
   b. **Spell:** Have a study partner read the terms aloud. Write the spelling of the terms on a separate sheet of paper.

2. **Practice Online**
   a. **Access** online learning resources. Go to evolve.elsevier.com > Evolve Resources > Student Resources.
   b. **Pronounce:** Select Audio Glossary > Chapter 13 > Exercise 15. Select a term to hear its pronunciation and repeat aloud.
   c. **Spell:** Select Activities > Chapter 13 > Spell Terms > Exercise 15. Select the audio icon and type the correct spelling of the term.

❏ Check the box when complete.

EXERCISE 16 ■ Analyze and Define

Analyze and define the following diagnostic terms.

1. otoscope

2. audiometry

3. audiogram

4. otoscopy

522 Chapter 13 Ear

5. audiometer

_____

_____

6. tympanometry

_____

_____

7. tympanometer

_____

_____

8. electrocochleography

_____

_____

EXERCISE 17 ■ Build

A Label

Build terms pictured by writing word parts above definitions.

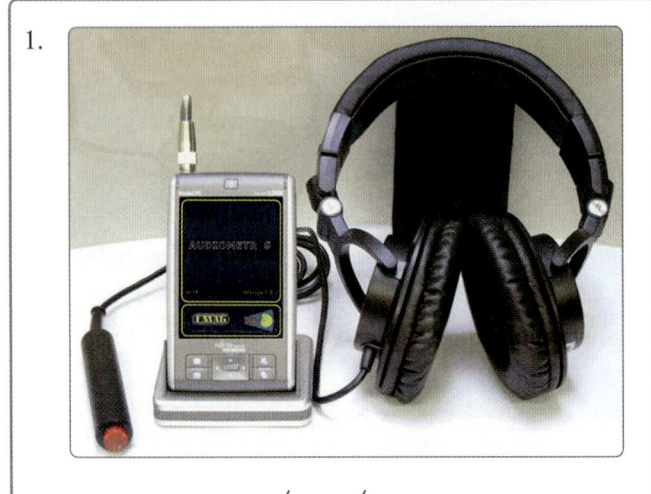

1. _____ / ____ / _____
    hearing   CV   instrument used to measure

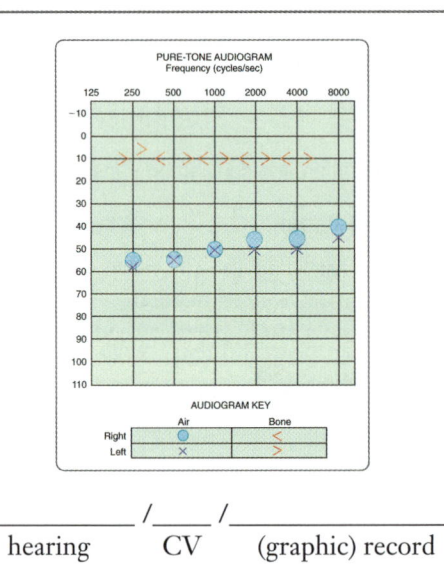

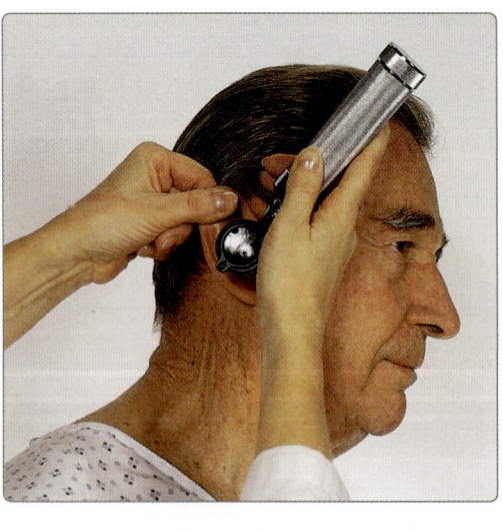

2. _____ / ____ / _____
    hearing   CV   (graphic) record

3. _____ / ____ / _____
    ear   CV   visual examination

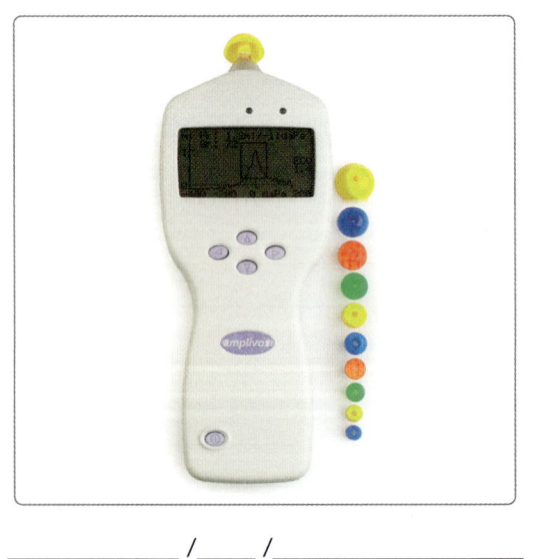

4. _____ / ____ / _____
    middle ear   CV   instrument used to measure

B Fill In

Build diagnostic terms for the following definitions by using the word parts you have learned.

1. measurement of middle ear (function) _____ / ___ / _____
   WR   CV   S

2. instrument used for visual examination of the ear _____ / ___ / _____
   WR   CV   S

3. measurement of hearing _____ / ___ / _____
   WR   CV   S

4. process of recording the electrical activity in the cochlea _____ / __ / _____ / __ / _____
   WR   CV   WR   CV   S

EXERCISE 18 ■ Review of Diagnostic Terms

Can you define, pronounce, and spell the following terms?

audiogram	audiometry	otoscope	tympanometer
audiometer	electrocochleography	otoscopy	tympanometry

Complementary Terms
BUILT FROM WORD PARTS

The following terms can be translated using definitions of word parts. Further explanation is provided within parentheses as needed.

MEDICAL SPECIALTIES

TERM	DEFINITION	TERM	DEFINITION
1. **audiologist** (aw-dē-OL-o-jist)	specialist who studies and treats (impaired) hearing	4. **otolaryngology** (ō-tō-lar-ing-GOL-o-jē)	study of the ear, (nose), and larynx (throat) (branch of medicine that treats diseases of the ear, nose, and throat); also called **otorhinolaryngology**)
2. **audiology** (aw-dē-OL-o-jē)	study of hearing		
3. **otolaryngologist (ENT)** (ō-tō-lar-ing-GOL-o-jist)	physician who studies and treats diseases of the ear, (nose), and larynx (throat); (also called **otorhinolaryngologist**)		

DESCRIPTIVE TERMS

TERM	DEFINITION	TERM	DEFINITION
5. **aural** (AW-rul)	pertaining to the ear	7. **vestibular** (ves-TIB-ū-lar)	pertaining to the vestibule
6. **cochlear** (KOK-lē-ar)	pertaining to the cochlea	8. **vestibulocochlear** (ves-tib-ū-lō-KOK-lē-ar)	pertaining to the vestibule and the cochlea

Refer to **Appendix E** for pharmacology terms related to the ear.

524 Chapter 13 Ear

EXERCISE 19 ■ Pronounce and Spell

Practice pronunciation and spelling on paper and online.

1. **Practice on Paper**
    a. **Pronounce:** Read the phonetic spelling and say aloud the terms listed in the previous table. Refer to Table 2.2 Pronunciation Key as needed.
    b. **Spell:** Have a study partner read the terms aloud. Write the spelling of the terms on a separate sheet of paper.
2. **Practice Online**
    a. **Access** online learning resources. Go to evolve.elsevier.com > Evolve Resources > Student Resources.
    b. **Pronounce:** Select Audio Glossary > Chapter 13 > Exercise 19. Select a term to hear its pronunciation and repeat aloud.
    c. **Spell:** Select Activities > Chapter 13 > Spell Terms > Exercise 19. Select the audio icon and type the correct spelling of the term.

❏ Check the box when complete.

EXERCISE 20 ■ Analyze and Define

Analyze and define the following complementary terms.

1. otolaryngology

2. audiologist

3. otolaryngologist

4. audiology

5. aural

6. cochlear

7. vestibular

8. vestibulocochlear

EXERCISE 21 ■ Build

A Label

Build terms pictured by writing word parts above definitions.

1. _____ / _____ 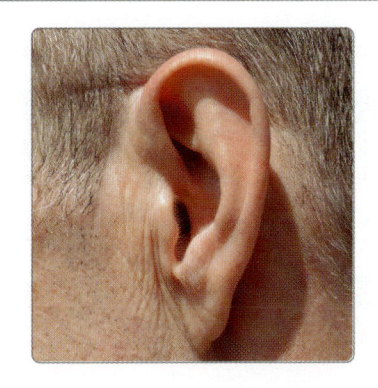
    ear / pertaining to

2. _____ / _____ 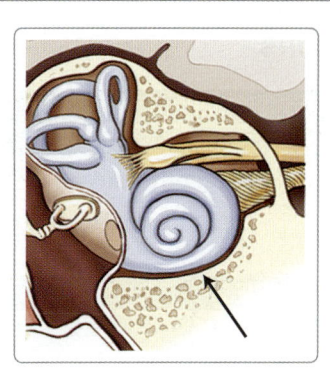
    cochlea / pertaining to

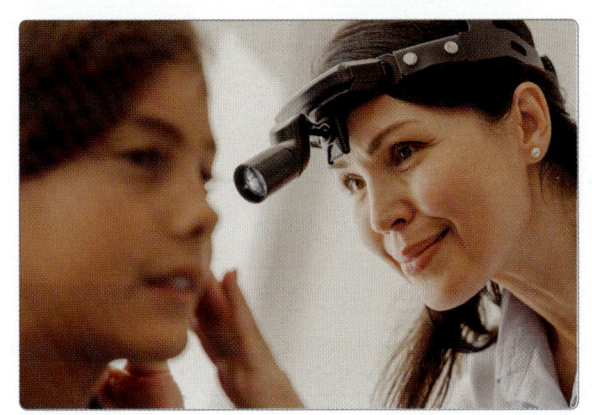

3. ___ / ___ / ___ / ___ / _____
    ear / CV / larynx / CV / physician who studies and treats

4. _____ / ___ / _____ 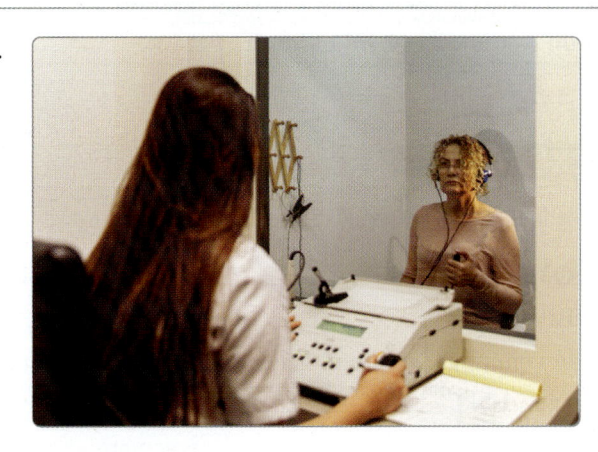
    hearing / CV / specialist who studies and treats

B Fill In

Build complementary terms for the following definitions by using the word parts you have learned.

1. study of hearing   _____ / ___ / _____
                        WR   CV   S

2. study of the ear, (nose), and larynx (throat)   _____ / ___ / _____ / ___ / _____
                                                    WR   CV   WR   CV   S

3. pertaining to the vestibule and the cochlea   _____ / ___ / _____ / _____
                                                  WR   CV   WR   S

4. pertaining to the vestibule   _____ / _____
                                  WR   S

EXERCISE 22 ■ Review of Complementary Terms

Can you define, pronounce, and spell the following terms?

audiologist	aural	otolaryngologist (ENT)	vestibular
audiology	cochlear	otolaryngology	vestibulocochlear

Abbreviations

DISEASES AND DISORDERS

ABBREVIATION	TERM	ABBREVIATION	TERM
AOM	acute otitis media	OE	otitis externa
BPPV	benign paroxysmal positional vertigo	OM	otitis media

MEDICAL SPECIALTIES

ABBREVIATION	TERM
ENT	ears, nose, throat; otolaryngologist

DESCRIPTIVE

ABBREVIATION	TERM
HOH	hard of hearing

EXERCISE 23 ■ Abbreviations

Write the terms abbreviated.

1. **OM** _____ _____ may be acute, abbreviated as **AOM** _____ _____ _____, or chronic.
2. **BPPV** _____ _____ _____ _____ symptoms may include dizziness, vertigo, nausea, or vomiting. Symptoms generally come and go, but patients with prolonged or worsening episodes may need referral to an **ENT** _____ _____ _____ doctor or _____.
3. **OE** _____ _____ is sometimes called "swimmer's ear" because repeated exposure to water can make the ear canal more prone to inflammation.
4. **HOH** _____ _____ _____ generally describes a person with mild to moderate hearing loss.

Chapter 13 Ear

PRACTICAL APPLICATION

EXERCISE 24 ■ Case Study: Translate Between Everyday Language and Medical Language

CASE STUDY: Marisol Montoya

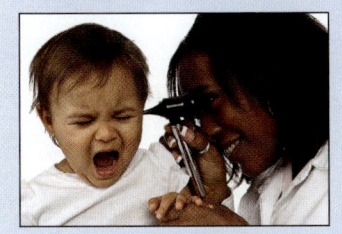

Marisol Montoya is only 13 months old, and she has already had five episodes of middle ear infections (inflammation). For the last few days she has had a fever and she keeps pulling on her ear as if it is painful. Today her mother noticed a pus-like liquid coming out of her left ear. Now her mother is seeing redness and swelling on her skull behind Marisol's earlobe. She calls her pediatrician, who arranges an immediate referral to an ear, nose, and throat physician.

Now that you have worked through Chapter 13, consider the medical terms that might be used to describe Marisol's experience. See the Chapter at a Glance section at the end of the chapter for a list of terms that might apply.

A. Underline phrases in the case study that could be substituted with medical terms.

B. Write the medical term and its definition for three of the phrases you underlined.

MEDICAL TERM	DEFINITION
1. _____	_____
2. _____	_____
3. _____	_____

DOCUMENTATION: Excerpt from Otolaryngology Visit

Marisol was examined by an otolaryngologist; an excerpt from the medical record is documented below.

Marisol Montoya is a 13-month-old female referred by her pediatrician for possible mastoiditis. Her mother reports a history of frequent episodes of otitis media, and she currently has symptoms of fever, otalgia, and otopyorrhea. Today her mother noted inflammation in the left mastoid region. Physical exam reveals an unhappy child with a temperature of 101.7°F. Otoscopy is difficult due to pain but shows both otitis externa in the left ear and otitis media bilaterally. Tympanometry shows evidence of poor mobility and suggests a collection of fluid and pressure in the middle ear. Examination of the left mastoid region reveals erythema, edema, and severe tenderness. Impression: acute mastoiditis. Bilateral myringotomies will be performed and fluid obtained will be sent for cultures. In the meantime, antibiotics will be started and a CT scan of the affected area will be obtained. If she worsens or does not improve, mastoidectomy will be considered.

C. Underline medical terms presented in Chapter 13 used in the previous excerpt from Marisol's medical record. See the Chapter at a Glance section at the end of the chapter for a complete list.

D. Select and define three of the medical terms you underlined. To check your answers, go to Appendix A.

MEDICAL TERM	DEFINITION
1. _____	_____
2. _____	_____
3. _____	_____

Chapter 13 Ear

EXERCISE 25 — Interact with Medical Documents

A

Read the report and complete it by writing medical terms on answer lines within the document. Definitions of terms to be written appear after the document.

99665-AUD TOHE, Jimmy

Name: **TOHE, Jimmy** MR#: **99665-AUD** Sex: **M** Allergies: **Demerol**
DOB: **03/09/19XX** Age: **62** PCP: **Unknown**

ENT Clinic Visit
Date: 04 September 20XX 10:00

Subjective: Jimmy Tohe is a 62-year-old male, appearing younger than his stated age. He was brought into the 1. _____ clinic by his daughter, who states that he is unable to hear what is being said to him by family members. She states that this problem has existed for at least 30 years but that it appears to be getting markedly worse. The patient states he had several episodes of ear infections as a child and young adult. He denies any 2. _____ or 3. _____.

Objective: Temperature, 99.4. Pulse, 72. Respirations, 20. Blood pressure, 136/76 mm Hg. Weight, 162 pounds. Patient ambulates without difficulty. Alert and oriented ×3. 4. _____ reveals scarring of the tympanic membranes bilaterally. Auditory canals appear normal bilaterally.

Assessment:
1. Mild loss of hearing bilaterally, probably caused by 5. _____ as a child.
2. Recent exacerbation of hearing loss most likely attributable to 6. _____.

Plan:
1. Patient referred to 7. _____ for complete 8. _____ workup.

Electronically signed: McKeegan, Bridey MD, 09/04/20XX 10:30

Definitions of Medical Terms to Complete the Document

Write the medical terms defined on corresponding answer lines in the document.

1. abbreviation for ears, nose, and throat
2. ringing in the ears
3. sense of one's own body or the environment revolving
4. visual examination of the ear
5. inflammation of the middle ear
6. hearing impairment occurring with age
7. specialist who studies and treats impaired hearing
8. measurement of hearing

EXERCISE 25 — Interact with Medical Documents—cont'd

B

Read the medical report and answer the questions below it.

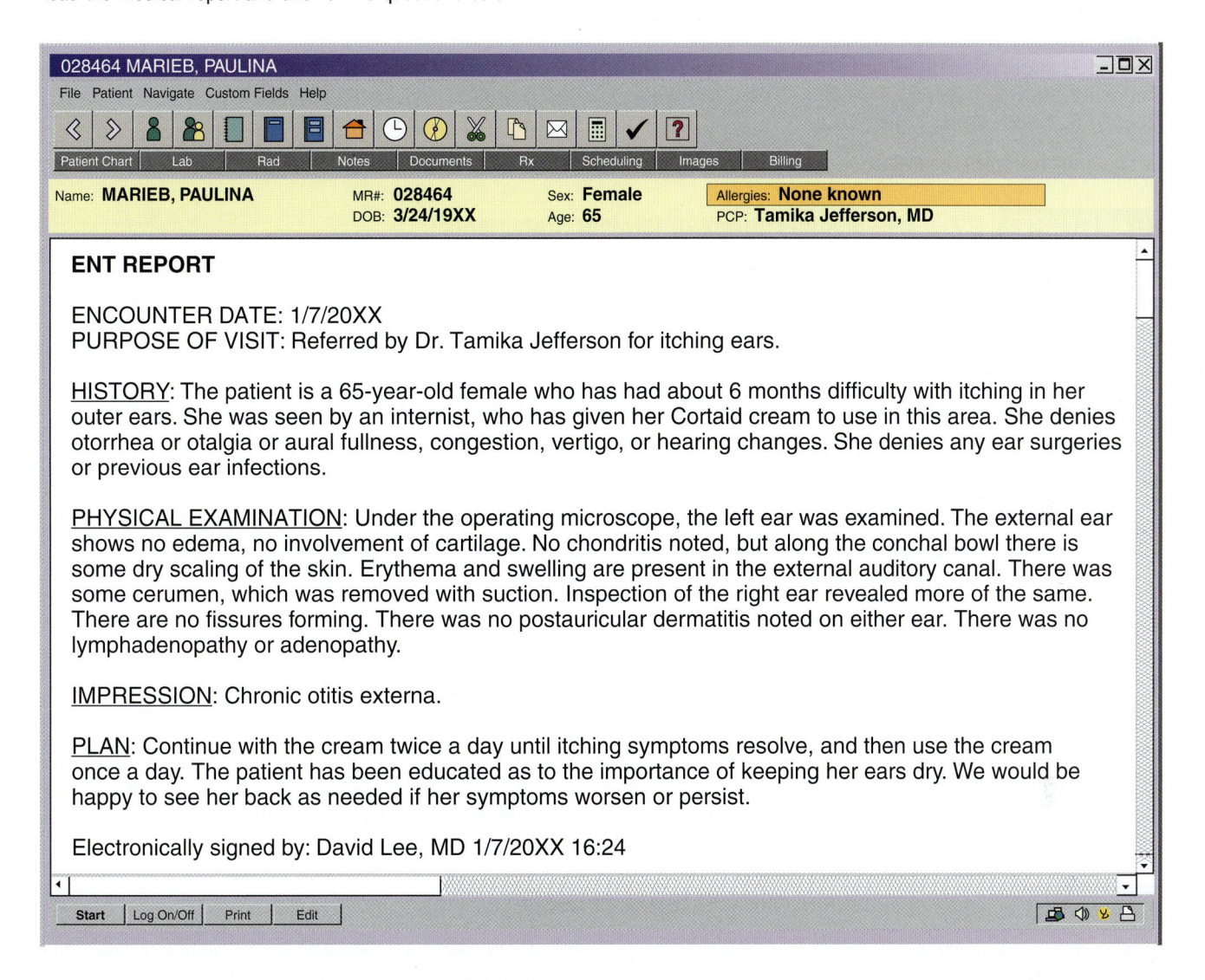

028464 MARIEB, PAULINA

File Patient Navigate Custom Fields Help

| Patient Chart | Lab | Rad | Notes | Documents | Rx | Scheduling | Images | Billing |

Name: **MARIEB, PAULINA** MR#: **028464** Sex: **Female** Allergies: **None known**
DOB: **3/24/19XX** Age: **65** PCP: **Tamika Jefferson, MD**

ENT REPORT

ENCOUNTER DATE: 1/7/20XX
PURPOSE OF VISIT: Referred by Dr. Tamika Jefferson for itching ears.

HISTORY: The patient is a 65-year-old female who has had about 6 months difficulty with itching in her outer ears. She was seen by an internist, who has given her Cortaid cream to use in this area. She denies otorrhea or otalgia or aural fullness, congestion, vertigo, or hearing changes. She denies any ear surgeries or previous ear infections.

PHYSICAL EXAMINATION: Under the operating microscope, the left ear was examined. The external ear shows no edema, no involvement of cartilage. No chondritis noted, but along the conchal bowl there is some dry scaling of the skin. Erythema and swelling are present in the external auditory canal. There was some cerumen, which was removed with suction. Inspection of the right ear revealed more of the same. There are no fissures forming. There was no postauricular dermatitis noted on either ear. There was no lymphadenopathy or adenopathy.

IMPRESSION: Chronic otitis externa.

PLAN: Continue with the cream twice a day until itching symptoms resolve, and then use the cream once a day. The patient has been educated as to the importance of keeping her ears dry. We would be happy to see her back as needed if her symptoms worsen or persist.

Electronically signed by: David Lee, MD 1/7/20XX 16:24

Use the medical report above to answer the questions.

1. The patient has been experiencing:
   a. pruritus
   b. hearing loss
   c. otalgia
   d. vertigo

2. In the patient's left ear, suction removed:
   a. scaling
   b. cerumen
   c. chondritis
   d. otorrhea

3. The patient's condition has been diagnosed as chronic:
   a. abnormal condition of fungus in the ear
   b. inflammation of the tympanic membrane
   c. hardening of the stapes
   d. inflammation of the outer ear, specifically the external auditory canal

530 Chapter 13 Ear

EXERCISE 26 ■ Use Medical Language in Online Electronic Health Records

Select the correct medical terms to complete three medical records in one patient's electronic file.

🌐 Access online resources at evolve.elsevier.com > Evolve Resources > Student Resources > Activities > Chapter 13 > Electronic Health Records

Topic: Acoustic Neuroma
Record 1, Referrals: Audiology Assessment
Record 2, Notes: Urgent Care Clinic Note
Record 3, Encounters: Office Visit

❏ Check the box when complete.

EXERCISE 27 ■ Use Medical Terms in Clinical Statements

For each phrase printed in bold, circle the medical term or abbreviation defined. Answers are listed in Appendix A. For pronunciation practice, read the answers aloud.

1. A **cystlike mass composed of epithelial cells and cholesterol occurring in the middle ear** (acoustic neuroma, cholesteatoma, otitis media) may destroy adjacent bones, including the ossicles.

2. **Inflammation of the labyrinth** (labyrinthitis, mastoiditis, myringitis) is an infection of the inner ear and may cause sudden intense **sensation of revolving** (tinnitus, vertigo, presbycusis), nausea, vomiting, and imbalance.

3. The **process of recording electrical activity in the cochlea in response to sound** (audiology, electrocochleography, otoscopy) may be used in the diagnosis of Ménière disease.

4. The **instrument used to visually examine the ear** is called an (otoscope, ophthalmoscope, audiometer). The **instrument used to measure hearing** is called an (otoscope, ophthalmoscope, audiometer).

5. **Surgical repair of the eardrum** (myringotomy, myringitis, myringoplasty) is one form of **surgical repair of the middle ear** (tympanostomy, tympanoplasty, otoplasty).

6. **Hearing loss occurring with age** (tinnitus, presbyopia, presbycusis) may be diagnosed and treated by a(n) **specialist who studies and treats impaired hearing** (otolaryngologist, optometrist, audiologist).

7. Untreated **inflammation of the middle ear** (otitis externa, otitis media, labyrinthitis) can lead to **inflammation of the mastoid bone** (mastoiditis, myringitis, otorrhea), which is characterized by otalgia, fever, and redness and swelling behind the ear. In acute cases, **excision of the mastoid bone** (labyrinthectomy, stapedectomy, mastoidectomy) may be performed to remove infected tissue and prevent the infection from spreading.

EXERCISE 28 ■ Pronounce Medical Terms in Use

Practice pronunciation of terms by reading aloud the following paragraph. Use the phonetic spellings to assist with pronunciation. The script also contains medical terms not presented in the chapter. If interested, research their meanings in a medical dictionary or a reliable online source.

ACUTE OTITIS MEDIA

Acute **otitis media** (ō-TĪ-tis) (MĒ-dē-a) is one of the most common pediatric infections. Most middle ear infections are caused by bacteria, and some by viruses. Symptoms include **otalgia** (ō-TAL-ja), **otorrhea** (ō-tō-RĒ-a), ear pulling, and irritability. The tympanic membrane will be bulging, red in color, with a thickened appearance and reduced translucency. Antibiotics may be ordered if the infection does not resolve on its own. If unresponsive to antibiotic treatment, a **myringotomy** (mir-ing-GOT-o-mē) may be performed to identify the causative pathogen, allowing for the appropriate antibiotic treatment to be prescribed.

CHAPTER REVIEW

EXERCISE 29 ■ Chapter Content Quiz

Test your understanding of terms and abbreviations introduced in this chapter. Circle the letter for the medical term or abbreviation related to the words in italics.

1. The vestibular nerve and the auditory nerve are branches of the *pertaining to the vestibule and the cochlea* nerve.
    a. aural
    b. cochlear
    c. vestibulocochlear

2. The abbreviation *ENT*, meaning "ears, nose, and throat," can also refer to the following:
    a. otolaryngologist
    b. audiologist
    c. otoscopy

3. A *specialist who studies and treats impaired hearing* has completed a doctoral program and earned a certificate of competence.
    a. otolaryngology
    b. otolaryngologist
    c. audiologist

4. The patient reported being bothered by *ringing in the ears* for the last three weeks.
    a. tinnitus
    b. vertigo
    c. presbycusis

5. Vertigo, tinnitus, and fluctuating hearing loss in *chronic disease of the inner ear* usually occur in episodes that can last for several days.
    a. mastoiditis
    b. presbycusis
    c. Ménière disease

6. *Process of recording electrical activity in the cochlea in response to sound*, may be used in the diagnosis of Ménière disease.
    a. electrocochleography
    b. tympanometry
    c. audiometry

7. Thought to be caused by a viral infection, labyrinthitis may cause sudden intense *sensation of revolving*, nausea, vomiting, and imbalance.
    a. tinnitus
    b. vertigo
    c. aural fullness

8. A *cystlike mass composed of epithelial cells and cholesterol* may destroy adjacent bones, including the ossicles.
    a. cholesteatoma
    b. otosclerosis
    c. otitis media

9. Manifestations of *benign tumor within the auditory canal growing from the vestibulocochlear nerve* often begin with tinnitus and gradual hearing loss.
    a. otitis externa
    b. mastoiditis
    c. acoustic neuroma

10. Typical presentation of *abnormal condition of fungus in the ear* is with inflammation, pruritus, scaling, and extreme discomfort.
    a. otomycosis
    b. otalgia
    c. otopyorrhea

11. Mild *hardening of the ear* may be treated with a hearing aid.
    a. otalgia
    b. otomycosis
    c. otosclerosis

12. A(n) *instrument used to measure middle ear function* changes the air pressure in the ear, causing the eardrum to move back and forth.
    a. tympanometer
    b. audiometer
    c. otoscope

13. *Surgical repair of the middle ear* may include placement of a graft to close perforation of the eardrum and improve hearing.
    a. myringotomy
    b. myringoplasty
    c. tympanoplasty

14. A *surgically implanted electronic device that converts sound into electrical impulses* has internal and external components.
    a. cochlear implant
    b. audiogram
    c. electrocochleography

15. The abbreviation for *inflammation of the outer ear* is
    a. OM
    b. OE
    c. AOM

16. Gentamicin is a powerful antibiotic that may cause *adverse pharmacologic reaction causing damage to the vestibulocochlear nerve*.
    a. acoustic neuroma
    b. ototoxicity
    c. cholesteatoma

17. Children with multiple episodes of otitis media may require *creation of an artificial opening in the middle ear* for the placement of tubes.
    a. stapedectomy
    b. myringotomy
    c. tympanostomy

18. *Surgical repair of the (outer) ear* is usually performed for cosmetic reasons and involves changing the shape, position, or size of the ears.
    a. otoplasty
    b. tympanoplasty
    c. myringoplasty

19. *Visual examination of the ear* would be the best method for determining the presence of a foreign body in the ear canal.
    a. audiometry
    b. tympanometry
    c. otoscopy

20. Hearing aids may be prescribed for people who have *hearing impairment occurring with age*.
    a. tinnitus
    b. presbycusis
    c. cochlear implant

CHAPTER AT A GLANCE — Word Parts New to This Chapter

COMBINING FORMS

audi/o	cochle/o	mastoid/o	ot/o	tympan/o
aur/i	labyrinth/o	myring/o	staped/o	vestibul/o

CHAPTER AT A GLANCE — Ear Terms Built from Word Parts

DISEASE AND DISORDER	SURGICAL	DIAGNOSTIC	COMPLEMENTARY
labyrinthitis	cochlear implant	audiogram	audiologist
mastoiditis	labyrinthectomy	audiometer	audiology
myringitis	mastoidectomy	audiometry	aural
otalgia	mastoidotomy	electrocochleography	cochlear
otomycosis	myringoplasty	otoscope	otolaryngologist (ENT)
otopyorrhea	myringotomy	otoscopy	otolaryngology
otorrhea	otoplasty	tympanometer	vestibular
otosclerosis	stapedectomy	tympanometry	vestibulocochlear
	tympanoplasty		
	tympanostomy		

CHAPTER AT A GLANCE — Ear Terms NOT Built from Word Parts

DISEASE AND DISORDER			
acoustic neuroma	Ménière disease	ototoxicity	tinnitus
cholesteatoma	otitis externa (OE)	presbycusis	vertigo
	otitis media (OM)		

PART 2 BODY SYSTEMS

Musculoskeletal System

14

Outline

ANATOMY, 534
Function, 534
Bone Structure, 534
Skeletal Bones, 535
Joints, 539
Muscles, 540

WORD PARTS, 544
Bone Combining Forms, 544
Muscle and Joint Combining Forms, 544
Combining Forms Used with Musculoskeletal System Terms, 545
Prefixes, 545
Suffixes, 545

MEDICAL TERMS, 552
Disease and Disorder Terms, 552
 Built from Word Parts, 552
 NOT Built from Word Parts, 558
Surgical Terms, 565
 Built from Word Parts, 565
Diagnostic Terms, 570
 Built from Word Parts and
  NOT Built from Word Parts, 570
Complementary Terms, 575
 Built from Word Parts, 575
 NOT Built from Word Parts, 579
Abbreviations, 584

PRACTICAL APPLICATION, 586
CASE STUDY Translate Between Everyday Language and Medical Language, 586
Interact with Medical Documents, 587
Use Medical Language in Online Electronic Health Records, 588
Use Medical Terms in Clinical Statements, 588
Pronounce Medical Terms in Use, 589
Use Plural Endings, 589

CHAPTER REVIEW, 590
Chapter Content Quiz, 590
Chapter at a Glance, 591

Answers to Chapter Exercises, Appendix A

Objectives

Upon completion of this chapter, you will be able to:

1. Pronounce anatomic structures of the musculoskeletal system.
2. Define and spell word parts related to the musculoskeletal system.
3. Define, pronounce, and spell disease and disorder terms related to the musculoskeletal system.
4. Define, pronounce, and spell surgical terms related to the musculoskeletal system.
5. Define, pronounce, and spell diagnostic terms related to the musculoskeletal system.
6. Define, pronounce, and spell complementary terms related to the musculoskeletal system.
7. Interpret the meaning of abbreviations related to the musculoskeletal system.
8. Apply medical language in clinical contexts.

TABLE 14.1 Types of Arthroplasty, 566
TABLE 14.2 Procedures for Treatment of Compression Fractures Caused by Osteoporosis, 567
TABLE 14.3 Diagnostic Imaging Procedures Used for the Musculoskeletal System, 571

ANATOMY

The musculoskeletal system consists of muscles, bones, bone marrow, joints, cartilage, tendons, ligaments, and bursae. The adult human skeleton contains 206 bones and more than 600 muscles. Joints form the union between bones and often allow for movement, although some do not. Most of the joints in the skeleton are freely moving and contain cartilage and bursae.

Function

The functions of the muscular system are movement, posture, joint stability, and heat production. The functions of the skeletal system are to provide a framework for the body, protect the soft body parts such as the brain, store calcium, and support and protect bone marrow (where blood cells are produced). The organs and structures of the musculoskeletal system work together to protect, support, and move the body.

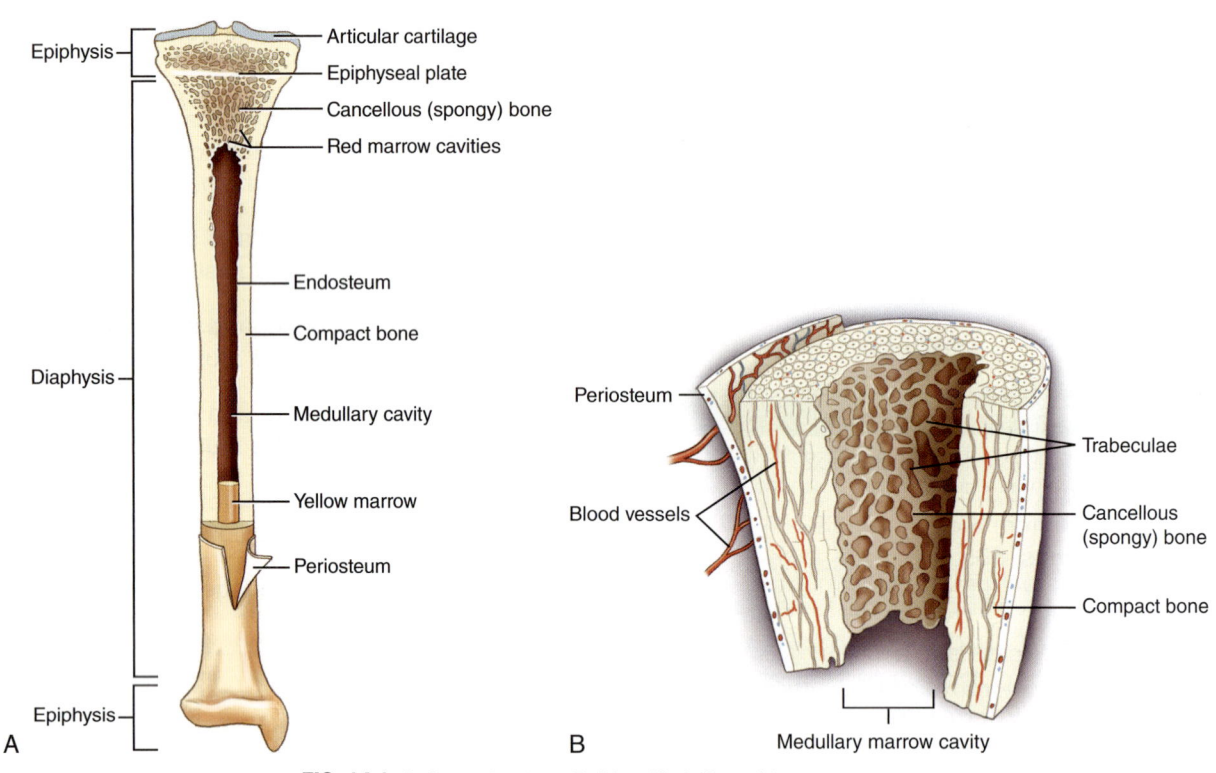

FIG. 14.1 **A,** Bone structure. **B,** Magnified view of bone structure.

Bone Structure

TERM	DEFINITION
bone (bōn)	organ made up of hard connective tissue with a dense outer layer and spongy inner layer
periosteum (per-ē-OS-tē-um)	outermost layer of the bone, made up of fibrous tissue
PERIOSTEUM is composed of the prefix **peri-**, meaning **surrounding**, and the word root **oste**, meaning **bone**.	
compact bone (KOM-pakt) (bōn)	dense, hard layers of bone tissue that lie underneath the periosteum
cancellous bone (KAN-sel-us) (bōn)	tissue encased within compact bone that contains little spaces like a sponge; provides structural support and houses bone marrow that produces blood cells (also called **spongy bone**)
endosteum (en-DOS-tē-um)	membranous lining of the hollow cavity of the bone
ENDOSTEUM is composed of the prefix **endo-**, meaning **within**, and the word root **oste**, meaning **bone**.	

Chapter 14 Musculoskeletal System 535

TERM	DEFINITION
diaphysis (dī-AF-i-sis)	middle section (shaft) of the long bones (Fig. 14.1)
🏛 **DIAPHYSIS** comes from the Greek *diaphusis*, meaning state of growing between.	
epiphysis (*pl.* epiphyses) (e-PIF-i-sis), (e-PIF-i-sēz)	end of each long bone (Fig. 14.1)
🏛 **EPIPHYSIS** has been used in the English language since the 1600s and retains the meaning given to it by a Greco-Roman physician. It means a **portion of bone attached for a time to another bone** by cartilage, but that later combines with the principal bone. During the period of growth, the epiphysis is separated from the main portion of the bone by cartilage.	
bone marrow (bōn) (MAR-ō)	material found in the cavities of bones
red marrow (red) (MAR-ō)	thick, bloodlike material found in flat bones and the ends of long bones; location of blood cell formation
yellow marrow (YEL-ō) (MAR-ō)	soft, fatty material found in the medullary cavity of long bones

Skeletal Bones

TERM	DEFINITION
maxilla (mak-SIL-a)	upper jawbone
mandible (MAN-di-bul)	lower jawbone

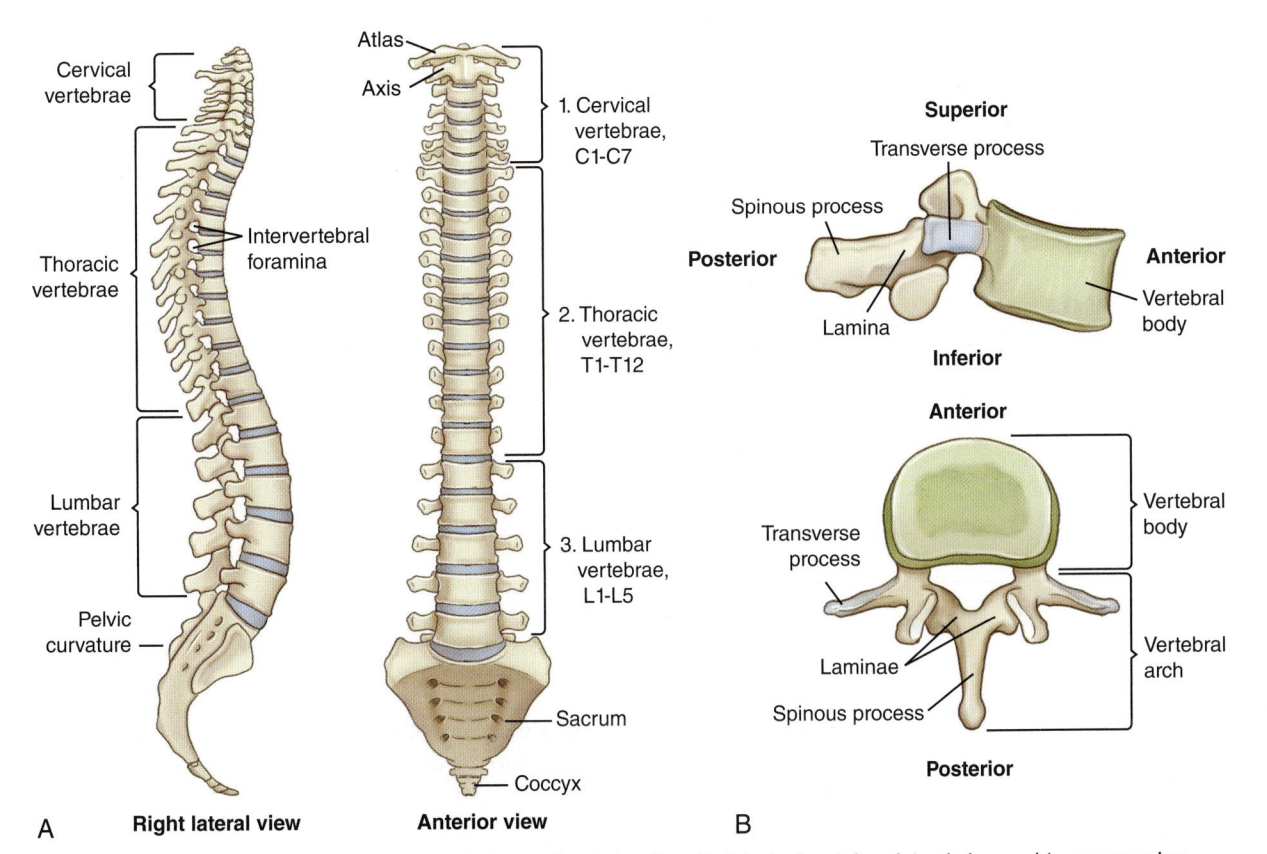

FIG. 14.2 A, Vertebral column, right lateral view and anterior view. **B,** A typical vertebra, lateral view and transverse view.

Skeletal Bones—cont'd

TERM	DEFINITION
vertebral column (ver-TĒ-brel) (KOL-em)	curved structure made up of bones called vertebrae *(pl.)* or vertebra *(s.)* through which the spinal cord runs. The vertebral column protects the spinal cord, supports the head, and provides points of attachment for ribs and muscles. (Fig. 14.2)
cervical vertebrae (C1 to C7) (SUR-vi-kal) (VER-te-bray)	first set of seven vertebrae, forming the neck (contains the first anterior curve of the spine)
thoracic vertebrae (T1 to T12) (tha-RAS-ik) (VER-te-bray)	second set of 12 vertebrae. They articulate with the 12 pairs of ribs to form the outward (posterior) curve of the spine.
lumbar vertebrae (L1 to L5) (LUM-bar) (VER-te-brāy)	third set of five larger vertebrae, which forms the inward curve of the spine (lower anterior curve)
sacrum (SĀ-krum)	next five vertebrae, which fuse together to form a triangular bone positioned between the two hip bones, forming joints called the sacroiliac joints
coccyx (KOK-siks)	four vertebrae fused together to form the tailbone
laminae (*s.* **lamina**) (LAM-i-nā) (LAM-i-na)	flat plates of bone that form the vertebral arch, the posterior portion of the spinal canal
clavicle (KLAV-i-kul)	collarbone
scapula (SKAP-ū-la)	shoulder blade
acromion process (a-KRŌ-mē-on) (PRA-ses)	extension of the scapula, which forms the superior point of the shoulder
sternum (STUR-num)	breastbone
xiphoid process (ZĪ-foid) (PRA-ses)	lower portion of the sternum
humerus (HŪ-mer-us)	upper arm bone
ulna and radius (UL-na), (RĀ-dē-us)	lower arm bones
olecranon process (ō-LEK-ra-non) (PRA-ses)	projection at the proximal end of the ulna that forms the bony point of the elbow
carpal bones (KAR-pal) (bōnz)	wrist bones; there are 8 carpal bones in each wrist
metacarpal bones (*met*-a-KAR-pal) (bōnz)	hand bones (also called **metacarpus**)

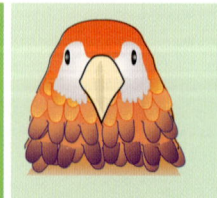

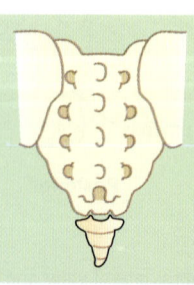

Coccyx is derived from the Greek word *cuckoo* because of its resemblance to a cuckoo's beak.

Chapter 14 Musculoskeletal System   537

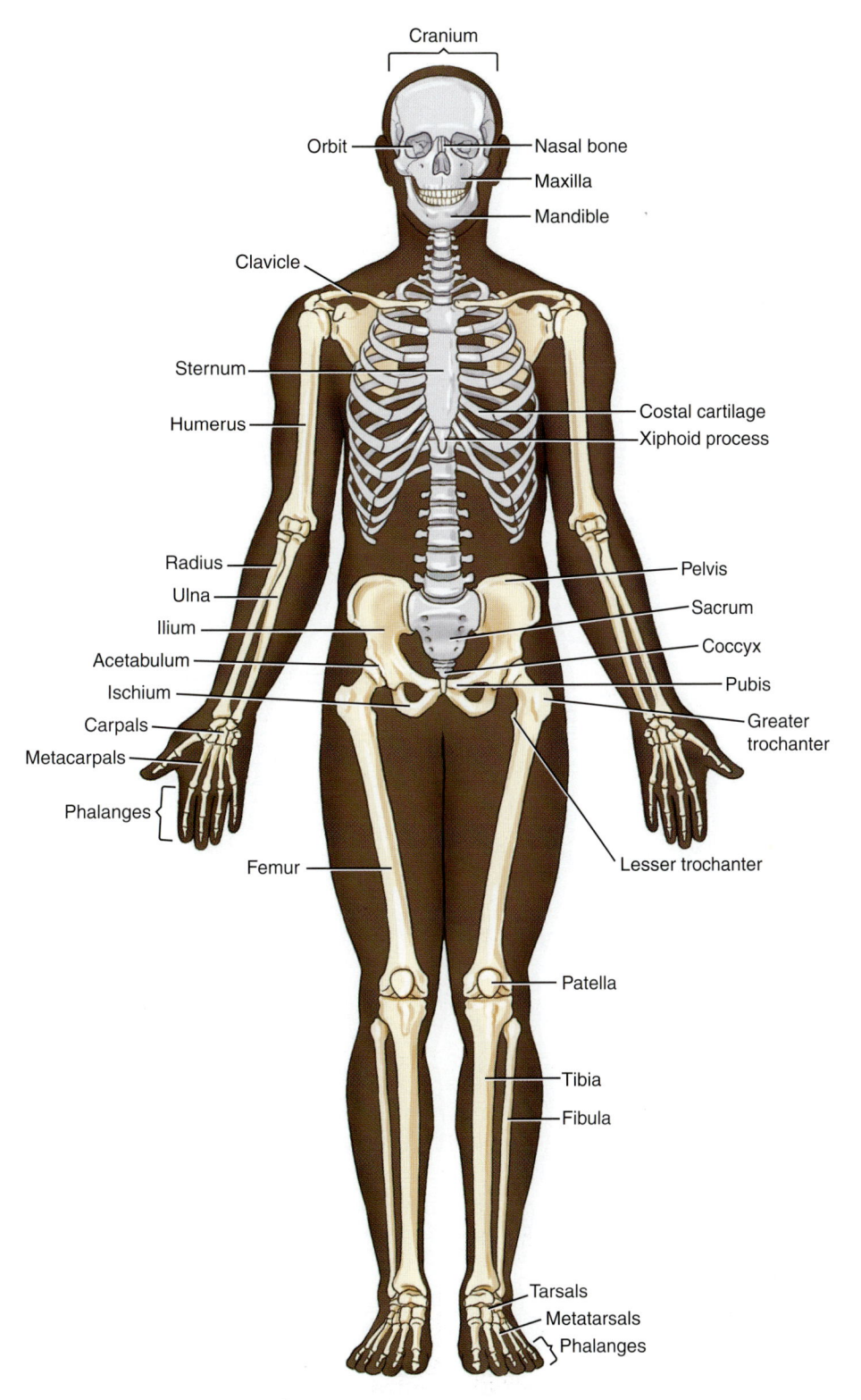

FIG. 14.3 Anterior view of the skeleton.

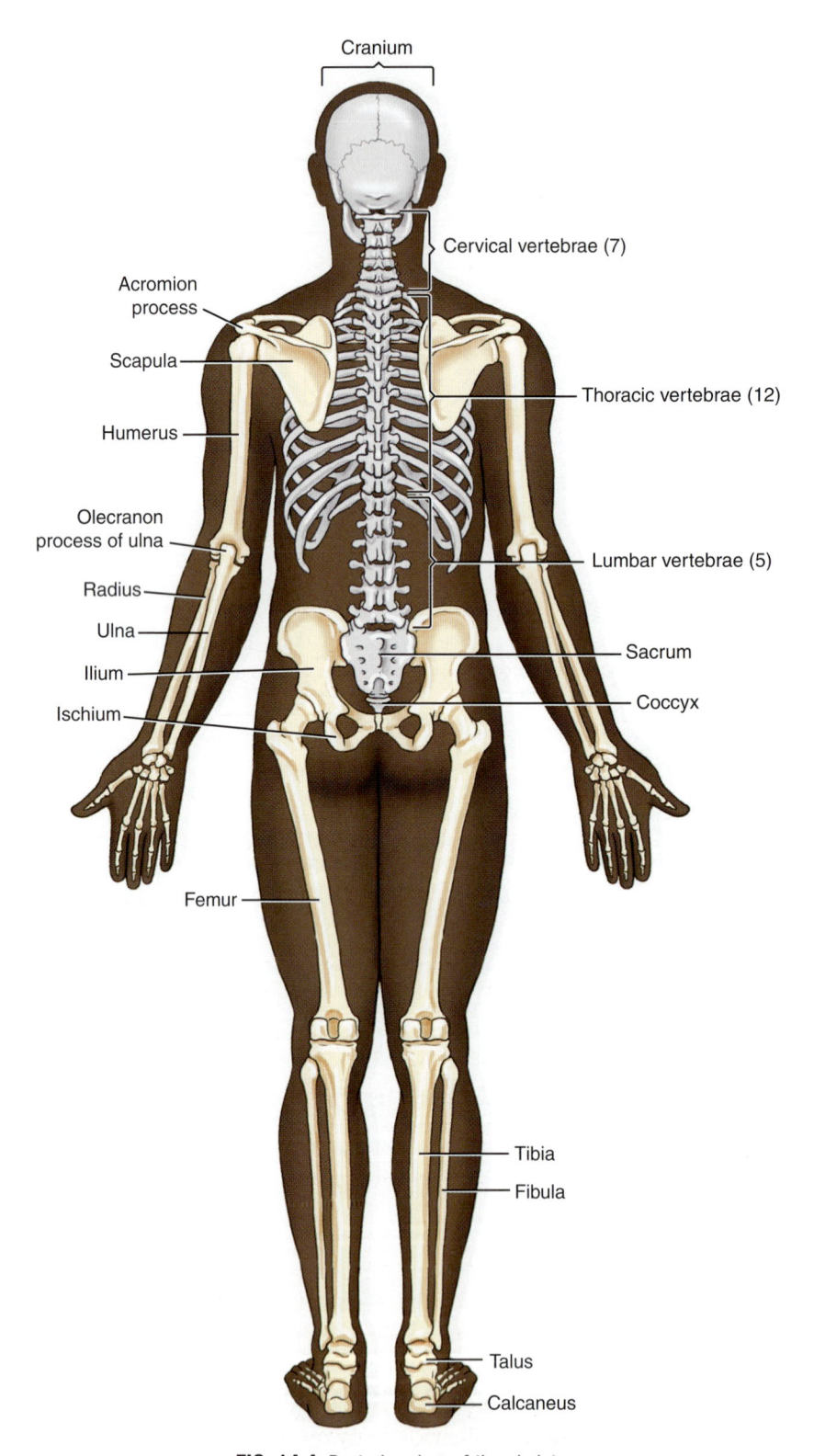

FIG. 14.4 Posterior view of the skeleton.

Skeletal Bones—cont'd

TERM	DEFINITION
METACARPUS is composed of the prefix **meta-**, meaning **beyond**, and **carpus**, meaning **wrist**.	
phalanx (*pl.* phalanges) (FĀ-lanks) (fa-LAN-jēz)	finger and toe bones
pelvis (PEL-vis)	bowl-like structure made up of three bones fused together (also called **pelvic bones** and **hip bones**)
ischium (IS-kē-um)	lower, posterior portion of the pelvis on which one sits
ilium (IL-ē-um)	upper, wing-shaped part on each side of the pelvis
pubis (PŪ-bis)	anterior portion of the pelvis
acetabulum (*as*-a-TAB-ū-lum)	large socket in the pelvis for the head of the femur
femur (FĒ-mer)	upper leg bone
tibia and fibula (TIB-ē-a), (FIB-ū-la)	lower leg bones
patella (*pl.* patellae) (pa-TEL-a) (pa-TEL-ē)	kneecap
tarsal bones (TAR-sal) (bōnz)	ankle bones; there are 7 tarsal bones in each ankle
calcaneus (kal-KĀ-nē-us)	heel bone
metatarsal bones (*met*-a-TAHR-sal) (bōnz)	foot bones

Joints

TERM	DEFINITION
joint (joint)	junction of two or more bones, which often allows for movement of these bones (also called **articulation**) (Fig. 14.5)
cartilage (KAR-ti-lej)	firm connective tissue primarily found in joints. Articular cartilage covers the contacting surfaces of bones.
meniscus (me-NIS-kus)	crescent-shaped cartilage found in some joints, including the knee
intervertebral disk (*in*-ter-VUR-tē-bral) (disk)	cartilaginous pad found between the vertebrae in the spine (also called **intervertebral disc**)
pubic symphysis (PŪ-bik) (SIM-fi-sis)	cartilaginous joint at which two pubic bones come together anteriorly at the midline
synovia (si-NŌ-vē-a)	fluid secreted by the synovial membrane and found in joint cavities, bursae, and around tendons (also called **synovial fluid**)
bursa (*pl.* bursae) (BUR-sa) (BUR-sā)	fluid-filled sac that allows for easy movement of one part of a joint over another

FIG. 14.5 Knee joint.

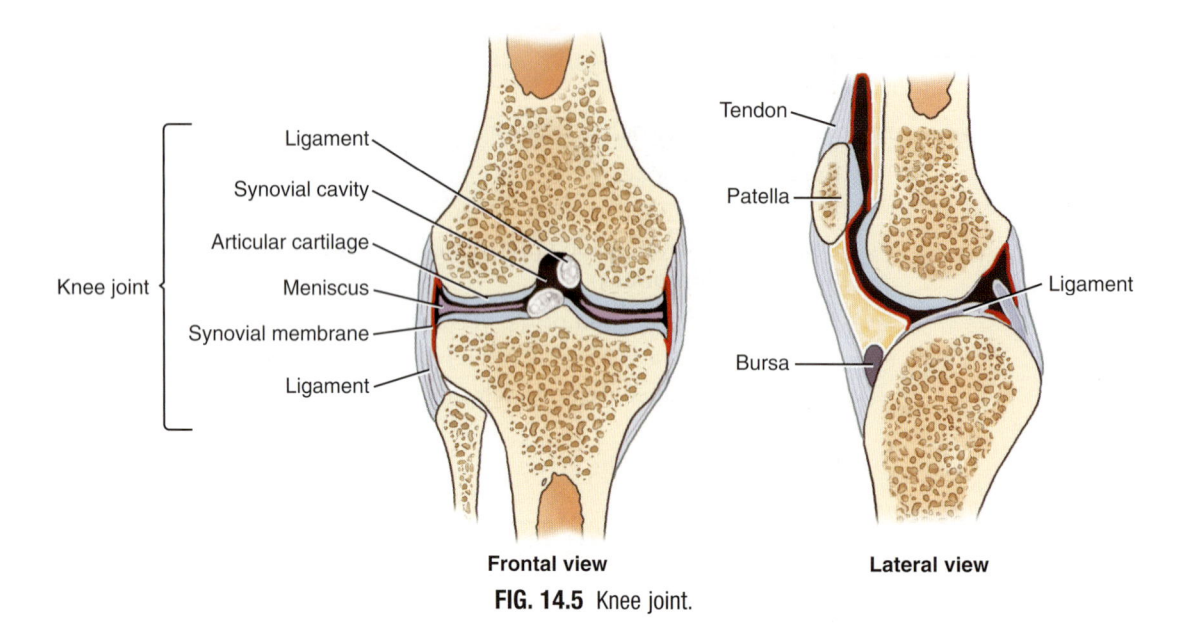

Joints—cont'd

TERM	DEFINITION
ligament (LIG-a-ment)	flexible, tough band of fibrous connective tissue that attaches one bone to another at a joint
tendon (TEN-don)	band of fibrous connective tissue that attaches muscle to bone
aponeurosis (ap-ō-noo-RŌ-sis)	strong sheet of tissue that acts as a tendon to attach muscles to bone

Muscles

TERM	DEFINITION
muscle (MUS-el)	tissue composed of specialized cells with the ability to contract to produce movement; the three types of muscle tissue are skeletal, smooth, and cardiac
fascia (FASH-uh)	band or sheet of connective tissue that encloses muscles and separates their layers
skeletal muscles (SKEL-e-tal) (MUS-els)	attached to bones by tendons and make body movement possible. Skeletal muscles produce action by working in pairs and pulling on bones to which they connect. They are also known as voluntary muscles because we have control over these muscles. Alternating dark and light bands create striations (stripes). (also called **striated muscles**) (Figs. 14.6. 14.7, and 14.8A)
smooth muscles (smooth) (MUS-els)	located in internal organs such as the walls of blood vessels and the digestive tract. They are also known as involuntary muscles because they respond to impulses from the autonomic nerves and are not controlled voluntarily. (also called **unstriated muscles**) (Fig. 14.8B)
cardiac muscle (KAR-dē-ak) (MUS-el)	forms most of the wall of the heart. Its involuntary contraction produces the heartbeat. (also called **myocardium**) (Fig. 14.8C)

Chapter 14 Musculoskeletal System   541

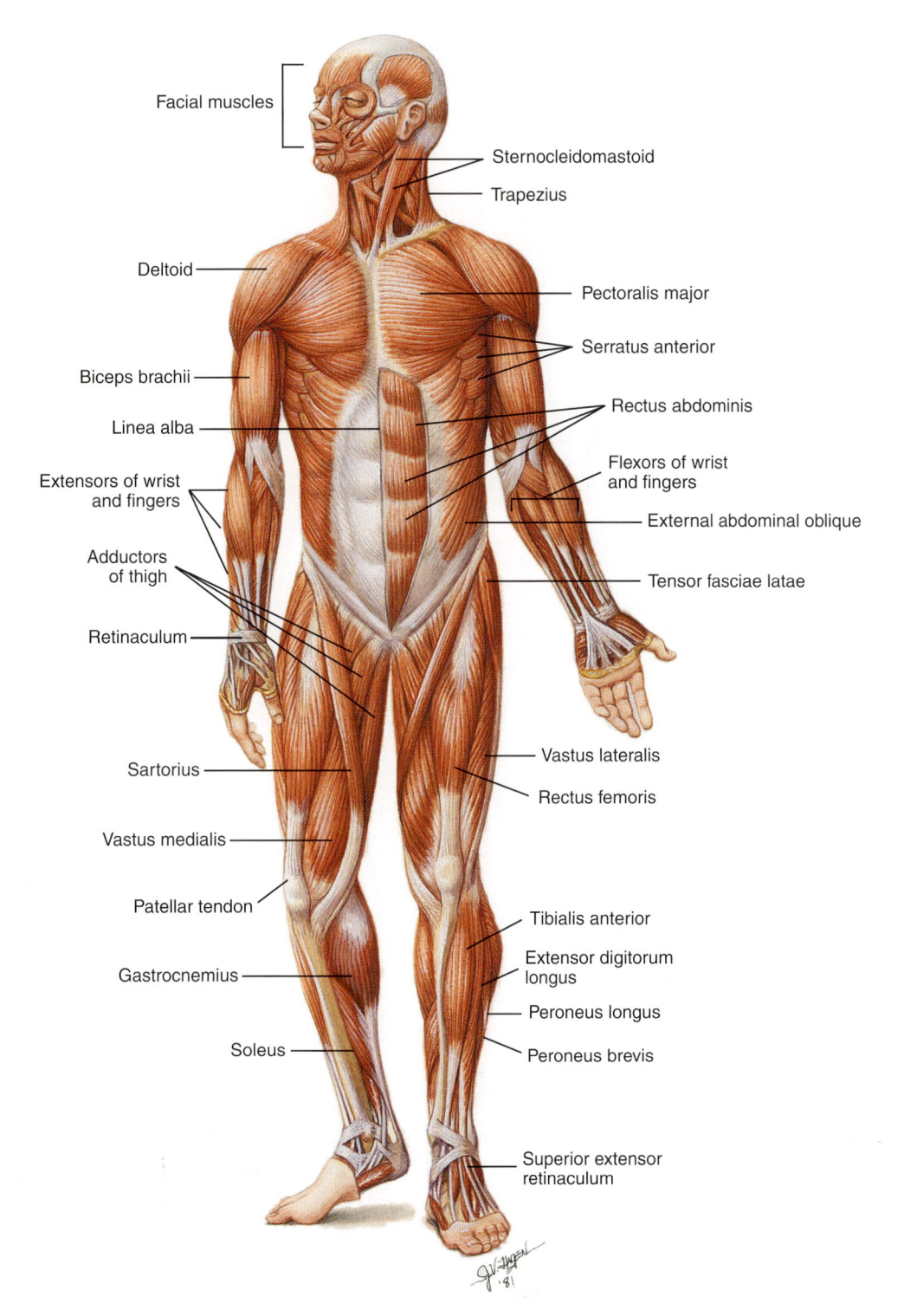

FIG. 14.6 Anterior view of the muscular system.

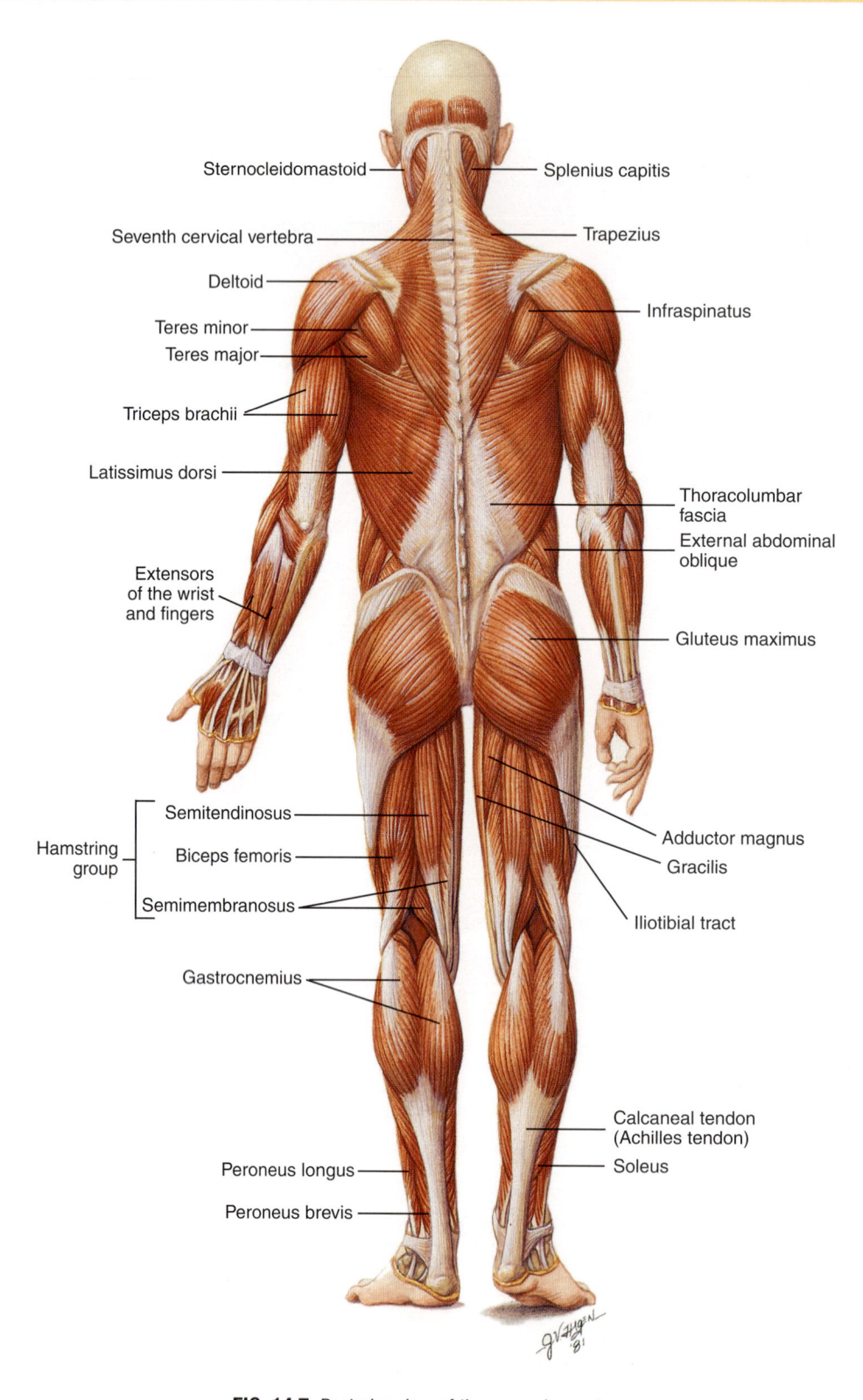

FIG. 14.7 Posterior view of the muscular system.

Chapter 14 Musculoskeletal System   543

Striations

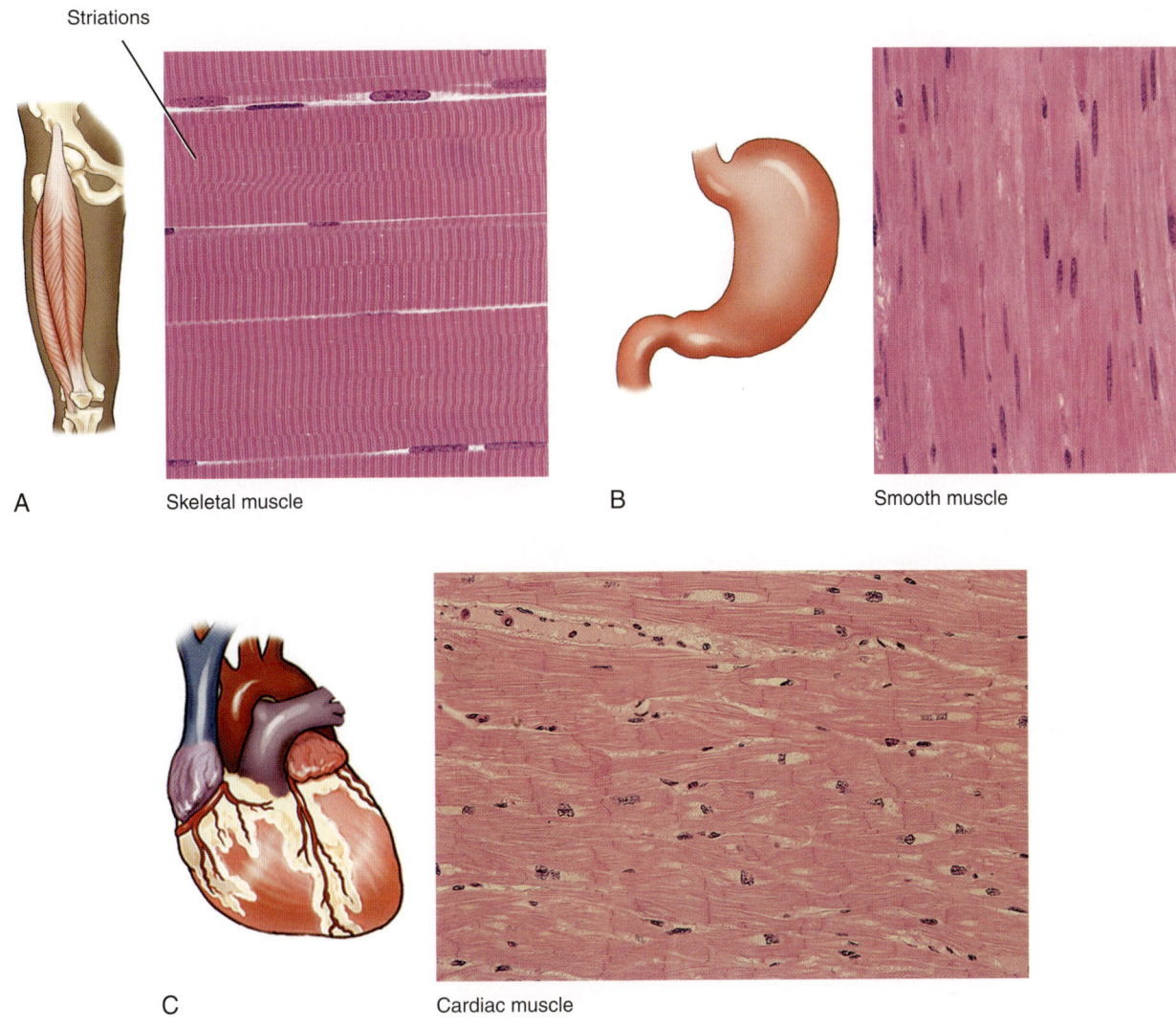

A Skeletal muscle

B Smooth muscle

C Cardiac muscle

FIG. 14.8 Types of muscle tissue, with their related histology views.

PRONOUNCE ANATOMIC STRUCTURES

Practice saying aloud each of the organs and specific structures on the previous pages.

To hear the terms, go to Evolve Resources at www.evolve.elsevier.com and select:
Student Resources > Chapter 14 > Audio Glossary > Anatomic Structures

❏ Check the box when complete.

Chapter 14   Musculoskeletal System

🔗 WORD PARTS

Use paper flashcards or electronic flashcards on Evolve to memorize word parts used to analyze, define, and build medical terms in this chapter. To reinforce learning, study one section of the Word Parts Table at a time, and then complete the corresponding exercise on the following pages.

1 ■ Bone Combining Forms

COMBINING FORM	DEFINITION	COMBINING FORM	DEFINITION
carp/o	carpals (wrist)	pelv/i	pelvis, pelvic cavity
clavicul/o	clavicle (collarbone)	phalang/o	phalanx (*pl.* phalanges) (any bone of the fingers or toes)
cost/o	rib		
crani/o	cranium (skull)	pub/o	pubis (anterior portion of the pelvis)
femor/o	femur (upper leg bone) (*Note:* The u in femur changes to an o in the word root femor/.)		
		rachi/o	vertebra (*pl.* vertebrae), spine, vertebral column
fibul/o	fibula (lower leg bone)	radi/o	radius (lower arm bone)
humer/o	humerus (upper arm bone)	sacr/o	sacrum (lower portion of the spine forming the posterior pelvic wall)
ili/o	ilium (upper, wing-shaped portion of the pelvis)		
ischi/o	ischium (lower posterior portion of the pelvis)	scapul/o	scapula (shoulder blade)
		spondyl/o	vertebra (*pl.* vertebrae), spine, vertebral column
lumb/o	loin, lumbar region of the spine		
mandibul/o	mandible (lower jawbone)	stern/o	sternum (breastbone)
maxill/o	maxilla (upper jawbone)	tars/o	tarsals (ankle bones)
		tibi/o	tibia (lower leg bone)
myel/o	bone marrow (*Note:* myel/o also means spinal cord; see Chapter 15)	uln/o	ulna (lower arm bone)
oste/o	bone	vertebr/o	vertebra (*pl.* vertebrae), spine, vertebral column
patell/o	patella (kneecap)		

> 💡 **ILIUM VS. ILEUM** Compare the combining form for ilium, **ili/o**, the portion of the pelvis, with the combining form for ileum, **ile/o**, the distal portion of the intestine. The pronunciation is the same. Think of il**i**um with an **i** and intestin**e** with an **e** to help distinguish the word roots.

2 ■ Muscle and Joint Combining Forms

COMBINING FORM	DEFINITION	COMBINING FORM	DEFINITION
arthr/o	joint	lamin/o	lamina (thin, flat plate or layer)
burs/o	bursa (cavity)	menisc/o	meniscus (crescent)
chondr/o	cartilage	my/o	muscle(s), muscle tissue
disc/o	intervertebral disk	myos/o	muscle(s), muscle tissue
fasci/o	fascia (connective tissue enclosing and separating muscle layers)	synovi/o	synovia, synovial membrane
		tendin/o	tendon
		ten/o	tendon

3 ■ Combining Forms Used with Musculoskeletal System Terms

COMBINING FORM	DEFINITION	COMBINING FORM	DEFINITION
ankyl/o	stiff, bent	necr/o	death (cells, body)
electr/o	electricity, electrical activity	rhabd/o	rod-shaped, striated
hem/o	blood	petr/o	stone *(Note: lith/o, also a combining form for stone, was introduced in Chapter 6.)*
kinesi/o	movement, motion		
kyph/o	hump (increased convexity of the spine)	sarc/o	flesh, connective tissue
		SARC When **sarc** appears with **oma** in a term, the suffix **-sarcoma** is used rather than the combining form **sarc/o**.	
lord/o	bent forward (increased concavity of the spine)		
		scoli/o	(lateral) curved (spine)

4 ■ Prefixes

PREFIX	DEFINITION	PREFIX	DEFINITION
a-	absence of, without	micro-	small
brady-	slow	poly-	many, much
dys-	painful, abnormal, difficult, labored	sub-	under, below
hyper-	above, excessive	supra-	above
inter-	between	syn-	together, joined
intra-	within		

5 ■ Suffixes

SUFFIX	DEFINITION	SUFFIX	DEFINITION
-a	noun suffix, no meaning	-ic	pertaining to
-ac	pertaining to	-itis	inflammation
-al	pertaining to	-malacia	softening
-algia	pain	-oma	tumor, swelling
-ar	pertaining to	-osis	abnormal condition (means increase when used with blood cell word roots)
-ary	pertaining to		
-asthenia	weakness		
-centesis	surgical puncture to aspirate fluid (with a sterile needle)	-penia	abnormal reduction in number
		-plasty	surgical repair
		-rrhaphy	suturing, repairing
-desis	surgical fixation, fusion	-sarcoma	malignant tumor
-eal	pertaining to	-schisis	split, fissure
-ectomy	excision, surgical removal		
-gram	the record, radiographic image	-scopy	visual examination
-graphy	process of recording, radiographic imaging	-tomy	cut into, incision
		-trophy	nourishment, development
-ia	diseased state, condition of		

🔍 Refer to **Appendix B** and **Appendix C** for alphabetical lists of word parts and their meanings.

546　Chapter 14　Musculoskeletal System

EXERCISE 1 ■ Bone Combining Forms

Refer to the first section of the word parts table.

A Label

Fill in the blanks with combining forms in this diagram of the skeleton, anterior view.
To check your answers, go to Appendix A.

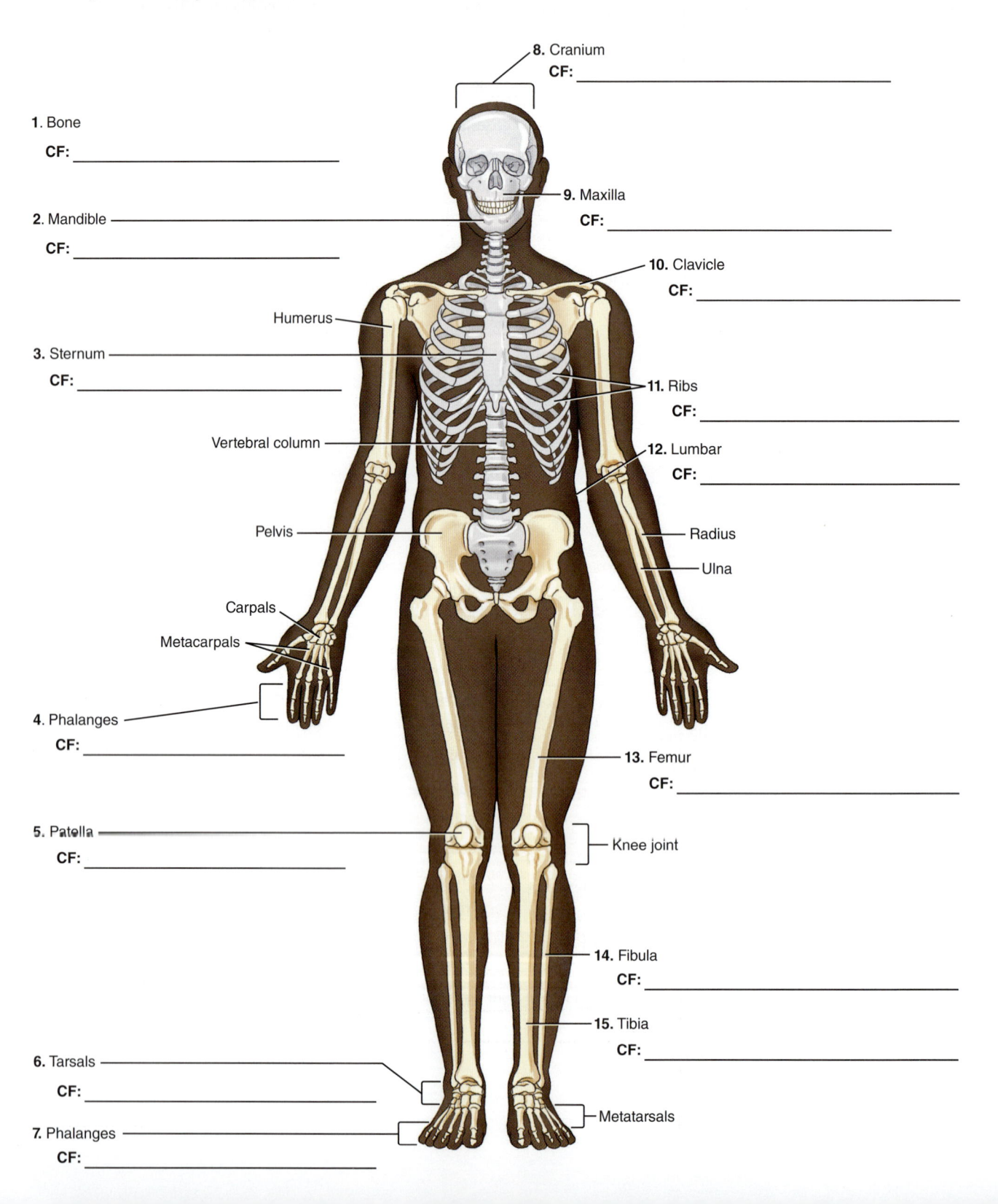

8. Cranium
   CF: _____

1. Bone
   CF: _____

9. Maxilla
   CF: _____

2. Mandible
   CF: _____

10. Clavicle
    CF: _____

Humerus

3. Sternum
   CF: _____

11. Ribs
    CF: _____

Vertebral column

12. Lumbar
    CF: _____

Pelvis

Radius

Ulna

Carpals

Metacarpals

4. Phalanges
   CF: _____

13. Femur
    CF: _____

5. Patella
   CF: _____

Knee joint

14. Fibula
    CF: _____

15. Tibia
    CF: _____

6. Tarsals
   CF: _____

Metatarsals

7. Phalanges
   CF: _____

Chapter 14   Musculoskeletal System   547

B   Label

Fill in the blanks with combining forms in this diagram of the skeleton, posterior view, and the pelvis.

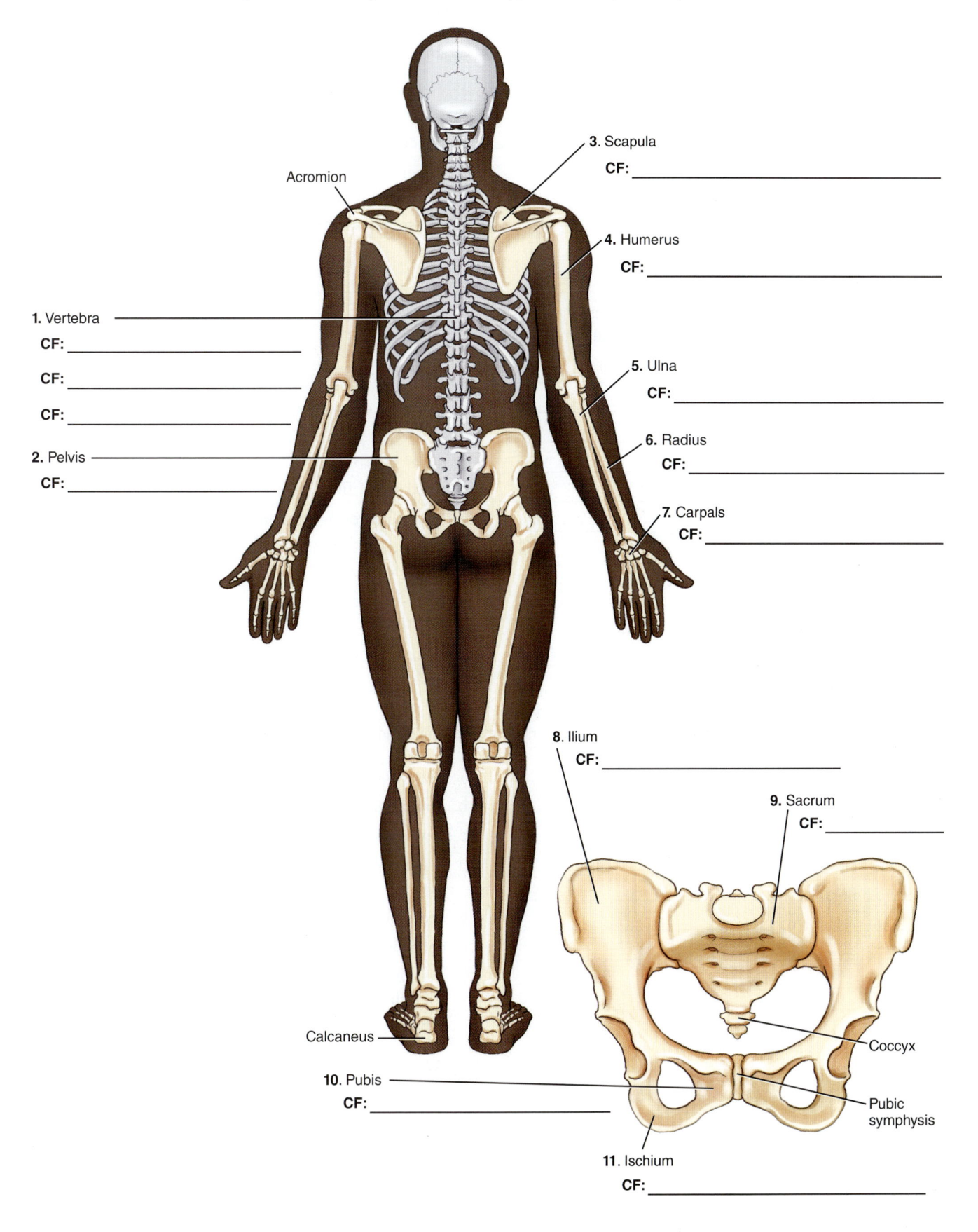

Acromion

3. Scapula
CF: _____

4. Humerus
CF: _____

1. Vertebra
CF: _____
CF: _____
CF: _____

5. Ulna
CF: _____

6. Radius
CF: _____

2. Pelvis
CF: _____

7. Carpals
CF: _____

8. Ilium
CF: _____

9. Sacrum
CF: _____

Calcaneus

10. Pubis
CF: _____

Coccyx

Pubic symphysis

11. Ischium
CF: _____

548 Chapter 14 Musculoskeletal System

C Define and Match

Step 1: Write the definitions after the following combining forms.
Step 2: Match the descriptions on the right with the combining forms and definitions.

_____ 1. rachi/o, _____
_____ 2. patell/o, _____
_____ 3. maxill/o, _____
_____ 4. phalang/o, _____
_____ 5. carp/o, _____
_____ 6. humer/o, _____

a. upper jawbone
b. finger and toe bones
c. wrist bones
d. kneecap
e. upper arm bone
f. made up of bones called vertebrae through which the spinal cord runs

D Define and Match

Step 1: Write the definitions after the following combining forms.
Step 2: Match the descriptions on the right with the combining forms and definitions.

_____ 1. lumb/o, _____
_____ 2. ischi/o, _____
_____ 3. pub/o, _____
_____ 4. spondyl/o, _____
_____ 5. scapul/o, _____
_____ 6. tars/o, _____
_____ 7. pelv/i, _____

a. anterior portion of the pelvis
b. made up of bones called vertebrae through which the spinal cord runs
c. ankle bones
d. third set of five larger vertebrae
e. lower, posterior portion of the pelvis on which one sits
f. shoulder blade
g. bowl-like structure made up of three bones fused together

E Define and Match

Step 1: Write the definitions after the following combining forms.
Step 2: Match the descriptions on the right with the combining forms and definitions.

_____ 1. mandibul/o, _____
_____ 2. sacr/o, _____
_____ 3. femor/o, _____
_____ 4. clavicul/o, _____
_____ 5. ili/o, _____
_____ 6. vertebr/o, _____
_____ 7. stern/o, _____

a. upper leg bone
b. upper, wing-shaped part on each side of the pelvis
c. lower jawbone
d. made up of bones called vertebrae through which the spinal cord runs
e. breastbone
f. collarbone
g. five vertebrae, which fuse together to form a triangular bone positioned between the two hip bones

Chapter 14 Musculoskeletal System   549

F Identify

Write the combining form for each of the following terms.

1. rib _____
2. radius (lower arm bone) _____
3. tibia (lower leg bone) _____
4. fibula (lower leg bone) _____
5. ulna (lower arm bone) _____
6. cranium (skull) _____
7. bone _____
8. bone marrow _____

EXERCISE 2 ■ Muscle and Joint Combining Forms

Refer to the second section of the word parts table.

A Label

Fill in the blanks with combining forms on these diagrams of the knee joint and vertebra.

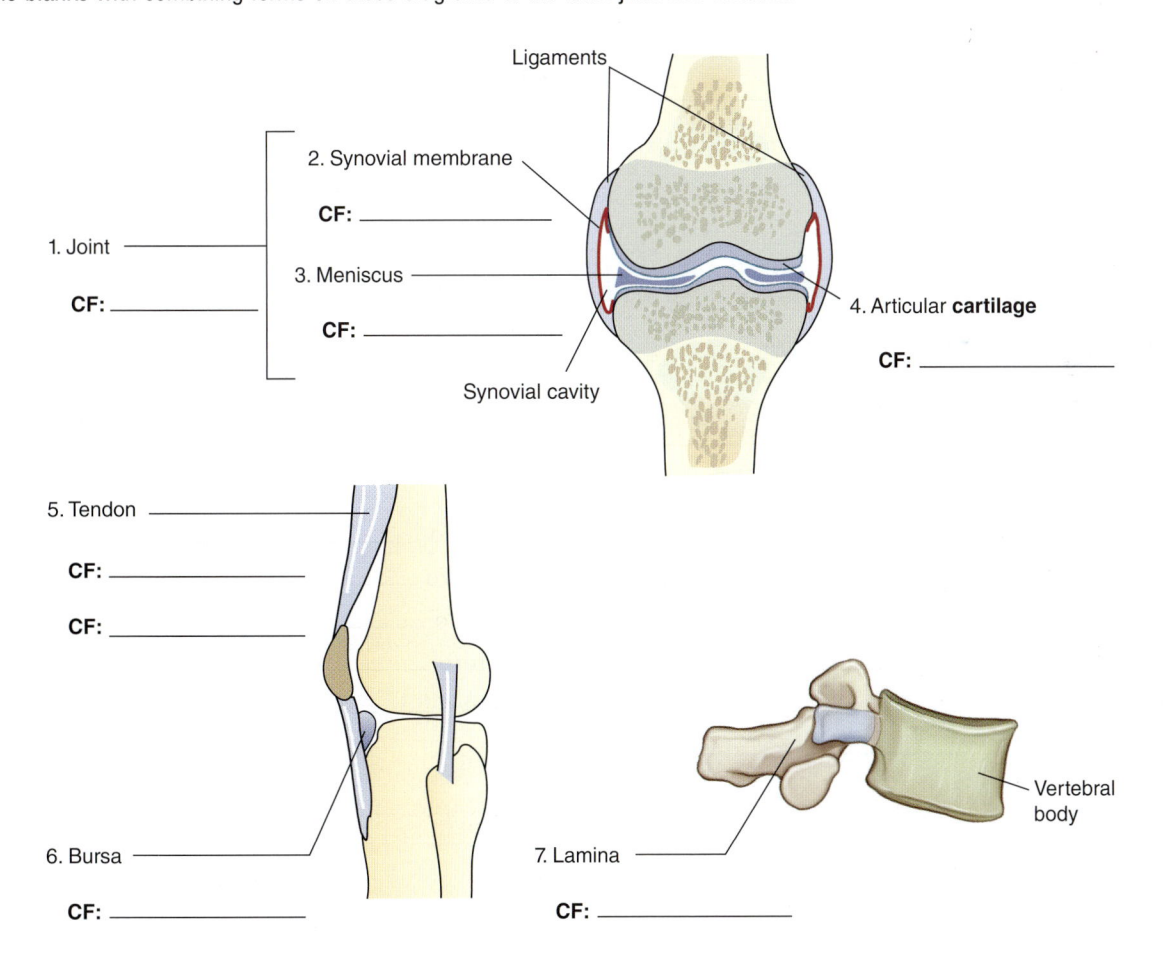

Ligaments

2. Synovial membrane
CF: _____

1. Joint
CF: _____

3. Meniscus
CF: _____

Synovial cavity

4. Articular **cartilage**
CF: _____

5. Tendon
CF: _____
CF: _____

6. Bursa
CF: _____

7. Lamina
CF: _____

Vertebral body

B Define and Match

Step 1: Write the definitions after the following combining forms.
Step 2: Match the descriptions on the right with the combining forms and definitions.

_____ 1. disc/o, _____
_____ 2. synovi/o, _____
_____ 3. fasci/o, _____
_____ 4. ten/o, _____
_____ 5. arthr/o, _____

a. band of fibrous connective tissue that attaches muscle to bone
b. junction of two or more bones, which often allows for movement of these bones
c. cartilaginous pad found between the vertebrae in the spine
d. fluid secreted by the synovial membrane
e. connective tissue enclosing and separating muscle layers

C Define and Match

Step 1: Write the definitions after the following combining forms.
Step 2: Match the descriptions on the right with the combining forms and definitions. Answers may be used more than once.

_____ 1. myos/o, _____
_____ 2. tendin/o, _____
_____ 3. burs/o, _____
_____ 4. menisc/o, _____
_____ 5. chondr/o, _____
_____ 6. my/o, _____

a. firm connective tissue primarily found in joints
b. band of fibrous connective tissue that attaches muscle to bone
c. fluid-filled sac that allows for easy movement of one part of a joint over another
d. crescent-shaped cartilage found in some joints, including the knee
e. tissue composed of specialized cells with the ability to contract

EXERCISE 3 ■ Combining Forms Used with Musculoskeletal System Terms

Refer to the third section of the word parts table.

A Define

Write the definitions of the following combining forms.

1. rhabd/o _____
2. petr/o _____
3. kinesi/o _____
4. necr/o _____
5. hem/o _____
6. electr/o _____
7. kyph/o _____
8. ankyl/o _____
9. scoli/o _____
10. lord/o _____
11. sarc/o _____

B Identify

Write the combining form for each of the following.

1. electricity, electrical activity _____
2. stone _____
3. movement, motion _____
4. rod-shaped, striated _____

5. blood _____
6. death (cells, body) _____
7. hump (increased convexity of the spine) _____
8. stiff, bent _____
9. (lateral) curved (spine) _____
10. bent forward (increased concavity of the spine) _____
11. flesh, connective tissue _____

EXERCISE 4 ■ Prefixes

Refer to the fourth section of the word parts table.

A Define

Write the definitions of the following prefixes.

1. supra- _____
2. syn- _____
3. inter- _____

B Identify

Write the prefix for each of the following definitions.

1. together, joined _____
2. between _____
3. above _____
4. under, below _____
5. absence of, without _____
6. many, much _____
7. slow _____
8. small _____
9. above, excessive _____
10. within _____
11. painful, abnormal, difficult, labored _____

EXERCISE 5 ■ Suffixes

Refer to the fifth section of the word parts table.

A Define

Write the definitions of the following suffixes.

1. -desis _____
2. -schisis _____
3. -asthenia _____
4. -trophy _____
5. -ac, -al, -ar, -ary, -eal, -ic, _____

B Identify

Write the suffix for each of the following definitions.

1. weakness _____
2. surgical fixation, fusion _____
3. split, fissure _____
4. nourishment, development _____
5. noun suffix, no meaning _____

C Match

Match the suffixes in the first column with their correct definitions in the second column.

_____ 1. -algia   a. diseased state, condition of
_____ 2. -penia   b. tumor, swelling
_____ 3. -oma   c. softening
_____ 4. -malacia   d. abnormal condition
_____ 5. -osis   e. malignant tumor
_____ 6. -itis   f. pain
_____ 7. -sarcoma   g. inflammation
_____ 8. -ia   h. abnormal reduction in number

D Match

Match the suffixes in the first column with their correct definitions in the second column.

_____ 1. -centesis   a. surgical fixation, fusion
_____ 2. -ectomy   b. cut into, incision
_____ 3. -plasty   c. excision, surgical removal
_____ 4. -rrhaphy   d. surgical puncture to aspirate fluid (with a sterile needle)
_____ 5. -tomy   e. surgical repair
_____ 6. -desis   f. suturing, repairing
_____ 7. -scopy   g. process of recording, radiographic imaging
_____ 8. -graphy   h. visual examination
_____ 9. -gram   i. the record, radiographic image

MEDICAL TERMS

Medical terms relevant to this chapter have been grouped by topics, such as Disease and Disorder, and are listed in tables designated as Built from Word Parts or *NOT* Built from Word Parts. The exercises following each table assist with learning term definitions, pronunciations, and spellings.

Disease and Disorder Terms

BUILT FROM WORD PARTS

The following terms can be translated using definitions of word parts. Further explanation is provided within parentheses as needed.

TERM	DEFINITION	TERM	DEFINITION
1. ankylosis (*ang*-ki-LŌ-sis)	abnormal condition of stiffness (often referring to fusion of a joint, such as the result of chronic rheumatoid arthritis)	3. bursitis (ber-SĪ-tis)	inflammation of a bursa
		4. chondromalacia (*kon*-drō-ma-LĀ-sha)	softening of cartilage
		5. chondrosarcoma (*kon*-dro-sar-KŌ-ma)	malignant tumor of cartilage
2. arthritis (ar-THRĪ-tis)	inflammation of a joint (The most common forms of arthritis are osteoarthritis and rheumatoid arthritis.) (Fig. 14.9)	6. cranioschisis (*krā*-nē-OS-ki-sis)	fissure (split) of the cranium (congenital)
		7. discitis (dis-KĪ-tis)	inflammation of an intervertebral disk

Chapter 14 Musculoskeletal System 553

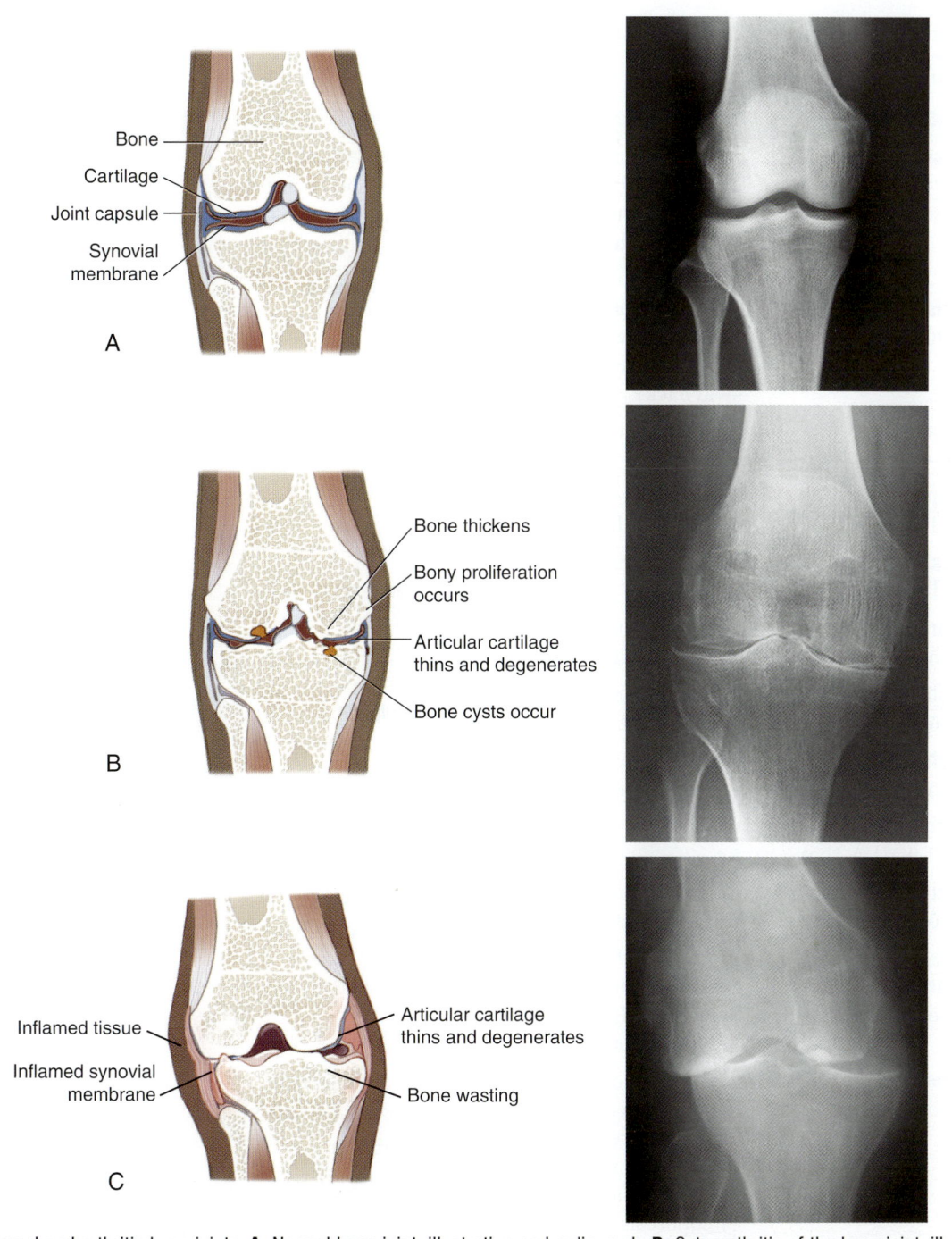

FIG. 14.9 Normal and arthritic knee joints. **A,** Normal knee joint, illustration and radiograph. **B,** Osteoarthritis of the knee joint, illustration and radiograph. **C,** Rheumatoid arthritis of the knee joint, illustration and radiograph.

TERM	DEFINITION	TERM	DEFINITION
8. **fasciitis** (fa-shē-Ī-tis)	inflammation of the fascia (connective tissue enclosing and separating muscle layers)	9. **fibromyalgia** (fī-brō-mī-AL-ja)	pain in the fibrous tissues and muscles (a common condition characterized by widespread pain and stiffness of muscles, fatigue, and disturbed sleep)

Disease and Disorder Terms—cont'd
BUILT FROM WORD PARTS

TERM	DEFINITION	TERM	DEFINITION
10. kyphosis (kī-FŌ-sis)	abnormal condition of a hump (in the thoracic spine) (also called **hunchback** or **humpback**)	23. osteosarcoma (os-tē-ō-sar-KŌ-ma)	malignant tumor of the bone
		24. polymyositis (PM) (pol-ē-mī-ō-SĪ-tis)	inflammation of many muscles
11. lordosis (lōr-DŌ-sis)	abnormal condition of bending forward (in the lumbar spine) (also called **swayback**)	25. rachischisis (ra-KIS-ki-sis)	fissure (split) of the vertebral column (congenital) (also called **spina bifida**)
12. meniscitis (men-i-SĪ-tis)	inflammation of a meniscus	26. rhabdomyolysis (rab-dō-mī-OL-i-sis)	dissolution of striated muscle (caused by trauma, extreme exertion, or drug toxicity; in severe cases renal failure can result)
13. myeloma (mī-e-LŌ-ma)	tumor of the bone marrow (malignant)		
14. osteitis (os-tē-Ī-tis)	inflammation of the bone		
15. osteoarthritis (OA) (os-tē-ō-ar-THRĪ-tis)	inflammation of the bone and joint (Fig. 14.9B)	27. sarcopenia (sar-kō-PĒ-nē-a)	abnormal reduction of connective tissue (such as loss of skeletal muscle mass in the elderly)
16. osteochondritis (os-tē-ō-kon-DRĪ-tis)	inflammation of the bone and cartilage		
17. osteochondroma (os-tē-ō-kon-DRŌ-ma)	tumor composed of bone and cartilage (benign)	28. scoliosis (skō-lē-Ō-sis)	abnormal condition of (lateral) curved (spine) (Fig. 14.10)
18. osteomalacia (os-tē-ō-ma-LĀ-sha)	softening of bone	29. spondylarthritis (spon-dil-ar-THRĪ-tis)	inflammation of the vertebral joints (also called **spondyloarthritis**)
19. osteomyelitis (os-tē-ō-mī-e-LĪ-tis)	inflammation of the bone and bone marrow (caused by bacterial infection)	30. spondylosis (spon-di-LŌ-sis)	abnormal condition of the vertebrae (a general term used to describe changes to the spine from osteoarthritis or ankylosis)
20. osteonecrosis (os-tē-ō-ne-KRŌ-sis)	abnormal condition of bone death (due to lack of blood supply)		
21. osteopenia (os-tē-ō-PĒ-nē-a)	abnormal reduction of bone mass (caused by inadequate replacement of bone lost to normal bone lysis and can lead to osteoporosis)	31. synoviosarcoma (si-nō-vē-ō-sar-KŌ-ma)	malignant tumor of the synovial membrane
		32. tendinitis (ten-di-NĪ-tis)	inflammation of a tendon (also spelled **tendonitis**)
22. osteopetrosis (os-tē-ō-pe-TRŌ-sis)	abnormal condition of stonelike bones (very dense bones caused by defective resorption of bone)	33. tenosynovitis (ten-ō-sin-ō-VĪ-tis)	inflammation of the tendon and synovial membrane *(Note: the i in synovi is dropped because the suffix begins with an i.)*

Chapter 14   Musculoskeletal System   555

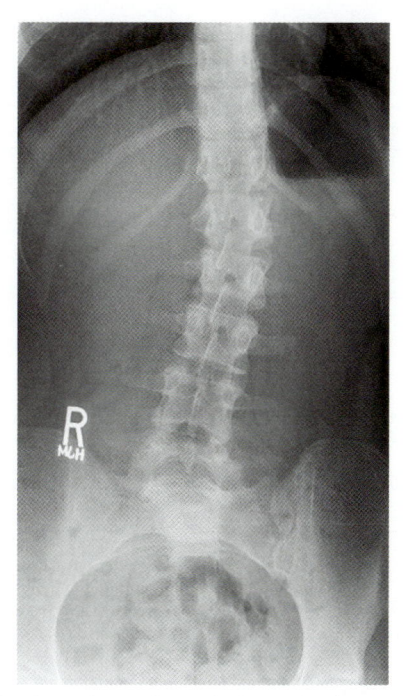

FIG. 14.10 AP lumbar spine radiograph demonstrating congenital scoliosis.

EXERCISE 6 ■ Pronounce and Spell

Practice pronunciation and spelling on paper and online.

1. **Practice on Paper**
   a. **Pronounce:** Read the phonetic spelling and say aloud the terms listed in the previous table. Refer to Table 2.2 Pronunciation Key as needed.
   b. **Spell:** Have a study partner read the terms aloud. Write the spelling of the terms on a separate sheet of paper.

2. **Practice Online**
   a. **Access** online learning resources. Go to evolve.elsevier.com > Evolve Resources > Student Resources.
   b. **Pronounce:** Select Audio Glossary > Chapter 14 > Exercise 6. Select a term to hear its pronunciation and repeat aloud.
   c. **Spell:** Select Activities > Chapter 14 > Spell Terms > Exercise 6. Select the audio icon and type the correct spelling of the term.

❏ Check the box when complete.

EXERCISE 7 ■ Analyze and Define

Analyze and define the following disease and disorder terms.

1. osteitis

2. tenosynovitis

3. osteopetrosis

4. osteomalacia

5. chondrosarcoma

6. osteochondroma

7. discitis

8. osteonecrosis

9. sarcopenia

10. synoviosarcoma

11. spondylosis

12. cranioschisis

13. chondromalacia

14. ankylosis

15. meniscitis

16. fibromyalgia

17. fasciitis

Chapter 14 Musculoskeletal System 557

EXERCISE 8 ■ Build

A Label

Build terms pictured by writing word parts above definitions.

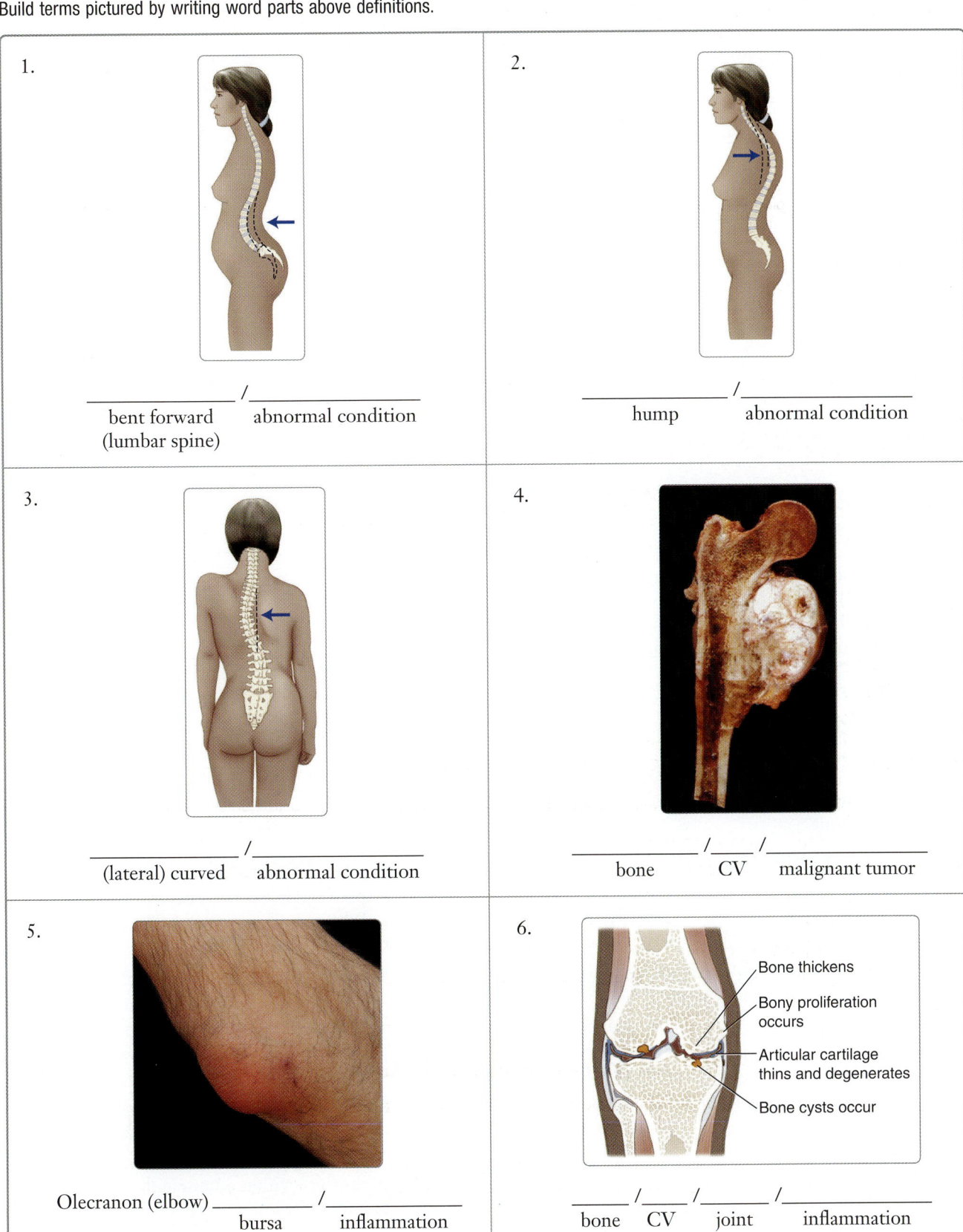

1. _____ / _____
   bent forward   abnormal condition
   (lumbar spine)

2. _____ / _____
   hump   abnormal condition

3. _____ / _____
   (lateral) curved   abnormal condition

4. _____ / ____ / _____
   bone   CV   malignant tumor

5. Olecranon (elbow) _____ / _____
                       bursa   inflammation

6. _____ / ____ / _____ / _____
   bone   CV   joint   inflammation

558 Chapter 14 Musculoskeletal System

B Fill In

Build disease and disorder terms for the following definitions with the word parts you have learned.

1. inflammation of the bone and cartilage _____ / _____ / _____ / _____
   WR / CV / WR / S

2. inflammation of the bone and bone marrow _____ / _____ / _____ / _____
   WR / CV / WR / S

3. inflammation of a joint _____ / _____
   WR / S

4. dissolution of striated muscle _____ / _____ / _____ / _____ / _____
   WR / CV / WR / CV / S

5. tumor of the bone marrow _____ / _____
   WR / S

6. inflammation of a tendon _____ / _____
   WR / S

7. abnormal condition of the vertebrae _____ / _____
   WR / S

8. abnormal reduction of bone mass _____ / _____ / _____
   WR / CV / S

9. fissure (split) of the vertebral column (congenital) _____ / _____
   WR / S

10. inflammation of the vertebral joints _____ / _____ / _____
    WR / WR / S

Disease and Disorder Terms
NOT BUILT FROM WORD PARTS

Word parts may be present in the following terms; however, their full meanings cannot be translated using definitions of word parts alone.

TERM	DEFINITION
1. **ankylosing spondylitis** (*ang*-ki-LŌ-sing) (*spon*-di-LI-tis)	form of arthritis that first affects the spine and adjacent structures and that, as it progresses, causes a forward bend of the spine (also called **Strümpell-Marie arthritis** or **disease**, or **rheumatoid spondylitis**)
🏛 **ANKYLOSING SPONDYLITIS** was first described in 1884 by Adolf von Strümpell (1853–1925). It became known as **Strümpell-Marie disease** after von Strümpell and French physician Pierre Marie.	
2. **bunion** (BUN-yun)	abnormal prominence of the joint at the base of the great toe, the metatarsal-phalangeal joint. It is a common problem, often hereditary or caused by poorly fitted shoes. (also called **hallux valgus**)
3. **carpal tunnel syndrome (CTS)** (KAR-pl) (TUN-el) (SIN-drōm)	common nerve entrapment disorder of the wrist caused by compression of the median nerve; symptoms include pain and tingling in portions of the hand and fingers
4. **compartment syndrome** (kom-PART-ment) (SIN-drōm)	painful condition caused by increased pressure within a muscle that can lead to ischemia; acute compartment syndrome is a medical emergency and is caused by severe injury

TERM	DEFINITION
5. dislocation (*dis*-lō-KĀ-shun)	displacement of bones in a joint from their normal alignment (also called **luxation**)
6. exostosis (*ek*-sos-TŌ-sis)	abnormal benign growth on the surface of a bone (also called **spur**)
7. fracture (fx) (FRAK-chūr)	broken bone
8. ganglion cyst (GANG-glē-on) (sist)	collection of jellylike fluid forming a benign mass arising from joints, most commonly appearing in the wrist, hand, and ankle
9. gout (gowt)	disease in which an excessive amount of uric acid in the blood causes sodium urate crystals (tophi) to be deposited in the joints, producing arthritis. The great toe is frequently affected.
10. herniated disk (HER-nē-*āt*-ed) (disk)	rupture of the intervertebral disk cartilage, which allows the contents to protrude through it, putting pressure on the spinal nerve roots (also called **slipped disk, ruptured disk, herniated intervertebral disk,** or **herniated nucleus pulposus [HNP]**)
11. Lyme disease (līm) (di-ZĒZ)	infection caused by a bite from a deer tick infected with *Borrelia burgdorferi*. This bacterium provokes an immune response in the body, the symptoms of which can mimic several musculoskeletal diseases. Patients may experience fever, headache, and joint pain. A rash (target lesion) may initially arise at the site of the tick bite.

LYME DISEASE was first reported in Lyme, Connecticut, in 1975.

TERM	DEFINITION
12. muscular dystrophy (MD) (MUS-kū-lar) (DIS-tro-fē)	group of hereditary diseases characterized by degeneration of muscle and weakness
13. myasthenia gravis (MG) (*mī*-as-THĒ-nē-a) (GRA-vis)	chronic disease characterized by muscle weakness and thought to be caused by a defect in the transmission of impulses from nerve to muscle cell. The face, larynx, and throat are frequently affected; no true paralysis of the muscles exists.
14. osteoporosis (*os*-tē-ō-po-RŌ-sis)	abnormal loss of bone density that may lead to an increase in fractures of the ribs, thoracic and lumbar vertebrae, hips, and wrists after slight trauma (occurs predominantly in postmenopausal women)
15. plantar fasciitis (PLAN-tar) (fas-ē-Ī-tis)	inflammation of the connective tissue of the sole of the foot (plantar fascia) due to repetitive injury; common cause of heel pain
16. repetitive strain injury (RSI) (rē-PET-i-tiv) (strān) (IN-ja-rē)	cumulative damage to joint, muscle, or other tissue caused by movements performed over and over again; characterized by pain, swelling, numbness, and lack of strength and flexibility, most commonly affecting the hands, wrists, elbows, and shoulders

REPETITIVE MOTION DISORDERS (RMDS) are a group of musculoskeletal disorders that can lead to repetitive strain injuries. They are caused by overuse and repetitive motions performed in the course of normal work or recreational activities and include **tendinitis, bursitis, tenosynovitis, ganglion cyst,** and **carpal tunnel syndrome**. The use of rest breaks and stretching, improved posture or ergonomics, antiinflammatory medications, and physical therapy provide the majority of treatment for RMDs. Surgery may be needed as treatment for permanent injuries.

TERM	DEFINITION
17. rheumatoid arthritis (RA) (RŪ-ma-toid) (ar-THRĪ-tis)	chronic systemic disease characterized by autoimmune inflammatory changes in the connective tissue throughout the body (Fig. 14.9C)
18. rotator cuff disease (RŌ-tā-tor) (kuf) (di-ZĒZ)	damage to one or more of the four muscles or tendons stabilizing the shoulder joint due to injury or degeneration; symptoms may include pain, limited range of motion, and muscle weakness
19. spinal stenosis (SPĪ-nal) (ste-NŌ-sis)	narrowing of the spinal canal with compression of nerve roots. The condition is either congenital or due to spinal degeneration. Symptoms are pain radiating to the thigh or lower legs and numbness or tingling in the lower extremities.
20. spondylolisthesis (*spon*-di-lō-lis-THĒ-sis)	forward slipping of one vertebra over another

Disease and Disorder Terms—cont'd
NOT BUILT FROM WORD PARTS

TERM	DEFINITION
21. **sprain** (sprān)	abnormal stretching or tearing of a ligament that supports a joint
22. **strain** (strān)	abnormal stretching or tearing of a muscle or tendon
23. **subluxation** (sub-luk-SĀ-shun)	partial dislocation of bones in a joint
24. **tarsal tunnel syndrome** (TĀR-sl) (TUN-el) (SIN-drōm)	painful foot disorder caused by compression of the posterior tibial nerve as it passes through the ankle

EXERCISE 9 ■ Pronounce and Spell

Practice pronunciation and spelling on paper and online.

1. **Practice on Paper**
   a. **Pronounce:** Read the phonetic spelling and say aloud the terms listed in the previous table. Refer to Table 2.2 Pronunciation Key as needed.
   b. **Spell:** Have a study partner read the terms aloud. Write the spelling of the terms on a separate sheet of paper.

2. **Practice Online**
   a. **Access** online learning resources. Go to evolve.elsevier.com > Evolve Resources > Student Resources.
   b. **Pronounce:** Select Audio Glossary > Chapter 14 > Exercise 9. Select a term to hear its pronunciation and repeat aloud.
   c. **Spell:** Select Activities > Chapter 14 > Spell Terms > Exercise 9. Select the audio icon and type the correct spelling of the term.

❑ Check the box when complete.

EXERCISE 10 ■ Match

Match the terms in the first column with their correct definitions in the second column.

_____ 1. muscular dystrophy
_____ 2. exostosis
_____ 3. ankylosing spondylitis
_____ 4. myasthenia gravis
_____ 5. tarsal tunnel syndrome
_____ 6. subluxation
_____ 7. strain
_____ 8. repetitive strain injury
_____ 9. compartment syndrome
_____ 10. sprain

a. abnormal benign growth on the surface of a bone
b. form of arthritis that first affects the spine and adjacent structures, eventually causing a forward bend of the spine
c. group of hereditary diseases characterized by degeneration of muscles and weakness
d. chronic disease characterized by muscle weakness and thought to be caused by a defect in the transmission of impulses from nerve to muscle cell
e. foot disorder caused by compression of the posterior tibial nerve as it passes through the ankle
f. abnormal stretching or tearing of a ligament that supports a joint
g. condition caused by increased pressure within a muscle that can lead to ischemia
h. cumulative damage to joint, muscle, or other tissue caused by movements performed over and over again
i. partial dislocation of bones in a joint
j. abnormal stretching or tearing of a muscle or tendon

Chapter 14 Musculoskeletal System   561

EXERCISE 11 ■ Label

Write the medical terms pictured and defined.

1. _____
rupture of the intervertebral disk cartilage, which allows the contents to protrude through it, putting pressure on the spinal nerve roots

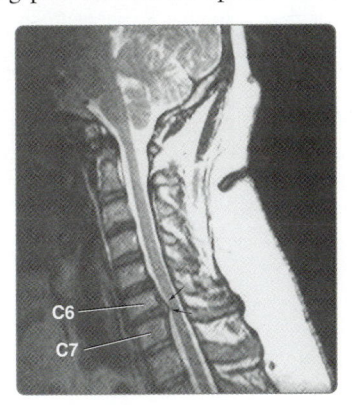

2. _____
chronic systemic disease characterized by autoimmune inflammatory changes in the connective tissue throughout the body

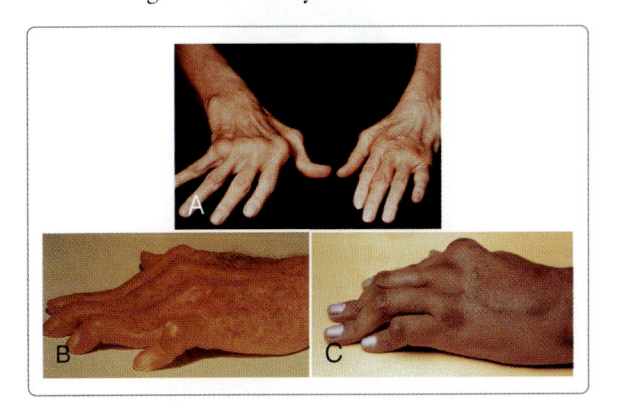

3. _____
common nerve entrapment disorder of the wrist caused by compression of the median nerve

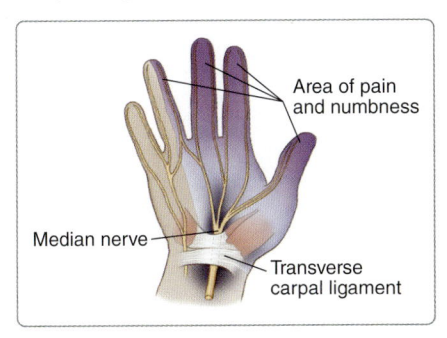

4. _____
forward slipping of one vertebra over the other

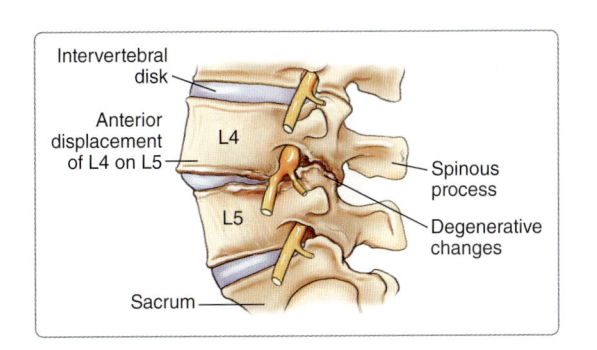

5. _____
disease in which an excessive amount of uric acid in the blood causes sodium urate crystals (tophi) to be deposited in the joints

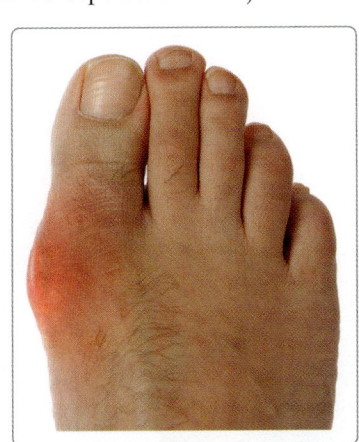

6. _____
abnormal loss of density that may lead to an increase in fractures

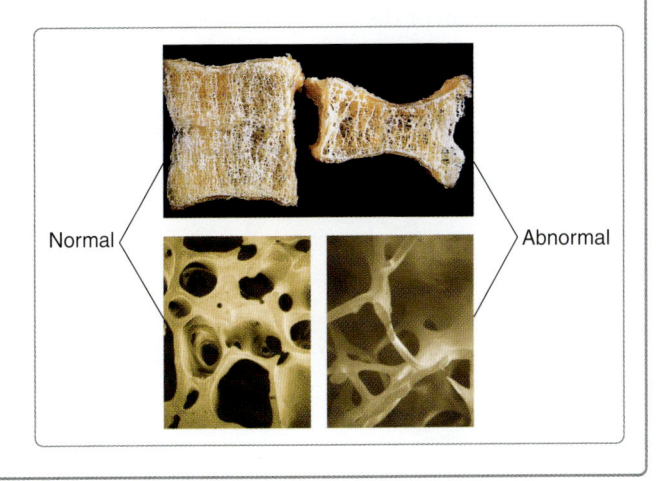

562 Chapter 14 Musculoskeletal System

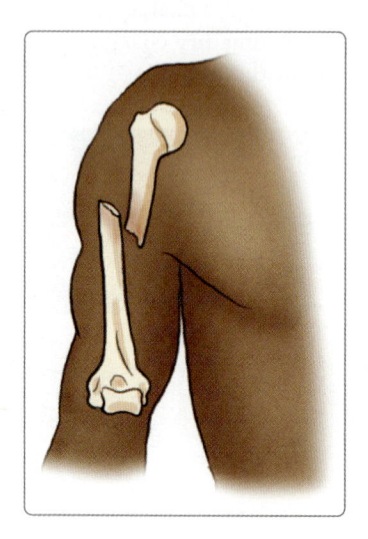

7. _____
broken bone

8. _____
infection caused by a bite from an infected deer tick, which provokes an immune response that can mimic several musculoskeletal diseases. A rash (target lesion) may be found at the site of the tick bite.

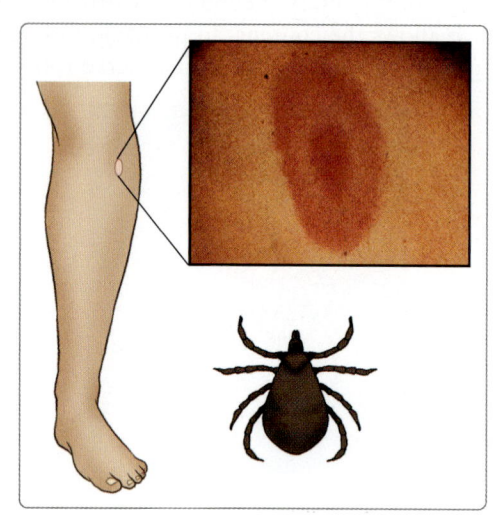

9. _____
abnormal prominence of the joint at the base of the great toe, the metatarsal-phalangeal joint

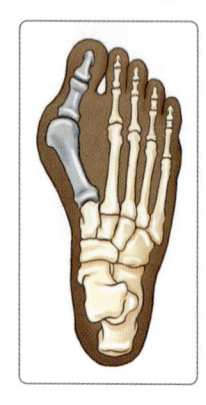

10. _____
narrowing of the spinal canal with compression of nerve roots

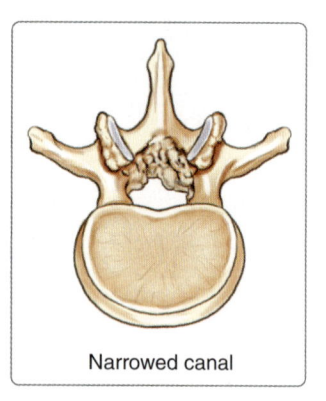

11. _____
inflammation of the connective tissue of the sole of the foot; common cause of heel pain

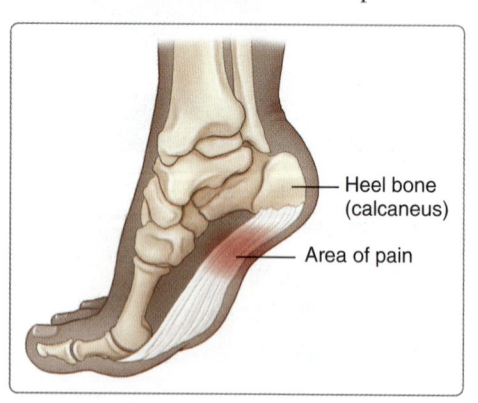

12. _____
collection of jellylike fluid forming a benign mass arising from joints

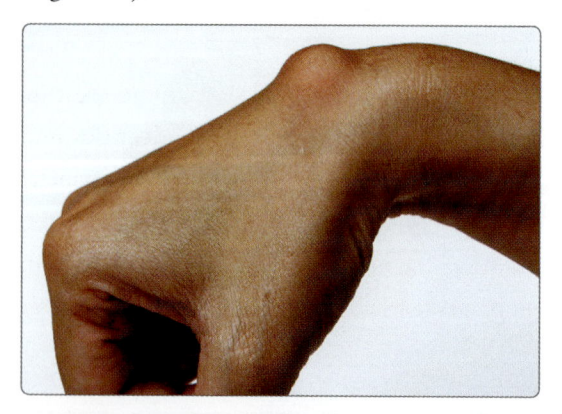

13. _____
damage to one or more of the four muscles or tendons stabilizing the shoulder joint due to injury or degeneration

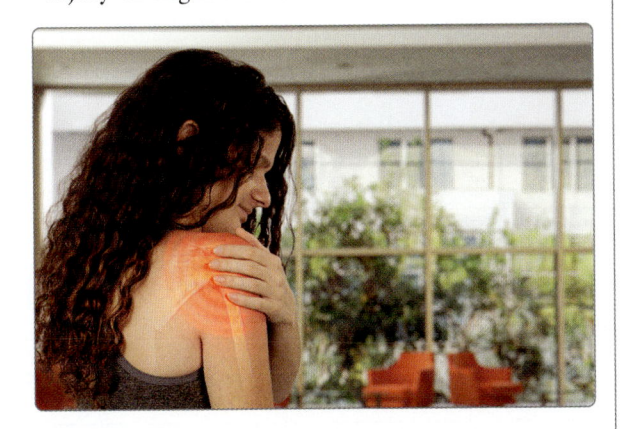

14. _____
displacement of bones in a joint from their normal alignment

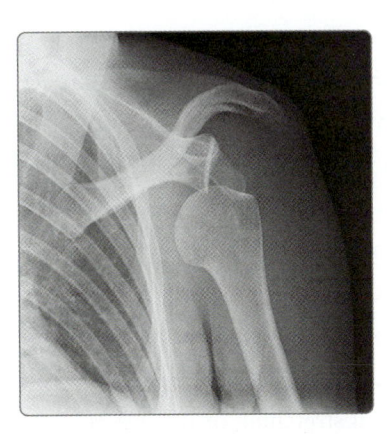

EXERCISE 12 ■ Identify

Write the medical terms defined.

1. Conditions affecting the spine:
   a. forward slipping of one vertebra over another _____
   b. rupture of the intervertebral disk cartilage, which allows the contents to protrude through it, putting pressure on the spinal nerve roots _____
   c. form of arthritis that first affects the spine and adjacent structures and that, as it progresses, causes a forward bend of the spine _____
   d. narrowing of the spinal canal with compression of nerve roots _____
2. Conditions involving joints:
   a. abnormal prominence of the joint at the base of the great toe, the metatarsal-phalangeal joint _____
   b. painful foot disorder caused by compression of the posterior tibial nerve as it passes through the ankle _____
   c. common nerve entrapment disorder of the wrist caused by compression of the median nerve _____
   d. collection of jellylike fluid forming a benign mass arising from joints, most commonly appearing in the wrist, hand, and ankle _____
   e. disease in which an excessive amount of uric acid in the blood causes sodium urate crystals (tophi) to be deposited in the joints, producing arthritis. The great toe is frequently affected. _____
   f. infection caused by a bite from a deer tick infected with *Borrelia burgdorferi*. This bacterium provokes an immune response in the body, the symptoms of which include joint pain. _____
   g. chronic systemic disease characterized by autoimmune inflammatory changes in the connective tissue throughout the body, including joint linings causing painful swelling _____
   h. displacement of bones in a joint from their normal alignment (also called luxation) _____

i. partial dislocation of bones in a joint _____

j. cumulative damage to joint, muscle, or other tissue caused by movements performed over and over again; characterized by pain, swelling, numbness, and lack of strength and flexibility, most commonly affecting the hands, wrists, elbows, and shoulders _____

3. Conditions affecting bone:
   a. abnormal benign growth on the surface of a bone (also called spur) _____
   b. broken bone _____
   c. abnormal loss of bone density that may lead to an increase in fractures of the ribs, thoracic and lumbar vertebrae, hips, and wrists after slight trauma _____

4. Conditions affecting muscle:
   a. damage to one or more of the four muscles or tendons stabilizing the shoulder joint due to injury or degeneration; symptoms may include pain, limited range of motion, and muscle weakness _____

   b. abnormal stretching or tearing of a muscle or tendon _____
   c. abnormal stretching or tearing of a ligament that supports a joint _____
   d. painful condition caused by increased pressure within a muscle that can lead to ischemia _____

   e. inflammation of the connective tissue of the sole of the foot due to repetitive injury; common cause of heel pain _____

   f. chronic disease characterized by muscle weakness and thought to be caused by a defect in the transmission of impulses from nerve to muscle cell _____
   g. group of hereditary diseases characterized by degeneration of muscle and weakness _____

EXERCISE 13 ■ Review of Disease and Disorder Terms

Can you define, pronounce, and spell the following terms?

ankylosing spondylitis	fracture (fx)	osteomalacia	sarcopenia
ankylosis	ganglion cyst	osteomyelitis	scoliosis
arthritis	gout	osteonecrosis	spinal stenosis
bunion	herniated disk	osteopenia	spondylarthritis
bursitis	kyphosis	osteopetrosis	spondylolisthesis
carpal tunnel syndrome (CTS)	lordosis	osteoporosis	spondylosis
	Lyme disease	osteosarcoma	sprain
chondromalacia	meniscitis	plantar fasciitis	strain
chondrosarcoma	muscular dystrophy (MD)	polymyositis (PM)	subluxation
compartment syndrome		rachischisis	synoviosarcoma
cranioschisis	myasthenia gravis (MG)	repetitive strain injury (RSI)	tarsal tunnel syndrome
discitis	myeloma		tendinitis
dislocation	osteitis	rhabdomyolysis	tenosynovitis
exostosis	osteoarthritis (OA)	rheumatoid arthritis (RA)	
fasciitis	osteochondritis		
fibromyalgia	osteochondroma	rotator cuff disease	

Chapter 14 Musculoskeletal System 565

Surgical Terms
BUILT FROM WORD PARTS

The following terms can be translated using definitions of word parts. Further explanation is provided within parentheses as needed.

TERM	DEFINITION
1. arthrocentesis (ar-thrō-sen-TĒ-sis)	surgical puncture to aspirate fluid from a joint
2. arthrodesis (ar-thrō-DĒ-sis)	surgical fixation of a joint (also called **joint fusion**)
3. arthroplasty (AR-thrō-plas-tē)	surgical repair of a joint (Table 14.1)
4. bursectomy (bur-SEK-to-mē)	excision of a bursa
5. carpectomy (kar-PEK-to-mē)	excision of a carpal bone
6. chondrectomy (kon-DREK-to-mē)	excision of cartilage
7. chondroplasty (KON-drō-plas-tē)	surgical repair of cartilage
8. costectomy (kos-TEK-to-mē)	excision of a rib
9. cranioplasty (KRĀ-nē-ō-plas-tē)	surgical repair of the skull
10. craniotomy (krā-nē-OT-o-mē)	incision into the cranium (as for surgery of the brain)
11. discectomy (dis-KEK-to-mē)	excision of an intervertebral disk (a portion of the herniated disk is removed to relieve pressure on nerve roots; uses a larger incision than microdiscectomy)
12. fasciotomy (fash-ē-OT-o-mē)	incision into the fascia (to relieve tension or pressure)
13. laminectomy (lam-i-NEK-to-mē)	excision of a lamina (often performed to relieve pressure on the nerve roots in the lower spine caused by a herniated disk and other conditions)
14. maxillectomy (mak-si-LEK-to-mē)	excision of the maxilla
15. meniscectomy (men-i-SEK-to-mē)	excision of a meniscus (performed for a torn cartilage)

TERM	DEFINITION
16. microdiscectomy (mī-kro-dis-KEK-to-mē)	small excision of an intervertebral disk (minimally invasive surgery to remove a portion of the herniated disk to relieve pressure on nerve roots)

MICROENDOSCOPIC DISCECTOMY (MED) uses a fluoroscope and special dilating instrumentation to create a small tunnel to the affected disk area. An endoscopic tool allows the surgeon to visualize and remove the thick, sticky nucleus of the herniated disk. The disk then softens and contracts, relieving severe low back and leg pain. Recovery time is significantly less than open discectomy because of a small incision and less trauma to surrounding tissues.

TERM	DEFINITION
17. myorrhaphy (mī-OR-a-fē)	suturing of a muscle
18. osteotomy (os-tē-OT-o-mē)	incision into a bone
19. phalangectomy (fal-an-JEK-to-mē)	excision of a finger or toe bone
20. rachiotomy (rā-kē-OT-o-mē)	incision into the vertebral column
21. spondylosyndesis (spon-di-lō-sin-DĒ-sis)	fusing together of the vertebrae (also called **spinal fusion**) (Note: the prefix syn- appears in the middle of the term.)
22. synovectomy (sin-ō-VEK-to-mē)	excision of the synovial membrane (of a joint) (Note: the i in synovi is dropped because the suffix begins with a vowel.)
23. tarsectomy (tar-SEK-to-mē)	excision of (one or more) tarsal bones
24. tenomyoplasty (ten-ō-MĪ-ō-plas-tē)	surgical repair of the tendon and muscle
25. tenorrhaphy (te-NOR-a-fē)	suturing of a tendon
26. vertebroplasty (VER-te-brō-plas-tē)	surgical repair of a vertebra (usually performed for compression fractures due to osteoporosis) (Table 14.2)

TABLE 14.1 Types of Arthroplasty

Total hip arthroplasty (THA) is indicated for degenerative joint disease or rheumatoid arthritis. The operation originally involved replacement of the hip joint with a metallic femoral head and a plastic-coated acetabulum. More recently, however, many different materials have been used in an attempt to prevent the artificial joint from wearing out too quickly. These materials include joints composed of metal, ceramics, polyethylene (plastic), and combinations of each.

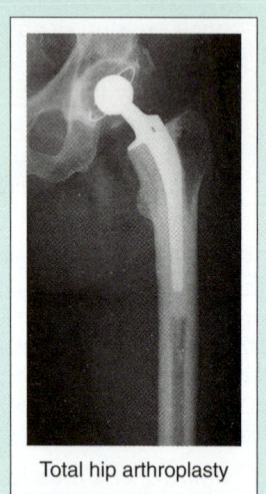

Total hip arthroplasty

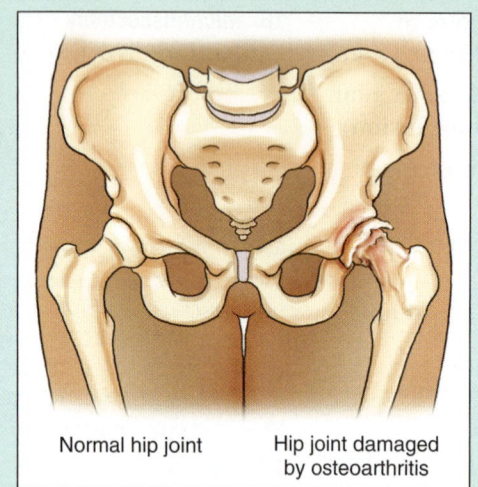

Normal hip joint | Hip joint damaged by osteoarthritis

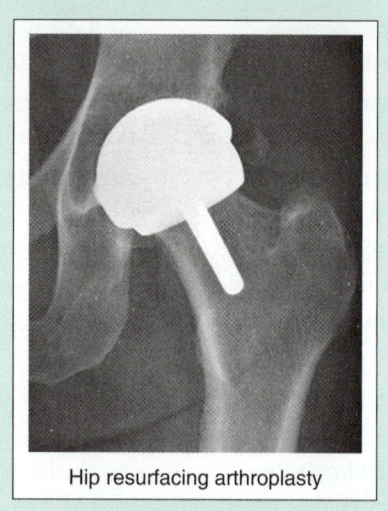

Hip resurfacing arthroplasty

Hip resurfacing arthroplasty (HRA) is a procedure that provides an option for younger, active patients needing a total hip arthroplasty. The procedure requires the removal of a few millimeters of bone from the femoral head instead of the removal of the entire femoral head required in total hip arthroplasty. A metal cap is then placed on top of the femur, and smooth metal is placed in the acetabulum. The risk of fracture of the neck of the femur is increased when smaller diameter components are used, making HRA less appropriate for women.

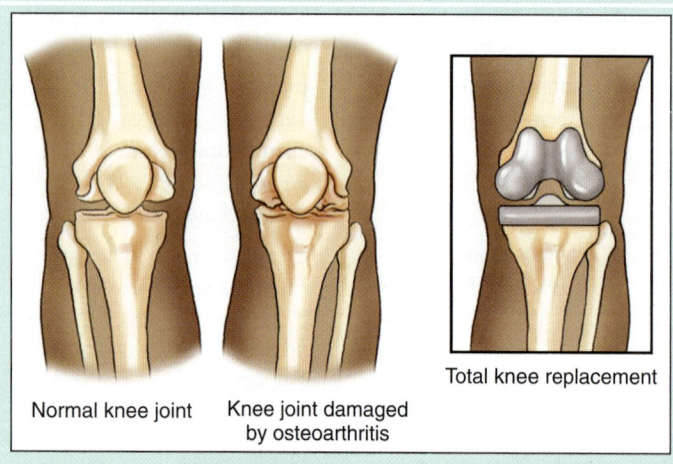

Normal knee joint | Knee joint damaged by osteoarthritis

Total knee replacement

Total knee arthroplasty (TKA) is designed to replace worn surfaces of the knee joint. Various prostheses (artificial parts) are used.

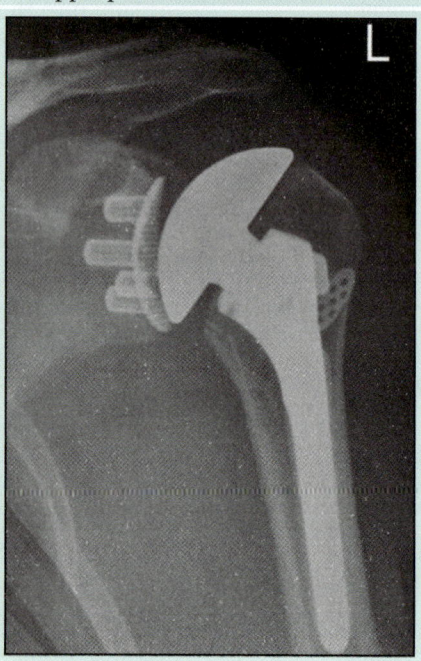

Shoulder arthroplasty is a procedure that restores the major functions of this ball and socket joint: motion, stability, strength, and smoothness. Prostheses are applied to the head of the humerus and the glenoid cavity (part of the scapula). Osteoarthritis, rheumatoid arthritis, and severe rotator cuff tears are some of the most common reasons for this surgery.

TABLE 14.2 Procedures for Treatment of Compression Fractures Caused by Osteoporosis

Percutaneous vertebroplasty (PV) is a minimally invasive operation in which an interventional radiologist places a needle through the skin into the damaged vertebra. A special liquid cement is injected into the area through the needle to fill the holes left by osteoporosis.

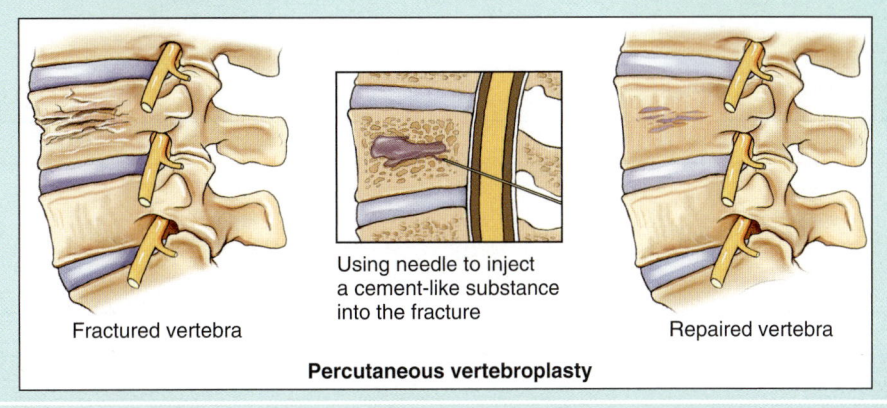

Fractured vertebra — Using needle to inject a cement-like substance into the fracture — Repaired vertebra

Percutaneous vertebroplasty

Kyphoplasty is similar to vertebroplasty except a balloonlike device is used to expand the compressed vertebra before the cement is injected. Recent studies have generated controversy as to whether these procedures are better than nonsurgical management, such as pain medication and physical therapy. In either case, it is important to treat the underlying osteoporosis to prevent future fractures.

EXERCISE 14 ■ Pronounce and Spell

Practice pronunciation and spelling on paper and online.

1. **Practice on Paper**
   a. **Pronounce:** Read the phonetic spelling and say aloud the terms listed in the previous table. Refer to Table 2.2 Pronunciation Key as needed.
   b. **Spell:** Have a study partner read the terms aloud. Write the spelling of the terms on a separate sheet of paper.

2. **Practice Online**
   a. **Access** online learning resources. Go to evolve.elsevier.com > Evolve Resources > Student Resources.
   b. **Pronounce:** Select Audio Glossary > Chapter 14 > Exercise 14. Select a term to hear its pronunciation and repeat aloud.
   c. **Spell:** Select Activities > Chapter 14 > Spell Terms > Exercise 14. Select the audio icon and type the correct spelling of the term.

❏ Check the box when complete.

EXERCISE 15 ■ Analyze and Define

Analyze and define the following surgical terms.

1. vertebroplasty

2. tarsectomy

3. arthrodesis

4. laminectomy

Chapter 14 Musculoskeletal System

5. synovectomy
   _____
   _____

6. fasciotomy
   _____
   _____

7. rachiotomy
   _____
   _____

8. bursectomy
   _____
   _____

9. discectomy
   _____
   _____

10. arthrocentesis
    _____
    _____

11. maxillectomy
    _____
    _____

12. cranioplasty
    _____
    _____

13. carpectomy
    _____
    _____

14. phalangectomy
    _____
    _____

EXERCISE 16 ■ Build

A Label

Build terms pictured by writing word parts above definitions.

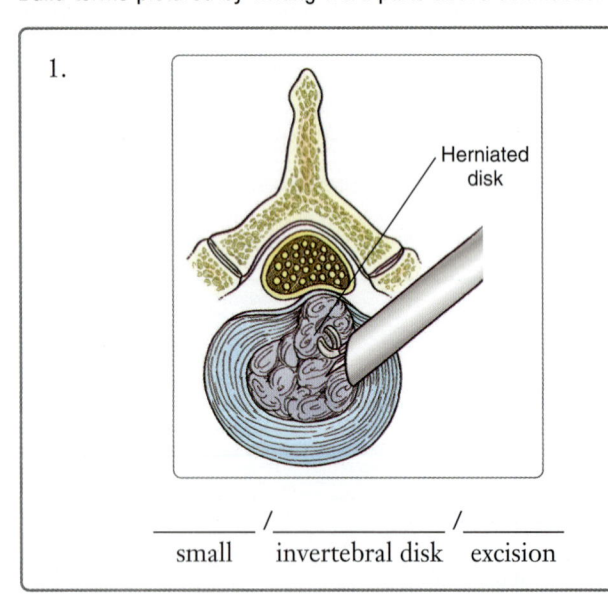

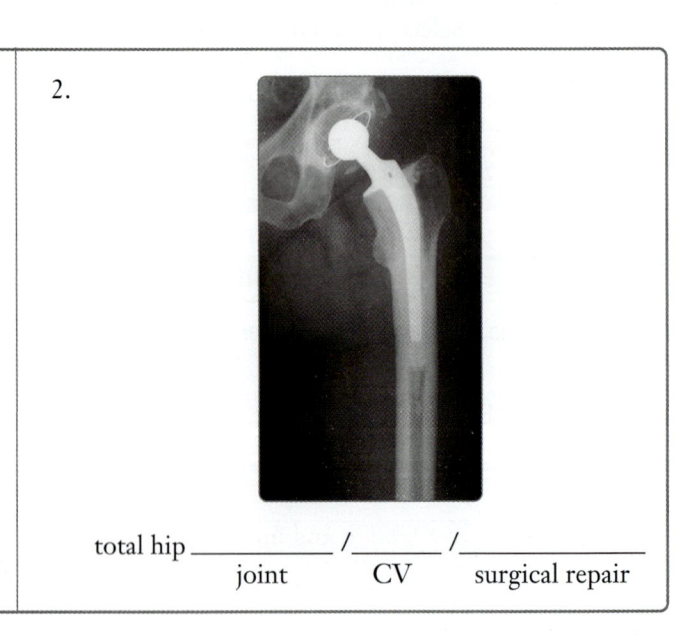

1. _____ / _____ / _____
   small   invertebral disk   excision

2. total hip _____ / _____ / _____
              joint   CV   surgical repair

3.

_____ / ____ / __syn__ / _____
vertebra   CV   together   fusion

4.

_____ / _____
meniscus   excision

5.

_____ / _____ / _____
cranium   CV   incision

6.

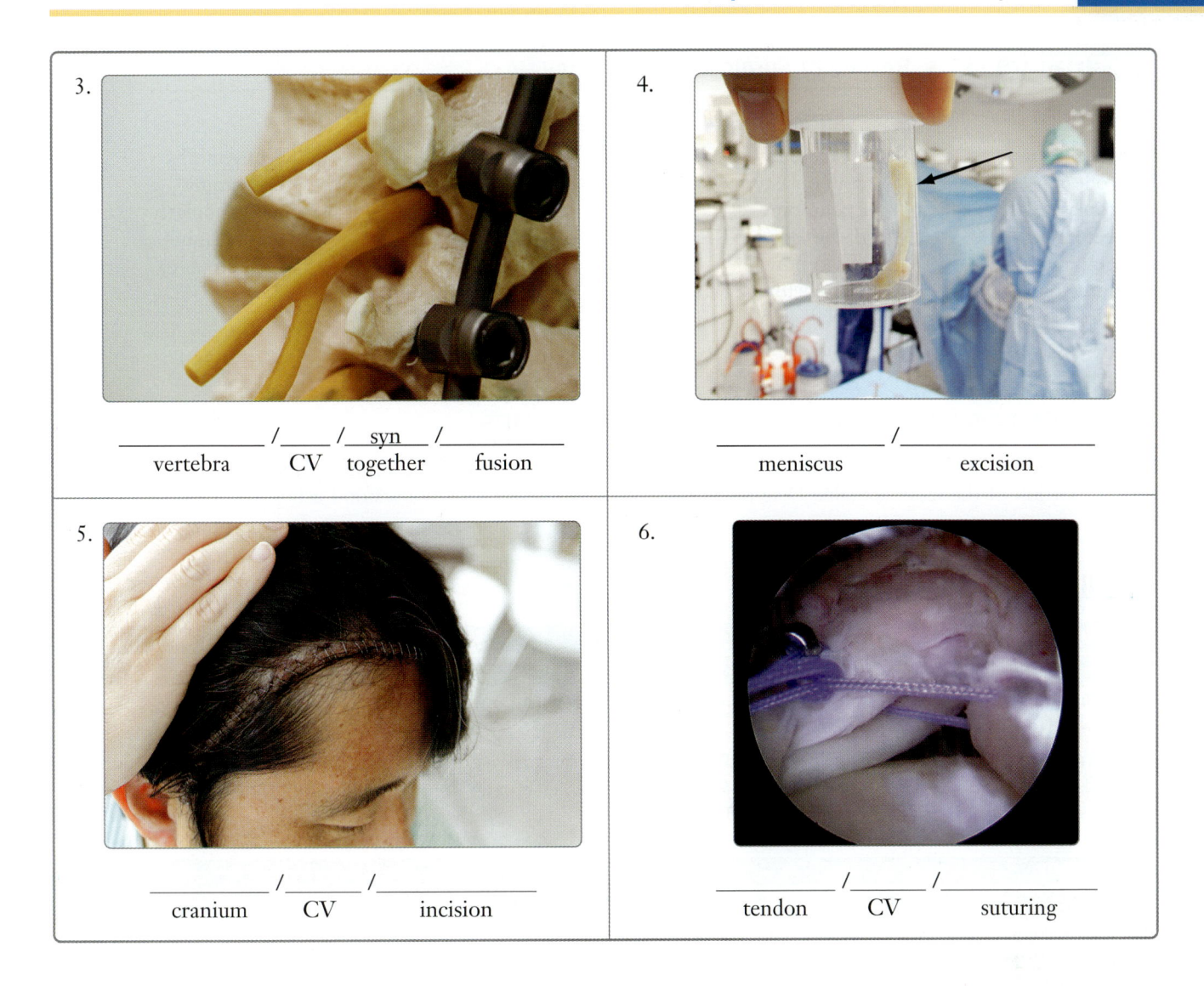

_____ / _____ / _____
tendon   CV   suturing

B Fill In

Build surgical terms for the following definitions by using the word parts you have learned.

1. incision into a bone

   _____ / ____ / _____
      WR   CV   S

2. excision of cartilage

   _____ / _____
      WR   S

3. surgical repair of cartilage

   _____ / ____ / _____
      WR   CV   S

4. suturing of a muscle

   _____ / ____ / _____
      WR   CV   S

5. surgical repair of a tendon and muscle

   _____ / ____ / _____ / ____ / _____
      WR   CV   WR   CV   S

6. excision of a rib

   _____ / _____
      WR   S

EXERCISE 17 ■ Review of Surgical Terms

Can you define, pronounce, and spell the following terms?

arthrocentesis	costectomy	meniscectomy	synovectomy
arthrodesis	cranioplasty	microdiscectomy	tarsectomy
arthroplasty	craniotomy	myorrhaphy	tenomyoplasty
bursectomy	discectomy	osteotomy	tenorrhaphy
carpectomy	fasciotomy	phalangectomy	vertebroplasty
chondrectomy	laminectomy	rachiotomy	
chondroplasty	maxillectomy	spondylosyndesis	

Diagnostic Terms

BUILT FROM WORD PARTS AND *NOT* BUILT FROM WORD PARTS

The first portion of the table contains Diagnostic Terms that can be translated using definitions of word parts. The second portion of the table contains Diagnostic Terms that cannot be fully understood using the definitions of word parts.

■ Built from Word Parts

DIAGNOSTIC IMAGING

TERM	DEFINITION
1. arthrography (ar-THROG-ra-fē)	radiographic imaging of a joint (with contrast materials)

MAGNETIC RESONANCE (MR) has mostly replaced conventional **arthrography** as the imaging technique for joints such as the knee, wrist, hip, and shoulder. Many of the remaining arthrograms are performed in conjunction with MR. A conventional arthrogram might be used in situations in which a patient cannot undergo MR, such as a person with a cardiac pacemaker.

ENDOSCOPY

TERM	DEFINITION
2. arthroscopy (ar-THROS-ko-pē)	visual examination of a joint

OTHER

TERM	DEFINITION
3. electromyogram (EMG) (ē-*lek*-trō-MĪ-ō-gram)	record of the (intrinsic) electrical activity in a (skeletal) muscle

■ *NOT* Built from Word Parts

DIAGNOSTIC IMAGING

TERM	DEFINITION
1. dual x-ray absorptiometry (DXA) (du-al) (EKS-rā) (ab-*sorp*-shē-OM-e-trē)	radiographic imaging, usually of the lumbar spine and hips, to measure bone loss and bone mineral density; the procedure utilizes low doses of radiation and is used in the diagnosis of osteoporosis and monitoring of treatment (also called **dual-energy x-ray absorptiometry [DEXA], bone densitometry,** and **bone density test**) (Fig. 14.11)

TABLE 14.3 Diagnostic Imaging Procedures Used for the Musculoskeletal System

In addition to **arthrography**, the following diagnostic imaging procedures are commonly used for diagnosing diseases, fractures, strains, and other conditions of the musculoskeletal system.

Bone densitometry is a method of determining the density of bone by radiographic techniques used to diagnose osteoporosis. **Dual X-ray absorptiometry (DXA)** is commonly used for this test. (Fig. 14.11)

Bone scan (nuclear medicine test) is used to detect the presence of metastatic disease of the bone and to monitor degenerative bone disease. (Fig. 14.13)

Magnetic resonance (MR) is used to evaluate the bones and soft tissue of the shoulders, hips, elbows, knees, ankles, feet, and spinal cord for stenosis, spinal cord defects, and degenerative disk changes. (Fig. 14.12)

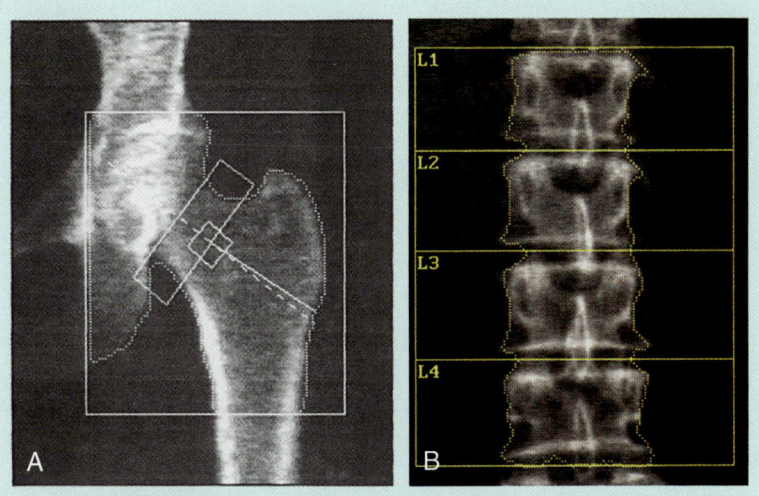

FIG. 14.11 DXA images of the (A) left hip and (B) spine.

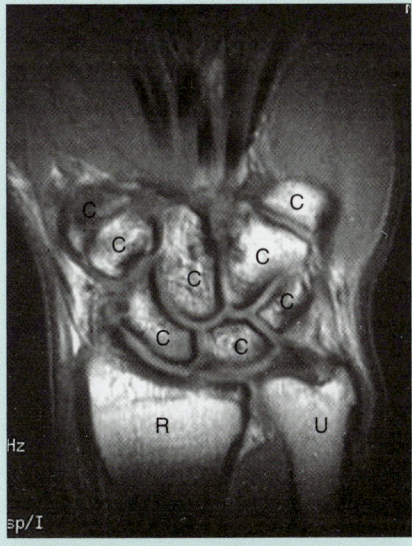

FIG. 14.12 Coronal MR scan of the wrist. Marrow within the carpal bones (C), radius (R), and ulna (U).

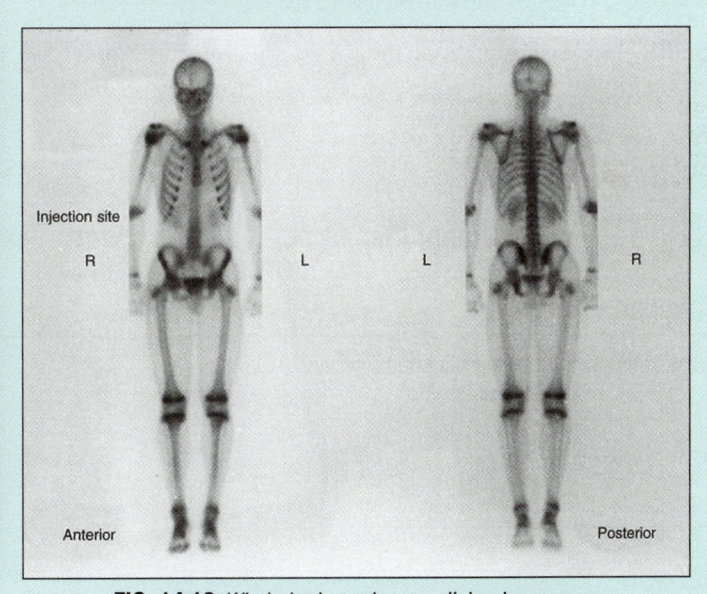

FIG. 14.13 Whole body nuclear medicine bone scan.

Radiography (radiographic imaging) of the bones and joints is used to identify fractures or tumors, monitor healing, or identify abnormal structures.

Single-photon emission computed tomography (SPECT) of the bone is an even more sensitive nuclear method for detecting bone abnormalities.

Diagnostic Terms—cont'd
BUILT FROM WORD PARTS AND *NOT* BUILT FROM WORD PARTS
- ***NOT* Built from Word Parts**

LABORATORY

TERM	DEFINITION
2. bone markers (bōn) (MAR-krs)	blood and urine tests to determine the rate of bone turnover (resorption and formation); often used with DXA to diagnose and monitor treatment of osteoporosis and other bone disorders
3. muscle biopsy (MUS-el) (BĪ-op-sē)	removal of muscle tissue using a needle or small incision; used to assess musculoskeletal abnormalities involving weakness or pain, such as muscular dystrophy, myasthenia gravis, and polymyositis

EXERCISE 18 ■ Pronounce and Spell

Practice pronunciation and spelling on paper and online.

1. **Practice on Paper**
   a. **Pronounce:** Read the phonetic spelling and say aloud the terms listed in the previous table. Refer to Table 2.2 Pronunciation Key as needed.
   b. **Spell:** Have a study partner read the terms aloud. Write the spelling of the terms on a separate sheet of paper.

2. **Practice Online**
   a. **Access** online learning resources. Go to evolve.elsevier.com > Evolve Resources > Student Resources.
   b. **Pronounce:** Select Audio Glossary > Chapter 14 > Exercise 18. Select a term to hear its pronunciation and repeat aloud.
   c. **Spell:** Select Activities > Chapter 14 > Spell Terms > Exercise 18. Select the audio icon and type the correct spelling of the term.

❏ Check the box when complete.

EXERCISE 19 ■ Diagnostic Terms Built from Word Parts

A Analyze and Define

Analyze and define the following diagnostic terms.

1. electromyogram

2. arthrography

3. arthroscopy

Chapter 14 Musculoskeletal System   573

B Build

Build diagnostic terms for the following definitions using word parts you have learned.

1. radiographic imaging of a joint   _____ / ___ / _____
                                        WR   CV   S

2. visual examination of a joint   _____ / ___ / _____
                                        WR   CV   S

C Label

Build terms pictured by writing word parts above definitions.

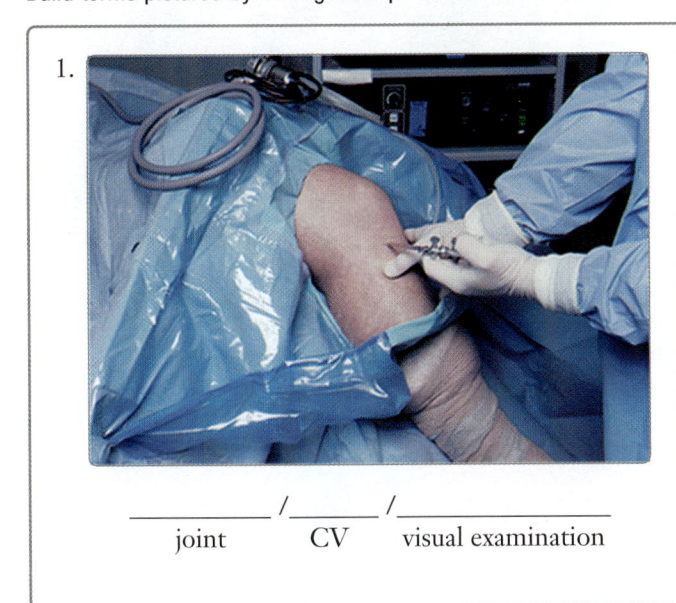

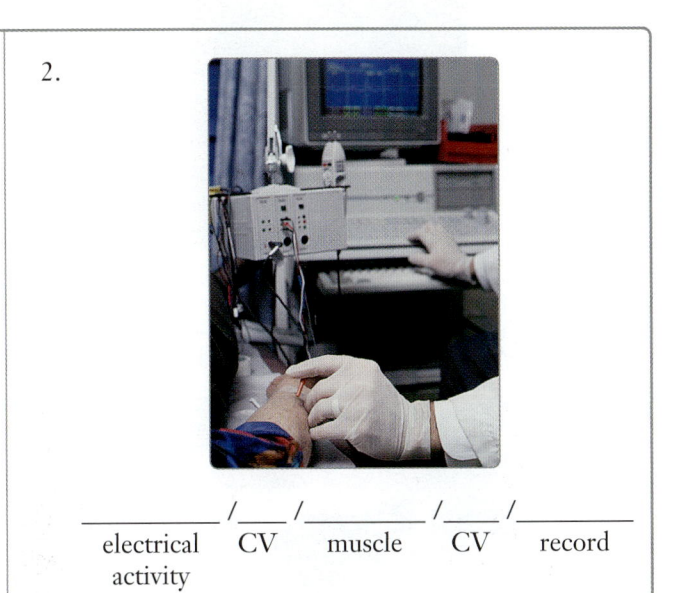

1.
_____ / ___ / _____
joint   CV   visual examination

2.
_____ / ___ / _____ / ___ / _____
electrical CV muscle CV record
activity

EXERCISE 20 ■ Diagnostic Terms NOT Built from Word Parts

A Match

Select the term described. Answers may be used more than once.

_____ 1. often used with DXA
_____ 2. also called bone density test
_____ 3. used to assess musculoskeletal abnormalities involving weakness or pain
_____ 4. collects a sample using a needle or small incision
_____ 5. determines the rate of bone turnover
_____ 6. measures bone loss and bone mineral density

a. dual x-ray absorptiometry
b. bone markers
c. muscle biopsy

574   Chapter 14   Musculoskeletal System

B   Label

Write the medical terms pictured and defined.

1. _____
radiographic imaging, usually of the lumbar spine and hips, to measure bone loss and bone mineral density

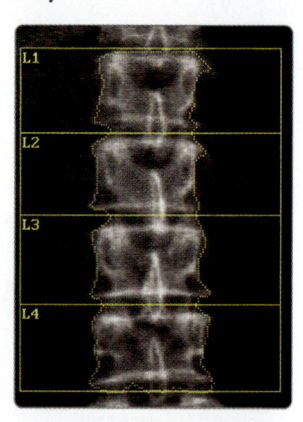

2. _____
removal of muscle tissue, using a needle or small incision, to assess musculoskeletal abnormalities involving weakness or pain

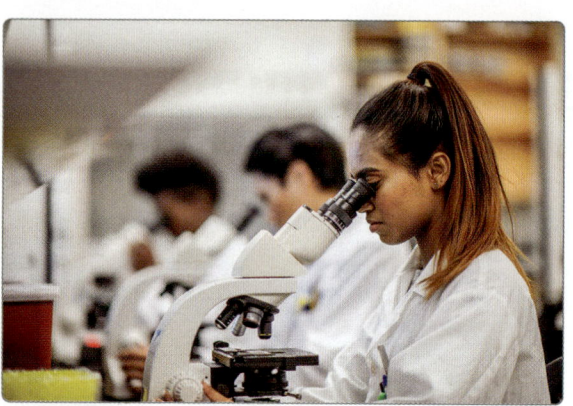

3. _____
blood and urine tests to determine the rate of bone turnover (resorption and formation)

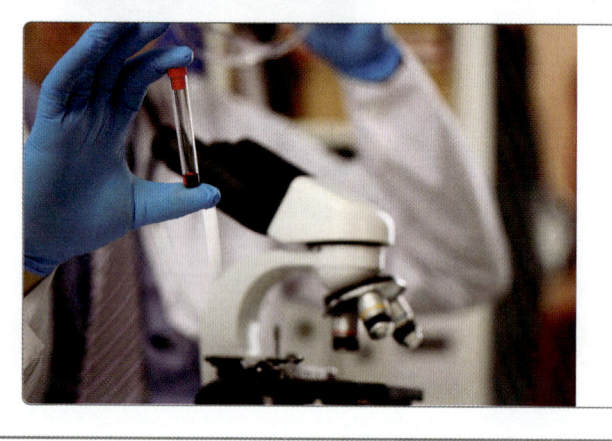

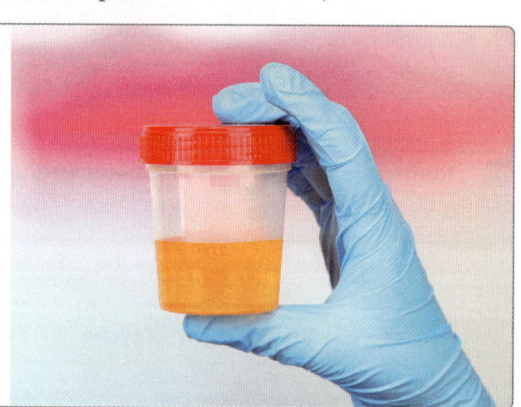

EXERCISE 21 ■ Review of Diagnostic Terms

Can you define, pronounce, and spell the following terms?

arthrography	dual x-ray absorptiometry (DXA)
arthroscopy	electromyogram (EMG)
bone markers	muscle biopsy

Complementary Terms
BUILT FROM WORD PARTS

The following terms can be translated using definitions of word parts. Further explanation is provided within parentheses as needed.

SIGNS AND SYMPTOMS

TERM	DEFINITION	TERM	DEFINITION
1. arthralgia (ar-THRAL-ja)	joint pain	7. hyperkinesia (hī-per-ki-NĒ-zha)	excessive movement (hyperactive)
2. atrophy (AT-ro-fē)	without development (process of wasting away)	*MOVEMENT DISORDERS are impairments in voluntary movement and are also known as dyskinesias. Bradykinesia is characterized by slowness of all voluntary movement and speech, while hyperkinesia describes excessive or involuntary movements. Parkinson disease and Tourette syndrome are some examples of movement disorders.*	
3. bradykinesia (brad-ē-ki-NĒ-zha)	slow movement		
4. dyskinesia (dis-ki-NĒ-zha)	difficult movement	8. hypertrophy (hī-PER-tro-fē)	excessive development
5. dystrophy (DIS-tro-fē)	abnormal development	9. myalgia (mī-AL-ja)	muscle pain
6. hemarthrosis (hē-mar-THRŌ-sis)	abnormal condition of blood in the joint (sign and lab finding)	10. myasthenia (mī-as-THĒ-nē-a)	muscle weakness

DESCRIPTIVE TERMS

TERM	DEFINITION	TERM	DEFINITION
11. carpal (CAR-pal)	pertaining to the carpals (wrist)	22. lumbar (LUM-bar)	pertaining to the loins (the part of the back between the thorax and pelvis)
12. clavicular (kla-VIK-ū-lar)	pertaining to the clavicle (collarbone)		
13. cranial (KRĀ-nē-al)	pertaining to the cranium (skull)	23. patellar (pa-TEL-lar)	pertaining to the patella (kneecap)
14. femoral (FEM-or-al)	pertaining to the femur (upper leg bone)	24. patellofemoral (pa-tel-ō-FEM-or-al)	pertaining to the patella and femur
15. fibular (FIB-ū-lar)	pertaining to the fibula (lower leg bone)	25. phalangeal (fa-LAN-jē-al)	pertaining to the phalanx (*pl.* phalanges) (any bone of the fingers or toes)
16. humeral (HŪ-mer-al)	pertaining to the humerus (upper arm bone)	26. pubic (PŪ-bik)	pertaining to the pubis (anterior portion of the pelvis)
17. iliac (IL-ē-ak)	pertaining to the ilium (upper, wing-shaped portion of the pelvis)		
18. intercostal (in-ter-KOS-tal)	pertaining to between the ribs	27. radial (RĀ-dē-al)	pertaining to the radius (lower arm bone)
19. intervertebral (in-ter-VER-te-bral)	pertaining to between the vertebrae	28. sacral (SĀ-kral)	pertaining to the sacrum (lower portion of the spine forming the posterior pelvic wall)
20. intracranial (in-tra-KRĀ-nē-al)	pertaining to within the cranium (skull)	29. scapular (SKAP-ū-lar)	pertaining to the scapula (shoulder blade)
21. ischial (IS-kē-al)	pertaining to the ischium (lower posterior portion of the pelvis)	30. sternal (STER-nal)	pertaining to the sternum (breastbone)

Chapter 14 Musculoskeletal System

TERM	DEFINITION	TERM	DEFINITION
31. **submandibular** (*sub*-man-DIB-ū-lar)	pertaining to below the mandible (lower jawbone)	36. **tarsal** (TAR-sal)	pertaining to the tarsals (ankle bones)
32. **submaxillary** (sub-MAK-si-*lar*-ē)	pertaining to below the maxilla (upper jawbone)	37. **tibial** (TIB-ē-al)	pertaining to the tibia (lower leg bone)
33. **substernal** (sub-STER-nal)	pertaining to under the sternum (breastbone)	38. **ulnar** (UL-nar)	pertaining to the ulna (lower arm bone)
34. **supraclavicular** (*sū*-pra-kla-VIK-ū-lar)	pertaining to above the clavicle (collarbone)	39. **vertebral** (VER-te-bral), (ver-TĒ-bral)	pertaining to the vertebrae
35. **suprapatellar** (*sū*-pra-pa-TEL-ar)	pertaining to above the patella (kneecap)		

🔍 Refer to **Appendix E** for pharmacology terms related to the musculoskeletal system.

EXERCISE 22 ▪ Pronounce and Spell

Practice pronunciation and spelling on paper and online.

1. **Practice on Paper**
   a. **Pronounce:** Read the phonetic spelling and say aloud the terms listed in the previous table. Refer to Table 2.2 Pronunciation Key as needed.
   b. **Spell:** Have a study partner read the terms aloud. Write the spelling of the terms on a separate sheet of paper.

2. **Practice Online** 🌐
   a. **Access** online learning resources. Go to evolve.elsevier.com > Evolve Resources > Student Resources.
   b. **Pronounce:** Select Audio Glossary > Chapter 14 > Exercise 22. Select a term to hear its pronunciation and repeat aloud.
   c. **Spell:** Select Activities > Chapter 14 > Spell Terms > Exercise 22. Select the audio icon and type the correct spelling of the term.

❏ Check the box when complete.

EXERCISE 23 ▪ Analyze and Define

Analyze and define the following complementary terms describing signs and symptoms.

1. myalgia

2. arthralgia

3. hypertrophy

4. atrophy

Chapter 14   Musculoskeletal System   577

5. hyperkinesia

8. hemarthrosis

6. dyskinesia

9. dystrophy

7. bradykinesia

10. myasthenia

EXERCISE 24 ■ Build

A Fill In

Build complementary descriptive terms for the following definitions by using the word parts you have learned.

1. pertaining to above the collarbone   ___ P / ___ WR / ___ S

2. pertaining to above the kneecap   ___ P / ___ WR / ___ S

3. pertaining to between the vertebrae   ___ P / ___ WR / ___ S

4. pertaining to below the upper jawbone   ___ P / ___ WR / ___ S

5. pertaining to below the lower jawbone   ___ P / ___ WR / ___ S

6. pertaining to under the breastbone   ___ P / ___ WR / ___ S

7. pertaining to within the cranium   ___ P / ___ WR / ___ S

8. pertaining to between the ribs   ___ P / ___ WR / ___ S

9. pertaining to the patella and femur   ___ WR / ___ CV / ___ WR / ___ S

578 Chapter 14 Musculoskeletal System

B Label

Build terms for the following definitions. Write the corresponding word parts above the abbreviations as shown in number 1.

12. pertaining to the cranium (skull)
 _____ / _____
  WR   S

1. pertaining to the scapula (shoulder blade)
 scapul / _ar_
   WR   S

2. pertaining to the humerus (upper arm bone)
 _____ / _____
  WR   S

3. pertaining to the sternum (breastbone)
 _____ / _____
  WR   S

4. pertaining to the vertebrae
 _____ / _____
  WR   S

5. pertaining to the ilium (upper, wing-shaped portion of the pelvis)
 _____ / _____
  WR   S

6. pertaining to the carpals (wrist)
 _____ / _____
  WR   S

7. pertaining to the phalanx (pl. phalanges) (any bone of the fingers or toes)
 _____ / _____
  WR   S

8. pertaining to the pubis (anterior portion of the pelvis)
 _____ / _____
  WR   S

9. pertaining to the patella (kneecap)
 _____ / _____
  WR   S

10. pertaining to the tarsals (ankle bones)
 _____ / _____
  WR   S

11. pertaining to the phalanx (pl. phalanges) (any bone of the fingers or toes)
 _____ / _____
  WR   S

13. pertaining to the clavicle (collarbone)
 _____ / _____
  WR   S

14. pertaining to the loins (the part of the back between the thorax and pelvis)
 _____ / _____
  WR   S

15. pertaining to the radius (lower arm bone)
 _____ / _____
  WR   S

16. pertaining to the ulna (lower arm bone)
 _____ / _____
  WR   S

17. pertaining to the sacrum (lower portion of the spine forming the posterior pelvic wall)
 _____ / _____
  WR   S

18. pertaining to the ischium (lower posterior portion of the pelvis)
 _____ / _____
  WR   S

19. pertaining to the femur (upper leg bone)
 _____ / _____
  WR   S

20. pertaining to the fibula (lower leg bone)
 _____ / _____
  WR   S

21. pertaining to the tibia (lower leg bone)
 _____ / _____
  WR   S

Complementary Terms
NOT BUILT FROM WORD PARTS

Word parts may be present in the following terms; however, their full meanings cannot be translated using definitions of word parts alone.

SIGNS & SYMPTOMS

TERM	DEFINITION
1. crepitus (KREP-i-tus)	crackling sensation heard or felt when two bones rub against each other or grating caused by the rubbing together of dry surfaces of a joint (also called **crepitation**)

CREPITUS is also used to describe the crackling sounds heard during auscultation of the lungs (with a stethoscope) in patients with pneumonia.

EQUIPMENT

TERM	DEFINITION
2. prosthesis (*pl.* prostheses) (pros-THĒ-sis), (pros-THĒ-sēz)	artificial substitute for a missing body part such as a limb, joint, or eye

MEDICAL SPECIALTIES

TERM	DEFINITION
3. chiropractic (kī-rō-PRAK-tik)	system of treatment that consists of manipulation of the vertebral column and other joints
4. chiropractor (DC) (KĪ-rō-*prak*-tor)	specialist in manipulation of the vertebral column and other joints
5. orthopedics (Ortho) (*or*-thō-PĒ-diks)	branch of medicine dealing with the study and treatment of diseases and abnormalities of the musculoskeletal system
6. orthopedist (*or*-thō-PĒ-dist)	physician who specializes in the study and treatment of diseases and abnormalities of the musculoskeletal system
7. orthotics (or-THOT-iks)	making and fitting of orthopedic appliances used to support, align, prevent, or treat musculoskeletal deformities; examples of appliances include braces, splints, and arch supports
8. orthotist (or-THOT-ist)	specialist in making and fitting appliances used to support, align, prevent or treat musculoskeletal deformities

ORTHOSIS the Greek word meaning **make straight** refers to the orthopedic appliance. The plural form is orthoses.

TERM	DEFINITION
9. osteopath (DO) (OS-tē-ō-*path*)	physician who specializes in a system of medicine placing emphasis on the relation between organs and the musculoskeletal system (osteopathy)
10. osteopathy (*os*-tē-OP-a-thē)	system of medicine that uses the usual forms of diagnosis and treatment but places greater emphasis on the relation between body organs and the musculoskeletal system; manipulation may be used in addition to other treatments
11. podiatrist (pō-DĪ-a-trist)	specialist in treating and diagnosing diseases and disorders of the foot, including medical and surgical treatment
12. rheumatologist (*roo*-ma-TOL-ō-jist)	physician who specializes in the study and treatment of musculoskeletal disorders characterized by inflammation and degeneration of structures (rheumatic diseases)
13. rheumatology (*roo*-ma-TOL-ō-jē)	study and treatment of musculoskeletal disorders characterized by inflammation and degeneration of structures (rheumatic diseases)

RHEUMATOLOGY AND ORTHOPEDICS: WHAT IS THE DIFFERENCE? While both medical specialties focus on the diagnosis and treatment of disease and disorders of the musculoskeletal system, **rheumatology** focuses on medical management for chronic conditions while **orthopedics** focuses on surgical treatment for acute or chronic conditions. For example, a patient with **rheumatoid arthritis** would see a **rheumatologist** for medications to manage symptoms of the disease and would be referred to an **orthopedist** if joint replacement surgery was warranted.

TYPES OF BODY MOVEMENT (FIG. 14.14)

TERM	DEFINITION
14. abduction (ab-DUK-shun)	moving away from the midline
15. adduction (ad-DUK-shun)	moving toward the midline
💡 **MIDLINE VS. MIDDLE** The two terms are synonyms, both describing an imaginary line that separates the body, or body part, into equal halves. In medical language, *midline* is the preferred term and is used as a common reference point.	
16. inversion (in-VER-zhun)	turning inward
17. eversion (ē-VER-zhun)	turning outward
18. extension (ek-STEN-shun)	movement in which a limb is placed in a straight position, increasing the angle between the bones on either side of the joint
19. flexion (FLEK-shun)	movement in which a limb is bent, decreasing the angle between the bones on either side of the joint
20. pronation (prō-NĀ-shun)	movement that turns the palm down
21. supination (sū-pi-NĀ-shun)	movement that turns the palm up
22. rotation (rō-TĀ-shun)	turning around its own axis

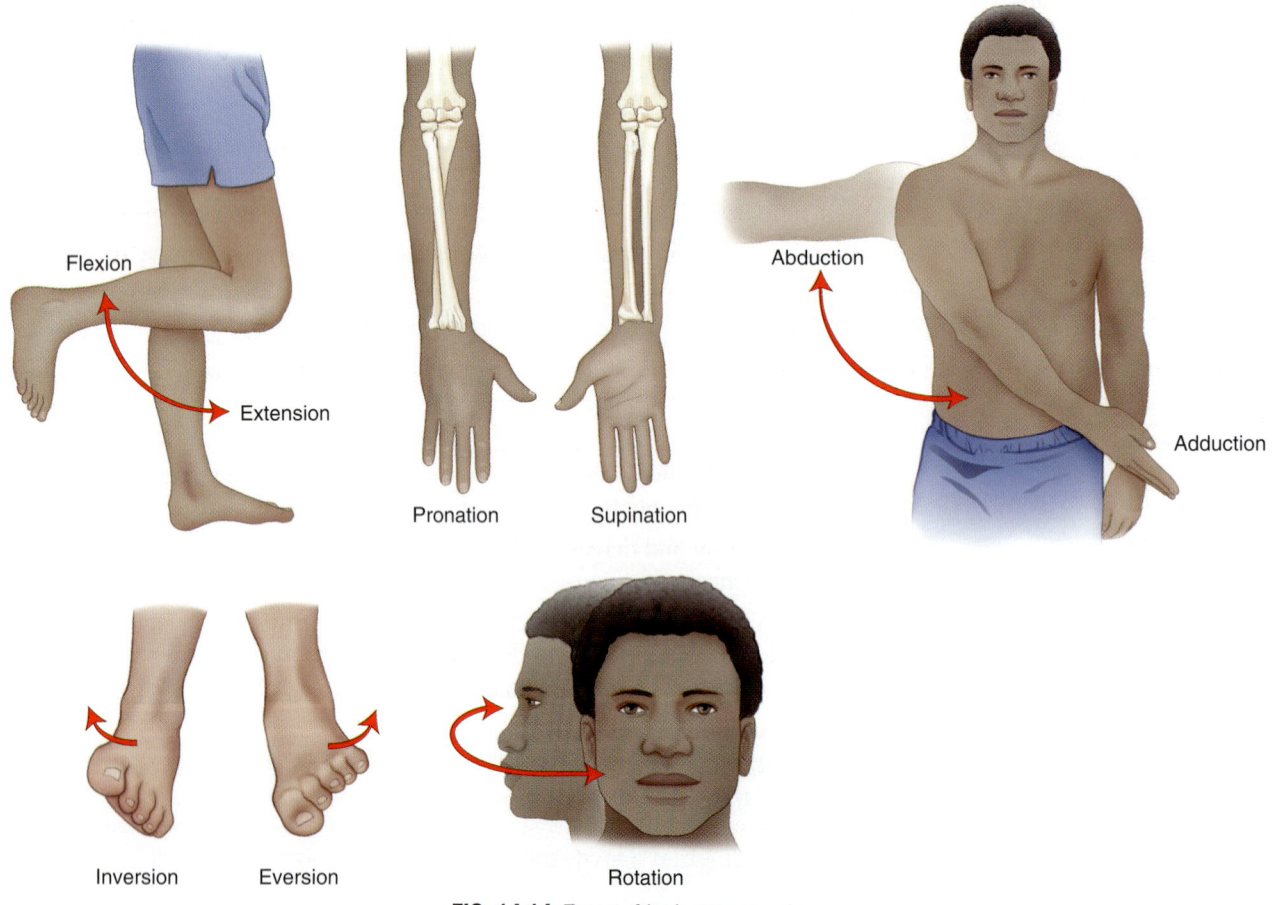

Flexion
Extension
Pronation
Supination
Abduction
Adduction
Inversion
Eversion
Rotation

FIG. 14.14 Types of body movements.

Chapter 14 Musculoskeletal System 581

EXERCISE 25 ■ Pronounce and Spell

Practice pronunciation and spelling on paper and online.

1. **Practice on Paper**
   a. **Pronounce:** Read the phonetic spelling and say aloud the terms listed in the previous table. Refer to Table 2.2 Pronunciation Key as needed.
   b. **Spell:** Have a study partner read the terms aloud. Write the spelling of the terms on a separate sheet of paper.

2. **Practice Online**
   a. **Access** online learning resources. Go to evolve.elsevier.com > Evolve Resources > Student Resources.
   b. **Pronounce:** Select Audio Glossary > Chapter 14 > Exercise 25. Select a term to hear its pronunciation and repeat aloud.
   c. **Spell:** Select Activities > Chapter 14 > Spell Terms > Exercise 25. Select the audio icon and type the correct spelling of the term.

❏ Check the box when complete.

EXERCISE 26 ■ Fill In

A Identify

Fill in the blanks with the correct terms.

1. The study and treatment of musculoskeletal disorders characterized by inflammation and degeneration of structures is the medical specialty called _____.
2. The making and fitting of appliances used to support, align, prevent, or treat musculoskeletal deformities (examples include braces, splints, and arch supports) is called _____.
3. The crackling sensation heard or felt when two bones rub against each other or grating caused by the rubbing together of dry surfaces of a joint is called _____.
4. The system of treatment that consists of manipulation of the vertebral column is called _____.
5. The branch of medicine dealing with the study and treatment of diseases and abnormalities of the musculoskeletal system is called _____.
6. The system of medicine that uses the usual forms of diagnosis and treatment, considers the relation between body organs and the musculoskeletal system, and may use manipulation of the musculoskeletal system in addition to other treatments is called _____.
7. An artificial substitute for a missing body part such as limb, joint, or eye is called a _____.

B Label

Write the medical terms pictured and defined.

1. _____
physician who specializes in the study and treatment of diseases and abnormalities of the musculoskeletal system

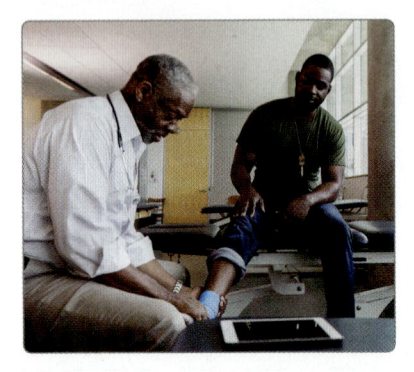

2. _____
physician who specializes in the study and treatment of musculoskeletal disorders characterized by inflammation and degeneration of structures

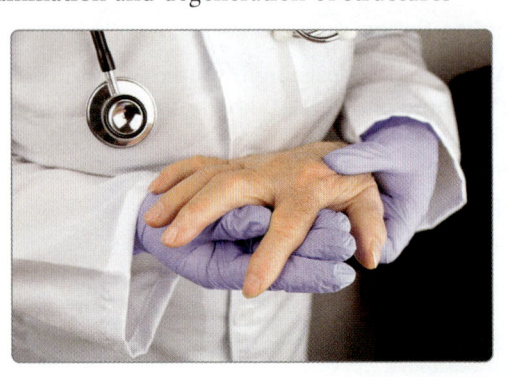

3. _____
specialist in treating and diagnosing diseases and disorders of the foot, including medical and surgical treatment

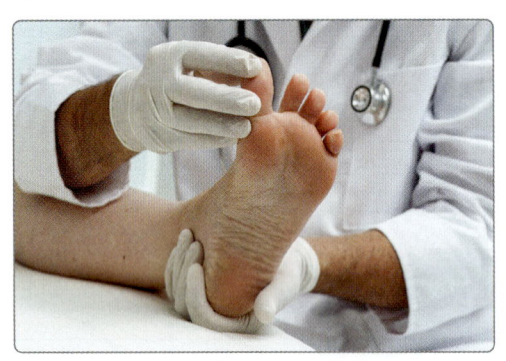

4. _____
specialist in making and fitting appliances used to support, align, prevent or treat musculoskeletal deformities

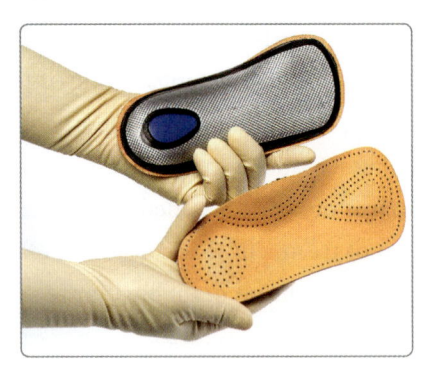

5. _____
specialist in the manipulation of the vertebral column

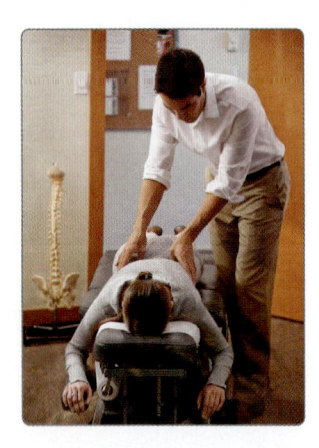

6. _____
physician specializing in a system of medicine placing emphasis on the relation between organs and the musculoskeletal system; manipulation may be used in addition to other treatments

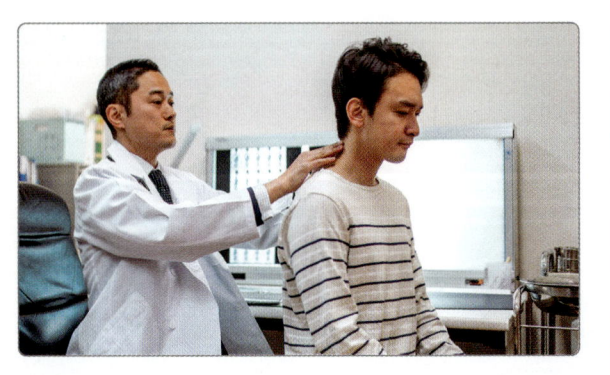

EXERCISE 27 ■ Match

Match the descriptions in the first column with the correct terms in the second column.

_____ 1. replaces a body part
_____ 2. the making of supports for body parts responsible for motion
_____ 3. manages the treatment of RA
_____ 4. performs joint replacement surgery
_____ 5. performs foot surgery
_____ 6. physician trained in manipulation of the musculoskeletal system as well as allopathic treatment and diagnosis
_____ 7. trained in the manipulation of the vertebral column and is not a physician
_____ 8. crackling sensation or sound

a. rheumatologist
b. chiropractor
c. osteopath
d. prosthesis
e. crepitus
f. orthopedist
g. podiatrist
h. orthotics

EXERCISE 28 ■ Types of Body Movement

Match the terms in the first column with their correct definitions in the second column.

_____ 1. abduction
_____ 2. adduction
_____ 3. pronation
_____ 4. rotation
_____ 5. eversion
_____ 6. extension
_____ 7. flexion
_____ 8. inversion
_____ 9. supination

a. movement in which a limb is placed in a straight position
b. movement that turns the palm up
c. turning outward
d. moving toward the midline
e. turning around its own axis
f. turning inward
g. movement in which a limb is bent
h. moving away from the midline
i. movement that turns the palm down

EXERCISE 29 ■ Review of Complementary Terms

Can you define, pronounce, and spell the following terms?

abduction	fibular	orthopedist	rotation
adduction	flexion	orthotics	sacral
arthralgia	hemarthrosis	orthotist	scapular
atrophy	humeral	osteopath (DO)	sternal
bradykinesia	hyperkinesia	osteopathy	submandibular
carpal	hypertrophy	patellar	submaxillary
chiropractic	iliac	patellofemoral	substernal
chiropractor (DC)	intercostal	phalangeal	supination
clavicular	intervertebral	podiatrist	supraclavicular
cranial	intracranial	pronation	suprapatellar
crepitus	inversion	prosthesis	tarsal
dyskinesia	ischial	(*pl.* prostheses)	tibial
dystrophy	lumbar	pubic	ulnar
eversion	myalgia	radial	vertebral
extension	myasthenia	rheumatologist	
femoral	orthopedics (Ortho)	rheumatology	

Abbreviations

DISEASE AND DISORDER

ABBREVIATION	TERM	ABBREVIATION	TERM
CTS	carpal tunnel syndrome	OA	osteoarthritis
fx	fracture	PM	polymyositis
HNP	herniated nucleus pulposus	RA	rheumatoid arthritis
MD	muscular dystrophy	RSI	repetitive strain injury
MG	myasthenia gravis		

DIAGNOSTIC

ABBREVIATION	TERM	ABBREVIATION	TERM
DEXA	dual-energy x-ray absorptiometry (bone density test); spoken as a whole word (de-ksa)	DXA	dual x-ray absorptiometry (bone density test); spoken as a whole word (de-ksa)
		EMG	electromyogram

TREATMENT

ABBREVIATION	TERM	ABBREVIATION	TERM
THA	total hip arthroplasty	TKA	total knee arthroplasty

MEDICAL SPECIALTIES

ABBREVIATION	TERM	ABBREVIATION	TERM
DC	Doctor of Chiropractic	Ortho	orthopedics; spoken as a whole word (or-thō)
DO	Doctor of Osteopathy		

DESCRIPTIVE

ABBREVIATION	TERM	ABBREVIATION	TERM
C1-C7	cervical vertebrae	T1-T12	thoracic vertebrae
L1-L5	lumbar vertebrae		

Refer to **Appendix D** for a complete list of abbreviations.

EXERCISE 30 ■ Abbreviations

Write the terms abbreviated.

1. Vertebrae make up the bones of the spinal column. **C1 to C7** _____ _____ are the first set that form the neck. The second set **T1 to T12** _____ _____ articulate with the 12 pairs of ribs that form the outward curve of the spine. **L1 to L5** _____ _____, the third set, are larger and form the inward curve of the spine.

2. Patients with **RA** _____ _____ may experience muscle atrophy and weakness because of inactivity.

3. Water exercise or gentle movement, such as Tai Chi, is recommended for many patients with **OA** _____, the most common joint disease.

4. **MG** _____ _____ most often affects women and the onset occurs at any age. It is an acquired autoimmune disorder.

5. **EMG** _____ is used to evaluate patients with localized or diffuse muscle weakness, such as **PM** _____.
6. **CTS** _____ is a common condition in which, for various reasons, the median nerve in the wrist becomes compressed, causing numbness and pain. A patient with symptoms of CTS that didn't improve with splints and physical therapy might be referred to **Ortho** _____ for possible surgery.
7. Nine types of **MD** _____ have been identified. Because symptoms of the disease are similar to other muscular disorders, diagnosis is often difficult.
8. **HNP** _____ may also be referred to as slipped disk, ruptured disk, or herniated intervertebral disk.
9. **THA** _____ is used to treat severe osteoarthritis of the hip joints.
10. Taking a holistic view of medicine, the **DO** _____ evaluates the patient's musculoskeletal system in relation to overall health.
11. Knee replacement surgery, also called **TKA** _____, is used in patients who have disabling pain due to arthritis.
12. Movements performed over and over again may lead to **RSI**, _____, the cumulative damage to a joint, muscle, or other tissue.
13. Various **fx** _____ types describe the nature of the break and include transverse, spiral, oblique, comminuted, and compression.
14. **DXA** _____ and **DEXA** _____ name the same diagnostic procedure measuring bone loss and bone mineral density.
15. A **DC** _____ is not a medical doctor, but has received graduate-level training in the treatment of some musculoskeletal disorders with a primary focus on pain reduction.

Chapter 14 Musculoskeletal System

PRACTICAL APPLICATION

EXERCISE 31 ■ Case Study: Translate Between Everyday Language and Medical Language

CASE STUDY: Shanti Mehra

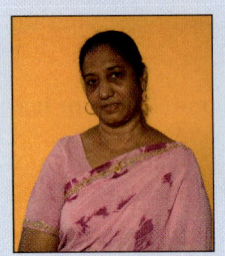

Shanti Mehra was walking to the store to buy more cigarettes. It was cold and icy and unfortunately, she slipped on some ice on the pavement. Her hand and wrist buckled under her when she fell. Now she is worried she may have broken some finger or wrist bones. She goes to the emergency department and an x-ray is done. She is told that she has broken one of her lower arm bones and is referred to a musculoskeletal specialist. She is also told that her bones are not dense enough and that she needs to have additional tests done.

Now that you have worked through Chapter 14, consider the medical terms that might be used to describe Mrs. Mehra's experience. See the Chapter at a Glance Section at the end of the chapter for a list of terms that might apply.

A. Underline phrases in the case study that could be substituted with medical terms.

B. Write the medical term and its definition for three of the phrases you underlined.

MEDICAL TERM   DEFINITION
1. _____   _____
2. _____   _____
3. _____   _____

DOCUMENTATION: Excerpt from Orthopedic Clinic Visit

Mrs. Mehra made an appointment with an orthopedist; a portion of the report is documented below.

Progress Note

Physical Examination: She has prominent dorsal kyphosis in the thoracic vertebral column. AP and lateral radiographs of the right wrist reveal a distal radial fracture. Her bones show evidence of osteoporosis.
Assessment and Plan: A DXA test is recommended to assess bone mineral density. She was advised to continue immobilization of the radiocarpal joint for at least 4 weeks.

C. Underline medical terms presented in Chapter 14 used in the previous excerpt from Mrs. Mehra's medical record. See the Chapter at a Glance Section at the end of the chapter for a complete list.

D. Select and define three of the medical terms you underlined. To check your answers, go to Appendix A.

MEDICAL TERM   DEFINITION
1. _____   _____
2. _____   _____
3. _____   _____

Chapter 14 Musculoskeletal System 587

EXERCISE 32 ■ Interact With Medical Documents

A

Read the report and complete it by writing medical terms on answer lines within the document. Definitions of terms to be written appear after the document.

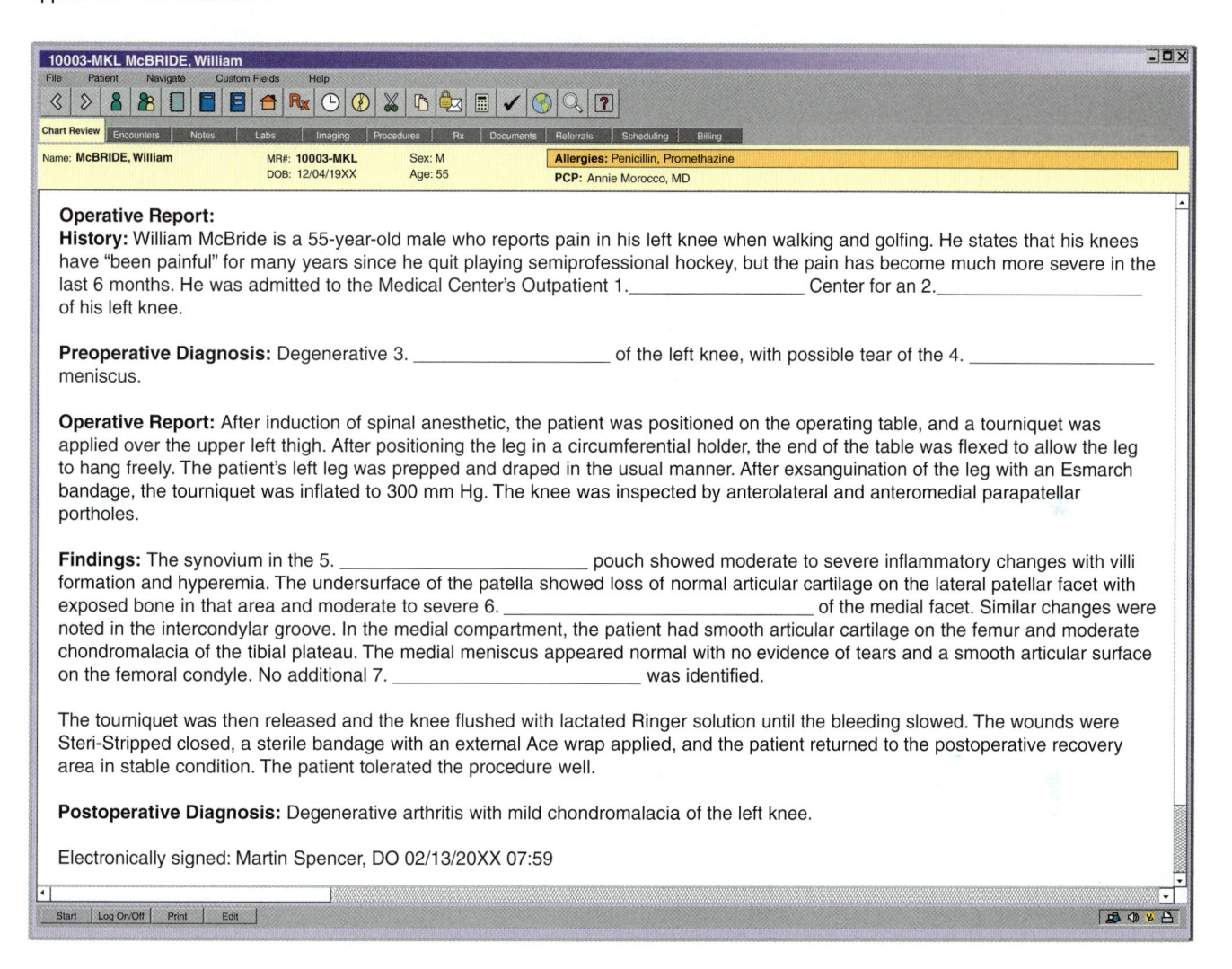

10003-MKL McBRIDE, William

Name: McBRIDE, William MR#: 10003-MKL Sex: M Allergies: Penicillin, Promethazine
DOB: 12/04/19XX Age: 55 PCP: Annie Morocco, MD

Operative Report:
History: William McBride is a 55-year-old male who reports pain in his left knee when walking and golfing. He states that his knees have "been painful" for many years since he quit playing semiprofessional hockey, but the pain has become much more severe in the last 6 months. He was admitted to the Medical Center's Outpatient 1._____ Center for an 2._____ of his left knee.

Preoperative Diagnosis: Degenerative 3._____ of the left knee, with possible tear of the 4._____ meniscus.

Operative Report: After induction of spinal anesthetic, the patient was positioned on the operating table, and a tourniquet was applied over the upper left thigh. After positioning the leg in a circumferential holder, the end of the table was flexed to allow the leg to hang freely. The patient's left leg was prepped and draped in the usual manner. After exsanguination of the leg with an Esmarch bandage, the tourniquet was inflated to 300 mm Hg. The knee was inspected by anterolateral and anteromedial parapatellar portholes.

Findings: The synovium in the 5._____ pouch showed moderate to severe inflammatory changes with villi formation and hyperemia. The undersurface of the patella showed loss of normal articular cartilage on the lateral patellar facet with exposed bone in that area and moderate to severe 6._____ of the medial facet. Similar changes were noted in the intercondylar groove. In the medial compartment, the patient had smooth articular cartilage on the femur and moderate chondromalacia of the tibial plateau. The medial meniscus appeared normal with no evidence of tears and a smooth articular surface on the femoral condyle. No additional 7._____ was identified.

The tourniquet was then released and the knee flushed with lactated Ringer solution until the bleeding slowed. The wounds were Steri-Stripped closed, a sterile bandage with an external Ace wrap applied, and the patient returned to the postoperative recovery area in stable condition. The patient tolerated the procedure well.

Postoperative Diagnosis: Degenerative arthritis with mild chondromalacia of the left knee.

Electronically signed: Martin Spencer, DO 02/13/20XX 07:59

Definitions of Medical Terms to Complete the Document

Write the medical terms defined on corresponding answer lines in the document.

1. branch of medicine dealing with the study and treatment of diseases and abnormalities of the musculoskeletal system
2. visual examination of a joint
3. inflammation of a joint
4. toward the middle or midline
5. pertaining to above the patella
6. softening of cartilage
7. study of (body changes caused by) disease

588　Chapter 14　Musculoskeletal System

B

Read the medical report and answer the questions below it.

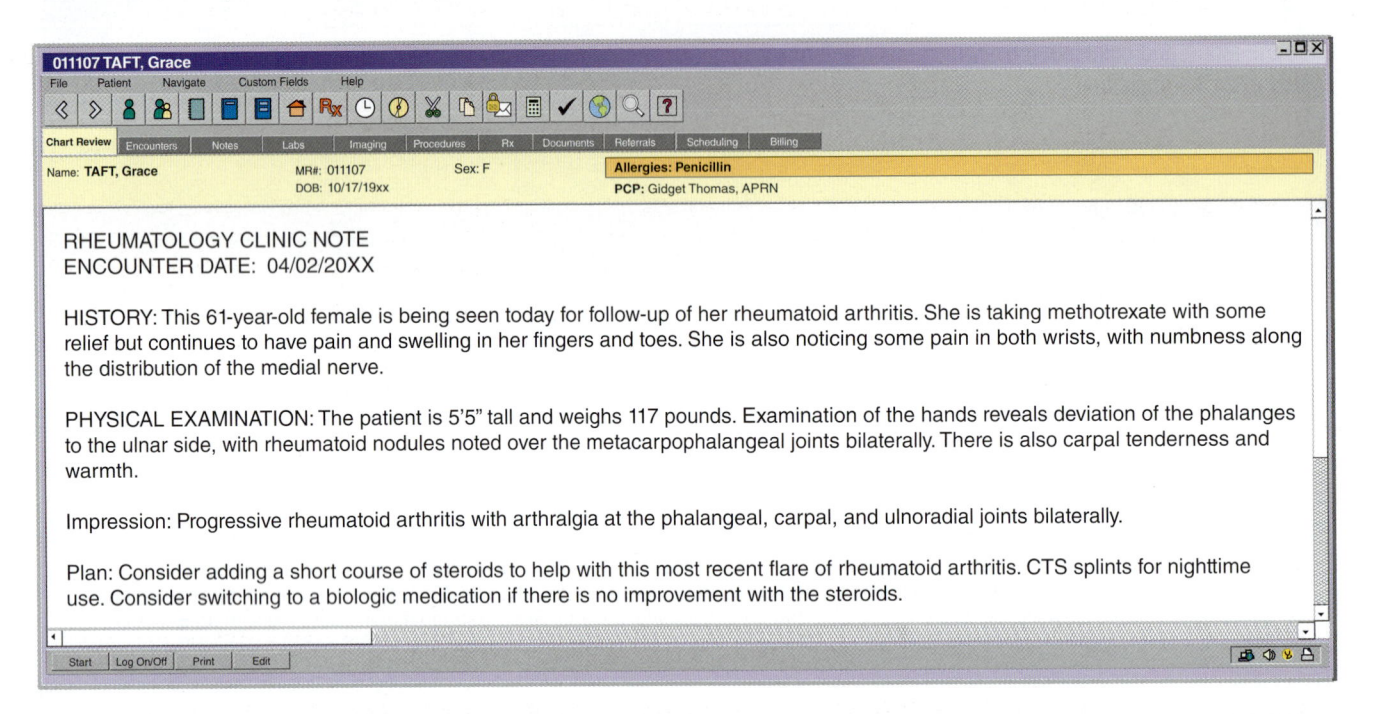

011107 TAFT, Grace

Name: TAFT, Grace　　MR#: 011107　　Sex: F　　Allergies: Penicillin
　　　　　　　　　　　　DOB: 10/17/19xx　　　　　　PCP: Gidget Thomas, APRN

RHEUMATOLOGY CLINIC NOTE
ENCOUNTER DATE: 04/02/20XX

HISTORY: This 61-year-old female is being seen today for follow-up of her rheumatoid arthritis. She is taking methotrexate with some relief but continues to have pain and swelling in her fingers and toes. She is also noticing some pain in both wrists, with numbness along the distribution of the medial nerve.

PHYSICAL EXAMINATION: The patient is 5'5" tall and weighs 117 pounds. Examination of the hands reveals deviation of the phalanges to the ulnar side, with rheumatoid nodules noted over the metacarpophalangeal joints bilaterally. There is also carpal tenderness and warmth.

Impression: Progressive rheumatoid arthritis with arthralgia at the phalangeal, carpal, and ulnoradial joints bilaterally.

Plan: Consider adding a short course of steroids to help with this most recent flare of rheumatoid arthritis. CTS splints for nighttime use. Consider switching to a biologic medication if there is no improvement with the steroids.

Use the medical report above to answer the questions.

1. Pain and numbness in the wrist with compression of the medial nerve could indicate
   a. ankylosing spondylitis
   b. gout
   c. carpal tunnel syndrome
   d. plantar fasciitis

2. The patient is exhibiting tenderness and warmth over the
   a. ankles
   b. wrists
   c. elbows
   d. knees

EXERCISE 33 ■ Use Medical Language in Online Electronic Health Records

Select the correct medical terms to complete three medical records in one patient's electronic file.

  Access online resources at evolve.elsevier.com > Evolve Resources > Student Resources > Activities > Chapter 14 > Electronic Health Records

Topic: Fracture, Parkinson Disease
Record 1, Chart Review: Admission Note
Record 2, Imaging: Radiology Report
Record 3, Referrals: Neurology Consultation

❏ Check the box when complete.

EXERCISE 34 ■ Use Medical Terms in Clinical Statements

For each phrase printed in bold, circle the medical term or abbreviation defined. Answers are listed in Appendix A. For pronunciation practice, read the answers aloud.

1. About a month after Mrs. Torres began taking statins to lower her cholesterol levels, she began experiencing **muscle pain** (arthralgia, myalgia, osteomyelitis) and **muscle weakness** (myasthenia, fibromyalgia, myelitis). A series of creatinine kinase blood tests confirmed a diagnosis of **dissolution of striated muscle**, or (fasciitis, polymyositis, rhabdomyolysis).

2. During an examination of the patient's left knee, a **crackling sound** (osteopenia, exostosis, crepitus) was noted during **movement in which a limb is bent, decreasing the angle between the bones on either side of the joint** (inversion, flexion, extension), and **movement in which a limb is placed in a straight position, increasing the angle between the bones on either side of the joint** (eversion, flexion, extension).

3. Shortly after Aqsa started training for a 5k race, she noticed pain in the bottom of her feet and heels, especially in the morning just after getting up. It was so painful, she made an appointment with a **specialist in treating and diagnosing diseases and disorders of the foot, including medical and surgical treatment** (orthopedist, osteopath, podiatrist).

4. After ruling out **inflammation of a tendon** (osteitis, tendinitis, tenosynovitis) and **inflammation of a bursa** (bursitis, arthritis, meniscitis), Aqsa was diagnosed with **inflammation of the connective tissue of the sole of the foot due to repetitive injury** (tarsal tunnel syndrome, gout, plantar fasciitis).

5. Aqsa was referred to physical therapy to help with stretching and for **making and fitting of orthopedic appliances used to support, align, prevent, or treat musculoskeletal deformities** (orthotics, chiropractic, rheumatology) for splints to be worn at night.

EXERCISE 35 ■ Pronounce Medical Terms in Use

Practice pronunciation of terms by reading aloud the following sentences. Use the phonetic spellings to assist with pronunciation. The script also contains medical terms not presented in the chapter. If interested, research their meanings in a medical dictionary or a reliable online source.

1. The **orthopedist** (or-thō-PĒ-dist) recommended Mr. Shah have an **arthrodesis** (ar-thrō-DĒ-sis) to reduce pain caused from an ankle **fracture** (FRAK-chur) he sustained several years ago.
2. Mrs. Diaz severed a tendon by accidentally walking through a glass patio door. A **tenorrhaphy** (te-NOR-a-fē) was performed to repair the tendon.
3. An **electromyogram** (e-lek-trō-MĪ-ō-gram) can assist the physician in diagnosing **muscular dystrophy** (MUS-kū-lar) (DIS-trō-fē). **Atrophy** (AT-rō-fē) frequently occurs in patients with this disease.
4. Adjective forms of medical terms are used by health professionals to indicate areas of the body that describe anatomic locations, areas of pain, sites of injections, locations of lesions, and so forth. Below are some examples.
    a. **cranial** (KRĀ-nē-al) laceration
    b. **intercostal** (in-ter-KOS-tal) muscles
    c. pain in the **supraclavicular** (sū-pra-kla-VIK-ū-lar) region
    d. herniation of an **intervertebral** (in-ter-VER-te-bral) disk
    e. **intracranial** (in-tra-KRĀ-nē-al) pressure
    f. **femoral** (FEM-or-al) artery
    g. strain of the **patellofemoral** (pa-tel-ō-FEM-or-al) ligament
    h. degenerative disease of the **vertebral** (ver-TĒ-bral) joints

EXERCISE 36 ■ Use Plural Endings

Circle the correct singular or plural term to match the context of the sentence.

1. The (**epiphysis, epiphyses**) are the enlarged ends of the long bone.
2. The distal (**phalanx, phalanges**) of the ring finger was fractured.
3. Osteoporosis was present in four lumbar (**vertebrae, vertebra**).
4. A (**prosthesis, prostheses**) was implanted in the left hip.
5. Many synovial joints contain (**bursa, bursae**).
6. Two (**lamina, laminae**) make up the vertebral arch in a single vertebra.

CHAPTER REVIEW

EXERCISE 37 — Chapter Content Quiz

Test your understanding of terms and abbreviations introduced in this chapter. Circle the letter for the medical term or abbreviation related to the words in italics.

1. Jessie Steinbach was diagnosed with *an infection caused by a bite from a deer tick infected with Borrelia burgdorferi* after noting symptoms of fever, headache, and joint pain. Her symptoms started after a camping trip last summer.
   a. rheumatoid arthritis
   b. Lyme disease
   c. rhabdomyolysis

2. Tommy John surgery, named after the first professional baseball player to have it performed, involves *suturing of a tendon* of the ulnar collateral ligament, usually with a graft from a different tendon in the body.
   a. tenomyoplasty
   b. myorrhaphy
   c. tenorrhaphy

3. Orthopedists may perform *visual examination of a joint* to diagnose and sometimes treat problems in the knee, shoulder, or elbow.
   a. arthroscopy
   b. arthrography
   c. arthrocentesis

4. Ever since his initial diagnosis of ankylosing spondylitis, James Montoya has been seeing a *physician who specializes in the study and treatment of musculoskeletal disorders characterized by inflammation and degeneration of structures*.
   a. podiatrist
   b. rheumatologist
   c. chiropractor

5. Dr. Lu ordered an electromyogram (EMG) for Mr. Borunda when he suspected *chronic disease characterized by muscle weakness and thought to be caused by a defect in the transmission of impulses from nerve to muscle*.
   a. muscular dystrophy
   b. meniscitis
   c. myasthenia gravis

6. A total hip *surgical repair of a joint* was recommended for Mrs. Jiang when she could no longer tolerate the pain from her osteoarthritis.
   a. arthrodesis
   b. arthroplasty
   c. chondroplasty

7. Ayaz Ismail noticed ulnoradial pain whenever he was asked to put his forearm into *movement that turns the palm up*.
   a. pronation
   b. eversion
   c. supination

8. While training for the National Guard, Jayla experienced unusual achy, cramping pain in her lower legs that increased as she ran. She also felt a tingling sensation and noticed swelling in both legs. She was diagnosed with chronic exertional *condition caused by increased pressure within a muscle that can lead to ischemia*, and fasciotomy was performed when nonsurgical treatments did not provide relief.
   a. repetitive strain injury
   b. myasthenia gravis
   c. compartment syndrome

9. A(n) *excision of a lamina* was performed on Mr. Lopez, who had been experiencing spinal stenosis for many years.
   a. laminectomy
   b. synovectomy
   c. vertebroplasty

10. Dawn Labenz met with a *specialist in making and fitting of appliances used to support, align, prevent, or treat musculoskeletal deformities* to have arch supports made for her shoes after experiencing plantar fasciitis for the second time.
    a. orthopedist
    b. osteopath
    c. orthotist

11. Mr. O'Rourke had a radiograph of his knee to determine how much *inflammation of the bone and joint* was present.
    a. OA
    b. RA
    c. DO

12. Mrs. Jerue developed *abnormal condition of bone death* of the jaw after a rather difficult tooth extraction.
    a. osteomalacia
    b. osteopetrosis
    c. osteonecrosis

13. Natalie Pageau experienced *pertaining to under the sternum* pain after eating; she was relieved to find indigestion to be the cause rather than angina.
    a. supraclavicular
    b. substernal
    c. submandibular

14. Mr. Sadowsky's symptoms of *slow movement* worsened as his Parkinson disease progressed.
    a. bradykinesia
    b. hyperkinesia
    c. hypertrophy

15. After his fall from a ladder, Adam Murphy had an emergency *incision into the cranium* to relieve intracranial pressure.
    a. cranioplasty
    b. craniotomy
    c. rachiotomy

16. Two-year-old Joshia presented to Urgent Care, crying and refusing to use his left arm. Prior to the injury, his teenage brother was swinging him around in a circle holding both wrists. Examination revealed radial head *partial dislocation of bones in a joint*, which was quickly treated with a gentle maneuver to slip the bone back in place.
    a. subluxation
    b. hemarthrosis
    c. sprain

17. Mr. Cohen complained of chronic wrist *pain in the joint*. A plain radiograph showed soft tissue swelling along with erosions in the carpal bones. Arthrocentesis revealed monosodium urate crystals and confirmed the diagnosis of gout.
    a. atrophy
    b. arthralgia
    c. myalgia

18. An osteotomy or partial phalangectomy may be required during *abnormal prominence of the joint at the base of the great toe* surgery to realign the metatarsal-phalangeal joint.
    a. carpal tunnel syndrome
    b. exostosis
    c. bunion

19. Lily Chakraborty developed severe *abnormal condition of (lateral) curved (spine)* as a teen; a partial costectomy and other corrective surgery was performed with good results.
    a. scoliosis
    b. kyphosis
    c. lordosis

20. Dr. Nair advised Melanie Chua to increase her calcium and vitamin D intake after radiographs showed *abnormal reduction of bone mass* at the distal radial portion of her wrist.
    a. osteosarcoma
    b. osteopetrosis
    c. osteopenia

CHAPTER AT A GLANCE Word Parts New to This Chapter

COMBINING FORMS

ankyl/o	fibul/o	menisc/o	scoli/o	
arthr/o	humer/o	myos/o	spondyl/o	
burs/o	ili/o	oste/o	stern/o	
carp/o	ischi/o	patell/o	synovi/o	
chondr/o	kinesi/o	petr/o	tars/o	
clavicul/o	kyph/o	phalang/o	ten/o	
cost/o	lamin/o	pub/o	tendin/o	
crani/o	lord/o	rachi/o	tibi/o	
disc/o	lumb/o	radi/o	uln/o	
fasci/o	mandibul/o	sacr/o	vertebr/o	
femor/o	maxill/o	scapul/o		

PREFIXES
inter-
supra-
syn-

SUFFIXES
-asthenia
-schisis
-trophy

CHAPTER AT A GLANCE Musculoskeletal System Terms Built From Word Parts

DISEASE AND DISORDER

ankylosis	fasciitis	osteomalacia	sarcopenia
arthritis	kyphosis	osteomyelitis	scoliosis
bursitis	lordosis	osteonecrosis	spondylarthritis
chondromalacia	meniscitis	osteopenia	spondylosis
chondrosarcoma	myeloma	osteopetrosis	synoviosarcoma
cranioschisis	osteitis	osteosarcoma	tendinitis
discitis	osteoarthritis (OA)	polymyositis (PM)	tenosynovitis
fibromyalgia	osteochondritis	rachischisis	
	osteochondroma	rhabdomyolysis	

SURGICAL
arthrocentesis
arthrodesis
arthroplasty
bursectomy
carpectomy
chondrectomy
chondroplasty
costectomy
cranioplasty
craniotomy
discectomy
fasciotomy
laminectomy
maxillectomy
meniscectomy
microdiscectomy
myorrhaphy
osteotomy
phalangectomy
rachiotomy
spondylosyndesis
synovectomy
tarsectomy
tenomyoplasty
tenorrhaphy
vertebroplasty

DIAGNOSTIC
arthroscopy
arthrography
electromyogram (EMG)

COMPLEMENTARY
arthralgia
atrophy
bradykinesia
carpal
clavicular
cranial
dyskinesia
dystrophy
femoral
fibular
hemarthrosis
humeral
hyperkinesia
hypertrophy
iliac
intercostal
intervertebral
intracranial
ischial
lumbar
myalgia
myasthenia
patellar
patellofemoral
phalangeal
pubic
radial
sacral
scapular
sternal
submandibular
submaxillary
substernal
supraclavicular
suprapatellar
tarsal
tibial
ulnar
vertebral

CHAPTER AT A GLANCE Musculoskeletal System Terms *NOT* Built from Word Parts

DISEASE AND DISORDER
ankylosing spondylitis
bunion
carpal tunnel syndrome (CTS)
compartment syndrome
dislocation
exostosis
fracture (fx)
ganglion cyst
gout
herniated disk
Lyme disease
muscular dystrophy (MD)
myasthenia gravis (MG)
osteoporosis
plantar fasciitis
repetitive strain injury (RSI)
rheumatoid arthritis (RA)
rotator cuff disease
spinal stenosis
spondylolisthesis
sprain
strain
subluxation
tarsal tunnel syndrome

DIAGNOSTIC
dual x-ray absorptiometry (DXA)
bone markers
muscle biopsy

COMPLEMENTARY
chiropractic
chiropractor (DC)
crepitus
orthopedics (Ortho)
orthopedist
orthotics
orthotist
osteopath (DO)
osteopathy
podiatrist
prosthesis (*pl.* prostheses)
rheumatologist
rheumatology

TYPES OF BODY MOVEMENT
abduction
adduction
inversion
eversion
extension
flexion
pronation
supination
rotation

PART 2 BODY SYSTEMS

Nervous System and Behavioral Health 15

Outline

ANATOMY, 594
Function, 594
Organs and Anatomic Structures of the Nervous System, 595

WORD PARTS, 598
Combining Forms of the Nervous System, 598
Combining Forms Used with Nervous System Terms, 598
Prefixes, 598
Suffixes, 599

MEDICAL TERMS, 603
Disease and Disorder Terms, 603
   Built from Word Parts, 603
   NOT Built from Word Parts, 608
Surgical Terms, 612
   Built from Word Parts, 612
Diagnostic Terms, 614
   Built from Word Parts and
     NOT Built from Word Parts, 614
Complementary Terms, 619
   Built from Word Parts, 619
   NOT Built from Word Parts, 622
Behavioral Health Terms, 626
   Built from Word Parts, 626
   NOT Built from Word Parts, 628
Abbreviations, 630

PRACTICAL APPLICATION, 632
CASE STUDY Translate Between Everyday Language and Medical Language, 632
Interact with Medical Documents, 633
Use Medical Language in Online Electronic Health Records, 635
Use Medical Terms in Clinical Statements, 635
Pronounce Medical Terms in Use, 636

CHAPTER REVIEW, 636
Chapter Content Quiz, 636
Chapter at a Glance, 638

Answers to Chapter Exercises, Appendix A

Objectives

Upon completion of this chapter, you will be able to:

1. Pronounce organs and anatomic structures of the nervous system.
2. Define and spell word parts related to the nervous system.
3. Define, pronounce, and spell disease and disorder terms related to the nervous system.
4. Define, pronounce, and spell surgical terms related to the nervous system.
5. Define, pronounce, and spell diagnostic terms related to the nervous system.
6. Define, pronounce, and spell complementary terms related to the nervous system.
7. Define, pronounce, and spell behavioral health terms.
8. Interpret the meaning of abbreviations related to the nervous system and behavioral health.
9. Apply medical language in clinical contexts.

TABLE 15.1 Types of Dementia, 609
TABLE 15.2 Types of Cognitive Impairment, 623

ANATOMY

The nervous system consists of the brain, spinal cord, and nerves and may be divided into two parts: the **central nervous system** (CNS) and the **peripheral nervous system** (PNS). The central nervous system consists of the brain and spinal cord. The peripheral nervous system is the collection of spinal and cranial nerves, whose branches infiltrate virtually all parts of the body, conveying messages to and from the CNS. (Figs. 15.1 and 15.2)

Function

The nervous system forms a complex communication system allowing for the coordination of body functions and activities. The nervous system can also be divided into two parts from a functional standpoint. The somatic nervous system is responsible for sending signals to the skeletal (voluntary) muscles and receives input from the senses. The autonomic nervous system generally operates on a "subconscious" level, meaning it governs itself outside of our awareness. It sends signals to the "involuntary" tissues, which include smooth muscles, cardiac muscle, glands, and fat. These tissues have receptors that send autonomic signals back to the brain and spinal cord. As a whole, the nervous system is designed to detect changes inside and outside the body, to evaluate this sensory information, and to send directions to muscles or glands in response. This system also provides for mental activities such as thought, memory, and emotions.

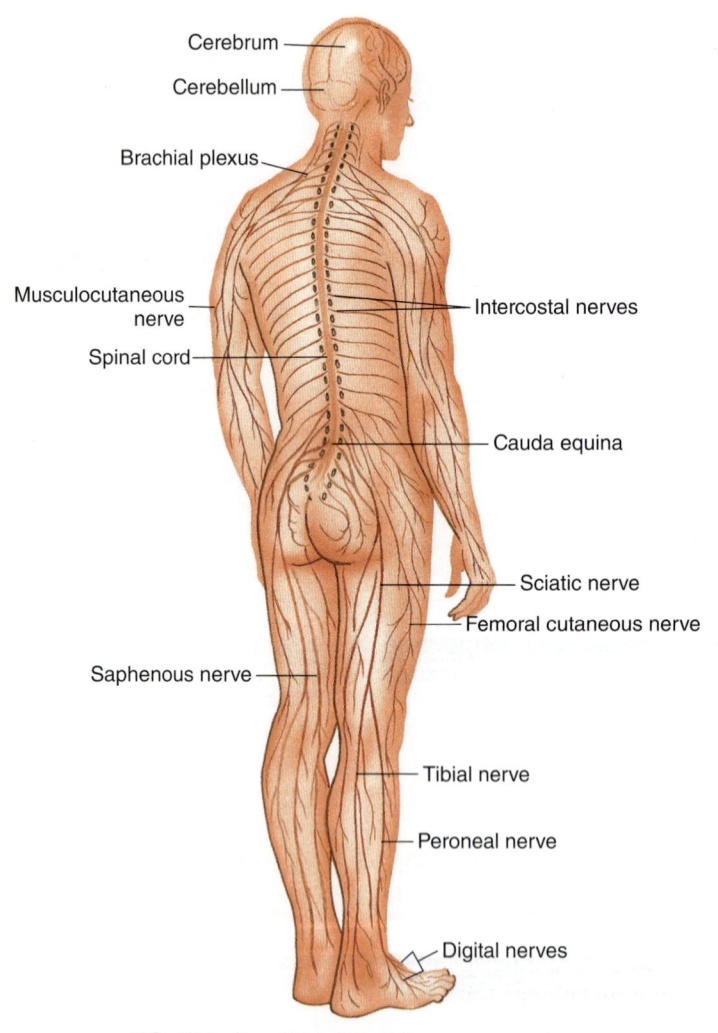

FIG. 15.1 Simplified view of the nervous system.

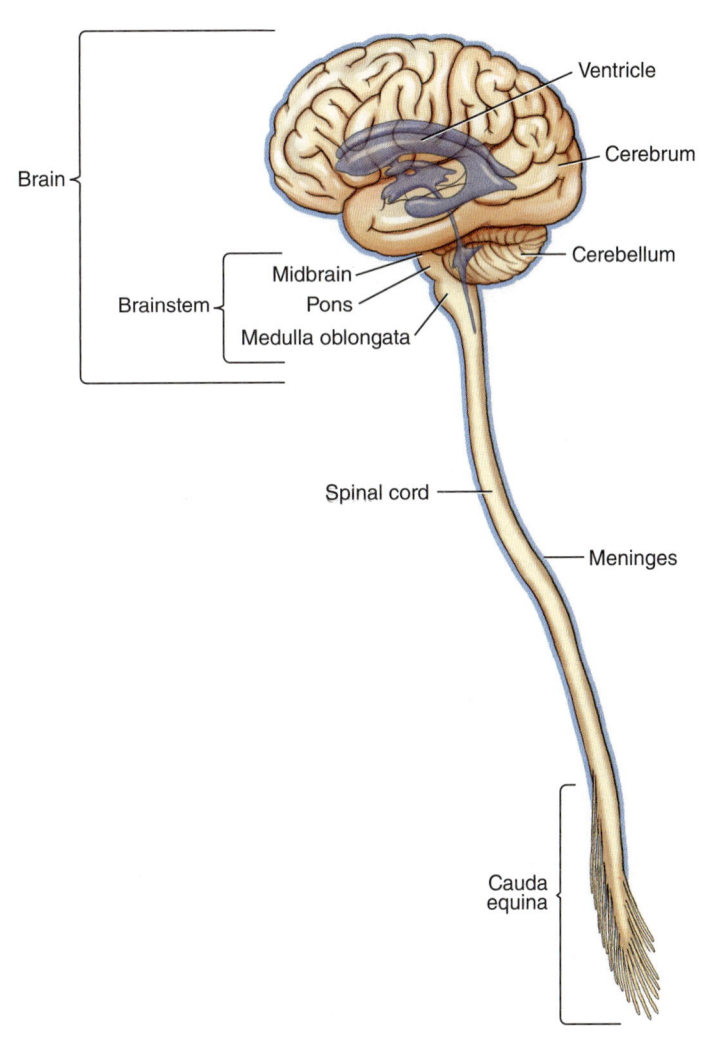

FIG. 15.2 Brain and spinal cord.

Organs and Anatomic Structures of the Nervous System

TERM	DEFINITION
brain (brān)	contained within the cranium, the center for coordinating body activities and comprises the cerebrum, cerebellum, and brainstem (Fig. 15.2).
cerebrum (se-RĒ-brum)	largest portion of the brain, divided into left and right hemispheres. The cerebrum controls the skeletal muscles, interprets general senses (such as temperature, pain, and touch), and contains centers for sight and hearing. Intellect, memory, and emotional reactions also take place in the cerebrum.
gray matter (grā) (MAT-ur)	outer portion of the cerebrum, contains neuron cell bodies that collect and process information. Gray matter forms the inner portion of the spinal cord (Fig 15.3).
white matter (wīt) (MAT-ur)	inner portion of the cerebrum, contains axons, long cords that extend from neurons; conveys information to different parts of the brain. White matter forms the outer portion of the spinal cord (Fig. 15.3).
ventricles (VEN-tri-kulz)	four interconnected cavities (spaces) within the brain that produce and circulate **cerebrospinal fluid (CSF)**

Organs and Anatomic Structures of the Nervous System—cont'd

TERM	DEFINITION
cerebellum (ser-a-BEL-um)	posterior portion of the brain located under the cerebrum; assists in the coordination of skeletal muscles to maintain balance (also called **hindbrain**)

🏛 **CEREBELLUM** was named in the third century BC by Erasistratus, who also named the cerebrum. **Cerebellum** literally means **little brain** and is the diminutive of **cerebrum**, meaning **brain**. Although it was named long ago, its function was not understood until the nineteenth century.

TERM	DEFINITION
brainstem (BRĀN-stem)	stemlike portion of the brain that connects with the spinal cord and relays information to and from the cerebrum; responsible for many vital functions, including breathing, blood pressure, heart rate, and sleep. Three structures comprise the brainstem: midbrain, pons, and medulla oblongata.
midbrain (MID-brān)	most superior portion of the brainstem; has multiple functions, including visual signal processing, coordination of movement, pain suppression, and production of the neurotransmitter dopamine
pons (ponz)	middle section of the brainstem (pons is the Latin term for "bridge"); serves as a message pathway between the cerebrum and the cerebellum. The pons is also an origin for nerves that are responsible for eye movements, hearing, facial sensation, and expressions.
medulla oblongata (ma-DŪL-a) (ob-long-GAH-ta)	lowest portion of the brainstem; located between the pons and spinal cord. It contains centers that control respiration, heart rate, and blood pressure. The medulla oblongata is responsible for involuntary reflexes such as swallowing and sneezing. It also serves as an origin for nerves that coordinate mouth and tongue movements, voice, gag reflex, and head and neck movements.
cerebrospinal fluid (CSF) (ser-ē-brō-SPĪ-nal) (FLOO-id)	clear, colorless fluid contained in the ventricles that flows through the subarachnoid space around the brain and spinal cord. It cushions the brain and spinal cord from shock, transports nutrients, and clears metabolic waste.
spinal cord (SPĪ-nal) (kord)	passes through the vertebral canal, extending from the medulla oblongata to the level of the second lumbar vertebra. The spinal cord conducts nerve impulses to and from the brain and initiates reflex action to sensory information without input from the brain.
meninges (me-NIN-jēz)	three layers of membrane that cover the brain and spinal cord (Fig. 15.3)

🏛 **MENINGES** were first named by a Persian physician in the tenth century. When translated into Latin, they became **dura mater**, meaning **hard mother** (because it is a tough membrane), and **pia mater**, meaning **soft mother** (because it is a delicate membrane). **Mater** was used because the Arabians believed that the meninges were the mother of all other body membranes.

TERM	DEFINITION
dura mater (DUR-a) (MĀ-ter)	tough outer layer of the meninges
arachnoid (a-RAK-noid)	delicate middle layer of the meninges. The arachnoid membrane is loosely attached to the pia mater by weblike fibers, which allow for the **subarachnoid space**.

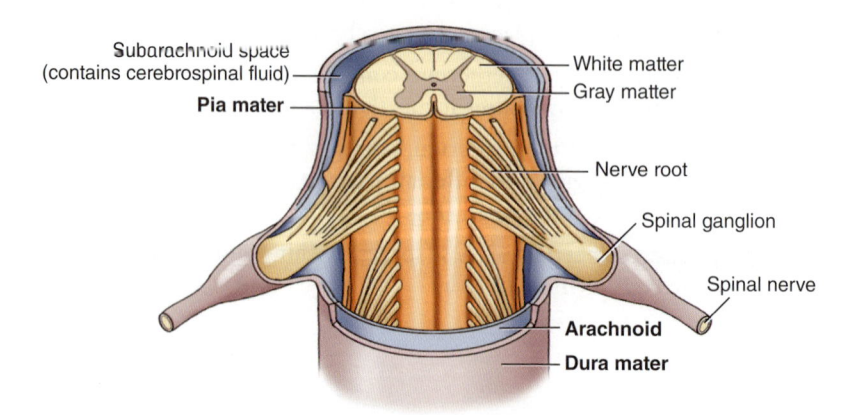

FIG. 15.3 Layers of meninges.

Chapter 15 Nervous System and Behavioral Health 597

TERM	DEFINITION
pia mater (PĒ-a) (MĀ-ter)	thin inner layer of the meninges
nerve (nurv)	cordlike structure made up of bundles of fibers composed of neurons; carries impulses from one part of the body to another. There are 12 pairs of cranial nerves and 31 pairs of spinal nerves. (Figs. 15.1 and 15.4)
ganglion (*pl.* ganglia) (GANG-glē-on) (GANG-glē-a)	group of nerve cell bodies located outside the central nervous system
glia (GLĒ-a)	specialized cells located throughout the nervous system that support and nourish nervous tissue. Some cells assist in the secretion of cerebrospinal fluid and others assist with phagocytosis. They do not conduct impulses. (also called **neuroglia**)

🏛 **GLIA** is the Greek word for **glue**; named in 1856 by the pathologist Rudolph Virchow. These gelatinous cells were originally credited with holding the nerves together. Today we know that they perform many more tasks in the brain and spinal cord.

| neuron
(NŪR-on) | nerve cell that conducts impulses to carry out the function of the nervous system. Destroyed neurons in the central nervous system cannot be replaced. |

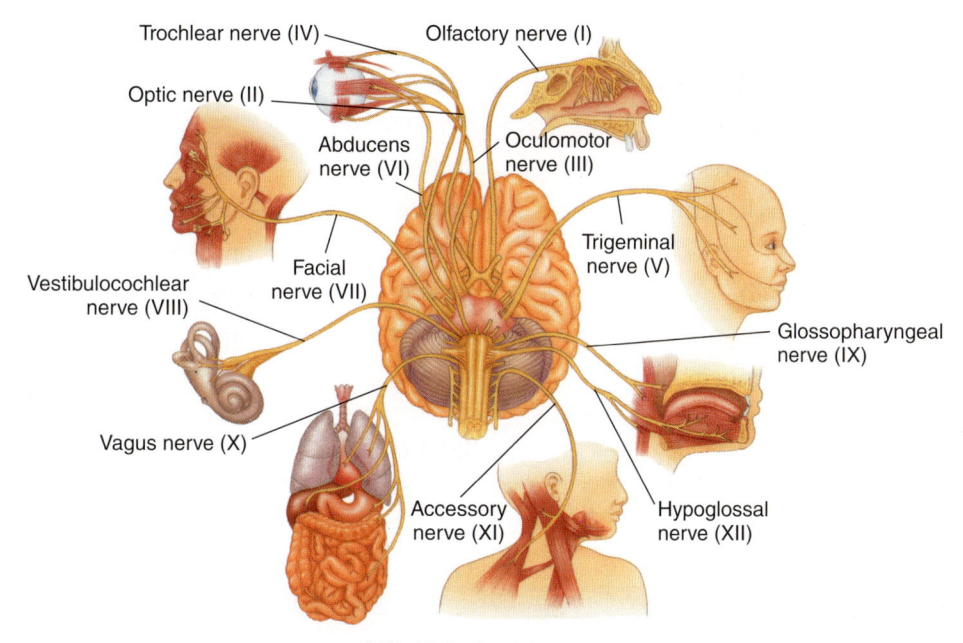

FIG. 15.4 Cranial nerves.

PRONOUNCE ANATOMIC STRUCTURES

Practice saying aloud each of the organs and specific structures on the previous pages.

To hear the terms, go to Evolve Resources at www.evolve.elsevier.com and select:
Student Resources > Audio Glossary > Chapter 15 > Anatomic Structures

❏ Check the box when complete.

WORD PARTS

Use paper flashcards or electronic flashcards on Evolve to memorize word parts used to analyze, define, and build medical terms in this chapter. To reinforce learning, study one section of the Word Parts Table at a time, and then complete the corresponding exercise on the following pages.

1 ■ Combining Forms of the Nervous System

COMBINING FORM	DEFINITION	COMBINING FORM	DEFINITION
cerebell/o	cerebellum	meningi/o	meninges
cerebr/o	cerebrum	myel/o	spinal cord
dur/o	hard, dura mater	**MYELO** refers to bone marrow when used with musculoskeletal terms.	
encephal/o	brain	neur/o	nerve(s), nerve tissue
gangli/o	ganglion	poli/o	gray matter
ganglion/o	ganglion	radicul/o	nerve root
gli/o	glia	rhiz/o	nerve root
mening/o	meninges	A **NERVE ROOT** is the proximal end of a peripheral nerve, closest to the spinal cord.	

2 ■ Combining Forms Used With Nervous System Terms

COMBINING FORM	DEFINITION	COMBINING FORM	DEFINITION
angi/o	vessel(s); blood vessel(s)	hydr/o	water
blast/o	developing cell, germ cell	ment/o	mind
cephal/o	head	mon/o	one, single
crani/o	cranium (skull)	phas/o	speech
embol/o	plug	psych/o	mind
esthesi/o	sensation, sensitivity, feeling	quadr/i	four (Note: an i is the combining vowel in quadr/i.)
hem/o	blood	thromb/o	blood clot
hemat/o	blood		

3 ■ Prefixes

PREFIX	DEFINITION	PREFIX	DEFINITION
a-	absence of, without	intra-	within
an-	absence of, without	para-	beside, around, abnormal
dys-	painful, abnormal, difficult, labored	poly-	many, much
hemi-	half	post-	after
hyper-	above, excessive	pre-	before
inter-	between	sub-	under, below

Chapter 15 Nervous System and Behavioral Health   599

4 ■ Suffixes

SUFFIX	DEFINITION	SUFFIX	DEFINITION
-a	noun suffix, no meaning	-logy	study of
-al	pertaining to	-lysis	loosening, dissolution, separating
-algia	pain	-malacia	softening
-cele	hernia, protrusion	-oma	tumor, swelling
-ectomy	excision, surgical removal	-osis	abnormal condition (means increase when used with blood cell word roots)
-genic	producing, originating, causing		
-graphy	process of recording, radiographic imaging	-paresis	slight paralysis
-ia	diseased state, condition of	-pathy	disease
-iatrist	specialist, physician	-plasty	surgical repair
-iatry	treatment, specialty	-plegia	paralysis
-ictal	seizure, attack	-rrhage	excessive flow
-ism	state of	-rrhaphy	suturing, repairing
-itis	inflammation	-tomy	cut into, incision
-logist	one who studies and treats (specialist, physician)	-us	noun suffix, no meaning

Refer to **Appendix B** and **Appendix C** for a complete list of word parts.

EXERCISE 1 ■ Nervous System Combining Forms

Refer to the first section of the word parts table.

A Label

Fill in the blanks with combining forms in this diagram of the brain and spinal cord.
To check your answers, go to Appendix A.

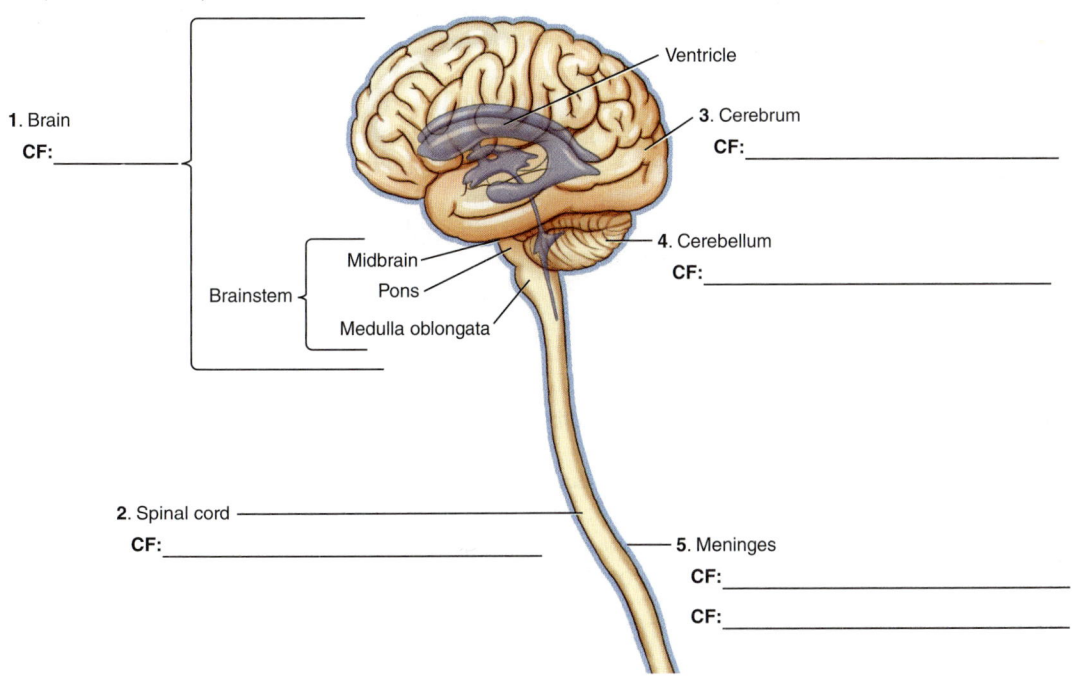

1. Brain
   CF: _____

2. Spinal cord
   CF: _____

3. Cerebrum
   CF: _____

4. Cerebellum
   CF: _____

5. Meninges
   CF: _____
   CF: _____

B Identify

Write the combining form for each of the following definitions.

1. glia _____   2. nerve _____

C Label

Fill in the blanks with combining forms in this diagram of the spinal cord and layers of meninges.

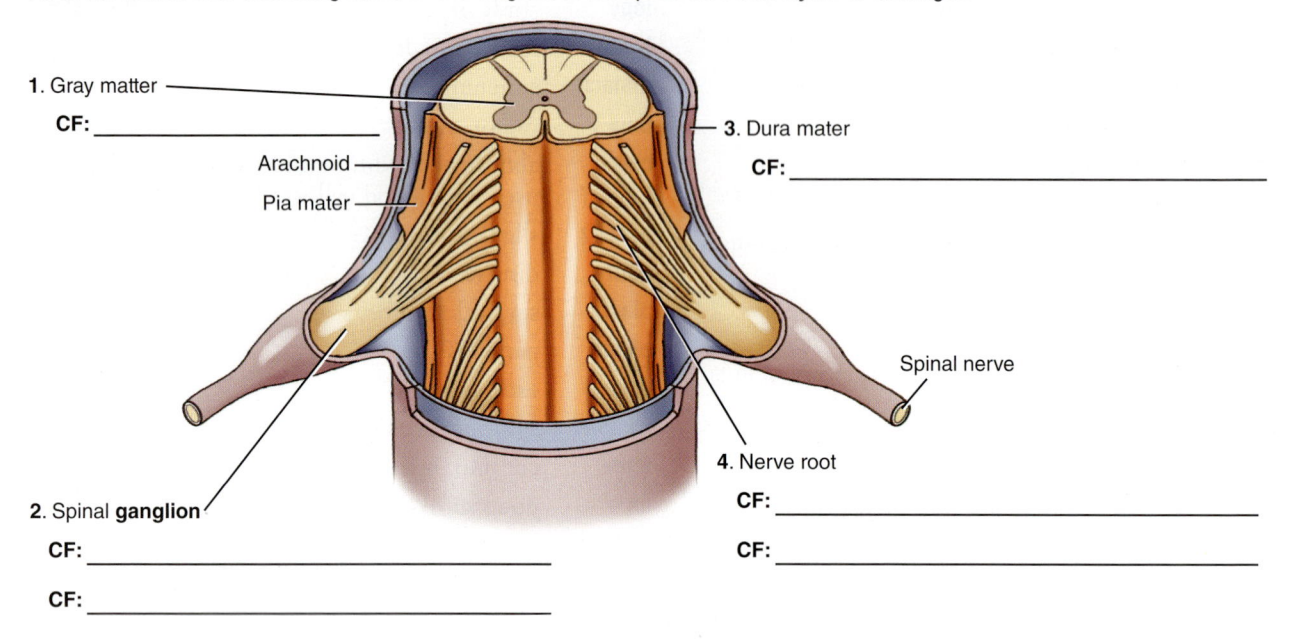

1. Gray matter
   CF: _____

2. Spinal **ganglion**
   CF: _____
   CF: _____

3. Dura mater
   CF: _____

4. Nerve root
   CF: _____
   CF: _____

D Define and Match

Step 1: Write the definitions after the following combining forms.
Step 2: Match the descriptions on the right with the combining forms and definitions.

_____ 1. gangli/o, _____
_____ 2. dur/o, _____
_____ 3. encephal/o, _____
_____ 4. cerebell/o, _____
_____ 5. meningi/o, _____
_____ 6. neur/o, _____

a. assists in the coordination of skeletal muscles to maintain balance
b. cordlike structure made up of bundles of fibers composed of neurons that carries impulses from one part of the body to another
c. contained within the cranium; the center for coordinating body activities
d. tough outer layer of the meninges
e. group of nerve cell bodies located outside the central nervous system
f. three layers of membrane that cover the brain and spinal cord

E Define and Match

Step 1: Write the definitions after the following combining forms.
Step 2: Match the descriptions on the right with the combining forms and definitions.

_____ 1. gli/o, _____
_____ 2. ganglion/o, _____
_____ 3. mening/o, _____
_____ 4. cerebr/o, _____
_____ 5. myel/o, _____
_____ 6. poli/o, _____

a. conducts impulses to and from the brain and initiates reflex action to sensory information
b. specialized cells that support and nourish nervous tissue
c. outer portion of cerebrum, inner portion of spinal cord; processes information
d. group of nerve cell bodies located outside the central nervous system
e. three layers of membrane that cover the brain and spinal cord
f. largest portion of the brain, divided into left and right hemispheres

F Identify

Write the combining forms for the following term.

1. nerve root
   a. _____
   b. _____

EXERCISE 2 ■ Combining Forms Used with Nervous System Terms

Refer to the second section of the word parts table.

A Define

Write the definitions of the following combining forms new to this chapter.

1. mon/o _____
2. psych/o _____
3. quadr/i _____
4. ment/o _____
5. phas/o _____
6. esthesi/o _____

B Match

Match the combining forms in the first column with their correct definitions in the second column. Answers may be used more than once.

_____ 1. thromb/o   a. blood
_____ 2. hydr/o   b. blood clot
_____ 3. hemat/o   c. skull
_____ 4. hem/o   d. developing cell, germ cell
_____ 5. embol/o   e. head
_____ 6. crani/o   f. plug
_____ 7. cephal/o   g. vessel(s); blood vessel(s)
_____ 8. blast/o   h. water
_____ 9. angi/o

EXERCISE 3 ■ Prefixes

Refer to the third section of the word parts table. Match the prefixes in the first column with their correct definitions in the second column.

_____ 1. sub-   a. above, excessive
_____ 2. pre-   b. absence of, without
_____ 3. post-   c. after
_____ 4. poly-   d. before
_____ 5. intra-   e. between
_____ 6. inter-   f. half
_____ 7. hyper-   g. beside, around, abnormal
_____ 8. hemi-   h. painful, abnormal, difficult, labored
_____ 9. dys-   i. under, below
_____ 10. a-, an-   j. within
_____ 11. para-   k. many, much

EXERCISE 4 ■ Suffixes

Refer to the fourth section of the word parts table.

A Define

Write the definitions of the following suffixes new to this chapter.

1. -paresis _____
2. -iatry _____
3. -ictal _____
4. -iatrist _____

B Match

Match the suffixes in the first column with their correct definitions in the second column.

____ 1. -al		a. suturing, repairing
____ 2. -ectomy		b. surgical repair
____ 3. -graphy		c. noun suffix, no meaning
____ 4. -genic		d. process of recording, radiographic imaging
____ 5. -logy		e. pertaining to
____ 6. -lysis		f. one who studies and treats (specialist, physician)
____ 7. -plasty		g. loosening, dissolution, separating
____ 8. -rrhaphy		h. excision, surgical removal
____ 9. -tomy		i. cut into, incision
____ 10. -a, -us		j. study of
____ 11. -logist		k. producing, originating, causing

C Match

Match the suffixes in the first column with their correct definitions in the second column.

____ 1. -algia		a. tumor, swelling
____ 2. -cele		b. state of
____ 3. -ia		c. softening
____ 4. -ism		d. paralysis
____ 5. -itis		e. pain
____ 6. -oma		f. inflammation
____ 7. -osis		g. hernia, protrusion
____ 8. -pathy		h. excessive flow
____ 9. -malacia		i. diseased state, condition of
____ 10. -plegia		j. disease
____ 11. -rrhage		k. abnormal condition (means increase when used with blood cell word roots)

Chapter 15 Nervous System and Behavioral Health

MEDICAL TERMS

Medical terms relevant to this chapter have been grouped by topics, such as Disease and Disorder, and are listed in tables designated as Built from Word Parts or *NOT* Built from Word Parts. The exercises following each table assist with learning term definitions, pronunciations, and spellings.

Disease and Disorder Terms

BUILT FROM WORD PARTS

The following terms can be translated using definitions of word parts. Further explanation is provided within parentheses as needed.

TERM	DEFINITION
1. cerebellitis (*ser*-e-bel-Ī-tis)	inflammation of the cerebellum
2. cerebral embolism (se-RĒ-bral) (EM-bō-lizm)	pertaining to the cerebrum, state of a plug (clot or piece of plaque from a distant site lodged in a cerebral artery, causing sudden blockage of blood supply to the brain tissue)
3. cerebral thrombosis (se-RĒ-bral) (throm-BŌ-sis)	pertaining to the cerebrum, abnormal condition of a blood clot (onset of symptoms may appear from minutes to days after an obstruction of a blood vessel in the brain)
CEREBRAL EMBOLISM and **THROMBOSIS** are both causes of ischemic stroke, which results from blocked vessels.	
4. duritis (dū-RĪ-tis)	inflammation of the dura mater
5. encephalitis (en-*sef*-a-LĪ-tis)	inflammation of the brain
6. encephalomalacia (en-*sef*-a-lō-ma-LĀ-sha)	softening of the brain
7. encephalopathy (en-*sef*-a-LOP-a-thē)	disease of the brain
8. encephalomyeloradiculitis (en-*sef*-a-lō-*mī*-e-lō-ra-*dik*-ū-LĪ-tis)	inflammation of the brain, spinal cord, and nerve roots
9. gangliitis (*gang*-glē-Ī-tis)	inflammation of a ganglion

TERM	DEFINITION
10. glioblastoma (*glī*-ō-blas-TŌ-ma)	tumor composed of developing glia (the most malignant primary tumor of the brain)
11. glioma (glī-Ō-ma)	tumor composed of glia
GLIOMA is a general term referring to brain and spinal cord tumors developing from any of the types of glial cells or their developing cells. **Glioblastoma** is the most aggressive form of glioma.	
12. hydrocephalus (*hī*-drō-SEF-a-lus)	water (increased amount of cerebrospinal fluid) in the head (brain)
HYDROCEPHALUS may be congenital or acquired and is caused by obstructed circulation of cerebrospinal fluid, which results in dilated cerebral ventricles and impaired brain function. For infants, hydrocephalus can cause enlargement of the cranium. The condition was first described around 30 AD in the book *De Medicina*.	
13. intracerebral hemorrhage (*in*-tra-SER-e-bral) (HEM-o-rij)	pertaining to within the cerebrum, excessive flow of blood (bleeding into the brain as a result of a ruptured blood vessel within the cerebrum)
INTRACEREBRAL HEMORRHAGE symptoms often develop suddenly and vary, depending on the location of the hemorrhage; acute symptoms include dyspnea, dysphagia, aphasia, diminished level of consciousness, and hemiparesis. Intracerebral hemorrhage is a cause of hemorrhagic stroke and is frequently associated with high blood pressure.	
14. meningioma (me-*nin*-jē-Ō-ma)	tumor of the meninges (usually benign and slow growing; most common tumor originating in the brain and surrounding tissues)
15. meningitis (*men*-in-JĪ-tis)	inflammation of the meninges

603

Disease and Disorder Terms—cont'd
BUILT FROM WORD PARTS

TERM	DEFINITION	TERM	DEFINITION
16. meningocele (me-NING-gō-sēl)	protrusion of the meninges (through a defect in the skull or vertebral arch)	24. polyneuritis (*pol*-ē-nū-RĪ-tis)	inflammation of many nerves
		25. polyneuropathy (*pol*-ē-nū-ROP-a-thē)	disease of many nerves
17. meningomyelocele (me-*ning*-gō-MĪ-e-lō-*sēl*)	protrusion of the meninges and spinal cord (through a vertebral arch defect); (also called **myelomeningocele**) (see Fig. 9.7)	**POLYNEUROPATHY** most often occurs as a complication of diabetes mellitus, but may also occur as a result of drug therapy, critical illness such as sepsis, or carcinoma; symptoms include weakness, distal sensory loss, and burning.	
		26. radiculitis (ra-*dik*-ū-LĪ-tis)	inflammation of the nerve roots
		27. radiculopathy (ra-*dik*-ū-LOP-a-thē)	disease of the nerve roots
18. mononeuropathy (*mon*-ō-nū-ROP-a-thē)	disease affecting a single nerve (such as carpal tunnel syndrome)	**PERIPHERAL NEUROPATHY** refers to disorders of the peripheral nervous system, including **radiculopathy, mononeuropathy,** and **polyneuropathy**.	
19. myelitis (*mī*-e-LĪ-tis)	inflammation of the spinal cord	28. rhizomeningomyelitis (*rī*-zō-me-*ning*-gō-*mī*-e-LĪ-tis)	inflammation of the nerve root, meninges, and spinal cord
20. myelomalacia (*mī*-e-lō-ma-LĀ-sha)	softening of the spinal cord		
21. neuralgia (nū-RAL-ja)	nerve pain	29. subdural hematoma (sub-DŪ-ral) (*hē*-ma-TŌ-ma)	pertaining to below the dura mater, tumor of blood (collection of blood that has leaked out of a broken vessel)
22. neuritis (nū-RĪ-tis)	inflammation of a nerve		
23. poliomyelitis (polio) (*pō*-lē-ō-*mī*-e-LĪ-tis)	inflammation of the gray matter of the spinal cord (This infectious disease, commonly referred to as *polio*, is caused by one of three polioviruses.)	**HEMATOMA,** though translated as *tumor of blood* from the meaning of its word parts, is a collection of blood resulting from a broken blood vessel.	

EXERCISE 5 ■ Pronounce and Spell

Practice pronunciation and spelling on paper and online.

1. **Practice on Paper**
   a. **Pronounce:** Read the phonetic spelling and say aloud the terms listed in the previous table. Refer to Table 2.2 Pronunciation Key as needed.
   b. **Spell:** Have a study partner read the terms aloud. Write the spelling of the terms on a separate sheet of paper.

2. **Practice Online**
   a. **Access** online learning resources. Go to evolve.elsevier.com > Evolve Resources > Student Resources.
   b. **Pronounce:** Select Audio Glossary > Chapter 15 > Exercise 5. Select a term to hear its pronunciation and repeat aloud.
   c. **Spell:** Select Activities > Chapter 15 > Spell Terms > Exercise 5. Select the audio icon and type the correct spelling of the term.

❏ Check the box when complete.

Chapter 15 Nervous System and Behavioral Health 605

EXERCISE 6 ■ Analyze and Define

Analyze and define the following terms.

1. myelitis

2. hydrocephalus

3. poliomyelitis

4. radiculopathy

5. encephalopathy

6. encephalitis

7. rhizomeningomyelitis

8. cerebral thrombosis

9. meningocele

10. myelomalacia

11. radiculitis

12. gangliitis

13. duritis

14. polyneuritis

EXERCISE 7 ■ Build

A Label

Build terms pictured by writing word parts above definitions.

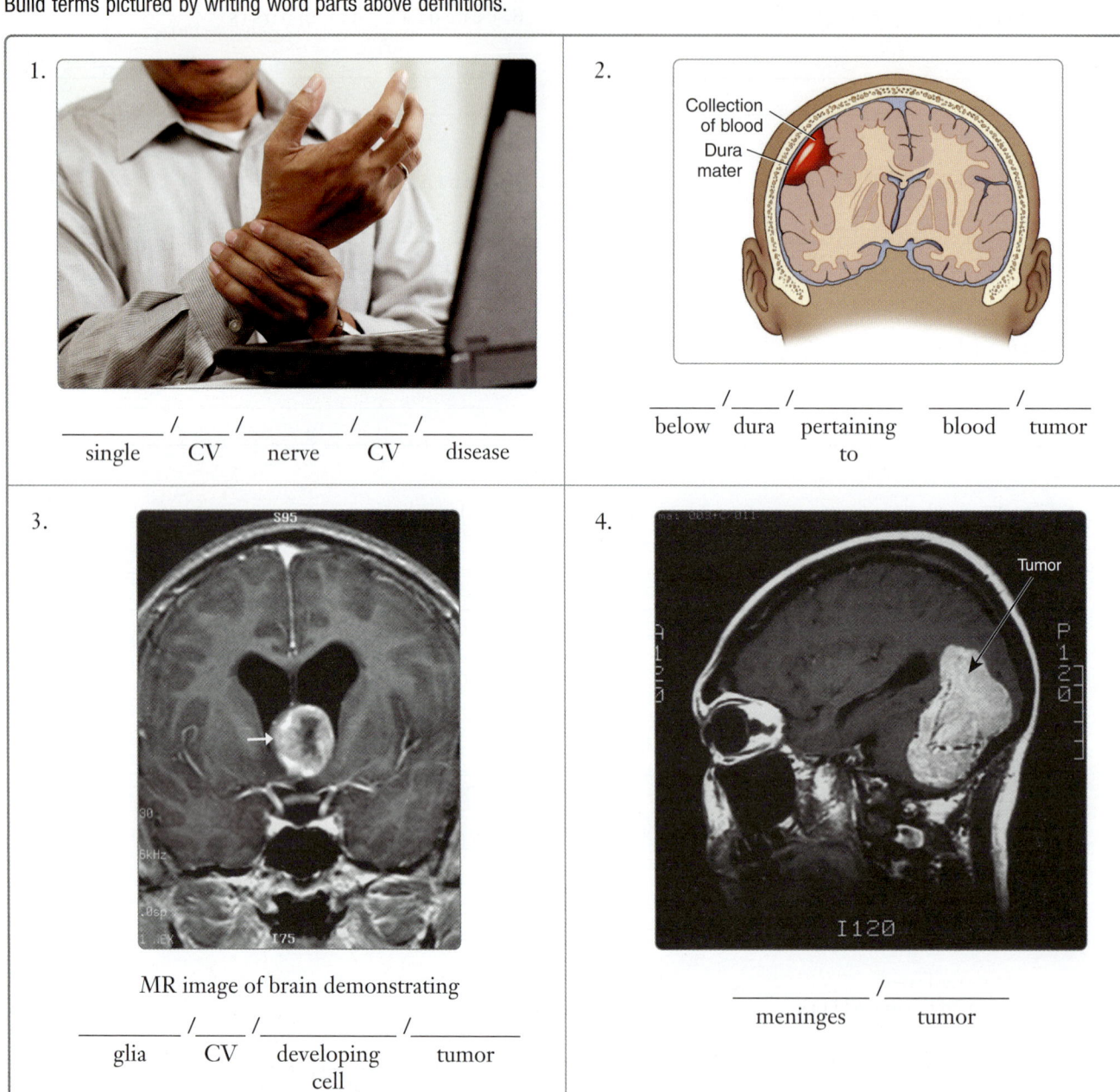

1. _____ / ____ / _____ / ____ / _____
   single   CV   nerve   CV   disease

2. _____ / ____ / _____   _____ / _____
   below   dura pertaining   blood   tumor
                    to

3. MR image of brain demonstrating
   _____ / ____ / _____ / _____
   glia   CV   developing   tumor
                      cell

4. _____ / _____
   meninges   tumor

Chapter 15 Nervous System and Behavioral Health 607

5.

_____ / _____ / _____   _____ / ___ / _____
within cerebrum pertaining   blood CV excessive
              to   flow

6.

_____ / _____   _____ / _____
cerebrum   pertaining to   plug   state of

7.

_____ / _____ / ____ / _____
  many   nerve   CV   disease

8.

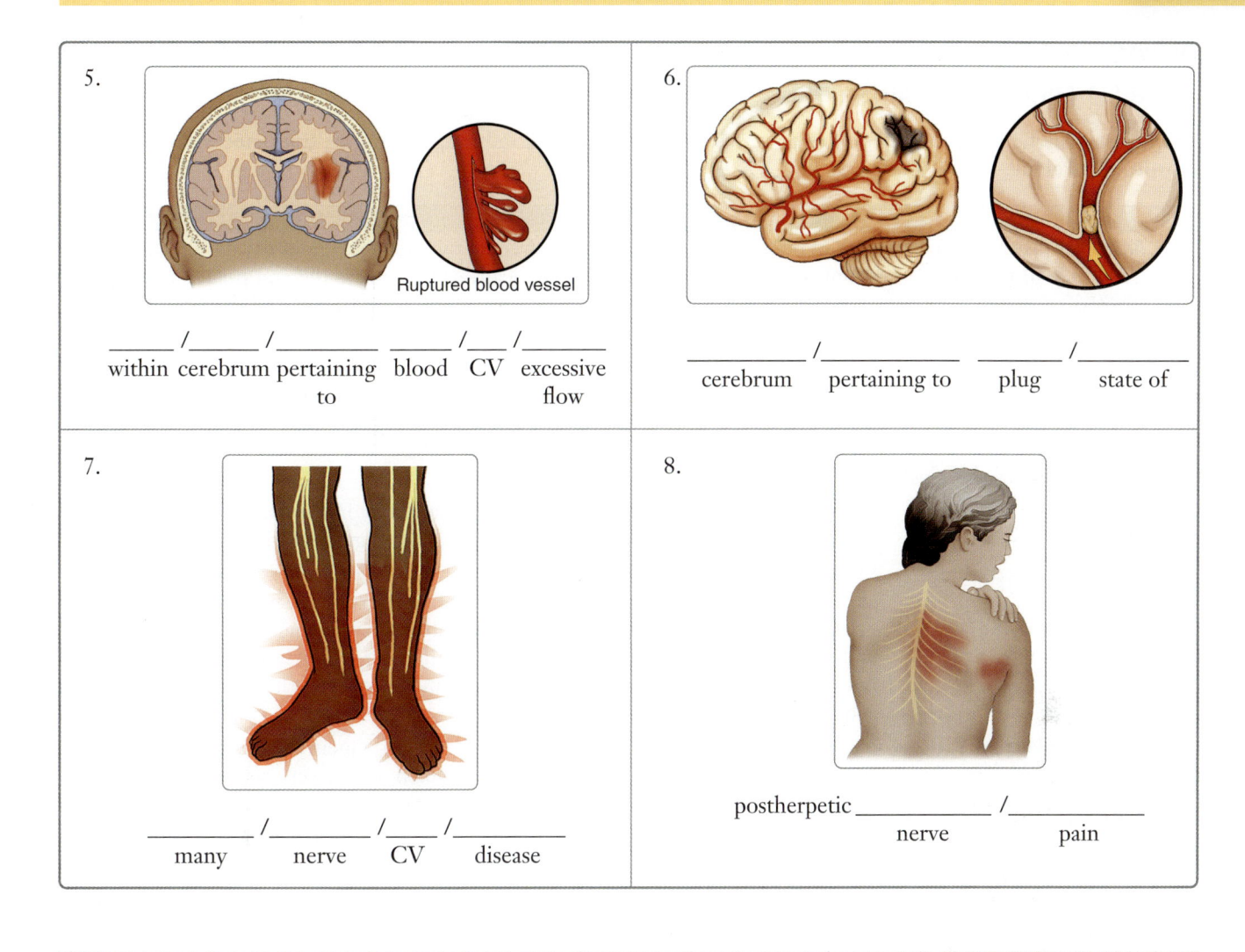

postherpetic _____ / _____
              nerve   pain

B Fill In

Build disease and disorder terms for the following definitions by using the word parts you have learned.

1. inflammation of the nerve

    _____ / _____
        WR   S

2. tumor composed of glia

    _____ / _____
        WR   S

3. softening of the brain

    _____ / ___ / _____
        WR   CV   S

4. inflammation of the cerebellum

    _____ / _____
        WR   S

5. inflammation of the brain, spinal cord, and nerve roots

    _____ / ___ / _____ / ___ / _____ / _____
      WR   CV   WR   CV   WR   S

6. inflammation of the meninges

    _____ / _____
        WR   S

7. protrusion of the meninges and spinal cord (through a vertebral arch defect)

    _____ / ___ / _____ / ___ / _____
      WR   CV   WR   CV   S

Disease and Disorder Terms
NOT BUILT FROM WORD PARTS

Word parts may be present in the following terms; however, their full meanings cannot be translated using definitions of word parts alone.

TERM	DEFINITION
1. **Alzheimer disease (AD)** (AWLTZ-hī-mer) (di-ZĒZ)	type of dementia that occurs more frequently after the age of 65, but can begin at any age. The brain shrinks dramatically as nerve cells die and tissues atrophy. The disease is slowly progressive and usually results in profound dementia in 5 to 10 years. A prominent feature of AD is the inability to remember the recent past, while memories of the distant past remain intact.
2. **amyotrophic lateral sclerosis (ALS)** (ā-*mī*-ō-TRŌ-fik) (LAT-er-al) (skle-RŌ-sis)	progressive muscle atrophy caused by degeneration and scarring of neurons along the lateral columns of the spinal cord that control muscles (also called **Lou Gehrig disease**)
3. **Bell palsy** (bel) (PAWL-zē)	paralysis of muscles on one side of the face caused by inflammation or compression of the facial nerve, cranial nerve VII. Signs include a sagging mouth on the affected side and nonclosure of the eyelid; paralysis is usually temporary.
4. **botulism** (BOCH-e-liz-um)	serious illness caused by a bacterial toxin that interferes with nerve conduction, causing skeletal muscle paralysis. Initial symptoms may include trouble seeing and muscle weakness leading to difficulty swallowing and breathing. Foodborne botulism, wound botulism, and infant botulism are types of the illness, all of which can be fatal and are medical emergencies.
5. **cerebral aneurysm** (se-RĒ-bral) (AN-ū-rizm)	ballooning of a weakened portion of an arterial wall (aneurysm) in the cerebrum. It is usually asymptomatic until it ruptures, which can be very serious and can result in death.
6. **cerebral palsy (CP)** (se-RĒ-bral) (PAWL-zē)	condition characterized by lack of muscle control and partial paralysis, caused by a brain defect or lesion present at birth or shortly after
7. **chronic traumatic encephalopathy (CTE)** (KRON-ik) (tra-MAT-ik) (en-*sef*-a-LOP-a-thē)	progressive degenerative disease of the brain that generally appears years or decades after repeated head trauma. Originally diagnosed in boxers (dementia pugilistica), it has now been found in other professional athletes who experienced repeated head trauma, such as football, ice hockey, soccer, wrestling, and basketball players. Signs and symptoms include memory loss, aggression, confusion, attention deficits, poor judgment, anxiety, and depression. Currently, CTE can only be definitively diagnosed after death by brain autopsy, but in the future, diagnostic imaging, chemical biomarkers, and neuropsychological tests may be helpful.
8. **dementia** (de-MEN-sha)	cognitive impairment characterized by loss of intellectual brain function. Patients have difficulty in various ways, including difficulty in performing complex tasks, reasoning, learning and retaining new information, orientation, word finding, and behavior. Dementia has several causes and is not considered part of normal aging. (Table 15.1)
9. **epilepsy** (EP-i-lep-se)	condition characterized by recurrent seizures; a general term given to a group of neurologic disorders, all characterized by abnormal electrical activity in the brain

🏛 **EPILEPSY** was written about by Hippocrates, in 400 BC, in a book titled **Sacred Disease**. It was believed at one time that epilepsy was a punishment for offending the gods. The Greek **epilepsia** meant **seizure** and is derived from **epi**, meaning **upon**, and **lambanein**, meaning **to seize**. The term literally means **seized upon** (by the gods).

| 10. **migraine** (MĪ-grān) | intense, throbbing headache; usually one-sided and often associated with nausea, vomiting, and extreme sensitivity to light or sound. Migraines may occur with or without auras (sensory symptoms preceding the headache, such as flashes of light, blind spots, or tingling in the arms or legs). |
| 11. **multiple sclerosis (MS)** (MUL-ti-pl) (skle-RŌ-sis) | chronic degenerative disease characterized by sclerotic patches along the brain and spinal cord; signs and symptoms fluctuate over the course of the disease; more common symptoms include fatigue, balance and coordination impairments, numbness, and vision problems |

TABLE 15.1 Types of Dementia

COMMON TYPES OF DEMENTIA

Alzheimer disease	most common type of dementia, responsible for 60% to 80% of all cases. The disease, which appears to be due to a variety of causes, is a progressive neurodegenerative disorder characterized by diffuse brain atrophy and the presence of senile plaques and neurofibrillary tangles within the brain cortex. Women are affected more than men, possibly because women tend to live longer, and because the chances of having AD double with every 5 additional years of life after age 65.
Vascular or multiple infarct dementia	affects approximately 10% of patients with dementia. It is secondary to cerebrovascular disease and usually occurs in older patients. Dementia usually worsens in a stepwise fashion, and other neurologic findings (such as paralysis or cranial nerve abnormalities) are often present.
Lewy body dementia	usually a rapidly progressive form of dementia; it is responsible for approximately 10% of all dementias. Lewy body dementia is characterized by hallucinations, fluctuations in severity, sleep disorders, and Parkinson symptoms, the latter of which occur less than 1 year before the dementia.
Parkinson dementia	generally does not develop until patients have advanced Parkinson disease; similar to Lewy body dementia
Frontotemporal dementia (Pick disease)	affects the anterior portions of the brain; most common symptoms are personality changes, disinhibition, and impulsiveness. Atrophy may be observed on brain CT or MR.

LESS COMMON FORMS OF DEMENTIA

Normal pressure hydrocephalus	imbalance of cerebrospinal fluid in the brain leads to a triad of dementia, urinary incontinence, and gait instability. Sometimes caused by trauma or subarachnoid hemorrhage; can be treated with a ventricular peritoneal shunt
Wernicke-Korsakoff syndrome	form of dementia found with chronic alcoholism; caused by thiamine deficiency and poor nutritional status
Infections	including Creutzfeldt-Jakob disease, HIV infection, syphilis, and tuberculosis
Tumors and chronic subdural hematomas	space-occupying lesions that prevent normal brain function

---

TERM	DEFINITION
12. **Parkinson disease (PD)** (PAR-kin-sun) (di-ZĒZ)	chronic degenerative disease of the central nervous system. Signs and symptoms include resting tremors of the hands and feet, rigidity, expressionless face, shuffling gait, and eventually dementia. It usually occurs after the age of 50 years (also called **parkinsonism**).

PARKINSON DISEASE was first described by James Parkinson, an English professor, in his **Essay on the Shaking Palsy** in 1817.

13. **sciatica** (sī-AT-i-ka)	inflammation of the sciatic nerve, causing pain that starts in the lower back and extends down the leg; can be caused by injury, infection, arthritis, herniated disk, or from prolonged pressure on the nerve from sitting for long periods
14. **shingles** (SHING-gelz)	viral disease that affects the peripheral nerves and causes blisters on the skin that follow the course of the affected nerves (also called **herpes zoster**)

POSTHERPETIC NEURALGIA is a complication of **shingles** (herpes zoster) and is caused by damage to the nerve fibers. Severe pain and hyperesthesia persist after the skin lesions disappear and may last months or even years.

15. **stroke** (strōk)	interruption of blood supply to a region of the brain, depriving nerve cells in the affected area of oxygen and nutrients. The cells cannot perform and may be damaged or die within minutes. The parts of the body controlled by the involved cells will experience dysfunction. Speech, movement, memory, and other CNS functions may be affected in varying degrees. **Ischemic stroke** is a result of a blocked blood vessel. **Hemorrhagic stroke** is a result of bleeding (also called **cerebrovascular accident [CVA]** or **brain attack**).

Disease and Disorder Terms—cont'd
NOT BUILT FROM WORD PARTS

TERM	DEFINITION
16. **subarachnoid hemorrhage (SAH)** (*sub*-e-RAK-noid) (HEM-o-rij)	bleeding between the pia mater and arachnoid layers of the meninges (subarachnoid space), caused by a ruptured blood vessel (usually a cerebral aneurysm). The patient may experience an intense, sudden headache accompanied by nausea, vomiting, and neck pain. SAH is a critical condition that must be recognized and treated immediately to prevent permanent brain damage or death (a cause of **hemorrhagic stroke**).
17. **transient ischemic attack (TIA)** (TRAN-sē-ent) (is-KĒ-mik) (a-TAK)	sudden deficient supply of blood to the brain lasting a short time. The symptoms may be similar to those of stroke, but with TIA the symptoms are temporary and the usual outcome is complete recovery. TIAs are often warning signs for eventual occurrence of a stroke.

EXERCISE 8 ■ Pronounce and Spell

Practice pronunciation and spelling on paper and online.

1. **Practice on Paper**
   a. **Pronounce:** Read the phonetic spelling and say aloud the terms listed in the previous table. Refer to Table 2.2 Pronunciation Key as needed.
   b. **Spell:** Have a study partner read the terms aloud. Write the spelling of the terms on a separate sheet of paper.

2. **Practice Online**
   a. **Access** online learning resources. Go to evolve.elsevier.com > Evolve Resources > Student Resources.
   b. **Pronounce:** Select Audio Glossary > Chapter 15 > Exercise 8. Select a term to hear its pronunciation and repeat aloud.
   c. **Spell:** Select Activities > Chapter 15 > Spell Terms > Exercise 8. Select the audio icon and type the correct spelling of the term.

❑ Check the box when complete.

EXERCISE 9 ■ Match

Match the terms in the first column with their definitions in the second column.

_____ 1. multiple sclerosis
_____ 2. migraine
_____ 3. cerebral palsy
_____ 4. Parkinson disease
_____ 5. amyotrophic lateral sclerosis
_____ 6. dementia
_____ 7. botulism
_____ 8. chronic traumatic encephalopathy
_____ 9. epilepsy

a. condition characterized by lack of muscle control and partial paralysis, caused by a brain defect or a lesion present at birth or shortly after
b. progressive muscle atrophy caused by degeneration and scarring of neurons along the lateral columns of the spinal cord
c. cognitive impairment characterized by loss of intellectual brain function; not considered part of normal aging
d. progressive degenerative disease of the brain that generally appears years or decades after repeated head trauma
e. serious illness caused by a bacterial toxin that interferes with nerve conduction, causing skeletal muscle paralysis
f. chronic degenerative disease of the central nervous system, characterized by resting tremors of the hands and feet, rigidity, expressionless face, shuffling gait, and dementia
g. condition characterized by recurrent seizures
h. chronic degenerative disease characterized by sclerotic patches along the brain and spinal cord
i. intense, throbbing headache; usually one-sided and often associated with nausea, vomiting, and extreme sensitivity to light or sound

Chapter 15 Nervous System and Behavioral Health   611

EXERCISE 10 ■ Label

Write the medical terms pictured and defined.

1. _____
inflammation of the sciatic nerve, causing pain that starts in the lower back and extends down the leg

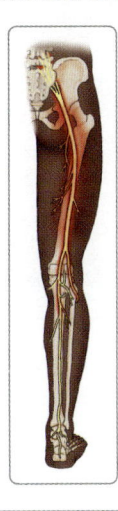

2. _____
type of dementia that occurs more frequently after the age of 65; the brain shrinks dramatically

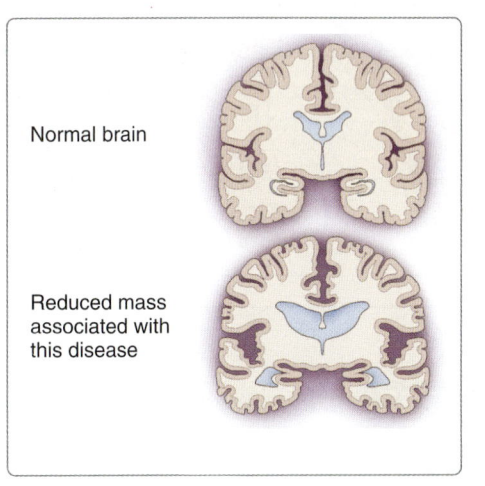

Normal brain

Reduced mass associated with this disease

3. _____
viral disease that affects the peripheral nerves and causes blisters on the skin that follow the course of the affected nerves

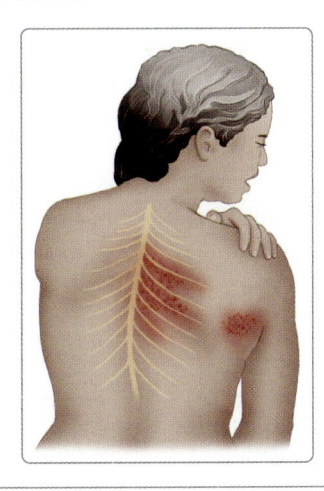

4. _____
ballooning of a weakened portion of an arterial wall in the cerebrum

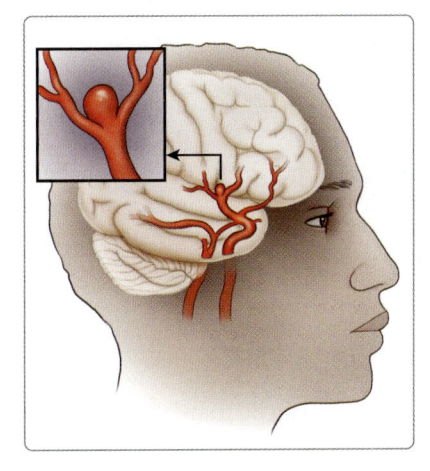

5. _____
bleeding between the pia mater and arachnoid layers of the meninges caused by a ruptured blood vessel

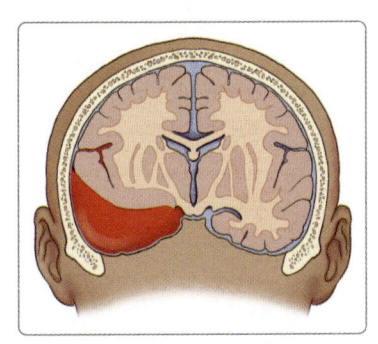

6. _____
interruption of blood supply to a region of the brain, depriving nerve cells in the affected area of oxygen and nutrients

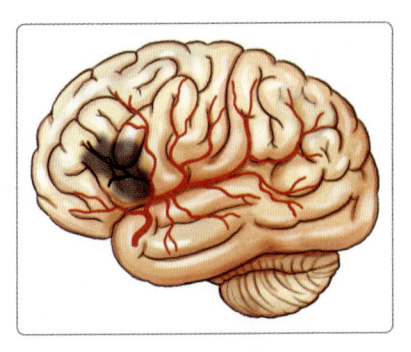

612 Chapter 15 Nervous System and Behavioral Health

7. _____
sudden deficient supply of blood to the brain lasting a short time

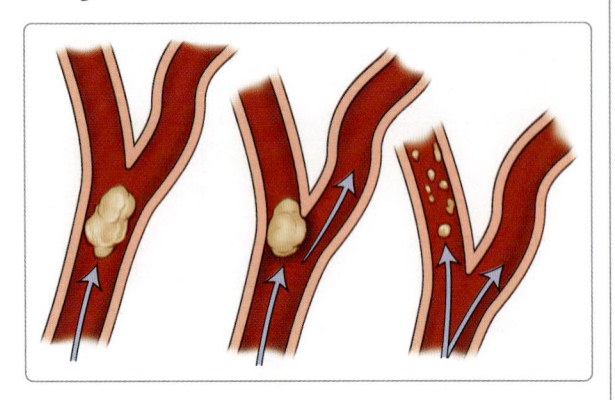

8. _____
paralysis of muscles on one side of the face caused by inflammation or compression of the facial nerve

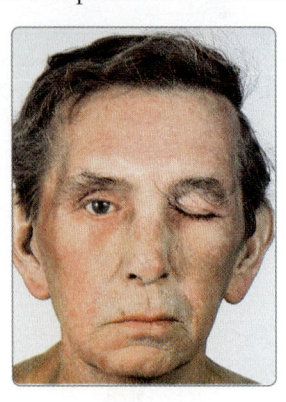

EXERCISE 11 ■ Review of Disease and Disorder Terms

Can you define, pronounce, and spell the following terms?

Alzheimer disease (AD)	dementia	meningioma	polyneuritis
amyotrophic lateral sclerosis (ALS)	duritis	meningitis	polyneuropathy
Bell palsy	encephalitis	meningocele	radiculitis
botulism	encephalomalacia	meningomyelocele	radiculopathy
cerebellitis	encephalomyeloradiculitis	migraine	rhizomeningomyelitis
cerebral aneurysm	encephalopathy	mononeuropathy	sciatica
cerebral embolism	epilepsy	multiple sclerosis (MS)	shingles
cerebral palsy (CP)	gangliitis	myelitis	stroke
cerebral thrombosis	glioblastoma	myelomalacia	subarachnoid hemorrhage (SAH)
chronic traumatic encephalopathy (CTE)	glioma	neuralgia	subdural hematoma
	hydrocephalus	neuritis	transient ischemic attack (TIA)
	intracerebral hemorrhage	Parkinson disease (PD)	
		poliomyelitis (polio)	

Surgical Terms
BUILT FROM WORD PARTS

The following terms can be translated using definitions of word parts. Further explanation is provided within parentheses as needed.

TERM	DEFINITION	TERM	DEFINITION
1. **ganglionectomy** (gang-glē-o-NEK-to-mē)	excision of a ganglion (also called **gangliectomy**)	4. **neuroplasty** (NŪR-ō-plas-tē)	surgical repair of a nerve
GANGLIONECTOMY may be performed to treat ganglion cysts that are painful, limit movement, or cause nerve entrapment.		5. **neurorrhaphy** (nū-ROR-a-fē)	suturing of a nerve
2. **neurectomy** (nū-REK-to-mē)	excision of a nerve	6. **neurotomy** (nū-ROT-o-mē)	incision into a nerve
		7. **rhizotomy** (rī-ZOT-o-mē)	incision into a nerve root
3. **neurolysis** (nū-ROL-i-sis)	loosening, separating a nerve (to release it from surrounding tissues)		

Chapter 15   Nervous System and Behavioral Health   613

EXERCISE 12 ■ Pronounce and Spell

Practice pronunciation and spelling on paper and online.

1. **Practice on Paper**
   a. **Pronounce:** Read the phonetic spelling and say aloud the terms listed in the previous table. Refer to Table 2.2 Pronunciation Key as needed.
   b. **Spell:** Have a study partner read the terms aloud. Write the spelling of the terms on a separate sheet of paper.

2. **Practice Online**
   a. **Access** online learning resources. Go to evolve.elsevier.com > Evolve Resources > Student Resources.
   b. **Pronounce:** Select Audio Glossary > Chapter 15 > Exercise 12. Select a term to hear its pronunciation and repeat aloud.
   c. **Spell:** Select Activities > Chapter 15 > Spell Terms > Exercise 12. Select the audio icon and type the correct spelling of the term.

❏ Check the box when complete.

EXERCISE 13 ■ Analyze and Define

Analyze and define the following surgical terms.

1. neurectomy

2. neurorrhaphy

3. ganglionectomy

4. neurotomy

5. neurolysis

6. neuroplasty

7. rhizotomy

EXERCISE 14 ■ Build

A Fill In

Build surgical terms for the following definitions by using the word parts you have learned.

1. excision of a nerve   _____ / _____
                                     WR   S

2. suturing of a nerve   _____ / ___ / _____
                                     WR   CV   S

614 Chapter 15 Nervous System and Behavioral Health

3. incision into a nerve _____ / _____ / _____
   WR / CV / S

4. loosening, separating a nerve (to release it from surrounding tissue) _____ / _____ / _____
   WR / CV / S

5. surgical repair of a nerve _____ / _____ / _____
   WR / CV / S

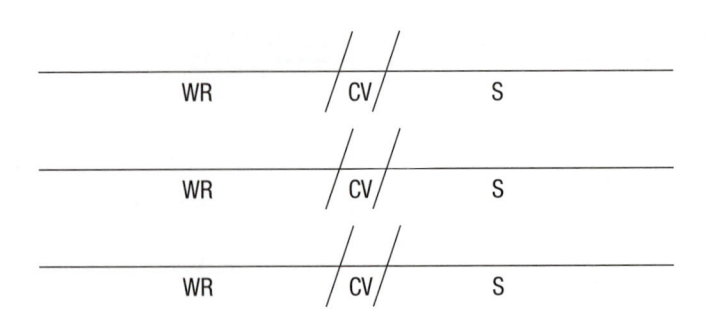

B Label

Build terms pictured by writing word parts above definitions.

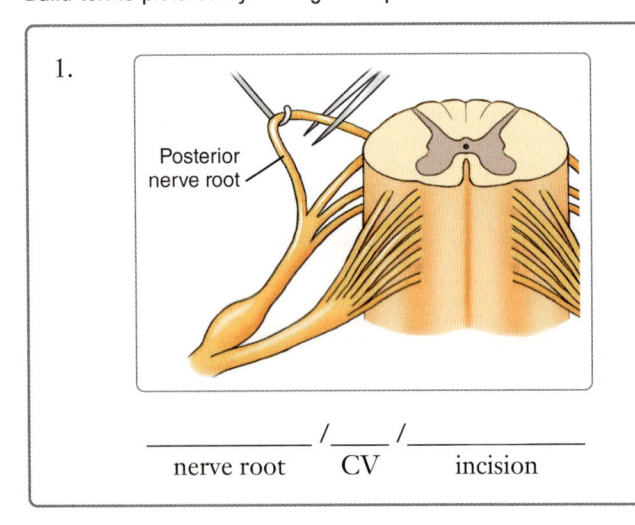

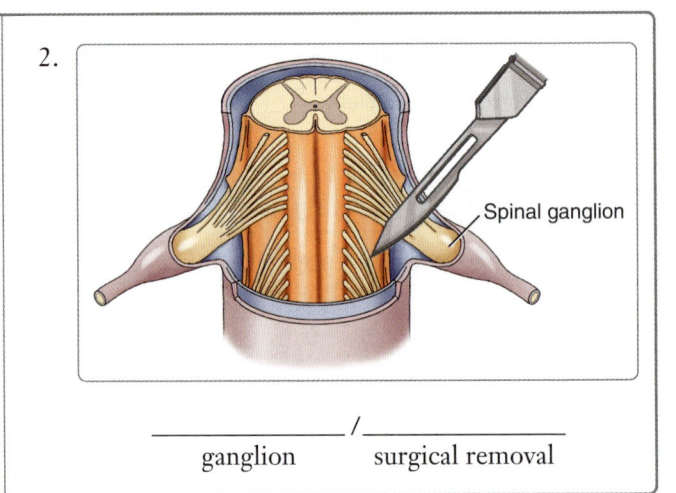

1. _____ / _____ / _____
   nerve root / CV / incision

2. _____ / _____
   ganglion / surgical removal

EXERCISE 15 ■ Review of Surgical Terms

Can you define, pronounce, and spell the following terms?

| ganglionectomy | neurolysis | neurorrhaphy | rhizotomy |
| neurectomy | neuroplasty | neurotomy | |

Diagnostic Terms

BUILT FROM WORD PARTS AND *NOT* BUILT FROM WORD PARTS

The first portion of the table contains nervous system diagnostic terms that can be translated using definitions of word parts. The second portion of the table contains terms that cannot be fully understood using the definitions of word parts.

■ **Terms Built from Word Parts**

DIAGNOSTIC IMAGING

TERM	DEFINITION	TERM	DEFINITION
1. **cerebral angiography** (se-RĒ-bral) (an-jē-OG-ra-fē)	process of recording (scan of) the blood vessels of the cerebrum (after an injection of contrast materials)	2. **CT myelography** (C-T) (mī-e-LOG-ra-fē)	process of recording (scan of) the spinal cord (after an injection of contrast materials into the subarachnoid space by lumbar puncture; size, shape, and position of the spinal cord and nerve roots are demonstrated)
		CT is the abbreviation for computed tomography.	

NEURODIAGNOSTIC PROCEDURES

TERM	DEFINITION	TERM	DEFINITION
3. electroencephalogram (EEG) (ē-*lek*-trō-en-SEF-a-lō-gram)	record of electrical activity of the brain	4. electroencephalograph (ē-*lek*-trō-en-SEF-a-lō-graf)	instrument used to record electrical activity of the brain
		5. electroencephalography (ē-*lek*-trō-en-*sef*-a-LOG-ra-fē)	process of recording the electrical activity of the brain

■ NOT Built from Word Parts

DIAGNOSTIC IMAGING

TERM	DEFINITION
1. positron emission tomography (PET) (POZ-i-tron) (ē-MISH-un) (tō-MOG-rah-fē)	nuclear medicine procedure creating computerized images of chemical changes, such as sugar metabolism in brain tissue. Radioactive materials called tracers are bound to molecules used in metabolism. Areas that are more active, such as cancers, will use more of these molecules, and the PET scan will detect higher activity there. PET is usually combined with CT imaging, which shows precise anatomic location of the abnormality.

NEURODIAGNOSTIC PROCEDURES

TERM	DEFINITION
2. evoked potential studies (EP studies) (i-VŌKD) (pō-TEN-shal) (STUD-ēz)	group of diagnostic tests that measure changes and responses in brain waves elicited by visual, auditory, or somatosensory stimuli
3. deep tendon reflexes (DTR) (dēp) (TEN-don) (RĒ-flek-suhs)	portion of the physical examination where gentle strikes at specific locations are performed to assess the possibility of potential neurologic abnormalities (also called **muscle stretch reflexes [MSR]**)

OTHER

TERM	DEFINITION
4. lumbar puncture (LP) (LUM-bar) (PUNK-chur)	diagnostic procedure performed by insertion of a needle into the subarachnoid space, usually between the third and fourth lumbar vertebrae; performed for many reasons, including the removal of cerebrospinal fluid (also called **spinal tap**)

EXERCISE 16 ■ Pronounce and Spell

Practice pronunciation and spelling on paper and online.

1. **Practice on Paper**
    a. **Pronounce:** Read the phonetic spelling and say aloud the terms listed in the previous table. Refer to Table 2.2 Pronunciation Key as needed.
    b. **Spell:** Have a study partner read the terms aloud. Write the spelling of the terms on a separate sheet of paper.

616 Chapter 15   Nervous System and Behavioral Health

2. **Practice Online** 🌐

   a. **Access** online learning resources. Go to evolve.elsevier.com > Evolve Resources > Student Resources.
   b. **Pronounce:** Select Audio Glossary > Chapter 15 > Exercise 16. Select a term to hear its pronunciation and repeat aloud.
   c. **Spell:** Select Activities > Chapter 15 > Spell Terms > Exercise 16. Select the audio icon and type the correct spelling of the term.

   ❏ Check the box when complete.

EXERCISE 17 ■ Diagnostic Terms Built from Word Parts

A   Analyze and Define

Analyze and define the following diagnostic terms.

1. electroencephalogram

2. electroencephalograph

3. electroencephalography

4. CT myelography

5. cerebral angiography

B   Label

Build terms pictured by writing word parts above definitions.

1. CT _____ / ____ / _____
       spinal cord   CV   process of recording

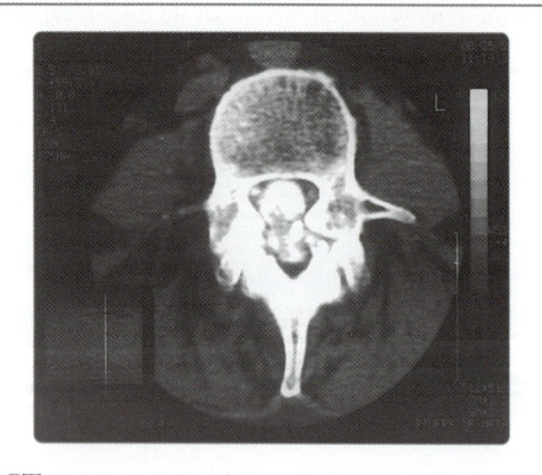

2. _____ / _____   _____ / ___ / _____ 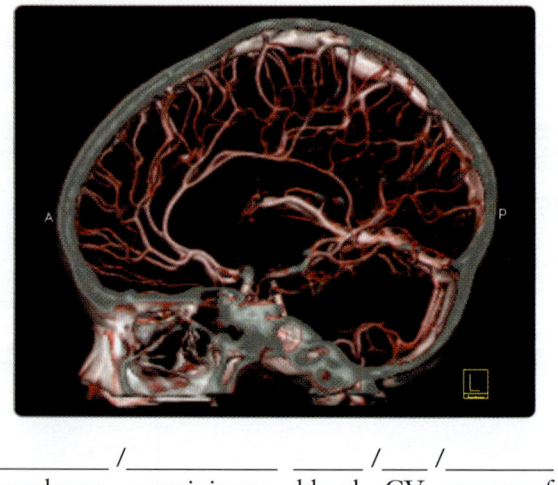
   cerebrum   pertaining to   blood   CV   process of
                              vessels   recording

Chapter 15   Nervous System and Behavioral Health   617

C Fill In

Build diagnostic terms that correspond to the following definitions by using the word parts you have learned.

1. record of electrical activity of the brain   _____ / __ / _____ / __ / ___
   WR   CV   WR   CV   S

2. instrument used to record electrical activity of the brain   _____ / __ / _____ / __ / ___
   WR   CV   WR   CV   S

3. process of recording the electrical activity of the brain   _____ / __ / _____ / __ / ___
   WR   CV   WR   CV   S

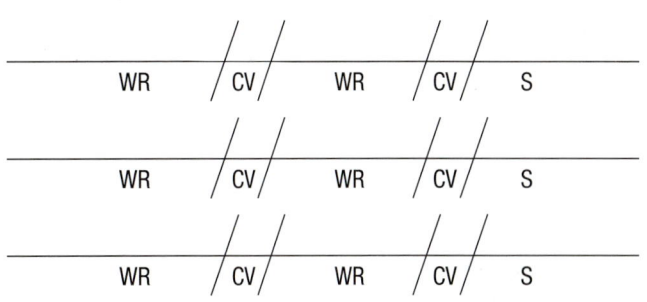

EXERCISE 18 ■ Diagnostic Terms NOT Built from Word Parts

A Match

Match the diagnostic terms in the first column with their correct definitions in the second column.

_____ 1. evoked potential studies
_____ 2. positron emission tomography
_____ 3. lumbar puncture
_____ 4. deep tendon reflexes

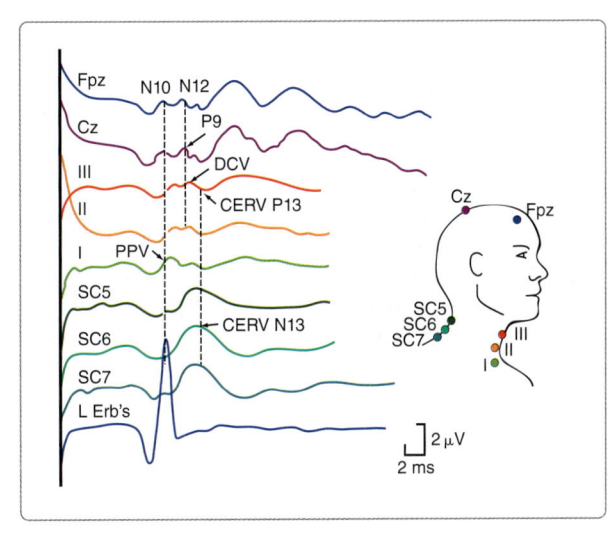

a. diagnostic procedure performed by insertion of a needle into the subarachnoid space, usually between the third and fourth lumbar vertebrae
b. portion of the physical examination where gentle strikes at specific locations are performed to assess the possibility of potential neurologic abnormalities
c. group of diagnostic tests that measure changes and responses in brain waves elicited by visual, auditory, or somatosensory stimuli
d. nuclear medicine procedure creating computerized images of chemical changes, such as sugar metabolism in brain tissue

B Label

Write the diagnostic terms pictured and defined.

1. _____
   group of diagnostic tests that measure changes and responses in brain waves elicited by visual, auditory, or somatosensory stimuli

618 Chapter 15 Nervous System and Behavioral Health

2. _____
diagnostic procedure performed by insertion of a needle into the subarachnoid space

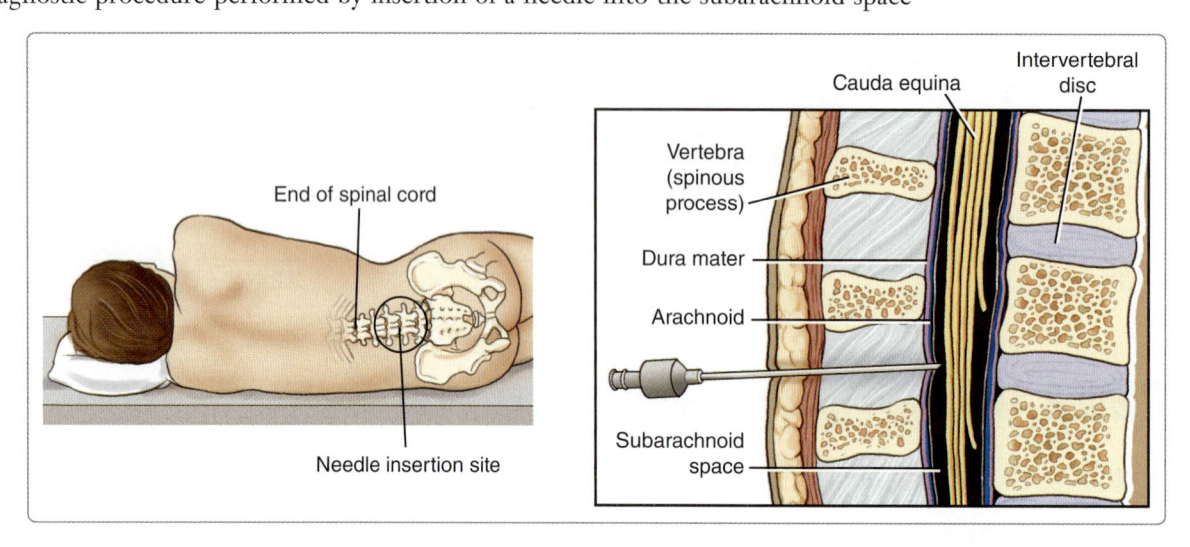

3. _____
portion of the physical examination where gentle strikes at specific locations are performed to assess the possibility of potential neurologic abnormalities

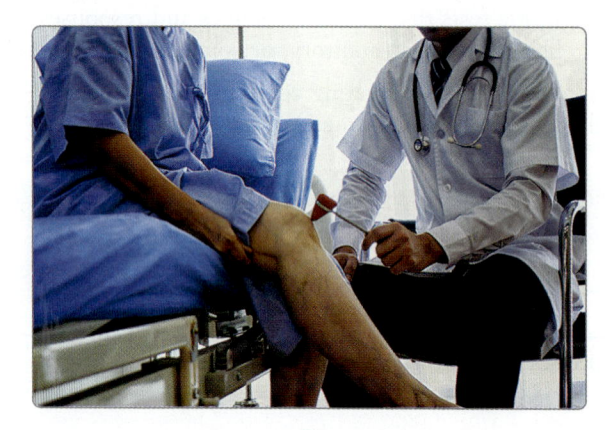

4. _____
nuclear medicine procedure creating computerized images of chemical changes; areas that are more active, such as cancers, will use more of these molecules and higher activity will be detected there

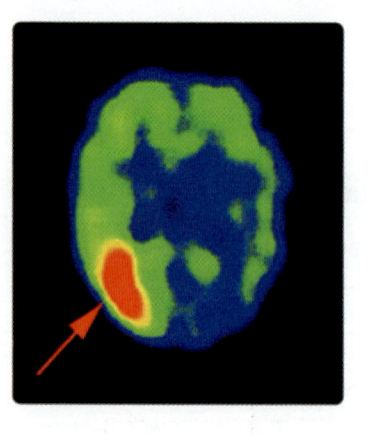

EXERCISE 19 ■ Review of Diagnostic Terms

Can you define, pronounce, and spell the following terms?

cerebral angiography
CT myelography
deep tendon reflexes (DTR)
electroencephalogram (EEG)
electroencephalograph
electroencephalography
evoked potential studies (EP studies)
lumbar puncture (LP)
positron emission tomography (PET)

Complementary Terms
BUILT FROM WORD PARTS

The following terms can be translated using definitions of word parts. Further explanation is provided within parentheses as needed.

SIGNS & SYMPTOMS

TERM	DEFINITION	TERM	DEFINITION
1. **anesthesia** (an-es-THĒ-zha)	without (loss of) feeling or sensation	7. **hemiplegia** (hem-ē-PLĒ-ja)	paralysis of half (right or left side of the body; stroke is the most common cause of hemiplegia)
2. **aphasia** (a-FĀ-zha)	condition of without speaking (loss or impairment of the ability to speak)	8. **hyperesthesia** (hī-per-es-THĒ-zha)	excessive sensitivity (to stimuli)
3. **cephalgia** (sef-AL-ja)	head pain (headache) (NOTE: the al is dropped from the combining form cephal/o)	9. **monoparesis** (mon-ō-pa-RĒ-sis)	slight paralysis of one (limb)
		10. **monoplegia** (mon-ō-PLĒ-ja)	paralysis of one (limb)
MIGRAINE, tension headache, and cluster headaches account for nearly 90% of all headaches.		11. **paresthesia** (par-es-THĒ-zha)	abnormal sensation (such as burning, prickling, or tingling sensation, often in the extremities; may be caused by nerve damage or peripheral neuropathy) (Note: the a is dropped from the prefix para.)
4. **dysesthesia** (dis-es-THĒ-zha)	painful sensation		
5. **dysphasia** (dis-FĀ-zha)	condition of difficulty speaking		
6. **hemiparesis** (hem-ē-pa-RĒ-sis)	slight paralysis of half (right or left side of the body)		
		12. **quadriplegia** (kwod-ri-PLĒ-ja)	paralysis of four (limbs)

MEDICAL SPECIALTIES

TERM	DEFINITION	TERM	DEFINITION
13. **neurologist** (nū-ROL-o-jist)	physician who studies and treats diseases of the nervous system	14. **neurology** (nū-ROL-o-jē)	study of nerves (branch of medicine dealing with diseases of the nervous system)

DESCRIPTIVE TERMS

TERM	DEFINITION	TERM	DEFINITION
15. **craniocerebral** (krā-nē-ō-su-RĒ-bral)	pertaining to the cranium and cerebrum	18. **postictal** (pōst-IK-tal)	(occurring) after a seizure or attack
16. **interictal** (in-ter-IK-tal)	(occurring) between seizures or attacks	19. **preictal** (prē-IK-tal)	(occurring) before a seizure or attack
17. **mental** (MEN-tel)	pertaining to the mind		

EXERCISE 20 ■ Pronounce and Spell

Practice pronunciation and spelling on paper and online.

1. Practice on Paper

   a. **Pronounce:** Read the phonetic spelling and say aloud the terms listed in the previous table. Refer to Table 2.2 Pronunciation Key as needed.
   b. **Spell:** Have a study partner read the terms aloud. Write the spelling of the terms on a separate sheet of paper.

620   Chapter 15   Nervous System and Behavioral Health

2. **Practice Online** 🌐
    a. **Access** online learning resources. Go to evolve.elsevier.com > Evolve Resources > Student Resources.
    b. **Pronounce:** Select Audio Glossary > Chapter 15 > Exercise 20. Select a term to hear its pronunciation and repeat aloud.
    c. **Spell:** Select Activities > Chapter 15 > Spell Terms > Exercise 20. Select the audio icon and type the correct spelling of the term.
❏ Check the box when complete.

EXERCISE 21 ■ Analyze and Define

Analyze and define the following complementary terms.

1. preictal

4. interictal

2. paresthesia

5. monoparesis

3. mental

6. dysesthesia

EXERCISE 22 ■ Build

A Label

Build terms pictured by writing word parts above definitions.

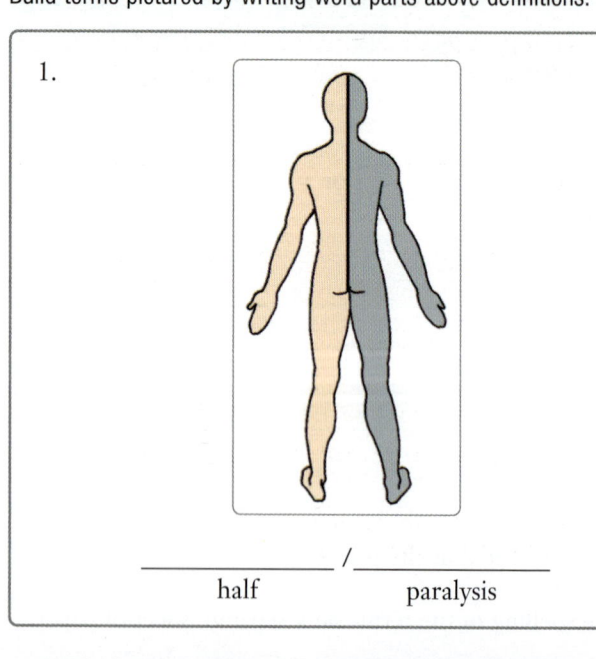

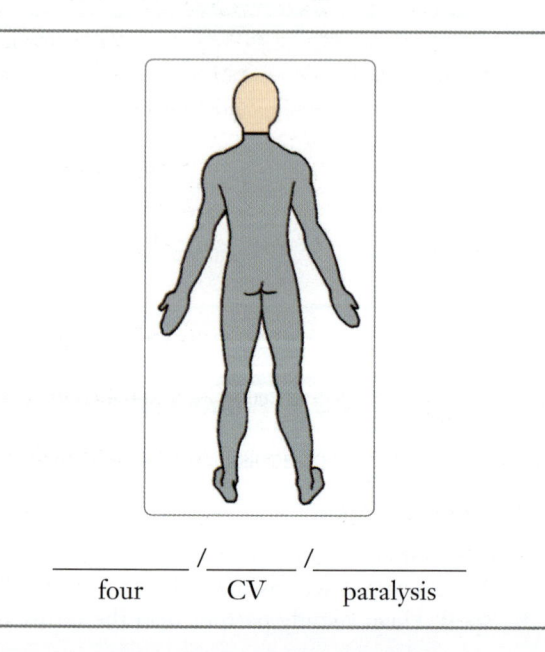

1.

_____ / _____
  half   paralysis

2.

_____ / _____ / _____
  four   CV   paralysis

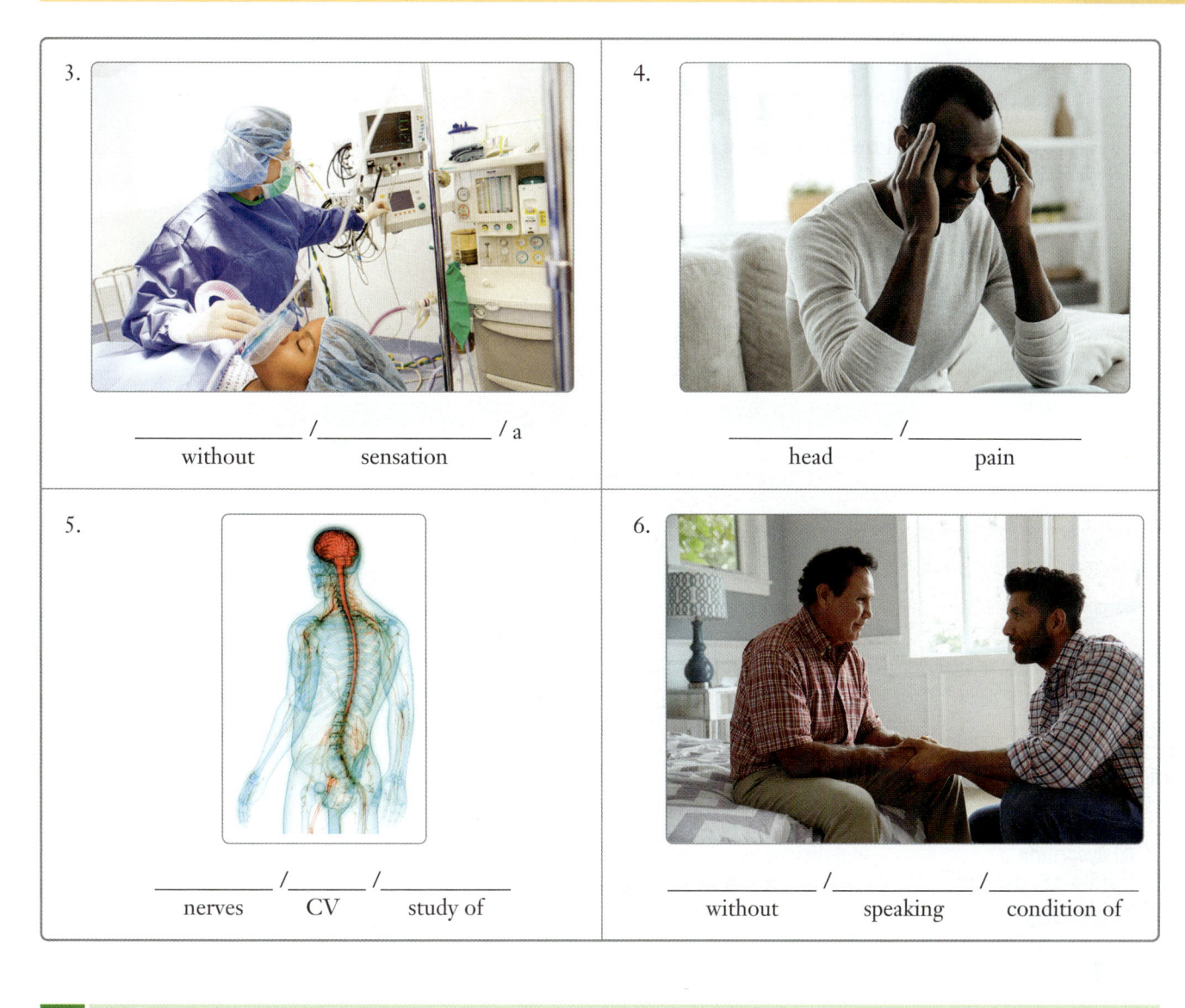

Chapter 15 Nervous System and Behavioral Health   621

3.

_____ / _____ / a
  without   sensation

4.

_____ / _____
  head   pain

5.

_____ / _____ / _____
 nerves   CV   study of

6.

_____ / _____ / _____
 without   speaking   condition of

B Fill In

Build complementary terms for the following definitions by using the word parts you have learned.

1. slight paralysis of half (right or left side of the body)

   _____ / _____
      P   S(WR)

2. condition of difficulty speaking

   _____ / _____ / _____
     P   WR   S

3. excessive sensitivity (to stimuli)

   _____ / _____ / _____
     P   WR   S

4. pertaining to the cranium and cerebrum

   _____ / ____ / _____ / _____
    WR   CV   WR   S

5. slight paralysis of one (limb)

   _____ / ____ / _____
    WR   CV   S

Chapter 15 Nervous System and Behavioral Health

6. (occurring) after a seizure or attack

    _____ / _____
    P   S(WR)

7. physician who studies and treats diseases of the nervous system

    _____ / ___ / _____
    WR   CV   S

Complementary Terms
NOT BUILT FROM WORD PARTS

Word parts may be present in the following terms; however, their full meanings cannot be translated using definitions of word parts alone.

SIGNS AND SYMPTOMS	
TERM	DEFINITION
1. ataxia (a-TAK-sē-a)	lack of muscle coordination
2. coma (KŌ-ma)	state of profound unconsciousness
3. concussion (kon-KUSH-un)	injury to the brain caused by minor or major head trauma; symptoms include vertigo, headache, and possible loss of consciousness

CONCUSSION is a common type of **traumatic brain injury (TBI)**, an umbrella term used to describe mild to severe damage to the brain sustained by a wide range of injuries. Falls, motor vehicle accidents, sports injuries, combat-related injuries or violence may all cause TBI.

4. convulsion (kun-VUL-zhun)	sudden, involuntary contraction of a group of muscles; may be present during a seizure
5. disorientation (dis-or-ē-en-TĀ-shun)	state of mental confusion as to time, place, or identity
6. dysarthria (dis-AR-thrē-a)	inability to use speech that is distinct and connected because of a loss of muscle control after damage to the peripheral or central nervous system
7. paraplegia (par-a-PLĒ-ja)	paralysis from the waist down caused by damage to the lower level of the spinal cord

PARAPLEGIA is composed of the Greek **para**, meaning **beside**, and **plegia**, meaning **paralysis**. It has been used since Hippocrates' time and at first meant paralysis of any limb or side of the body. Since the nineteenth century, it has been used to mean paralysis from the waist down.

8. seizure (SĒ-zher)	sudden, abnormal surge of electrical activity in the brain, resulting in involuntary body movements or behaviors
9. spasticity (spa-STIS-i-tē)	continued contraction of certain muscles due to damage of the brain or spinal cord controlling voluntary movement and causing tightness and stiffness that can interfere with normal movement, speech, and gait; associated with cerebral palsy, multiple sclerosis, and other neurologic disorders

SPASTICITY derives from the Greek word **spastikos** meaning *to pull*.

10. syncope (SINK-o-pē)	fainting or sudden loss of consciousness caused by lack of blood supply to the cerebrum
11. unconsciousness (un-KON-shus-nes)	state of being unaware of surroundings and incapable of responding to stimuli as a result of injury, shock, illness, or drugs

EQUIPMENT	
TERM	DEFINITION
12. shunt (shunt)	tube implanted in the body to redirect the flow of fluid

TABLE 15.2 Types of Cognitive Impairment

Mild cognitive impairment (MCI)	presence of significant memory changes when adjusted for age-related norms. The patient usually has little difficulty performing activities of daily living. This condition may be an early manifestation of Alzheimer disease or other forms of dementia.
Age-associated memory impairment	refers to a normal aging process in which the speed of mental processing and the performance of tasks decreases, and recent memory and learning are more difficult. Verbal intelligence is preserved, and this condition is not a forerunner of dementia.
Delirium	potentially reversible acute disturbance of consciousness with impairment of cognition. A number of conditions can cause delirium by interfering with brain metabolism. Drugs, alcohol, systemic infections, head trauma, hypoglycemia, and electrolyte disturbances are common examples.
Pseudodementia	behavioral disorder resembling dementia but is not caused by brain tissue abnormalities. This can be found in mental illness, such as major depression, and can be reversible with treatment.

DESCRIPTIVE TERMS

TERM	DEFINITION
13. **cognitive** (COG-ni-tiv)	pertaining to the mental processes of comprehension, judgment, memory, and reason (Table 15.2)
14. **conscious** (KON-shus)	awake, alert, aware of one's surroundings
15. **gait** (gāt)	manner or style of walking
16. **incoherent** (in-kō-HĒR-ent)	unable to express one's thoughts or ideas in an orderly, intelligible manner

EXERCISE 23 ■ Pronounce and Spell

Practice pronunciation and spelling on paper and online.

1. **Practice on Paper**
   a. **Pronounce:** Read the phonetic spelling and say aloud the terms listed in the previous table. Refer to Table 2.2 Pronunciation Key as needed.
   b. **Spell:** Have a study partner read the terms aloud. Write the spelling of the terms on a separate sheet of paper.

2. **Practice Online**
   a. **Access** online learning resources. Go to evolve.elsevier.com > Evolve Resources > Student Resources.
   b. **Pronounce:** Select Audio Glossary > Chapter 15 > Exercise 23. Select a term to hear its pronunciation and repeat aloud.
   c. **Spell:** Select Activities > Chapter 15 > Spell Terms > Exercise 23. Select the audio icon and type the correct spelling of the term.

❏ Check the box when complete.

624　Chapter 15　Nervous System and Behavioral Health

EXERCISE 24 ■ Fill In

A Label

Write the medical terms pictured and defined.

1. _____
paralysis from the waist down caused by damage to the lower level of the spinal cord

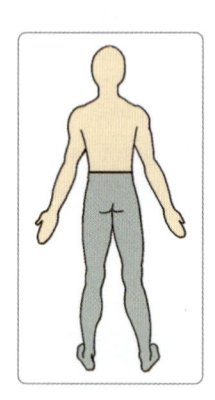

2. _____
injury to the brain caused by minor or major head trauma; symptoms include vertigo, headache, and possible loss of consciousness

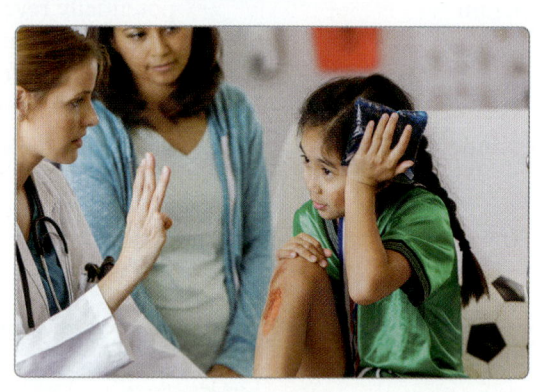

3. _____
fainting or sudden loss of consciousness caused by lack of blood supply to the cerebrum

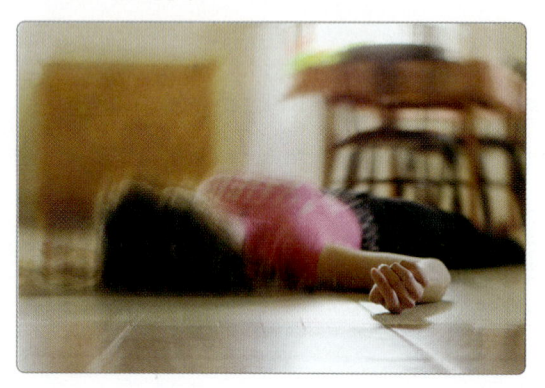

4. _____
lack of muscle coordination

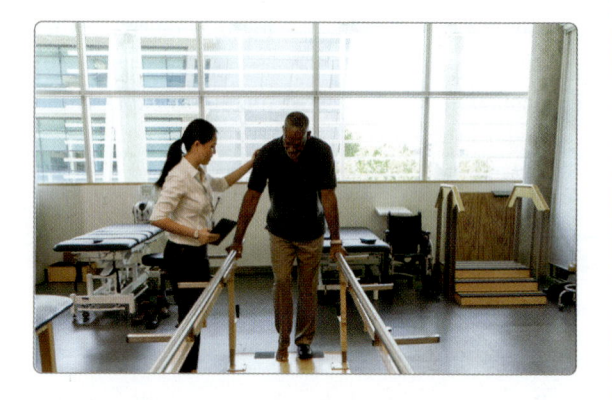

5. _____
inability to use speech that is distinct and connected because of a loss of muscle control after damage to the peripheral or central nervous system

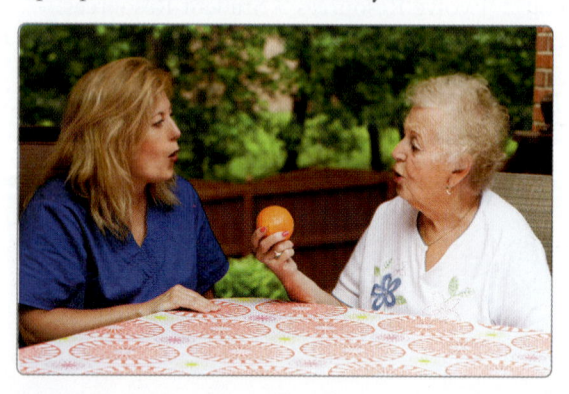

6. _____
state of profound unconsciousness

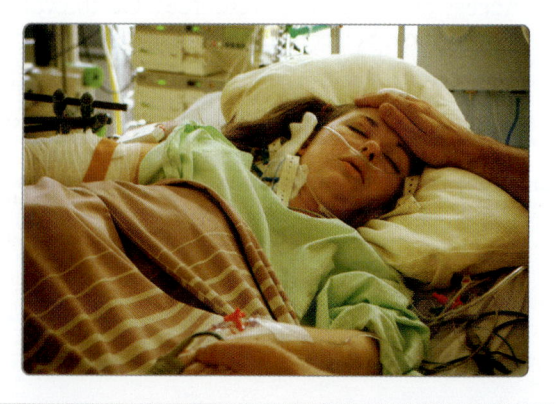

B Identify

Write the term for each of the following definitions.

1. Continued contraction of certain muscles due to damage of the brain or spinal cord is called _____.
2. The state of being unaware of surroundings and incapable of responding to stimuli as a result of injury, shock, illness, or drugs is referred to as _____.
3. _____ describes a person who is awake, alert, aware of one's surroundings.
4. The sudden, abnormal surge of electrical activity in the brain is called _____.
5. A _____ is the sudden, involuntary contraction of a group of muscles.
6. A tube implanted in the body to redirect the flow of fluid is a _____.
7. _____ describes a manner or style of walking.
8. The inability to express one's thoughts or ideas in an orderly, intelligible manner is called _____.
9. _____ is a state of mental confusion as to time, place, or identity.
10. _____ is the term that means pertaining to the mental processes of comprehension, judgment, memory, and reason.

EXERCISE 25 ■ Match

A. Match the definitions in the first column with the correct terms in the second column.

____ 1. state of profound unconsciousness	a.	shunt
____ 2. fainting or sudden loss of consciousness	b.	ataxia
____ 3. paralysis from the waist down caused by damage to the lower level of the spinal cord	c.	gait
	d.	coma
____ 4. lack of muscle coordination	e.	seizure
____ 5. tube implanted in the body to redirect the flow of fluid	f.	syncope
____ 6. manner or style of walking	g.	dysarthria
____ 7. inability to use speech that is distinctive and connected because of a loss of muscle control	h.	paraplegia
____ 8. sudden, abnormal surge of electrical activity in the brain		

B. Match the definitions in the first column with the correct terms in the second column.

____ 1. unable to express one's thoughts or ideas in an orderly, intelligible manner	a.	spasticity
____ 2. awake, alert, aware of one's surroundings	b.	unconsciousness
____ 3. continued contraction of certain muscles due to damage of the brain or spinal cord controlling voluntary movement	c.	cognitive
	d.	disorientation
____ 4. state of being unaware of surroundings and incapable of responding to stimuli as a result of injury, shock, illness, or drugs	e.	convulsion
	f.	incoherent
____ 5. pertaining to the mental processes of comprehension, judgment, memory, and reason	g.	concussion
	h.	conscious
____ 6. injury to the brain caused by head trauma		
____ 7. state of mental confusion as to time, place, or identity		
____ 8. sudden, involuntary contraction of a group of muscles		

> **EXERCISE 26 ■ Review of Complementary Terms**

Can you define, pronounce, and spell the following terms?

anesthesia	craniocerebral	incoherent	postictal
aphasia	disorientation	interictal	preictal
ataxia	dysarthria	mental	quadriplegia
cephalgia	dysesthesia	monoparesis	seizure
cognitive	dysphasia	monoplegia	shunt
coma	gait	neurologist	spasticity
concussion	hemiparesis	neurology	syncope
conscious	hemiplegia	paraplegia	unconsciousness
convulsion	hyperesthesia	paresthesia	

Behavioral Health Terms

Behavioral health is a wide-reaching field that includes mental health, interpersonal relationships, lifestyle, substance abuse, and other external forces. Mental health is part of behavioral health, but it is mainly focused on the biologic component of a person's state of mind. Behavioral health and physical health are closely connected.

BUILT FROM WORD PARTS

The following terms can be translated using definitions of word parts. Further explanation is provided within parentheses as needed.

TERM	DEFINITION	TERM	DEFINITION
1. **psychiatrist** (sī-KĪ-a-trist)	physician who studies and treats disorders of the mind (Psychiatrists have additional training and experience in prevention, diagnosis, and treatment of mental, emotional, and behavioral disorders. Psychiatrists often prescribe medications for patients with these disorders.)	5. **psychology** (sī-KOL-o-jē)	study of the mind (a profession that involves dealing with the mind and mental processes in relation to human behavior)
		6. **psychopathy** (sī-KOP-a-thē)	(any) disease of the mind
		7. **psychosis** (*pl.* **psychoses**) (sī-KO-sis), (sī-KO-sēz)	abnormal condition of the mind (major mental disorder characterized by extreme derangement, often with delusions and hallucinations)
2. **psychiatry** (sī-KĪ-a-trē)	specialty of the mind (branch of medicine that deals with the treatment of mental disorders)		
		8. **psychosomatic** (sī-kō-sō-MAT-ik)	pertaining to the mind and body (interrelations of)
3. **psychogenic** (sī-*kō*-JEN-ik)	originating in the mind		
4. **psychologist** (sī-KOL-o-jist)	specialist of the mind (Clinical psychologists have graduate training in clinical psychology, administer psychological tests, and treat individuals with disturbances of mental, emotional, and behavioral disorders by counseling therapy.)		

Chapter 15 Nervous System and Behavioral Health 627

EXERCISE 27 ■ Pronounce and Spell

Practice pronunciation and spelling on paper and online.

1. **Practice on Paper**
   a. **Pronounce:** Read the phonetic spelling and say aloud the terms listed in the previous table. Refer to Table 2.2 Pronunciation Key as needed.
   b. **Spell:** Have a study partner read the terms aloud. Write the spelling of the terms on a separate sheet of paper.

2. **Practice Online**
   a. **Access** online learning resources. Go to evolve.elsevier.com > Evolve Resources > Student Resources.
   b. **Pronounce:** Select Audio Glossary > Chapter 15 > Exercise 27. Select a term to hear its pronunciation and repeat aloud.
   c. **Spell:** Select Activities > Chapter 15 > Spell Terms > Exercise 27. Select the audio icon and type the correct spelling of the term.

❑ Check the box when complete.

EXERCISE 28 ■ Analyze and Define

Analyze and define the following terms.

1. psychosomatic

2. psychopathy

3. psychology

4. psychiatry

5. psychologist

6. psychogenic

7. psychiatrist

8. psychosis

EXERCISE 29 ■ Build

Build behavioral health terms for the following definitions by using the word parts you have learned.

1. specialty of the mind (branch of medicine that deals with the treatment of mental disorders) _____ / _____
   WR / S

2. abnormal condition of the mind _____ / _____
   WR / S

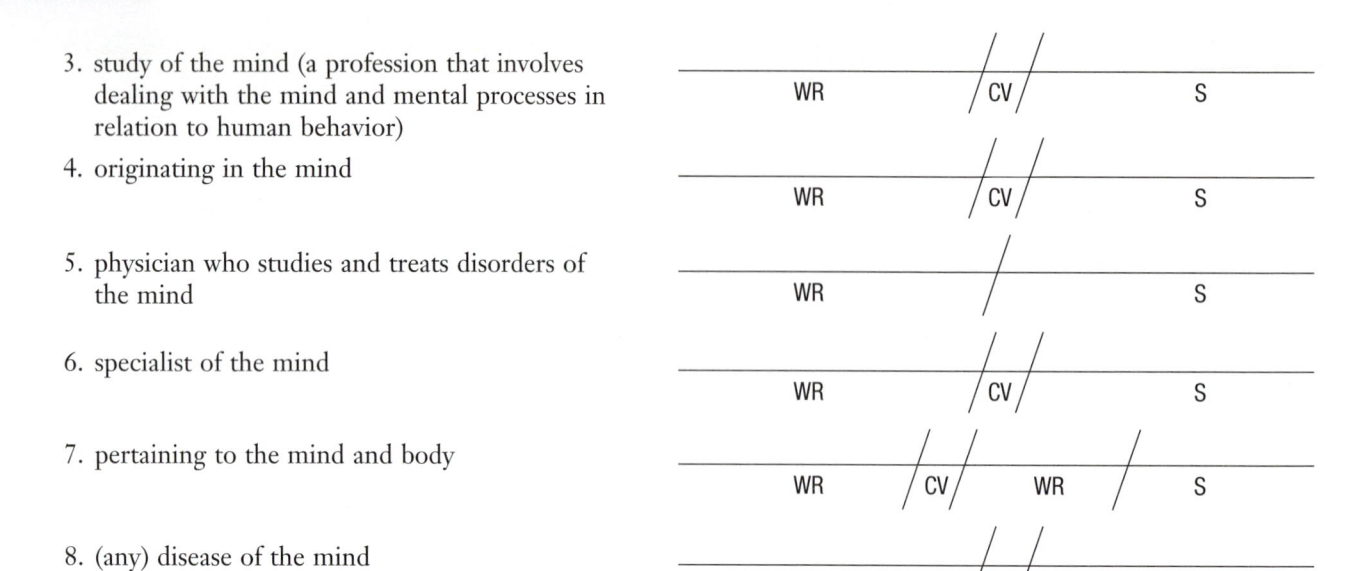

3. study of the mind (a profession that involves dealing with the mind and mental processes in relation to human behavior)

_____ / _____ / _____
WR   CV   S

4. originating in the mind

_____ / _____ / _____
WR   CV   S

5. physician who studies and treats disorders of the mind

_____ / _____
WR   S

6. specialist of the mind

_____ / _____ / _____
WR   CV   S

7. pertaining to the mind and body

_____ / _____ / _____ / _____
WR   CV   WR   S

8. (any) disease of the mind

_____ / _____ / _____
WR   CV   S

Behavioral Health Terms
NOT BUILT FROM WORD PARTS

Word parts may be present in the following terms; however, their full meanings cannot be translated using definitions of word parts alone.

TERM	DEFINITION
1. anorexia nervosa (an-ō-REK-sē-a) (ner-VŌ-sa)	eating disorder characterized by a disturbed perception of body image, resulting in failure to maintain body weight, intensive fear of gaining weight, pronounced desire for thinness, and, in females, amenorrhea
2. anxiety disorder (ang-ZĪ-e-tē) (dis-OR-der)	disorder characterized by feelings of apprehension, tension, or uneasiness arising typically from the anticipation of unreal or imagined danger
3. attention deficit/hyperactivity disorder (ADHD) (a-TEN-shun) (DEF-i-sit) (hī-per-ak-TIV-i-tē) (dis-OR-der)	disorder of learning and behavioral problems characterized by marked inattention, distractibility, impulsiveness, and hyperactivity
4. autism (AW-tizm)	spectrum of mental disorders, the features of which include onset during infancy or childhood, preoccupation with subjective mental activity, inability to interact socially, and impaired communication (also referred to as **autism spectrum disorders [ASD]**)
5. bipolar disorder (bī-PŌ-lar) (dis-OR-der)	major psychological disorder typified by a disturbance in mood. The disorder is manifested by manic (elevated or irritated mood, excessive energy, impulsiveness) and depressive episodes that may alternate; or elements of both may occur simultaneously.
6. bulimia nervosa (bū-LĒ-mē-a) (ner-VŌ-sa)	eating disorder characterized by uncontrolled binge eating followed by purging (induced vomiting)
7. major depression (MĀ-jor) (dē-PRESH-un)	mood disturbance characterized by feelings of sadness, despair, discouragement, hopelessness, lack of joy, altered sleep patterns, and difficulty with decision making and daily function. Depression ranges from normal feelings of sadness (resulting from and proportional to personal loss or tragedy), through dysthymia (chronic depressive neurosis), to major depression. (also referred to as **clinical depression, mood disorder**)

Chapter 15 Nervous System and Behavioral Health

TERM	DEFINITION
8. obsessive-compulsive disorder (OCD) (ob-SES-iv) (kom-PUL-siv) (dis-OR-der)	disorder characterized by intrusive, unwanted thoughts that result in the tendency to perform repetitive acts or rituals (compulsions), usually as a means of releasing tension or anxiety
9. panic attack (PAN-ik) (a-TAK)	episode of sudden onset of acute anxiety, occurring unpredictably, with feelings of acute apprehension, dyspnea, dizziness, sweating, chest pain, depersonalization, paresthesia, and fear of dying
10. phobia (FŌ-bē-a)	marked and persistent fear that is excessive or unreasonable cued by the presence or anticipation of a specific situation or object (such as claustrophobia, the abnormal fear of being in enclosed spaces)
11. pica (PĪ-ka)	compulsive eating of nonnutritive substances such as clay or ice. This condition may be a result of an iron deficiency. When iron deficiency is the cause of pica, the condition will disappear in 1 or 2 weeks when treated with iron therapy.
12. posttraumatic stress disorder (PTSD) (*pōst*-tra-MAT-ik) (stres) (dis-OR-der)	significant behavioral health disorder in which some people exposed to a traumatic event go on to develop a series of symptoms related to it. These include mentally reexperiencing the event, increased autonomic arousal (the fight-flight-freeze response), avoidance of thoughts or activities that are reminders of the trauma, social withdrawal, and difficulty making emotional contacts with family and friends. NOTE: *posttraumatic* also appears with a hyphen, as **post-traumatic**, and with a space, as **post traumatic**
13. schizophrenia (*skit*-sō-FRĒ-nē-a)	any one of a large group of psychotic disorders characterized by gross distortions of reality, disturbance of language and communication, withdrawal from social interaction, and the disorganization and fragmentation of thought, perception, and emotional reaction
14. somatoform disorders (sō-MAT-ō-form) (dis-OR-derz)	disorders characterized by physical symptoms for which no known physical cause exists

Refer to **Appendix E** for pharmacology terms related to the nervous system and behavioral health.

EXERCISE 30 ■ Pronounce and Spell

Practice pronunciation and spelling on paper and online.

1. **Practice on Paper**
   a. **Pronounce:** Read the phonetic spelling and say aloud the terms listed in the previous table. Refer to Table 2.2 Pronunciation Key as needed.
   b. **Spell:** Have a study partner read the terms aloud. Write the spelling of the terms on a separate sheet of paper.

2. **Practice Online**
   a. **Access** online learning resources. Go to evolve.elsevier.com > Evolve Resources > Student Resources.
   b. **Pronounce:** Select Audio Glossary > Chapter 15 > Exercise 30. Select a term to hear its pronunciation and repeat aloud.
   c. **Spell:** Select Activities > Chapter 15 > Spell Terms > Exercise 30. Select the audio icon and type the correct spelling of the term.

❏ Check the box when complete.

Chapter 15 Nervous System and Behavioral Health

EXERCISE 31 ■ Match

A. Match the definitions in the first column with the correct terms in the second column.

_____ 1. manifested by manic and depressive episodes
_____ 2. episode of acute anxiety; occurs unpredictably
_____ 3. characterized by feelings of apprehension and tension
_____ 4. disorder of learning and behavioral problems with distractibility
_____ 5. mood disturbance characterized by feelings of sadness, despair, and discouragement
_____ 6. marked and persistent fear that is excessive or unreasonable
_____ 7. binge eating followed by purging

a. panic attack
b. anxiety disorder
c. major depression
d. phobia
e. bulimia nervosa
f. attention deficit/hyperactivity disorder
g. bipolar disorder

B. Match the definitions in the first column with the correct terms in the second column.

_____ 1. physical symptoms for which no known physical cause exists
_____ 2. eating of nonnutritive substances, such as ice
_____ 3. disturbed perception of body image with failure to maintain body weight
_____ 4. characterized by gross distortions of reality and disturbance of language and communication
_____ 5. preoccupation with subjective mental activity, inability to interact socially, and impaired communication
_____ 6. mentally reexperiencing a traumatic event; avoidance of thoughts or activities that are reminders of the trauma
_____ 7. intrusive unwanted thoughts that result in rituals and/or repetitive acts

a. schizophrenia
b. pica
c. autism
d. posttraumatic stress disorder
e. obsessive-compulsive disorder
f. anorexia nervosa
g. somatoform disorders

EXERCISE 32 ■ Review of Behavioral Health Terms

Can you define, pronounce, and spell the following terms?

anorexia nervosa
anxiety disorder
attention deficit/hyperactivity disorder (ADHD)
autism
bipolar disorder
bulimia nervosa
major depression
obsessive-compulsive disorder (OCD)
panic attack
phobia
pica
posttraumatic stress disorder (PTSD)
psychiatrist
psychiatry
psychogenic
psychologist
psychology
psychopathy
psychosis (pl. psychoses)
psychosomatic
schizophrenia
somatoform disorders

Abbreviations

DISEASES AND DISORDERS

ABBREVIATION	TERM	ABBREVIATION	TERM
AD	Alzheimer disease	OCD	obsessive-compulsive disorder
ADHD	attention deficit/hyperactivity disorder	PD	Parkinson disease
ALS	amyotrophic lateral sclerosis	polio	poliomyelitis; spoken as a whole word (PŌL-ē-ō)
ASD	autism spectrum disorders	PTSD	posttraumatic stress disorder
CP	cerebral palsy	SAH	subarachnoid hemorrhage
CTE	chronic traumatic encephalopathy	TBI	traumatic brain injury
CVA	cerebrovascular accident	TIA	transient ischemic attack
MS	multiple sclerosis		

Chapter 15 Nervous System and Behavioral Health

DIAGNOSTIC

ABBREVIATION	TERM	ABBREVIATION	TERM
DTR	deep tendon reflexes	LP	lumbar puncture
EEG	electroencephalogram	PET	positron emission tomography; spoken as a whole word (pet)
EP studies	evoked potential studies		

DESCRIPTIVE

ABBREVIATION	TERM	ABBREVIATION	TERM
CNS	central nervous system	PNS	peripheral nervous system
CSF	cerebrospinal fluid		

Refer to **Appendix D** for a complete list of abbreviations.

EXERCISE 33 ■ Fill In

Write the terms abbreviated.

1. **DTR** _____ _____ _____ provide an objective sign of neurologic abnormality. **Polio** _____ frequently affects the spinal cord and can cause a decrease in these muscle stretch reflexes.

2. Diagnostic tests used to diagnose patients with diseases of the nervous system include **EEG** _____ _____, CT, MR, **PET** _____ _____ _____, **EP studies** _____ _____ _____, and **LP** _____ _____.

3. Diseases that affect the nervous system are **AD** _____ _____, **ALS** _____ _____ _____, **CP** _____ _____, **MS** _____ _____, and **PD** _____ _____.

4. Stroke is the disruption of normal blood supply to the brain; it often occurs suddenly. Because of this, Hippocrates used the term *apoplexy*, which literally means *struck down*, to describe the condition. The term *stroke* grew out of the term *apoplexy*. The term *brain attack* is used to signify that a stroke is in progress and an emergency situation exists. **CVA** _____ _____ is also used to describe a stroke. An ischemic stroke, which is caused by a thrombosis or embolus, is frequently preceded by a **TIA** _____ _____. A ruptured cerebral aneurysm is the most common cause of **SAH** _____ _____, a type of hemorrhagic stroke.

5. The examination of **CSF** _____ _____ may assist in the diagnosis of cerebral hemorrhage, meningitis, encephalitis, and other diseases.

6. Two common psychiatric disorders are **OCD** _____-_____ _____, and **ADHD** _____ _____ / _____ _____ _____. **ASD** _____ _____ _____ are usually diagnosed during childhood.

7. The nervous system may be divided into the **CNS** _____ _____ _____ and the **PNS** _____ _____ _____.

8. Psychiatric disorders related to trauma include **PTSD** _____ _____ _____ and **CTE** _____ _____ _____.

9. A concussion is a mild form of **TBI** _____ _____ _____. More severe TBI can lead to serious physical and psychological symptoms, coma, and death.

Chapter 15 Nervous System and Behavioral Health

PRACTICAL APPLICATION

EXERCISE 34 ■ Case Study: Translate Between Everyday Language and Medical Language

CASE STUDY: Koji Kaneshiro

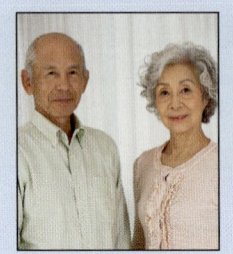

Kazuno Kaneshiro is worried about her husband, Koji. He was eating breakfast with her when he suddenly stopped speaking and dropped his spoon onto the table. "He never does that!" she thought. He seemed to be unable to speak. Also, his right arm was hanging limply by his side. She noticed that the left side of his face was also droopy. She had seen a billboard about strokes and was afraid he might be having one. She remembered the billboard saying that every minute counts, so she called 911 immediately.

Now that you have worked through Chapter 15, consider the medical terms that might be used to describe Mr. Kaneshiro's experience. See the Chapter at a Glance Section at the end of the chapter for a list of terms that might apply.

A. Underline phrases in the case study that could be substituted with medical terms.

B. Write the medical term and its definition for three of the phrases you underlined.

MEDICAL TERM	DEFINITION
1. _____	_____
2. _____	_____
3. _____	_____

DOCUMENTATION: Excerpt from Emergency Department Visit

Mr. Kaneshiro was evaluated in the local emergency department; an excerpt from the medical record is documented below.

This 78-year-old male presented to the emergency department after the sudden onset of aphasia, right hemiplegia, and facial droop. Physical exam reveals an elderly male who is alert and oriented ×3, but shows evidence of dysphasia. Focused neurologic exam is significant for right-sided facial drooping with paralysis of the seventh cranial nerve. The rest of the cranial nerves appear normal. Motor exam reveals hemiparesis on the right. Paresthesias are also present on the right. Cerebellar exam is normal, though difficult to test on the right. Gait is not assessed due to the patient's weakness. A CT of the head without contrast indicates no evidence of cerebral or subarachnoid hemorrhage. The patient appears to be experiencing a CVA. We will start him on the stroke protocol.

C. Underline medical terms presented in Chapter 15 used in the previous excerpt from Mr. Kaneshiro's medical record. See the Chapter at a Glance Section at the end of the chapter for a complete list.

D. Select and define three of the medical terms you underlined. To check your answers, go to Appendix A.

MEDICAL TERM	DEFINITION
1. _____	_____
2. _____	_____
3. _____	_____

Chapter 15 Nervous System and Behavioral Health

EXERCISE 35 — Interact with Medical Documents

A

Read the report and complete it by writing medical terms on answer lines within the document. Definitions of terms to be written appear after the document.

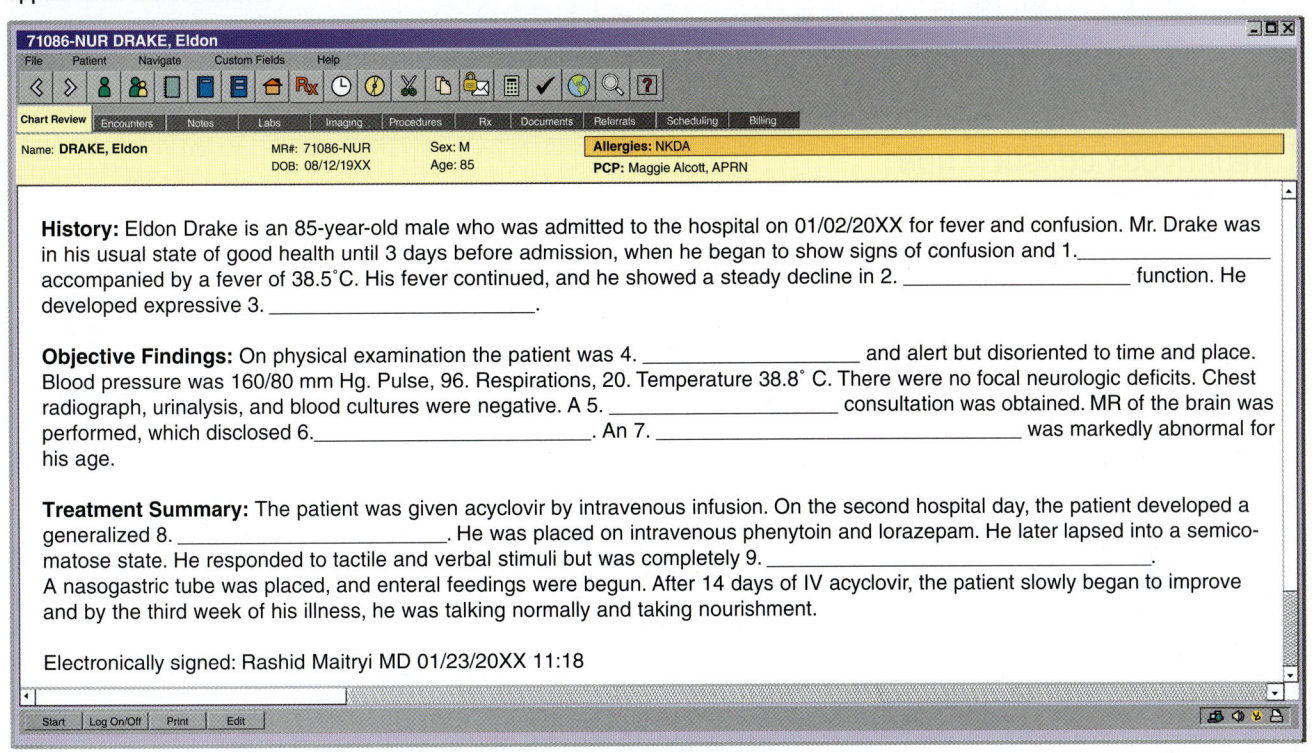

71086-NUR DRAKE, Eldon

Name: DRAKE, Eldon   MR#: 71086-NUR   Sex: M   Allergies: NKDA
                     DOB: 08/12/19XX   Age: 85   PCP: Maggie Alcott, APRN

History: Eldon Drake is an 85-year-old male who was admitted to the hospital on 01/02/20XX for fever and confusion. Mr. Drake was in his usual state of good health until 3 days before admission, when he began to show signs of confusion and 1._____ accompanied by a fever of 38.5°C. His fever continued, and he showed a steady decline in 2._____ function. He developed expressive 3._____.

Objective Findings: On physical examination the patient was 4._____ and alert but disoriented to time and place. Blood pressure was 160/80 mm Hg. Pulse, 96. Respirations, 20. Temperature 38.8° C. There were no focal neurologic deficits. Chest radiograph, urinalysis, and blood cultures were negative. A 5._____ consultation was obtained. MR of the brain was performed, which disclosed 6._____. An 7._____ was markedly abnormal for his age.

Treatment Summary: The patient was given acyclovir by intravenous infusion. On the second hospital day, the patient developed a generalized 8._____. He was placed on intravenous phenytoin and lorazepam. He later lapsed into a semicomatose state. He responded to tactile and verbal stimuli but was completely 9._____.
A nasogastric tube was placed, and enteral feedings were begun. After 14 days of IV acyclovir, the patient slowly began to improve and by the third week of his illness, he was talking normally and taking nourishment.

Electronically signed: Rashid Maitryi MD 01/23/20XX 11:18

Definitions of Medical Terms to Complete the Document
Write the medical terms defined on corresponding answer lines in the document.

1. a state of mental confusion as to time, place, or identity
2. pertaining to the mental processes of comprehension, judgment, memory, and reason
3. loss of the ability to speak
4. awake, alert, and aware of one's surroundings
5. study of nerves (branch of medicine dealing with diseases of the nervous system)
6. inflammation of the brain
7. record of electrical impulses of the brain
8. sudden, abnormal surge of electrical activity in the brain
9. unable to express one's thoughts or ideas in an orderly, intelligible manner

Chapter 15 Nervous System and Behavioral Health

B

Read the medical report and answer the questions below it.

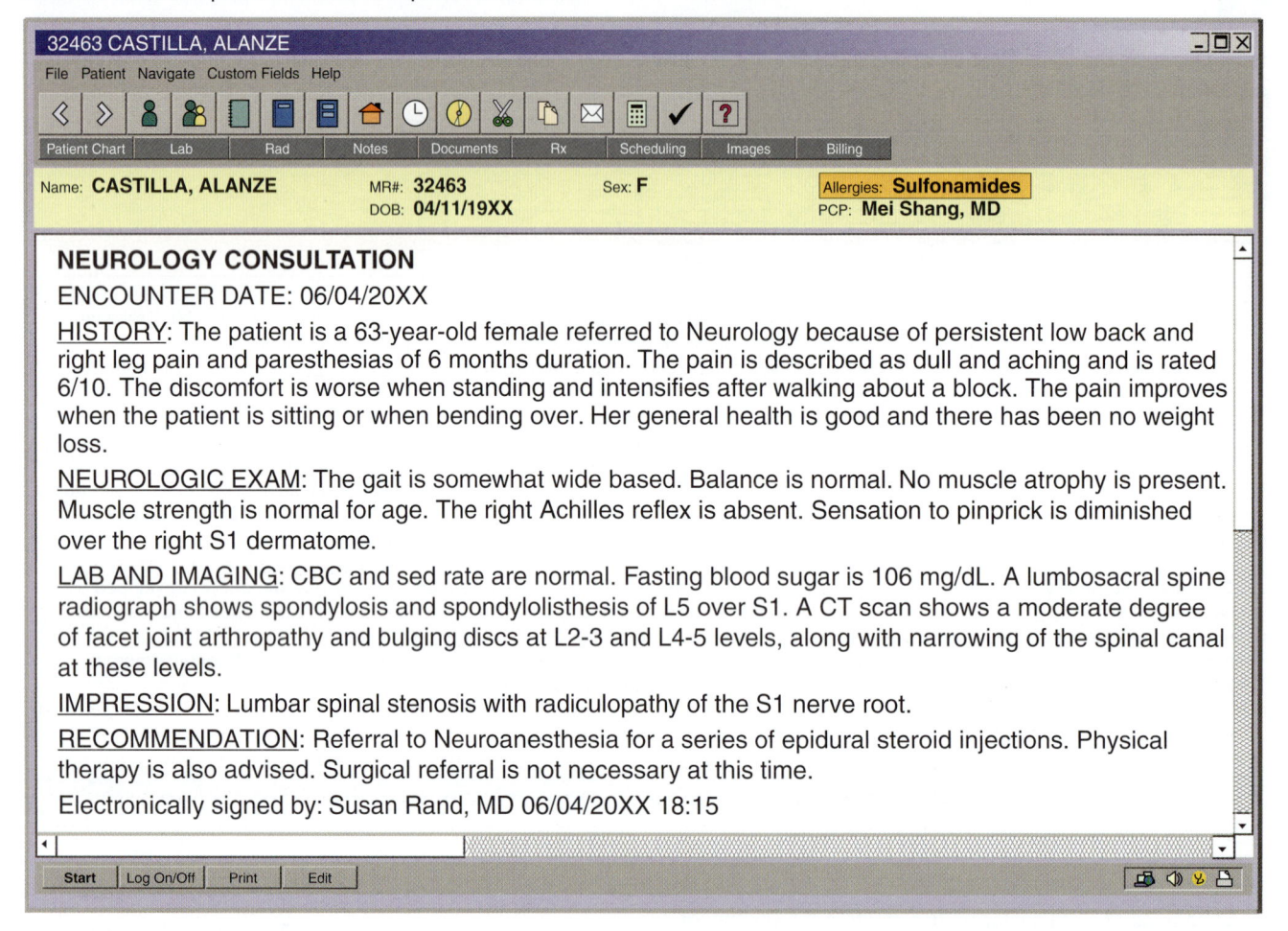

32463 CASTILLA, ALANZE

File Patient Navigate Custom Fields Help

| Patient Chart | Lab | Rad | Notes | Documents | Rx | Scheduling | Images | Billing |

Name: **CASTILLA, ALANZE** MR#: **32463** Sex: **F** Allergies: **Sulfonamides**
DOB: **04/11/19XX** PCP: **Mei Shang, MD**

NEUROLOGY CONSULTATION

ENCOUNTER DATE: 06/04/20XX

<u>HISTORY</u>: The patient is a 63-year-old female referred to Neurology because of persistent low back and right leg pain and paresthesias of 6 months duration. The pain is described as dull and aching and is rated 6/10. The discomfort is worse when standing and intensifies after walking about a block. The pain improves when the patient is sitting or when bending over. Her general health is good and there has been no weight loss.

<u>NEUROLOGIC EXAM</u>: The gait is somewhat wide based. Balance is normal. No muscle atrophy is present. Muscle strength is normal for age. The right Achilles reflex is absent. Sensation to pinprick is diminished over the right S1 dermatome.

<u>LAB AND IMAGING</u>: CBC and sed rate are normal. Fasting blood sugar is 106 mg/dL. A lumbosacral spine radiograph shows spondylosis and spondylolisthesis of L5 over S1. A CT scan shows a moderate degree of facet joint arthropathy and bulging discs at L2-3 and L4-5 levels, along with narrowing of the spinal canal at these levels.

<u>IMPRESSION</u>: Lumbar spinal stenosis with radiculopathy of the S1 nerve root.

<u>RECOMMENDATION</u>: Referral to Neuroanesthesia for a series of epidural steroid injections. Physical therapy is also advised. Surgical referral is not necessary at this time.

Electronically signed by: Susan Rand, MD 06/04/20XX 18:15

Start Log On/Off Print Edit

Use the medical report above to answer the questions.

1. Spinal stenosis causes compression of nerve roots demonstrated by which of the following symptoms for the patient?
   a. total paralysis
   b. abnormal sensation of burning, prickling, or tingling
   c. paralysis of one limb
   d. slight paralysis

2. The patient's diagnosis is spinal stenosis with:
   a. disease of the nerve roots
   b. disease of peripheral nerves
   c. disease affecting a single nerve
   d. disease of many nerves

Chapter 15 Nervous System and Behavioral Health   635

EXERCISE 36 ■ Use Medical Language in Online Electronic Health Records

Select the correct medical terms to complete three medical records in one patient's electronic file.

🌐 Access online resources at evolve.elsevier.com > Evolve Resources > Student Resources > Activities > Chapter 15 > Electronic Health Records

Topic: Migraine
Record 1, Encounters: Office Visit Report
Record 2, Report: Emergency Department Report
Record 3, Imaging: Diagnostic Imaging Report

❑ Check the box when complete.

EXERCISE 37 ■ Use Medical Terms in Clinical Statements

For each phrase printed in bold, circle the medical term or abbreviation defined. Answers are listed in Appendix A. For pronunciation practice read the answers aloud.

1. **Mood disturbance characterized by feelings of sadness, despair, discouragement, and hopelessness** (anxiety disorder, major depression, psychosis) is a diagnosis frequently encountered in the field of **study of the mind** (psychology, neurology, otolaryngology). It may be accompanied by **disorder characterized by feelings of apprehension, tension, or uneasiness** (bipolar disorder, dementia, anxiety disorder). Fortunately, there are medications that may be prescribed by a **physician with additional training and experience in the diagnosis, prevention, and treatment of mental disorders who can prescribe medications and direct therapy** (psychiatrist, psychologist, psych tech) that are helpful in treating both conditions. Psychotherapy performed by a **specialist of the mind** (psychologist, physiologist, neurologist) can also be helpful.

2. The most common type of **cognitive impairment characterized by loss of intellectual brain function** (dementia, dysphasia, psychopathy) is caused by **slowly progressive disease occurring more frequently after age 65** (Parkinson disease, multiple sclerosis, Alzheimer disease), accounting for 60% to 80% of all cases. Other types include vascular dementia, **chronic degenerative disease of the central nervous system** (Parkinson disease, encephalopathy, meningitis), normal pressure **water in the head (increased amount of cerebrospinal fluid in the brain)** (encephalitis, meningomyelitis, hydrocephalus), and Huntington disease.

3. Common symptoms of a(n) **interruption of blood supply to a region of the brain**, (stroke, syncope, concussion) include **condition of without speaking** (aphagia, dysphasia, aphasia), **paralysis of half (right or left side of the body)** (quadriplegia, hemiplegia, myalgia), and facial drooping. Prompt diagnosis and treatment are critical. While the majority of strokes are ischemic, resulting from **pertaining to the cerebrum, abnormal condition of a blood clot** (cerebral thrombosis, cerebral aneurysm, cerebral embolism), some are hemorrhagic, caused by intracranial bleeding. **Process of recording the blood vessels of the cerebrum** (CT myelography, cerebral angiography, electroencephalography) can help make the diagnosis. Prompt treatment with thrombolytic agents (which break up clots) can help save lives but can be extremely dangerous if given to a patient with a brain bleed. A **sudden deficient supply of blood to the brain lasting a short time** (SAH, CVA, TIA) usually does not require treatment.

4. **Head pain or headache** (neuralgia, arthralgia, cephalgia) is classified by type. **An intense, throbbing headache, usually one-sided** (sciatica, migraine, TIA), tension headache, and cluster headaches account for nearly 90% of all headaches. Other types of headaches include posttraumatic headaches, giant cell (temporal) arteritis, sinus headaches, brain tumor, and chronic daily headaches. Patients with **chronic degenerative disease characterized by sclerotic patches along the brain and spinal cord** (MS, PD, CP) often have headaches, and patients who experience migraines have an increased risk of **paralysis of muscles on one side of the face caused by inflammation or compression of the facial nerve** (botulism, Bell palsy, poliomyelitis). **Bleeding between the pia mater and arachnoid layers of the meninges caused by a ruptured blood vessel** (cerebral thrombosis, meningitis, subarachnoid hemorrhage) may cause a headache that the patient describes as "the worst in my entire life."

636 Chapter 15 Nervous System and Behavioral Health

EXERCISE 38 ■ Pronounce Medical Terms in Use

Practice pronunciation of terms by reading aloud the following paragraph. Use the phonetic spellings to assist with pronunciation. The script also contains medical terms not presented in the chapter. If interested, research their meanings in a medical dictionary or a reliable online source.

> A 36-year-old right-handed female presents to the emergency department for an episode of **monoparesis** (mon-ō-pa-RĒ-sis) of the right leg, which started earlier in the day. She has a history of **major depression** (MĀ-jor) (dē-PRESH-un), for which she sees a **psychiatrist** (sī-KĪ-a-trist), and is treated with medication. About 6 months ago, she had an episode of optic **neuritis** (nū-RĪ-tis), which was treated with steroids. She denies any history of **seizures** (SĒ-zherz). On examination, she was noted to have **gait** (gāt) difficulties due to the weakness of her right leg. There was no evidence of **paresthesia** (par-es-THĒ-zha) or **cognitive** (COG-ni-tiv) impairment. Because of her age, a diagnosis of **stroke** (strōk) or **TIA** (T-I-A) is unlikely. A **subdural hematoma** (sub-DŪ-ral) (hē-ma-TŌ-ma) or intracranial lesion, such as **meningioma** (me-nin-jē-Ō-ma) or **glioblastoma** (glī-ō-blas-TŌ-ma), must be ruled out. Her symptoms are suggestive of **multiple sclerosis** (MUL-ti-pl) (skle-RŌ-sis). We will order an MR of the brain with contrast to see if any characteristic lesions are present. If not, we will consider a **lumbar puncture** (LUM-bar) (PUNK-chur) and refer her to a **neurologist** (nū-ROL-o-jist) for **evoked potential studies** (i-VŌKD) (pō-TEN-shal) (STUD-ēz).

CHAPTER REVIEW

EXERCISE 39 ■ Chapter Content Quiz

Test your understanding of terms and abbreviations introduced in this chapter. Circle the letter for the medical term or abbreviation related to the words in italics.

1. Jack Cheng was in a serious motorcycle accident that resulted in *paralysis of all four limbs*.
   a. quadriplegia
   b. monoplegia
   c. hemiplegia

2. During her stroke, Mrs. Delgado had *inability to speak*.
   a. dysarthria
   b. aphasia
   c. dysphasia

3. Jacob Mamula experienced a brief period of being *unaware of his or her surroundings and unable to respond to stimuli* after suffering a concussion from a hard hit during the football game.
   a. convulsion
   b. incoherent
   c. unconsciousness

4. The newborn had *protrusion of the meninges* through a defect in his skull.
   a. myelomalacia
   b. myelomeningocele
   c. meningocele

5. Gabriella Moreno was advised to schedule an appointment with a *physician who studies and treats disorders of the mind* when she was diagnosed with bipolar disorder.
   a. neurologist
   b. psychologist
   c. psychiatrist

6. *Chronic degenerative disease characterized by sclerotic patches along the brain and spinal cord* is more common in women, and frequently presents in the fourth or fifth decade of life.
   a. multiple sclerosis
   b. schizophrenia
   c. amyotrophic lateral sclerosis

7. The *process of recording of electrical activity of the brain* was scheduled for Caleb Cook when he started experiencing seizures.
   a. electroencephalogram
   b. electroencephalography
   c. electroencephalograph

8. *Abnormal condition of a clot in the cerebrum* was the cause of the TIA that Mr. Hernandez experienced.
   a. cerebral thrombosis
   b. cerebral aneurysm
   c. cerebral embolism

9. Mrs. Patel was having headaches and blurred vision. Her doctor was concerned about a meningioma. She ordered a *diagnostic procedure to examine blood flow and metabolic activity*.
   a. evoked potential studies
   b. positron emission tomography
   c. lumbar puncture

10. Misha Sanov was diagnosed with *viral disease that affects the peripheral nerves and causes blisters on the skin that follow the course of the affected nerves* over her upper abdomen.
    a. shingles
    b. sciatica
    c. epilepsy

11. Because of scarring from a burn injury to her right hand, Emma Sammani had *loosening, separating a nerve to release it from surrounding tissues* to provide pain relief.
    a. neurolysis
    b. neuralgia
    c. rhizotomy

12. Mr. Rosenthal was taking medication to try to prevent rapid progression of his *type of dementia that occurs more frequently after the age of 65, with dramatic brain shrinkage*.
    a. PD
    b. CP
    c. AD

13. After his military service ended, Brandon O'Rourke experienced *significant behavioral disorder in which some people exposed to a traumatic event go on to develop a series of symptoms related to it*.
    a. somatoform disorder
    b. panic attacks
    c. posttraumatic stress disorder

14. James Robbins had poliomyelitis as a child and was left with *slight paralysis of one (limb)*, which made it difficult for him to walk without assistance.
    a. monoparesis
    b. monoplegia
    c. hemiparesis

15. The physician assistant thought that Mrs. Ng's complaints of headaches and abdominal pain, which started after she lost her job, might be *pertaining to the mind and body*.
    a. psychopathy
    b. psychogenic
    c. psychosomatic

16. Corrine Pageau was brought to the emergency department after experiencing a seizure. She was eventually diagnosed with herpes simplex *inflammation of the brain*.
    a. meningitis
    b. encephalitis
    c. radiculitis

17. Daniel Roth lost consciousness after complaining of severe cephalgia; a CT scan revealed *bleeding between the pia mater and arachnoid layers of the meninges caused by a ruptured blood vessel*.
    a. subarachnoid hemorrhage
    b. subdural hematoma
    c. hydrocephalus

18. Malia Williams has been receiving therapy in the psychology department for her *disorder characterized by intrusive, unwanted thoughts that result in the tendency to perform repetitive acts or rituals*.
    a. attention deficit/hyperactivity disorder
    b. bipolar disorder
    c. obsessive-compulsive disorder

19. Kevin, who has primary progressive multiple sclerosis, experiences painful bouts of *continued contraction of certain muscles due to damage of the brain or spinal cord controlling voluntary movement*.
    a. ataxia
    b. spasticity
    c. dysesthesia

20. Causes of transverse *inflammation of the spinal cord* include infections, immune system disorders, and other conditions that damage the insulating substance covering nerves.
    a. myelitis
    b. neuritis
    c. meningitis

Chapter 15 Nervous System and Behavioral Health

CHAPTER AT A GLANCE — Word Parts New to This Chapter

COMBINING FORMS

cerebell/o	esthesi/o	mening/o	myel/o	quadr/i	
cerebr/o	gangli/o	meningi/o	phas/o	radicul/o	
dur/o	ganglion/o	ment/o	poli/o	rhiz/o	
encephal/o	gli/o	mon/o	psych/o		

SUFFIXES

- -iatrist
- -iatry
- -ictal
- -paresis

CHAPTER AT A GLANCE — Nervous System Terms Built from Word Parts

DISEASE AND DISORDER
- cerebellitis
- cerebral embolism
- cerebral thrombosis
- duritis
- encephalitis
- encephalomalacia
- encephalopathy
- encephalomyeloradiculitis
- gangliitis
- glioblastoma
- glioma
- hydrocephalus
- intracerebral hemorrhage
- meningioma
- meningitis
- meningocele
- meningomyelocele
- mononeuropathy
- myelitis
- myelomalacia
- neuralgia
- neuritis
- poliomyelitis (polio)
- polyneuritis
- polyneuropathy
- radiculitis
- radiculopathy
- rhizomeningomyelitis
- subdural hematoma

SURGICAL
- ganglionectomy
- neurectomy
- neurolysis
- neuroplasty
- neurorrhaphy
- neurotomy
- rhizotomy

DIAGNOSTIC
- cerebral angiography
- CT myelography
- electroencephalogram (EEG)
- electroencephalograph
- electroencephalography

COMPLEMENTARY
- anesthesia
- aphasia
- cephalgia
- craniocerebral
- dysesthesia
- dysphasia
- hemiparesis
- hemiplegia
- hyperesthesia
- interictal
- mental
- monoparesis
- monoplegia
- neurologist
- neurology
- paresthesia
- postictal
- preictal
- quadriplegia

BEHAVIORAL HEALTH
- psychiatrist
- psychiatry
- psychogenic
- psychologist
- psychology
- psychopathy
- psychosis (*pl.* psychoses)
- psychosomatic

CHAPTER AT A GLANCE — Nervous System Terms NOT Built from Word Parts

DISEASE AND DISORDER
- Alzheimer disease (AD)
- amyotrophic lateral sclerosis (ALS)
- Bell palsy
- botulism
- cerebral aneurysm
- cerebral palsy (CP)
- chronic traumatic encephalopathy (CTE)
- dementia
- epilepsy
- migraine
- multiple sclerosis (MS)
- Parkinson disease (PD)
- sciatica
- shingles
- stroke
- subarachnoid hemorrhage (SAH)
- transient ischemic attack (TIA)

DIAGNOSTIC
- deep tendon reflexes (DTR)
- evoked potential studies (EP studies)
- lumbar puncture (LP)
- positron emission tomography (PET)

COMPLEMENTARY
- ataxia
- cognitive
- coma
- concussion
- conscious
- convulsion
- disorientation
- dysarthria
- gait
- incoherent
- paraplegia
- seizure
- shunt
- spasticity
- syncope
- unconsciousness

BEHAVIORAL HEALTH
- anorexia nervosa
- anxiety disorder
- attention deficit/hyperactivity disorder (ADHD)
- autism
- bipolar disorder
- bulimia nervosa
- major depression
- obsessive-compulsive disorder (OCD)
- panic attack
- phobia
- pica
- posttraumatic stress disorder (PTSD)
- schizophrenia
- somatoform disorders

PART 2 BODY SYSTEMS

Endocrine System 16

Outline

ANATOMY, 640
Function, 640
Endocrine Glands and Hormones, 641

WORD PARTS, 643
Endocrine System Combining Forms, 643
Combining Forms Used with Endocrine System Terms, 643
Prefixes, 643
Suffixes, 644

MEDICAL TERMS, 647
Disease and Disorder Terms, 647
　Built from Word Parts, 647
　NOT Built from Word Parts, 650
Surgical Terms, 656
　Built from Word Parts, 656
Diagnostic Terms, 657
　NOT Built from Word Parts, 657
Complementary Terms, 659
　Built from Word Parts and
　　NOT Built from Word Parts, 659
Abbreviations, 664

PRACTICAL APPLICATION, 666
CASE STUDY Translate Between Everyday Language and Medical Language, 666
Interact with Medical Documents, 667
Use Medical Language in Online Electronic Health Records, 669
Use Medical Terms in Clinical Statements, 669
Pronounce Medical Terms in Use, 670

CHAPTER REVIEW, 670
Chapter Content Quiz, 670
Chapter at a Glance, 672

CAPSTONE, 672
Scribe It, 672

Answers to Chapter Exercises, Appendix A

Objectives

Upon completion of this chapter, you will be able to:

1. Pronounce glands and hormones of the endocrine system.
2. Define and spell word parts related to the endocrine system.
3. Define, pronounce, and spell disease and disorder terms related to the endocrine system.
4. Define, pronounce, and spell surgical terms related to the endocrine system.
5. Define, pronounce, and spell diagnostic terms related to the endocrine system.
6. Define, pronounce, and spell complementary terms related to the endocrine system.
7. Interpret the meaning of abbreviations related to the endocrine system.
8. Apply medical language in clinical contexts.

TABLE 16.1 Diabetes Mellitus, 652

ANATOMY

The endocrine system is composed of endocrine glands distributed throughout the body. The endocrine glands are: pituitary, thyroid, parathyroid, adrenal, pancreas, gonads (ovaries and testes), and thymus.

Function

The endocrine system regulates body activities through the use of chemical messengers called **hormones**, which when released into the bloodstream influence metabolic activities, growth, and development (Fig. 16.1). The nervous system also regulates body activities by receiving electrical impulses that convey information about the state of the body, and then activating glandular secretions in response. Hormones secreted by the **endocrine glands** that make up the endocrine system go directly into the bloodstream and are transported throughout the body. They are referred to as **ductless glands** because they do not have ducts to carry their secretions. In contrast, the **exocrine** or **duct glands** have ducts that carry their secretions from the producing gland to other parts of the body. An example is the parotid gland, which produces saliva that flows through the parotid duct into the mouth. Only those terms related to the major endocrine glands—pituitary, thyroid, parathyroids, adrenals, and the islets of Langerhans in the pancreas—are presented in this chapter. The thymus primarily functions as part of the lymphatic system and was presented in Chapter 10. The male and female sex glands were also presented in previous chapters.

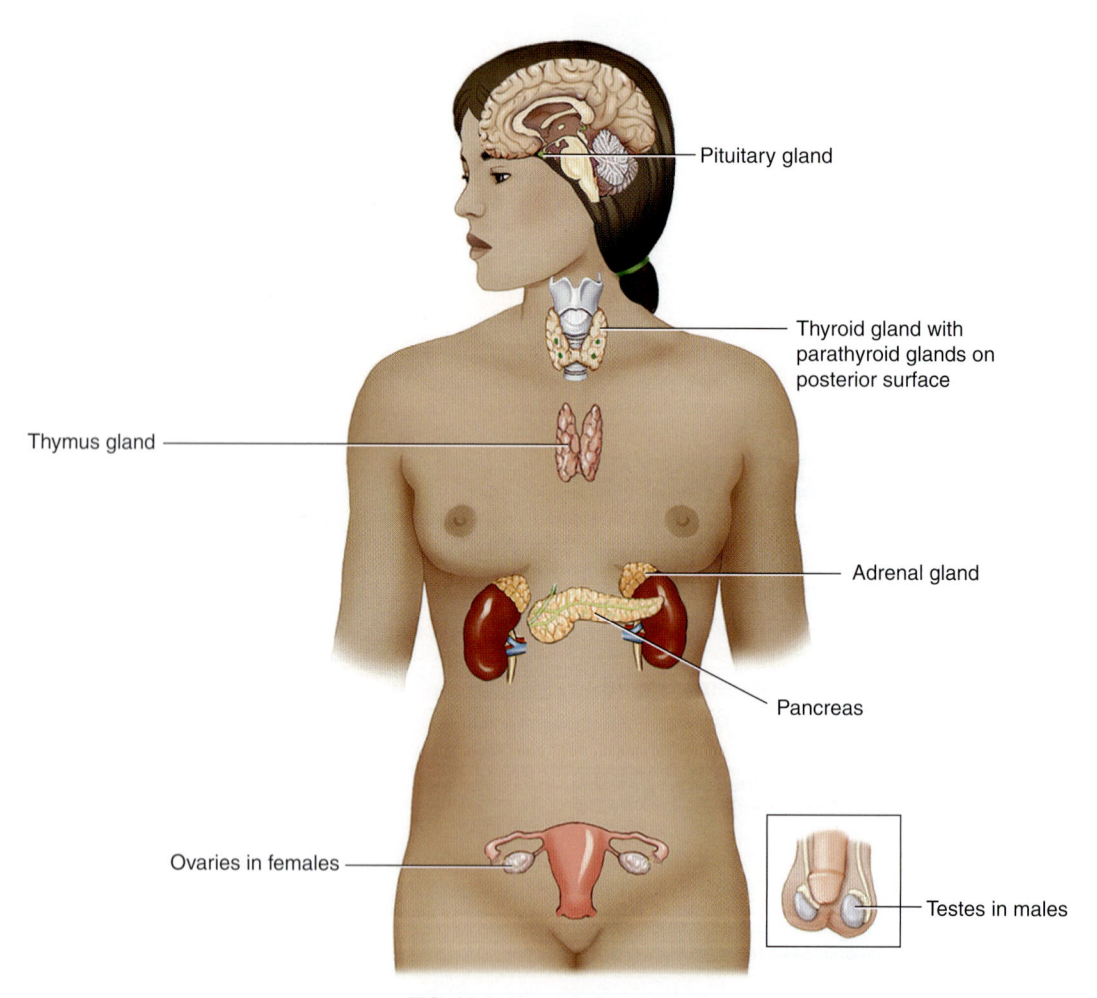

FIG. 16.1 The endocrine system.

Chapter 16 Endocrine System   641

Endocrine Glands and Hormones

TERM	DEFINITION
pituitary gland (pi-TOO-i-*tar*-ē) (gland)	pea-sized gland located at the base of the brain. The pituitary is divided into two lobes. It is often referred to as the **master gland** because it produces hormones that stimulate the function of other endocrine glands. (also called **hypophysis cerebri**) (Fig. 16.2 and Fig. 16.3A)
anterior lobe (ān-TĒR-ē-er) (lōb)	produces and secretes the following hormones (also called **adenohypophysis**):
growth hormone (GH) (grohth) (HŌR-mōn)	regulates the growth of the body
adrenocorticotropic hormone (ACTH) (a-*drē*-nō-*kōr*-ti-kō-TRŌ-pik) (HŌR-mōn)	stimulates the adrenal cortex
thyroid-stimulating hormone (TSH) (THĪ-royd) (STIM-yuh-lāt-ing) (HŌR-mōn)	stimulates the thyroid gland
gonadotropic hormones (gō-na-dō-TRŌ-pik) (HŌR-mōns)	stimulate the gonads (the testes in males and ovaries in females). **Follicle-stimulating hormone** (FSH) and **luteinizing hormone** (LH) are the gonadotropic hormones released from the adenohypophysis.
prolactin (PRL) (prō-LAK-tin)	promotes development of glandular tissue during pregnancy and stimulates milk production after birth of an infant
posterior lobe (po-STĒR-ē-er) (lōb)	stores and releases antidiuretic hormone and oxytocin (also called **neurohypophysis**)
antidiuretic hormone (ADH) (*an*-tē-*dī*-ū-RET-ik) (HŌR-mōn)	stimulates the kidney to reabsorb water and constricts blood vessels to help maintain blood pressure (also called **vasopressin**)
oxytocin (*ok*-sē-TŌ-sin)	stimulates uterine contractions during labor and postpartum, and milk letdown by the breasts postpartum

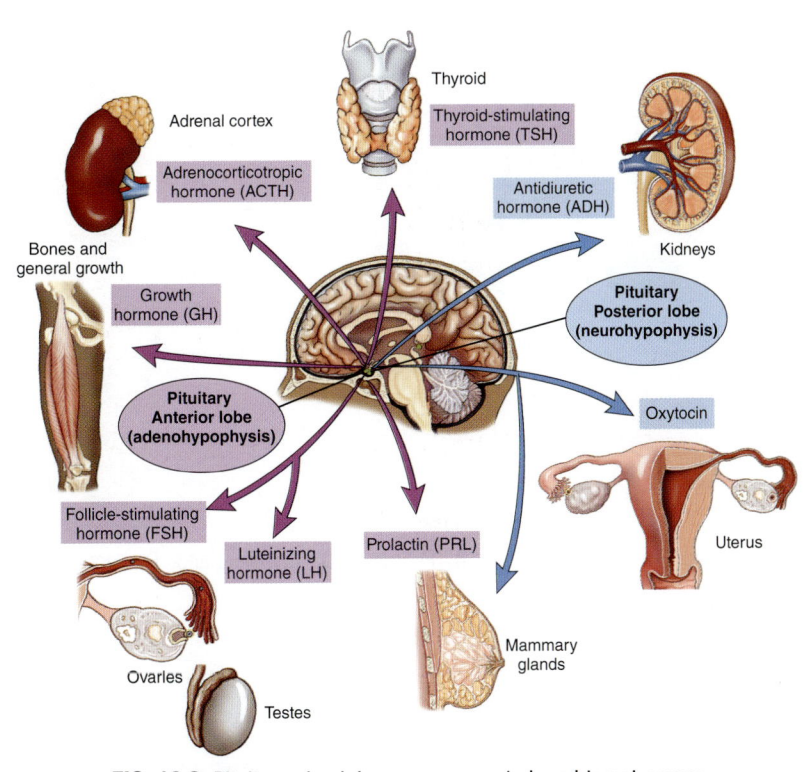

FIG. 16.2 Pituitary gland, hormones secreted, and target organs.

Chapter 16 Endocrine System

TERM	DEFINITION
hypothalamus (*hī*-pō-THAL-a-mus)	located superior to the pituitary gland in the brain. The hypothalamus secretes "releasing" hormones that function to stimulate or inhibit the release of pituitary gland hormones.
thyroid gland (THĪ-royd) (gland)	largest endocrine gland. It is located anteriorly in the neck below the larynx and comprises bilateral lobes connected by an isthmus (Fig. 16.3C). The thyroid gland secretes the hormones triiodothyronine (T_3) and thyroxine (T_4), which require iodine for their production. Thyroxine is necessary for body cell metabolism.
parathyroid glands (*par*-a-THĪ-royd) (glans)	four small bodies embedded in the posterior aspect of the lobes of the thyroid gland (Fig. 16.3D). Parathyroid hormone (PTH), the hormone produced by the glands, helps maintain the level of calcium in the blood by its effects on bone and kidneys.
islets of Langerhans (Ī-lets) (LAHNG-er-hahnz)	clusters of endocrine tissue found throughout the pancreas, made up of different cell types that secrete various hormones, including insulin and glucagon, which regulate blood sugar. Nonendocrine cells found throughout the pancreas produce enzymes that facilitate digestion (Fig. 16.4).
adrenal glands (a-DRĒ-nal) (glans)	paired glands, one of which is located superior to each kidney. The outer portion is called the **adrenal cortex**, and the inner portion is called the **adrenal medulla**. The following hormones are secreted by the adrenal glands:
cortisol (KOR-ti-sol)	secreted by the adrenal cortex. It aids the body during stress by increasing glucose levels to provide energy (also called **hydrocortisone**).
aldosterone (al-DOS-ter-ōn)	secreted by the adrenal cortex. Electrolytes (including sodium and potassium) that are necessary for normal body function are regulated by this hormone.
epinephrine, norepinephrine (*ep*-i-NEF-rin), (*nor*-ep-i-NEF-rin)	secreted by the adrenal medulla. These hormones help the body to deal with stress by increasing the blood pressure, heartbeat, and respirations. (also called **adrenaline** and **noradrenaline**, respectively)

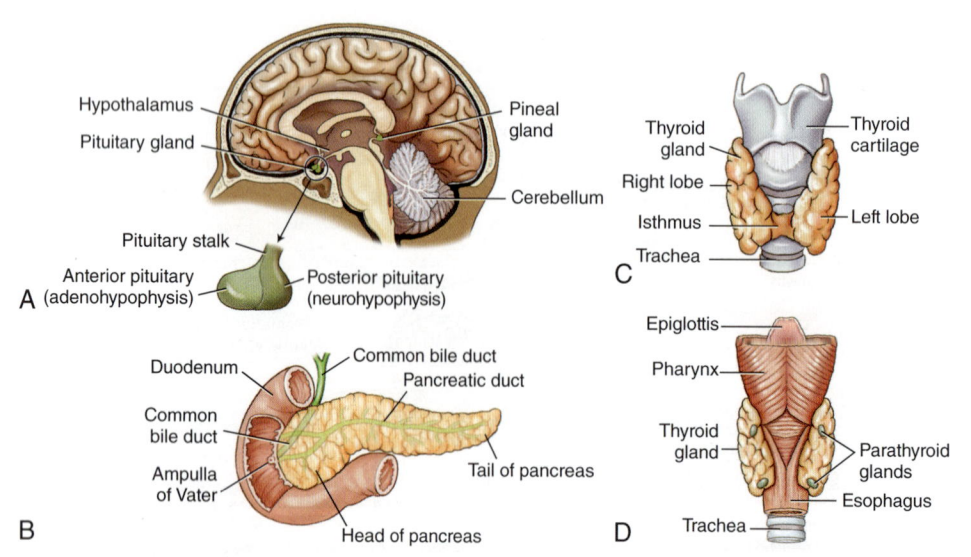

FIG. 16.3 A, Pituitary and pineal glands. **B,** Pancreas. **C,** Thyroid gland. **D,** Parathyroid glands, posterior view.

Chapter 16 Endocrine System 643

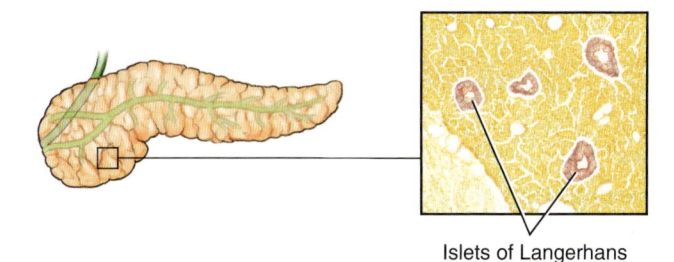

FIG. 16.4 Pancreas, with microscopic illustration of islets of Langerhans.

PRONOUNCE ANATOMIC STRUCTURES

Practice saying aloud each of the organs and specific structures on the previous pages.

To hear the terms, go to Evolve Resources at www.evolve.elsevier.com and select:

Student Resources > Audio Glossary > Chapter 16 > Anatomic Structures

❑ Check the box when complete.

WORD PARTS

Use paper flashcards or electronic flashcards on Evolve to memorize word parts used to analyze, define, and build medical terms in this chapter. To reinforce learning, study one section of the Word Parts Table at a time, and then complete the corresponding exercises on the following pages.

1 ■ Endocrine System Combining Forms

COMBINING FORM	DEFINITION	COMBINING FORM	DEFINITION
adren/o	adrenal glands	endocrin/o	endocrine
adrenal/o	adrenal glands	parathyroid/o	parathyroid glands
cortic/o	cortex (the outer layer of a body organ)	pituitar/o	pituitary gland
		thyroid/o	thyroid gland

2 ■ Combining Forms Used with Endocrine System Terms

COMBINING FORM	DEFINITION	COMBINING FORM	DEFINITION
acr/o	extremities, height	glyc/o	sugar
calc/i	calcium (Note: the combining vowel is i.)	kal/i	potassium (Note: the combining vowel is i.)
dips/o	thirst	natr/o	sodium

3 ■ Prefixes

PREFIX	DEFINITION	PREFIX	DEFINITION
eu-	normal, good	pan-	all, total
hyper-	above, excessive	poly-	many, much
hypo-	below, incomplete, deficient, under	syn-	together, joined

4 ■ Suffixes

SUFFIX	DEFINITION
-al	pertaining to
-drome	run, running
-ectomy	excision, surgical removal
-emia	in the blood
-ia	diseased state, condition of
-ism	state of
-itis	inflammation

SUFFIX	DEFINITION
-logist	one who studies and treats (specialist, physician)
-logy	study of
-megaly	enlargement
-oma	tumor, swelling
-pathy	disease
-plasia	condition of formation, development, growth

Refer to **Appendix B** and **Appendix C** for a complete list of word parts.

EXERCISE 1 ■ Endocrine System Combining Forms

Refer to the first section of the word parts table.

A Label

Fill in the blanks with combining forms in this diagram of the endocrine glands.
To check your answers, go to Appendix A at the back of the textbook.

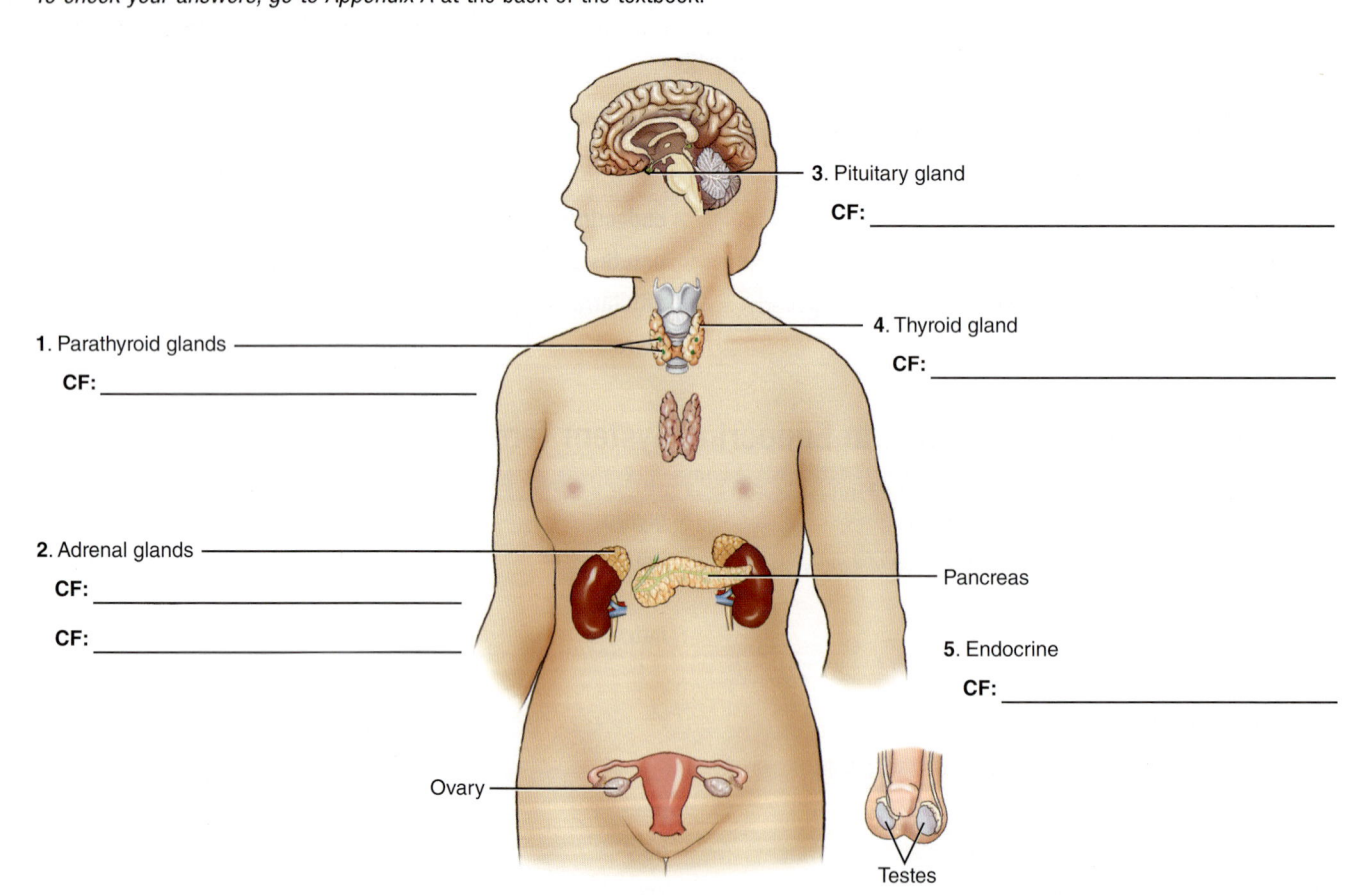

3. Pituitary gland
   CF: _____

1. Parathyroid glands
   CF: _____

4. Thyroid gland
   CF: _____

2. Adrenal glands
   CF: _____
   CF: _____

Pancreas

5. Endocrine
   CF: _____

Ovary

Testes

B Label

Fill in the blank with the combining form in this diagram of adrenal glands (with transverse cross-sectional view).

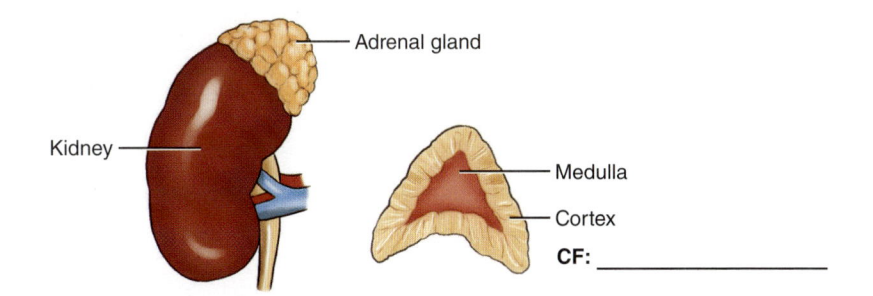

- Adrenal gland
- Kidney
- Medulla
- Cortex

CF: _____

C Define and Match

Step 1: Write the definitions after the following combining forms.
Step 2: Match the descriptions on the right with the combining forms and definitions. Answers may be used more than once; no answer line appears for those not described in a lettered item.

_____ 1. adrenal/o, _____
_____ 2. pituitar/o, _____
_____ 3. cortic/o, _____
_____ 4. parathyroid/o, _____
_____ 5. adren/o, _____
_____ 6. thyroid/o, _____
       7. endocrin/o, _____

a. referred to as the master gland because it produces hormones that stimulate the function of other endocrine glands
b. four small bodies embedded in the posterior aspect of the lobes of the thyroid gland
c. largest endocrine gland; secretes triiodothyronine (T_3) and thyroxine (T_4)
d. paired glands, one of which is located above each kidney
e. outer portion of adrenal gland

EXERCISE 2 ■ Combining Forms Used with Endocrine System Terms

Refer to the second portion of the word parts table.

A Define

Write the definitions of the following combining forms.

1. dips/o _____
2. kal/i _____
3. calc/i _____
4. acr/o _____
5. natr/o _____
6. glyc/o _____

B Identify

Write the combining form for each of the following.

1. extremities, height _____
2. calcium _____
3. thirst _____
4. sugar _____
5. potassium _____
6. sodium _____

Chapter 16 Endocrine System

EXERCISE 3 — Prefixes

Refer to the third section of the word parts table.

A Define

Write the definitions of the following prefixes.

1. syn- _____
2. hypo- _____
3. pan- _____
4. eu- _____
5. poly- _____
6. hyper- _____

B Identify

Write the prefix for each of the following.

1. all, total _____
2. normal, good _____
3. many, much _____
4. above, excessive _____
5. together, joined _____
6. below, incomplete, deficient, under _____

EXERCISE 4 — Suffixes

Refer to the fourth section of the word parts table.

A Identify

Write the suffix for each of the following.

1. state of _____
2. enlargement _____
3. in the blood _____
4. pertaining to _____
5. disease _____
6. one who studies and treats (specialist, physician) _____

B Label

Write the suffix pictured and defined.

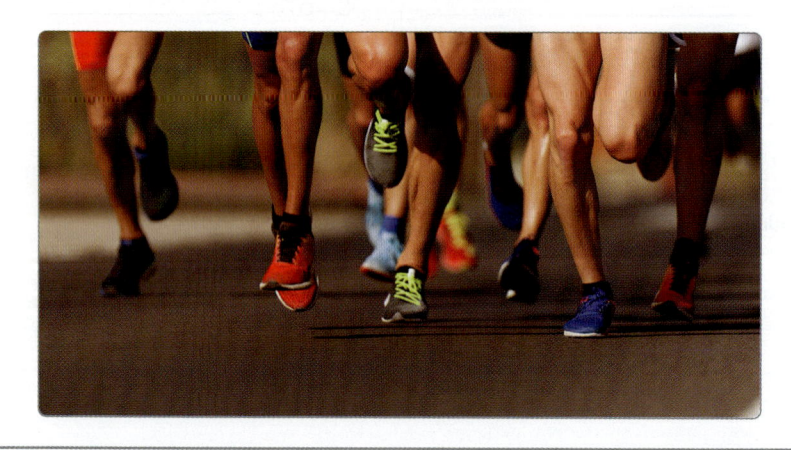

1. _____
   run, running

C Define

Write definitions for the following suffixes

1. -oma _____
2. -ectomy _____
3. -plasia _____
   _____
4. -logy _____
5. -itis _____
6. -drome _____
7. -ia _____

MEDICAL TERMS

Medical terms relevant to this chapter have been grouped by topics, such as Disease and Disorder, and are listed in tables designated as Built from Word Parts or *NOT* Built from Word Parts. The exercises following each table assist with learning term definitions, pronunciations, and spellings.

Disease and Disorder Terms
BUILT FROM WORD PARTS

The following terms can be translated using definitions of word parts. Further explanation is provided within parentheses as needed.

TERM	DEFINITION	TERM	DEFINITION
1. acromegaly (ak-rō-MEG-a-lē)	enlargement of the extremities (and face; due to increased soft tissue, bone, and cartilage; caused by excessive production of the growth hormone by the pituitary gland after puberty)	8. hyperparathyroidism (hī-per-par-a-THĪ-royd-izm)	state of excessive parathyroid gland (activity); (results in hypercalcemia and leads to osteoporosis, as well as symptoms of muscle weakness, abdominal pain, nausea, vomiting, and drowsiness)
2. adrenalitis (a-drē-nal-Ī-tis)	inflammation of the adrenal glands	9. hyperpituitarism (hī-per-pi-TOO-i-ta-rizm)	state of excessive pituitary gland (activity); (characterized by excessive secretion of pituitary hormones)
3. adrenomegaly (a-drē-nō-MEG-a-lē)	enlargement (of one or both) of the adrenal glands	10. hyperthyroidism (hī-per-THĪ-royd-izm)	state of excessive thyroid gland (activity); (characterized by excessive secretion of thyroid hormones; signs and symptoms include tachycardia, weight loss, irritability, and heat intolerance)
4. endocrinopathy (en-dō-kri-NOP-a-thē)	(any) disease of the endocrine (system)		
5. hypercalcemia (hī-per-kal-SĒ-mē-a)	excessive calcium in the blood		
6. hyperglycemia (hī-per-glī-SĒ-mē-a)	excessive sugar in the blood		
7. hyperkalemia (hī-per-ka-LĒ-mē-a)	excessive potassium in the blood		

Disease and Disorder Terms—cont'd
BUILT FROM WORD PARTS

TERM	DEFINITION	TERM	DEFINITION
11. **hypocalcemia** (hī-pō-kal-SĒ-mē-a)	deficient calcium in the blood	16. **hypothyroidism** (hī-pō-THĪ-royd-izm)	state of deficient thyroid gland (activity); (characterized by decreased secretion of thyroid hormones; signs and symptoms include fatigue, weight gain, and cold intolerance)
12. **hypoglycemia** (hī-pō-glī-SĒ-mē-a)	deficient sugar in the blood		
13. **hypokalemia** (hī-pō-ka-LĒ-mē-a)	deficient potassium in the blood		
14. **hyponatremia** (hī-pō-na-TRĒ-mē-a)	deficient sodium in the blood	17. **panhypopituitarism** (pan-hī-pō-pi-TŪ-i-ta-rizm)	state of total deficient pituitary gland (activity); (characterized by decreased secretion of all the anterior pituitary hormones; this is a more serious condition than hypopituitarism in that it affects the function of all the other endocrine glands)
15. **hypopituitarism** (hī-pō-pi-TŪ-i-ta-rizm)	state of deficient pituitary gland (activity); (characterized by decreased secretion of one or more of the pituitary hormones, which can affect the function of the target endocrine gland; for example, hypothyroidism can result from decreased secretion of thyroid-stimulating hormone by the pituitary gland)		
		PANHYPOPITUITARISM contains two prefixes, **pan-** meaning *total* and **hypo-** meaning *deficient.*	
		18. **parathyroidoma** (par-a-thī-royd-Ō-ma)	tumor of a parathyroid gland
		19. **thyroiditis** (thī-royd-Ī-tis)	inflammation of the thyroid gland

EXERCISE 5 ■ Pronounce and Spell

Practice pronunciation and spelling on paper and online.

1. **Practice on Paper**
   a. **Pronounce:** Read the phonetic spelling and say aloud the terms listed in the previous table. Refer to Table 2.2 Pronunciation Key as needed.
   b. **Spell:** Have a study partner read the terms aloud. Write the spelling of the terms on a separate sheet of paper.

2. **Practice Online**
   a. **Access** online learning resources. Go to evolve.elsevier.com > Evolve Resources > Student Resources.
   b. **Pronounce:** Select Audio Glossary > Chapter 16 > Exercise 5. Select a term to hear its pronunciation and repeat aloud.
   c. **Spell:** Select Activities > Chapter 16 > Spell Terms > Exercise 5. Select the audio icon and type the correct spelling of the term.

❏ Check the box when complete.

Chapter 16 Endocrine System 649

EXERCISE 6 ■ Analyze and Define

Analyze and define the following terms.

1. adrenalitis

2. hypocalcemia

3. hyperthyroidism

4. hyperkalemia

5. hyperpituitarism

6. adrenomegaly

7. endocrinopathy

8. hyponatremia

9. parathyroidoma

10. panhypopituitarism

EXERCISE 7 ■ Build

A Label

Build terms pictured by writing word parts above definitions.

1.

_____ / _____ / _____
extremities   CV   enlargement

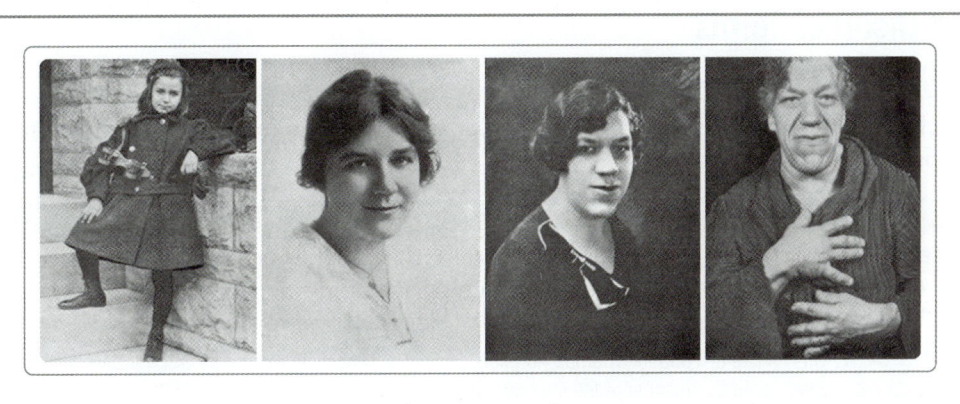

650 Chapter 16 Endocrine System

2.

_____ / _____ / _____
excessive   sugar   in the blood

3.

_____ / _____ / _____
deficient   sugar   in the blood

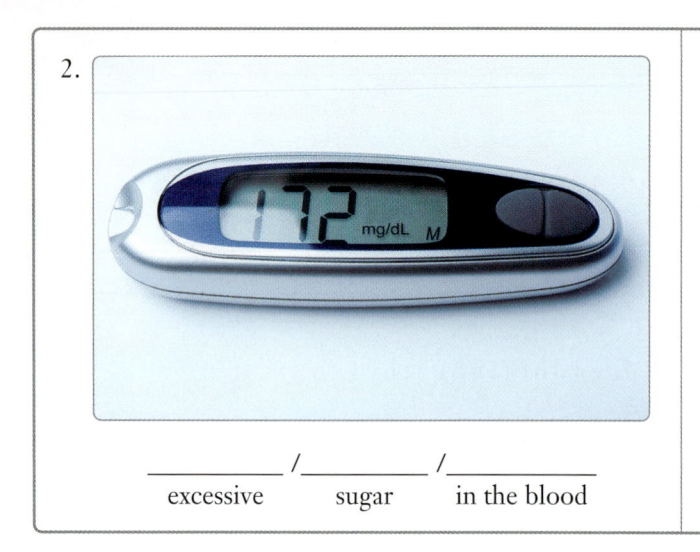

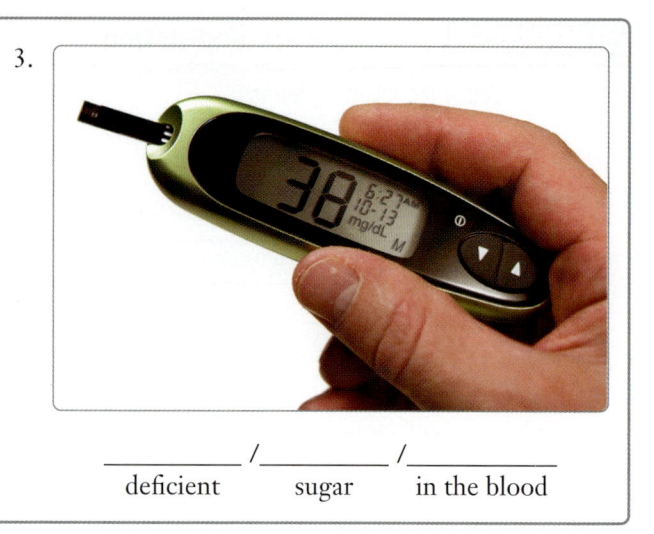

B Fill In

Build disease and disorder terms for the following definitions by using the word parts you have learned.

1. state of deficient thyroid gland activity

   _____ / _____ / _____
   P   WR   S

2. deficient potassium in the blood

   _____ / _____ / _____
   P   WR   S

3. state of excessive parathyroid gland activity

   _____ / _____ / _____
   P   WR   S

4. state of deficient pituitary gland activity

   _____ / _____ / _____
   P   WR   S

5. excessive calcium in the blood

   _____ / _____ / _____
   P   WR   S

6. thyroid inflammation

   _____ / _____
   WR   S

Disease and Disorder Terms
NOT BUILT FROM WORD PARTS

Word parts may be present in the following terms; however, their full meanings cannot be translated using definitions of word parts alone.

TERM	DEFINITION
1. Addison disease (AD-i-sun) (di-ZĒZ)	chronic syndrome resulting from a deficiency in the hormonal secretion of the adrenal cortex. Signs and symptoms may include weakness, weight loss, hypotension, darkening of skin, and loss of appetite.
🏛 **ADDISON DISEASE** was named in **1855** for **Thomas Addison**, an English physician and pathologist. He described the disease as a "morbid state with feeble heart action, anemia, irritability of the stomach, and a peculiar change in the color of the skin."	
2. congenital hypothyroidism (kon-JEN-i-tal) (hī-pō-THĪ-royd-izm)	condition caused by congenital absence or atrophy (wasting away) of the thyroid gland, resulting in hypothyroidism. The disease is characterized by puffy features, mental deficiency, large tongue, and short stature.

TERM	DEFINITION
3. **Cushing syndrome** (KOOSH-ing) (SIN-drōm)	group of signs and symptoms attributed to the excessive production of cortisol by the adrenal cortices (*pl.* of cortex). This syndrome may be the result of a pituitary tumor that produces ACTH or a primary adrenal cortex hypersecretion. Signs include abnormally pigmented skin, "moon face," pads of fat on the chest and abdomen, "buffalo hump" (fat on the upper back), wasting away of muscle, and hypertension.

🏛 **CUSHING SYNDROME** was named for an American neurosurgeon, **Harvey Williams Cushing** (1869-1939), after he described adrenocortical hyperfunction.

4. **diabetes insipidus (DI)** (dī-a-BĒ-tēz) (in-SIP-i-dus)	result of decreased secretion of antidiuretic hormone by the posterior lobe of the pituitary gland. Symptoms include excessive thirst (polydipsia), large amounts of urine (polyuria), and water being excreted from the body.
5. **diabetes mellitus (DM)** (dī-a-BĒ-tēz) (MEL-li-tus)	chronic disease involving a disorder of carbohydrate metabolism characterized by elevated blood sugar (hyperglycemia); caused by underactivity of the insulin-producing islets of Langerhans or poor cellular response to insulin. DM can lead to chronic renal disease, retinopathy, and neuropathy. In extreme cases the patient may develop ketosis, acidosis, and finally coma. (Table 16.1)
6. **gigantism** (jī-GAN-tizm)	condition brought about by hypersecretion of growth hormone by the pituitary gland before puberty

GIGANTISM AND ACROMEGALY are both caused by overproduction of growth hormone. **Gigantism** occurs before puberty and before the growing ends of the bones have closed. If untreated, an individual may reach 8 feet tall in adulthood. **Acromegaly** occurs after puberty. The body parts most affected are those in the hands, feet, and jaw.

7. **Graves disease** (grāvz) (di-ZĒZ)	autoimmune disorder of the thyroid gland characterized by the production of more thyroid hormone than the body needs (hyperthyroidism), goiter, and exophthalmos (abnormal protrusion of the eyeballs)
8. **Hashimoto thyroiditis** (*hah*-she-MŌ-tō) (thī-royd-Ī-tis)	disease in which thyroid gland cells are destroyed by autoimmune processes. Characterized by hypothyroidism and goiter; more common in females.
9. **ketoacidosis** (kē-tō-*as*-i-DŌ-sis)	serious condition resulting from uncontrolled diabetes mellitus in which acid ketones accumulate from fat metabolism in the absence of adequate insulin. If not promptly controlled by adequate insulin and hydration, can progress to coma and death.
10. **metabolic syndrome** (*met*-a-BOL-ik) (SIN-drōm)	group of signs and symptoms including insulin resistance, obesity characterized by excessive fat around the area of the waist and abdomen, hypertension, hyperglycemia, elevated triglycerides, and low levels of HDL, the "good" cholesterol. Risks include development of type 2 diabetes mellitus, coronary heart disease, or stroke. (also called **syndrome X** and **insulin resistance syndrome**)
11. **myxedema** (*mik*-se-DĒ-ma)	condition resulting from an extreme deficiency of the thyroid hormone thyroxine; a severe form of hypothyroidism in an adult. Signs include puffiness of the face and hands, coarse and thickened skin, enlarged tongue, slow speech, and anemia.
12. **neuroblastoma** (*nū*-rō-blas-TŌ-ma)	malignant cancer that often starts in the adrenal medulla; composed of immature nerve cells. Primarily affects children.
13. **obesity** (ō-BĒS-i-tē)	excess of body fat, which increases body weight; a condition in which body mass index (BMI) is greater than 30 kg/m². Overweight is defined as BMI between 25 and 29.9 kg/m².
14. **pheochromocytoma** (fē-ō-*krō*-mō-sī-TŌ-ma)	tumor of the adrenal medulla, which is usually nonmalignant and characterized by hypertension, headaches, palpitations, diaphoresis, chest pain, and abdominal pain. Surgical removal of the tumor is the most common treatment. Though usually curable with early detection, it can be fatal if untreated.
15. **thyrotoxicosis** (*thī*-rō-*tok*-si-KŌ-sis)	condition caused by excessive thyroid hormones

TABLE 16.1 Diabetes Mellitus

Two major forms of diabetes mellitus are **type 1**, previously called insulin-dependent diabetes mellitus (IDDM) or juvenile-onset diabetes, and **type 2**, previously called noninsulin-dependent diabetes mellitus (NIDDM) or adult-onset diabetes mellitus (AODM). Type 2 diabetes mellitus has reached epidemic proportions and is a major cause of cardiovascular disease.

TYPE 1 DIABETES MELLITUS

Cause	autoimmune disease in which the beta cells of the pancreas that produce insulin are destroyed and eventually no insulin is produced
Characteristics	abrupt onset, occurs primarily in childhood or adolescence; patients often are thin
Signs and Symptoms	polyuria, polydipsia, weight loss, and hyperglycemia; these are present if blood sugar is not controlled and can progress to ketoacidosis if not promptly treated
Treatment	insulin injections and diet

TYPE 2 DIABETES MELLITUS

Cause	resistance of body cells to the action of insulin, coupled with a decrease in the ability of the pancreas to make sufficient insulin to overcome this resistance
Characteristics	slow onset, usually occurs in middle-aged or elderly adults; most patients are obese
Signs and Symptoms	fatigue, blurred vision, thirst, and hyperglycemia; these may be present if blood sugar is not controlled
Treatment	diet, exercise, oral or injected medication, and sometimes insulin

LONG-TERM COMPLICATIONS OF DIABETES MELLITUS
MACROVASCULAR COMPLICATIONS
- coronary artery disease → myocardial infarction
- cerebrovascular disease → stroke
- peripheral artery disease → leg pain when walking (intermittent vascular claudication)

MICROVASCULAR COMPLICATIONS
- diabetic retinopathy → loss of vision
- diabetic nephropathy → chronic renal disease, kidney failure
- neuropathy → loss of feeling in the distal extremities (feet, hands), which can lead to amputation

---

EXERCISE 8 ■ Pronounce and Spell

Practice pronunciation and spelling on paper and online.

1. **Practice on Paper**

    a. **Pronounce:** Read the phonetic spelling and say aloud the terms listed in the previous table. Refer to Table 2.2 Pronunciation Key as needed.

    b. **Spell:** Have a study partner read the terms aloud. Write the spelling of the terms on a separate sheet of paper.

2. **Practice Online**

    a. **Access** online learning resources. Go to evolve.elsevier.com > Evolve Resources > Student Resources.

    b. **Pronounce:** Select Audio Glossary > Chapter 16 > Exercise 8. Select a term to hear its pronunciation and repeat aloud.

    c. **Spell:** Select Activities > Chapter 16 > Spell Terms > Exercise 8. Select the audio icon and type the correct spelling of the term.

❏ Check the box when complete.

EXERCISE 9 ■ Match

Match the terms in the first column with their correct definitions in the second column.

_____ 1. diabetes insipidus
_____ 2. neuroblastoma
_____ 3. pheochromocytoma
_____ 4. thyrotoxicosis
_____ 5. diabetes mellitus
_____ 6. ketoacidosis
_____ 7. Graves disease
_____ 8. obesity

a. serious condition resulting from uncontrolled diabetes mellitus in which acid ketones accumulate from fat metabolism in the absence of adequate insulin
b. tumor of the adrenal medulla, characterized by hypertension, headaches, palpitations, diaphoresis, chest pain, and abdominal pain
c. result of decreased secretion of antidiuretic hormone by the posterior lobe of the pituitary gland
d. excess of body fat, which increases body weight
e. autoimmune disorder characterized by hyperthyroidism, goiter, and exophthalmos
f. chronic disease involving a disorder of carbohydrate metabolism characterized by elevated blood sugar (hyperglycemia)
g. childhood cancer that often starts in the adrenal medulla
h. condition caused by excessive thyroid hormones

EXERCISE 10 ■ Match

Match the terms in the first column with their correct definitions in the second column.

_____ 1. metabolic syndrome
_____ 2. congenital hypothyroidism
_____ 3. myxedema
_____ 4. Addison disease
_____ 5. gigantism
_____ 6. Cushing syndrome
_____ 7. Hashimoto thyroiditis

a. severe form of hypothyroidism in an adult
b. excessive production of cortisol by the adrenal cortices
c. condition brought about by hypersecretion of growth hormone by the pituitary gland before puberty
d. condition caused by absence or atrophy (wasting away) of the thyroid gland in childhood
e. also called syndrome X and insulin resistance syndrome
f. autoimmune disease characterized by hypothyroidism and goiter
g. associated with weakness, weight loss, hypotension, darkening of skin, and loss of appetite.

EXERCISE 11 ■ Fill In

A Identify

Fill in the blanks with the correct terms

1. _____ is a condition in which body mass index (BMI) is greater than 30 kg/m^2.
2. A condition caused by excessive thyroid hormones, or _____, can become a medical emergency.
3. A disease in which thyroid gland cells are destroyed by autoimmune processes, or _____ _____, differs from Graves disease in that it usually presents with hypothyroidism.
4. _____ _____ is associated with excessive thirst and excessive urine output.
5. If not promptly controlled by insulin and hydration, _____ can progress to coma and death.
6. A chronic disease involving a disorder of carbohydrate metabolism, _____ _____, can cause renal disease, retinopathy, and neuropathy.
7. _____ is a malignant cancer that often starts in the adrenal medulla.

B Label

Write the medical terms pictured and defined.

1. _____
   condition brought about by hypersecretion of growth hormone by the pituitary gland before puberty

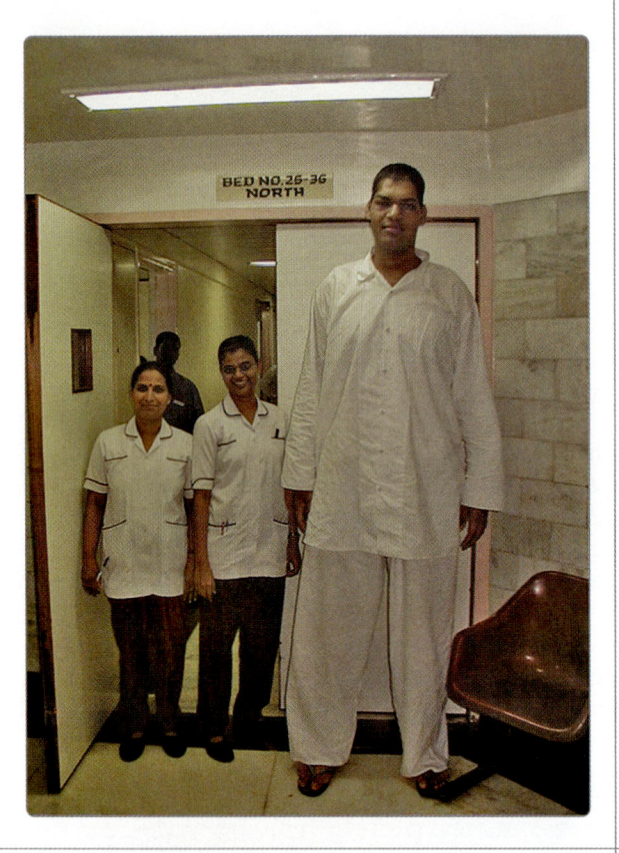

2. _____
   chronic syndrome resulting from a deficiency in the hormonal secretion of the adrenal cortex with symptoms of weight loss, hypotension, and skin darkening

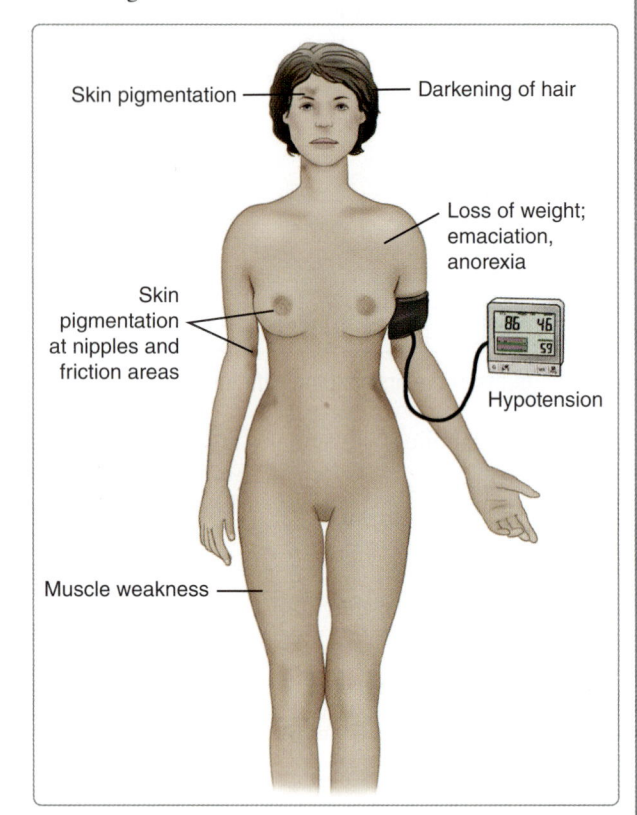

3. _____
   autoimmune disorder of the thyroid gland characterized by hyperthyroidism, goiter, and protrusion of the eyeballs

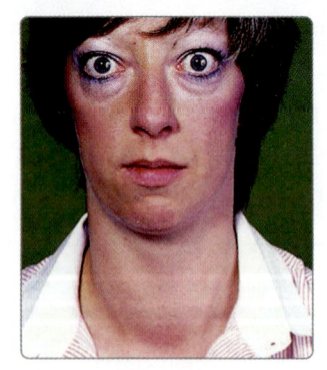

4. _____
   condition resulting from a deficiency of the thyroid hormone thyroxine; a severe form of hypothyroidism in an adult, characterized by puffiness of the face and hands, coarse and thickened skin, enlarged tongue, slow speech, and anemia

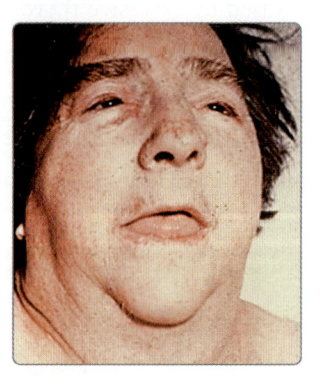

Chapter 16 Endocrine System   655

5. _____
   A. group of signs and symptoms attributed to the excessive production of cortisol by the adrenal cortices
   B. same child after treatment for this condition

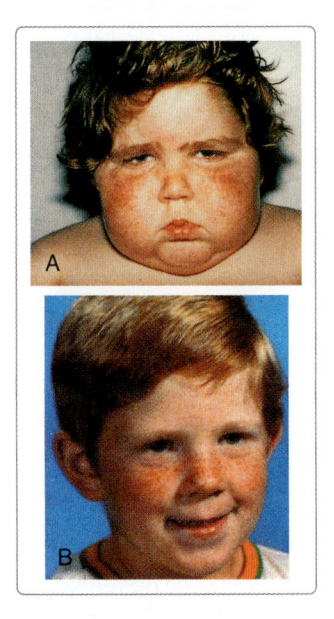

6. _____
   group of signs and symptoms including insulin resistance, obesity characterized by excessive fat around the area of the waist, hypertension, hyperglycemia, elevated triglycerides, and low levels of HDL, the "good" cholesterol

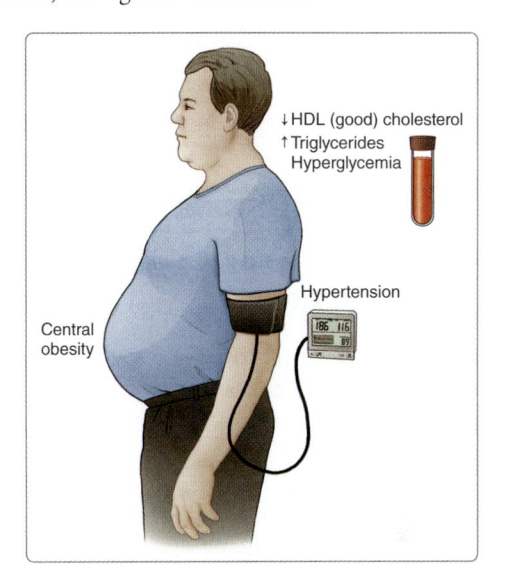

7. _____
   tumor of the adrenal medulla characterized by hypertension, headaches, palpitations, and other symptoms

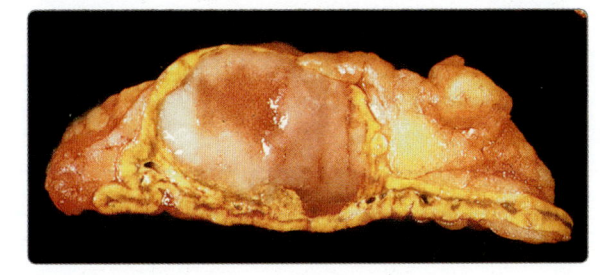

8. _____
   A. condition caused by congenital absence or atrophy of the thyroid gland, resulting in hypothyroidism; characterized by puffy features, mental deficiency, large tongue, and short stature
   B. same child after treatment for this condition

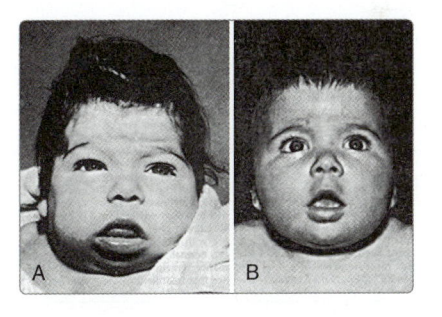

EXERCISE 12 ■ Review of Disease and Disorder Terms

Can you define, pronounce, and spell the following terms?

acromegaly
Addison disease
adrenalitis
adrenomegaly
congenital hypothyroidism
Cushing syndrome
diabetes insipidus (DI)
diabetes mellitus (DM)
endocrinopathy
gigantism
Graves disease
Hashimoto thyroiditis
hypercalcemia
hyperglycemia
hyperkalemia
hyperparathyroidism
hyperpituitarism
hyperthyroidism
hypocalcemia
hypoglycemia
hypokalemia
hyponatremia
hypopituitarism
hypothyroidism
ketoacidosis
metabolic syndrome
myxedema
neuroblastoma
obesity
panhypopituitarism
parathyroidoma
pheochromocytoma
thyroiditis
thyrotoxicosis

Surgical Terms

BUILT FROM WORD PARTS

The following terms can be translated using definitions of word parts. Further explanation is provided within parentheses as needed.

TERM	DEFINITION	TERM	DEFINITION
1. adrenalectomy (ad-rē-nal-EK-to-mē)	excision of (one or both) adrenal glands	3. thyroidectomy (thī-royd-EK-to-mē)	excision of the thyroid gland
2. parathyroidectomy (par-a-thī-royd-EK-to-mē)	excision of (one or more) parathyroid glands		

EXERCISE 13 ■ Pronounce and Spell

Practice pronunciation and spelling on paper and online.

1. **Practice on Paper**
   a. **Pronounce:** Read the phonetic spelling and say aloud the terms listed in the previous table. Refer to Table 2.2 Pronunciation Key as needed.
   b. **Spell:** Have a study partner read the terms aloud. Write the spelling of the terms on a separate sheet of paper.

2. **Practice Online**
   a. **Access** online learning resources. Go to evolve.elsevier.com > Evolve Resources > Student Resources.
   b. **Pronounce:** Select Audio Glossary > Chapter 16 > Exercise 13. Select a term to hear its pronunciation and repeat aloud.
   c. **Spell:** Select Activities > Chapter 16 > Spell Terms > Exercise 13. Select the audio icon and type the correct spelling of the term.

❏ Check the box when complete.

EXERCISE 14 ■ Analyze and Define

Analyze and define the following terms.

1. adrenalectomy

   _____

   _____

2. thyroidectomy

   _____

   _____

3. parathyroidectomy

   _____

   _____

EXERCISE 15 ■ Build

Build surgical terms for the following definitions by using the word parts you have learned.

1. excision of the thyroid gland   _____ / _____
                                        WR   S

2. excision of (one or both) adrenal glands   _____ / _____
                                                   WR   S

3. excision of (one or more) parathyroid glands   _____ / _____
                                                       WR   S

EXERCISE 16 ■ Review of Surgical Terms

Can you define, pronounce, and spell the following terms?

adrenalectomy
parathyroidectomy
thyroidectomy

Diagnostic Terms
NOT BUILT FROM WORD PARTS

Word parts may be present in the following terms; however, their full meanings cannot be translated using definitions of word parts alone.

DIAGNOSTIC IMAGING	
TERM	**DEFINITION**
1. **radioactive iodine uptake (RAIU)** (rā-dē-ō-AK-tiv) (Ī-ō-dīn) (UP-tāk)	nuclear medicine scan that measures thyroid function, particularly when distinguishing different causes of hyperthyroidism. Radioactive iodine is given to the patient orally, after which the amount of its uptake into the thyroid gland is measured. Images of the gland can also be obtained using this procedure.
2. **sestamibi parathyroid scan** (ses-ta-MIB-ē) (par-a-THĪ-royd) (skan)	nuclear medicine procedure used to localize hyperactive parathyroid glands. The glands that take up an abnormal amount of radioactive substance are identified and selected for surgical removal; the other parathyroid glands may be left in place.
3. **thyroid sonography** (THĪ-royd) (so-NOG-ra-fē)	ultrasound test of the thyroid gland used to help determine whether a thyroid nodule is likely benign or possibly malignant, including whether it is cystic or solid. Also used to help guide a fine needle aspiration (FNA) biopsy.

LABORATORY	
TERM	**DEFINITION**
4. **fasting blood sugar (FBS)** (FAST-ing) (blud) (SHOOG-er)	blood test to determine the amount of glucose (sugar) in the blood after fasting for 8 to 10 hours. Elevation may indicate diabetes mellitus.
5. **fine needle aspiration (FNA)** (FĪN) (NĒ-del) (as-pi-RĀ-shen)	biopsy technique that uses a narrow hollow needle to obtain tiny amounts of tissue for pathologic examination. Thyroid nodules are frequently biopsied using FNA.
6. **glycosylated hemoglobin (HbA1c)** (glī-KŌ-sa-lāt-ad) (HĒ-mō-glō-bin)	blood test used to diagnose diabetes and monitor its treatment by measuring the amount of glucose (sugar) bound to hemoglobin in the blood. HbA1c provides an indication of blood sugar level over the past three months, covering the 120-day lifespan of the red blood cell (also called **glycated hemoglobin, hemoglobin A1c, and A1c test**).
7. **thyroid-stimulating hormone level (TSH)** (THĪ-royd) (STIM-yuh-lāt-ing) (HŌR-mōn) (LEV-el)	blood test that measures the amount of thyroid-stimulating hormone in the blood; used to diagnose thyroid disorders (hyperthyroidism and hypothyroidism) and to monitor patients on thyroid replacement therapy
8. **thyroxine level (T_4)** (thī-ROK-sin) (LEV-el)	blood test that gives the direct measurement of the amount of thyroxine in the patient's blood. A greater-than-normal amount indicates hyperthyroidism; a less-than-normal amount indicates hypothyroidism.

658 Chapter 16 Endocrine System

EXERCISE 17 ■ Pronounce and Spell

Practice pronunciation and spelling on paper and online.

1. **Practice on Paper**
   a. **Pronounce:** Read the phonetic spelling and say aloud the terms listed in the previous table. Refer to Table 2.2 Pronunciation Key as needed.
   b. **Spell:** Have a study partner read the terms aloud. Write the spelling of the terms on a separate sheet of paper.

2. **Practice Online**
   a. **Access** online learning resources. Go to evolve.elsevier.com > Evolve Resources > Student Resources.
   b. **Pronounce:** Select Audio Glossary > Chapter 16 > Exercise 17. Select a term to hear its pronunciation and repeat aloud.
   c. **Spell:** Select Activities > Chapter 16 > Spell Terms > Exercise 17. Select the audio icon and type the correct spelling of the term.

❏ Check the box when complete.

EXERCISE 18 ■ Fill In

A Label

Write the diagnostic terms pictured and defined.

1. _____
   ultrasound test of the thyroid gland used to help determine whether a thyroid nodule is likely benign or possibly malignant

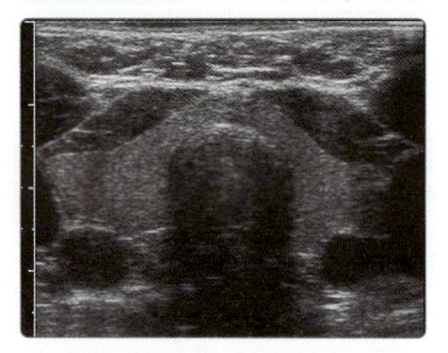

2. _____
   nuclear medicine scan that measures thyroid function, particularly when distinguishing different causes of hyperthyroidism

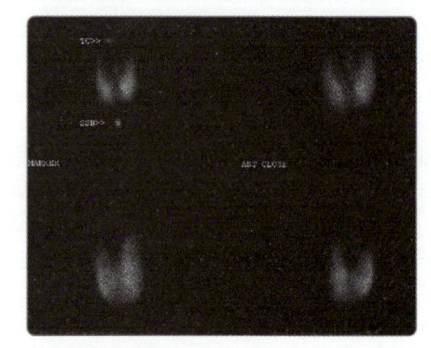

3. _____
   nuclear medicine procedure used to localize hyperactive parathyroid glands

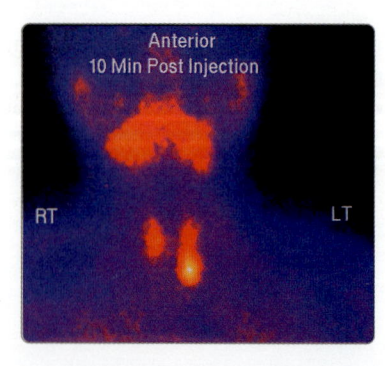

4. _____
   biopsy technique that uses a narrow hollow needle to obtain tiny amounts of tissue for pathologic examination

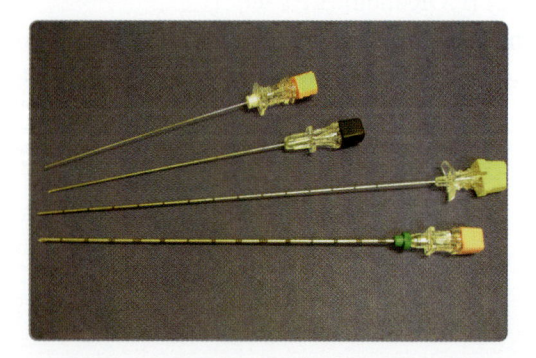

B Identify

Fill in the blanks with the correct terms

1. _____ _____ is a blood test that measures the direct amount of that hormone in the blood; higher-than-normal values represent hyperthyroidism.
2. A glucometer is a device that is frequently used to measure the amount of glucose in the blood after not eating for 8-10 hours, referred to as _____ _____ _____.
3. A test that provides an idea of blood sugar levels over the past three months, or _____ _____, is related to the lifespan of red blood cells, about 120 days.
4. A blood test that is used to diagnose thyroid disorders and to monitor patients on thyroid replacement therapy is called _____-_____ _____ _____.

EXERCISE 19 ■ Match

Match the terms in the first column with their correct definitions in the second column.

_____ 1. fasting blood sugar
_____ 2. sestamibi parathyroid scan
_____ 3. thyroxine level
_____ 4. radioactive iodine uptake
_____ 5. thyroid-stimulating hormone level
_____ 6. glycosylated hemoglobin
_____ 7. thyroid sonography
_____ 8. fine needle aspiration

a. nuclear medicine procedure used to localize hyperactive parathyroid glands
b. determines the amount of glucose in the blood after fasting for 8 to 10 hours
c. uses a hollow needle to obtain tiny amounts of tissue for pathologic examination
d. uses radioactive iodine to measure thyroid function
e. used to indicate whether a thyroid nodule is likely benign or possibly malignant
f. used to diagnose thyroid disorders and to monitor thyroid replacement therapy
g. measures the amount of thyroxine in the blood
h. provides an indication of blood sugar level over the past 3 months

EXERCISE 20 ■ Review of Diagnostic Terms

Can you define, pronounce, and spell the following terms?

fasting blood sugar (FBS)
fine needle aspiration (FNA)
glycosylated hemoglobin (HbA1c)
radioactive iodine uptake (RAIU)
sestamibi parathyroid scan
thyroid sonography
thyroid-stimulating hormone level (TSH)
thyroxine level (T$_4$)

Complementary Terms

BUILT FROM WORD PARTS AND *NOT* BUILT FROM WORD PARTS

■ Built from Word Parts

The first portion of the table contains Endocrine System Complementary Terms that can be translated using definitions of word parts. The second portion of the table contains Endocrine System Complementary Terms that cannot be fully understood using the definitions of word parts.

SIGNS AND SYMPTOMS

TERM	DEFINITION	TERM	DEFINITION
1. adrenocorticohyperplasia (a-drē-nō-kōr-ti-kō-hī-per-PLĀ-zha)	excessive development of the adrenal cortex (Note: hyper, a prefix, appears within this term.)	2. euglycemia (ū-glī-SĒ-mē-a)	normal (level of) sugar in the blood (within normal range)

TERM	DEFINITION	TERM	DEFINITION
3. euthyroid (ū-THĪ-royd)	normal thyroid gland activity	5. polydipsia (pol-ē-DIP-sē-a)	condition of much thirst
4. glycemia (glī-SĒ-mē-a)	sugar in the blood		

MEDICAL SPECIALTIES

TERM	DEFINITION	TERM	DEFINITION
6. endocrinologist (en-dō-kri-NOL-o-jist)	physician who studies and treats diseases of the endocrine (system)	7. endocrinology (en-dō-kri-NOL-o-jē)	study of the endocrine (system) (a branch of medicine dealing with diseases of the endocrine system)

DESCRIPTIVE TERMS

TERM	DEFINITION
8. cortical (KOR-ti-kal)	pertaining to the cortex

OTHER

TERM	DEFINITION
9. syndrome (SIN-drōm)	run together (signs and symptoms occurring together that are characteristic of a specific disorder)

■ NOT Built from Word Parts

SIGNS AND SYMPTOMS

TERM	DEFINITION
1. exophthalmos (ek-sof-THAL-mos)	abnormal protrusion of the eyeball
2. goiter (GOY-ter)	enlargement of the thyroid gland. May be caused by autoimmune diseases of the thyroid (Graves disease or Hashimoto thyroiditis), iodine deficiency, or the presence of multiple nodules.
3. tetany (TET-a-nē)	condition affecting nerves, causing muscle spasms as a result of low amounts of calcium in the blood; caused by a deficiency of the parathyroid hormone

OTHER

TERM	DEFINITION
4. hormone (HOR-mōn)	chemical substance secreted by an endocrine gland that is carried in the blood to a target tissue
5. incretins (in-KRĒ-tins)	group of hormones produced by the gastrointestinal system that stimulate the release of insulin from the pancreas and help preserve the beta cells. *Incretin mimetics* are medications that copy this action and help control blood sugar in patients with type 2 diabetes mellitus.
6. metabolism (me-TAB-ō-*lizm*)	sum total of all the chemical processes that take place in a living organism

Chapter 16 Endocrine System   661

EXERCISE 21 ■ Pronounce and Spell

Practice pronunciation and spelling on paper and online.

1. **Practice on Paper**
   a. **Pronounce:** Read the phonetic spelling and say aloud the terms listed in the previous table. Refer to Table 2.2 Pronunciation Key as needed.
   b. **Spell:** Have a study partner read the terms aloud. Write the spelling of the terms on a separate sheet of paper.

2. **Practice Online**
   a. **Access** online learning resources. Go to evolve.elsevier.com > Evolve Resources > Student Resources.
   b. **Pronounce:** Select Audio Glossary > Chapter 16 > Exercise 21. Select a term to hear its pronunciation and repeat aloud.
   c. **Spell:** Select Activities > Chapter 16 > Spell Terms > Exercise 21. Select the audio icon and type the correct spelling of the term.

❑ Check the box when complete.

EXERCISE 22 ■ Complementary Terms Built from Word Parts

A Analyze and Define

Analyze and define the following terms.

1. syndrome

2. endocrinologist

3. polydipsia

4. euglycemia

5. adrenocorticohyperplasia

6. euthyroid

7. cortical

8. endocrinology

9. glycemia

662   Chapter 16   Endocrine System

B Label

Build terms pictured by writing word parts above definitions.

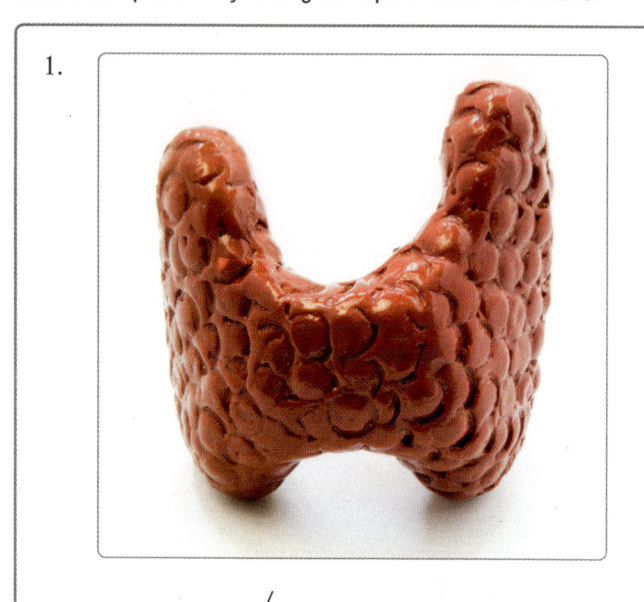

1.

_____ / _____
 normal   thyroid gland (activity)

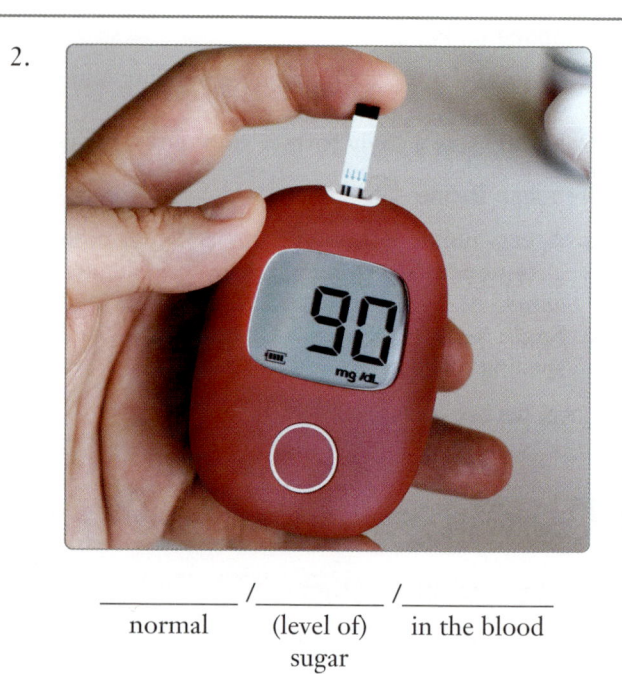

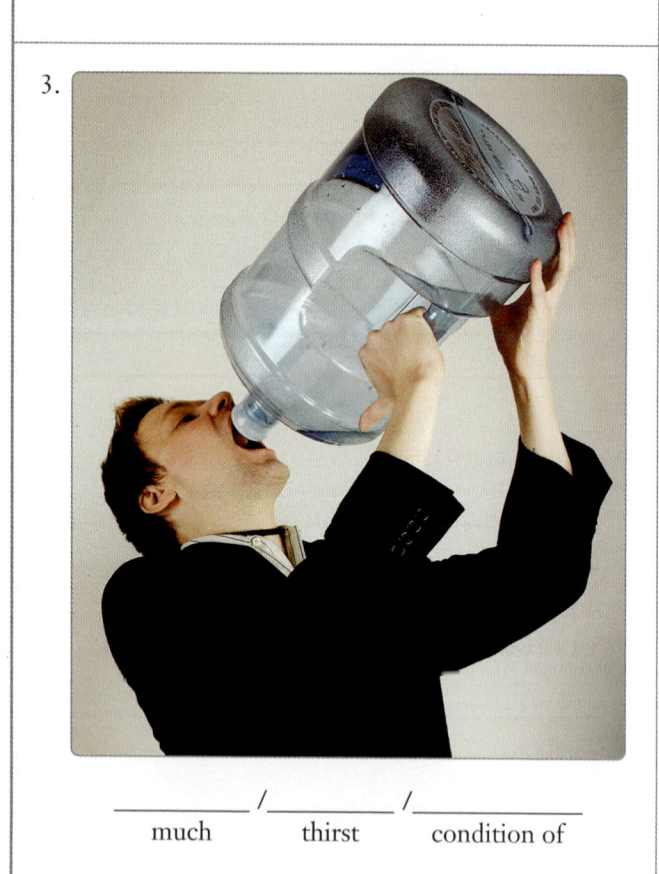

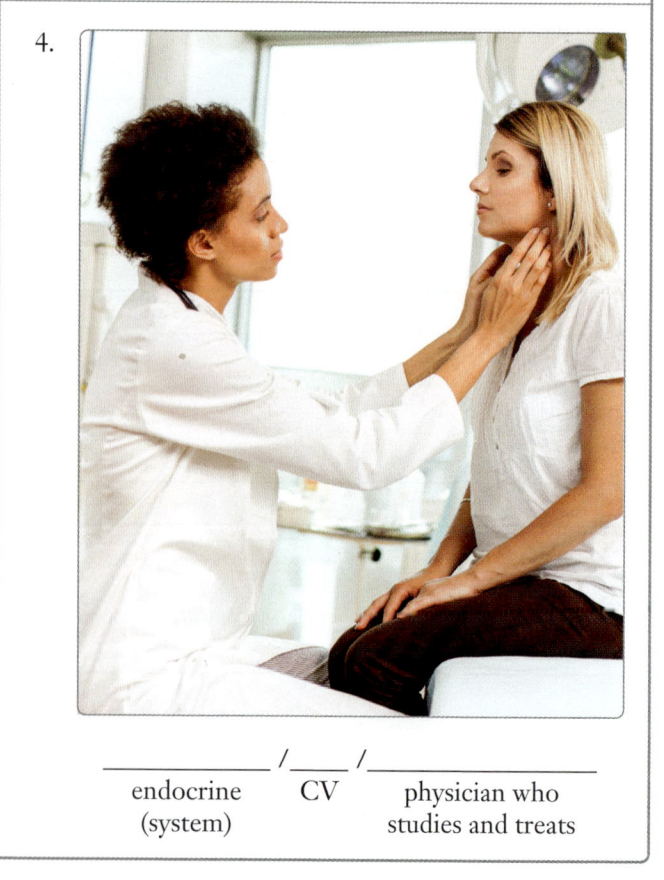

2.

_____ / _____ / _____
 normal   (level of)   in the blood
              sugar

3.

_____ / _____ / _____
 much   thirst   condition of

4.

_____ / ____ / _____
 endocrine   CV   physician who
 (system)   studies and treats

C Fill In

Build complementary terms for the following definitions by using the word parts you have learned.

1. sugar in the blood

   _____ / _____
   WR   S

2. run together (signs and symptoms occurring together)

   _____ / _____
   P   S(WR)

3. excessive development of the adrenal cortex

   _____ / CV / _____ / CV / ___ / ___
   WR   WR   P   S

4. study of the endocrine (system)

   _____ / CV / _____
   WR   S

5. pertaining to the cortex

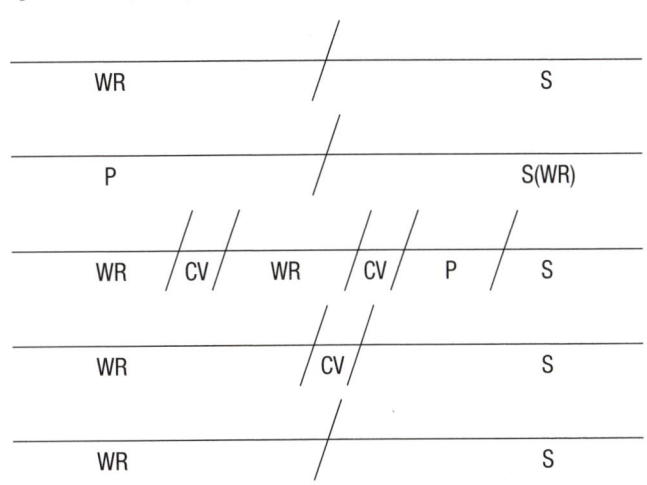

   _____ / _____
   WR   S

EXERCISE 23 ■ Complementary Terms NOT Built from Word Parts

A Match

Match the terms in the first column with their correct definitions in the second column

_____ 1. tetany
_____ 2. incretins
_____ 3. goiter
_____ 4. exophthalmos
_____ 5. metabolism
_____ 6. hormone

a. chemical substance secreted by an endocrine gland that is carried in the blood to a target tissue
b. nerve condition causing muscle spasms due to low amounts of calcium in the blood
c. sum total of all the chemical processes that take place in a living organism
d. may be caused by autoimmune diseases of the thyroid, iodine deficiency, or the presence of multiple nodules
e. abnormal protrusion of the eyeball
f. group of hormones that stimulate the release of insulin from the pancreas and help preserve the beta cells

B Label

Write the terms pictured and defined.

1. _____
   enlargement of the thyroid gland

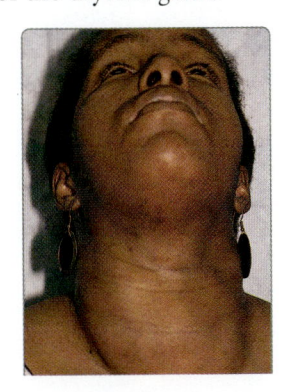

2. _____
   abnormal protrusion of the eyeball

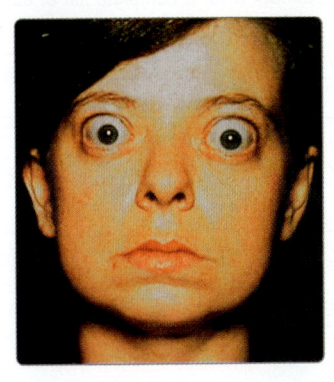

C Identify

Fill in the blanks with the correct terms.

1. The sum total of all the chemical processes that take place in a living organism is called its _____.
2. A chemical substance secreted by an endocrine gland is called a(n) _____.
3. _____ describes muscle spasms that result from low calcium due to parathyroid hormone deficiency.
4. Hormones produced by the gastrointestinal system that stimulate insulin release are called _____.

EXERCISE 24 ■ Review of Complementary Terms

Can you define, pronounce, and spell the following terms?

adrenocorticohyperplasia	cortical	glycemia	polydipsia
endocrinologist	euglycemia	hormone	syndrome
endocrinology	euthyroid	incretins	tetany
exophthalmos	goiter	metabolism	

Abbreviations

DISEASE AND DISORDERS

ABBREVIATION	TERM	ABBREVIATION	TERM
DI	diabetes insipidus	T1DM	type 1 diabetes mellitus (also abbreviated **T1D**)
DKA	diabetic ketoacidosis		
DM	diabetes mellitus	T2DM	type 2 diabetes mellitus (also abbreviated **T2D**)
SIADH	syndrome of inappropriate ADH (secretion)		

DIAGNOSTIC

ABBREVIATION	TERM	ABBREVIATION	TERM
ACTH	adrenocorticotropic hormone	LH	luteinizing hormone
ADH	antidiuretic hormone	PRL	prolactin
FBS	fasting blood sugar	PTH	parathyroid hormone
FNA	fine needle aspiration	RAIU	radioactive iodine uptake
FSH	follicle-stimulating hormone	TSH	thyroid-stimulating hormone
GH	growth hormone	T_4	thyroxine level
HbA1c	glycosylated hemoglobin		

Refer to **Appendix D** for a complete list of abbreviations.

EXERCISE 25 ■ Abbreviations

Write the terms abbreviated.

1. **DM** _____ _____ is a chronic disease characterized by elevated blood sugar. **T1DM** _____ _____ _____ is an autoimmune disease that generally starts in childhood or adolescence. It is important to monitor **FBS** _____ _____ _____, as episodes of severe hyperglycemia can lead to **DKA** _____ _____, which can be fatal.

2. **T2DM** _____ _____ _____ _____ has a slower onset, and is associated with obesity. **HbA1c** _____ _____ is used for both diagnosis and monitoring of treatment.

3. Patients presenting with Graves disease will likely have a high **T₄** _____ _____ and a low **TSH** _____-_____ _____. **RAIU** _____ _____ _____ testing can help differentiate this from other forms of thyrotoxicosis. **FNA** _____ _____ _____ of the thyroid may be needed if ultrasound reveals any nodules. If thyroidectomy is required, it is important to try to leave at least one parathyroid gland intact. A low level of **PTH** _____ _____ can reveal inadvertent removal of all four glands.

4. In addition to a semen analysis for their male partners, an infertility workup for women would include **FSH** _____-_____ _____ and **LH** _____ _____ levels.

5. **ADH** _____ _____ evaluation may be performed along with other blood and urine tests to help diagnose **DI** _____ _____, which results from too little ADH (or a lack of response to it), and **SIADH** _____ of _____ _____ (secretion), which results from too much ADH.

6. Functional pituitary tumors most commonly cause overproduction of specific hormones, including **GH** _____ _____, which leads to acromegaly, **ACTH** _____ _____ _____, which causes Cushing syndrome, and **PRL** _____, which can cause galactorrhea, infertility, and menstrual irregularities in women.

Chapter 16 Endocrine System

PRACTICAL APPLICATION

EXERCISE 26 — Case Study: Translate Between Everyday Language and Medical Language

CASE STUDY: Lily Macabal

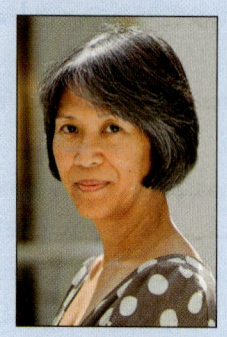

Lily Macabal has not been feeling well. She feels restless all the time and feels more irritable. Her appetite is increased, but she has been losing weight. She seems to always feel warm, and sometimes her heart races. Her hair seems thin and brittle. Recently she has noticed a lump in the front of her neck, and her husband says that her eyes seem to stick out more than they used to. She remembers her mother having a condition caused by too much thyroid hormone, and she wonders if she is going through the same thing. She sees her family doctor, who recommends a referral to an endocrine specialist.

Now that you have worked through Chapter 16 on the endocrine system, consider the medical terms that might be used to describe Mrs. Macabal's experience. See the Chapter at a Glance section at the end of the chapter for a list of terms that might apply.

A. Underline phrases in the case study that could be substituted with medical terms.

B. Write the medical term and its definition for three of the phrases you underlined.

MEDICAL TERM	DEFINITION
1. _____	_____
2. _____	_____
3. _____	_____

DOCUMENTATION: Excerpt from Endocrinology Clinic Visit

Mrs. Macabal saw an endocrinologist; an excerpt from her medical record is presented below.

This 56-year-old female was referred by her PCP for evaluation of a thyroid endocrinopathy. She has had multiple symptoms of hyperthyroidism and appears to be experiencing thyrotoxicosis. Her exophthalmos is suggestive of Graves disease. Thyroid sonography performed in our office showed no discrete nodules, with increased vascularity and diffuse hypoechoic tissue throughout. A TSH and free T_4 level have been ordered to assess her thyroid function. A radioactive iodine uptake test will be performed to assess her thyroid function. Consider treatment with either radioiodine therapy or near-total thyroidectomy, with the understanding that either treatment may result in hypothyroidism and require thyroid hormone replacement therapy.

C. Underline medical terms presented in Chapter 16 used in the previous excerpt from Mrs. Macabal's medical record. See the Chapter at a Glance section at the end of the chapter for a complete list.

D. Select and define three of the medical terms you underlined. To check your answers, go to Appendix A.

MEDICAL TERM	DEFINITION
1. _____	_____
2. _____	_____
3. _____	_____

Chapter 16 Endocrine System   667

EXERCISE 27 ■ Interact with Medical Documents

A

Read the report and complete it by writing medical terms on answer lines within the document. Definitions of terms to be written appear after the document.

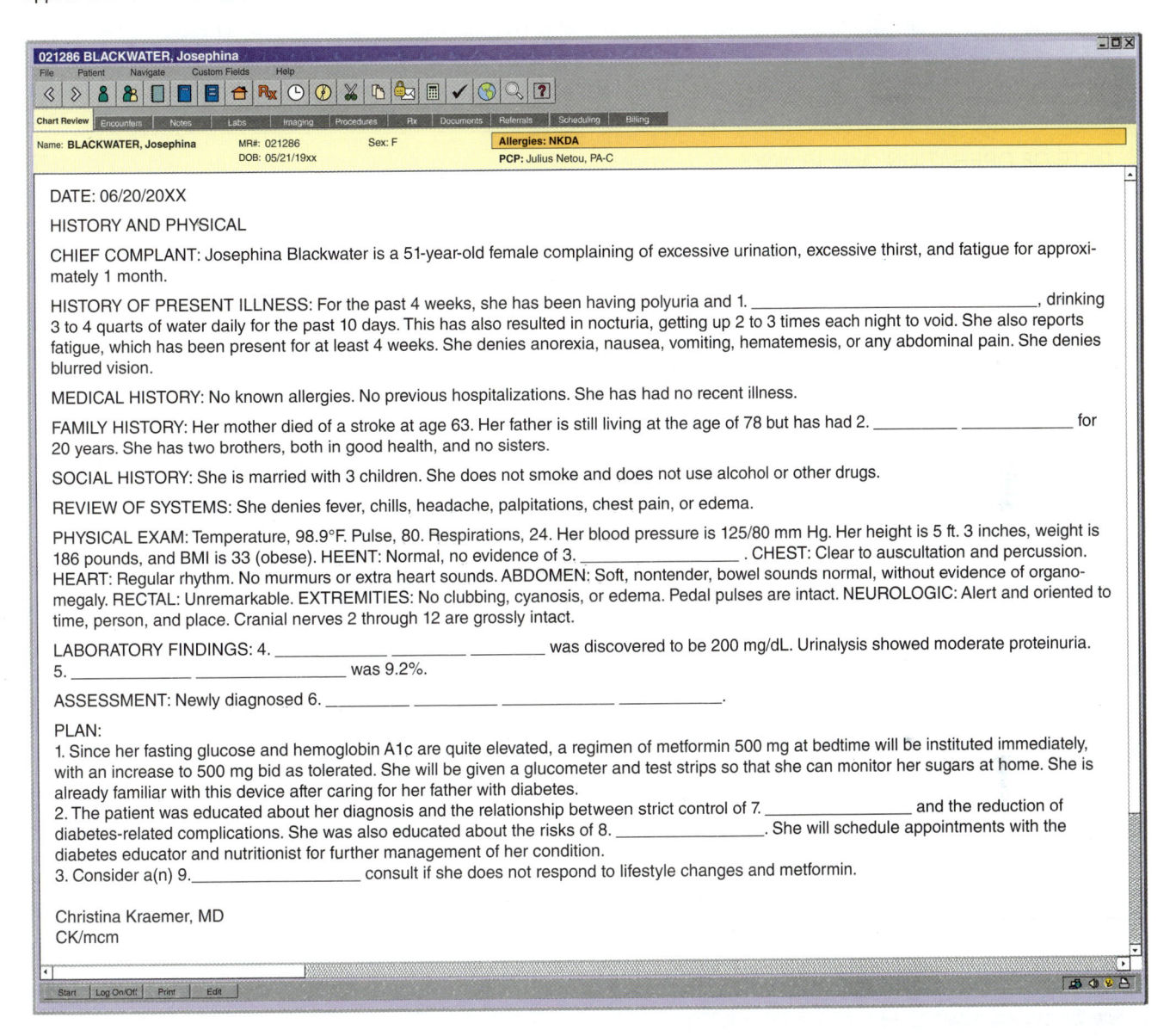

021286 BLACKWATER, Josephina

Name: BLACKWATER, Josephina MR#: 021286 Sex: F Allergies: NKDA
DOB: 05/21/19xx PCP: Julius Netou, PA-C

DATE: 06/20/20XX
HISTORY AND PHYSICAL
CHIEF COMPLAINT: Josephina Blackwater is a 51-year-old female complaining of excessive urination, excessive thirst, and fatigue for approximately 1 month.
HISTORY OF PRESENT ILLNESS: For the past 4 weeks, she has been having polyuria and 1. _____, drinking 3 to 4 quarts of water daily for the past 10 days. This has also resulted in nocturia, getting up 2 to 3 times each night to void. She also reports fatigue, which has been present for at least 4 weeks. She denies anorexia, nausea, vomiting, hematemesis, or any abdominal pain. She denies blurred vision.
MEDICAL HISTORY: No known allergies. No previous hospitalizations. She has had no recent illness.
FAMILY HISTORY: Her mother died of a stroke at age 63. Her father is still living at the age of 78 but has had 2. _____ _____ for 20 years. She has two brothers, both in good health, and no sisters.
SOCIAL HISTORY: She is married with 3 children. She does not smoke and does not use alcohol or other drugs.
REVIEW OF SYSTEMS: She denies fever, chills, headache, palpitations, chest pain, or edema.
PHYSICAL EXAM: Temperature, 98.9°F. Pulse, 80. Respirations, 24. Her blood pressure is 125/80 mm Hg. Her height is 5 ft. 3 inches, weight is 186 pounds, and BMI is 33 (obese). HEENT: Normal, no evidence of 3. _____. CHEST: Clear to auscultation and percussion. HEART: Regular rhythm. No murmurs or extra heart sounds. ABDOMEN: Soft, nontender, bowel sounds normal, without evidence of organomegaly. RECTAL: Unremarkable. EXTREMITIES: No clubbing, cyanosis, or edema. Pedal pulses are intact. NEUROLOGIC: Alert and oriented to time, person, and place. Cranial nerves 2 through 12 are grossly intact.
LABORATORY FINDINGS: 4. _____ _____ _____ was discovered to be 200 mg/dL. Urinalysis showed moderate proteinuria.
5. _____ _____ was 9.2%.
ASSESSMENT: Newly diagnosed 6. _____ _____ _____ _____.
PLAN:
1. Since her fasting glucose and hemoglobin A1c are quite elevated, a regimen of metformin 500 mg at bedtime will be instituted immediately, with an increase to 500 mg bid as tolerated. She will be given a glucometer and test strips so that she can monitor her sugars at home. She is already familiar with this device after caring for her father with diabetes.
2. The patient was educated about her diagnosis and the relationship between strict control of 7. _____ and the reduction of diabetes-related complications. She was also educated about the risks of 8. _____. She will schedule appointments with the diabetes educator and nutritionist for further management of her condition.
3. Consider a(n) 9. _____ consult if she does not respond to lifestyle changes and metformin.

Christina Kraemer, MD
CK/mcm

Definitions of Medical Terms to Complete the Document

Write the medical terms defined on corresponding answer lines in the document.

1. excessive thirst
2. chronic disease involving a disorder of carbohydrate metabolism and characterized by elevated blood sugar
3. abnormal protrusion of the eyeball
4. blood test to determine the amount of glucose (sugar) in the blood after fasting for 8 to 10 hours
5. the test measuring the amount of hemoglobin coated in sugar over the lifespan of the red blood cell
6. T2DM
7. excessive sugar in the blood
8. deficient sugar in the blood
9. study of the endocrine (system)

668 Chapter 16 Endocrine System

B

Read the medical report and answer the questions below it.

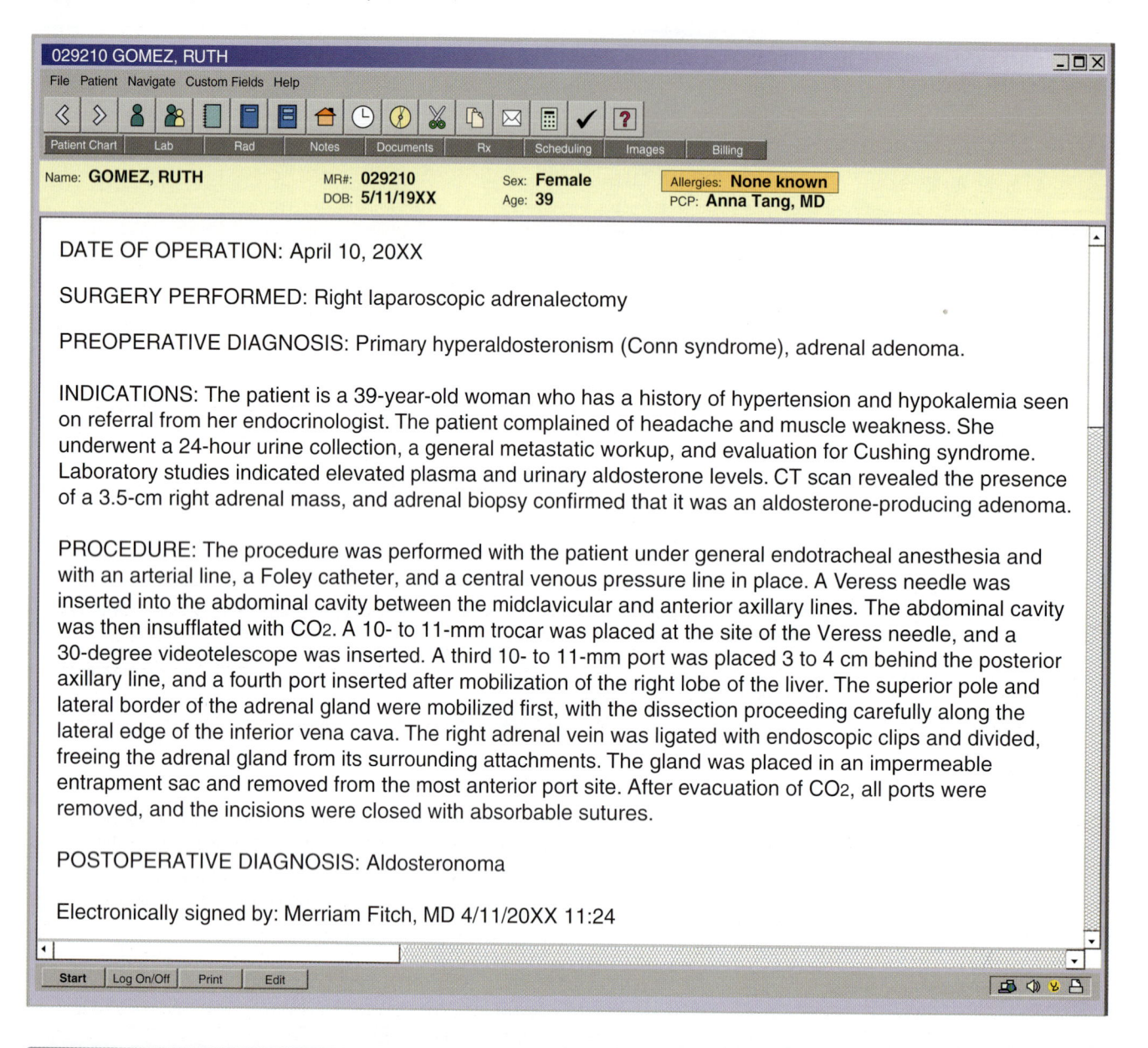

029210 GOMEZ, RUTH

File Patient Navigate Custom Fields Help

Patient Chart | Lab | Rad | Notes | Documents | Rx | Scheduling | Images | Billing

Name: **GOMEZ, RUTH**   MR#: **029210**   Sex: **Female**   Allergies: **None known**
DOB: **5/11/19XX**   Age: **39**   PCP: **Anna Tang, MD**

DATE OF OPERATION: April 10, 20XX

SURGERY PERFORMED: Right laparoscopic adrenalectomy

PREOPERATIVE DIAGNOSIS: Primary hyperaldosteronism (Conn syndrome), adrenal adenoma.

INDICATIONS: The patient is a 39-year-old woman who has a history of hypertension and hypokalemia seen on referral from her endocrinologist. The patient complained of headache and muscle weakness. She underwent a 24-hour urine collection, a general metastatic workup, and evaluation for Cushing syndrome. Laboratory studies indicated elevated plasma and urinary aldosterone levels. CT scan revealed the presence of a 3.5-cm right adrenal mass, and adrenal biopsy confirmed that it was an aldosterone-producing adenoma.

PROCEDURE: The procedure was performed with the patient under general endotracheal anesthesia and with an arterial line, a Foley catheter, and a central venous pressure line in place. A Veress needle was inserted into the abdominal cavity between the midclavicular and anterior axillary lines. The abdominal cavity was then insufflated with CO_2. A 10- to 11-mm trocar was placed at the site of the Veress needle, and a 30-degree videotelescope was inserted. A third 10- to 11-mm port was placed 3 to 4 cm behind the posterior axillary line, and a fourth port inserted after mobilization of the right lobe of the liver. The superior pole and lateral border of the adrenal gland were mobilized first, with the dissection proceeding carefully along the lateral edge of the inferior vena cava. The right adrenal vein was ligated with endoscopic clips and divided, freeing the adrenal gland from its surrounding attachments. The gland was placed in an impermeable entrapment sac and removed from the most anterior port site. After evacuation of CO_2, all ports were removed, and the incisions were closed with absorbable sutures.

POSTOPERATIVE DIAGNOSIS: Aldosteronoma

Electronically signed by: Merriam Fitch, MD 4/11/20XX 11:24

Start | Log On/Off | Print | Edit

Use the medical report above to answer the questions.

1. Which procedure was performed during surgery:
   a. excision of a parathyroid gland
   b. surgical repair of the thyroid gland
   c. excision of an adrenal gland
   d. surgical repair of the thymus

2. The patient had a history of:
   a. excessive sugar in the blood
   b. deficient potassium in the blood
   c. deficient sodium in the blood
   d. deficient calcium in the blood

3. The patient was evaluated for a:
   a. group of symptoms from the excessive production of cortisol
   b. condition caused by congenital absence of the thyroid gland
   c. syndrome caused by deficient secretion from the adrenal cortex
   d. condition causing muscle spasms resulting from low amounts of calcium

Chapter 16 Endocrine System   669

EXERCISE 28 ■ Use Medical Language in Online Electronic Health Records

Select the correct medical terms to complete three medical records in one patient's electronic file.

Access online resources at evolve.elsevier.com > Evolve Resources > Student Resources > Activities > Chapter 16 > Electronic Health Records

Topic: Hyperparathyroidism
Record 1, Chart Review: Preoperative Note
Record 2, Imaging: Nuclear Medicine Report
Record 3, Encounters: Office Visit Report

❏ Check the box when complete.

EXERCISE 29 ■ Use Medical Terms in Clinical Statements

For each phrase printed in bold, circle the medical term or abbreviation defined. Answers are listed in Appendix A. For pronunciation practice, read the answers aloud.

1. A **biopsy technique that uses a narrow hollow needle to obtain tiny amounts of tissue for pathologic examination** (glycosylated hemoglobin, fine needle aspiration, fasting blood sugar) is frequently performed on thyroid nodules. **Ultrasound test of the thyroid gland used to help determine whether a thyroid nodule is likely benign or possibly malignant** (sestamibi parathyroid scan, radioactive iodine uptake, thyroid sonography) is often used to localize the lesion. The procedure may be performed by a(n) **physician who studies and treats diseases of the endocrine system** (endocrinologist, pathologist, hematologist) or by a radiologist.

2. Unlike the **blood test to determine the amount of glucose (sugar) in the blood after fasting for 8–10 hours** (fasting blood sugar, glycosylated hemoglobin, radioactive iodine uptake test), **blood test used to diagnose diabetes and monitor its treatment by measuring the amount of glucose (sugar) bound to hemoglobin in the blood** (fasting blood sugar, glycosylated hemoglobin, radioactive iodine uptake test) results are not altered by eating habits the day before the test.

3. The primary treatment for **tumor of the adrenal medulla** (pheochromocytoma, adrenomegaly, thyrotoxicosis) is surgical removal of the tumor by laparoscopic **excision of an adrenal gland** (adenectomy, adrenalectomy, thyroidectomy).

4. **Excess of body fat, which increases body weight** (obesity, metabolic syndrome, gigantism) is associated with type 2 **chronic disease involving a disorder of carbohydrate metabolism characterized by elevated blood sugar** (Cushing syndrome, ketoacidosis, diabetes mellitus), hypertension, and coronary artery disease. The cornerstone of treatment is lifestyle modification, which includes counseling on diet, exercise, and goals for weight loss. Pharmacologic therapy (medication) may be considered in patients with a body mass index of 30-39 kg/m^2. Bariatric surgery is often used in patients with a BMI of ≥35 kg/m^2 or those with a lower BMI and other conditions, such as **group of signs and symptoms including insulin resistance, obesity characterized by excessive fat around the area of the waist and abdomen, hypertension, hyperglycemia, elevated triglycerides, and low levels of the "good" cholesterol HDL** (Addison disease, metabolic syndrome, Graves disease).

EXERCISE 30 ■ Pronounce Medical Terms in Use

Practice pronunciation of terms by reading aloud the following paragraph. Use the phonetic spellings to assist with pronunciation. The script also contains medical terms not presented in the chapter. If interested, research their meanings in a medical dictionary or a reliable online source.

> A 65-year-old female patient presented to her doctor because of a 10-pound weight gain, fatigue, hair loss, dry skin, and cold intolerance. She was referred to an **endocrinologist** (en-dō-kri-NOL-o-jist) who established a diagnosis of **hypothyroidism** (hī-pō-THĪ-royd-izm) after test results indicated an elevated **thyroid-stimulating hormone level** (THĪ-royd) (STIM-yuh-lāt-ing) (HŌR-mōn) (LEV-el) and a low **thyroxine level** (thī-ROK-sin) (LEV-el). Approximately 20 years ago she had a painless thyroid nodule. At that time, **thyroid sonography** (THĪ-royd) (so-NOG-ra-fē) and **fine needle aspiration** (FĪN) (NĒ-del) (as-pi-RĀ-shen) were performed; a diagnosis of thyroid cancer was confirmed, but it had not spread beyond the gland. She underwent a **thyroidectomy** (thī-royd-EK-to-mē) and received thyroid hormone replacement therapy thereafter. She remained in a **euthyroid** (ū-THĪ-royd) state until she stopped taking the medication 6 months ago. Consequently, she became hypothyroid and could have easily developed **myxedema** (mik-se-DĒ-ma) if she had not sought treatment.

CHAPTER REVIEW

EXERCISE 31 ■ Chapter Content Quiz

Test your understanding of terms and abbreviations introduced in this chapter. Circle the letter for the medical term or abbreviation related to the words in italics.

1. Inez Villalvazo was diagnosed with Hashimoto thyroiditis after she presented to her doctor with *enlargement of the thyroid gland*.
   a. myxedema
   b. tetany
   c. goiter

2. An episode of *serious condition resulting from uncontrolled diabetes mellitus in which acid ketones accumulate* resulted in admission to the intensive care unit for Mr. Khalile.
   a. ketoacidosis
   b. tetany
   c. euglycemia

3. Diana Worthington complained of weight loss and muscle aches, as well as darkening of her skin. She was diagnosed with *chronic syndrome resulting from a deficiency in hormonal secretion from the adrenal cortex*.
   a. Cushing syndrome
   b. Graves disease
   c. Addison disease

4. Malini Sobel noticed polydipsia and polyuria and found herself drinking a lot of water. This was related to *decreased secretion of antidiuretic hormone by the posterior lobe of the pituitary gland*.
   a. diabetes mellitus
   b. diabetes insipidus
   c. diabetic retinopathy

5. Ryan McAvoy had *condition brought about by hypersecretion of growth hormone by the pituitary gland before puberty* and was over 6 feet tall as an 11-year-old.
   a. gigantism
   b. acromegaly
   c. metabolic syndrome

6. *Deficient sodium in the blood* and *excessive potassium in the blood* are two laboratory findings in Addison disease.
   a. hypoglycemia and hypercalcemia
   b. hyponatremia and hyperkalemia
   c. hypocalcemia and hyperglycemia

7. A(n) *excision of (one or both) adrenal glands* was performed on Mr. Rockov after a tumor was discovered.
   a. thyroidectomy
   b. adrenalectomy
   c. parathyroidectomy

8. Mrs. Lucio has been working hard to help control her diabetes mellitus with diet and exercise. Her recent *blood test used to diagnose diabetes and monitor its treatment by measuring the amount of glucose (sugar) bound to hemoglobin in the blood* showed marked improvement since the last test 3 months ago.
   a. FSH
   b. FBS
   c. HbA1c

9. Dr. Chen told Mrs. Onwubiko that weight loss, regular exercise, and healthy eating are central in the treatment and prevention of *a group of health problems including insulin resistance, obesity, hypertension, hyperglycemia, elevated triglycerides, and low levels of HDL*.
   a. metabolic syndrome
   b. Cushing syndrome
   c. irritable bowel syndrome

10. Congenital hypothyroidism is a(n) *any disease of the endocrine system* that is characterized by puffy features, mental deficiency, large tongue, and short stature.
    a. adrenopathy
    b. neuropathy
    c. endocrinopathy

11. Dr. Turecki performed a *biopsy technique that uses a narrow hollow needle to obtain tiny amounts of tissue for pathologic examination* on the patient who had been found to have a multinodular goiter on thyroid sonography.
    a. thyroid-stimulating hormone level (TSH)
    b. thyroxine level (T_4)
    c. fine needle aspiration (FNA)

12. *Excessive development of the adrenal cortex* was the cause of Cushing syndrome in Mr. Lim when he presented with "moon face," "buffalo hump," and hypertension.
    a. pheochromocytoma
    b. thyrotoxicosis
    c. adrenocorticohyperplasia

13. The pharmacist told Mrs. Tranh that her new diabetes medication acted in the same way as *a group of hormones produced by the gastrointestinal system that stimulate the release of insulin from the pancreas*.
    a. hormones
    b. incretins
    c. corticoids

14. Mrs. Webber had *nuclear medicine scan that measures thyroid function using radioactive iodine* and was diagnosed with Graves disease. Since she had her thyroid removed, she has been on thyroid hormone replacement therapy and had periodic measurements of her *blood test that measures the amount of thyroid-stimulating hormone in the blood*.
    a. thyroid scan, T_4
    b. RAIU, TSH
    c. thyroid sonography, LH

15. Dr. Nair performed a parathyroidectomy on Mrs. Chaugary to treat her *state of excessive parathyroid gland activity*.
    a. hyperpituitarism
    b. hyperthyroidism
    c. hyperparathyroidism

16. Rodrigo Garcia was diagnosed during infancy with *malignant cancer that often starts in the adrenal medulla, composed of immature nerve cells*; luckily, it had not metastasized.
    a. neuroblastoma
    b. pheochromocytoma
    c. parathyroidoma

17. Jianna Roberts had a goiter and a high TSH level; she was eventually diagnosed with *disease in which thyroid gland cells are destroyed by autoimmune processes*.
    a. Graves disease
    b. Hashimoto thyroiditis
    c. Cushing syndrome

18. *Result of decreased secretion of antidiuretic hormone by the posterior lobe of the pituitary gland* was the cause of Max Mazet's polydipsia.
    a. DI
    b. SIADH
    c. DKA

19. Sheehan syndrome is a rare cause of *state of total deficient pituitary gland activity* that results from severe blood loss or low blood pressure during pregnancy or delivery.
    a. hypopituitarism
    b. panhypopituitarism
    c. hypothyroidism

20. *Nuclear medicine procedure used to localize hyperactive parathyroid glands* would be useful in diagnosing a parathyroidoma.
    a. parathyroidectomy
    b. sestamibi parathyroid scan
    c. fine needle aspiration

Chapter 16   Endocrine System

CHAPTER AT A GLANCE — Word Parts New to This Chapter

COMBINING FORMS

acr/o	calc/i	endocrin/o	natr/o	pituitar/o	
adren/o	cortic/o	glyc/o	parathyroid/o	thyroid/o	
adrenal/o	dips/o	kal/i			

SUFFIXES

-drome

CHAPTER AT A GLANCE — Endocrine System Terms Built from Word Parts

DISEASE AND DISORDER
- acromegaly
- adrenalitis
- adrenomegaly
- endocrinopathy
- hypercalcemia
- hyperglycemia
- hyperkalemia
- hyperparathyroidism
- hyperpituitarism
- hyperthyroidism
- hypocalcemia
- hypoglycemia
- hypokalemia
- hyponatremia
- hypopituitarism
- hypothyroidism
- panhypopituitarism
- parathyroidoma
- thyroiditis

SURGICAL
- adrenalectomy
- parathyroidectomy
- thyroidectomy

COMPLEMENTARY
- adrenocorticohyperplasia
- cortical
- endocrinologist
- endocrinology
- euglycemia
- euthyroid
- glycemia
- polydipsia
- syndrome

CHAPTER AT A GLANCE — Endocrine System Terms NOT Built from Word Parts

DISEASE AND DISORDER
- Addison disease
- congenital hypothyroidism
- Cushing syndrome
- diabetes insipidus (DI)
- diabetes mellitus (DM)
- gigantism
- Graves disease
- Hashimoto thyroiditis
- ketoacidosis
- metabolic syndrome
- myxedema
- neuroblastoma
- obesity
- pheochromocytoma
- thyrotoxicosis

DIAGNOSTIC
- fasting blood sugar (FBS)
- fine needle aspiration (FNA)
- glycosylated hemoglobin (HbA1c)
- radioactive iodine uptake (RAIU)
- sestamibi parathyroid scan
- thyroid sonography
- thyroid-stimulating hormone level (TSH)
- thyroxine level (T$_4$)

COMPLEMENTARY
- exophthalmos
- goiter
- hormone
- incretins
- metabolism
- tetany

△ CAPSTONE

EXERCISE 32 ■ Scribe It

Drawing on what you have learned from studying chapters 1–16, practice scribing notes from a patient encounter by completing medical documentation. *Note: the following abbreviations are used, MD = medical doctor and Pt = patient.*

> **Setting:** Triage room in the Emergency Department of an urban hospital
> **Patient Information:** Adele Sun, 32-year-old female
> **Provider:** Dr. Laja Sharma, Emergency Physician

MD: Hello, my name is Dr. Sharma, and this is my scribe, Connor. He will be taking notes. Can I please confirm your name and age?
Pt: Adele Sun. I am 32 years old.
MD: How would you like to be addressed?
Pt: Please call me Addy.
MD: First, can you tell me why you came to the Emergency Department today?
Pt: I can't catch my breath.
MD: I'm sorry to hear that. Can you walk me through from when this started until now?
Pt: About 5 days ago, I started having a dry cough. I also felt like I had a fever, but sometimes I felt very cold. For the last two days, I have been coughing up green phlegm. I have been having sudden attacks of coughing so often that I have difficulty breathing.

Chapter 16 Endocrine System 673

MD: I'd like to ask you some more focused questions about your symptoms. Have you had any pain with this fever and cough?
Pt: Yes, I've had pain in my back, on the right, under my ribs.
MD: Have you passed out or felt as if you might pass out?
Pt: I have passed out a few times before, and now it feels like I might.
MD: Have you had any headaches or muscle aches?
Pt: Yes, but I have also had those for years.
MD: Have you had weakness or excessive tiredness?
Pt: I have had that for years also, but it seems worse in the last few days.
MD: How about vomiting or frequent, loose stools?
Pt: No.
MD: Thanks for answering those questions; now I'd like to ask you some questions about any conditions you have been diagnosed with in the past.
Pt: Okay.
MD: Can you tell me about any medical conditions you have, and when they were diagnosed?
Pt: I have low thyroid that was diagnosed 3 years ago. I also have been dealing with depression and anxiety for about 4 years.
MD: Okay, thanks. Have you had any surgeries?
Pt: I had my thyroid removed about 3 years ago.
MD: And what was the reason for the thyroid removal?
Pt: They said I had a condition where the thyroid gland is overactive; I also had an enlarged thyroid gland, and my eyes seemed to stick out too much.
MD: Are you taking any medications?
Pt: Yes, I take levothyroxine and sertraline.
MD: Do you have any allergies to medications?
Pt: Sulfa drugs
MD: What happens when you take them?
Pt: I get a rash.
MD: Have you ever been pregnant?
Pt: No, I haven't.
MD: When was your last menstrual period?
Pt: About 5 months ago.
MD: Are your periods regular? If not, how long have they been irregular?
Pt: I don't have regular periods; they are infrequent and I don't have much flow. It has been this way for about 3 years.
MD: Are you up to date on vaccinations? Specifically, have you had a COVID-19 vaccine and a flu shot?
Pt: I am up to date on all vaccinations, including COVID, but I haven't had a flu shot.

A Subjective

Fill in portions of the medical record based on the previous dialogue. See underlined phrases for reference. Use Appendix A to check your answers.

Chief Complaint (CC): "I can't _____."

History of Present Illness (HPI): Adele Sun is a ___- year-old female with a history of _____ disease, major _____, and _____, who presents with dyspnea. 5 days ago, she became _____ and had a dry cough. 2 days ago, she began producing green _____ and started having _____ of coughing. She has been coughing so much that she is now having _____. She also reports posterior thoracic pain, under her ribs. Associated symptoms include chills, near _____, worsening weakness, and worsening _____. Other symptoms include _____ and _____, although she states these have been present for "years." She denies _____ or _____.

Past Medical History (PMH): _____ after surgery for _____, diagnosed 3 years ago; major depression and anxiety, diagnosed _____ years ago

Surgeries: _____ 3 years ago

OB/GYN hx: _____ 0 _____ 0 (gravida/para), LMP _____ months ago, _____ last 3 years

Medications: L_____ 0.75 µg (microgram) po qd, S_____ 150 mg po qd

Allergies: sulfa medications cause a rash

Vaccination Status: up to date on all required _____ and _____-19. Has not received a _____ shot this year.

B Objective

Write the medical terms and abbreviations defined in parentheses.

Physical Examination (PE)

Vital signs: BP: 90/60 mm Hg, P: 116, R: 24, T: 39.4 deg C, BMI: 22, Pulse oximetry: 90%

Gen: Thin, ill-appearing female in moderate distress, alert and conversant, with some limitations due to (rapid breathing) _____.

Skin: appears unusually tanned, with areas of hyperpigmentation noted on the elbows, knees, and palmar creases. (white patches on the skin caused by the destruction of melanocytes) _____ on the face is also noted. Hair pattern is more sparse than expected for patient's age.

Throat: mucous membranes moist, hyperpigmentation noted, no (redness) _____

Neck: without (disease of lymph nodes/enlarged lymph nodes) _____; midline scar noted at level of thyroid

Respiratory: dullness to (tapping of body surface to determine density) _____ right posterior chest, with decreased breath sounds, (whistling noises with a high pitch) _____, and (discontinuous sounds heard during inspiration that resemble the sound of the rustling of cellophane) _____ in that area. Otherwise, clear to (listening through a stethoscope for sounds) _____ and percussion. (Pertaining to the chest) _____ expansion normal.

Cardiac: (condition of rapid heart rate) _____, regular rhythm. No (unusual sounds heard during auscultation of the heart caused by turbulent blood flow) _____

Abdomen: normal bowel sounds without (sounds heard over an artery during auscultation resulting from vibration in the vessel wall caused by turbulent blood flow) _____. Mild diffuse tenderness in RUQ and LUQ. No masses. Liver and spleen normal size by percussion.

Musculoskeletal: diffuse (without development/process of wasting away) _____ noted in larger muscles bilaterally. Tenderness noted at the (pertaining to the patella and femur) _____ joints, (pertaining to the wrist) _____ joints, and over the (pertaining to the loins) _____ and (pertaining to the sacrum) _____ vertebrae.

Neurologic: muscle strength is 4 out of 5 bilaterally for upper and lower extremities. Sensation is intact. (abbreviation for deep tendon reflexes) _____s intact bilaterally. (Pertaining to the skull) _____ nerves 2-12 intact.

Extremities: (abnormal condition of blue) _____ noted at fingertips, no (puffy swelling of tissue from the accumulation of fluid) _____.

Pulses: (pertaining to the radius) _____, (pertaining to the back, starting with a "p") _____ tibial, and (pertaining to the back, starting with a "d") _____ pedal pulses are diminished bilaterally

C Assessment and Plan

Write the medical terms and abbreviations defined in parentheses.

This 32-year-old female with a history of Graves disease, major depression, and anxiety disorder, presented to the emergency department with a 5-day history of fever and (periodic, sudden attack, plural) _____ of coughing, and a 2-day history of dyspnea with a cough productive of green (mucus from the lungs, bronchi, and trachea expelled through the mouth) _____. Other significant symptoms include posterior thoracic pain and a longer history of (muscle pain, plural) _____, (head pain, plural) _____, (persistent, excessive tiredness and lack of energy that interferes with daily activities unrelated to exertion or lack of sleep) _____, weakness, and near (fainting) _____.

On physical exam she was found to be (having a fever) _____, with (rapid breathing) _____ and (condition of rapid heart rate) _____, and she had borderline (blood pressure that is below normal) _____. Pulse oximetry was 90%. Lung findings were suspicious for (diseased state of the lung) _____, and the (pertaining to away) _____ cyanosis supported the impression of (condition of deficient oxygen) _____. 2 liters oxygen by nasal cannula was immediately started after (noninvasive method of measuring oxygen in the blood) _____ was performed, and her values came up to 95%.

Given the acute nature of her respiratory symptoms, her vitals, and the (pertaining to the lungs) _____ physical exam findings, we believe she may have pneumonia, likely of viral or bacterial (study of causes of diseases) _____. (Incision into a vein with a needle to remove blood for testing) _____ was performed, an (pertaining to within the vein) _____ line was placed, and the following labs have been ordered: (abbreviation, laboratory test for basic blood screening that measures various aspects of erythrocytes, leukocytes, and thrombocytes) _____, chemistry panel, sputum (abbreviation for test performed on a sample to determine the presence of pathogenic bacteria) _____, rapid influenza diagnosis test, COVID-19 test, and a (abbreviation, blood test measuring the amount of thyroid-stimulating hormone) _____ level.

Diagnostic imaging: an (abbreviation, pertaining to the front and to the back) _____ portable (record of x-rays) _____ was ordered, and we are awaiting results.

D Emergency Department Course

Write the medical terms and abbreviations defined in parentheses.

While waiting for diagnostic imaging and lab results, Addy became nonresponsive/ (state of being unaware of surroundings and incapable of responding to stimuli) _____ and her (pressure exerted by the blood against blood vessel walls) _____ dropped to 66/26 mm Hg. A large infusion of intravenous isotonic saline was given. Her lab results came back and indicated (deficient sodium in the blood) _____ and (excessive potassium in the blood) _____. Based on these findings, the treatment team suspected adrenal crisis and treated her with 100 mg of IV hydrocortisone. (Abbreviation, adrenocorticotropic hormone) _____ and cortisol levels were also requested. Rapid influenza and COVID-19 tests were negative. Chest x-ray revealed a right lower lobe pneumonia with a small (fluid in the pleural cavity) _____. She received (abbreviation, intravenous) _____ antibiotics to treat the pneumonia. Her blood pressure returned to the normal range, and she became (awake, alert, aware of one's surroundings) _____. She was admitted to the inpatient floor of the hospital with a (state of complete knowledge/identifying a disease) _____ of adrenal crisis, likely caused by (chronic syndrome resulting from a deficiency in the hormonal secretion of the adrenal cortex) _____, precipitated by pneumonia.

Appendix A

Answer Key

ANSWERS TO CHAPTER 1 EXERCISES

Exercise 1
1. b
2. a
3. c
4. d
5. a
6. d
7. c
8. b

Exercise 2
Built from Word Parts; NOT Built from Word Parts

Exercise 3
1. a word part that is the core of the word
2. a word part attached to the end of the word root to modify its meaning
3. a word part attached to the beginning of a word root to modify its meaning

Exercise 4
1. a word part, usually an o, used to ease pronunciation
2. used
3. vowel
4. word roots
5. not

Exercise 5
a word root with the combining vowel attached, separated by a slash

Exercise 6
1. b
2. a
3. d
4. e
5. c

Exercise 7
1. *F*, a medical term may begin with the word root and have no prefix.
2. *F*, if the suffix begins with a vowel, the combining vowel is usually not used.
3. *T*
4. *T*
5. *F*, o is the combining vowel most often used.
6. *T*
7. *F*, a combining vowel is used between two word roots or between a word root and a suffix to ease pronunciation.
8. *F*, a combining form is a word root with a combining vowel attached and is not one of the four word parts.
9. *T*

Exercise 8
A
1. Divide the term into word parts with slashes.
2. Label each word part with abbreviations.
3. Identify each combining form by underlining the word root and combining vowel, and then writing the abbreviation CF below the underlined combining form.

B
WR CV S
oste/o/pathy
  CF

Exercise 9
A
apply the meaning of each word part

B
disease of the bone and joint

Exercise 10
1. WR   S
   arthr/itis
   inflammation of a joint
2. WR   S
   hepat/itis
   inflammation of the liver
3. P   WR   S
   sub/hepat/ic
   pertaining to under the liver
4. P   WR   S
   intra/ven/ous
   pertaining to within the vein
5. WR CV S
   arthr/o/pathy
     CF
   disease of a joint
6. WR   S
   oste/itis
   inflammation of the bone
7. WR CV S
   hepat/o/megaly
     CF
   enlargement of the liver
8. WR   S
   hepat/ic
   pertaining to the liver

Exercise 11
A
to place word parts together to form terms

B
arthr/o/pathy

Exercise 12
A
oste/o/arthr/itis

B
1. arthr/itis
2. hepat/ic
3. sub/hepat/ic
4. intra/ven/ous
5. oste/itis
6. hepat/itis
7. oste/o/arthr/o/pathy
8. hepat/o/megaly

Exercise 13
Check marks for numbers 2, 3, 4, 5, 7, 8, 10

677

ANSWERS TO CHAPTER 2 EXERCISES

Exercise 1
A *Label*
1. neur/o
2. epitheli/o
3. sarc/o
4. my/o
5. aden/o
6. fibr/o

B *Label*
1. tissue: hist/o
2. cell: cyt/o
3. organ: organ/o
4. system: system/o
5. internal organs: viscer/o

C *Define and Match*
1. d, flesh, connective tissue
2. e, fat, fat tissue
3. c, internal organs
4. f, cell(s)
5. b, tissue(s)
6. a, muscle(s), muscle tissue

D *Define and Match*
1. c, nerve(s), nerve tissue
2. f, organ
3. d, system
4. a, epithelium, epithelial tissue
5. b, fiber(s), fibrous tissue
6. e, gland, glandular tissue
7. g, blood

Exercise 2
A *Define*
1. tumor, mass
2. cancer
3. cause (of disease)
4. disease
5. body
6. cancer
7. rod-shaped, striated
8. smooth
9. knowledge
10. physician, medicine
11. life
12. virus
13. self
14. death (cells, body)

B *Identify*
1. path/o
2. onc/o
3. eti/o
4. a. cancer/o
   b. carcin/o
5. somat/o
6. lei/o
7. rhabd/o
8. gno/o
9. iatr/o
10. aut/o
11. vir/o
12. bi/o
13. necr/o

Exercise 3
A *Define*
1. blue
2. red
3. white
4. yellow
5. black

B *Identify*
1. cyan/o
2. erythr/o
3. leuk/o
4. melan/o
5. xanth/o

Exercise 4
A *Define*
1. new
2. above, excessive
3. after, beyond, change
4. below, incomplete, deficient, under
5. painful, abnormal, difficult, labored
6. through, complete
7. before
8. small

B *Identify*
1. neo-
2. hyper-
3. hypo-
4. meta-
5. dys-
6. dia-
7. pro-
8. micro-

Exercise 5
A *Label*
1. -cyte
2. -plasia
3. -logist
4. -logy
5. -megaly
6. -oma

B *Match*
1. g
2. j
3. b
4. c
5. e
6. d
7. f
8. i
9. a
10. h
11. k

C *Define*
1. one who studies and treats (specialist, physician)
2. disease
3. study of
4. pertaining to
5. control, stop, standing
6. cell
7. abnormal condition
8. pertaining to
9. growth, substance, formation
10. pertaining to
11. condition of formation, development, growth
12. resembling
13. substance or agent that produces or causes
14. producing, originating, causing
15. tumor, swelling
16. malignant tumor
17. state of
18. enlargement
19. view of, viewing

Exercise 6
Pronounce and Spell

Exercise 7
1. WR CV S
   cyt/o/logy
   CF
   study of cells
2. WR CV S
   hist/o/logy
   CF
   study of tissue
3. WR S
   viscer/al
   pertaining to internal organs
4. P S(WR)
   hypo/plasia
   incomplete development (of an organ or tissues); *Note: the word root is embedded in the suffix and is labeled as S(WR)*
5. WR CV S
   neur/o/pathy
   CF
   disease of the nerves
6. WR S
   system/ic
   pertaining to a (body) system
7. WR S
   somat/ic
   pertaining to the body
8. WR CV S
   somat/o/genic
   CF
   originating in the body
9. WR S
   epitheli/al
   pertaining to the epithelium
10. WR CV WR S
    erythr/o/cyt/osis
    CF
    increase in the number of red (blood) cells
11. WR CV WR S
    leuk/o/cyt/osis
    CF
    increase in the number of white (blood) cells

12. WR CV S
    my/o/pathy
       CF
    disease of the muscle
13. WR CV S
    erythr/o/cyte
        CF
    red (blood) cell
14. WR CV S
    leuk/o/cyte
        CF
    white (blood) cell

Exercise 8
A *Fill In*
1. neur/o/pathy
2. cyt/o/logy
3. somat/ic
4. my/o/pathy
5. dys/plasia
6. viscer/al
7. somat/o/genic
8. organ/o/megaly
9. lip/oid
10. system/ic

B *Label*
1. leuk/o/cyte
2. hyper/plasia
3. erythr/o/cyte
4. necr/osis

Exercise 9
Review of Body Structure Terms

Exercise 10
Pronounce and Spell

Exercise 11
1. WR S
   sarc/oma
   tumor composed of connective tissue
2. WR S
   melan/oma
   black tumor
3. WR S
   epitheli/oma
   tumor composed of epithelial tissue
4. WR S
   lip/oma
   tumor composed of fat tissue
5. P S(WR)
   neo/plasm
   new growth; *Note: the word root is embedded in the suffix and is labeled as S(WR)*
6. WR S
   my/oma
   tumor composed of muscle

7. WR S
   neur/oma
   tumor composed of nerve
8. WR S
   carcin/oma
   cancerous tumor
9. WR CV WR S
   aden/o/carcin/oma
        CF
   cancerous tumor of glandular tissue
10. WR CV WR CV S
    rhabd/o/my/o/sarcoma
         CF   CF
    malignant tumor of striated muscle
11. WR S
    aden/oma
    tumor composed of glandular tissue (benign)
12. WR CV WR S
    rhabd/o/my/oma
         CF
    tumor composed of striated muscle
13. WR S
    fibr/oma
    tumor composed of fibrous tissue
14. WR CV S
    lip/o/sarcoma
        CF
    malignant tumor of fat tissue
15. WR CV S
    fibr/o/sarcoma
        CF
    malignant tumor of fibrous tissue
16. P S(WR)
    meta/stasis
    beyond control (transfer of disease); *Note: the word root is embedded in the suffix and is labeled as S(WR)*

Exercise 12
A *Label*
1. carcin/oma
2. sarc/oma
3. melan/oma
4. rhabd/o/my/o/sarcoma
5. lei/o/my/oma
6. neur/oma

B *Fill In*
1. rhabd/o/my/oma
2. lip/o/sarcoma
3. neo/plasm
4. epitheli/oma
5. fibr/oma
6. aden/oma
7. meta/stasis
8. my/oma
9. fibr/o/sarcoma
10. aden/o/carcin/oma

Exercise 13
Pronounce and Spell

Exercise 14
A *Label*
1. encapsulated
2. radiation therapy
3. benign
4. malignant
5. chemotherapy
6. carcinoma in situ

B *Identify*
1. biological therapy
2. palliative
3. remission
4. hospice

C *Match*
1. h   6. j
2. i   7. c
3. g   8. d
4. b   9. e
5. a   10. f

Exercise 15
Review of Oncology Terms

Exercise 16
Pronounce and Spell

Exercise 17
A *Analyze and Define*
1. WR CV WR CV S
   cyt/o/path/o/logy
       CF   CF
   study of (changes in) cells in disease
2. WR CV WR CV S
   hist/o/path/o/logy
        CF   CF
   study of tissue in disease (study of tissue samples taken from patients)
3. WR CV S
   vir/o/logy
       CF
   study of viruses (branch of microbiology that is concerned with viruses and viral diseases)
4. WR CV WR CV S
   micr/o/bi/o/logy
        CF   CF
   study of small life (study of microorganisms, such as bacteria, fungi, viruses, and parasites)
5. WR S
   aut/opsy
   view of self (postmortem examination to determine the cause of death or obtain evidence)

6. WR   S
   bi/opsy
   view of life (the removal of living tissue from the body to be viewed under the microscope)

B *Fill In*
1. hist/o/path/o/logy
2. vir/o/logy
3. cyt/o/path/o/logy

C *Label*
1. hemat/o/logy
2. aut/opsy
3. micro/bi/o/logy
4. bi/opsy

Exercise 18

A *Identify*
1. genetic testing
2. Chemistry panel
3. complete blood count with differential
4. Specimen
5. culture and sensitivity

B *Label*
1. specimen
2. chemistry panel
3. genetic testing
4. culture and sensitivity

Exercise 19
Review of Laboratory Terms

Exercise 20
Pronounce and Spell

Exercise 21
1. WR CV S
   path/o/logy
       CF
   study of disease
2. WR CV S
   path/o/logist
       CF
   physician who studies diseases
3. P WR S
   dia/gno/sis
   state of complete knowledge (the art of identifying a disease based on the patient's signs, symptoms, and test results)
4. WR CV S
   onc/o/genic
       CF
   causing tumors
5. WR CV S
   onc/o/logy
       CF
   study of tumors

6. WR   S
   cancer/ous
   pertaining to cancer
7. WR CV S
   carcin/o/genic
       CF
   producing cancer
8. WR   S
   cyan/osis
   abnormal condition of blue (bluish discoloration of the skin)
9. WR CV S
   eti/o/logy
       CF
   study of causes (of disease)
10. WR   S
    xanth/osis
    abnormal condition of yellow
11. WR   S
    carcin/oid
    resembling cancer
12. WR CV S
    carcin/o/gen
        CF
    substance that causes cancer
13. WR CV S
    onc/o/logist
        CF
    physician who studies and treats tumors
14. P WR S
    pro/gno/sis
    state of before knowledge

Exercise 22

A *Label*
1. carcin/o/gen
2. cyan/osis
3. onc/o/logist
4. path/o/logist

B *Fill In*
1. dia/gno/sis
2. iatr/o/genic
3. eti/o/logy
4. onc/o/logy
5. path/o/logy
6. carcin/o/genic
7. xanth/osis
8. onc/o/genic
9. cancer/ous
10. pro/gno/sis

Exercise 23
Pronounce and Spell

Exercise 24

A *Label*
1. febrile
2. virus
3. inflammation
4. bacteria

B *Identify*
1. organism that feeds from a host it lives on or within
2. organism that feeds by absorbing organic molecules from its surroundings and may cause infection by invading body tissue
3. without fever
4. a form of life that is too small to be seen without a microscope
5. redness
6. invasion of pathogens in body tissue.
7. persistent, excessive tiredness and lack of energy that interferes with daily activities and is unrelated to exertion or lack of sleep
8. pertaining to disease of unknown origin
9. increase in the severity of a disease or its symptoms
10. disease that continues for a long time
11. sharp, sudden, short, or severe type of disease

Exercise 25

A
1. f   5. b
2. e   6. d
3. a   7. g
4. c

B
1. f   5. h
2. d   6. g
3. e   7. a
4. c   8. b

Exercise 26
Review of Complementary Terms

Exercise 27
1. etiologies
2. staphylococci
3. cyanoses
4. bacteria
5. nuclei
6. pharynges
7. sarcomata
8. carcinomata
9. anastomoses
10. pubes
11. prognoses
12. spermatozoa
13. fimbriae
14. thoraces
15. appendices

Exercise 28
1. diverticula
2. bronchus
3. testes
4. melanoma

5. emboli
6. diagnoses
7. metastases

Exercise 29
biopsy; diagnosis; carcinoma; metastases; prognosis; red blood cell; white blood cell; chemotherapy; radiation therapy; complete blood count with differential; culture and sensitivity

Exercise 30
A. disease was identified; not a cancerous tumor; did not have a fever; it looked like a positive outcome; more tired than usual
B. Answers may vary and may include: diagnosis, benign, afebrile, prognosis, and fatigue, along with their respective definitions.
C. biopsy, cytology, specimen, dysplasia, inflammation, pathologist, diagnosis, carcinoma
D. Answers may vary and may include: biopsy, cytology, specimen, dysplasia, inflammation, pathologist, diagnosis, and carcinoma, along with their respective definitions.

Exercise 31
A
1. chemotherapy
2. adenocarcinoma
3. pathology
4. malignant
5. radiation therapy
6. organomegaly
7. cyanosis
8. metastases

B
1. b
2. b
3. d
4. a. prognoses
   b. lipomata
   c. histologies

Exercise 32
1. diagnosis, CA, oncologist
2. neoplasm, cytology, benign, malignant
3. specimen, microbiology, C&S
4. pathology, sarcoma, metastasis, oncology, Px
5. infection, fatigue, febrile, leukocytosis, virus

Exercise 33
Pronunciation Exercise

Exercise 34
1. a
2. b
3. a
4. b
5. c
6. b
7. b
8. a
9. b
10. c
11. b
12. b
13. b
14. c
15. b
16. a
17. c
18. a
19. b
20. a

ANSWERS TO CHAPTER 3 EXERCISES

Exercise 1
A *Define*
1. belly (front)
2. head (upward)
3. side
4. middle
5. below
6. near (the point of attachment)
7. above
8. away (from the point of attachment)
9. back
10. tail (downward)
11. front
12. back, behind

B *Label*
1. head: cephal/o
2. back: dors/o
3. back, behind: poster/o
4. tail: caud/o
5. front: anter/o
6. belly (front): ventr/o
7. side: later/o
8. above: super/o
9. middle: medi/o
10. near: proxim/o
11. away: dist/o
12. below: infer/o

Exercise 2
A *Match*
1. c
2. a
3. b

B *Label*
1. tom/o
2. radi/o
3. son/o

Exercise 3
A *Label*
1. uni-
2. bi-

B *Define*
1. two
2. one

Exercise 4
A *Label*
1. -graphy
2. -graph
3. -gram

B *Define*
1. process of recording, radiographic imaging
2. instrument used to record; the record
3. the record, radiographic image
4. pertaining to
5. pertaining to
6. one who studies and treats (specialist, physician)
7. study of
8. pertaining to

Exercise 5
Pronounce and Spell

Exercise 6
1. WR   S
   proxim/al
   pertaining to near
2. WR   S
   later/al
   pertaining to a side
3. P   WR   S
   uni/later/al
   pertaining to one side
4. WR CV WR   S
   anter/o/poster/ior
   ─── CF
   pertaining to the front and to the back
5. WR   S
   cephal/ic
   pertaining to the head
6. WR   S
   super/ior
   pertaining to above
7. WR   S
   anter/ior
   pertaining to the front
8. WR   S
   dist/al
   pertaining to away
9. WR   S
   medi/al

pertaining to the middle
10. P WR S
    bi/later/al
    pertaining to two sides
11. WR CV WR S
    poster/o/anter/ior
         CF
    pertaining to the back and to the front
12. WR S
    caud/al
    pertaining to the tail
13. WR S
    infer/ior
    pertaining to below
14. WR S
    poster/ior
    pertaining to the back
15. WR S
    dors/al
    pertaining to the back
16. WR S
    ventr/al
    pertaining to the belly (front)

Exercise 7
A *Label*
1. a. super/ior
   b. cephal/ic
   c. poster/ior, dors/al
   d. infer/ior
   e. caud/al
   f. anter/ior
   g. ventr/al
2. dist/al
3. proxim/al
4. later/al
5. medi/al
6. a. poster/o/anter/ior
   b. anter/o/poster/ior

B *Fill In*
1. proxim/al
2. dist/al
3. bi/later/al
4. medi/al
5. poster/o/anter/ior
6. medi/o/later/al
7. uni/later/al
8. anter/o/poster/ior

Exercise 8
Review of Directional Terms

Exercise 9
Pronounce and Spell

Exercise 10
A *Label*
1. right hypochondriac
2. right lumbar
3. right iliac
4. hypogastric
5. epigastric
6. left hypochondriac
7. umbilical
8. left lumbar
9. left iliac

B *Match*
1. b   4. e
2. d   5. c
3. a   6. f

Exercise 11
Review of Abdominopelvic Regions Terms

Exercise 12
Pronounce and Spell

Exercise 13
A *Label*
1. coronal
2. axial
3. midsagittal
4. oblique

B *Fill In*
1. axial
2. midsagittal
3. coronal
4. sagittal
5. parasagittal
6. oblique

Exercise 14
Review of Anatomic Planes

Exercise 15
Pronounce and Spell

Exercise 16
A *Match*
1. e   4. c
2. a   5. b
3. d

B *Label*
1. supine
2. prone
3. sitting
4. orthopnea
5. lateral
6. semiprone

C *Fill In*
1. sitting
2. semiprone
3. Trendelenburg
4. lithotomy
5. orthopnea

Exercise 17
Review of Body Position Terms

Exercise 18
Pronounce and Spell

Exercise 19
A *Analyze and Define*
1. WR CV S
   tom/o/graphy
        CF
   process of recording slices (anatomical cross-sections)
2. WR CV S
   son/o/gram
        CF
   record of sound
3. WR CV S
   radi/o/graphy
        CF
   process of recording x-rays
4. WR CV S
   son/o/graphy
        CF
   process of recording sound
5. WR CV S
   radi/o/graph
        CF
   record of x-rays
6. WR CV S
   radi/o/logist
        CF
   physician who specializes in x-rays

B *Label*
1. radi/o/graphy
2. radi/o/graph
3. son/o/graphy
4. son/o/gram

C *Fill In*
1. tom/o/graphy
2. radi/o/logist
3. radi/o/logy

Exercise 20
A *Identify*
1. scan
2. Nuclear medicine
3. fluoroscopy
4. magnetic resonance imaging
5. Computed tomography

B *Label*
1. fluoroscopy
2. computed tomography
3. nuclear medicine
4. magnetic resonance imaging

Exercise 21
Review of Diagnostic Imaging Terms

Appendix A   Answer Key   683

Exercise 22
A *Fill In*
1. superior
2. anterior
3. inferior
4. posteroanterior
5. anteroposterior
6. medial
7. lateral
8. ultrasonography
9. nuclear medicine
10. magnetic resonance imaging
11. computed tomography
12. magnetic resonance

B *Label*
1. right upper quadrant (RUQ)
2. left upper quadrant (LUQ)
3. right lower quadrant (RLQ)
4. left lower quadrant (LLQ)

Exercise 23
A. near (her shoulder); belly near the navel; lower back near her waist; on her back facing upward, x-ray department, x-ray doctors, cross sections.
B. Answers will vary and may include proximal, ventral, umbilical region, lumbar region, supine, recumbent, radiology, radiologist, and computed tomography, along with their respective definitions.
C. medial, lateral, proximal, radiograph, AP, CT.
D. Answers will vary and may include medial, lateral, proximal, radiograph, AP, and CT, along with their respective definitions.

Exercise 24
A
1. anteroposterior
2. lateral
3. posterior (dorsal is used for head, trunk, and surfaces of hand and foot)
4. medial
5. anterior
6. radiology

B
1. b
2. a
3. a
4. answers may vary: the upper surface of the foot; the surface opposite the sole; the top of the foot

Exercise 25
1. lateral, distal, proximal
2. radiology, oblique plane, radiography, nuclear medicine
3. hypochondriac region, RUQ, umbilical region, RLQ
4. supine position, prone position

Exercise 26
Pronunciation Exercise

Exercise 27
Chapter Content Quiz
1. c
2. a
3. c
4. a
5. c
6. a
7. c
8. a
9. b
10. c
11. a
12. b
13. c
14. a
15. b
16. c
17. b
18. c
19. a
20. a. superior
    b. inferior
    c. medial
    d. lateral

ANSWERS TO CHAPTER 4 EXERCISES

Exercise 1
A *Label*
1. hornlike tissue: kerat/o
2. skin: cutane/o, derm/o, dermat/o
3. sebum: seb/o
4. hair: trich/o
5. sweat: hidr/o
6. nail: onych/o, ungu/o

B *Define and Match*
1. d, skin
2. b, sebum (oil)
3. c, nail
4. d, skin
5. e, hornlike tissue (keratin), hard
6. c, nail
7. a, sweat
8. f, hair
9. d, skin

Exercise 2
A *Define*
1. yellow
2. grapelike clusters
3. hidden
4. thick
5. white
6. fungus
7. red
8. hard
9. twisted chains
10. dry, dryness
11. wrinkle
12. gland glandular tissue
13. swallowing, eating

B *Identify*
1. myc/o
2. leuk/o
3. xanth/o
4. xer/o
5. pachy/o
6. strept/o
7. rhytid/o
8. staphyl/o
9. erythr/o
10. crypt/o
11. scler/o
12. phag/o
13. aden/o

Exercise 3
A *Define*
1. under, below
2. beside, around, abnormal
3. on, upon, over
4. within
5. through
6. through, across, beyond
7. below, incomplete, deficient, under
8. above, excessive

B *Identify*
1. intra-
2. sub-
3. epi-
4. para-
5. per-
6. trans-
7. hyper-
8. hypo-

Exercise 4
A *Match*
1. e
2. c
3. a
4. b
5. d

B *Label*
1. -coccus
2. -rrhea
3. -malacia
4. -itis
5. -plasty
6. -ectomy

C *Define*
1. pertaining to
2. study of
3. pertaining to
4. abnormal condition
5. pertaining to

Exercise 5
Pronounce and Spell

Exercise 6
1. WR CV WR S
   scler/o/derm/a
      CF
   hard skin (chronic hardening or induration of the connective tissue of the skin and other organs)
2. WR WR S
   hidr/aden/itis
   inflammation of a sweat gland
3. WR S
   dermat/itis
   inflammation of the skin
4. WR WR S
   pachy/derm/a
   thickening of the skin
5. WR CV S
   onych/o/malacia
      CF
   softening of the nails
6. WR S
   kerat/osis
   abnormal condition (growth) of hornlike tissue (keratin)
7. WR CV WR S
   dermat/o/fibr/oma
      CF
   fibrous tumor of the skin
8. P WR S
   par/onych/ia
   diseased state around the nail
   Note: the a from para- has been dropped because the following word root begins with a vowel.
9. WR CV WR S
   onych/o/crypt/osis
      CF
   abnormal condition of a hidden nail
10. WR CV S
    seb/o/rrhea
       CF
    discharge of sebum (excessive)
11. WR CV WR S
    onych/o/phag/ia
       CF
    condition of eating the nails, nail biting
12. WR CV WR S
    xer/o/derm/a
       CF
    dry skin (a mild form of a cutaneous disorder characterized by keratinization and noninflammatory scaling)
13. WR S
    xanth/oma
    yellow tumor (benign, primarily in the skin)

Exercise 7
A Label
1. dermat/itis
2. kerat/osis
3. onych/o/myc/osis
4. par/onych/ia

B Fill In
1. pachy/derm/a
2. xer/o/derm/a
3. seb/o/rrhea
4. xanth/oma
5. dermat/o/fibr/oma
6. onych/o/malacia
7. hidr/aden/itis
8. onych/o/crypt/osis
9. scler/o/derm/a
10. onych/o/phag/ia

Exercise 8
Pronounce and Spell

Exercise 9
A Identify
1. systemic lupus erythematosus
2. abrasion
3. pediculosis
4. contusion
5. gangrene
6. carbuncle
7. acne
8. laceration
9. pilonidal cyst
10. pressure injury
11. albinism
12. MRSA infection
13. abscess

B Label
1. a. fissure b. eczema
2. cellulitis
3. psoriasis
4. herpes
5. tinea
6. Kaposi sarcoma
7. actinic keratosis
8. furuncle
9. squamous cell carcinoma
10. basal cell carcinoma
11. impetigo
12. scabies
13. urticaria
14. candidiasis
15. vitiligo
16. rosacea
17. measles
18. keloid

Exercise 10
1. p
2. j
3. h
4. l
5. k
6. c
7. n
8. b
9. e
10. i
11. g
12. a
13. f
14. m
15. o
16. d

Exercise 11
1. d
2. b
3. f
4. p
5. m
6. l
7. o
8. a
9. n
10. e
11. i
12. g
13. k
14. c
15. j
16. h

Exercise 12
Review of Disease and Disorder Terms

Exercise 13
Pronounce and Spell

Exercise 14
A Analyze and Define
1. WR S
   rhytid/ectomy
   excision of wrinkles
2. WR CV S
   dermat/o/plasty
      CF
   surgical repair of the skin

B Build
1. rhytid/ectomy
2. dermat/o/plasty

Exercise 15
A Fill In
1. Mohs surgery
2. incision
3. cauterization
4. suturing
5. incision and drainage
6. debridement
7. excision
8. laser surgery
9. cryosurgery
10. dermabrasion
11. skin graft

B Match
1. i
2. h
3. g
4. d
5. a
6. e
7. b
8. f
9. j
10. c
11. k

Exercise 16
Review of Surgical Terms

Exercise 17
Pronounce and Spell

Appendix A Answer Key   685

Exercise 18
1. WR S
   ungu/al
   pertaining to the nail
2. P WR S
   trans/derm/al
   pertaining to through the skin
3. WR CV S
   strept/o/coccus
   CF
   berry-shaped (bacterium) in twisted chains
4. P WR S
   hypo/derm/ic
   pertaining to under the skin
5. WR CV S
   dermat/o/logy
   CF
   study of the skin
6. P WR S
   sub/cutane/ous
   pertaining to under the skin
7. WR CV S
   staphyl/o/coccus
   CF
   berry-shaped (bacterium) in grapelike clusters
8. WR CV S
   kerat/o/genic
   CF
   producing hornlike tissue
9. WR CV S
   dermat/o/logist
   CF
   physician who studies and treats skin (diseases)
10. WR S
    cutane/ous
    pertaining to the skin
11. P WR S
    epi/derm/al
    pertaining to upon the skin
12. WR CV WR S
    xanth/o/derm/a
    CF
    yellow skin
13. WR CV WR S
    erythr/o/derm/a
    CF
    red skin
14. P WR S
    per/cutane/ous
    pertaining to through the skin
15. WR S
    xer/osis
    abnormal condition of dryness
16. P WR S
    sub/ungu/al
    pertaining to under the nail
17. WR CV WR S
    leuk/o/derm/a
    CF
    white skin
18. P WR S
    hyper/trich/osis
    abnormal condition of excessive hair (growth)

Exercise 19
A *Label*
1. xanth/o/derm/a
2. leuk/o/derm/a
3. erythr/o/derm/a
4. hyper/trich/osis
5. strept/o/cocci
6. staphyl/o/cocci
7. intra/derm/al
8. sub/cutane/ous, hypo/derm/ic
9. trans/derm/al

B *Fill In*
1. dermat/o/logy
2. xer/osis
3. ungu/al
4. cutane/ous
5. dermat/o/logist
6. sub/ungu/al
7. epi/derm/al
8. per/cutane/ous
9. kerat/o/genic

Exercise 20
Pronounce and Spell

Exercise 21
A *Identify*
1. diaphoresis
2. macule
3. jaundice
4. leukoplakia
5. petechiae
6. pallor
7. ecchymosis
8. nodule
9. cyst
10. pruritus
11. purpura
12. papule
13. wheal
14. pustule
15. vesicle
16. induration
17. edema
18. lesion

B *Label*
1. ulcer
2. nevus
3. verruca
4. alopecia

Exercise 22
1. e   6. d
2. a   7. b
3. i   8. c
4. f   9. h
5. g

Exercise 23
1. d   8. e
2. i   9. f
3. a   10. m
4. k   11. c
5. j   12. g
6. l   13. h
7. b

Exercise 24
Review of Complementary Terms

Exercise 25
1. basal cell carcinoma
2. split-thickness skin grafts
3. full-thickness skin grafts
4. squamous cell carcinoma
5. systemic lupus erythematosus
6. subcutaneous
7. staphylococcus
8. streptococcus
9. incision and drainage
10. transdermal
11. intradermal
12. dermatology
13. methicillin-resistant *Staphylococcus aureus*, healthcare-associated MRSA infection, community-associated MRSA infection

Exercise 26
A. pale; very itchy; (lips beginning to) swell; (cheeks and arms covered with) different-sized red and white bumps
B. Answers will vary and may include pallor, pruritus, edema, erythema, urticaria.
C. pallor, pruritus, edema, urticaria
D. Answers will vary and may include pallor, pruritus, edema, and urticaria, along with their respective definitions.

Exercise 27
A
1. dermatology
2. nodule
3. medial
4. actinic keratosis
5. eczema
6. lesion
7. Mohs surgery
8. subcutaneous

Copyright © 2026 by Elsevier Inc. All rights are reserved, including those for text and data mining, AI training, and similar technologies.

9. excision
10. pathology
11. dermatologist
12. cauterization
13. suturing
14. basal cell carcinoma

B
1. a. s
   b. p
   c. p
   d. s
   e. s
   f. p
   g. s
   h. p
2. b
3. dictionary exercise

Exercise 28
1. lesions, impetigo
2. Mohs surgery, squamous cell carcinoma
3. MRSA, cellulitis, abscess
4. leukoderma, albinism, vitiligo
5. erythroderma, dermatologist, dermatitis

Exercise 29
Pronunciation Exercise

Exercise 30
1. b   11. a
2. b   12. c
3. c   13. c
4. b   14. b
5. a   15. a
6. c   16. b
7. a   17. b
8. a   18. b
9. c   19. a
10. b   20. b

ANSWERS TO CHAPTER 5 EXERCISES

Exercise 1
A Define and Match
1. d, adenoids
2. h, diaphragm
3. e, epiglottis
4. b, lobe(s)
5. a, nose
6. g, pharynx
7. c, lung, air
8. c, lung, air
9. a, nose
10. f, septum

B Label
1. sinus: sinus/o
2. nose: nas/o, rhin/o
3. tonsil: tonsill/o
4. epiglottis: epiglott/o
5. larynx: laryng/o
6. trachea: trache/o
7. pleura: pleur/o
8. lobe: lob/o
9. diaphragm: diaphragmat/o
10. adenoids: adenoid/o
11. pharynx: pharyng/o
12. lung: pneum/o, pneumon/o, pulmon/o
13. thorax, chest, chest cavity: thorac/o
14. bronchus: bronch/o, bronchi/o
15. mediastinum: mediastin/o
16. alveolus: alveol/o

C Define and Match
1. h, alveolus *(s.)*, alveoli *(pl.)*
2. j, bronchus *(s.)*, bronchi *(pl.)*
3. c, lung
4. g, larynx
5. d, pleura
6. i, thorax, chest, chest cavity
7. b, trachea
8. e, tonsil(s)
9. f, sinus(es)
10. a, mediastinum

Exercise 2
A Define
1. oxygen
2. breathe, breathing
3. mucus
4. imperfect, incomplete
5. straight
6. pus
7. blood
8. sleep
9. carbon dioxide
10. sound, voice
11. cancer
12. fungus
13. dust

B Identify
1. spir/o
2. ox/i
3. atel/o
4. orth/o
5. py/o
6. muc/o
7. hem/o
8. somn/o
9. phon/o
10. capn/o
11. coni/o
12. carcin/o
13. myc/o

Exercise 3
A Define
1. within
2. absence of, without
3. normal, good
4. many, much
5. fast, rapid
6. painful, abnormal, difficult, labored
7. below, incomplete, deficient, under
8. within
9. above, excessive
10. new

B Identify
1. a. endo-
   b. intra-
2. eu-
3. a. a-
   b. an-
4. poly-
5. tachy-
6. neo-
7. hyper-
8. hypo-
9. dys-

Exercise 4
A Match
1. g
2. c
3. d
4. e
5. a
6. f
7. i
8. k
9. l
10. b
11. h
12. m
13. j

B Label
1. -scope
2. -scopy
3. -tomy
4. -stomy
5. -meter
6. -metry
7. -rrhagia
8. -ptysis
9. -ectomy
10. -emia

C Define
1. flow, discharge
2. resembling
3. one who studies and treats (specialist, physician)
4. growth, substance, formation
5. pertaining to
6. tumor, swelling
7. study of
8. surgical repair
9. abnormal condition

Exercise 5
Pronounce and Spell

Exercise 6
1. WR   S
   trache/itis
   inflammation of the trachea
2. WR CV   WR   S
   nas/o/pharyng/itis
   ‾‾‾
   CF
   inflammation of the nose and pharynx
3. WR   S
   alveol/itis
   inflammation of the alveoli
4. WR CV   S
   py/o/thorax
   ‾‾‾
   CF
   pus in the chest cavity (pleural cavity)

Appendix A   Answer Key

5. WR S
   atel/ectasis
   incomplete expansion (of the lung or portion of the lung)
6. WR CV WR S
   rhin/o/myc/osis
   ⎯CF⎯
   abnormal condition of fungus in the nose
7. WR CV S
   trache/o/stenosis
   ⎯CF⎯
   narrowing of the trachea
8. WR S
   epiglott/itis
   inflammation of the epiglottis
9. WR S
   laryng/itis
   inflammation of the larynx
10. WR S P S(WR)
    pulmon/ary neo/plasm
    pertaining to (in) the lung, new growth (tumor); *Note: the word root is embedded in the suffix and is labeled as S(WR)*
11. WR S
    pneumon/ia
    diseased state of the lung
12. WR S
    rhin/itis
    inflammation of the nose (mucous membranes)
13. WR CV WR S
    pneum/o/coni/osis
    ⎯CF⎯
    abnormal condition of dust in the lungs
14. WR CV WR S
    bronch/o/pneumon/ia
    ⎯CF⎯
    diseased state of bronchi and lungs
15. WR CV WR CV WR S
    laryng/o/trache/o/bronch/itis
    ⎯CF⎯ ⎯CF⎯
    inflammation of the larynx, trachea, and bronchi
16. WR CV S
    bronch/o/spasm
    ⎯CF⎯
    involuntary muscle contraction of the bronchi

Exercise 7
A Label
1. bronchi/ectasis
2. hem/o/thorax
3. pneum/o/thorax
4. sinus/itis
5. pleur/itis
6. tonsill/itis

B Fill In
1. pharyng/itis
2. bronch/o/genic carcin/oma
3. lob/ar pneumon/ia
4. laryng/o/spasm
5. diaphragmat/o/cele
6. adenoid/itis
7. bronch/itis
8. rhin/o/rrhagia
9. pneumon/itis

Exercise 8
Pronounce and Spell

Exercise 9
A Identify
1. Cystic fibrosis
2. influenza
3. chronic obstructive pulmonary disease
4. pertussis
5. Croup
6. pulmonary edema
7. Epistaxis
8. idiopathic pulmonary fibrosis
9. Diphtheria
10. asphyxia
11. tuberculosis
12. Acute respiratory distress syndrome
13. coronavirus disease

B Label
1. pulmonary embolism
2. obstructive sleep apnea
3. deviated septum
4. pleural effusion
5. asthma
6. coccidioidomycosis
7. emphysema
8. upper respiratory infection

Exercise 10
1. j   6. c
2. i   7. a
3. d   8. e
4. g   9. b
5. f   10. h

Exercise 11
1. d   7. h
2. k   8. i
3. c   9. a
4. e   10. j
5. f   11. b
6. g

Exercise 12
Review of Disease and Disorder Terms

Exercise 13
Pronounce and Spell

Exercise 14
1. WR CV S
   trache/o/plasty
   ⎯CF⎯
   surgical repair of the trachea
2. WR CV S
   sept/o/plasty
   ⎯CF⎯
   surgical repair of the septum
3. WR CV S
   laryng/o/stomy
   ⎯CF⎯
   creation of an artificial opening into the larynx
4. WR CV S
   sinus/o/tomy
   ⎯CF⎯
   incision into a sinus
5. WR CV S
   laryng/o/plasty
   ⎯CF⎯
   surgical repair of the larynx
6. WR CV S
   thorac/o/tomy
   ⎯CF⎯
   incision into the chest cavity

Exercise 15
A Label
1. adenoid/ectomy
2. lob/ectomy
3. pneumon/ectomy
4. trache/o/stomy
5. thora/centesis *(Note: "co" is removed from the combining form in common usage)*
6. trache/o/tomy

B Fill In
1. laryng/o/trache/o/tomy
2. pleur/o/desis
3. tonsill/ectomy
4. bronch/o/plasty
5. laryng/ectomy
6. rhin/o/plasty

Exercise 16
Review of Surgical Terms

Exercise 17
Pronounce and Spell

Exercise 18
1. WR CV S
   spir/o/meter
   ⎯CF⎯
   instrument used to measure breathing

688 Appendix A Answer Key

2. WR CV S
   laryng/o/scope
   ___CF___
   instrument used for visual examination of the larynx
3. WR CV S
   capn/o/meter
   ___CF___
   instrument used to measure carbon dioxide
4. WR CV S
   spir/o/metry
   ___CF___
   measurement of breathing
5. WR CV S
   ox/i/meter
   ___CF___
   instrument used to measure oxygen
6. WR CV S
   laryng/o/scopy
   ___CF___
   visual examination of the larynx
7. WR CV S
   bronch/o/scope
   ___CF___
   instrument used for visual examination of the bronchi
8. WR CV S
   thorac/o/scope
   ___CF___
   instrument used for visual examination of the chest cavity
9. P S(WR)
   endo/scope
   instrument used for visual examination within (a hollow organ or body cavity); *Note: the word root is embedded in the suffix and is labeled as S(WR)*
10. WR CV S
    thorac/o/scopy
    ___CF___
    visual examination of the chest cavity
11. P S(WR)
    endo/scopic
    pertaining to visual examination within (a hollow organ or body cavity); *Note: the word root is embedded in the suffix and is labeled as S(WR)*
12. P S(WR)
    endo/scopy
    visual examination within (a hollow organ or body cavity); *Note: the word root is embedded in the suffix and is labeled as S(WR)*
13. P WR CV S
    poly/somn/o/graphy
    ___CF___
    process of recording many (tests) during sleep

14. WR CV S
    mediastin/o/scopy
    ___CF___
    visual examination of the mediastinum

Exercise 19
A Label
1. laryng/o/scope
2. spir/o/meter
3. capn/o/meter
4. ox/i/meter
5. poly/somn/o/graphy

B Fill In
1. laryng/o/scopy
2. mediastin/o/scopy
3. endo/scopic
4. thorac/o/scopy
5. bronch/o/scopy
6. spir/o/metry
7. bronch/o/scope
8. endo/scopy
9. thorac/o/scope
10. endo/scope

Exercise 20
Pronounce and Spell

Exercise 21
A Label
1. PPD (purified protein derivative) skin test
2. peak flow meter
3. arterial blood gas
4. pulse oximetry
5. stethoscope
6. lung ventilation/perfusion scan
7. chest radiograph
8. chest computed tomography (CT) scan
9. auscultation
10. percussion

B Identify
1. acid-fast bacilli smear
2. Pulmonary function tests

Exercise 22
1. f   7. g
2. e   8. h
3. a   9. k
4. d   10. i
5. b   11. j
6. c   12. l

Exercise 23
Review of Diagnostic Terms

Exercise 24
Pronounce and Spell

Exercise 25
1. WR S
   mediastin/al
   pertaining to the mediastinum
2. WR CV S
   pulmon/o/logy
   ___CF___
   study of the lung
3. WR S
   muc/ous
   pertaining to mucus
4. P S(WR)
   a/pnea
   absence of breathing; *Note: the word root is embedded in the suffix and is labeled as S(WR)*
5. P WR S
   hyp/ox/ia
   condition of deficient oxygen (to tissues)
6. WR CV WR S
   nas/o/pharyng/eal
   ___CF___
   pertaining to the nose and pharynx
7. P WR S
   intra/pleur/al
   pertaining to within the pleura
8. P WR S
   a/capn/ia
   condition of absence of carbon dioxide (in the blood)
9. P WR S
   dys/phon/ia
   condition of difficulty in speaking (voice)
10. P WR S
    hyp/ox/emia
    deficient oxygen in the blood
11. WR S
    thorac/ic
    pertaining to the chest
12. WR S
    diaphragmat/ic
    pertaining to the diaphragm
13. WR CV WR S
    bronch/o/alveol/ar
    ___CF___
    pertaining to the bronchi and alveoli
14. P S(WR)
    hypo/pnea
    deficient breathing; *Note: the word root is embedded in the suffix and is labeled as S(WR)*

Exercise 26
A Label
1. hem/o/ptysis
2. orth/o/pnea
3. pulmon/o/logist
4. alveol/ar

5. dys/pnea
6. endo/trache/al

B *Fill In*
1. tachy/pnea
2. muc/oid
3. rhin/o/rrhea
4. hyper/capn/ia
5. an/ox/ia
6. hyper/pnea
7. laryng/eal
8. hypo/capn/ia
9. eu/pnea
10. a/phon/ia
11. pulmon/ary
12. sept/al

Exercise 27
Pronounce and Spell

Exercise 28
A *Label*
1. airway
2. bronchodilator
3. nebulizer
4. ventilator

B *Identify*
1. hyperventilation
2. wheeze
3. sputum
4. aspirate
5. stridor
6. rhonchi
7. mucopurulent
8. Hypoventilation
9. nosocomial infection
10. paroxysm
11. patent
12. bronchoconstrictor
13. Effusion
14. crackles

Exercise 29
1. b
2. g
3. c
4. h
5. a
6. d
7. f
8. e
9. i

Exercise 30
1. e
2. g
3. h
4. c
5. i
6. a
7. b
8. d
9. f

Exercise 31
Review of Complementary Terms

Exercise 32
1. chronic obstructive pulmonary disease; pulmonary function tests, chest radiograph, arterial blood gas, venous blood gas
2. shortness of breath
3. A. left upper lobe; left lower lobe
   B. right upper lobe, right middle lobe, right lower lobe
4. acid-fast bacilli; tuberculosis
5. polysomnography; obstructive sleep apnea; continuous positive airway pressure
6. oxygen; carbon dioxide
7. peak flow meter
8. idiopathic pulmonary fibrosis
9. influenza; coronavirus disease; upper respiratory infection
10. hospital-acquired pneumonia
11. lung ventilation/perfusion scan; pulmonary embolism
12. acute respiratory distress syndrome
13. cystic fibrosis
14. laryngotracheobronchitis
15. community-acquired pneumonia
16. coccidioidomycosis
17. vital signs; temperature; blood pressure; pulse; respiration
18. respiratory syncytial virus

Exercise 33
A. difficulty breathing; runny nose; her throat was very sore; thick yellow mucus; cold
B. Answer will vary and may include dyspnea, rhinorrhea, pharyngitis, sputum, and/or upper respiratory infection.
C. dyspnea, mucoid, sputum, rhinorrhea, auscultation, percussion, crackles, rhonchi
D. Answer will vary and may include dyspnea, mucoid, sputum, rhinorrhea, auscultation, percussion, crackles, and/or rhonchi along with their respective definitions.

Exercise 34
A
1. sputum
2. hemoptysis
3. dyspnea
4. paroxysms
5. tuberculosis
6. R
7. SOB
8. pleural effusion
9. crackles
10. bronchogenic carcinoma
11. coccidioidomycosis
12. radiology

B
1. a
2. F
3. F
4. T

Exercise 35
Online Exercise

Exercise 36
1. dyspnea, SOB, orthopnea
2. crackles, hypoxemia
3. sinusitis, rhinitis, rhinorrhea, endoscopic
4. ABG, O_2, CO_2, COPD, acute respiratory distress syndrome, cystic fibrosis
5. PPD skin test, chest radiograph, tuberculosis

Exercise 37
Pronunciation Exercise

Exercise 38
1. b
2. c
3. a
4. c
5. a
6. a
7. b
8. c
9. c
10. b
11. a
12. c
13. b
14. c
15. b
16. c
17. a
18. c
19. c
20. a

ANSWERS TO CHAPTER 6 EXERCISES

Exercise 1
A *Label*
1. kidney: nephr/o, ren/o
2. meatus: meat/o
3. ureter: ureter/o
4. bladder: cyst/o, vesic/o
5. urethra: urethr/o

B *Define and Match*
1. g, kidney
2. a, bladder
3. g, kidney
4. d, glomerulus
5. f, renal pelvis
6. c, ureter
7. a, bladder
8. b, meatus
9. e, urethra

C *Label*
1. renal pelvis: pyel/o
2. glomerulus: glomerul/o

Exercise 2
A *Define*
1. water
2. urea, nitrogen
3. night
4. stone(s), calculus (*pl.* calculi)
5. albumin
6. urine, urinary tract
7. developing cell, germ cell
8. scanty, few
9. urine, urinary tract
10. sugar
11. sound
12. blood

B *Identify*
1. glycos/o
2. a. urin/o
   b. ur/o
3. hydr/o
4. blast/o
5. albumin/o
6. noct/i
7. azot/o
8. lith/o
9. olig/o
10. hem/o
11. son/o

Exercise 3
A *Define*
1. painful, abnormal, difficult, labored
2. through, across, beyond
3. absence of, without
4. many, much
5. within

B *Identify*
1. trans-
2. a-
3. dys-
4. intra-
5. poly-

Exercise 4
A *Label*
1. -lysis
2. -ptosis
3. -tripsy
4. -lith
5. -pexy
6. -uria

B *Match*
1. f
2. i
3. h
4. a
5. e
6. b
7. d
8. g
9. j
10. c

C *Define*
1. constriction or narrowing
2. inflammation
3. condition
4. study of
5. in the blood
6. the record, radiographic image
7. pertaining to
8. cut into, incision
9. abnormal condition
10. visual examination

Exercise 5
Pronounce and Spell

Exercise 6
1. WR CV WR S
   nephr/o/blast/oma
       CF
   kidney tumor containing developing cells
2. WR CV S
   ureter/o/stenosis
      CF
   narrowing of the ureter
3. WR S
   ur/emia
   urine (urea nitrogen) in the blood (presence of azotemia and wide range of signs and symptoms associated with chronic kidney disease)
4. WR CV S
   nephr/o/ptosis
     CF
   drooping kidney
5. WR CV S
   cyst/o/cele
     CF
   protrusion of the bladder
6. WR S
   nephr/itis
   inflammation of a kidney
7. WR S
   pyel/itis
   inflammation of the renal pelvis
8. WR CV WR S
   ureter/o/lith/iasis
      CF
   condition of stone(s) in the ureter
9. WR CV WR S
   pyel/o/nephr/itis
     CF
   inflammation of the renal pelvis and the kidney
10. WR S
    ureter/itis
    inflammation of a ureter

Exercise 7
A *Fill In*
1. ureter/o/cele
2. urethr/o/cyst/itis
3. vesic/o/ureter/al reflux
4. glomerul/o/nephr/itis
5. nephr/oma

B *Label*
1. urethr/itis
2. nephr/o/megaly
3. hydr/o/nephr/osis
4. cyst/o/lith
5. cyst/itis
6. nephr/o/lith/iasis

Exercise 8
Pronounce and Spell

Exercise 9
A *Label*
1. hypospadias
2. polycystic kidney disease

B *Identify*
1. renal calculus
2. urinary retention
3. renal hypertension
4. acute kidney injury
5. epispadias
6. urinary tract infection
7. chronic kidney disease
8. end-stage kidney disease

Exercise 10
1. i
2. f
3. j
4. h
5. a
6. e
7. c
8. g
9. b
10. d

Exercise 11
Review of Disease and Disorder Terms

Exercise 12
Pronounce and Spell

Exercise 13
A *Analyze and Define*
1. WR CV S
   ureter/o/stomy
      CF
   creation of an artificial opening into the ureter
2. WR CV WR CV S
   nephr/o/lith/o/tomy
     CF   CF
   incision into the kidney to remove stone(s)
3. WR CV S
   nephr/o/stomy
     CF
   creation of an artificial opening into the kidney
4. WR CV S
   nephr/o/lysis
     CF
   separating the kidney (from other body structures)
5. WR S
   cyst/ectomy
   excision of the bladder
6. WR CV WR CV S
   pyel/o/lith/o/tomy
     CF   CF
   incision into the renal pelvis to remove stone(s)

Appendix A   Answer Key   691

7. WR CV S
   nephr/o/pexy
       CF
   surgical fixation of the kidney
8. WR CV WR CV S
   cyst/o/lith/o/tomy
     CF   CF
   incision into the bladder to remove stone(s)
9. WR S
   nephr/ectomy
   excision of the kidney
10. WR S
    ureter/ectomy
    excision of the ureter
11. WR CV S
    cyst/o/stomy
      CF
    creation of an artificial opening into the bladder
12. WR CV S
    pyel/o/plasty
      CF
    surgical repair of the renal pelvis
13. WR CV S
    ur/o/stomy
     CF
    creation of an artificial opening into the urinary system
14. WR CV S
    meat/o/tomy
      CF
    incision into the meatus
15. WR CV S
    lith/o/tripsy
     CF
    surgical crushing of stone(s)
16. WR CV S
    urethr/o/plasty
       CF
    surgical repair of the urethra
17. WR CV WR CV S
    nephr/o/lith/o/tripsy
      CF   CF
    surgical crushing of stone(s) in the kidney (using shock waves)
18. WR CV WR S
    vesic/o/urethr/al suspension
      CF
    suspension pertaining to the bladder and urethra

B *Label*
1. cyst/o/stomy
2. nephr/o/stomy
3. pyel/o/lith/o/tomy
4. nephr/o/lith/o/tomy
5. lith/o/tripsy

Fill In
1. ureter/o/stomy
2. nephr/ectomy

3. nephr/o/lith/o/tripsy
4. ur/o/stomy
5. nephr/o/lysis
6. pyel/o/plasty
7. urethr/o/plasty
8. cyst/ectomy
9. meat/o/tomy
10. nephr/o/pexy
11. ureter/ectomy
12. cyst/o/lith/o/tomy
13. vesico/urethr/al (suspension)

Exercise 14
A *Identify*
1. renal transplant
2. fulguration
3. extracorporeal shock wave lithotripsy

B *Match*
1. b
2. a
3. c

Exercise 15
Review of Surgical Terms

Exercise 16
Pronounce and Spell

Exercise 17
A *Analyze and Define*
1.   WR CV WR CV S
   (voiding) cyst/o/urethr/o/graphy
            CF   CF
   radiographic imaging of the bladder and the urethra
2. WR CV S
   cyst/o/graphy
    CF
   radiographic imaging of the bladder
3. WR CV WR CV S
   nephr/o/son/o/graphy
     CF   CF
   process of recording the kidney using sound
4. WR CV S
   cyst/o/scope
    CF
   instrument used for visual examination of the bladder
5. WR CV S
   cyst/o/gram
    CF
   radiographic image of the bladder
6. WR CV S
   cyst/o/scopy
    CF
   visual examination of the bladder
7. WR CV S
   pyel/o/gram
    CF

   radiographic image of the renal pelvis
8. WR CV S
   ren/o/gram
    CF
   radiographic record of the kidney
9. WR CV S
   nephr/o/scopy
     CF
   visual examination of the kidney
10. WR CV S
    ureter/o/scopy
       CF
    visual examination of the ureter

B *Label*
1. cyst/o/gram
2. (retrograde) ur/o/gram
3. nephr/o/scopy
4. cyst/o/scopy

C *Fill In*
1. ureter/o/scopy
2. pyel/o/gram
3. nephr/o/son/o/graphy
4. cyst/o/scope
5. (voiding) cyst/o/urethr/o/graphy
6. cyst/o/graphy
7. ren/o/gram

Exercise 18
A *Label*
1. blood urea nitrogen
2. urinalysis
3. KUB
4. specific gravity

B *Match*
1. c   5. h
2. g   6. b
3. d   7. f
4. a   8. e

Exercise 19
Review of Diagnostic Terms

Exercise 20
Pronounce and Spell

Exercise 21
1. WR S
   noct/uria
   night urination
2. WR CV S
   ur/o/logist
    CF
   physician who studies and treats diseases of the urinary tract

3. WR S
   olig/uria
   condition of scanty urine (amount)
4. WR CV S
   nephr/o/logist
       CF
   physician who studies and treats diseases of the kidney
5. WR S
   hemat/uria
   blood in the urine
6. WR CV S
   ur/o/logy
     CF
   study of the urinary tract
7. P S(WR)
   poly/uria
   much (excessive) urine; *Note: the word root is embedded in the suffix and is labeled as S(WR)*
8. WR S
   albumin/uria
   albumin in the urine
9. P S(WR)
   an/uria
   absence of urine; *Note: the word root is embedded in the suffix and is labeled as S(WR)*
10. WR S
    azot/emia
    nitrogen in the blood
11. WR S
    py/uria
    pus in the urine
12. WR S
    urin/ary
    pertaining to urine
13. WR S
    glycos/uria
    sugar in the urine
14. P S(WR)
    dys/uria
    difficult or painful urination; *Note: the word root is embedded in the suffix and is labeled as S(WR)*
15. WR CV S
    nephr/o/logy
      CF
    study of the kidney
16. P WR S
    intra/vesic/al
    pertaining to within the (urinary) bladder
17. WR S
    meat/al
    pertaining to the meatus
18. P WR S
    trans/urethr/al
    pertaining to through the urethra

Exercise 22
A *Fill In*
1. noct/uria
2. olig/uria
3. py/uria
4. ur/o/logist
5. poly/uria
6. nephr/o/logy
7. urin/ary
8. azot/emia
9. ur/o/logy
10. trans/urethr/al
11. glycos/uria
12. intra/vesic/al
13. an/uria
14. albumin/uria

B *Label*
1. meat/al
2. nephr/o/logist
3. dys/uria
4. hemat/uria

Exercise 23
Pronounce and Spell

Exercise 24
A *Label*
1. hemodialysis
2. catheter
3. distended
4. enuresis
5. urinal
6. peritoneal dialysis

B *Identify*
1. electrolytes
2. diuretic
3. prolapse
4. urinary incontinence
5. urinary catheterization
6. void
7. stricture

Exercise 25
A
1. d   4. a
2. f   5. c
3. e   6. b

B
1. a   5. f
2. d   6. c
3. g   7. e
4. b

Exercise 26
Review of Complementary Terms

Exercise 27
1. kidneys ureters (and) bladder; voiding cystourethrography; vesicoureteral reflux
2. specific gravity; urinalysis
3. blood urea nitrogen; glomerular filtration rate
4. extracorporeal shock wave lithotripsy
5. catheterization; acute urinary retention; chronic urinary retention; urinary tract infection
6. hemodialysis
7. acute renal failure; acute kidney injury; chronic kidney disease, chronic renal failure; end-stage kidney disease, end-stage renal disease
8. overactive bladder
9. polycystic kidney disease

Exercise 28
A. blood when he urinated; infection of his bladder; difficulty urinating; physician who treats diseases of the urinary tract
B. Answers will vary and may include hematuria; cystitis; dysuria; urologist
C. and D. hematuria; renal calculi; UTI; end-stage kidney disease; hemodialysis along with their respective definitions

Exercise 29
A
1. nephrolithiasis
2. hematuria
3. urology
4. KUB
5. calculi
6. cystoscopy
7. pyelogram
8. nephrolithotomy
9. catheter

B
1. c
2. d
3. F, calculus is singular for stone
4. a. pertaining to the ureter
   b. instrument used for visual examination of the ureter

Exercise 30
Online Exercise

Exercise 31
1. nephrologist, CKD, hemodialysis, ureterostomy
2. dysuria, urinalysis, pyuria, cystitis

Appendix A Answer Key 693

3. urethrocystitis, retrograde urogram, cystourethrography
4. hematuria, ureterolithiasis, urology, ESWL

Exercise 32
Pronunciation Exercise

Exercise 33
1. c
2. b
3. c
4. b
5. a
6. a
7. b
8. c
9. b
10. c
11. b
12. c
13. a
14. b
15. b
16. c
17. a
18. a
19. c
20. b

ANSWERS TO CHAPTER 7 EXERCISES

Exercise 1
A *Label*
1. male: andr/o
2. seminal vesicle: vesicul/o
3. prostate gland: prostat/o
4. epididymis: epididym/o
5. testis: orch/o, orchi/o, orchid/o
6. vas deferens or ductus deferens: vas/o
7. glans penis: balan/o
8. sperm, spermatozoon: sperm/o, spermat/o

B *Define and Match*
1. g, sperm, spermatozoon
2. a, vessel, duct
3. g, sperm, spermatozoon
4. b, glans penis
5. f, prostate gland
6. d, testis, testicle
7. c, seminal vesicle(s)
8. d, testis, testicle
9. e, epididymis
10. d, testis, testicle
11. male

Exercise 2
A *Define*
1. scanty, few
2. hidden
3. stone(s), calculus (*pl.* calculi)
4. bladder, sac

B *Identify*
1. lith/o
2. cyst/o
3. crypt/o
4. olig/o

Exercise 3
A *Identify*
1. a. an-
   b. a-
2. hyper-

B *Define*
1. above, excessive
2. absence of, without
3. absence of, without

Exercise 4
A *Match*
1. d
2. g
3. f
4. b
5. a
6. e
7. c

B *Match*
1. g
2. f
3. c
4. e
5. a
6. d
7. b

Exercise 5
Pronounce and Spell

Exercise 6
1. WR CV S
   prostat/o/lith
      CF
   stone(s) in the prostate gland
2. WR S
   balan/itis
   inflammation of the glans penis
3. WR S
   orch/itis
   inflammation of the testis
4. WR CV WR S
   prostat/o/vesicul/itis
      CF
   inflammation of the prostate gland and the seminal vesicles
5. WR CV WR S
   prostat/o/cyst/itis
      CF
   inflammation of the prostate gland and the (urinary) bladder
6. WR WR S
   orchi/epididym/itis
   inflammation of the testis and the epididymis
7. WR CV S
   prostat/o/rrhea
      CF
   discharge from the prostate gland
8. WR S
   epididym/itis
   inflammation of the epididymis
9. WR S P S(WR)
   (benign) prostat/ic hyper/plasia
   excessive development pertaining to the prostate gland; *Note: the word root is embedded in the suffix and is labeled as S(WR)*
10. WR WR S
    crypt/orchid/ism
    state of hidden testis
11. WR S
    prostat/itis
    inflammation of the prostate gland
12. P WR S
    an/orch/ism
    state of absence of testis (unilateral or bilateral)
13. WR CV S
    andr/o/pathy
       CF
    disease of the male

Exercise 7
A *Label*
1. crypt/orchid/ism
2. balan/itis
3. benign prostat/ic hyper/plasia

B *Fill In*
1. prostat/o/cyst/itis
2. prostat/o/lith
3. orch/itis
4. epididym/itis
5. prostat/o/rrhea
6. prostat/o/vesicul/itis
7. an/orch/ism
8. prostat/itis
9. orchi/epididym/itis
10. andr/o/pathy

Exercise 8
Pronounce and Spell

Exercise 9
A *Identify*
1. testicular cancer
2. erectile dysfunction
3. priapism
4. testicular torsion
5. spermatocele
6. infertility

B Label
1. prostate cancer
2. phimosis
3. hydrocele
4. varicocele

Exercise 10
1. d
2. c
3. e
4. b
5. j
6. f
7. i
8. h
9. g
10. a

Exercise 11
Review of Disease and Disorder Terms

Exercise 12
Pronounce and Spell

Exercise 13
1. WR S
   vas/ectomy
   excision of a duct
2. WR CV WR CV S
   prostat/o/cyst/o/tomy
   CF   CF
   incision into the prostate gland and (urinary) bladder
3. WR CV S
   orchi/o/tomy
   CF
   incision into the testis
4. WR S
   epdidym/ectomy
   excision of the epididymis
5. WR CV S
   orchi/o/pexy
   CF
   surgical fixation of the testicle
6. WR CV WR S
   prostat/o/vesicul/ectomy
   CF
   excision of the prostate gland and the seminal vesicles
7. WR CV S
   orchi/o/plasty
   CF
   surgical repair of the testis
8. WR S
   vesicul/ectomy
   excision of the seminal vesicle(s)
9. WR S
   prostat/ectomy
   excision of the prostate gland
10. WR CV S
    balan/o/plasty
    CF
    surgical repair of the glans penis
11. WR CV WR CV S
    vas/o/vas/o/stomy
    CF   CF
    creation of artificial openings between ducts
12. WR S
    orchi/ectomy
    excision of the testis

Exercise 14
A Label
1. vas/ectomy
2. prostat/ectomy
3. orchi/o/pexy
4. epididym/ectomy

B Fill In
1. orchi/ectomy
2. balan/o/plasty
3. prostat/o/cyst/o/tomy
4. vesicul/ectomy
5. prostat/o/lith/o/tomy
6. orchi/o/tomy
7. prostat/o/vesicul/ectomy
8. orchi/o/plasty
9. vas/o/vas/o/stomy

Exercise 15
Pronounce and Spell

Exercise 16
A Label
1. robotic surgery
2. transurethral resection of the prostate gland
3. minimally invasive surgical treatments
4. circumcision
5. enucleation

B Identify
1. sterilization
2. ablation
3. hydrocelectomy
4. transurethral incision of the prostate gland
5. laser surgery
6. morcellation

Exercise 17
1. g
2. k
3. h
4. j
5. i
6. f
7. b
8. a
9. d
10. c
11. e

Exercise 18
Review of Surgical Terms

Exercise 19
Pronounce and Spell

Exercise 20
1. digital rectal examination
2. prostate-specific antigen
3. transrectal ultrasound
4. semen analysis
5. multiparametric MRI
6. total testosterone
7. MRI ultrasound fusion biopsy

Exercise 21
1. e
2. d
3. f
4. c
5. g
6. b
7. a

Exercise 22
Review of Diagnostic Terms

Exercise 23
Pronounce and Spell

Exercise 24
A Analyze and Define
1. WR S
   orchi/algia
   pain in the testis
2. WR CV WR S
   olig/o/sperm/ia
   CF
   condition of scanty sperm (in the semen)
3. P WR S
   a/sperm/ia
   condition of without sperm (or semen or ejaculation)
4. WR CV S
   balan/o/rrhea
   CF
   discharge from the glans penis

B Build
1. a/sperm/ia
2. olig/o/sperm/ia
3. orchi/algia
4. balan/o/rrhea

Exercise 25
A Match
1. c
2. f
3. b
4. g
5. a
6. e
7. d

B Match
1. a
2. g
3. d
4. b
5. c
6. h
7. e
8. f

Exercise 26
Review of Complementary Terms

Appendix A Answer Key   695

Exercise 27
1. lower urinary tract symptoms; bladder outlet obstruction
2. digital rectal examination; benign prostatic hyperplasia
3. transurethral incision; transurethral resection; robot-assisted simple prostatectomy
4. holmium laser enucleation of the prostate gland; photoselective vaporization of the prostate gland
5. minimally invasive surgical treatments; prostatic urethral lift; water vapor thermal therapy
6. human immunodeficiency virus
7. human papillomavirus
8. sexually transmitted infection; sexually transmitted disease
9. prostate-specific antigen
10. radical prostatectomy, robot-assisted radical prostatectomy
11. erectile dysfunction
12. transrectal ultrasound

Exercise 28
A. pain in his testicle; twisting of the spermatic cord with decreased blood flow to the testis; surgical fixation of the testis; surgical removal of the testis; reduced or absent ability to achieve pregnancy
B. Answers will vary and may include orchialgia, testicular torsion, orchiopexy, orchiectomy, infertility, and their respective definitions.
C. orchialgia, orchiectomy, infertility, testicular torsion, orchiopexy
D. Answers will vary and may include orchialgia, orchiectomy, infertility, testicular torsion, orchiopexy, and their respective definitions.

Exercise 29
A
1. nocturia
2. hematuria
3. BOO
4. urinary
5. benign prostatic hyperplasia
6. urology

B
1. c
2. b
3. c
4. a

Exercise 30
Online exercise

Exercise 31
1. PSA, urologist, MRI ultrasound fusion biopsy
2. cryptorchidism, testicular cancer, orchiopexy
3. benign prostatic hyperplasia, TURP, laser surgery, prostatectomy
4. STI, human immunodeficiency virus, syphilis, trichomoniasis

Exercise 32
Pronunciation Exercise

Exercise 33
1. a
2. b
3. a
4. c
5. a
6. c
7. b
8. a
9. c
10. c
11. b
12. a
13. c
14. a
15. c
16. a
17. b
18. a
19. c
20. b

ANSWERS TO CHAPTER 8 EXERCISES

Exercise 1
A *Label*
1. ovary: oophor/o
2. uterus: hyster/o, metr/o
3. fallopian (uterine) tube: salping/o
4. endometrium: endometri/o
5. cervix: cervic/o, trachel/o
6. vagina: colp/o, vagin/o
7. hymen: hymen/o

B *Label*
1. vulva: episi/o, vulv/o
2. perineum: perine/o

C *Identify*
1. men/o
2. gynec/o
3. mamm/o, mast/o
4. pelv/i

D *Define and Match*
1. f: fallopian tube (uterine tube)
2. e: uterus
3. a: perineum
4. c: cervix
5. b: vagina
6. c: cervix
7. d: breast
8. pelvis, pelvic cavity

E *Define and Match*
1. b: vagina
2. a: hymen
3. d: vulva
4. f: uterus
5. e: breast
6. g: ovary
7. d: vulva
8. c: endometrium
9. men/o: menstruation
10. gynec/o: woman

Exercise 2
A *Define*
1. scanty, few
2. blood
3. muscle(s), muscle tissue
4. white
5. pus
6. water

B *Identify*
1. py/o
2. hydr/o
3. hemat/o
4. my/o
5. olig/o
6. leuk/o

Exercise 3
A *Define*
1. within
2. absence of, without
3. surrounding (outer)
4. painful, abnormal, difficult, labored

B *Identify*
1. dys-
2. endo-
3. a-
4. peri-

Exercise 4
A *Match*
1. c
2. h
3. f
4. a
5. e
6. d
7. b
8. g

B *Define*
1. the record, radiographic image
2. abnormal condition

Copyright © 2026 by Elsevier Inc. All rights are reserved, including those for text and data mining, AI training, and similar technologies.

3. pain
4. flow, discharge
5. visual examination
6. pertaining to
7. excision, surgical removal
8. surgical repair
9. excessive bleeding
10. instrument used for visual examination
11. cut into, incision
12. one who studies and treats (specialist, physician)

C *Label*
1. -salpinx
2. -cleisis

Exercise 5
Pronounce and Spell

Exercise 6
1. WR   S
   vagin/osis
   abnormal condition of the vagina (caused by a bacterial imbalance)
2. WR CV   S
   hemat/o/salpinx
         CF
   blood in the fallopian tube
3. WR CV   S
   metr/o/rrhagia
        CF
   excessive bleeding from the uterus (irregular, out-of-cycle bleeding ranging from heavy to light, including spotting)
4. WR   S
   oophor/itis
   inflammation of the ovary
5. P WR   S
   peri/metr/itis
   inflammation surrounding the uterus (outer layer)
6. WR CV WR   S
   vulv/o/vagin/itis
        CF
   inflammation of the vulva and vagina
7. WR CV   S
   salping/o/cele
          CF
   hernia of the fallopian tube
8. WR CV WR CV   S
   men/o/metr/o/rrhagia
       CF   CF
   excessive bleeding from the uterus at menstruation (and between menstrual cycles; heavy and irregular bleeding)

Exercise 7
A *Label*
1. hydr/o/salpinx
2. mast/itis
3. vagin/osis
4. endometri/osis
5. salping/itis
6. endometr/itis

B *Fill In*
1. my/o/metr/itis
2. men/o/rrhagia
3. py/o/salpinx
4. cervic/itis

Exercise 8
Pronounce and Spell

Exercise 9
1. a   5. c
2. d   6. f
3. b   7. e
4. g

Exercise 10
1. h   5. e
2. f   6. g
3. b   7. a
4. c   8. d

Exercise 11
A *Identify*
1. ovarian cancer
2. Adenomyosis
3. toxic shock syndrome
4. Cervical cancer
5. premenstrual syndrome
6. abnormal uterine bleeding
7. Fibrocystic breast changes

B *Label*
1. uterovaginal prolapse
2. uterine fibroid
3. endometrial cancer
4. breast cancer
5. pelvic inflammatory disease
6. vaginal fistula
7. polycystic ovary syndrome
8. Bartholin cyst

Exercise 12
Review of Disease and Disorder Terms

Exercise 13
Pronounce and Spell

Exercise 14
1. WR CV   S
   colp/o/plasty
        CF
   surgical repair of the vagina
2. WR CV   S
   hymen/o/tomy
         CF
   incision into the hymen
3. WR   S
   vulv/ectomy
   excision of the vulva
4. WR CV   S
   perine/o/rrhaphy
          CF
   suturing of the perineum (tear)
5. WR CV   S
   salping/o/stomy
          CF
   creation of an artificial opening in the fallopian tube
6. WR   S
   oophor/ectomy
   excision of the ovary
7. WR CV   S
   mast/o/pexy
        CF
   surgical fixation of the breast
8. WR CV WR CV   S
   colp/o/perine/o/rrhaphy
        CF   CF
   suturing of the vagina and the perineum

Exercise 15
A *Label*
1. hyster/ectomy
2. salping/ectomy
3. salping/o/-oophor/ectomy
4. episi/o/rrhaphy
5. mast/ectomy
6. mamm/o/plasty

B *Fill In*
1. colp/o/rrhaphy
2. trachel/ectomy
3. colp/o/cleisis
4. hyster/o/pexy

Exercise 16
Pronounce and Spell

Exercise 17
A *Label*
1. tubal ligation
2. dilation and curettage
3. endometrial ablation
4. myomectomy

B *Identify*
1. anterior and posterior colporrhaphy
2. uterine artery embolization
3. conization

Appendix A Answer Key 697

C *Match*
1. c
2. a
3. b
4. c
5. g
6. c
7. c

Exercise 18
Review of Surgical Terms

Exercise 19
Pronounce and Spell

Exercise 20
A *Analyze and Define*
1. WR CV S
   colp/o/scopy
      CF
   visual examination of the vagina
2. WR CV S
   mamm/o/gram
      CF
   radiographic image of the breast
3. WR CV S
   colp/o/scope
      CF
   instrument used for visual examination of the vagina
4. WR CV S
   hyster/o/scopy
      CF
   visual examination of the uterus
5. WR CV WR CV S
   hyster/o/salping/o/gram
      CF   CF
   radiographic image of the uterus and fallopian tubes
6. WR CV S
   pelv/i/scopic
      CF
   pertaining to visual examination of the pelvic cavity
7. WR CV S
   pelv/i/scopy
      CF
   visual examination of the pelvic cavity
8. WR CV S
   mamm/o/graphy
      CF
   radiographic imaging of the breast
9. WR CV S
   hyster/o/scope
      CF
   instrument used for visual examination of the uterus
10. WR CV WR CV S
    son/o/hyster/o/graphy
       CF   CF
    process of recording the uterus with sound

B *Build*
1. mamm/o/graphy
2. mamm/o/gram
3. colp/o/scope
4. hyster/o/salping/o/gram

C *Build*
1. colp/o/scopy
2. hyster/o/scopy
3. pelv/i/scopic
4. pelv/i/scopy
5. hyster/o/scope
6. son/o/hyster/o/graphy

Exercise 21
A *Label*
1. transvaginal sonography
2. Pap test

B *Match*
1. c
2. d
3. e
4. f
5. a
6. b

C *Identify*
1. Sentinel lymph node biopsy
2. stereotactic breast biopsy
3. CA-125 test
4. HPV test

Exercise 22
Review of Diagnostic Terms

Exercise 23
Pronounce and Spell

Exercise 24
A *Analyze and Define*
1. WR CV S
   gynec/o/logist
      CF
   physician who studies and treats (female reproductive system) women
2. WR CV S
   gynec/o/logy
      CF
   study of women (branch of medicine dealing with health and diseases of the female reproductive system)
3. WR CV WR S
   vulv/o/vagin/al
      CF
   pertaining to the vulva and vagina
4. WR S
   mast/algia
   pain in the breast
5. WR S
   pelv/ic
   pertaining to the pelvis
6. WR CV S
   leuk/o/rrhea
      CF
   white discharge (from the vagina)
7. WR CV WR S
   vesic/o/vagin/al
      CF
   pertaining to the (urinary) bladder and the vagina
8. WR S
   vagin/al
   pertaining to the vagina
9. P WR S
   endo/cervic/al
   pertaining to within the cervix
10. WR CV WR CV S
    olig/o/men/o/rrhea
       CF   CF
    scanty menstrual flow (infrequent menstrual flow)

B *Build*
1. leuk/o/rrhea
2. pelv/ic
3. mast/algia
4. vulv/o/vagin/al
5. gynec/o/logist
6. gynec/o/logy
7. vesic/o/vagin/al
8. vagin/al
9. endo/cervic/al
10. a/men/o/rrhea
11. dys/men/o/rrhea

Exercise 25
A *Match*
1. g
2. d
3. i
4. b
5. c
6. e
7. a
8. h
9. f

B *Label*
1. speculum
2. contraception

C *Fill In*
1. fistula
2. menarche
3. dyspareunia
4. menopause
5. hormone replacement therapy
6. anovulation
7. oligoovulation

Exercise 26
Review of Complementary Terms

Exercise 27
1. anterior and posterior colporrhaphy
2. total abdominal hysterectomy and bilateral salpingo-oophorectomy; hormone replacement therapy
3. sonohysterography; transvaginal sonography
4. vaginal hysterectomy; laparoscopically assisted vaginal hysterectomy; total laparoscopic hysterectomy
5. dilation and curettage; cervix; loop electrosurgical excision procedure
6. fibrocystic breast changes
7. pelvic inflammatory disease; gynecology
8. premenstrual syndrome
9. uterine artery embolization
10. intrauterine device; intrauterine system; birth control
11. polycystic ovary syndrome
12. abnormal uterine bleeding

Exercise 28
A. trying for over a year to get pregnant; menstruating is very painful; she bleeds a lot; may have given her a disease; only one of his testicles was down; surgery to fix the other one
B. Answers will vary and may include infertility, dysmenorrhea, menorrhagia, sexually transmitted disease, sexually transmitted infection, cryptorchidism, orchiopexy, along with their respective definitions.
C. infertility, cryptorchidism, orchiopexy, menarche, dysmenorrhea, menorrhagia, Pap test, cervicitis, chlamydia, pelvic inflammatory disease, semen analysis, hysterosalpingogram
D. Answers will vary and may include infertility, cryptorchidism, orchiopexy, menarche, dysmenorrhea, menorrhagia, Pap test, cervicitis, chlamydia, pelvic inflammatory disease, semen analysis, hysterosalpingogram, along with their respective definitions

Exercise 29
A
1. mammography
2. carcinoma
3. hysterectomy
4. adenomyosis
5. endometriosis
6. hormone therapy
7. stereotactic breast biopsy
8. mediolateral
9. mastectomy
10. sentinel lymph node biopsy

B
1. c
2. a
3. d

Exercise 30
Use Medical Language in Online Electronic Health Records

Exercise 31
1. vaginal, leukorrhea, vaginitis
2. colposcopy, Pap test, conization, cervical cancer
3. mammography, mammogram, mastectomy, mammoplasty
4. amenorrhea, menopause, hormone therapy, dyspareunia, uterovaginal prolapse

Exercise 32
Pronunciation Exercise

Exercise 33
1. a
2. c
3. a
4. c
5. b
6. a
7. b
8. b
9. a
10. a
11. b
12. a
13. c
14. b
15. b
16. a
17. c
18. b
19. a
20. c

ANSWERS TO CHAPTER 9 EXERCISES

Exercise 1
A *Label*
1. umbilicus: omphal/o
2. fetus: fet/o
3. amnion, amniotic fluid: amni/o, amnion/o
4. chorion: chori/o

B *Identify*
1. puerper/o
2. a. par/o
   b. part/o
3. gravid/o
4. lact/o
5. nat/o

C *Define and Match*
1. c: amnion, amniotic fluid
2. d: umbilicus, navel
3. c: amnion, amniotic fluid
4. b: fetus, unborn offspring
5. a: chorion

D *Define*
1. milk
2. bear, give birth to, labor, childbirth
3. childbirth
4. pregnancy
5. birth

Exercise 2
A *Define*
1. first
2. scanty, few
3. pylorus, pyloric sphincter
4. water
5. head
6. vulva
7. uterus
8. esophagus
9. cancer
10. false
11. malformations
12. trachea
13. sound
14. pelvis, pelvic cavity

B *Identify*
1. cephal/o
2. olig/o
3. prim/i
4. hyster/o
5. pylor/o
6. pelv/i
7. pseud/o
8. episi/o
9. terat/o
10. esophag/o
11. carcin/o
12. trache/o
13. hydr/o
14. son/o

Exercise 3
A *Define*
1. before
2. small
3. new
4. many
5. after
6. painful, abnormal, difficult, labored
7. before
8. many, much
9. within
10. none

B *Identify*
1. nulli-
2. post-
3. micro-
4. intra-
5. a. ante-
   b. pre-
6. poly-
7. multi-
8. neo-
9. dys-

Exercise 4
A *Define*
1. study of
2. substance or agent that produces or causes
3. tumor, swelling
4. pertaining to
5. cut into, incision
6. one who studies and treats (specialist, physician)
7. hernia, protrusion
8. producing, orginating, causing
9. softening
10. inflammation
11. flow discharge
12. process of recording, radiographic imaging

B *Label*
1. -tocia
2. -rrhexis
3. -cyesis
4. -amnios

C *Identify*
1. -a
2. -e
3. -um
4. -us

Exercise 5
Pronounce and Spell

Exercise 6
A *Analyze and Define*
1. WR CV WR S
   chori/o/amnion/itis
   CF
   inflammation of the chorion and amnion
2. WR CV WR S
   chori/o/carcin/oma
   CF
   cancerous tumor of the chorion
3. WR CV S
   pseud/o/cyesis
   CF
   false pregnancy (a woman who believes she is pregnant)
4. WR S
   amnion/itis
   inflammation of the amnion
5. WR CV S
   hyster/o/rrhexis
   CF
   rupture of the uterus
6. WR CV WR S
   olig/o/hydr/amnios
   CF
   scanty amnion water (less than the normal amount of amniotic fluid)
7. P WR S
   poly/hydr/amnios
   much amnion water (more than the normal amount of amniotic fluid)
8. P S(WR)
   dys/tocia
   difficult labor

B *Label*
1. poly/hydr/amnios
2. olig/o/hydr/amnios
3. hyster/o/rrhexis
4. dys/tocia

C *Fill In*
1. chori/o/carcin/oma
2. amnion/itis
3. chori/o/amnion/itis
4. pseud/o/cyesis

Exercise 7
A *Match*
1. e
2. g
3. f
4. b
5. a
6. c
7. d

B *Label*
1. ectopic pregnancy
2. abruptio placentae
3. placenta previa

C *Identify*
1. placenta accreta spectrum
2. eclampsia
3. abortion
4. preeclampsia

Exercise 8
Review of Obstetric Disease and Disorder Terms

Exercise 9
Pronounce and Spell

Exercise 10
A *Analyze and Define*
1. WR S
   pylor/ic (stenosis)
   narrowing pertaining to the pyloric sphincter
2. WR CV S
   omphal/o/cele
   CF
   hernia at the umbilicus
3. WR S
   omphal/itis
   inflammation of the umbilicus
4. P WR S
   micro/cephal/us
   (fetus with a very) small head
5. WR CV WR S
   trache/o/esophag/eal (fistula)
   CF
   abnormal passageway pertaining to the trachea and the esophagus (between the trachea and esophagus)
6. WR CV S
   laryng/o/malacia
   CF
   softening of the larynx

B *Label*
1. micro/cephal/us
2. omphal/o/cele

C *Fill In*
1. laryng/o/malacia
2. pylor/ic (stenosis)
3. trache/o/esophag/eal (fistula)
4. omphal/itis

Exercise 11
A *Match*
1. i
2. c
3. j
4. f
5. k
6. b
7. g
8. e
9. h
10. a
11. d

B *Label*
1. esophageal atresia
2. coarctation of the aorta
3. spina bifida
4. gastroschisis

C *Identify*
1. Erythroblastosis fetalis
2. congenital heart disease
3. respiratory distress syndrome
4. congenital cytomegalovirus infection
5. Fetal alcohol syndrome
6. cleft lip or palate
7. Down syndrome

Exercise 12
Review of Neonatology Disease and Disorder Terms

Exercise 13
Pronounce and Spell

Exercise 14
A *Analyze and Define*
1. WR CV S
   episi/o/tomy

CF
incision into the vulva (perineum)
2. WR CV S
amni/o/tomy
CF
incision into the amnion (rupture of the fetal membrane to induce labor)

B *Build*
1. amni/o/tomy
2. episi/o/tomy

Exercise 15
A *Label*
1. cervical cerclage
2. in vitro fertilization
3. cesarean section

B *Match*
1. b
2. c
3. a

Exercise 16
Review of Obstetric Surgical Terms

Exercise 17
Pronounce and Spell

Exercise 18
A *Analyze and Define*
1. WR CV S
amni/o/centesis
CF
surgical puncture to aspirate amniotic fluid
2. WR S WR CV S
pelv/ic son/o/graphy
CF
pertaining to the pelvis, process of recording sound

B *Build*
1. pelv/ic son/o/graphy
2. amni/o/centesis

Exercise 19
A *Match*
1. c   3. d
2. a   4. b

B *Identify*
1. Apgar score
2. Chorionic villus sampling
3. quad screen
4. Nuchal translucency screening

Exercise 20
Review of Obstetric and Neonatology Diagnostic Terms

Exercise 21
Pronounce and Spell

Exercise 22
A *Analyze and Define*
1. P WR S
multi/gravid/a
many pregnancies
2. WR CV S
lact/o/rrhea
CF
(spontaneous) discharge of milk
3. WR S
puerper/al
pertaining to childbirth (immediately after childbirth and the time until reproductive organs return to normal)
4. WR CV S
amni/o/rrhea
CF
discharge (escape) of amniotic fluid
5. P WR S
nulli/par/a
no births
6. WR CV S
amni/o/rrhexis
CF
rupture of the amnion
7. P WR S
post/part/um
after childbirth
8. WR CV WR S
prim/i/par/a
CF
first birth
9. WR S
gravid/a
pregnant (woman)

B *Label*
1. ante/part/um
2. intra/part/um
3. lact/o/genic
4. multi/par/a

C *Fill In*
1. gravid/o/puerper/al
2. prim/i/gravid/a
3. par/a
4. nulli/gravid/a

Exercise 23
A *Identify*
1. parturition
2. Midwifery
3. puerperium
4. Quickening
5. obstetrics (OB)
6. In vivo
7. colostrum
8. Lochia

B *Label*
1. cephalic presentation
2. breech presentation
3. lactation
4. in vitro
5. midwife
6. obstetrician

C *Match*
1. e   5. c
2. g   6. d
3. a   7. f
4. b

D *Match*
1. d   5. b
2. f   6. g
3. c   7. e
4. a

Exercise 24
Review of Obstetric Complementary Terms

Exercise 25
Pronounce and Spell

Exercise 26
A *Analyze and Define*
1. WR CV S
terat/o/genic
CF
producing malformations
2. P WR CV S
neo/nat/o/logy
CF
study of the newborn
3. P WR S
neo/nat/e
new birth
4. WR S
fet/al
pertaining to the fetus
5. P WR S
pre/nat/al
pertaining to before birth (reference to the newborn)
6. WR CV S
terat/o/logy
CF
study of malformations
7. WR S
nat/al
pertaining to birth
8. P WR CV S
neo/nat/o/logist
CF
physician who studies and treats disorders of the newborn

Appendix A   Answer Key

9. WR CV S
   terat/o/gen
   ___CF___
   (any agent) producing malformations (in the developing embryo)
10. P   WR S
    post/nat/al
    pertaining to after birth (reference to the newborn)

B *Label*
1. neo/nat/e
2. neo/nat/o/logist
3. fet/al
4. terat/o/gen

C *Fill In*
1. post/nat/al
2. terat/o/logy
3. neo/nat/o/logy
4. terat/o/genic
5. nat/al
6. pre/nat/al

Exercise 27
A *Identify*
1. congenital anomaly
2. Stillborn
3. meconium

B *Label*
1. gavage
2. premature infant

C *Match*
1. d   4. a
2. e   5. b
3. c

Exercise 28
Review of Neonatology Complementary Terms

Exercise 29
1. expected (estimated) date of delivery, last menstrual period, date of birth
2. obstetrics, newborn
3. primipara, multipara
4. chorionic villus sampling, abortion
5. fetal alcohol syndrome
6. cytomegalovirus
7. respiratory distress syndrome
8. Cesarean section
9. vaginal birth after cesarean
10. in vitro fertilization
11. placenta accreta spectrum, antepartum hemorrhage, postpartum hemorrhage

Exercise 30
A. pregnant for the third time, born dead, ultrasound test, genetic condition that causes physical and mental problems, needle to take fluid out
B. Answers will vary and may include multigravida, para, stillborn, pelvic sonography, Down syndrome, and amniocentesis, and their respective definitions.
C. gravida, para, EDD, prenatal, Down syndrome, amniocentesis, abortion, congenital anomalies, tracheoesophageal fistula, neonatologist
D. Answers will vary and may include gravida, para, EDD, prenatal, Down syndrome, amniocentesis, abortion, congenital anomalies, tracheoesophageal fistula, neonatologist, and their respective definitions.

Exercise 31
A
1. gravida
2. para
3. EDD
4. prenatal
5. pelvic sonography
6. cephalic presentation

B
1. c
2. T
3. F, sonography was used

Exercise 32
1. nulligravida; nullipara
2. placenta previa; abruptio placentae; placenta accreta spectrum
3. puerperium; lochia
4. esophageal atresia; gavage
5. postpartum

Exercise 33
Online Exercise

Exercise 34
Pronunciation Exercise

Exercise 35
1. b   11. b
2. b   12. a
3. a   13. c
4. a   14. b
5. c   15. a
6. b   16. b
7. a   17. c
8. c   18. a
9. b   19. c
10. b   20. b

ANSWERS TO CHAPTER 10 EXERCISES

Exercise 1
A *Label*
1. heart: cardi/o
2. muscle: my/o
3. valve: valvul/o
4. ventricle: ventricul/o
5. aorta: aort/o
6. atrium: atri/o

B *Define and Match*
1. d, heart
2. e, atrium
3. a, valve
4. b, ventricle
5. c, aorta
6. f, muscle(s), muscle tissue

C *Label*
1. blood vessel: angi/o
2. vein: phleb/o, ven/o
3. artery: arteri/o
4. blood: hem/o, hemat/o
5. bone marrow: myel/o
6. plasma: plasm/o
7. cells: cyt/o

D *Define and Match*
1. c, artery *(s)*, arteries *(pl)*
2. d, bone marrow
3. a, blood
4. e, vein(s)
5. f, vessel, blood vessel
6. e, vein(s)
7. b, plasma
8. a, blood

E *Label*
1. lymph, lymph tissue: lymph/o
2. thymus gland: thym/o
3. lymph node(s): lymphaden/o
4. spleen: splen/o

Copyright © 2026 by Elsevier Inc. All rights are reserved, including those for text and data mining, AI training, and similar technologies.

F Define and Match
1. c, spleen
2. d, lymph
3. b, thymus gland
4. a, lymph node

Exercise 2
A Define
1. sound
2. blood clot
3. deficiency, blockage
4. red
5. yellowish, fatty plaque
6. electricity, electrical activity
7. white
8. immune system
9. plug

B Identify
1. thromb/o
2. ech/o
3. isch/o
4. ather/o
5. immun/o
6. electr/o
7. embol/o
8. leuk/o
9. erythr/o

Exercise 3
A Define
1. slow
2. all, total
3. many, much
4. fast, rapid
5. within
6. surrounding (outer)
7. within

B Identify
1. tachy-
2. brady-
3. poly-
4. peri-
5. pan-
6. endo-, intra-

Exercise 4
A Identify
1. -rrhage
2. -genic
3. -sclerosis
4. -lysis
5. -penia
6. -stasis
7. -apheresis
8. -logy
9. -logist
10. -us
11. -ar, -ic, -ous

B Match
1. f
2. l
3. g
4. i
5. c
6. k
7. j
8. b
9. d
10. a
11. h
12. e

C Match
1. d
2. f
3. g
4. a
5. c
6. b
7. e

Exercise 5
Pronounce and Spell

Exercise 6
1. WR CV WR S
   atri/o/ventricul/ar
       CF
   pertaining to the atrium and ventricle
2. WR CV WR CV S
   electr/o/cardi/o/graphy
       CF   CF
   process of recording the electrical activity of the heart
3. WR CV S
   cardi/o/logist
       CF
   physician who studies and treats diseases of the heart
4. WR CV S
   aort/o/gram
       CF
   radiographic image of the aorta (after an injection of contrast materials)
5. WR S
   valvul/itis
   inflammation of a valve (of the heart)
6. WR S
   phleb/ectomy
   excision of a vein
7. P WR S
   tachy/card/ia
   condition of a rapid heart (rate)
   Note: the "i" in cardi/o has been dropped because the suffix starts with an "i"
8. WR CV S
   angi/o/scopy
       CF
   visual examination (of the inside) of a blood vessel
9. WR CV S
   angi/o/graphy
       CF
   radiographic imaging of a blood vessel
10. WR CV S
    cardi/o/genic
        CF
    originating in the heart
11. WR S
    isch/emia
    deficiency in blood (flow); (caused by constriction or obstruction of a blood vessel)
12. WR CV WR S
    thromb/o/phleb/itis
        CF
    inflammation of a vein associated with a blood clot
13. WR S
    ather/ectomy
    excision of fatty plaque
14. WR CV S
    valvul/o/plasty
        CF
    surgical repair of a valve
15. WR S
    angi/oma
    tumor composed of blood vessels
16. WR CV WR S
    my/o/card/itis
        CF
    inflammation of the muscle of the heart; Note: the "i" in cardi/o has been dropped because the suffix starts with an "i"

Exercise 7
A Label
1. aort/ic stenosis Note: the suffix -stenosis stands as an independent word in this instance
2. cardi/o/megaly
3. ather/o/sclerosis
4. endarterectomy Note: the "o" in the prefix endo- and the "i" in the combining form arteri/o have been dropped because the following word parts begin with a vowel
5. arteri/o/gram
6. ven/o/gram
7. peri/card/itis Note: the "i" in cardi/o is dropped because the suffix starts with an "i"
8. peri/cardi/o/centesis
9. intra/ven/ous
10. ech/o/cardi/o/gram
11. electr/o/cardi/o/gram

B Fill In
1. phleb/itis
2. angi/o/plasty
3. endo/card/itis Note: the "i" in cardi/o has been dropped
4. brady/card/ia Note: the "i" in cardi/o has been dropped

Appendix A Answer Key

5. arteri/o/sclerosis
6. embol/ectomy
7. cardi/o/my/o/pathy
8. angi/o/stenosis
9. poly/arter/itis *Note: the "i" in arteri/o has been dropped*
10. cardi/o/logy

Exercise 8
Pronounce and Spell

Exercise 9
A *Disease and Disorder Terms*
1. cardiac arrest
2. varicose veins
3. Aneurysm
4. Coronary artery disease
5. Angina pectoris
6. myocardial infarction
7. fibrillation; arrhythmia
8. hypertensive
9. Heart failure
10. Peripheral artery disease
11. Intermittent claudication
12. cardiac tamponade
13. mitral valve stenosis; rheumatic heart disease
14. Deep vein thrombosis
15. Acute coronary syndrome
16. cor pulmonale

B *Surgical Terms*
1. artificial cardiac pacemaker
2. thrombolytic therapy
3. coronary artery bypass graft
4. catheter ablation
5. coronary stent
6. percutaneous transluminal coronary angioplasty
7. automatic implantable cardiac defibrillator
8. femoropopliteal bypass

Exercise 10
A *Label*
1. Doppler ultrasound
2. lipid profile
3. exercise stress test
4. sestamibi test
5. digital subtraction angiography
6. sphygmomanometer
7. cardiac catheterization

B *Fill In*
1. Transesophageal echocardiogram
2. single-photon emission computed tomography
3. creatine phosphokinase
4. C-reactive protein

5. Pulse
6. Troponin
7. blood pressure

Exercise 11
A *Match*
1. j   6. i
2. g   7. a
3. h   8. e
4. b   9. c
5. d   10. f

B *Label*
1. defibrillation
2. cardiopulmonary resuscitation

Exercise 12
Review of Cardiovascular Terms

Exercise 13
Pronounce and Spell

Exercise 14
1. WR CV S
   hem/o/stasis
       CF
   stoppage of bleeding
2. WR CV S
   hemat/o/logist
        CF
   physician who studies and treats diseases of the blood
3. WR CV S
   hem/o/lysis
       CF
   dissolution of blood (cells)
4. WR CV WR S
   lymph/o/cyt/osis
         CF
   increase in the number of lymphocytes
5. P WR CV S
   pan/cyt/o/penia
           CF
   abnormal reduction of all (blood) cells
6. WR CV WR CV S
   erythr/o/cyt/o/penia
          CF   CF
   abnormal reduction of red (blood) cells
7. WR S
   embol/ism
   state of a plug (blood clot, fat, or air lodged in a blood vessel)
8. WR S
   thromb/us
   blood clot

Exercise 15
A *Fill In*
1. leuk/o/cyt/o/penia
2. hem/o/rrhage
3. thromb/o/lysis
4. thromb/o/cyt/o/penia
5. embol/us *Note: the suffix -us is a noun ending with no meaning*
6. multiple myel/oma

B *Label*
1. phleb/o/tomy
2. plasm/apheresis
3. hemat/oma
4. thromb/osis

Exercise 16
Pronounce and Spell

Exercise 17
1. e   5. d
2. g   6. c
3. f   7. a
4. b

Exercise 18
1. bone marrow aspiration
2. bone marrow biopsy
3. phlebotomist
4. perfusionist

Exercise 19
1. blood dyscrasias
2. anticoagulant
3. venipuncture; extravasation
4. bone marrow transplant; peripheral blood stem cell transplant
5. complete blood count with differential
6. hematocrit; hemoglobin
7. bleeding profile, prothrombin time, activated partial thromboplastin time

Exercise 20
Review of Blood Terms

Exercise 21
Pronounce and Spell

Exercise 22
A *Analyze and Define*
1. WR WR CV S
   lymph/angi/o/graphy
             CF
   radiographic imaging of lymph vessels
2. WR S
   thym/ectomy
   excision of the thymus gland

3. WR CV S
   splen/o/rrhaphy
        CF
   suturing, repairing of the spleen
4. WR CV S
   splen/o/megaly
        CF
   enlargement of the spleen
5. WR S
   lymph/oma
   tumor of lymphatic tissue
6. WR S
   lymphaden/itis
   inflammation of lymph nodes

B *Build*
1. lymph/ang/itis Note: the "i" in angi/o is dropped because the suffix starts with an "i"
2. lymphaden/o/pathy
3. thym/oma
4. splen/ectomy

Exercise 23
A *Label*
1. infectious mononucleosis
2. lymphedema

B *Fill in*
1. lymphoma
2. lymphangiography
3. thymoma; thymectomy
4. splenectomy; splenomegaly
5. splenorrhaphy
6. lymphadenopathy
7. lymphadenitis
8. lymphangitis

Exercise 24
Review of Lymphatic Terms

Exercise 25
Pronounce and Spell

Exercise 26
1. WR CV S
   lymph/o/cyte
        CF
   lymph cell
2. WR CV S
   immun/o/logy
        CF
   study of the immune system
3. WR CV S
   immun/o/logist
        CF
   physician who studies and treats diseases of the immune system

Exercise 27
A *Match*
1. e   5. c
2. h   6. g
3. b   7. d
4. f   8. a

B *Match*
1. g   5. f
2. c   6. e
3. a   7. d
4. b

Exercise 28
1. allergen; antigen; antibody
2. anaphylaxis
3. Sarcoidosis
4. erythrocyte sedimentation rate; ESR
5. lymphocyte
6. vaccine; immunity
7. acquired immunodeficiency syndrome; AIDS; opportunistic infections
8. immunosuppression
9. immunology; immunodeficiency; allergy
10. immunologist; autoimmune disease; allergist

Exercise 29
Review of Immune Terms

Exercise 30
1. coronary artery disease; electrocardiogram; single-photon emission computed tomography; echocardiogram
2. deep vein thrombosis
3. complete blood count; differential; red blood cell; white blood cell; hemoglobin; hematocrit
4. coronary artery bypass graft; percutaneous transluminal coronary angioplasty; percutaneous coronary intervention
5. myocardial infarction; coronary care unit
6. blood pressure; pulse
7. heart failure
8. cardiopulmonary resuscitation
9. hypertensive heart disease
10. prothrombin time
11. atrioventricular
12. acute coronary syndrome
13. peripheral artery disease
14. digital subtraction angiography
15. transesophageal echocardiogram
16. C-reactive protein; creatine phosphokinase
17. atrial fibrillation
18. automatic implantable cardiac defibrillator; ventricular fibrillation
19. intravenous
20. hypertension
21. peripheral blood stem cell transplant; bone marrow transplant
22. erythrocyte sedimentation rate

Exercise 31
A. high blood pressure, pain in chest, heart was racing, breathing faster
B. answers will vary and may include hypertension, angina pectoris, tachycardia, tachypnea (from Chapter 5)
C. coronary artery disease, hypertension, hypercholesterolemia, varicose veins, cardiologist, coronary artery bypass grafts, aneurysm, along with their respective definitions
D. answers will vary and may include coronary artery disease, hypertension, hypercholesterolemia varicose veins, cardiologist, coronary artery bypass grafts. aneurysm, along with their respective definitions

Exercise 32
A
1. infectious mononucleosis
2. splenomegaly
3. splenectomy
4. lymphoma
5. vaccines
6. lymphadenopathy
7. arrhythmia
8. CBC with diff
9. leukemia
10. bone marrow biopsy
11. hematologist

B
1. b
2. c
3. b
4. F, no indication of hemolysis
5. T

Exercise 33
Online Exercise

Exercise 34
1. coronary artery disease, angioplasty, coronary artery bypass graft
2. tachycardia, pulse, hypotension
3. CBC with diff, leukemia, hematologist
4. thrombocytopenia, hemorrhage, hemostasis, anemia

Appendix A   Answer Key

5. autoimmune disease, thymoma, immunologist

Exercise 35
Pronunciation Exercise

Exercise 36
1. c	6. a	11. c	16. a
2. a	7. b	12. c	17. b
3. b	8. c	13. c	18. c
4. c	9. a	14. a	19. a
5. b	10. b	15. b	20. b

ANSWERS TO CHAPTER 11 EXERCISES

Exercise 1
A *Label*
1. mouth: or/o, stomat/o
2. esophagus: esophag/o
3. duodenum: duoden/o
4. colon: col/o, colon/o
5. cecum: cec/o
6. anus: an/o
7. stomach: gastr/o
8. antrum: antr/o
9. jejunum: jejun/o
10. ileum: ile/o
11. sigmoid colon: sigmoid/o
12. rectum: proct/o, rect/o

B *Define and Match*
1. e, jejunum
2. g, anus
3. h, stomach
4. b, rectum
5. a, mouth
6. c, colon
7. f, sigmoid colon
8. d, intestines (usually the small intestine)

C *Define and Match*
1. d, ileum
2. g, mouth
3. h, rectum
4. e, esophagus
5. a, antrum
6. f, colon
7. b, duodenum
8. c, cecum

Exercise 2
A *Identify*
1. peritone/o
2. chol/e
3. herni/o
4. diverticul/o
5. polyp/o
6. steat/o

B *Define*
1. hernia
2. abdomen, abdominal cavity
3. saliva, salivary gland
4. gall, bile
5. diverticulum, *pl.* diverticula (pouch extending from a hollow organ)
6. gum(s)
7. appendix
8. tongue
9. liver
10. lip(s)
11. peritoneum
12. palate
13. pancreas
14. abdomen, abdominal cavity
15. tongue
16. common bile duct
17. pylorus, pyloric sphincter
18. uvula
19. bile duct(s)
20. polyp, small growth
21. abdomen, abdominal cavity
22. fat
23. appendix
24. pharynx
25. bladder, sac
26. eating, swallowing

C *Label*
1. palate: palat/o
2. pharynx: pharyng/o
3. uvula: uvul/o
4. tongue: gloss/o, lingu/o
5. gallbladder: chol/e (gall), cyst/o (bladder)
6. pyloric sphincter: pylor/o
7. appendix: append/o, appendic/o
8. gum(s): gingiv/o
9. lip(s): cheil/o
10. salivary glands: sial/o
11. liver: hepat/o
12. bile duct(s): cholangi/o
13. common bile duct: choledoch/o
14. pancreas: pancreat/o
15. abdomen, abdominal cavity: abdomin/o, celi/o, lapar/o

Exercise 3
A *Define*
1. painful, abnormal, difficult, labored
2. half
3. absence of, without

B *Identify*
1. a-
2. hemi-
3. dys-

Exercise 4
A *Define*
1. digestion
2. pertaining to
3. noun suffix, no meaning
4. abnormal condition (means increase when used with blood cell word roots)
5. condition
6. diseased state, condition of

B *Identify*
1. -scope
2. -graphy
3. -logist
4. -logy
5. -gram
6. -scopy

C *Match*
1. c
2. a
3. f
4. b
5. g
6. e
7. d

D *Match*
1. d
2. c
3. g
4. f
5. a
6. b
7. e

Exercise 5
Pronounce and Spell

Exercise 6
1. WR CV WR   S
   steat/o/hepat/itis
   ──
   CF
   inflammation of the liver associated with (excess) fat
2. WR   S
   diverticul/osis
   abnormal condition of having diverticula
3. WR   S
   cholangi/oma
   tumor of the bile duct
4. WR   S
   hepat/oma
   tumor of the liver

5. WR S
   uvul/itis
   inflammation of the uvula
6. WR S
   pancreat/itis
   inflammation of the pancreas
7. WR S
   proct/itis
   inflammation of the rectum
8. WR S
   cheil/itis
   inflammation of the lips
9. WR S
   gastr/itis
   inflammation of the stomach
10. WR CV S
    rect/o/cele
      CF
    hernia of the rectum
11. WR CV S
    enter/o/pathy
      CF
    disease of the intestines
12. WR S
    periton/itis
    inflammation of the peritoneum
13. WR S
    enter/itis
    inflammation of the intestines
14. WR S
    gloss/itis
    inflammation of the tongue

Exercise 7
A *Label*
1. stomat/itis
2. gingiv/itis
3. dys/enter/y
4. appendic/itis
5. chol/e/lith/iasis, choledoch/o/lith/iasis

B *Fill in*
1. hepat/itis
2. col/itis
3. sial/o/lith
4. esophag/itis
5. diverticul/itis
6. chol/e/cyst/itis
7. polyp/osis
8. gastr/o/enter/itis

Exercise 8
Pronounce and Spell

Exercise 9
1. e   5. f
2. g   6. h
3. c   7. d
4. b   8. a

Exercise 10
1. peptic ulcer
2. volvulus
3. polyp
4. gastroesophageal reflux disease
5. adhesions
6. intussusception
7. hemorrhoids

Exercise 11
Review of Disease and Disorder Terms

Exercise 12
Pronounce and Spell

Exercise 13
1. WR CV S
   herni/o/rrhaphy
      CF
   suturing of a hernia
2. WR CV S
   gastr/o/plasty
      CF
   surgical repair of the stomach
3. P WR S
   hemi/col/ectomy
   excision of half of the colon
4. WR S
   antr/ectomy
   excision of the antrum
5. WR CV S
   enter/o/rrhaphy
      CF
   suturing of the (small) intestine
6. WR S
   uvul/ectomy
   excision of the uvula
7. WR CV WR CV S
   gastr/o/jejun/o/stomy
      CF   CF
   creation of an artificial opening between the stomach and the jejunum
8. WR CV WR S
   chol/e/cyst/ectomy
      CF
   excision of the gallbladder
9. WR CV S
   abdomin/o/plasty
      CF
   surgical repair of the abdomen
10. WR S
    pancreat/ectomy
    excision of the pancreas
11. WR CV S
    pylor/o/plasty
      CF
    surgical repair of the pylorus
12. WR CV WR CV S
    choledoch/o/lith/o/tomy
       CF   CF
    incision into the common bile duct to remove a stone
13. WR CV WR CV WR CV S
    uvul/o/palat/o/pharyng/o/plasty
       CF   CF   CF
    surgical repair of the uvula, palate, and pharynx
14. WR CV S
    abdomin/o/centesis
       CF
    surgical puncture to aspirate fluid from the abdominal cavity

Exercise 14
A *Label*
1. append/ectomy
2. col/ectomy
3. palat/o/plasty
4. polyp/ectomy
5. ile/o/stomy
6. col/o/stomy
7. gastr/o/stomy
8. gastr/ectomy

B *Fill In*
1. gloss/o/rrhaphy
2. esophag/o/gastr/o/plasty
3. diverticul/ectomy
4. gingiv/ectomy
5. lapar/o/tomy
6. an/o/plasty
7. chol/e/cyst/ectomy

Exercise 15
Pronounce and Spell

Exercise 16
1. vagotomy
2. anastomosis
3. abdominoperineal resection
4. bariatric surgery
5. hemorrhoidectomy

Exercise 17
Review of Surgical Terms

Exercise 18
Pronounce and Spell

Exercise 19
1. WR CV S
   proct/o/scope
      CF
   instrument used for visual examination of the rectum
2. WR CV S
   proct/o/scopy
      CF
   visual examination of the rectum

Appendix A Answer Key   707

3. WR CV S
   sigmoid/o/scopy
        CF
   visual examination of the sigmoid colon
4. WR CV S
   cholangi/o/graphy
        CF
   radiographic imaging of the bile ducts
5. WR CV S
   colon/o/scope
        CF
   instrument used for visual examination of the colon
6. WR CV S
   lapar/o/scope
        CF
   instrument used for visual examination of the abdominal cavity
7. WR CV S
   lapar/o/scopy
        CF
   visual examination of the abdominal cavity
8. WR S
   esopha/gram
   radiographic image of the esophagus
   Note: the combining vowel "o" and the "g" in esopha/o are dropped in the term esophagram

Exercise 20
A Fill In
1. esophag/o/scopy
2. cholangi/o/gram
3. esophag/o/gastr/o/duoden/o/scopy

B Label
1. colon/o/scopy
2. CT colon/o/graphy
3. capsule endo/scopy
4. gastr/o/scope
5. gastr/o/scopy

Exercise 21
Pronounce and Spell

Exercise 22
1. d   6. g
2. f   7. c
3. i   8. a
4. b   9. h
5. e

Exercise 23
A Label
1. endoscopic retrograde cholangiopancreatography
2. barium enema

B Identify
1. *Helicobacter pylori* stool antigen
2. fecal immunochemical test
3. abdominal sonography
4. endoscopic ultrasound
5. upper GI series
6. modified barium swallow
7. guaiac-based fecal occult blood test

Exercise 24
Review of Diagnostic Terms

Exercise 25
Pronounce and Spell

Exercise 26
1. WR S
   rect/al
   pertaining to the rectum
2. P S(WR)
   dys/pepsia
   difficult digestion
3. WR S
   palat/al
   pertaining to the palate
4. WR S
   esophag/eal
   pertaining to the esophagus
5. WR CV S
   steat/o/rrhea
        CF
   discharge of fat
6. WR S
   duoden/al
   pertaining to the duodenum
7. WR S
   or/al
   pertaining to the mouth
8. WR CV WR CV S
   gastr/o/enter/o/logist
      CF   CF
   physician who studies and treats diseases of the stomach and intestines
9. WR S
   steat/osis
   abnormal condition of fat
10. WR S
    pancreat/ic
    pertaining to the pancreas

Exercise 27
1. hepat/o/megaly
2. a/phag/ia
3. sub/lingu/al
4. nas/o/gastr/ic
5. or/o/gastr/ic
6. an/al
7. peritone/al
8. celi/ac
9. dys/phag/ia
10. ile/o/cec/al
11. col/o/rect/al

Exercise 28
Pronounce and Spell

Exercise 29
1. m   8. a
2. e   9. d
3. h   10. j
4. f   11. b
5. l   12. c
6. i   13. g
7. k

Exercise 30
A Label
1. stoma   3. reflux
2. palpate   4. ascites

B Identify
1. feces   6. melena
2. diarrhea   7. nausea
3. flatus   8. malabsorption
4. emesis   9. hematemesis
5. hematochezia

Exercise 31
Review of Complementary Terms

Exercise 32
1. modified barium swallow, upper gastrointestinal
2. *Helicobacter pylori*, gastroesophageal reflux disease, fecal immunochemical test, guaiac-based fecal occult blood test
3. esophagogastroduodenoscopy, percutaneous endoscopic gastrostomy
4. endoscopic retrograde cholangiopancreatography, endoscopic ultrasound
5. barium enema, ulcerative colitis, irritable bowel syndrome, gastrointestinal
6. nausea and vomiting, nonalcoholic steatohepatitis, nonalcoholic fatty liver disease
7. abdominoperineal resection, uvulopalatopharyngoplasty

Exercise 33
A. felt sick to her stomach, throwing up, difficult to eat, stomach doctor
B. Answers will vary and may include nausea, emesis, dysphagia, and gastroenterologist, along with their respective definitions.
C. esophagogastroduodenoscopy (EGD), gastroscope, *H. pylori*, peptic ulcer

Copyright © 2026 by Elsevier Inc. All rights are reserved, including those for text and data mining, AI training, and similar technologies.

D. Answers will vary and may include esophagogastroduodenoscopy (EGD), gastroscope, *Helicobacter pylori*, peptic ulcer, along with their respective definitions.

Exercise 34
A
1. hematochezia
2. diarrhea
3. nausea
4. emesis
5. gastroesophageal reflux disease (GERD)
6. *Helicobacter pylori* stool antigen
7. peptic ulcer
8. Crohn disease
9. ulcerative colitis
10. colorectal
11. esophagitis
12. ascites
13. hepatomegaly
14. hemorrhoids
15. colonoscopy

B
1. d
2. b
3. a
4. d

Exercise 35
Online Exercise

Exercise 36
1. esophagogastroduodenoscopy, gastroenterologist, peptic ulcer
2. oral, gingivitis, glossitis, sublingual
3. gastrectomy, pyloroplasty, vagotomy
4. hepatomegaly, hepatitis, hepatoma, cirrhosis

Exercise 37
Pronunciation Exercise

Exercise 38
1. b
2. b
3. a
4. a
5. c
6. a
7. c
8. a
9. b
10. c
11. c
12. a
13. a
14. b
15. c
16. a
17. c
18. b
19. b
20. c

ANSWERS TO CHAPTER 12 EXERCISES

Exercise 1
A *Label*
1. eye: ocul/o, ophthalm/o
2. eyelid: blephar/o
3. tear(s): dacry/o, lacrim/o
4. pupil: cor/o, pupill/o
5. sclera: scler/o
6. iris: ir/o, irid/o
7. vision: opt/o
8. conjunctiva: conjunctiv/o
9. uvea: uve/o
10. cornea: corne/o, kerat/o
11. lens: phac/o, phak/o
12. retina: retin/o

B *Define and Match*
1. e, sclera
2. a, pupil
3. j, cornea
4. h, conjunctiva
5. f, tear(s)
6. k, uvea
7. b, lens
8. c, eye
9. d, iris
10. a, pupil
11. j, cornea
12. c, eye
13. f, tear(s)
14. g, retina
15. i, eyelid
16. vision

Exercise 2
A *Define*
1. tension, pressure
2. light
3. cold
4. two, double
5. equal
6. bladder, sac
7. dry, dryness
8. vessel(s); blood vessel(s)
9. nose
10. fungus
11. developing cell, germ cell
12. white
13. false
14. nose

B *Identify*
1. cry/o
2. ton/o
3. cyst/o
4. dipl/o
5. phot/o
6. is/o
7. leuk/o
8. pseud/o
9. blast/o
10. myc/o
11. xer/o
12. angi/o
13. nas/o, rhin/o

Exercise 3
A *Define*
1. within
2. absence of, without
3. within
4. absence of, without
5. two

B *Identify*
1. bin-
2. a-, an-
3. endo-, intra-

Exercise 4
A *Identify*
1. -al
2. -ar
3. -ary
4. -eal
5. -ic
(answers may be in any order)

B *Match*
1. g
2. h
3. f
4. i
5. j
6. d
7. e
8. b
9. c
10. a

C *Label*
1. -opia
2. -phobia
3. -plegia

D *Define*
1. visual examination
2. inflammation
3. softening
4. surgical repair

E *Identify*
1. -logy
2. -metry
3. -tomy
4. -oma
5. -pexy
6. -ia

Exercise 5
Pronounce and Spell

Exercise 6
1. WR S
   scler/itis
   inflammation of the sclera
2. WR CV S
   ophthalm/o/plegia
       CF
   paralysis of the eye (muscles)
3. WR CV S
   retin/o/pathy
       CF
   disease of the retina

Copyright © 2026 by Elsevier Inc. All rights are reserved, including those for text and data mining, AI training, and similar technologies.

Appendix A   Answer Key   709

4. P   WR   S
    end/ophthalm/itis
    inflammation within the eye *Note: the o in the prefix endo- is dropped.*
5. WR   WR   S
    xer/ophthalm/ia
    condition of dry eye *Note: the o in the combining form xer/o is dropped.*
6. P   WR   S
    a/phak/ia
    condition of without a lens
7. WR   CV   S
    ophthalm/o/pathy
       CF
    disease of the eye
8. WR   CV   S
    scler/o/malacia
       CF
    softening of the sclera
9. WR   S
    uve/itis
    inflammation of the uvea
10. WR   CV   S
    kerat/o/malacia
       CF
    softening of the cornea

Exercise 7
A *Label*
1. retin/o/blast/oma
2. scler/itis
3. blephar/itis
4. blephar/o/ptosis
5. conjunctiv/itis
6. dacry/o/cyst/itis

B *Fill In*
1. ir/itis
2. ocul/o/myc/osis
3. ophthalm/algia
4. dipl/opia
5. kerat/itis
6. uve/o/scler/itis
7. irid/o/plegia
8. phac/o/malacia

Exercise 8
Pronounce and Spell

Exercise 9
A *Identify*
1. myopia
2. presbyopia
3. anisometropia
4. astigmatism
5. Nystagmus
6. glaucoma
7. hyperopia
8. Retinitis pigmentosa

9. nyctalopia
10. amblyopia

B *Label*
1. drusen
2. macular degeneration
3. pterygium
4. pinguecula
5. chalazion
6. sty
7. cataract
8. hyphema
9. strabismus
10. retinal detachment
11. glaucoma
12. keratoconus

C *Match*
1. h   6. c
2. e   7. j
3. a   8. d
4. g   9. f
5. b   10. i

D *Match*
1. i   6. c
2. b   7. d
3. f   8. j
4. h   9. e
5. a   10. g

Exercise 10
Review of Disease and Disorder Terms

Exercise 11
Pronounce and Spell

Exercise 12
A *Analyze and Define*
1. WR   CV   S
    kerat/o/plasty
       CF
    surgical repair of the cornea
2. WR   CV   S
    scler/o/tomy
       CF
    incision into the sclera
3. WR CV WR CV   S
    cry/o/retin/o/pexy
      CF   CF
    surgical fixation of the retina by using extreme cold
4. WR   CV   S
    blephar/o/plasty
       CF
    surgical repair of the eyelid
5. WR   S
    irid/ectomy
    excision (of part) of the iris

6. WR CV WR CV WR CV   S
    dacry/o/cyst/o/rhin/o/stomy
       CF   CF   CF
    creation of an artificial opening between the tear (lacrimal) sac and the nose
7. WR   CV   S
    irid/o/tomy
       CF
    incision into the iris

B *Label*
1. kerat/o/plasty
2. irid/o/tomy
3. cry/o/retin/o/pexy

C *Fill In*
1. dacry/o/cyst/o/rhin/o/stomy
2. irid/ectomy
3. scler/o/tomy
4. blephar/o/plasty

Exercise 13
A *Label*
1. photorefractive keratectomy
2. LASIK
3. scleral buckling
4. phacoemulsification

B *Identify*
1. Retinal photocoagulation
2. posterior capsulotomy
3. enucleation
4. Trabeculectomy
5. vitrectomy

C *Match*
1. e   6. i
2. g   7. h
3. b   8. c
4. a   9. f
5. d

Exercise 14
Review of Surgical Terms

Exercise 15
Pronounce and Spell

Exercise 16
A *Fill In*
1. ton/o/metry
2. kerat/o/meter
3. opt/o/metry
4. ton/o/meter
5. pupill/o/scope
6. retin/o/scopy

Appendix A Answer Key

B *Label*
1. fluorescein angi/o/graphy
2. pupill/o/meter
3. ophthalm/o/scopy
4. ophthalm/o/scope

C *Analyze and Define*
1. WR CV S
   pupill/o/scope
   CF
   instrument used for visual examination of the pupil
2. WR CV S
   opt/o/metry
   CF
   measurement of vision
3. WR CV S
   ophthalm/o/scope
   CF
   instrument used for visual examination of the eye
4. WR CV S
   ton/o/metry
   CF
   measurement of pressure (within the eye)
5. WR CV S
   pupill/o/meter
   CF
   instrument used to measure the pupil (diameter)
6. WR CV S
   ton/o/meter
   CF
   instrument used to measure pressure (within the eye)
7. WR CV S
   kerat/o/meter
   CF
   instrument used to measure (the curvature of) the cornea
8. WR CV S
   ophthalm/o/scopy
   CF
   visual examination of the eye
9. WR CV S
   (fluorescein) angi/o/graphy
   CF
   radiographic imaging of the blood vessels (of the eye with fluorescing dye)
10. WR CV S
    retin/o/scopy
    CF
    visual examination of the retina

Exercise 17
A *Label*
1. slit lamp
2. optical coherence tomography
3. fundus exam
4. phoropter

B *Identify*
1. Optical coherence tomography
2. slit lamp
3. phoropter
4. fundus examination

Exercise 18
Review of Diagnostic Terms

Exercise 19
Pronounce and Spell

Exercise 20
A *Analyze and Define*
1. WR CV S
   ophthalm/o/logy
   CF
   study of the eye
2. P WR S
   bin/ocul/ar
   pertaining to two or both eyes
3. WR S
   lacrim/al
   pertaining to tears
4. WR S
   pupill/ary
   pertaining to the pupil
5. WR CV S
   ophthalm/o/logist
   CF
   physician (surgeon) who studies and treats diseases of the eye
6. WR S
   corne/al
   pertaining to the cornea
7. WR S
   ophthalm/ic
   pertaining to the eye
8. WR CV WR S
   nas/o/lacrim/al
   CF
   pertaining to the nose and tear (ducts)
9. WR S
   opt/ic
   pertaining to vision
10. P WR S
    intra/ocul/ar
    pertaining to within the eye
11. WR S
    retin/al
    pertaining to the retina
12. WR CV S
    phot/o/phobia
    CF
    abnormal fear of (sensitivity to) light
13. WR CV WR S
    is/o/cor/ia
    CF
    condition of equal pupil (size)
14. P WR CV WR S
    an/is/o/cor/ia
    CF
    condition of absence of equal pupil (size)
15. WR CV WR S
    pseud/o/phak/ia
    CF
    condition of false lens
16. WR CV WR S
    leuk/o/cor/ia
    CF
    condition of white pupil

B *Label*
1. bin/ocul/ar
2. retin/al
3. lacrim/al
4. an/is/o/cor/ia
5. leuk/o/cor/ia
6. ophthalm/o/logist

C *Fill In*
1. ophthalm/o/logy
2. pseud/o/phak/ia
3. is/o/cor/ia
4. intra/ocul/ar
5. phot/o/phobia
6. pupill/ary
7. ophthalm/ic
8. corne/al
9. nas/o/lacrim/al
10. opt/ic

Exercise 21
A *Label*
1. mydriatic
2. miotic
3. intraocular lens
4. visual acuity

B *Identify*
1. optometrist
2. optician
3. emmetropia

C *Match*
1. d   5. g
2. e   6. b
3. a   7. c
4. f

Exercise 22
Review of Complementary Terms

Exercise 23
1. fluorescein angiography, optical coherence tomography, age-related macular degeneration

2. visual acuity, phacoemulsification, intraocular lens
3. photorefractive keratectomy, laser-assisted in situ keratomileusis, astigmatism, emmetropia
4. intraocular pressure, ophthalmology
5. retinitis pigmentosa, peripheral vision loss
6. doctor of optometry
7. right eye, left eye, both eyes

Exercise 24
A. one of his eyes seemed to move more slowly and to look in a different direction; white part of the same eye seemed to be irritated and looked red and inflamed; pupil looked white; eye physician
B. Answers will vary and may include amblyopia, strabismus, scleritis, leukocoria, and ophthalmologist, along with their respective definitions.
C. ophthalmologist; leukocoria; strabismus; amblyopia; scleritis; ophthalmoscopy; visual acuity; retinal; retinoblastoma
D. Answers will vary and may include ophthalmologist, leukocoria, strabismus, amblyopia, scleritis, ophthalmoscopy, visual acuity, retinal, and retinoblastoma, along with their respective definitions.

Exercise 25
A
1. ophthalmology
2. glaucoma
3. pterygium
4. blepharoptosis
5. astigmatism
6. presbyopia
7. retinopathy
8. cataract

B
1. b
2. d
3. b
4. c

Exercise 26
Online Exercise

Exercise 27
1. ophthalmologist
2. LASIK; hyperopia
3. iridectomy; glaucoma
4. blepharoplasty; blepharoptosis
5. keratometer
6. presbyopia; optometrist
7. iritis
8. retinopathy; vitrectomy; retinal photocoagulation

Exercise 28
Pronunciation Exercise

Exercise 29
1. b
2. a
3. b
4. c
5. a
6. a
7. b
8. a
9. c
10. c
11. b
12. a
13. b
14. a
15. c
16. b
17. c
18. a
19. b
20. c

ANSWERS TO CHAPTER 13 EXERCISES

Exercise 1
A *Label*
1. ear: aur/i, ot/o
2. hearing: audi/o
3. middle ear: tympan/o
4. stapes: staped/o
5. tympanic membrane: myring/o
6. mastoid bone: mastoid/o

B *Label*
1. labyrinth: labyrinth/o
2. cochlea: cochle/o
3. vestibule: vestibul/o

C *Define and Match*
1. g, stapes
2. d, vestibule
3. a, ear
4. f, cochlea
5. e, labyrinth
6. b, tympanic membrane (eardrum)
7. h, middle ear
8. a, ear
9. c, mastoid bone
10. hearing

Exercise 2
A *Define*
1. fungus
2. pus
3. electricity, electrical activity

B *Identify*
1. electr/o
2. myc/o
3. py/o

Exercise 3
A *Match*
1. d
2. g
3. a
4. e
5. c
6. j
7. f
8. b
9. h
10. i

B *Define*
1. creation of an artificial opening
2. visual examination
3. measurement
4. study of

C *Identify*
1. -graphy
2. -itis
3. -al, -ar
4. -gram

Exercise 4
Pronounce and Spell

Exercise 5
1. WR CV WR S
ot/o/myc/osis
CF
abnormal condition of fungus in the ear
2. WR S
ot/algia
pain in the ear
3. WR S
labyrinth/itis
inflammation of the labyrinth
4. WR S
myring/itis
inflammation of the tympanic membrane
5. WR CV S
ot/o/sclerosis
CF
hardening of the ear (stapes)
6. WR S
mastoid/itis
inflammation of the mastoid bone

7. WR CV WR CV   S
   ot/o/py/o/rrhea
   ‾CF‾ ‾CF‾
   discharge of pus from the ear
8. WR CV   S
   ot/o/rrhea
   ‾CF‾
   discharge from the ear

Exercise 6
A *Label*
1. ot/o/py/o/rrhea
2. myring/itis

B *Fill In*
1. mastoid/itis
2. ot/algia
3. ot/o/sclerosis
4. ot/o/myc/osis
5. labyrinth/itis
6. ot/o/rrhea

Exercise 7
Pronounce and Spell

Exercise 8
A *Identify*
1. vertigo; tinnitus
2. Ménière
3. Presbycusis
4. ototoxicity

B *Label*
1. otitis externa
2. otitis media
3. cholesteatoma
4. acoustic neuroma

Exercise 9
1. d   6. a
2. e   7. g
3. i   8. h
4. f   9. b
5. c

Exercise 10
Review of Disease and Disorder Terms

Exercise 11
Pronounce and Spell

Exercise 12
1. WR   S
   mastoid/ectomy
   excision of the mastoid bone
2. WR CV S
   myring/o/tomy
   ‾CF‾
   incision into the tympanic membrane
3. WR   S
   labyrinth/ectomy
   excision of the labyrinth
4. WR CV S
   mastoid/o/tomy
   ‾CF‾
   incision into the mastoid bone
5. WR CV S
   tympan/o/plasty
   ‾CF‾
   surgical repair of the middle ear
6. WR CV S
   myring/o/plasty
   ‾CF‾
   surgical repair of the tympanic membrane
7. WR   S
   staped/ectomy
   excision of the stapes
8. WR   S
   cochle/ar (implant)
   pertaining to the cochlea (implant)
9. WR CV S
   ot/o/plasty
   ‾CF‾
   surgical repair of the (outer) ear
10. WR CV S
    tympan/o/stomy
    ‾CF‾
    creation of an artificial opening into the middle ear

Exercise 13
A *Fill In*
1. mastoid/o/tomy
2. labyrinth/ectomy
3. tympan/o/plasty
4. mastoid/ectomy
5. ot/o/plasty
6. myring/o/plasty

B *Label*
1. myring/o/tomy
2. cochle/ar implant
3. staped/ectomy
4. tympan/o/stomy

Exercise 14
Review of Surgical Terms

Exercise 15
Pronounce and Spell

Exercise 16
1. WR CV   S
   ot/o/scope
   ‾CF‾
   instrument used for visual examination of the ear
2. WR CV   S
   audi/o/metry
   ‾CF‾
   measurement of hearing
3. WR CV S
   audi/o/gram
   ‾CF‾
   (graphic) record of hearing
4. WR CV S
   ot/o/scopy
   ‾CF‾
   visual examination of the ear
5. WR CV S
   audi/o/meter
   ‾CF‾
   instrument used to measure hearing
6. WR CV S
   tympan/o/metry
   ‾CF‾
   measurement of middle ear (function)
7. WR CV S
   tympan/o/meter
   ‾CF‾
   instrument used to measure middle ear (function)
8. WR CV WR CV S
   electro/o/cochle/o/graphy
   ‾CF‾   ‾CF‾
   process of recording the electrical activity in the cochlea

Exercise 17
A *Label*
1. audi/o/meter
2. audi/o/gram
3. ot/o/scopy
4. tympan/o/meter

B *Fill In*
1. tympan/o/metry
2. ot/o/scope
3. audi/o/metry
4. electr/o/cochle/o/graphy

Exercise 18
Review of Diagnostic Terms

Exercise 19
Pronounce and Spell

Exercise 20
1. WR CV WR CV S
   ot/o/laryng/o/logy
   ‾CF‾   ‾CF‾
   study of the ear, (nose), and larynx (throat)

Appendix A   Answer Key   713

2. WR CV S
   audi/o/logist
       CF
   specialist who studies and treats (impaired) hearing
3. WRCV WR CV S
   ot/o/laryng/o/logist
    CF   CF
   physician who studies and treats diseases of the ear, (nose), and larynx (throat)
4. WR CV S
   audi/o/logy
      CF
   study of hearing
5. WR S
   aur/al
   pertaining to the ear
6. WR S
   cochle/ar
   pertaining to the cochlea
7. WR S
   vestibul/ar
   pertaining to the vestibule
8. WR CV WR S
   vestibul/o/cochle/ar
      CF
   pertaining to the vestibule and the cochlea

Exercise 21

A *Label*
1. aur/al
2. cochle/ar
3. ot/o/laryng/o/logist
4. audi/o/logist

B *Fill In*
1. audi/o/logy
2. ot/o/laryng/o/logy
3. vestibul/o/cochle/ar
4. vestibul/ar

Exercise 22
Review of Complementary Terms

Exercise 23
1. otitis media; acute otitis media
2. benign paroxysmal positional vertigo; ears, nose, throat; otolaryngologist
3. otitis externa
4. hard of hearing

Exercise 24
A. middle ear infections (inflammation); ear as if it is painful; pus-like liquid coming out of her left ear; redness and swelling on her skull behind Marisol's earlobe; ear, nose, and throat physician
B. Answers will vary and may include otitis media, otalgia, otopyorrhea, mastoiditis, and otolaryngologist, along with their respective definitions.
C. mastoiditis, otitis media, otalgia, otopyorrhea, otoscopy, otitis externa, tympanometry, mastoiditis, myringotomies, and mastoidectomy
D. Answers will vary and may include mastoiditis, otitis media, otalgia, otopyorrhea, otoscopy, otitis externa, tympanometry, mastoiditis, myringotomies, and mastoidectomy, along with their respective definitions.

Exercise 25

A
1. ENT
2. tinnitus
3. vertigo
4. otoscopy
5. otitis media
6. presbycusis
7. audiologist
8. audiometry

B
1. a
2. b
3. d

Exercise 26
Online Exercise

Exercise 27
1. cholesteatoma
2. labyrinthitis; vertigo
3. electrocochleography
4. otoscope; audiometer
5. myringoplasty; tympanoplasty
6. presbycusis; audiologist
7. otitis media; mastoiditis; mastoidectomy

Exercise 28
Pronunciation Exercise

Exercise 29
1. c   11. c
2. a   12. a
3. c   13. c
4. a   14. a
5. c   15. b
6. a   16. b
7. b   17. c
8. a   18. a
9. c   19. c
10. a   20. b

ANSWERS TO CHAPTER 14 EXERCISES

Exercise 1

A *Label*
1. bone: oste/o
2. mandible: mandibul/o
3. sternum: stern/o
4. phalanges: phalang/o
5. patella: patell/o
6. tarsals: tars/o
7. phalanges: phalang/o
8. cranium: crani/o
9. maxilla: maxill/o
10. clavicle: clavicul/o
11. ribs: cost/o
12. lumbar: lumb/o
13. femur: femor/o
14. fibula: fibul/o
15. tibia: tibi/o

B *Label*
1. vertebra: rachi/o, spondyl/o, vertebr/o
2. pelvis: pelv/i
3. scapula: scapul/o
4. humerus: humer/o
5. ulna: uln/o
6. radius: radi/o
7. carpals: carp/o
8. ilium: ili/o
9. sacrum: sacr/o
10. pubis: pub/o
11. ischium: ischi/o

C *Define and Match*
1. f: vertebra, spine, vertebral column
2. d: patella
3. a: maxilla
4. b: phalanx
5. c: carpals
6. e: humerus

D *Define and Match*
1. d: loin, lumbar spine
2. e: ischium
3. a: pubis
4. b: vertebra, spine, vertebral column
5. f: scapula
6. c: tarsals
7. g: pelvis, pelvic cavity

E *Define and Match*
1. c: mandible
2. g: sacrum

Copyright © 2026 by Elsevier Inc. All rights are reserved, including those for text and data mining, AI training, and similar technologies.

3. a: femur
4. f: clavicle
5. b: ilium
6. d: vertebra, spine, vertebral column
7. e: sternum

F *Identify*
1. rib: cost/o
2. radius: radi/o
3. tibia: tibi/o
4. fibula: fibul/o
5. ulna: uln/o
6. cranium: crani/o
7. bone: oste/o
8. bone marrow: myel/o

Exercise 2
A *Label*
1. joint: arthr/o
2. synovial membrane: synovi/o
3. meniscus: menisc/o
4. cartilage: chondr/o
5. tendon: ten/o, tendin/o
6. bursa: burs/o
7. lamina: lamin/o

B *Define and Match*
1. c: intervertebral disk
2. d: synovia, synovial membrane
3. e: fascia
4. a: tendon
5. b: joint

C *Define and Match*
1. e: muscle
2. b: tendon
3. c: bursa
4. d: meniscus
5. a: cartilage
6. e: muscle

Exercise 3
A *Define*
1. rod-shaped, striated
2. stone
3. movement, motion
4. death
5. blood
6. electricity, electrical activity
7. hump (increased convexity of the spine)
8. stiff, bent
9. (lateral) curved (spine)
10. bent forward (increased concavity of the spine)
11. flesh, connective tissue

B *Identify*
1. electr/o
2. petr/o
3. kinesi/o
4. rhabd/o
5. hem/o
6. necr/o
7. kyph/o
8. ankyl/o
9. scoli/o
10. lord/o
11. sarc/o

Exercise 4
A *Define*
1. above
2. together, joined
3. between

B *Identify*
1. syn-
2. inter-
3. supra-
4. sub-
5. a-
6. poly-
7. brady-
8. micro-
9. hyper-
10. intra-
11. dys-

Exercise 5
A *Define*
1. surgical fixation, fusion
2. split, fissure
3. weakness
4. nourishment, development
5. pertaining to

B *Identify*
1. -asthenia
2. -desis
3. -schisis
4. -trophy
5. -a

C *Match*
1. f
2. h
3. b
4. c
5. d
6. g
7. e
8. a

D *Match*
1. d
2. c
3. e
4. f
5. b
6. a
7. h
8. g
9. i

Exercise 6
Pronounce and Spell

Exercise 7
1. WR S
   oste/itis
   inflammation of the bone
2. WR CV WR S
   ten/o/synov/itis
         CF
   inflammation of the tendon and synovial membrane
3. WR CV WR S
   oste/o/petr/osis
        CF
   abnormal condition of stonelike bones (very dense bones caused by defective resorption of bone)
4. WR CV S
   oste/o/malacia
        CF
   softening of bone
5. WR CV S
   chondr/o/sarcoma
          CF
   malignant tumor of cartilage
6. WR CV WR S
   oste/o/chondr/oma
        CF
   tumor composed of bone and cartilage (benign)
7. WR S
   disc/itis
   inflammation of an intervertebral disk
8. WR CV WR S
   oste/o/necr/osis
        CF
   abnormal condition of bone death
9. WR CV S
   sarc/o/penia
        CF
   abnormal reduction of connective tissue
10. WR CV S
    synovi/o/sarcoma
           CF
    malignant tumor of the synovial membrane
11. WR S
    spondyl/osis
    abnormal condition of the vertebrae
12. WR CV S
    crani/o/schisis
         CF
    fissure (split) of the cranium
13. WR CV S
    chondr/o/malacia
           CF
    softening of cartilage
14. WR S
    ankyl/osis
    abnormal condition of stiffness
15. WR S
    menisc/itis
    inflammation of the meniscus
16. WR CV WR S
    fibr/o/my/algia
        CF
    pain in the fibrous tissues and muscles
17. WR CV
    fasci/itis
    inflammation of the fascia (connective tissue enclosing and separating muscle layers)

Appendix A   Answer Key   715

Exercise 8
A *Label*
1. lord/osis
2. kyph/osis
3. scoli/osis
4. oste/o/sarcoma
5. burs/itis
6. oste/o/arthr/itis

B *Fill In*
1. oste/o/chondr/itis
2. oste/o/myel/itis
3. arthr/itis
4. rhabd/o/my/o/lysis
5. myel/oma
6. tendin/itis
7. spondyl/osis
8. oste/o/penia
9. rachi/schisis
10. spondyl/arthr/itis

Exercise 9
Pronounce and Spell

Exercise 10
1. c
2. a
3. b
4. d
5. e
6. i
7. j
8. h
9. g
10. f

Exercise 11
1. herniated disk
2. rheumatoid arthritis
3. carpal tunnel syndrome
4. spondylolisthesis
5. gout
6. osteoporosis
7. fracture
8. Lyme disease
9. bunion
10. spinal stenosis
11. plantar fasciitis
12. ganglion cyst
13. rotator cuff disease
14. dislocation

Exercise 12
1. Spine:
   a. spondylolisthesis
   b. herniated disk
   c. ankylosing spondylitis
   d. spinal stenosis
2. Joints:
   a. bunion
   b. tarsal tunnel syndrome
   c. carpal tunnel syndrome
   d. ganglion cyst
   e. gout
   f. Lyme disease
   g. rheumatoid arthritis
   h. dislocation
   i. subluxation
   j. repetitive strain injury
3. Bone:
   a. exostosis
   b. fracture
   c. osteoporosis
4. Muscle:
   a. rotator cuff disease
   b. strain
   c. sprain
   d. compartment syndrome
   e. plantar fasciitis
   f. myasthenia gravis
   g. muscular dystrophy

Exercise 13
Review of Terms

Exercise 14
Pronounce and Spell

Exercise 15
1. WR CV S
   vertebr/o/plasty
   CF
   surgical repair of a vertebra
2. WR S
   tars/ectomy
   excision of (one or more) tarsal bones
3. WR CV S
   arthr/o/desis
   CF
   surgical fixation of a joint
4. WR S
   lamin/ectomy
   excision of a lamina
5. WR S
   synov/ectomy
   excision of the synovial membrane
6. WR CV S
   fasci/o/tomy
   CF
   incision into the fascia (to relieve tension or pressure)
7. WR CV S
   rachi/o/tomy
   CF
   incision into the vertebral column
8. WR S
   burs/ectomy
   excision of a bursa
9. WR S
   disc/ectomy
   excision of an intervertebral disk
10. WR CV S
    arthr/o/centesis
    CF
    surgical puncture to aspirate fluid from a joint
11. WR S
    maxill/ectomy
    excision of the maxilla
12. WR CV S
    crani/o/plasty
    CF
    surgical repair of the skull
13. WR S
    carp/ectomy
    excision of a carpal bone
14. WR S
    phalang/ectomy
    excision of a finger or toe bone

Exercise 16
A *Label*
1. micro/disc/ectomy
2. arthr/o/plasty
3. spondyl/o/syn/desis
4. menisc/ectomy
5. crani/o/tomy
6. ten/o/rrhaphy

B *Fill In*
1. oste/o/tomy
2. chondr/ectomy
3. chondr/o/plasty
4. my/o/rrhaphy
5. ten/o/my/o/plasty
6. cost/ectomy

Exercise 17
Review of Terms

Exercise 18
Pronounce and Spell

Exercise 19
A *Analyze and Define*
1. WR CV WR CV S
   electr/o/my/o/gram
   CF   CF
   record of the electrical activity in a muscle
2. WR CV S
   arthr/o/graphy
   CF
   radiographic imaging of a joint
3. WR CV S
   arthr/o/scopy
   CF
   visual examination of a joint

B *Build*
1. arthr/o/graphy
2. arthr/o/scopy

Copyright © 2026 by Elsevier Inc. All rights are reserved, including those for text and data mining, AI training, and similar technologies.

C Label
1. arthr/o/scopy
2. electr/o/my/o/gram

Exercise 20
A *Match*
1. b
2. a
3. c
4. c
5. b
6. a

B *Label*
1. dual x-ray absorptiometry
2. muscle biopsy
3. bone markers

Exercise 21
Review of Terms

Exercise 22
Pronounce and Spell

Exercise 23
Note: the abbreviation S(WR) indicates a suffix with an embedded word root.
1. WR   S
   my/algia
   muscle pain
2. WR   S
   arthr/algia
   joint pain
3. P   S(WR)
   hyper/trophy
   excessive development
4. P   S(WR)
   a/trophy
   without development
5. P   WR   S
   hyper/kinesi/a
   excessive movement (hyperactivity)
6. P   WR   S
   dys/kinesi/a
   difficult movement
7. P   WR   S
   brady/kinesi/a
   slow movement
8. WR   WR   S
   hem/arthr/osis
   abnormal condition of blood in the joint
9. P   S(WR)
   dys/trophy
   abnormal development
10. WR   S
    my/asthenia
    muscle weakness

Exercise 24
A *Fill in*
1. supra/clavicul/ar
2. supra/patell/ar
3. inter/vertebr/al
4. sub/maxill/ary
5. sub/mandibul/ar
6. sub/stern/al
7. intra/crani/al
8. inter/cost/al
9. patell/o/femor/al

B *Label*
1. scapul/ar
2. humer/al
3. stern/al
4. vertebr/al
5. ili/ac
6. carp/al
7. phalang/eal
8. pub/ic
9. patell/ar
10. tars/al
11. phalang/eal
12. crani/al
13. clavicul/ar
14. lumb/ar
15. radi/al
16. uln/ar
17. sacr/al
18. ischi/al
19. femor/al
20. fibul/ar
21. tibi/al

Exercise 25
Pronounce and Spell

Exercise 26
A *Identify*
1. rheumatology
2. orthotics
3. crepitus
4. chiropractic
5. orthopedics
6. osteopathy
7. prosthesis (*pl.* prostheses)

B *Label*
1. orthopedist
2. rheumatologist
3. podiatrist
4. orthotist
5. chiropractor
6. osteopath

Exercise 27
1. d
2. h
3. a
4. f
5. g
6. c
7. b
8. e

Exercise 28
1. h
2. d
3. i
4. e
5. c
6. a
7. g
8. f
9. b

Exercise 29
Review of Terms

Exercise 30
1. cervical vertebrae; thoracic vertebrae; lumbar vertebrae
2. rheumatoid arthritis
3. osteoarthritis
4. myasthenia gravis
5. electromyogram; polymyositis
6. carpal tunnel syndrome; orthopedics
7. muscular dystrophy
8. herniated nucleus pulposus
9. total hip arthroplasty
10. Doctor of Osteopathy
11. total knee arthroplasty
12. repetitive strain injury
13. fracture
14. dual x-ray absorptiometry; dual-energy x-ray absorptiometry
15. Doctor of Chiropractic

Exercise 31
A. finger and wrist bones, broken, musculoskeletal specialist, bones are not dense enough
B. Answers will vary and may include carpal, fracture, orthopedist, osteoporosis, along with their respective definitions.
C. kyphosis, fracture, radial, osteoporosis, dual x-ray absorptiometry (DXA)
D. Answers will vary and may include kyphosis, fracture, radial, osteoporosis, dual x-ray absorptiometry (DXA), along with their respective definitions.

Exercise 32
A
1. orthopedic
2. arthroscopy
3. arthritis
4. medial
5. suprapatellar
6. chondromalacia
7. pathology

B
1. c
2. b

Exercise 33
Electronic Health Records Online

Exercise 34
1. myalgia; myasthenia; rhabdomyolysis
2. crepitus; flexion; extension
3. podiatrist
4. tendinitis; bursitis; plantar fasciitis
5. orthotics

Exercise 35
Pronunciation Exercise

Appendix A   Answer Key   717

Exercise 36
1. epiphyses
2. phalanx
3. vertebrae
4. prosthesis
5. bursae
6. laminae

Exercise 37
1. b
2. c
3. a
4. b
5. c
6. b
7. c
8. c
9. a
10. c
11. a
12. c
13. b
14. a
15. b
16. a
17. b
18. c
19. a
20. c

ANSWERS TO CHAPTER 15 EXERCISES

Exercise 1
A *Label*
1. brain: encephal/o
2. spinal cord: myel/o
3. cerebrum: cerebr/o
4. cerebellum: cerebell/o
5. meninges: meningi/o, mening/o

B *Identify*
1. glia: gli/o
2. nerve: neur/o

C *Label*
1. gray matter: poli/o
2. ganglion: gangli/o, ganglion/o
3. dura mater: dur/o
4. nerve root: radicul/o, rhiz/o

D *Define and Match*
1. e, ganglion
2. d, dura mater
3. c, brain
4. a, cerebellum
5. f, meninges
6. b, nerve

E *Define and Match*
1. b, glia
2. d, ganglion
3. e, meninges
4. f, cerebrum
5. a, spinal cord
6. c, gray matter

F *Identify*
1. radicul/o, rhiz/o

Exercise 2
A *Define*
1. one, single
2. mind
3. four
4. mind
5. speech
6. sensation, sensitivity, feeling

B *Match*
1. b
2. h
3. a
4. a
5. f
6. c
7. e
8. d
9. g

Exercise 3
1. i
2. d
3. c
4. k
5. j
6. e
7. a
8. f
9. h
10. b
11. g

Exercise 4
A *Define*
1. slight paralysis
2. treatment, specialty
3. seizure, attack
4. specialist, physician

B *Match*
1. e
2. h
3. d
4. k
5. j
6. g
7. b
8. a
9. i
10. c
11. f

C *Match*
1. e
2. g
3. i
4. b
5. f
6. a
7. k
8. j
9. c
10. d
11. h

Exercise 5
Pronounce and Spell

Exercise 6
1. WR   S
   myel/itis
   inflammation of the spinal cord
2. WR CV WR   S
   hydr/o/cephal/us
       CF
   water (increased amount of cerebrospinal fluid) in the head (brain)
3. WR CV WR   S
   poli/o/myel/itis
       CF
   inflammation of the gray matter of the spinal cord
4. WR CV S
   radicul/o/pathy
       CF
   disease of the nerve roots
5. WR CV S
   encephal/o/pathy
       CF
   disease of the brain
6. WR   S
   encephal/itis
   inflammation of the brain
7. WR CV WR CV WR   S
   rhiz/o/mening/o/myel/itis
     CF   CF
   inflammation of the nerve root, meninges, and spinal cord
8. WR   S   WR   S
   cerebr/al thromb/osis
   pertaining to the cerebrum, abnormal condition of a blood clot
9. WR CV S
   mening/o/cele
       CF
   protrusion of the meninges
10. WR CV S
    myel/o/malacia
        CF
    softening of the spinal cord
11. WR   S
    radicul/itis
    inflammation of the nerve roots
12. WR   S
    gangli/itis
    inflammation of a ganglion
13. WR   S
    dur/itis
    inflammation of the dura mater
14. P WR   S
    poly/neur/itis
    inflammation of many nerves

Exercise 7
A *Label*
1. mon/o/neur/o/pathy
2. sub/dur/al hemat/oma
3. gli/o/blast/oma
4. meningi/oma
5. intra/cerebr/al hem/o/rrhage

6. cerebr/al embol/ism
7. poly/neur/o/pathy
8. neur/algia

B *Fill In*
1. neur/itis
2. gli/oma
3. encephal/o/malacia
4. cerebell/itis
5. encephal/o/myel/o/radicul/itis
6. mening/itis
7. mening/o/myel/o/cele

Exercise 8
Pronounce and Spell

Exercise 9
1. h
2. i
3. a
4. f
5. b
6. c
7. e
8. d
9. g

Exercise 10
1. sciatica
2. Alzheimer disease
3. shingles
4. cerebral aneurysm
5. subarachnoid hemorrhage
6. stroke
7. transient ischemic attack
8. Bell palsy

Exercise 11
Review of Disease and Disorder Terms

Exercise 12
Pronounce and Spell

Exercise 13
1. WR S
   neur/ectomy
   excision of a nerve
2. WR CV S
   neur/o/rrhaphy
      CF
   suturing of a nerve
3. WR S
   ganglion/ectomy
   excision of a ganglion
4. WR CV S
   neur/o/tomy
      CF
   incision into a nerve
5. WR CV S
   neur/o/lysis
      CF
   loosening, separating a nerve (to release it from surrounding tissue)
6. WR CV S
   neur/o/plasty
      CF
   surgical repair of a nerve
7. WR CV S
   rhiz/o/tomy
      CF
   incision into a nerve root

Exercise 14
A *Fill In*
1. neur/ectomy
2. neur/o/rrhaphy
3. neur/o/tomy
4. neur/o/lysis
5. neur/o/plasty

B *Label*
1. rhiz/o/tomy
2. ganglion/ectomy

Exercise 15
Review of Surgical Terms

Exercise 16
Pronounce and Spell

Exercise 17
A *Analyze and Define*
1. WR CV WR CV S
   electr/o/encephal/o/gram
      CF   CF
   record of the electrical activity of the brain
2. WR CV WR CV S
   electr/o/encephal/o/graph
      CF   CF
   instrument used to record the electrical activity of the brain
3. WR CV WR CV S
   electr/o/encephal/o/graphy
      CF   CF
   process of recording the electrical activity of the brain
4. WR CV S
   CT myel/o/graphy
         CF
   process of recording (scan of) the spinal cord
5. WR S WR CV S
   cerebr/al angi/o/graphy
             CF
   process of recording (scan of) the blood vessels of the cerebrum

B *Label*
1. CT myel/o/graphy
2. cerebr/al angi/o/graphy

C *Fill In*
1. electr/o/encephal/o/gram
2. electr/o/encephal/o/graph
3. electr/o/encephal/o/graphy

Exercise 18
A *Match*
1. c
2. d
3. a
4. b

B *Label*
1. evoked potential studies
2. lumbar puncture
3. deep tendon reflexes
4. positron emission tomography

Exercise 19
Review of Diagnostic Terms

Exercise 20
Pronounce and Spell

Exercise 21
1. P S(WR)
   pre/ictal
   (occurring) before a seizure or attack
2. P WR S
   par/esthesi/a
   abnormal sensation *(Note: the a is dropped from the prefix para.)*
3. WR S
   ment/al
   pertaining to the mind
4. P S(WR)
   inter/ictal
   (occurring) between seizures or attacks
5. WR CV S
   mon/o/paresis
      CF
   slight paralysis of one (limb)
6. P WR S
   dys/esthesi/a
   painful sensation

Exercise 22
A *Label*
1. hemi/plegia
2. quadr/i/plegia
3. an/esthesi/a
4. ceph/algia *(NOTE: the al is dropped from the combining form cephal/o)*
5. neur/o/logy
6. a/phas/ia

B *Fill In*
1. hemi/paresis
2. dys/phas/ia
3. hyper/esthesi/a
4. crani/o/cerebr/al
5. mon/o/paresis

6. post/ictal
7. neur/o/logist

Exercise 23
Pronounce and Spell

Exercise 24
A *Label*
1. paraplegia
2. concussion
3. syncope
4. ataxia
5. dysarthria
6. coma

B *Identify*
1. spasticity
2. unconsciousness
3. conscious
4. seizure
5. convulsion
6. shunt
7. gait
8. incoherent
9. disorientation
10. cognitive

Exercise 25
A.
1. d   5. a
2. f   6. c
3. h   7. g
4. b   8. e

B.
1. f   5. c
2. h   6. g
3. a   7. d
4. b   8. e

Exercise 26
Review of Complementary Terms

Exercise 27
Pronounce and Spell

Exercise 28
1. WR CV WR S
   psych/o/somat/ic
       CF
   pertaining to the mind and body
2. WR CV S
   psych/o/pathy
      CF
   (any) disease of the mind
3. WR CV S
   psych/o/logy
      CF
   study of the mind
4. WR S
   psych/iatry
   specialty of the mind (branch of medicine that deals with the treatment of mental disorders)
5. WR CV S
   psych/o/logist
      CF
   specialist of the mind
6. WR CV S
   psych/o/genic
      CF
   originating in the mind
7. WR S
   psych/iatrist
   physician who studies and treats disorders of the mind
8. WR S
   psych/osis
   abnormal condition of the mind

Exercise 29
1. psych/iatry
2. psych/osis
3. psych/o/logy
4. psych/o/genic
5. psych/iatrist
6. psych/o/logist
7. psych/o/somat/ic
8. psych/o/pathy

Exercise 30
Pronounce and Spell

Exercise 31
A.
1. g   5. c
2. a   6. d
3. b   7. e
4. f

B.
1. g   5. c
2. b   6. d
3. f   7. e
4. a

Exercise 32
Review of Behavioral Health Terms

Exercise 33
1. deep tendon reflexes, poliomyelitis
2. electroencephalogram, positron emission tomography, evoked potential studies, lumbar puncture
3. Alzheimer disease, amyotrophic lateral sclerosis, cerebral palsy, multiple sclerosis, Parkinson disease
4. cerebrovascular accident, transient ischemic attack, subarachnoid hemorrhage
5. cerebrospinal fluid
6. obsessive-compulsive disorder, attention deficit/hyperactivity disorder, autism spectrum disorders
7. central nervous system, peripheral nervous system
8. posttraumatic stress disorder, chronic traumatic encephalopathy
9. traumatic brain injury

Exercise 34
A. unable to speak, right arm was hanging limply by his side, left side of his face was also droopy, strokes
B. Answers will vary and may include aphasia, hemiplegia, Bell palsy, stroke or cerebrovascular accident, and their respective definitions.
C. aphasia, hemiplegia, dysphasia, hemiparesis, paresthesias, gait, cerebral, subarachnoid hemorrhage, CVA
D. Answers will vary and may include aphasia, hemiplegia, dysphasia, hemiparesis, paresthesias, gait, cerebral, subarachnoid hemorrhage, CVA and their respective definitions.

Exercise 35
A
1. disorientation
2. cognitive
3. aphasia
4. conscious
5. neurology
6. encephalitis
7. electroencephalogram
8. seizure
9. incoherent

B
1. b
2. a

Exercise 36
Electronic Health Record

Exercise 37
1. major depression, psychology, anxiety disorder, psychiatrist, psychologist
2. dementia, Alzheimer disease, Parkinson disease, hydrocephalus
3. stroke, aphasia, hemiplegia, cerebral thrombosis, cerebral angiography, TIA

4. cephalgia, migraine, MS, Bell palsy, subarachnoid hemorrhage

Exercise 38
Pronunciation Exercise

Exercise 39
1. a
2. b
3. c
4. c
5. c
6. a
7. b
8. a
9. b
10. a
11. a
12. c
13. c
14. a
15. c
16. b
17. a
18. c
19. b
20. a

ANSWERS TO CHAPTER 16 EXERCISES

Exercise 1
A *Label*
1. parathyroid glands: parathyroid/o
2. adrenal glands: adren/o, adrenal/o
3. pituitary gland: pituitar/o
4. thyroid gland: thyroid/o
5. endocrine: endocrin/o

B *Label*
cortex: cortic/o

C *Define and Match*
1. d, adrenal glands
2. a, pituitary gland
3. e, cortex
4. b, parathyroid glands
5. d, adrenal glands
6. c, thyroid gland
7. endocrine

Exercise 2
A *Define*
1. thirst
2. potassium
3. calcium
4. extremities, height
5. sodium
6. sugar

B *Identify*
1. acr/o
2. calc/i
3. dips/o
4. glyc/o
5. kal/i
6. natr/o

Exercise 3
A *Define*
1. together, joined
2. below, incomplete, deficient, under
3. all, total
4. normal, good
5. many, much
6. above, excessive

B *Identify*
1. pan-
2. eu-
3. poly-
4. hyper-
5. syn-
6. hypo-

Exercise 4
A *Identify*
1. -ism
2. -megaly
3. -emia
4. -al
5. -pathy
6. -logist

B *Label*
1. -drome

C *Define*
1. tumor, swelling
2. excision, surgical removal
3. condition of formation, development, growth
4. study of
5. inflammation
6. run, running
7. diseased state, condition of

Exercise 5
Pronounce and Spell

Exercise 6
1. WR S
   adrenal/itis
   inflammation of the adrenal glands
2. P WR S
   hypo/calc/emia
   deficient calcium in the blood
3. P WR S
   hyper/thyroid/ism
   state of excessive thyroid gland activity
4. P WR S
   hyper/kal/emia
   excessive potassium in the blood
5. P WR S
   hyper/pituitar/ism
   state of excessive pituitary gland activity
6. WR CV S
   adren/o/megaly
      CF
   enlargement of the adrenal glands
7. WR CV S
   endocrin/o/pathy
      CF
   (any) disease of the endocrine (system)
8. P WR S
   hypo/natr/emia
   deficient sodium in the blood
9. WR S
   parathyroid/oma
   tumor of a parathyroid gland
10. P P WR S
    pan/hypo/pituitar/ism
    state of total deficient pituitary gland activity

Exercise 7
A *Label*
1. acr/o/megaly
2. hyper/glyc/emia
3. hypo/glyc/emia

B *Fill In*
1. hypo/thyroid/ism
2. hypo/kal/emia
3. hyper/parathyroid/ism
4. hypo/pituitar/ism
5. hyper/calc/emia
6. thyroid/itis

Exercise 8
Pronounce and Spell

Exercise 9
1. c
2. g
3. b
4. h
5. f
6. a
7. e
8. d

Exercise 10
1. e
2. d
3. a
4. g
5. c
6. b
7. f

Exercise 11
A *Identify*
1. Obesity
2. thyrotoxicosis
3. Hashimoto thyroiditis
4. Diabetes insipidus
5. ketoacidosis
6. diabetes mellitus
7. Neuroblastoma

Appendix A Answer Key

B *Label*
1. gigantism
2. Addison disease
3. Graves disease
4. myxedema
5. Cushing syndrome
6. metabolic syndrome
7. pheochromocytoma
8. congenital hypothyroidism

Exercise 12
Review of Disease and Disorder Terms

Exercise 13
Pronounce and Spell

Exercise 14
1. WR   S
   adrenal/ectomy
   excision of (one or both) adrenal glands
2. WR   S
   thyroid/ectomy
   excision of the thyroid gland
3. WR   S
   parathyroid/ectomy
   excision of (one or more) parathyroid glands

Exercise 15
1. thyroid/ectomy
2. adrenal/ectomy
3. parathyroid/ectomy

Exercise 16
Review of Surgical Terms

Exercise 17
Pronounce and Spell

Exercise 18
A *Label*
1. thyroid sonography
2. radioactive iodine uptake
3. sestamibi parathyroid scan
4. fine needle aspiration

B *Identify*
1. Thyroxine level
2. fasting blood sugar
3. glycosylated hemoglobin
4. thyroid-stimulating hormone level

Exercise 19
1. b
2. a
3. g
4. d
5. f
6. h
7. e
8. c

Exercise 20
Review of Diagnostic Terms

Exercise 21
Pronounce and Spell

Exercise 22
A *Analyze and Define*
1. P S(WR)
   syn/drome
   run together
2. WR   CV   S
   endocrin/o/logist
         CF
   physician who studies and treats diseases of the endocrine (system)
3. P   WR   S
   poly/dips/ia
   condition of much thirst
4. P   WR   S
   eu/glyc/emia
   normal (level of) sugar in the blood
5. WR CV WR CV P   S
   adren/o/cortic/o/hyper/plasia
        CF   CF
   excessive development of the adrenal cortex
6. P   WR
   eu/thyroid
   normal thyroid gland activity
7. WR   S
   cortic/al
   pertaining to the cortex
8. WR   CV   S
   endocrin/o/logy
         CF
   study of the endocrine (system)
9. WR   S
   glyc/emia
   sugar in the blood

B *Label*
1. eu/thyroid
2. eu/glyc/emia
3. poly/dips/ia
4. endocrin/o/logist

C *Fill In*
1. glyc/emia
2. syn/drome
3. adren/o/cortic/o/hyper/plasia
4. endocrin/o/logy
5. cortic/al

Exercise 23
A *Match*
1. b
2. f
3. d
4. e
5. c
6. a

B *Label*
1. goiter
2. exophthalmos

C *Identify*
1. metabolism
2. hormone
3. Tetany
4. incretins

Exercise 24
Review of Complementary Terms

Exercise 25
1. diabetes mellitus, type 1 diabetes mellitus, fasting blood sugar, diabetic ketoacidosis
2. type 2 diabetes mellitus, glycosylated hemoglobin
3. thyroxine level, thyroid-stimulating hormone, radioactive iodine uptake, fine needle aspiration, parathyroid hormone
4. follicle-stimulating hormone, luteinizing hormone
5. antidiuretic hormone, diabetes insipidus, syndrome of inappropriate ADH (secretion)
6. growth hormone, adrenocorticotropic hormone, prolactin

Exercise 26
A. a lump in the front of her neck, eyes seem to stick out more, too much thyroid hormone, endocrine specialist
B. Answers will vary and may include goiter, exophthalmos, hyperthyroidism or thyrotoxicosis, endocrinologist, and their respective definitions.
C. endocrinopathy, hyperthyroidism, thyrotoxicosis, exophthalmos, Graves disease, thyroid sonography, TSH, T$_4$, radioactive iodine uptake, thyroidectomy, hypothyroidism
D. Answers will vary and may include endocrinopathy, hyperthyroidism, thyrotoxicosis, exophthalmos, Graves disease, thyroid sonography, TSH, T$_4$, radioactive iodine uptake, thyroidectomy, hypothyroidism, and their respective definitions.

Exercise 27
A
1. polydipsia
2. diabetes mellitus
3. exophthalmos
4. fasting blood sugar

5. glycosylated hemoglobin
6. type 2 diabetes mellitus
7. hyperglycemia
8. hypoglycemia
9. endocrinology

B
1. c
2. b
3. a

Exercise 28
Online Exercise

Exercise 29
1. fine needle aspiration, thyroid sonography, endocrinologist
2. fasting blood sugar, glycosylated hemoglobin
3. pheochromocytoma, adrenalectomy
4. obesity, diabetes mellitus, metabolic syndrome

Exercise 30
Pronunciation Exercise

Exercise 31
1. c
2. a
3. c
4. b
5. a
6. b
7. b
8. c
9. a
10. c
11. c
12. c
13. b
14. b
15. c
16. a
17. b
18. a
19. b
20. b

Exercise 32
Fill-in answers appear in bold.

1. *Subjective*
Chief Complaint (CC): "I can't **catch my breath**."
History of Present Illness (HPI): Adele Sun is a **32**-year-old female with a history of **Graves** disease, major **depression,** and **anxiety,** who presents with dyspnea. 5 days ago, she became **febrile** and had a dry cough. 2 days ago, she began producing green **sputum** and started having **paroxysms** of coughing. She has been coughing so much that she is now having **dyspnea**. She also reports posterior thoracic pain, under her ribs. Associated symptoms include chills, near **syncope**, worsening weakness, and worsening **fatigue**. Other symptoms include **myalgia** and **cephalgia**, although she states these have been present for "years." She denies **emesis** or **diarrhea**.
Past Medical History (PMH): **Hypothyroidism** after surgery for **Graves disease,** diagnosed 3 years ago; major depression and anxiety, diagnosed **4** years ago
Surgeries: **Thyroidectomy** 3 years ago
OB/GYN hx: **G$_0$P$_0$**, LMP **5** months ago, **oligomenorrhea** last 3 years
Medications: **Levothyroxine** 0.75 μg (microgram) po qd, **Sertraline** 150 mg po qd
Allergies: sulfa medications cause a rash
Vaccination Status: up to date on all required **vaccinations** and **COVID**-19. Has not received a **flu** shot this year.

2. *Objective*
Physical Examination (PE)
Vital signs: BP: 90/60 mm Hg, P: 116, R: 24, T: 39.4 deg C, BMI: 22, Pulse oximetry: 90%
Gen: Thin, ill-appearing female in moderate distress, alert and conversant, with some limitations due to **tachypnea**
Skin: appears unusually tanned, with areas of hyperpigmentation noted on the elbows, knees, and palmar creases. **Vitiligo** on the face is also noted. Hair pattern is more sparse than expected for patient's age.
Throat: mucous membranes moist, hyperpigmentation noted, no **erythema**
Neck: without **lymphadenopathy;** midline scar noted at level of thyroid
Respiratory: dullness to **percussion** right posterior chest, with decreased breath sounds, **wheezes**, and **crackles** in that area. Otherwise, clear to **auscultation** and percussion. **Thoracic** expansion normal
Cardiac: **tachycardia**, regular rhythm. No **murmurs**
Abdomen: normal bowel sounds without **bruits**. Mild diffuse tenderness in RUQ and LUQ. No masses. Liver and spleen normal size by percussion.
Musculoskeletal: diffuse **atrophy** noted in larger muscles bilaterally. Tenderness noted at the **patellofemoral** joints, **carpal** joints, and over the **lumbar** and **sacral** vertebrae.
Neurologic: muscle strength is 4 out of 5 bilaterally for upper and lower extremities. Sensation is intact. **DTR**s intact bilaterally. **Cranial** nerves 2-12 intact.
Extremities: **Cyanosis** noted at fingertips, no **edema**
Pulses: **radial**, **posterior** tibial, and **dorsal** pedal pulses are diminished bilaterally

3 *Assessment and Plan*
This 32-year-old female with a history of Graves disease, major depression, and anxiety disorder, presented to the emergency department with a 5-day history of fever and **paroxysms** of coughing, and a 2-day history of dyspnea with a cough productive of green **sputum**. Other significant symptoms include posterior thoracic pain and a longer history of **myalgias, cephalgias, fatigue,** weakness, and near **syncope**.
On physical exam she was found to be **febrile**, with **tachypnea** and **tachycardia**, and she had borderline **hypotension**. Pulse oximetry was 90%. Lung findings were suspicious for **pneumonia**, and the **distal** cyanosis supported the impression of **hypoxia**. 2 liters oxygen by nasal cannula was immediately started after **pulse oximetry** was performed, and her values came up to 95%.

Given the acute nature of her respiratory symptoms, her vitals, and the **pulmonary** physical exam findings, we believe she may have pneumonia, likely of viral or bacterial **etiology**. **Phlebotomy** was performed, an **intravenous** line was placed, and the following labs have been ordered: **CBC with diff**, chemistry panel, sputum **C&S**, rapid influenza diagnosis test, COVID-19 test, and a **TSH** level.

Diagnostic imaging: an **AP** portable **radiograph** was ordered, and we are awaiting results.

4 Emergency Department Course

While waiting for diagnostic imaging and lab results, Addy became nonresponsive/**unconscious** and her **blood pressure** dropped to 66/26 mm Hg. A large infusion of intravenous isotonic saline was given. Her lab results came back and indicated **hyponatremia** and **hyperkalemia**. Based on these findings, the treatment team suspected adrenal crisis and treated her with 100 mg of IV hydrocortisone. **ACTH** and cortisol levels were also requested. Rapid influenza and COVID-19 tests were negative. Chest x-ray revealed a right lower lobe pneumonia with a small **pleural effusion**. She received **IV** antibiotics to treat the pneumonia. Her blood pressure returned to the normal range, and she became **conscious**. She was admitted to the inpatient floor of the hospital with a **diagnosis** of adrenal crisis, likely caused by **Addison disease**, precipitated by pneumonia.

Combining Forms, Prefixes, and Suffixes Alphabetized by Word Part

Appendix B

COMBINING FORMS	DEFINITION	CHAPTER
A		
abdomin/o	abdomen, abdominal cavity	11
acr/o	extremities, height	16
aden/o	gland, glandular tissue	2
adenoid/o	adenoids	5
adren/o	adrenal glands	16
adrenal/o	adrenal glands	16
albumin/o	albumin	6
alveol/o	alveolus (s.), alveoli (pl.)	5
amni/o	amnion, amniotic fluid	9
amnion/o	amnion, amniotic fluid	9
andr/o	male	7
angi/o	vessel(s); blood vessel(s)	10
ankyl/o	stiff, bent	14
an/o	anus	11
anter/o	front	3
antr/o	antrum	11
aort/o	aorta	10
appendic/o	appendix	11
append/o	appendix	11
arteri/o	artery (s), arteries (pl)	10
arthr/o	joint	14
atel/o	imperfect, incomplete	5
ather/o	yellowish, fatty plaque	10
atri/o	atrium	10
audi/o	hearing	13
aur/i	ear	13
aut/o	self	2
azot/o	urea, nitrogen	6
B		
balan/o	glans penis	7
bi/o	life	2

COMBINING FORMS	DEFINITION	CHAPTER
blast/o	developing cell, germ cell	6
blephar/o	eyelid	12
bronch/o	bronchus	5
bronchi/o	bronchus	5
burs/o	bursa (cavity)	14
C		
calc/i	calcium	16
cancer/o	cancer	2
capn/o	carbon dioxide	5
carcin/o	cancer	2
cardi/o	heart	10
carp/o	carpals (wrist)	14
caud/o	tail (downward)	3
cec/o	cecum	11
celi/o	abdomen, abdominal cavity	11
cephal/o	head	3
cerebell/o	cerebellum	15
cerebr/o	cerebrum	15
cervic/o	cervix	8
cheil/o	lip(s)	11
cholangi/o	bile duct	11
chol/e	gall, bile	11
choledoch/o	common bile duct	11
chondr/o	cartilage	14
chori/o	chorion	9
clavicul/o	clavicle (collarbone)	14
cochle/o	cochlea	13
col/o	colon (large intestine)	11
colon/o	colon (large intestine)	11
colp/o	vagina	8
coni/o	dust	5
conjunctiv/o	conjunctiva	12
cor/o	pupil	12

725

Appendix B Combining Forms, Prefixes, and Suffixes Alphabetized by Word Part

COMBINING FORMS	DEFINITION	CHAPTER
corne/o	cornea	12
cortic/o	cortex (outer layer of body organ)	16
cost/o	rib	14
crani/o	cranium (skull)	14
cry/o	cold	12
crypt/o	hidden	4
cutane/o	skin	4
cyan/o	blue	2
cyst/o	bladder, sac	6
cyt/o	cell(s)	2
D		
dacry/o	tear(s)	12
dermat/o	skin	4
derm/o	skin	4
diaphragmat/o	diaphragm	5
dipl/o	two, double	12
dips/o	thirst	16
disc/o	intervertebral disk	14
dist/o	away (from the point of attachment)	3
diverticul/o	diverticulum	11
dors/o	back	3
duoden/o	duodenum	11
dur/o	hard, dura mater	15
E		
ech/o	sound	10
electr/o	electricity, electrical activity	10
embol/o	plug	10
encephal/o	brain	15
endocrin/o	endocrine	16
endometri/o	endometrium	8
enter/o	intestines (usually the small intestine)	11
epididym/o	epididymis	7
epiglott/o	epiglottis	5
episi/o	vulva	8
epitheli/o	epithelium, epithelial tissue	2
erythr/o	red	2
esophag/o	esophagus	9

COMBINING FORMS	DEFINITION	CHAPTER
esthesi/o	sensation, sensitivity, feeling	15
eti/o	cause (of disease)	2
F		
fasci/o	fascia (connective tissue enclosing and separating muscle layers)	14
femor/o	femur (upper leg bone)	14
fet/o	fetus, unborn offspring	9
fibr/o	fiber(s), fibrous tissue	2
fibul/o	fibula (lower leg bone)	14
G		
gangli/o	ganglion	15
ganglion/o	ganglion	15
gastr/o	stomach	11
gingiv/o	gum	11
gli/o	glia	15
glomerul/o	glomerulus	6
gloss/o	tongue	11
glycos/o	sugar	6
gno/o	knowledge	2
gravid/o	pregnancy	9
gynec/o	woman, female reproductive organs	8
gyn/o	woman, female reproductive organs	8
H		
hem/o	blood	5
hemat/o	blood	2
hepat/o	liver	11
herni/o	hernia (protrusion of an organ through a membrane or cavity wall)	11
hidr/o	sweat	4
hist/o	tissue(s)	2
humer/o	humerus (upper arm bone)	14
hydr/o	water	6
hymen/o	hymen	8
hyster/o	uterus	8

Appendix B Combining Forms, Prefixes, and Suffixes Alphabetized by Word Part

COMBINING FORMS	DEFINITION	CHAPTER
I		
iatr/o	physician, medicine (also means treatment)	2
ile/o	ileum	11
ili/o	ilium (upper, wing-shaped portion of the pelvis)	14
immun/o	immune system	10
infer/o	below	3
irid/o	iris	12
ir/o	iris	12
is/o	equal	12
ischi/o	ischium (lower posterior portion of the pelvis)	14
isch/o	deficiency, blockage	10
J		
jejun/o	jejunum	11
K		
kal/i	potassium	16
kerat/o	cornea	12
kerat/o	hornlike tissue (keratin), hard	4
kinesi/o	movement, motion	14
kyph/o	hump (increased convexity of the spine)	14
L		
labyrinth/o	labyrinth	13
lacrim/o	tear(s)	12
lact/o	milk	9
lamin/o	lamina (thin, flat plate or layer)	14
lapar/o	abdomen, abdominal cavity	11
laryng/o	larynx	5
later/o	side	3
lei/o	smooth	2
leuk/o	white	2
lingu/o	tongue	11
lip/o	fat, fat tissue	2
lith/o	stone(s), calculus (*pl.* calculi)	6
lob/o	lobe(s)	5

COMBINING FORMS	DEFINITION	CHAPTER
lord/o	bent forward (increased concavity of the spine)	14
lumb/o	loin, lumbar region of the spine	14
lymphaden/o	lymph node	10
lymph/o	lymph, lymph tissue	10
M		
mamm/o	breast	8
mandibul/o	mandible (lower jawbone)	14
mast/o	breast	8
mastoid/o	mastoid bone	13
maxill/o	maxilla (upper jawbone)	14
meat/o	meatus (opening)	6
medi/o	middle	3
mediastin/o	mediastinum	5
melan/o	black	2
meningi/o	meninges	15
mening/o	meninges	15
menisc/o	meniscus (crescent)	14
men/o	menstruation	8
ment/o	mind	15
metr/o	uterus	8
mon/o	one, single	15
muc/o	mucus	5
myc/o	fungus	4
myel/o	bone marrow	10
myel/o	spinal cord	15
my/o	muscle(s), muscle tissue	2
myos/o	muscle(s), muscle tissue	14
myring/o	tympanic membrane (eardrum)	13
N		
nas/o	nose	5
nat/o	birth	9
natr/o	sodium	16
necr/o	death (cells, body)	2
nephr/o	kidney	6

Appendix B Combining Forms, Prefixes, and Suffixes Alphabetized by Word Part

COMBINING FORMS	DEFINITION	CHAPTER
neur/o	nerve(s), nerve tissue	2
noct/i	night	6
O		
ocul/o	eye	12
olig/o	scanty, few	6
omphal/o	umbilicus, navel	9
onc/o	tumor, mass	2
onych/o	nail	4
oophor/o	ovary	8
ophthalm/o	eye	12
opt/o	vision	12
orchid/o	testis, testicle	7
orchi/o	testis, testicle	7
orch/o	testis, testicle	7
organ/o	organ	2
or/o	mouth	11
orth/o	straight	5
oste/o	bone	14
ot/o	ear	13
ox/i	oxygen	5
P		
pachy/o	thick	4
palat/o	palate	11
pancreat/o	pancreas	11
parathyroid/o	parathyroid glands	16
par/o	bear, give birth to, labor, childbirth	9
part/o	bear, give birth to, labor, childbirth	9
patell/o	patella (kneecap)	14
path/o	disease	2
pelv/i	pelvis, pelvic cavity	8
perine/o	perineum	8
peritone/o	peritoneum	11
petr/o	stone	14
phac/o	lens	12
phag/o	eating, swallowing	4
phak/o	lens	12
phalang/o	phalanx (*pl.* phalanges) (any bone of the fingers or toes)	14
pharyng/o	pharynx	5
phas/o	speech	15

COMBINING FORMS	DEFINITION	CHAPTER
phleb/o	vein(s)	10
phon/o	sound, voice	5
phot/o	light	12
pituitar/o	pituitary gland	16
plasm/o	plasma	10
pleur/o	pleura	5
pneum/o	lung, air	5
pneumon/o	lung, air	5
poli/o	gray matter	15
polyp/o	polyp, small growth	11
poster/o	back, behind	3
prim/i	first	9
proct/o	rectum	11
prostat/o	prostate gland	7
proxim/o	near (the point of attachment)	3
pseud/o	false	9
psych/o	mind	15
pub/o	pubis (anterior portion of the pelvis)	14
puerper/o	childbirth	9
pulmon/o	lung	5
pupill/o	pupil	12
pyel/o	renal pelvis	6
pylor/o	pylorus, pyloric sphincter	9
py/o	pus	5
Q		
quadr/i	four	15
R		
rachi/o	vertebra (*pl.* vertebrae), spine, vertebral column	14
radicul/o	nerve root	15
radi/o	radius (lower arm bone)	14
radi/o	x-rays, ionizing radiation	3
rect/o	rectum	11
ren/o	kidney	6
retin/o	retina	12
rhabd/o	rod-shaped, striated	2
rhin/o	nose	5
rhiz/o	nerve root	15
rhytid/o	wrinkles	4

Appendix B — Combining Forms, Prefixes, and Suffixes Alphabetized by Word Part

COMBINING FORMS	DEFINITION	CHAPTER
S		
sacr/o	sacrum (lower portion of the spine forming the posterior pelvic wall)	14
salping/o	fallopian tube (uterine tube)	8
sarc/o	flesh, connective tissue	2
scapul/o	scapula (shoulder blade)	14
scler/o	hard	4
scler/o	sclera	12
scoli/o	(lateral) curved (spine)	14
seb/o	sebum (oil)	4
sept/o	septum	5
sial/o	saliva, salivary gland	11
sigmoid/o	sigmoid colon	11
sinus/o	sinus(es)	5
somat/o	body	2
somn/o	sleep	5
son/o	sound	3
sperm/o	sperm, spermatozoon (*pl.* spermatozoa)	7
spermat/o	sperm, spermatozoon (*pl.* spermatozoa)	7
spir/o	breathe, breathing	5
splen/o	spleen	10
spondyl/o	vertebra (*pl.* vertebrae), spine, vertebral column	14
staped/o	stapes	13
staphyl/o	grapelike clusters	4
steat/o	fat	11
stern/o	sternum (breastbone)	14
stomat/o	mouth	11
strept/o	twisted chains	4
super/o	above	3
synovi/o	synovia, synovial membrane	14
system/o	system	2
T		
tars/o	tarsals (ankle bones)	14
tendin/o	tendon	14
ten/o	tendon	14
terat/o	malformations	9

COMBINING FORMS	DEFINITION	CHAPTER
thorac/o	thorax, chest, chest cavity	5
thromb/o	blood clot	10
thym/o	thymus gland	10
thyroid/o	thyroid gland	16
thyr/o	thyroid gland	16
tibi/o	tibia (lower leg bone)	14
tom/o	to cut, section, or slice	3
ton/o	tension, pressure	12
tonsill/o	tonsil(s)	5
trachel/o	cervix	8
trache/o	trachea	5
trich/o	hair	4
tympan/o	middle ear	13
U		
uln/o	ulna (lower arm bone)	14
ungu/o	nail	4
ureter/o	ureter	6
urethr/o	urethra	6
ur/o	urine, urinary tract	6
urin/o	urine, urinary tract	6
uve/o	uvea	12
uvul/o	uvula	11
V		
vagin/o	vagina	8
valvul/o	valve	10
vas/o	vessel, duct	7
ven/o	vein	10
ventricul/o	ventricle	10
ventr/o	belly (front)	3
vertebr/o	vertebra (*pl.* vertebrae), spine, vertebral column	14
vesic/o	bladder, sac	6
vesicul/o	seminal vesicle(s)	7
vestibul/o	vestibule	13
vir/o	virus	2
viscer/o	internal organs	2
vulv/o	vulva	8
X		
xanth/o	yellow	2
xer/o	dry, dryness	4

Appendix B Combining Forms, Prefixes, and Suffixes Alphabetized by Word Part

PREFIX	DEFINITION	CHAPTER
a-	absence of, without	5
an-	absence of, without	5
ante-	before	9
bi-	two	3, 12
bin-	two	12
brady-	slow	10
dia-	through, complete	2
dys-	painful, abnormal, difficult, labored	2
endo-	within	5
epi-	on, upon, over	4
eu-	normal, good	5
hemi-	half	11
hyper-	above, excessive	2
hypo-	below, incomplete, deficient, under	2
inter-	between	14
intra-	within	4
meta-	after, beyond, change	2

PREFIX	DEFINITION	CHAPTER
micro-	small	2
multi-	many	9
neo-	new	2
nulli-	none	9
pan-	all, total	10
para-	beside, around, abnormal	4
per-	through	4
peri-	surrounding (outer)	8
poly-	many, much	5
post-	after	9
pre-	before	9
pro-	before	2
sub-	under, below	4
supra-	above	14
sym-	together, joined	14
syn-	together, joined	14
tachy-	fast, rapid	5
trans-	through, across, beyond	4
uni-	one	3

SUFFIX	DEFINITION	CHAPTER
-a	no meaning	4
-ac	pertaining to	11
-al	pertaining to	2
-algia	pain	7
-amnios	amnion, amniotic fluid	9
-apheresis	removal	10
-ar	pertaining to	5
-ary	pertaining to	5
-asthenia	weakness	14
-cele	hernia, protrusion	5
-centesis	surgical puncture to aspirate fluid	5
-cleisis	surgical closure	8
-coccus (*pl.* -cocci)	berry-shaped (form of bacterium)	4
-cyesis	pregnancy	9
-cyte	cell	2
-desis	surgical fixation, fusion	5

SUFFIX	DEFINITION	CHAPTER
-drome	run, running	16
-e	no meaning	9
-eal	pertaining to	5
-ectasis	stretching out, dilation, expansion	5
-ectomy	excision, surgical removal	4
-emia	in the blood	5
-gen	substance or agent that produces or causes	2
-genic	producing, originating, causing	2
-gram	the record, radiographic image	3
-graph	instrument used to record; the record	3
-graphy	process of recording, radiographic imaging	3
-ia	diseased state, condition of	4
-iasis	condition	6
-iatrist	specialist, physician	15
-iatry	treatment, specialty	15

Appendix B Combining Forms, Prefixes, and Suffixes Alphabetized by Word Part

SUFFIX	DEFINITION	CHAPTER
-ic	pertaining to	2
-ictal	seizure, attack	15
-ior	pertaining to	3
-ism	state of	7
-itis	inflammation	4
-lith	stone(s), calculus (pl. calculi)	6
-logist	one who studies and treats (specialist, physician)	2
-logy	study of	2
-lysis	loosening, dissolution, separating	6
-malacia	softening	4
-megaly	enlargement	2
-meter	instrument used to measure	5
-metry	measurement	5
-oid	resembling	2
-oma	tumor, swelling	2
-opia	vision (condition)	12
-opsy	view of, viewing	2
-osis	abnormal condition (means increase when used with blood cell word roots)	2
-ous	pertaining to	2
-paresis	slight paralysis	15
-pathy	disease	2
-penia	abnormal reduction in number	10
-pepsia	digestion	11
-pexy	surgical fixation, suspension	6
-phobia	abnormal fear of or aversion to specific things	12
-physis	growth	14
-plasia	condition of formation, development, growth	2
-plasm	growth, substance, formation	2

SUFFIX	DEFINITION	CHAPTER
-plasty	surgical repair	4
-plegia	paralysis	12
-pnea	breathing	5
-ptosis	drooping, sagging, prolapse	6
-ptysis	spitting, coughing	5
-rrhage	excessive flow	10
-rrhagia	excessive bleeding	5
-rrhaphy	suturing, repairing	8
-rrhea	flow, discharge	4
-rrhexis	rupture	9
-salpinx	fallopian tube (uterine tube)	8
-sarcoma	malignant tumor	2
-schisis	split, fissure	14
-sclerosis	hardening	10
-scope	instrument used for visual examination	5
-scopic	pertaining to visual examination	5
-scopy	visual examination	5
-sis	state of	2
-spasm	sudden, involuntary muscle contraction	5
-stasis	control, stop, standing	2
-stenosis	constriction or narrowing	5
-stomy	creation of an artificial opening	5
-thorax	chest, chest cavity	5
-tocia	birth, labor	9
-tomy	cut into, incision	5
-tripsy	surgical crushing	6
-trophy	nourishment, development	14
-um	no meaning	9
-uria	urine, urination	6
-us	no meaning	9

Combining Forms, Prefixes, and Suffixes Alphabetized by Definition

Appendix C

DEFINITION	COMBINING FORM	CHAPTER
A		
abdomen, abdominal cavity	abdomin/o, lapar/o, celi/o	11
above	super/o	3
adenoids	adenoid/o	5
adrenal glands	adren/o, adrenal/o	16
albumin	albumin/o	6
alveolus *(s.)*, alveoli *(pl.)*	alveol/o	5
amnion, amniotic fluid	amni/o, amnion/o	9
antrum	antr/o	11
anus	an/o	11
aorta	aort/o	10
appendix	append/o, appendic/o	11
artery *(s)*, arteries *(pl)*	arteri/o	10
atrium	atri/o	10
away (from the point of attachment)	dist/o	3
B		
back	dors/o	3
back, behind	poster/o	3
bear, give birth to, labor, childbirth	par/o, part/o	9
belly (front)	ventr/o	3
below	infer/o	3
bent forward (increased concavity of the spine)	lord/o	14
bile duct(s)	cholangi/o	11
birth	nat/o	9
black	melan/o	2
bladder, sac	cyst/o, vesic/o	6
blood	hem/o, hemat/o	5, 2
blood clot	thromb/o	10
blue	cyan/o	2
body	somat/o	2

DEFINITION	COMBINING FORM	CHAPTER
bone	oste/o	14
bone marrow	myel/o	10
brain	encephal/o	15
breast	mamm/o, mast/o	8
breathe, breathing	spir/o	5
bronchus *(s.)*, bronchi *(pl.)*	bronch/o, bronchi/o	5
bursa (cavity)	burs/o	14
C		
calcium	calc/i	16
cancer	cancer/o, carcin/o	2
carbon dioxide	capn/o	5
carpals (wrist)	carp/o	14
cartilage	chondr/o	14
cause (of disease)	eti/o	2
cecum	cec/o	11
cell(s)	cyt/o	2
cerebellum	cerebell/o	15
cerebrum	cerebr/o	15
cervix	cervic/o, trachel/o	8
childbirth	puerper/o	9
chorion	chori/o	9
clavicle (collarbone)	clavicul/o	14
cochlea	cochle/o	13
cold	cry/o	12
colon	col/o, colon/o	11
common bile duct	choledoch/o	11
conjunctiva	conjunctiv/o	12
cornea	corne/o, kerat/o	12
cortex	cortic/o	16
cranium (skull)	crani/o	14
(lateral) curved (spine)	scoli/o	14
D		
death (cells, body)	necr/o	2
deficiency, blockage	isch/o	10

Appendix C — Combining Forms, Prefixes, and Suffixes Alphabetized by Definition

DEFINITION	COMBINING FORM	CHAPTER
developing cell, germ cell	blast/o	6
diaphragm	diaphragmat/o	5
disease	path/o	2
diverticulum	diverticul/o	11
dry, dryness	xer/o	4
duodenum	duoden/o	11
dust	coni/o	5
E		
ear	aur/i, ot/o	13
eating, swallowing	phag/o	4
electricity, electrical activity	electr/o	10
endocrine	endocrin/o	16
endometrium	endometri/o	8
epididymis	epididym/o	7
epiglottis	epiglott/o	5
epithelium, epithelial tissue	epitheli/o	2
equal	is/o	12
esophagus	esophag/o	9, 11
extremities, height	acr/o	16
eye	ocul/o, ophthalm/o	12
eyelid	blephar/o	12
F		
fallopian tube (uterine tube)	salping/o	8
false	pseud/o	9
fascia (connective tissue enclosing and separating muscle layers)	fasci/o	14
fat, fat tissue	lip/o	2
fat	steat/o	11
femur (upper leg bone)	femor/o	14
fetus, unborn offspring	fet/o	9
fiber(s), fibrous tissue	fibr/o	2
fibula (lower leg bone)	fibul/o	14
first	prim/i	9
flesh, connective tissue	sarc/o	2, 14
four	quadr/i	15
front	anter/o	3

DEFINITION	COMBINING FORM	CHAPTER
fungus	myc/o	3
G		
gall, bile	chol/e	11
ganglion	gangli/o, ganglion/o	15
gland, glandular tissue	aden/o	2
glans penis	balan/o	7
glia	gli/o	15
glomerulus	glomerul/o	6
grapelike clusters	staphyl/o	4
gray matter	poli/o	15
gum(s)	gingiv/o	11
H		
hard	scler/o	4
hard, dura mater	dur/o	15
head	cephal/o	3
hearing	audi/o	13
heart	cardi/o	10
hernia	herni/o	11
hidden	crypt/o	4
hornlike tissue (keratin), hard	kerat/o	4
humerus (upper arm bone)	humer/o	14
hump (increased convexity of the spine)	kyph/o	14
hymen	hymen/o	8
I		
ileum	ile/o	11
ilium (upper, wing-shaped portion of the pelvis)	ili/o	14
immune system	immun/o	10
imperfect, incomplete	atel/o	5
internal organs	viscer/o	2
intervertebral disk	disc/o	14
intestines (usually the small intestine)	enter/o	11
iris	ir/o, irid/o	12
ischium (lower posterior portion of the pelvis)	ischi/o	14
J		
jejunum	jejun/o	11
joint	arthr/o	14

Appendix C Combining Forms, Prefixes, and Suffixes Alphabetized by Definition

DEFINITION	COMBINING FORM	CHAPTER
K		
kidney	nephr/o, ren/o	6
knowledge	gno/o	2
L		
labyrinth	labyrinth/o	13
lamina (thin, flat plate or layer)	lamin/o	14
larynx	laryng/o	5
lens	phac/o, phak/o	12
life	bi/o	2
light	phot/o	12
lip(s)	cheil/o	11
liver	hepat/o	11
lobe(s)	lob/o	5
loin, lumbar region of the spine	lumb/o	14
lung	pulmon/o	5
lung, air	pneum/o, pneumon/o	5
lymph node	lymphaden/o	10
lymph, lymph tissue	lymph/o	10
M		
male	andr/o	7
malformations	terat/o	9
mandible (lower jawbone)	mandibul/o	14
mastoid bone	mastoid/o	13
maxilla (upper jawbone)	maxill/o	14
meatus (opening)	meat/o	6
mediastinum	mediastin/o	5
meninges	mening/o, meningi/o	15
meniscus (crescent)	menisc/o	14
menstruation	men/o	8
middle	medi/o	3
middle ear	tympan/o	13
milk	lact/o	9
mind	ment/o, psych/o	15
mouth	or/o, stomat/o	11
movement, motion	kinesi/o	14
mucus	muc/o	5
muscle(s), muscle tissue	my/o, myos/o	2, 14

DEFINITION	COMBINING FORM	CHAPTER
N		
nail	onych/o, ungu/o	4
near (the point of attachment)	proxim/o	3
nerve(s), nerve tissue	neur/o	2, 15
nerve root	radicul/o, rhiz/o	15
night	noct/i	6
nose	nas/o, rhin/o	5
O		
one, single	mon/o	15
organ	organ/o	2
ovary	oophor/o	8
oxygen	ox/i	5
P		
palate	palat/o	11
pancreas	pancreat/o	11
parathyroid glands	parathyroid/o	16
patella (kneecap)	patell/o	14
pelvis, pelvic cavity	pelv/i	8
perineum	perine/o	8
peritoneum	peritone/o	11
phalanx (any bone of the fingers or toes)	phalang/o	14
pharynx	pharyng/o	5
physician, medicine (also means treatment)	iatr/o	2
plasma	plasm/o	10
pleura	pleur/o	5
plug	embol/o	10
polyp, small growth	polyp/o	11
potassium	kal/i	16
pregnancy	gravid/o	9
prostate gland	prostat/o	7
pubis (anterior portion of the pelvis)	pub/o	14
pupil	cor/o, pupill/o	12
pus	py/o	5
pylorus, pyloric sphincter	pylor/o	9, 11
R		
radius (lower arm bone)	radi/o	14
rectum	proct/o, rect/o	11

DEFINITION	COMBINING FORM	CHAPTER	DEFINITION	COMBINING FORM	CHAPTER
red	erythr/o	2	sugar	glycos/o	6
renal pelvis	pyel/o	6	sweat	hidr/o	4
retina	retin/o	12	synovia, synovial membrane	synovi/o	14
rib	cost/o	14	system	system/o	2
rod-shaped, striated	rhabd/o	2			
S			**T**		
sacrum (lower portion of the spine forming the posterior pelvic wall)	sacr/o	14	tail (downward)	caud/o	3
			tarsals (ankle bones)	tars/o	14
saliva, salivary gland	sial/o	11	tear(s)	dacry/o, lacrim/o	12
			tendon	ten/o, tendin/o	14
scanty, few	olig/o	6	tension, pressure	ton/o	12
scapula (shoulder blade)	scapul/o	14	testis, testicle	orch/o, orchi/o, orchid/o	7
sclera	scler/o	12	thick	pachy/o	4
sebum (oil)	seb/o	4	thirst	dips/o	16
self	aut/o	2	thorax, chest, chest cavity	thorac/o	5
seminal vesicle(s)	vesicul/o	7			
sensation, sensitivity, feeling	esthesi/o	15	thymus gland	thym/o	10
			thyroid gland	thyr/o, thyroid/o	16
septum	sept/o	5	tibia (lower leg bone)	tibi/o	14
side	later/o	3			
sigmoid colon	sigmoid/o	11	tissue(s)	hist/o	2
sinus(es)	sinus/o	5	to cut, section, or slice	tom/o	3
skin	cutane/o, derm/o, dermat/o	4			
			tongue	gloss/o, lingu/o	11
sleep	somn/o	5	tonsil(s)	tonsill/o	5
smooth	lei/o	2	trachea	trache/o	5
sodium	natr/o	16	tumor, mass	onc/o	2
sound	son/o, ech/o	3, 10	twisted chains	strept/o	4
sound, voice	phon/o	5	two, double	dipl/o	12
speech	phas/o	15	tympanic membrane (eardrum)	myring/o	13
sperm, spermatozoon	sperm/o, spermat/o	7			
spinal cord	myel/o	15	**U**		
spleen	splen/o	10	ulna (lower arm bone)	uln/o	14
stapes	staped/o	13	umbilicus, navel	omphal/o	9
sternum (breastbone)	stern/o	14	urea, nitrogen	azot/o	6
			ureter	ureter/o	6
stiff, bent	ankyl/o	14	urethra	urethr/o	6
stomach	gastr/o	11	urine, urinary tract	ur/o, urin/o	6
stone	petr/o	14	uterus	hyster/o, metr/o	8
stone(s), calculus (*pl.* calculi)	lith/o	6	uvea	uve/o	12
straight	orth/o	5	uvula	uvul/o	11

Appendix C Combining Forms, Prefixes, and Suffixes Alphabetized by Definition

DEFINITION	COMBINING FORM	CHAPTER
V		
vagina	colp/o, vagin/o	8
valve	valvul/o	10
vein(s)	phleb/o, ven/o	10
ventricle	ventricul/o	10
vertebra (*pl.* vertebrae), spine, vertebral column	rachi/o, spondyl/o, vertebr/o	14
vessel(s); blood vessel(s)	angi/o	10
vessel, duct	vas/o	7
vestibule	vestibul/o	13
vision	opt/o	12
vulva	episi/o, vulv/o	8

DEFINITION	COMBINING FORM	CHAPTER
W		
water	hydr/o	6
white	leuk/o	2
woman, female reproductive organs	gyn/o, gynec/o	8
wrinkles	rhytid/o	4
X		
x-rays, ionizing radiation	radi/o	3
Y		
yellow	xanth/o	2
yellowish, fatty plaque	ather/o	10

DEFINITION	PREFIX	CHAPTER
above	supra-	14
above, excessive	hyper-	2
absence of, without	a-, an-	5
after	post-	9
after, beyond, change	meta-	2
all, total	pan-	10
before	ante-, pre-	9
before	pro-	2
below, incomplete, deficient, under	hypo-	2
beside, around, abnormal	para-	4
between	inter-	14
fast, rapid	tachy-	5
half	hemi-	11
many	multi-	9
many, much	poly-	5
new	neo-	2

DEFINITION	PREFIX	CHAPTER
none	nulli-	9
normal, good	eu-	5
on, upon, over	epi-	4
one	uni-	3
painful, abnormal, difficult, labored	dys-	2
slow	brady-	10
small	micro-	2
surrounding (outer)	peri-	8
through	per-	4
through, across, beyond	trans-	4
through, complete	dia-	2
together, joined	sym-, syn-	14
two	bin-	12
two	bi-	3, 12
under, below	sub-	4
within	intra-	4
within	endo-	5

Appendix C — Combining Forms, Prefixes, and Suffixes Alphabetized by Definition

DEFINITION	SUFFIX	CHAPTER
abnormal condition (means increase when used with blood cell word roots)	-osis	2
abnormal fear of or aversion to specific things	-phobia	12
abnormal reduction in number	-penia	10
amnion, amniotic fluid	-amnios	9
berry-shaped (form of bacterium)	-coccus (pl. -cocci)	4
birth, labor	-tocia	9
breathing	-pnea	5
cell	-cyte	2
chest, chest cavity	-thorax	5
condition	-iasis	6
condition of formation, development, growth	-plasia	2
constriction or narrowing	-stenosis	5
control, stop, standing	-stasis	2
creation of an artificial opening	-stomy	5
cut into, incision	-tomy	5
digestion	-pepsia	11
disease	-pathy	2
diseased state, condition of	-ia	4
drooping, sagging, prolapse	-ptosis	6
enlargement	-megaly	2
excessive bleeding	-rrhagia	5
excessive flow	-rrhage	10
excision, surgical removal	-ectomy	4
fallopian tube (uterine tube)	-salpinx	8
flow, discharge	-rrhea	4
growth	-physis	14
growth, substance, formation	-plasm	2
hardening	-sclerosis	10
hernia, protrusion	-cele	5
in the blood	-emia	5

DEFINITION	SUFFIX	CHAPTER
inflammation	-itis	4
instrument used for visual examination	-scope	5
instrument used to measure	-meter	5
instrument used to record; the record	-graph	3
loosening, dissolution, separating	-lysis	6
malignant tumor	-sarcoma	2
measurement	-metry	5
no meaning	-a, -e, -um, -us	4, 9
nourishment, development	-trophy	14
one who studies and treats (specialist, physician)	-logist	2
pain	-algia	7
paralysis	-plegia	12
pertaining to	-ac	11
pertaining to	-ous	2, 6
pertaining to	-ar, -ary, -eal	5
pertaining to	-al, -ic	2
pertaining to	-ior	3
pertaining to visual examination	-scopic	5
pregnancy	-cyesis	9
process of recording, radiographic imaging	-graphy	3
producing, originating, causing	-genic	2
removal	-apheresis	10
resembling	-oid	2
run, running	-drome	16
rupture	-rrhexis	9
seizure, attack	-ictal	15
slight paralysis	-paresis	15
softening	-malacia	4
specialist, physician	-iatrist	15
spitting, coughing	-ptysis	5
split, fissure	-schisis	14
state of	-ism	7
state of	-sis	2
stone(s), calculus (pl. calculi)	-lith	6

Appendix C Combining Forms, Prefixes, and Suffixes Alphabetized by Definition

DEFINITION	SUFFIX	CHAPTER	DEFINITION	SUFFIX	CHAPTER
stretching out, dilation, expansion	-ectasis	5	surgical puncture to aspirate fluid	-centesis	5
study of	-logy	2	surgical repair	-plasty	4
substance or agent that produces or causes	-gen	2	suturing, repairing	-rrhaphy	8
			the record, radiographic image	-gram	3
sudden, involuntary muscle contraction	-spasm	5	treatment, specialty	-iatry	15
surgical closure	-cleisis	8	tumor, swelling	-oma	2
surgical crushing	-tripsy	6	urine, urination	-uria	6
surgical fixation, fusion	-desis	5	view of, viewing	-opsy	2
			vision (condition)	-opia	12
surgical fixation, suspension	-pexy	6	visual examination	-scopy	5
			weakness	-asthenia	14

Appendix D

Abbreviations

Topics include:
Common Medical Abbreviations, p. 741
Institute for Safe Medication Practices' (ISMP) List of Error-Prone Abbreviations, Symbols, and Dose Designations; includes The Joint Commission's "Do Not Use" list, p. 750

Abbreviations are written as they appear most commonly in the medical and healthcare environment. Some may also appear in both capital and small letters and with or without periods. To make a plural, add "s" to uppercase abbreviations (e.g., BPs for blood pressures) and apostrophe ('s) for lower case abbreviations (e.g., cm's for centimeters).

COMMON MEDICAL ABBREVIATIONS	DEFINITIONS
A1c	glycosylated hemoglobin
AAA	abdominal aortic aneurysm
AAD	antibiotic-associated diarrhea
AB	abortion
ABD	abdomen
ABE	acute bacterial endocarditis
ABG	arterial blood gas
ABX	antibiotics
AC	acromioclavicular
ac	acute
a.c.	before meals
ACS	acute coronary syndrome
ACTH	adrenocorticotropic hormone
AD	Alzheimer disease
ADC	AIDS dementia complex
ADH	antidiuretic hormone
ADHD	attention deficit/hyperactivity disorder
ADLs	activities of daily living
ad lib	as desired
Adm	admission
AER	auditory evoked response
AF	atrial fibrillation
AFB	acid-fast bacilli
AFib	atrial fibrillation
AFP	alpha-fetoprotein
AHD	arteriosclerotic heart disease
AI	aortic insufficiency

COMMON MEDICAL ABBREVIATIONS	DEFINITIONS
AICD	automatic implantable cardiac defibrillator
AIDS	acquired immunodeficiency syndrome
AK	actinic keratosis
AKA	above-knee amputation
AKI	acute kidney injury
alk phos	alkaline phosphatase
ALL	acute lymphoblastic leukemia
ALS	amyotrophic lateral sclerosis
ALT	alanine aminotransferase
AM (or a.m.)	between midnight and noon
AMA	against medical advice; American Medical Association
AMB	ambulate; ambulatory
AMI	acute myocardial infarction
AML	acute myeloid leukemia
AMP (or amp)	ampule
amt	amount
angio	angiogram; angiography
ant	anterior
A&O	alert and oriented
AODM	adult-onset diabetes mellitus
AOM	acute otitis media
AP	anteroposterior; angina pectoris
A&P	anatomy and physiology; auscultation and percussion; anterior and posterior
A&P repair	anterior and posterior colporrhaphy

741

COMMON MEDICAL ABBREVIATIONS	DEFINITIONS
APH	antepartum hemorrhage
APR	abdominoperineal resection
aPTT	activated partial thromboplastin time
ARDS	acute respiratory distress syndrome
ARF	acute renal failure
ARM	artificial rupture of membranes
AMD, ARMD	age-related macular degeneration
ART	assisted reproductive technology
ASA	aspirin (acetylsalicylic acid)
ASCVD	arteriosclerotic cardiovascular disease
ASD	atrial septal defect; autism spectrum disorder
ASHD	arteriosclerotic heart disease
Ast (or AST)	astigmatism
as tol	as tolerated
AUB	abnormal uterine bleeding
AUL	acute undifferentiated leukemia
AUR	acute urinary retention
AV	atrioventricular; arteriovenous
AVM	arteriovenous malformation
AVR	aortic valve replacement
ax	axillary
BA	bronchial asthma
BBB	bundle branch block
BC	birth control
BCC	basal cell carcinoma
BE	barium enema
b.i.d.	twice a day
BK	below knee
BKA	below-knee amputation
BM	bowel movement
BMI	body mass index
BMP	basic metabolic panel
BMT	bone marrow transplant
BOM	bilateral otitis media
BOO	bladder outlet obstruction
BP	blood pressure
BPH	benign prostatic hyperplasia
BPPV	benign paroxysmal positional vertigo
BR	bed rest
BRBPR	bright red blood per rectum

COMMON MEDICAL ABBREVIATIONS	DEFINITIONS
BRM	biological response modifier
BRP	bathroom privileges
BS	blood sugar; bowel sounds; breath sounds
BSO	bilateral salpingo-oophorectomy
BUN	blood urea nitrogen
Bx	biopsy
$\bar{c}$	with
C	Celsius
C1-C7 or C_1-C_7	cervical vertebrae
Ca (or Ca^{2+})	calcium
CA	cancer; carcinoma
CABG	coronary artery bypass graft
CAD	coronary artery disease
CAL (or cal)	calorie
CA-MRSA	community-associated MRSA (methicillin-resistant *Staphylococcus aureus*) infection
CAP	capsule (or cap); community-acquired pneumonia
CAPD	continuous ambulatory peritoneal dialysis
cath	catheterization, catheter
CBC with diff	complete blood count with differential
CBR	complete bed rest
CBS	chronic brain syndrome
CC	chief complaint; colony count
CCU	coronary care unit
CDC	Centers for Disease Control and Prevention
CDH	congenital dislocation of the hip
CDI	*Clostridium difficile* infection
C. diff or C. difficile	*Clostridium difficile* (bacteria)
CEA	carcinoembryonic antigen
CF	cystic fibrosis
CHB	complete heart block
CHD	coronary heart disease
chemo	chemotherapy
CHF	congestive heart failure
CHO	carbohydrate
chol	cholesterol
CI	coronary insufficiency

Appendix D Abbreviations

COMMON MEDICAL ABBREVIATIONS	DEFINITIONS
circ	circumcision
CIS	carcinoma in situ
CJD	Creutzfeldt-Jakob disease
Cl (or Cl⁻)	chloride
CKD	chronic kidney disease
CLBSI	central line bloodstream infection
CLD	chronic liver disease
CLL	chronic lymphocytic leukemia
cl liq	clear liquid
cm	centimeter
CML	chronic myelogenous leukemia
CMP	comprehensive metabolic panel
CMV	cytomegalovirus
CNS	central nervous system
c/o	complains of
CO	carbon monoxide
CO_2	carbon dioxide
COB	coordination of benefits
cocci	coccidioidomycosis
COLD	chronic obstructive lung disease
comp	compound
cond	condition
COPD	chronic obstructive pulmonary disease
COVID-19	coronavirus disease
CP	cerebral palsy
CPAP	continuous positive airway pressure
CPD	cephalopelvic disproportion
CPK	creatine phosphokinase
CPN	chronic pyelonephritis
CPR	cardiopulmonary resuscitation
CRD	chronic respiratory disease
creat	creatinine
CRF	chronic renal failure
crit	hematocrit (also HCT, Hct)
CRP	C-reactive protein
C&S	culture and sensitivity
C/S, CS, C-section	cesarean section
CSF	cerebrospinal fluid
CT	computed tomography
CTE	chronic traumatic encephalopathy
CTS	carpal tunnel syndrome

COMMON MEDICAL ABBREVIATIONS	DEFINITIONS
Cu	copper
CUR	chronic urinary retention
CVA	cerebrovascular accident (stroke)
CVD	cardiovascular disease
CVP	central venous pressure
CVS	chorionic villus sampling
Cx	cervix
CXR	chest radiograph (x-ray)
DAT	diet as tolerated
D&C	dilation and curettage
DC	Doctor of Chiropractic
D&E	dilation and evacuation
DCIS	ductal carcinoma in situ
decub	pressure ulcer
del	delivery
derm	dermatology
DI	diabetes insipidus
DIC	diffuse intravascular coagulation
diff	differential (part of complete blood count)
disch	discharge
DISH	diffuse idiopathic skeletal hyperostosis
DKA	diabetic ketoacidosis
DLE	discoid lupus erythematosus
DM	diabetes mellitus
DNA	deoxyribonucleic acid
DND	died natural death
DO	Doctor of Osteopathy
DOA	dead on arrival
DOB	date of birth
DOD	date of death
Dr	dram
DRE	digital rectal examination
DRG	diagnosis-related group
DSA	digital subtraction angiography
DTR	deep tendon reflexes
DVT	deep vein thrombosis
DW	distilled water
D/W	dextrose in water
Dx	diagnosis
E	enema

COMMON MEDICAL ABBREVIATIONS	DEFINITIONS
EBL	estimated blood loss
ECG	electrocardiogram
ECHO	echocardiogram
ECT	electroconvulsive therapy
ED	erectile dysfunction, emergency department
EDD	expected (estimated) date of delivery
EEG	electroencephalogram
EGD	esophagogastroduodenoscopy
EKG	electrocardiogram
Elix (or elix)	elixir
Em	emmetropia
EMG	electromyogram
ENG	electronystagmography
ENT	ears, nose, throat; otolaryngologist
EP	ectopic pregnancy
EP studies	evoked potential studies
ER	emergency room
ERCP	endoscopic retrograde cholangiopancreatography
ERT	estrogen replacement therapy
ESKD	end-stage kidney disease
ESR	erythrocyte sedimentation rate
ESRD	end-stage renal disease
ESWL	extracorporeal shock wave lithotripsy
etio	etiology
EUS	endoscopic ultrasound
exam	examination
ext	extract; external
F	Fahrenheit
FA	fluorescein angiography
FAS	fetal alcohol syndrome
FBD	fibrocystic breast disease
FBS	fasting blood sugar
FCC	fibrocystic (breast) changes
FDA	Food and Drug Administration
Fe	iron
FHT	fetal heart tones
FIT	fecal immunochemical test
flu	influenza

COMMON MEDICAL ABBREVIATIONS	DEFINITIONS
FNA	fine needle aspiration
Fr	French (catheter size)
FS	frozen section
FSH	follicle-stimulating hormone
FTD	frontotemporal dementia
FTSG	full-thickness skin graft
FTT	failure to thrive
FUO	fever of undetermined origin
fx	fracture
g	gram
GC	gonorrhea
GERD	gastroesophageal reflux disease
GFR	glomerular filtration rate
gFOBT	guaiac-based fecal occult blood test
GH	growth hormone
GI	gastrointestinal
GSW	gunshot wound
gtt	drops
GTT	glucose tolerance test
GU	genitourinary
GYN	gynecology; gynecologist
h	hour
H	hypodermic
HAART	highly active antiretroviral therapy
HAI	healthcare-associated infection
HA-MRSA	healthcare-associated MRSA infection
HAND	HIV-associated neurocognitive disorder
HAP	hospital-acquired pneumonia
HB	heart block
HbA1c	glycosylated hemoglobin
HBV	hepatitis B virus
HCl	hydrochloric acid
HCO$_3$	bicarbonate
Hct	hematocrit
HCVD	hypertensive cardiovascular disease
HD	hemodialysis
HDL	high-density lipoprotein
HF	heart failure
Hg	mercury
Hgb	hemoglobin

COMMON MEDICAL ABBREVIATIONS	DEFINITIONS
H&H	hemoglobin and hematocrit
HHD	hypertensive heart disease
HIV	human immunodeficiency virus
HMD	hyaline membrane disease
HME	heat and moisture exchanger
HNP	herniated nucleus pulposus
H$_2$O	water
H$_2$O$_2$	hydrogen peroxide (hydrogen dioxide)
HOB	head of bed
HOH	hard of hearing
HoLEP	holmium laser enucleation of the prostate gland
H&P	history and physical examination
H. pylori	*Helicobacter pylori*
HPV	human papillomavirus
HRT	hormone replacement therapy
HSG	hysterosonography; hysterosalpingogram
ht	height
HTN	hypertension
Hx	history
hypo	hypodermic
IBD	inflammatory bowel disease
IBS	irritable bowel syndrome
ICD	implantable cardiac defibrillator
ICU	intensive care unit
ID	intradermal
I&D	incision and drainage
IDDM	insulin-dependent diabetes mellitus
IHD	ischemic heart disease
IM	intramuscular
inf	inferior
INR	international normalized ratio
I&O	intake and output
IOL	intraocular lens
IOP	intraocular pressure
IPF	idiopathic pulmonary fibrosis
IPPB	intermittent positive pressure breathing
IR	interventional radiology
irrig	irrigation

COMMON MEDICAL ABBREVIATIONS	DEFINITIONS
isol	isolation
IUD	intrauterine device
IUS	intrauterine system
IV	intravenous
IVC	intravenous cholangiogram
IVF	in vitro fertilization
IVU	intravenous urogram
K	potassium
KCl	potassium chloride
kg	kilogram
KO	keep open
KUB	kidney, ureter, bladder (radiograph)
KVO	keep vein open
L	liter
L1-L5 or L$_1$-L$_5$	lumbar vertebrae
lab	laboratory
LAC (or lac)	laceration
LAD	left anterior descending (coronary artery)
LAGB	laparoscopic adjustable gastric banding
LAP	laparotomy
LAR	low anterior resection
LARC	long-acting reversible contraception
LASIK	laser-assisted in situ keratomileusis
lat	lateral
LAVH	laparoscopically assisted vaginal hysterectomy
L&D	labor and delivery
LDH	lactic dehydrogenase
LDL	low-density lipoprotein
LE	lupus erythematosus
LEEP	loop electrosurgical excision procedure
lg	large
LH	luteinizing hormone
LLL	left lower lobe (of lung)
LLQ	left lower quadrant
LMP	last menstrual period
LOC	loss of consciousness; level of consciousness

Appendix D Abbreviations

COMMON MEDICAL ABBREVIATIONS	DEFINITIONS
LP	lumbar puncture
LPM	liters per minute (oxygen)
LPN	licensed practical nurse
LPR	laryngopharyngeal reflux
LR	lactated Ringer (IV solution)
lt	left
LTB	laryngotracheobronchitis
LUL	left upper lobe (of lung)
LUQ	left upper quadrant
LUTS	lower urinary tract symptoms
lytes	electrolytes
MBS	modified barium swallow
mcg	microgram
MCH	mean corpuscular hemoglobin
MCV	mean corpuscular volume
MD	muscular dystrophy; medical doctor
med	medial
mEq	milliequivalent
MET (or met)	metastasis
METS (or mets)	metastases
mg	milligram
MG	myasthenia gravis
MI	myocardial infarction
MISTs	minimally invasive surgical treatments
mL	milliliter
mm	millimeter
MM	multiple myeloma
MOM	milk of magnesia
MR	magnetic resonance; mitral regurgitation
MRI	magnetic resonance imaging
MRCP	magnetic resonance cholangiopancreatography
MRSA	methicillin-resistant *Staphylococcus aureus*
MS	multiple sclerosis
multip	multipara
MVP	mitral valve prolapse
Na	sodium
NaCl	sodium chloride (salt)
NAFLD	nonalcoholic fatty liver disease

COMMON MEDICAL ABBREVIATIONS	DEFINITIONS
NAS	no added salt
NASH	nonalcoholic steatohepatitis
NB	newborn
NCD	neurocognitive disorder
neg	negative
neuro	neurology
NG	nasogastric
NG	nasogastric
NICU	neonatal intensive care unit
NIDDM	noninsulin-dependent diabetes mellitus
NIH	National Institutes of Health
NIVA	noninvasive vascular assessment
NK	natural killer (immune system cells)
NKDA	no known drug allergies
NM	nuclear medicine
noc, noct	night
NPH	normal pressure hydrocephalus
NPO	nothing by mouth
NPPV	noninvasive positive-pressure ventilator
NS	normal saline
NSAID	nonsteroidal antiinflammatory drug
NSR	normal sinus rhythm
N&V	nausea and vomiting
NVS	neurologic vital signs
O_2	oxygen
OA	osteoarthritis
OAB	overactive bladder
OB	obstetrics
OCD	obsessive-compulsive disorder
OCT	optical coherence tomography
OD	Doctor of Optometry; overdose
OE	otitis externa
OIC	opioid-induced constipation
oint	ointment
OM	otitis media
OOB	out of bed
OP	outpatient
Ophth	ophthalmic or ophthalmology
OR	operating room
Ortho or ortho	orthopedics

COMMON MEDICAL ABBREVIATIONS	DEFINITIONS
OSA	obstructive sleep apnea
OT	occupational therapy
OTC	over-the-counter drugs
oto	otology
oz	ounce
$\bar{p}$	after
P	phosphorus; pulse
PA	physician's assistant or posteroanterior
PAC	premature atrial complex
PaCO₂	carbon dioxide partial pressure (measure of amount of carbon dioxide in arterial blood)
PAD	peripheral artery disease
PAE	prostatic artery embolization
PAF	paroxysmal atrial fibrillation
PaO₂	oxygen partial pressure (measure of amount of oxygen in arterial blood)
PAS	placenta accreta spectrum
PAT	paroxysmal atrial tachycardia
PBSCT	peripheral blood stem cell transplant
pc (or p.c.)	after meals
PCI	percutaneous coronary intervention
PCOS	polycystic ovary syndrome
PCP	primary care physician; *Pneumocystis* pneumonia
PCU	progressive care unit
PCV	packed cell volume
PD	Parkinson disease
PDA	patent ductus arteriosus
PDR	*Physicians' Desk Reference*
PE	pulmonary embolism; pulmonary edema
Peds (or peds)	pediatrics
PEEP	positive end-expiratory pressure
PEG	percutaneous endoscopic gastrostomy
PEP	positive expiratory pressure
per	by
PERRLA	pupils equal, round, reactive to light and accommodation
PET	positron emission tomography

COMMON MEDICAL ABBREVIATIONS	DEFINITIONS
PFM	peak flow meter
PFTs	pulmonary function tests
PHACO	phacoemulsification
PICC	peripherally inserted central catheter
PICU	pediatric intensive care unit
PID	pelvic inflammatory disease
PJP	*Pneumocystis jiroveci* pneumonia
PKD	polycystic kidney disease
PKU	phenylketonuria
PM	polymyositis; between noon and midnight
PMDD	premenstrual dysphoric disorder
PMS	premenstrual syndrome
PNS	peripheral nervous system
po (or PO)	orally; postoperative; phone order
polio	poliomyelitis
post-op	postoperatively
PP	postpartum; postprandial (after meals)
PPD	purified protein derivative
PPH	postpartum hemorrhage
pr	per rectum
PRBC	packed red blood cells
pre-op	preoperatively
PRH	prolactin-releasing hormone
primip	primipara
PRK	photorefractive keratectomy
PRL	prolactin
PRN	as needed (whenever necessary)
PSA	prostate-specific antigen
PSG	polysomnography
pt	patient; pint
PT	prothrombin time; physical therapy
PTCA	percutaneous transluminal coronary angioplasty
PTH	parathyroid hormone
PT/INR	prothrombin time/international normalized ratio
PTSD	posttraumatic stress disorder
PTT	partial thromboplastin time
PUL	percutaneous ultrasound lithotripsy; prostatic urethral lift
PVC	premature ventricular complex

Common Medical Abbreviations	Definitions
PVD	peripheral vascular disease
PVL	peripheral vision loss (tunnel vision)
PVP	photoselective vaporization of the prostate gland
Px	prognosis
q	every
q_h	every (number) hour (e.g., q2h)
qt	quart
R	rectal; respiration
RA	rheumatoid arthritis
RAD	reactive airway disease
RAIU	radioactive iodine uptake
RALP	robot-assisted laparoscopic prostatectomy
RARP	robot-assisted radical prostatectomy
RASP	robot-assisted simple prostatectomy
RBC	red blood cell (erythrocyte)
RDS	respiratory distress syndrome
reg	regular
REM	rapid eye movement
resp	respirations
RHD	rheumatic heart disease
RLL	right lower lobe (of lung)
RLQ	right lower quadrant
RML	right middle lobe (of lung)
RN	registered nurse
R/O	rule out
ROM	range of motion; rupture of membranes
RP	radical prostatectomy; retinitis pigmentosa
RR	recovery room
RSV	respiratory syncytial virus infection
rt	right; routine
RT	respiratory therapy
RUL	right upper lobe (of lung)
RUQ	right upper quadrant
Rx	prescription
RYGB	Roux-en-Y gastric bypass
$\bar{s}$	without
SAB	spontaneous abortion
SABA	short-acting beta agonist (relief of asthma symptoms)

Common Medical Abbreviations	Definitions
SAH	subarachnoid hemorrhage
SARS	severe acute respiratory syndrome
SBE	subacute bacterial endocarditis; self-breast examination
SCC	squamous cell carcinoma
SCLC	small cell lung cancer
SG	specific gravity
SHG	sonohysterography
SI	sacroiliac
SIADH	syndrome of inappropriate ADH secretion
SICU	surgical intensive care unit
SIDS	sudden infant death syndrome
SLE	systemic lupus erythematosus
SMAC	Sequential Multiple Analyzer Computer
SMR	submucous resection
SNF	skilled nursing facility
SOB	shortness of breath
SPECT	single-photon emission computed tomography
SSE	soapsuds enema
SSER	somatosensory evoked response
STAPH or staph	staphylococcus
stat	immediately
STD	sexually transmitted disease
STI	sexually transmitted infection
STREP or strep	streptococcus
STSG	split-thickness skin graft
subcut	subcutaneous
subling	sublingual
sup	superior
supp	suppository
surg	surgical
SVD	spontaneous vaginal delivery
SVN	small-volume nebulizer
SWL	shock wave lithotripsy
T	temperature
T1-T12 or T_1-T_{12}	thoracic vertebrae
T1D	type 1 diabetes (mellitus)
T1DM	type 1 diabetes mellitus
T2D	type 2 diabetes (mellitus)
T2DM	type 2 diabetes mellitus
T_3	triiodothyronine

COMMON MEDICAL ABBREVIATIONS	DEFINITIONS
T_4	thyroxine
tab	tablet
TAB	therapeutic abortion
T&A	tonsillectomy and adenoidectomy
TAH	total abdominal hysterectomy
TAH/BSO	total abdominal hysterectomy/bilateral salpingo-oophorectomy
TAT	tetanus antitoxin
TB	tuberculosis
TBI	traumatic brain injury
TCDB	turn, cough, deep breathe
TCT	thrombin clotting time
TD	transdermal
TEE	transesophageal echocardiogram
temp	temperature
TENS	transcutaneous electrical nerve stimulation
TGs	triglycerides
THA	total hip arthroplasty
THR	total hip replacement
TIA	transient ischemic attack
tid	three times per day
tinct	tincture
TKA	total knee arthroplasty
TLC	total lung capacity
TLH	total laparoscopic hysterectomy
TPN	total parenteral nutrition
tr	tincture
trach	tracheostomy
TRUS	transrectal ultrasound
TSH	thyroid-stimulating hormone
TSS	toxic shock syndrome
TUIP	transurethral incision of the prostate gland
TULIP	transurethral laser incision of the prostate gland
TUNA	transurethral needle ablation
TURP	transurethral resection of the prostate gland
TVS	transvaginal sonography
TWE	tap water enema
Tx	treatment; traction
UA	urinalysis

COMMON MEDICAL ABBREVIATIONS	DEFINITIONS
UAE	uterine artery embolization
UC	ulcerative colitis
UGI	upper gastrointestinal
UGI-SBFT	upper gastrointestinal [series] with small bowel follow-through [radiograph]
ung	ointment
UPPP	uvulopalatopharyngoplasty
URI	upper respiratory infection
US	ultrasound
UTI	urinary tract infection
UV	ultraviolet
UVR	ultraviolet radiation
V_1	tidal volume
VA	visual acuity
vag	vaginal
VATS	video-assisted thoracic surgery
VBAC	vaginal birth after cesarean section
VBG	venous blood gas
VC	vital capacity
VCUG	voiding cystourethrogram
VD	venereal disease
VDRL	Venereal Disease Research Laboratory
vent	ventilator
VER	visual evoked response
VF	ventricular fibrillation
VFib	ventricular fibrillation
VH	vaginal hysterectomy
VLAP	visual laser ablation of the prostate
VLDL	very-low-density lipoprotein
V/Q scan	lung ventilation/perfusion scan
VRE	vancomycin-resistant enterococci
VS	vital signs
VUR	vesicoureteral reflux
WA	while awake
WBC	white blood cell (leukocyte)
W/C	wheelchair
wt	weight
WVTT	water vapor thermal therapy
XRT	radiation therapy; x-ray radiotherapy; x-ray therapy

Appendix D Abbreviations

Institute for Safe Medication Practices' List of Error-Prone Abbreviations, Symbols, and Dose Designations

The abbreviations, symbols, and dose designations found in this table have been reported to ISMP through the ISMP National Medication Errors Reporting Program (ISMP MERP) as being frequently misinterpreted and involved in harmful medication errors. They should **NEVER** be used when communicating medical information. This includes internal communications, telephone/verbal prescriptions, computer-generated labels, labels for drug storage bins, medication administration records, as well as pharmacy and prescriber computer order entry screens.

ABBREVIATIONS	INTENDED MEANING	MISINTERPRETATION	CORRECTION
μg	Microgram	Mistaken as "mg"	Use "mcg"
AD, AS, AU	Right ear, left ear, each ear	Mistaken as OD, OS, OU (right eye, left eye, each eye)	Use "right ear," "left ear," or "each ear"
OD, OS, OU	Right eye, left eye, each eye	Mistaken as AD, AS, AU (right ear, left ear, each ear)	Use "right eye," "left eye," or "each eye"
BT	Bedtime	Mistaken as "BID" (twice daily)	Use "bedtime"
cc	Cubic centimeters	Mistaken as "u" (units)	Use "mL"
D/C	Discharge or discontinue	Premature discontinuation of medications if D/C (intended to mean "discharge") has been misinterpreted as "discontinued" when followed by a list of discharge medications	Use "discharge" and "discontinue"
IJ	Injection	Mistaken as "IV" or "intrajugular"	Use "injection"
IN	Intranasal	Mistaken as "IM" or "IV"	Use "intranasal" or "NAS"
HS	Half-strength	Mistaken as bedtime	Use "half-strength" or "bedtime"
hs	At bedtime, hours of sleep	Mistaken as half-strength	
IU**	International unit	Mistaken as IV (intravenous) or 10 (ten)	Use "units"
o.d. or OD	Once daily	Mistaken as "right eye" (OD-oculus dexter), leading to oral liquid medications administered in the eye	Use "daily"
OJ	Orange juice	Mistaken as OD or OS (right or left eye); drugs meant to be diluted in orange juice may be given in the eye	Use "orange juice"
Per os	By mouth, orally	The "os" can be mistaken as "left eye" (OS-oculus sinister)	Use "PO," "by mouth," or "orally"
q.d. or QD**	Every day	Mistaken as q.i.d., especially if the period after the "q" or the tail of the "q" is misunderstood as an "i"	Use "daily"
qhs	Nightly at bedtime	Mistaken as "qhr" or every hour	Use "nightly"
qn	Nightly or at bedtime	Mistaken as "qh" (every hour)	Use "nightly" or "at bedtime"
q.o.d. or QOD**	Every other day	Mistaken as "q.d." (daily) or "q.i.d." (four times daily) if the "o" is poorly written	Use "every other day"
q1d	Daily	Mistaken as q.i.d. (four times daily)	Use "daily"

Appendix D Abbreviations

ABBREVIATIONS	INTENDED MEANING	MISINTERPRETATION	CORRECTION
q6PM, etc.	Every evening at 6 PM	Mistaken as every 6 hours	Use "daily at 6 PM" or "6 PM daily"
SC, SQ, sub q	Subcutaneous	SC mistaken as SL (sublingual); SQ mistaken as "5 every"; the "q" in "sub q" has been mistaken as "every" (e.g., a heparin dose ordered "sub q 2 hours before surgery" misunderstood as every 2 hours before surgery)	Use "subcut" or "subcutaneously"
ss	Sliding scale (insulin) or ½ (apothecary)	Mistaken as "55"	Spell out "sliding scale"; use "one half" or "½"
SSRI	Sliding scale regular insulin	Mistaken as "selective-serotonin reuptake inhibitor"	Spell out "sliding scale (insulin)"
SSI	Sliding scale insulin	Mistaken as "Strong Solution of Iodine" (Lugol's)	
i/d	One daily	Mistaken as "tid"	Use "1 daily"
TIW or tiw	3 times a week	Mistaken as "3 times a day" or "twice in a week"	Use "3 times weekly"
U or u**	Unit	Mistaken as the number 0 or 4, causing a 10-fold overdose or greater (e.g., 4U seen as "40" or 4u seen as "44"); mistaken as "cc" so dose given in volume instead of units (e.g., 4u seen as 4cc)	Use "unit"
UD	As directed ("ut dictum")	Mistaken as unit dose (e.g., diltiazem 125 mg IV infusion "UD" misinterpreted as meaning to give the entire infusion as a unit [bolus] dose)	Use "as directed"

DOSE DESIGNATIONS AND OTHER INFORMATION	INTENDED MEANING	MISINTERPRETATION	CORRECTION
Trailing zero after decimal point (e.g., 1.0 mg)**	1 mg	Mistaken as 10 mg if the decimal point is not seen	Do not use trailing zeros for doses expressed in whole numbers
"Naked" decimal point (e.g., .5 mg)**	0.5 mg	Mistaken as 5 mg if the decimal point is not seen	Use zero before a decimal point when the dose is less than a whole unit
Abbreviations such as mg. or mL. with a period following the abbreviation	mg mL	The period is unnecessary and could be mistaken as the number 1 if written poorly	Use mg, mL, etc., without a terminal period
Drug name and dose run together (especially problematic for drug names that end in "l" such as Inderal40 mg; Tegretol300 mg)	Inderal 40 mg Tegretol 300 mg	Mistaken as Inderal 140 mg Mistaken as Tegretol 1300 mg	Place adequate space between the drug name, dose, and unit of measure

Appendix D Abbreviations

ABBREVIATIONS	INTENDED MEANING	MISINTERPRETATION	CORRECTION
Numerical dose and unit of measure run together (e.g., 10mg, 100mL)	10 mg 100 mL	The "m" is sometimes mistaken as a zero or two zeros, risking a 10- to 100-fold overdose	Place adequate space between the dose and unit of measure
Large doses without properly placed commas (e.g., 100000 units; 1000000 units)	100,000 units 1,000,000 units	100000 has been mistaken as 10,000 or 1,000,000; 1000000 has been mistaken as 100,000	Use commas for dosing units at or above 1,000, or use words such as 100 "thousand" or 1 "million" to improve readability

ABBREVIATIONS	INTENDED MEANING	MISINTERPRETATION	CORRECTION
To avoid confusion, do not abbreviate drug names when communicating medical information. Examples of drug name abbreviations involved in medication errors include:			
APAP	acetaminophen	Not recognized as acetaminophen	Use complete drug name
ARA A	vidarabine	Mistaken as cytarabine (ARA C)	Use complete drug name
AZT	zidovudine (Retrovir)	Mistaken as azathioprine or aztreonam	Use complete drug name
CPZ	Compazine (prochlorperazine)	Mistaken as chlorpromazine	Use complete drug name
DPT	Demerol-Phenergan-Thorazine	Mistaken as diphtheria-pertussis-tetanus (vaccine)	Use complete drug name
DTO	Diluted tincture of opium, or deodorized tincture of opium (Paregoric)	Mistaken as tincture of opium	Use complete drug name
HCl	hydrochloric acid or hydrochloride	Mistaken as potassium chloride (the "H" is misinterpreted as "K")	Use complete drug name unless expressed as a salt of a drug
HCT	hydrocortisone	Mistaken as hydrochlorothiazide	Use complete drug name
HCTZ	hydrochlorothiazide	Mistaken as hydrocortisone (seen as HCT 250 mg)	Use complete drug name
MgSO4**	magnesium sulfate	Mistaken as morphine sulfate	Use complete drug name
MS, MSO4**	morphine sulfate	Mistaken as magnesium sulfate	Use complete drug name
MTX	methotrexate	Mistaken as mitoxantrone	Use complete drug name
NoAC	novel/new anticoagulant	No anticoagulant	Use complete drug name
PCA	procainamide	Mistaken as patient-controlled analgesia	Use complete drug name
PTU	propylthiouracil	Mistaken as mercaptopurine	Use complete drug name

Appendix D Abbreviations

ABBREVIATIONS	INTENDED MEANING	MISINTERPRETATION	CORRECTION
T3	Tylenol with codeine No. 3	Mistaken as liothyronine	Use complete drug name
TAC	triamcinolone	Mistaken as tetracaine, Adrenalin, cocaine	Use complete drug name
TNK	TNKase	Mistaken as "TPA"	Use complete drug name
TPA or tPA	tissue plasminogen activator, Activase (alteplase)	Mistaken as TNKase (tenecteplase), or less often as another tissue plasminogen activator, Retavase (retaplase)	Use complete drug name
ZnSO4	zinc sulfate	Mistaken as morphine sulfate	Use complete drug name

STEMMED DRUG NAMES	INTENDED MEANING	MISINTERPRETATION	CORRECTION
"Nitro" drip	nitroglycerin infusion	Mistaken as sodium nitroprusside infusion	Use complete drug name
"Norflox"	norfloxacin	Mistaken as Norflex	Use complete drug name
"IV Vanc"	intravenous vancomycin	Mistaken as Invanz	Use complete drug name

SYMBOLS	INTENDED MEANING	MISINTERPRETATION	CORRECTION
ʒ	Dram	Symbol for dram mistaken as "3"	Use metric system
ɱ	Minim	Symbol for minim mistaken as "mL"	
×3d	For three days	Mistaken as "3 doses"	Use "for three days"
> and <	More than and less than	Mistaken as opposite of intended; mistakenly use incorrect symbol; "< 10" mistaken as "40"	Use "more than" or "less than"
/ (slash mark)	Separates two doses or indicates "per"	Mistaken as the number 1 (e.g., "25 units/10 units" misread as "25 units and 110" units)	Use "per" rather than a slash mark to separate doses
@	At	Mistaken as "2"	Use "at"
&	And	Mistaken as "2"	Use "and"
+	Plus or and	Mistaken as "4"	Use "and"
°	Hour	Mistaken as a zero (e.g., q2° seen as q 20)	Use "hr," "h," or "hour"
Φ or ∅	zero, null sign	Mistaken as numerals 4, 6, 8, and 9	Use 0 or zero, or describe intent using whole words

**These abbreviations are included on The Joint Commission's "minimum list" of dangerous abbreviations, acronyms, and symbols that must be included on an organization's "Do Not Use" list, effective Jan. 1, 2004. Visit www.jointcommission.org for more information about this Joint Commission requirement.
© ISMP 2015. Used with permission from the Institute for Safe Medication Practices. Report actual or potential medication errors to the ISMP Medication Errors Reporting Program (MERP) via the Web at www.ismp.org or by calling 1-800-FAIL-SAFE.

Appendix E

Pharmacology Terms

Topics include:
General Pharmacy Terms, p. 755
Routes of Administration, p. 757
General Drug Categories, p. 757
Terms related to body systems introduced in Chapters 2, 4–16, p. 758

GENERAL PHARMACY TERMS	
absorption	process in which a drug is taken up into the body, organ, tissue, or cell
adverse drug reaction (ADR)	any unintended harmful reaction from a drug administered at a normal dose
ampule (or ampoule)	small, sterile glass or plastic container that usually holds a single dose of a liquid medication
aseptic technique	method used to minimize the microbial contamination of compounded sterile drugs
bar code medication administration (BCMA)	hardware and software used to provide electronic verification that the "five rights" (right patient, right drug, right dose, right route, and right time) are achieved for the administration of medications; designed for patient safety and to decrease errors. Hardware consists of a bar code printer, reader, and mobile computer.
bioavailability	percentage of administered drug available to affect the body and target site(s) after absorption, metabolism, and other factors
biologic	drug produced from living sources, such as human, animal, or microorganisms such as bacteria and yeast. According to the FDA, "biologics can be composed of sugars, proteins, or nucleic acids or complex combinations of these substances, or may be living entities such as cells and tissues." (also called **biological, biological product**)
biosimilar	drug that is made from the same sources, such as living cells or microorganisms, as an original biologic approved by the FDA
capsule (cap)	small, digestible container (made of gelatin or plant cellulose) used to hold a dose of medication for oral administration
chemotherapy	treatment of cancer with medications that target all cells reproducing at a fast rate; destroys both tumor cells and healthy cells that have rapid production rates **(also called chemo)**
compounding	act of combining drug ingredients to prepare a customized prescription or drug order for a patient
contraindication	factor that prohibits administration of a drug
controlled substance	drug that has been identified as having the potential for abuse or addiction; designated as schedule I, II, III, IV, or V under the federal Controlled Substance Act
cream	water-based, semisolid preparation that is applied topically to external parts of the body
dietary supplement	any vitamin, mineral, amino acid, botanical, herbal, or natural nondrug agent that may be taken orally for general well-being; these agents are not approved by the FDA to diagnose, cure, treat, or prevent any disease
distribution	uptake pattern of a drug throughout the body to various tissues
dose	amount of a drug or other substance to be administered at one time
drug	any substance taken by mouth; injected into a muscle, the skin, a blood vessel, or a cavity of the body; or applied topically to treat, cure, prevent, or diagnose a disease or condition
drug-drug interaction (DDI)	modification of the effect of a drug when administered with another drug; food, diseases, and conditions can also interact with a drug to cause a modification of the drug's effect

elimination	removal of a substance from the body by any route, including the kidneys, liver, lungs, and sweat glands
elixir	liquid containing sweeteners, flavorings, water, and/or alcohol in which an oral medication may be dispersed
emulsion	stable mixture that contains one component suspended within another component that it cannot normally dissolve in or mix with
Food and Drug Administration (FDA)	U.S. federal agency responsible for the enforcement of federal regulations regarding the manufacturing and distribution of food, drugs, and cosmetics as protection against the sale of impure or dangerous substances
formulary	listing of drugs and drug information used by health practitioners within an institution to prescribe treatment that is medically appropriate
generic name	official, established nonproprietary name assigned to a drug
inhaler	device containing a drug to be breathed in nasally or by mouth
mechanism of action (MOA)	means by which a drug exerts a desired effect
metabolism	chemical changes that a drug or other substance undergoes in the body
ointment	oil-based, semisolid preparation that is applied topically to external parts of the body
over-the-counter (OTC) drug	drug that may be purchased without a prescription (also called **nonprescription drug**)
pharmaceutical	drug synthesized from molecular components through chemical reactions and used for medicinal purposes
pharmacist	person formally trained to formulate and dispense medications and provide drug information
pharmacodynamics	study of the actions of drugs on the body
pharmacogenomics	study of the correlation between genetics and responses to drugs
pharmacokinetics (PK)	study of the actions of the body on drugs or the movement of drugs in the body
pharmacology	study of the preparation, properties, uses, and actions of drugs
pharmacy	place for preparing and dispensing drugs
placebo	inactive substance, prescribed as if it were an effective dose of a needed medication
prescription (Rx)	order for a medication, therapy, or a therapeutic device given by a properly authorized person for a specified patient
preservative	substance included in some parenteral and topical medications used to prevent the growth of microorganisms in the product
route of administration	method in which a drug or agent is given to a patient
side effect	any reaction or result from a medication other than what is the primary intended effect
solution	homogenous mixture of one or more substances dissolved into another substance
state board of pharmacy	agency responsible for regulating the practice of pharmacy within the state
suppository	topical form of a drug that is inserted into the rectum, vagina, or penis
suspension	liquid in which particles of a solid are dispersed, but not dissolved, and in which the dispersal is maintained by stirring or shaking
tablet	small, solid dose form of a medication
toxicity	level at which a drug's concentration within the body produces serious adverse effects
trade name	proprietary name assigned to a drug by its manufacturer that is registered as part of the drug's identity (also called **brand name**)
United States Pharmacopeia (USP)	compendium, recognized officially by the federal Food and Drug Administration, that contains descriptions, uses, strengths, and standards of purity for selected drugs and guidance for related standards of practice

ROUTES OF ADMINISTRATION

buccal	administration of drug by absorption through the inner cheek tissue
enteral	administration of a medication through the digestive tract, including oral ingestion
epidural	injection of drug into the epidural space of the spinal cord
infusion	prolonged administration of a fluid substance directly into a vein, artery, or under the skin in which the flow rate is driven by gravity or a mechanical pump
inhalation	method of drug administration that involves the breathing in of a spray, vapor, or powder via the nose or mouth
injection	introduction of a liquid substance directly into the body, bypassing natural routes of entry by using a needle
intramuscular (IM)	administration of a medication directly into a muscle
intrathecal	administration of drug into the subarachnoid space of the meninges in the spine
intravenous (IV)	administration of a medication directly into a vein using a needle or tube
jet injection	administration of a liquid substance through intact skin without a needle, using a narrow, high-pressure stream
oral	administration of a medication by mouth
parenteral	administration of a medication via a route that bypasses the digestive tract; most commonly used to refer to injection methods
rectal	administration of drug by absorption through the rectum
subcutaneous	introduction of a medication into the tissue just beneath the skin
sublingual	administration of drug by absorption through tissue under the tongue
topical	administration of a medication to an external area of the body
transdermal	method of applying drug to unbroken skin so that it is continuously absorbed through the skin to produce a systemic effect; a transdermal patch is a drug delivery system that controls the rate of absorption through the skin

GENERAL DRUG CATEGORIES

antibacterial	drug that targets bacteria to kill or halt growth
antibiotic	drug that targets bacteria, fungi, or protozoa to kill or halt growth; commonly used as synonym for antibacterial
antifungal	drug that targets fungi to kill or halt growth
antihistamine	drug that treats allergic and hypersensitivity reactions by blocking histamine-1 receptors
antiinflammatory	drug that reduces inflammation
antimicrobial	drug that targets microorganisms to kill or halt growth
antineoplastic agent	drug used to destroy or slow the rapid replication of cancer cells
antiretroviral	drug that suppresses the replication of the human immunodeficiency virus (HIV); highly active antiretroviral therapy (HAART) is the combination of three or more of these drugs to treat HIV infection
antiviral	drug that targets viruses to kill or halt growth
antiadrenergic agent	drug that blocks adrenergic receptors to reduce sympathetic nervous system activity in the body
bactericidal	designation for an antimicrobial agent that kills or destroys bacteria
bacteriostatic	the designation for an antimicrobial agent that halts the growth or replication of bacteria but does not kill them
cytotoxic	agent that causes cell death
dietary supplement	product that provides nutrients that may be missing from the diet; dietary supplements are not strictly regulated for safety and efficacy
disinfectant	chemical agent that can be applied to inanimate objects to destroy microorganisms

Appendix E Pharmacology Terms

herbal supplement	naturally derived, often plant-based, dietary supplement that is touted to improve health; herbal supplements are not strictly regulated for safety and efficacy
immunosuppressant	drug that reduces the response of the immune system; used in autoimmune diseases and to prepare a patient for an organ transplant (also called **immunomodulator**)
narcotic	drug that has opium-like effects to cause drowsiness, pain relief, and sedation; can be habit-forming and is regulated as a controlled substance
nonsteroidal antiinflammatory drug (NSAID)	drug that reduces pain, inflammation, and fever
parasympatholytic	agent that blocks the actions of the parasympathetic nervous system
parasympathomimetic	agent that enhances the actions of the parasympathetic nervous system
puberty inhibitor	gonadotropin-releasing hormone (GnRH) agonists used to temporarily suppress the release of sex-specific hormones
radiopharmaceutical	drug with a radioactive component; used for diagnosis or treatment
smoking cessation agent	drug that helps a patient quit smoking; may be a behavioral deterrent or a nicotine substitute
sympatholytic	agent that blocks the actions of the sympathetic nervous system
sympathomimetic	agent that enhances the actions of the sympathetic nervous system
vaccine	substance that is used to stimulate the body's immune response against infectious disease; may be administered by injection, mouth, or nasal spray (also called **immunization**)
vitamin	organic compound essential in small quantities for normal physiologic and metabolic functioning

CHAPTER 2: BODY STRUCTURE, COLOR, AND ONCOLOGY

alkylating agent	type of antineoplastic agent that binds to cellular DNA to interfere with replication
antimetabolite	type of antineoplastic agent that interferes with a cell's normal metabolism
antineoplastic agent	drug used to destroy or slow the replication of cancer cells
chemotherapeutic agent	drug used to destroy or slow the replication of cancer cells
kinase inhibitor	type of antineoplastic agent that interferes with protein phosphorylation
mitotic inhibitor	type of antineoplastic agent that interrupts cellular division

CHAPTER 4: INTEGUMENTARY SYSTEM

antibacterial	drug used to combat an infection caused by bacteria
antifungal	drug used to combat an infection caused by fungi
antihistamine	drug used to minimize allergy symptoms by blocking histamine-1 receptors
antipruritic	agent that reduces itching
antipsoriatic	drug that treats psoriasis
antiseptic	chemical agent that can safely be applied to external tissues to kill or halt the growth of microorganisms
astringent	agent that reduces inflammation and irritation and provides a protective barrier on mucosa and skin by contracting the surface tissue
emollient	external agent that softens or soothes the skin
keratolytic	agent that augments the shedding of the top layer of dead skin
pediculicide	agent that kills lice
retinoid	derivative of vitamin A that regulates the growth of epithelial cells
rubefacient	topical agent that increases blood flow to the area to treat muscle aches
scabicide	agent that kills scabies

Appendix E Pharmacology Terms

CHAPTER 5: RESPIRATORY SYSTEM

antitussive	drug that suppresses coughing
bronchodilator	drug that expands the airways by relaxing smooth muscle in the lungs
decongestant	drug that relieves nasal congestion by reducing swelling of mucous membranes
expectorant	drug that promotes expulsion of mucus from the lungs
leukotriene receptor antagonist (LTRA)	drug that blocks late-stage regulators of allergic and hypersensitivity reactions to treat allergy-induced asthma
mucolytic	drug that thins out mucus in the lungs so that it can be expelled more easily

CHAPTER 6: URINARY SYSTEM

aldosterone receptor antagonist (ARA)	drug that decreases reabsorption of water and sodium by the kidneys to treat edema or high blood pressure
alpha-1 blocker	drug that relaxes the muscles in the prostate and bladder neck to improve urination in men with an enlarged prostate
antispasmodic	drug that prevents or relieves bladder muscle spasms associated with incontinence
diuretic	drug that promotes the formation and excretion of urine to reduce the volume of extracellular fluid; used to reduce high blood pressure or edema; commonly referred to as a "water pill"
muscle relaxant	drug that reduces bladder muscle contractility to relieve spasm-induced pain or uncontrolled urination
urinary alkalinizer	agent that increases the urine pH
vasopressin	drug that increases water retention by the kidneys (also called **antidiuretic hormone** or **ADH**)

CHAPTER 7: MALE REPRODUCTIVE SYSTEM

androgen	natural or synthetic hormone involved in male reproduction and secondary gender attributes
antiandrogen	drug that blocks the effects of androgen hormones in the body
phosphodiesterase-5 inhibitor (PDE5 inhibitor)	drug that blocks the inactivation of cyclic guanosine monophosphate to increase vasodilation in the penis; used to treat erectile dysfunction
spermicide	contact agent that kills sperm

CHAPTER 8: FEMALE REPRODUCTIVE SYSTEM

antiestrogen	drug used to block the action of estrogen hormones in the body
contraceptive	agent (drug or barrier) used to prevent conception or pregnancy
contraceptive implant	small, flexible rod that releases a hormone to pause ovulation and is placed under the skin of the upper arm; lasts for up to 5 years
emergency contraceptive	pill that delays ovulation and can be taken up to 5 days after having sex; pills contain ulipristal acetate (prescription) or levonorgestrel (over-the-counter); (also called **morning-after pill**)
estrogen	natural or synthetic hormone involved in female reproduction and secondary gender characteristics
fertility drugs	drugs that enhance a female's ability to conceive a child
hormone replacement therapy (HRT)	regimen that mimics the body's normal levels of female hormones when they are no longer produced; typically used during menopause
intrauterine device (IUD)	hormonal or nonhormonal implant placed directly in the uterus to prevent pregnancy; may be left in place for 5 years or longer
long-acting reversible contraception (LARC)	nonpermanent birth control methods that last for a period of time, including hormonal and nonhormonal IUDs, implants, and injections
medication abortion	administration of mifepristone to stop the release of progesterone, followed by misoprostol for contractions to expel the contents of the uterus

oral contraceptive	exogenous hormones taken by mouth to prevent pregnancy
ovulation stimulant	drug that enhances the release of an egg from the ovary to promote pregnancy
progestin	synthetic or natural hormone involved in female reproduction and secondary gender characteristics
vaginal ring	device containing estrogen and progestin hormones that is inserted in the vagina to prevent pregnancy

CHAPTER 9 : OBSTETRICS AND NEONATOLOGY

abortifacient	drug that causes uterine muscles to contract with subsequent abortion of the fetus
oxytocic	hormone that stimulates the uterine muscles to contract, thereby inducing labor in a pregnant woman
pregnancy category	level of risk the Food and Drug Administration assigns a drug based on documented problems with the use of that drug during pregnancy
tocolytic	agent that suppresses labor contractions

CHAPTER 10 : CARDIOVASCULAR, IMMUNE, AND LYMPHATIC SYSTEMS AND BLOOD

angiotensin-converting enzyme inhibitor (ACE inhibitor)	drug that prevents the formation of angiotensin-II, which is a strong vasoconstrictor and major contributor to high blood pressure
angiotensin receptor blocker (ARB)	drug that blocks the angiotensin-II molecule from binding to its receptors throughout the body to prevent its effects and reduce high blood pressure
antianginal	drug that relieves the chest pain paroxysms caused by lack of oxygen delivery to the heart; typically involves vasodilation
antiarrhythmic	drug that treats abnormal heart rhythm
anticoagulant	drug that prevents blood clotting and coagulation; commonly referred to as a blood thinner
antihypertensive	drug that lowers blood pressure
antiplatelet agent	drug that prevents platelet formation or aggregation or causes platelet destruction
beta-blocker (BB)	drug that inhibits beta-adrenergic receptors to decrease heart rate and force of contractility; used to treat arrhythmias, hypertension, heart failure, and more
calcium channel blocker (CCB)	drug that regulates the entry of calcium into muscle cells of the heart and blood vessels; used to treat heart failure, arrhythmias, angina, and hypertension
colony-stimulating factor (CSF)	agent that promotes the replication of blood cells in the bone marrow
direct thrombin inhibitor (DTI)	drug that blocks the action of thrombin, thereby reducing blood coagulation
erythropoiesis stimulating agent (ESA)	agent that stimulates red blood cell production in the bone marrow
hemostatic	drug that stops bleeding or hemorrhaging
inotropic agent	drug that strengthens or weakens the contraction of the heart muscles
nitrate	drug that dilates the blood vessels
platelet aggregation inhibitor	drug that stops platelets from adhering together
renin inhibitor	drug that blocks renin activity to reduce high blood pressure; renin is the first step in the renin-angiotensin-aldosterone system (RAAS), which is a common contributor to chronic high blood pressure
thrombolytic	drug that dissolves blood clots

vasodilator	drug that expands blood vessels to lower blood pressure
vasopressor	drug that contracts blood vessels to raise blood pressure (also called **vasoconstrictor**)
CHAPTER 11 : DIGESTIVE SYSTEM	
antacid	drug that neutralizes acid in the stomach
antidiarrheal	drug that treats diarrhea by increasing water absorption, decreasing muscle contraction of the intestines, altering electrolyte exchange, or absorbing toxins or microorganisms
antiemetic	drug that reduces or prevents nausea and vomiting
antihyperlipidemic agent	drug used to reduce high levels of bad cholesterol and/or raise levels of good cholesterol by affecting levels of low-density lipoproteins, high-density lipoproteins, total cholesterol, and/or triglycerides, which are collectively called lipids (also called **hypolipidemic agent**)
bile acid sequestrant	type of antihyperlipidemic agent used to lower high cholesterol levels by increasing the excretion of bile acids
cathartic	agent that aids the evacuation of the bowels by accelerating defecation
enema	liquid agent administered rectally to clear the contents of the bowel
fibrate	type of antihyperlipidemic agent that affects lipid levels by facilitating lipid metabolism
histamine-2 receptor antagonist (H2RA)	drug that reduces production of stomach acid by blocking the H2 receptors on gastric parietal cells (also called **H2 blocker**)
laxative	drug that aids the evacuation of the bowel
proton pump inhibitor (PPI)	drug that reduces production of stomach acid by blocking the proton pump on gastric parietal cells
statin	type of antihyperlipidemic agent that treats dyslipidemia by inhibiting 3-hydroxy-3-methylglutaryl coenzyme A reductase (also called **HMG-CoA reductase inhibitor**)
CHAPTER 12 : EYE	
antiglaucoma agent	drug that treats glaucoma of the eye
miotic	agent that contracts the pupil
mydriatic	agent that dilates the pupil
ophthalmic	agent that is intended to be used in the eye; must be sterile
CHAPTER 13 : EAR	
ceruminolytic	agent that breaks down ear wax
otic	agent intended to be used in the ear
CHAPTER 14 : MUSCULOSKELETAL SYSTEM	
antiarthritic agent	drug used in the treatment of arthritis
antigout agent	drug that opposes the buildup of uric acid crystals in the joints to prevent and treat gout attacks
antispasmodic	drug that prevents or relieves muscle spasms
biologic	genetically engineered protein that targets a specific hyperfunctioning component of the immune system to treat diseases such as rheumatoid arthritis
bisphosphonate	drug that binds to bone matrix to treat osteoporosis
disease-modifying antirheumatic drug (DMARD)	drug that slows the progression of rheumatoid arthritis
muscle relaxant	drug that reduces muscle contractility to relieve tension- or spasm-induced pain
neuromuscular blocking agent (NMBA)	drug that blocks all nerve stimulation of the skeletal muscles to cause paralysis

CHAPTER 15 : NERVOUS SYSTEM AND BEHAVIORAL HEALTH

Term	Definition
adrenergic agonist	drug that stimulates aspects of the sympathetic nervous system
amphetamine	drug that stimulates the central nervous system
anticonvulsant	drug that reduces the incidence and severity of seizures and convulsions (also called **antiepileptic drug**)
analgesic	drug that relieves pain
anesthetic	drug that causes numbness or a loss of feeling that can be used locally or systemically; often used systemically to put a patient "to sleep" during extensive procedures
anticholinergic	drug that blocks the action of acetylcholine and therefore suppresses the parasympathetic nervous system
anticholinesterase	drug that prevents the breakdown of acetylcholine to yield a cholinergic or parasympathetic effect
antidepressant	drug used to treat depression and other disorders related to chemical imbalances of the central nervous system
antiparkinsonian agent	drug that treats Parkinson disease and parkinsonism by affecting levels of dopamine or acetylcholine in the brain
antipsychotic	drug that treats psychosis disorders by inducing a calming or tranquilizing effect or by adjusting neurotransmitter levels in the brain (also called **neuroleptic**)
antipyretic	drug that reduces fever
anxiolytic	drug that relieves anxiety
benzodiazepine (BZD)	type of drug that binds to receptors in the brain to calm and sedate the central nervous system
central nervous system stimulant	drug that excites the central nervous system; can be used for many brain disorders
cholinergic	agent that acts like acetylcholine to activate the parasympathetic nervous system
dopaminergic	drug that acts like dopamine, a neurotransmitter in the brain
hypnotic	drug used to induce sleep; many hypnotic agents may also induce sedative effects
mood stabilizer	drug that balances neurotransmitters in the brain to lessen the mood swings of bipolar disorder
monoamine oxidase inhibitor (MAOI)	type of antidepressant that prevents the breakdown of many active neurotransmitters in the brain
nonsteroidal antiinflammatory drug (NSAID)	drug that reduces pain, inflammation, and fever
opioid antagonist	drug that can treat opioid or narcotic overdose
sedative	drug that depresses the central nervous system to calm a patient; many sedative agents may also induce sleep
selective serotonin reuptake inhibitor (SSRI)	type of antidepressant that maintains a higher level of serotonin in the central nervous system
tranquilizer	drug that reduces anxiety or agitation
tricyclic antidepressant (TCA)	type of antidepressant that maintains a higher level of various neurotransmitters in the central nervous system

CHAPTER 16 : ENDOCRINE SYSTEM	
antidiabetic agent	drug that treats diabetes by controlling blood sugar levels
antithyroid agent	drug that counters hyperthyroidism by reducing the production of thyroid hormones
corticosteroid	drug that mimics hormones produced by the adrenal glands and has antiinflammatory and immunosuppressive effects
hypoglycemic agent	drug that lowers blood sugar levels (also called **antihyperglycemic**)
thyroid hormone	replacement hormone to regulate metabolism and endocrine functions

Illustration Credits

Chapter 1
Fig. 1.1 From Magee D: *Orthopedic physical assessment*, ed 5, St. Louis, 2008, Saunders.
Ex 5 From iStock.com/SDI Productions.
Ex 12.B From iStock.com/Jacob Ammentorp Lund.
Ex 13 From iStock.com/SDI Productions.

Chapter 2
Ex 5.A,3 From iStock.com/digitalskillet.
Ex 5.A,4 From iStock.com/Savushkin.
Ex 5.A,6 From Swartz M: *Textbook of physical diagnosis*, ed 5, St. Louis, 2006, Saunders/Elsevier.
Ex 8.B,4 From Kumar V, Abbas AK, Fausto M: *Robbins and Cotran pathologic basis of disease*, ed 7, Philadelphia, WB Saunders, 2005.
Ex 12.A,1 From Mace JD, Kowalczyk N: *Radiographic pathology for technologists*, ed 4, St Louis, 2004, Mosby/Elsevier.
Ex 12.A,2 From Bullough P: *Orthopaedic pathology*, ed 5, St. Louis, 2010, Elsevier.
Ex 12.A,3 From Habif TP: *Clinical dermatology*, ed 4, St. Louis, 2004, Elsevier Mosby.
Ex 12.A,4 From Damanjov I, Linder J: *Anderson's pathology*, ed 10, St. Louis, 1996, Mosby.
Ex 14.A,1 Wenig B: *Atlas of head and neck pathology*, ed 3, St. Louis, 2016, Elsevier.
Ex 14.A,2 From iStock.com/JCPJR.
Ex 14.A,5 From Rhoda Baer.
Ex 17.C,1 From iStock.com/dmbaker.
Ex 17.C,2 From iStock.com/fstop123.
Ex 17.C,3 From iStock.com/sturti.
Ex 17.C,4 From iStock.com/Gumpanat.
Ex 18.B,1 From iStock.com/Radevich Tatiana.
Ex 18.B,2 From iStock.com/ThamKC.
Ex 18.B,3 From iStock.com/KTS.
Ex 18.B,4 From iStock.com/jarun011.
Ex 22.A,1 From iStock.com/Ljupco.
Ex 22.A,2 From Kamal A, Brockelhurst JC: *Color atlas of geriatric medicine*, ed 2, St. Louis, 1991, Mosby.
Ex 22.A,3 From iStock.com/FatCamera.
Ex 22.A,4 From iStock.com/PeopleImages.
Ex 24.A,1 From iStock.com/chas53.
Ex 24.A,2 From iStock.com/Chiari_VFX.
Ex 24.A,3 From iStock.com/praisaeng.
Ex 24.A,4 From iStock.com/image_jungle.
Ex 30 From Thinkstock.com/Jack Hollingsworth.

Chapter 3
Ex 2 B (1) From iStock.com/nimon_t.
Ex 2 B (2) From iStock.com/Fabianodp.
Ex 2 B (3) From iStock.com/hudiemm.
Ex 3 A (1) From iStock.com/mosabua.
Ex 3 A (2) From iStock.com/IlexImage.
Ex 4 A (1A) From iStock.com/andresr.
Ex 4 A (1B) From iStock.com/xavierarnau.
Ex 4 A (2A) From iStock.com/RASimon.
Ex 4 A (2B) From Ruppel GL: *Manual pulmonary function testing*, ed 7, St. Louis, 1998, Mosby.
Ex 4 A (3A) From Patton KT, Thibodeau GA: *Anatomy and physiology*, ed 7, St. Louis, 2010, Mosby.
Ex 4A (3B) From Pagana KD, Pagana TJ: *Mosby's manual of diagnostic and laboratory test reference*, ed 7, St. Louis, 2004, Elsevier Mosby.
Ex 7A (6) From Bontrager KL: *Radiographic positioning and related anatomy*, ed 5, St. Louis, 2002, Mosby.
Table 3.2, Bottom images from Bontrager KL: *Radiographic positioning and related anatomy*, ed 5, St. Louis, 2002, Mosby.
Ex 13A From Williamson P: *The human body in health and disease*, ed 8, St. Louis, 2024, Elsevier.
Ex 19B (1) From Ruppel GL: *Manual pulmonary function testing*, ed 7, St. Louis, 1998, Mosby.
Ex 19B (2) From Ruppel GL: *Manual pulmonary function testing*, ed 7, St. Louis, 1998, Mosby.
Ex 19B (3) From Pagana KD, Pagana TJ: *Mosby's manual of diagnostic and laboratory test reference*, ed 7, St. Louis, 2004, Elsevier Mosby.
Ex 19B (4) From Pagana KD, Pagana TJ: *Mosby's manual of diagnostic and laboratory test reference*, ed 7, St. Louis, 2004, Elsevier Mosby.
Ex 20B (1) From iStock.com/3alexd.
Ex 20B (2) From iStock.com/Morsa Images.
Ex 20B (3) From Ballinger PW, Frank ED: *Merrill's atlas of radiographic positions and radiologic procedures*, ed 10, St. Louis, 2003, Mosby.
Ex 20B,4 (A) From Siemens Medical Systems, Inc., New Jersey. (B) From Bontrager KL, Lampignano JP: *Radiographic positioning and related anatomy*, ed 8, St. Louis, 2014, Mosby.
Ex 23 From Siri Stafford: Thinkstock.

Chapter 4
Ex 4.B,1 From iStock.com/SciePro.
Ex 4.B,2 From iStock.com/ GOLFX.
Ex 4.B,3 From iStock.com/mvp64.
Ex 4.B,4 From iStock.com/praisaeng.
Ex 4.B,5 From iStock.com/izusek.
Ex 4.B,6 From iStock.com/SDI Productions.
Fig 4.2 From Frazier M: *Essentials of human diseases and conditions*, ed 3, St. Louis, 2004, Elsevier Mosby.

Illustration Credits

Ex. 7.A,1 From Frazier M, *Essentials of human disease and conditions*, ed 3, St. Louis, 2004, Mosby.

Ex. 7. A,2 From Schwarzenberger K, et al: *General dermatology*, ed 1, Philadelphia, 2009, Saunders.

Ex. 7. A,3 From Bologina JL, et al: *Dermatology*, ed 2, St. Louis, 2008, Mosby.

Fig. 4.3B (1) Copyright Richar P. Usatine, MD.

Fig. 4.3B (2) From James WD, et al: *Andrews' diseases of the skin*, ed 12, Philadelphia, 2016, Elsevier.

Fig. 4.3B (3) From Habif TP, Dinulos JG, Chapman MS, Zung KA: *Skin disease*, ed 4, 2018, Elsevier.

Table 4.1 (1) From Frazier M: *Essentials of human disease and conditions*, ed 3, St. Louis, 2004, Elsevier Mosby.

Table 4.1 (2) From Perry A, Potter P, Elkin M: *Nursing interventions & clinical skills*, ed 4, St. Louis, 2008, Mosby/Elsevier.

Table 4.1(3) From Habif TP, et al: *Skin disease: diagnosis and treatment*, ed 4, 2018, Elsevier Inc.

Table 4.1 (4) From Marks JG, Miller JJ: *Lookingbill and Marks' principles of dermatology*, ed 5, St. Louis, 2019, Elsevier.

Table 4.1 (5) From Gawkrodger D, Ardern-Jones M: *Dermatology*, ed 5, Oxford, 2012, Churchill Livingstone.

Fig. 4.5 Inset photo from: Potter PA, Perry AG: *Fundamentals of nursing*, ed 4, St. Louis, 1997, Mosby.

Ex 9B (1) From Goering R, et al: *Mims' medical microbiology*, ed 4, Edinburgh, 2008, Mosby Ltd.

Ex 9B (2) From Weston W, et al: *Color textbook of pediatric dermatology*, ed 4, St. Louis, 2007, Mosby.

Ex 9B (3) From Weston W, et al: *Color textbook of pediatric dermatology*, ed 4, St. Louis, 2007, Mosby.

Ex 9B (4) From Habif TP: *Clinical dermatology*, ed 4, St. Louis, 2004, Elsevier Mosby.

Ex 9B (5) From Christensen B, Kockrow E: *Adult health nursing*, ed 5, St. Louis, 2006, Elsevier Mosby.

Ex 9 B (6) From Habif TP: *Clinical dermatology*, ed 4, St. Louis, 2004, Elsevier Mosby.

Ex 9B (7) From Bork K, Brauninger W: *Skin diseases in clinical practice*, ed 2, Philadelphia, 1998, WB Saunders.

Ex 9B (8) From Callen JP: *Color atlas of dermatology*, ed 2, Philadelphia, 2000, Saunders.

Ex 9B (9) From Callen JP: *Color atlas of dermatology*, ed 2, Philadelphia, 2000, Saunders.

Ex 9B (10) From Wilson S, Giddens J: *Health assessment for nursing practice*, ed 4, St. Louis, 2009, Mosby. Courtesy Gary Monheit, MD, University of Alabama at Birmingham School of Medicine.

Ex 9B (11) From Frazier M: *Essentials of human disease and conditions*, ed 3, St. Louis, 2004, Elsevier Mosby.

Ex 9B (12) From Bork K, Brauninger W: *Skin diseases in clinical practice*, ed 2, Philadelphia, 1998, WB Saunders.

Ex 9B (13) From Cohen J: *Infectious diseases*, ed 3, St. Louis, 2010, Mosby.

Ex 9B (14) From Echenfield LF, Freiden IJ, Mathes E, Zenglein A: *Neonatal and infant dermatology*, ed 3, 2015, Elsevier Inc.

Ex 9B (15) From Cohen BA: *Pediatric dermatology*, ed 3, St. Louis, 2005, Mosby.

Ex 9B (16) From *Dorland's illustrated medical dictionary*, ed 31, Philadelphia, 2007, Saunders.

Ex 9B (17) From istock.com/andriano_cz.

Ex 9B (18) From Bork K, Brauninger W: *Skin diseases in clinical practice*, ed 2, Philadelphia, 1998, WB Saunders.

Fig. 4.6 From Habif TP: *Clinical dermatology*, ed 4, St. Louis, 2004, Elsevier Mosby.

Ex 19A (1) From Haught JM, Patel S, English JC: *Xanthoderma: a clinical review*, J Amer Acad Derm 57(6):1051-1058, 2007.

Ex 19A (2) From Goldman L, Schafer AI: *Goldman-Cecil medicine*, ed 26, Philadelphia, 2020, Elsevier.

Ex 19A (3) From Dinulos JGH: *Habif's clinical dermatology: a color guide to diagnosis and therapy*, ed 7, Philadelphia, 2021, Elsevier.

Ex 19A (4) From Ball J, et al: *Seidel's guide to physical examination*, ed 8, St. Louis, 2014, Elsevier.

Ex 19A (7) From Shiland B: *Mastering healthcare terminology*, ed 2, St. Louis, 2006, Elsevier Mosby.

Ex 19A (8) From Shiland B: *Mastering healthcare terminology*, ed 2, St. Louis, 2006, Elsevier Mosby.

Fig. 4.8A From James WD, et al: *Andrews' disease of the skin: clinical dermatology*, 2020, Elsevier.

Fig. 4.8B From James WD, et al: *Andrews' disease of the skin: clinical dermatology*, 2020, Elsevier.

Fig. 4.8C From iStock.com/HaraldBiebel.

Ex 21B (1) From iStock.com/phokin.

Ex 21B (2) From Bork K, Brauninger W: *Skin diseases in clinical practice*, ed 2, Philadelphia, 1998, WB Saunders.

Ex 21B (3) From Bork K, Brauninger W: *Skin diseases in clinical practice*, ed 2, Philadelphia, 1998, WB Saunders.

Ex 21B (4) From Bork K, Brauninger W: *Skin diseases in clinical practice*, ed 2, Philadelphia, 1998, WB Saunders.

Ex 26 From iStock.com/AndreyPopov.

Chapter 5

Ex 4B 1 From Olympus America.

Ex 4B 3 From iStock.com/BanksPhotos.

Ex 4B 5 From iStock.com/inkit.

Ex 4B 6 From iStock.com/agrobacter.

Ex 4B 7 From iStock.com/KatarzynaBialasiewicz.

Ex 4B 8 From iStock.com/AaronAmat.

Ex 4B 9 From iStock.com/redhumv.

Ex 4B 10 From iStock.com/serezniy.

Fig. 5.3 From Eisenberg RL, Johnson NM: *Comprehensive radiographic pathology*, ed 3, St. Louis, 2003, Mosby.

Ex 7.A 6 From iStock.com/phichet_c.

Fig. 5.7 C From Kumar V, et al: *Robbins' basic pathology*, ed 7, Philadelphia, 2003, Saunders.

Ex 9B 1 From Kumar V, et al: *Robbins' basic pathology*, ed 7, Philadelphia, 2003, Saunders.

Ex 9B 5 From istock.com/Dr_Microbe.

Ex 19A 2 From iStock.com/inkit.

Ex 19A 3 Courtesy Nonin Medical, Inc. Reprinted with permission of Nonin Medical, Inc. Copyright 2013.

Ex 19A 4 Courtesy Nonin Medical, Inc. Reprinted with permission of Nonin Medical, Inc. Copyright 2013.

Ex 19A 5 From iStock.com/Devilkae.

Ex 21A 1 From Centers for Disease Control and Prevention Public Health Image Library, Atlanta, Ga. Photo credit: Greg Knobloch. Permission note: public domain no permission needed. https://phil.cdc.gov/Details.aspx?pid56806.

Ex 21A 2 From Cummings N: *Perspectives in athletic training*, St. Louis, 2009, Mosby.

Ex 21A 3 From Wilson SF, Thompson JM: *Respiratory disorders*, St. Louis, 1990, Mosby.

Ex 21A 4 From istock.com/gawrav.

Ex 21A 5 Nelcor Puritan Bennett.

Ex 21A 6 From Ballinger PW, Frank ED: *Merrill's atlas of radiographic positions and radiologic procedures*, ed 10, St. Louis, 2003, Mosby.

Ex 21A 7 From Ruppel GL: *Manual pulmonary function testing*, ed 7, St. Louis, 1998, Mosby.

Ex 21A 8 From Paulino A: *PET_CT in radiotherapy treatment planning*, Philadelphia, 2008, Saunders/Elsevier.

Ex 21A 9 From Seidel H, et al: *Mosby's guide to physical examination*, ed 5, St. Louis, 2003, Mosby.

Ex 21A 10 From Seidel H, et al: *Mosby's guide to physical examination*, ed 5, St. Louis, 2003, Mosby.

Ex 26A 1 From iStock.com/Osobystist.

Ex 26A 2 From iStock.com/Branimir76.

Ex 26A 3 From iStock.com/stevanovicigor.

Ex 26A 5 From iStock.com/AaronAmat.

Ex 26 A 6 From iStock.com/Ariyathailand.

Fig. 5.13 A, From Lewis SM, et al: *Medical-surgical nursing*, ed 6, St. Louis, 2004, Elsevier Mosby.

Ex 28A 1 From iStock.com/Mykhailo Pervak.

Ex 28A 2 From iStock.com/Fahroni.

Ex 28A 3 From Cummings N: *Perspectives in athletic training*, St. Louis, 2009, Mosby.

Ex 28A 4 Lewis SM, et al: *Medical-surgical nursing*, ed 6, St. Louis, 2004, Elsevier Mosby.

Ex 33 From Thinkstock.com/kolino_tanya.

Chapter 6

Ex 4A 2 From Stein, HA, Skatt BJ, Stein RM: *The ophthalmic assistant: fundamentals and clinical practice*, ed 5, St. Louis, 1998, Mosby.

Ex 4A 3 From iStock.com/omyos.

Ex 4A 4 From iStock.com/alex-mit.

Ex 4A 5 From iStock.com/andrewsafonov.

Fig. 6.5A From Damjanov I: *Pathology, a color atlas*, ed 2, St. Louis, 2000, Mosby.

Fig. 6.6 From Damjanov I: *Pathology, a color atlas*, ed 2, St. Louis, 2000, Mosby.

Ex 7B 2 From Damjanov I: *Pathology, a color atlas*, ed 2, St. Louis, 2000, Mosby.

Ex 7B 5 From Damjanov I: *Pathology, a color atlas*, ed 2, St. Louis, 2000, Mosby.

Ex 7B 6 From Wein A, et al: *Campbell-Walsh urology*, ed 10, Philadelphia, 2012, Saunders.

Ex 9A 2 From Brundage D: *Renal disorders*, St. Louis, 1992, Mosby.

Ex 13B 5 (1) From Dornier Medical Systems, Kennesaw, GA.

Fig. 6.10 From Wein A, et al: *Campbell-Walsh urology*, ed 10, Philadelphia, 2012, Saunders.

Fig. 6.11 From Wein A, et al: *Campbell-Walsh urology*, ed 10, Philadelphia, 2012, Saunders.

Fig. 6.12 From Bontrager KL: *Textbook of radiographic positioning and related anatomy*, ed 6, St. Louis, 2002, Mosby.

Ex 17B 1 From Ballinger PW, Frank ED: *Merrill's atlas of radiographic positions and radiologic procedures*, ed 10, St. Louis, 2003, Mosby.

Ex 17B 2 From Ballinger PW, Frank ED: *Merrill's atlas of radiographic positions and radiologic procedures*, ed 10, St. Louis, 2003, Mosby.

Ex 18A 1 From iStock.com/SDI Productions.

Ex 18A 2 From iStock.com/Radevich Tatiana.

Ex 18A 3 From Wein A, et al: *Campbell-Walsh urology*, ed 10, 2012, Saunders.

Ex 22B 2 From iStock.com/SvetaZi.

Ex 22B 3 From iStock.com/vchal.

Ex 22B 4 From iStock.com.

Ex 24A 1 From iStock.com/Picsfive.

Ex 24A 2 From iStock.com/Andrii Pohranychnyi.

Ex 24A 3 From iStock.com/digitalskillet.

Ex 24A 4 From iStock.com/goodmoments.

Ex 24A 5 From iStock.com/jedsadabodin.

Ex 24A 6 From iStock.com/Jakovo.

Ex 28 From iStock.com/viafilms.

Chapter 7

Fig. 7.4A, From Zitelli BM, David HW: *Atlas of pediatric physical diagnosis*, ed 2, St. Louis, 1992, Mosby.

Ex 7A 1 From Bork K, Brauninger W: *Skin diseases in clinical practice*, ed 2, Philadelphia, 1998, WB Saunders.

Fig. 7.7 Courtesy EDAP Technomed, Inc., Vaulx-en-Velin, France.

Ex 16.A 1 From Courtesy EDAP Technomed, Inc., Vaulx-en-Velin, France.

Fig. 7.10A From Murray P, et al: *Medical microbiology*, ed 5, St. Louis, 2005, Mosby.

Fig. 7.10B From Mahon C, et al: *Textbook of diagnostic microbiology*, ed 4, Philadelphia, 2011, Elsevier.

Fig. 7.10C From Goldman L, Schafer A: *Goldman's Cecil medicine*, ed 24, Philadelphia, 2012, Saunders.

Ex 28 From iStock.com/numbeos.

Chapter 8

Fig. 8.2 From Patton KT, Thibodeau GA: *The human body in health and disease*, ed 6, St. Louis, 2014, Mosby.

Ex 1B From Patton KT, Thibodeau GA: *The human body in health and disease*, ed 6, St. Louis, 2014, Mosby.

Ex 4A (2) Rohrer, TE Cook JL, Kaufman A: *Flaps and grafts in dermatologic surgery*, ed 2, St. Louis, 2017, Elsevier.

Ex 7A, 3 From iStock.com/Dr_Microbe.

Fig. 8.10 From Black J, Hawks J: *Medical-surgical nursing*, ed 8, St. Louis, 2009, Elsevier.

Ex 15A (5) From Black J, Hawks J: *Medical-surgical nursing*, ed 8, St. Louis, 2009, Elsevier.

Ex 15A (6) From Black J, Hawks J: *Medical-surgical nursing*, ed 8, St. Louis, 2009, Elsevier.

Ex 17A (4) From Baggish MS, Karram MM: *Atlas of pelvic anatomy and gynecologic surgery*, ed 4, Philadelphia, 2016, Elsevier.

Fig 8.15 A From Biopsys Medical, Inc, Irvine, Calif.

Fig 8.15B From Pagana KD, Pagana TJ: *Mosby's manual of diagnostic and laboratory test reference*, ed 7, St. Louis, 2004, Elsevier Mosby.

Fig 8.15C From Bassett LW, et al: *Breast imaging: expert radiology series*, Philadelphia, 2010, Saunders.

Fig 8.16B From Ballinger PW, Frank ED: *Merrill's atlas of radiographic positions and radiologic procedures*, ed 10, St. Louis, 2003, Mosby.

Ex, 20B (1) From Bontrager KL, Lampignano JP: *Radiographic positioning and related anatomy*, ed 8, St. Louis, 2014, Mosby.

Ex 20B (2) From Bontrager KL, Lampignano JP: *Radiographic positioning and related anatomy*, ed 8, St. Louis, 2014, Mosby.

Ex 20B (3) From iStock.com/peakSTOCK.

Ex 20B (4) From Bontrager KL, Lampignano JP: *Radiographic positioning and related anatomy*, ed 8, St. Louis, 2014, Mosby.

Ex 21A (1) From Ballinger PW, Frank ED: *Merrill's atlas of radiographic positions and radiologic procedures*, ed 10, St. Louis, 2003, Mosby.

Ex 25B (1) From iStock.com/praisaeng.

Ex 25B (2) From iStock.com/areeya_ann, CopterAnansak, Lalocracio.

Ex 28 Case study from: iStock.com/IPGGutenbergUKLtd.

Chapter 9

Fig. 9.4 From iStock.com/Anastasiia Krasavina.

Ex 6B From Smith RP: *Netter's obstetrics and gynecology*, ed 3, St. Louis, 2018, Elsevier.

Ex 6B 2 From Smith RP: *Netter's obstetrics and gynecology*, ed 3, St. Louis, 2018, Elsevier.

Fig. 9.5 From Zitelli BJ, David HW: *Atlas of pediatric physical diagnosis*, ed 4, St. Louis, 2002, Mosby.

Fig. 9.6 From Lowdermilk DL, et al: *Maternity and women's health care*, ed 10, St. Louis, 2012, Mosby.

Fig. 9.7B From Hockenberry M, et al: *Wong's nursing care of infants and children*, ed 9, St. Louis, 2011, Elsevier.

Ex 10B 1 From iStock.com/corbac40.

Ex 10B 2 From Hockenberry M, et al: *Wong's nursing care of infants and children*, ed 9, St. Louis, 2011, Elsevier.

Ex 11B 4 From Hockenberry M, et al: *Wong's nursing care of infants and children*, ed 9, St. Louis, 2011, Elsevier.

Ex 15A 1 From Gabbe SH, Niebyl JR, Simpson JL, et al: *Obstetrics: normal and problem pregnancies*, ed 7, St. Louis, 2016, Elsevier.

Fig. 9.14 From *Dorland's illustrated medical dictionary*, ed 32, Philadelphia, 2012, Saunders-Elsevier.

Ex 18B 1 From Bontrager KL, Lampignano JP: *Radiographic positioning and related anatomy*, ed 8, St. Louis, 2014, Mosby.

Ex 22B 1 From iStock.com/Antonio_Diaz.

Ex 22B 2 From iStock.com/gorodenkoff.

Ex 22B 3 From iStock.com/Tatiana Foxy.

Ex 22B 4 From iStock.com/kate_sept2004.

Ex 23B 3 From iStock.com/szeyuen.

Ex 23B 4 From iStock.com/wildpixel.

Ex 23B 5 From iStock.com/Gewoldi.

Ex 23B 6 From iStock.com/FatCamera.

Ex 24B 1 From iStock.com/FatCamera.

Ex 24B 2 From iStock.com/FatCamera.

Ex 24B 3 From Bontrager KL, Lampignano JP: *Radiographic positioning and related anatomy*, ed 8, St. Louis, 2014, Mosby.

Ex 24B 4 From iStock.com/draghicich.

Ex 27.B 1 From iStock.com/Andesign101.

Ex 27.B 2 From iStock.com/Yobro10.

Ex 30 From iStock.com/LindaYolanda.

Chapter 10

Ex 7A 2 From Otto CM: *Textbook of clinical echocardiography*, ed 6, Philadelphia, 2018, Elsevier.

Ex 7A 5 From Ballinger PW, Frank ED: *Merrill's atlas of radiographic positions and radiologic procedures*, ed 10, St. Louis, 2003, Mosby.

Ex 7A 6 From Patton KT, Thibodeau GA: *Anatomy and physiology*, ed 7, St. Louis, 2010, Mosby.

Ex 7A 9 From Ignatavicius DM, Workman L: *Medical-surgical nursing*, ed 6, St. Louis, 2010, Saunders.

Ex 7A 10 From iStock.com/kalus.

Ex 7A 11 From Patton KT, Thibodeau GA: *Anatomy and physiology*, ed 7, St. Louis, 2010, Mosby.

Fig. 10.12A From Thibodeau GA, Patton KT: *Anatomy and physiology*, ed 4, St. Louis, 2001, Mosby.

Fig. 10.12B From Bork K, Brauninger W: *Skin diseases in clinical practice*, ed 2, Philadelphia, 1998, WB Saunders.
Ex 9B 1 From iStock.com/ Lightstar59m.
Ex 9B 2 From iStock.com/agrobacter.
Ex 9B 3 From Leonard PC: *Building a medical vocabulary with spanish translations*, ed 7, 2009, Saunders.
Ex 9B 6 From Ballinger PW, Frank ED: *Merrill's atlas of radiographic positions and radiologic procedures*, ed 10, St. Louis, 2003.
Ex 9B 7 From Herring W: Learning *Radiology: Recognizing the Basics*, ed3, Saunders.
Ex 10A 2 From iStock.com/ blueshot.
Ex 10A 3 From Yates D, Caldicott L: Preoperative assessment of vascular patients, *Anaesthesia & Intensive Care Medicine*, June 2007, Elsevier.
Ex 10A 4 From Herring W: *Learning radiology: Recognizing the basics*, ed 3, Philadelphia, Saunders, 2005.
Ex 10A 5 From Ballinger PW, Frank ED: *Merrill's atlas of radiographic positions and radiologic procedures*, ed 10, St. Louis, 2003, Mosby.
Ex 10A 6 From iStock.com/ AndreyPopov.
Ex 11B 1 From iStock.com/thelinke.
Ex 11B 2 From iStock.com/Pixel_away.
Ex 15B 1 From iStock.com/Casanowe.
Ex 15B 2 From iStock.com/Zilli.
Ex 15B 3 From Bolognia JL et al: *Dermatology*, ed 2, St. Louis, 2008, Mosby.
Ex 183 From iStock.com/choja.
Ex 184 From iStock.com/kadmy.
Ex 23A 1 From iStock.com/jarun011.
Ex 23A 2 From Swartz MH: *Textbook of physical diagnosis: history and examination*, ed 7, Philadelphia, 2014, Saunders.
Ex 31 From Thinkstock.com/KatarzynaBialasiewicz.

Chapter 11
Ex 7 A 1 From iStock.com/canbedone.
Ex 7A 2 From iStock.com/Lighthaunter.
Ex 7A 3 From iStock.com/lovelyday12.
Ex 10 1 From Damjanov I, Linder J, eds. *Anderson's pathology*, ed 10, St. Louis, 1996, Mosby.
Ex 10 6 From *Dorland's illustrated medical dictionary*, ed 32, Philadelphia, 2012, Saunders-Elsevier.
Fig. 11.10 From Anderson KN: *Mosby's medical, nursing and allied health dictionary*, St. Louis, 2003, Mosby.
Ex 14A 1 From iStock.com/Mohammed Haneefa Nizamudeen.
Ex 14A 2 From iStock.com/wildpixel.
Ex 14A 3 From iStock.com/Maos.
Fig. 11.13A Permission from Olympus obtained with the 7th edition.
Fig. 11.13B From White RA, Klein SR: *Endoscopic surgery*, St. Louis, 1991, Mosby.
Fig. 11.15 From White RA, Klein SR: *Endoscopic surgery*, St. Louis, 1991, Mosby.
Ex 20B 1 From White RA, Klein SR: *Endoscopic surgery*, St. Louis, 1991, Mosby.
Ex 20B 2 From Bontrager KL, Lampignano JP: *Textbook of radiographic positioning and related anatomy*, ed 8, St. Louis, 2014, Mosby.
Ex 20B 3 Permission from Olympus obtained with the 7th edition.
Ex 20B 4 From Ignatavicius DM, Workman L: *Medical-surgical nursing*, ed 6, St. Louis, 2010, Saunders.
Table 11.1 From Hagen-Ansert S: *Textbook of diagnostic ultrasonography*, ed 5, St. Louis, 2001, Mosby.
Fig. 11.16 From Kowalczyk N: *Radiographic pathology for technologists*, ed 6, St. Louis, 2014, Elsevier.
Ex 23A 1 From Ballinger PW, Frank ED: *Merrill's atlas of radiographic positions and radiologic procedures*, ed 10, St. Louis, 2003, Mosby.
Ex 23A 2 From Kowalczyk N: *Radiographic pathology for technologists*, ed 6, St. Louis, 2014, Elsevier.
Ex 30A 2 From iStock.com/YakobchukOlena.
Ex 20A 4 From Lewis SM: *Medical-surgical nursing*, ed 7, St. Louis, 2007, Mosby.
Fig. 11.17 From iStock.com/PaulMaguire.
Ex 33 From Thinkstock.com/Christopher Robbins.
Fig. 11.18 From iStock.com/undefined undefined.

Chapter 12
Fig. 12.3 From Zitelli BJ, David HW: *Atlas of pediatric physical diagnosis*, ed 2, St. Louis, 1992, Mosby.
Ex 4C From iStock.com/SlayStorm.
Ex 4C From iStock.com/AaronAmat.
Ex 4C From iStock.com/Nikola Ilic.
Ex 7A 1 From Kumar V, et al: *Robbins & Cotran pathologic basis of disease*, ed 10, Philadelphia, 2021, Elsevier.
Ex 7A 2 From Scheie HG, Albert DM: *Textbook of ophthalmology*, ed 9, Philadelphia, 1977, WB Saunders.
Ex 7A 3 From Zitelli BJ, David HW: *Atlas of pediatric physical diagnosis*, ed 2, St. Louis, 1992, Mosby.
Ex 7A 4 From Stein HA, Slatt BJ, Stein RM: *The ophthalmic assistant: fundamentals and clinical practice*, ed 5, St. Louis, 1998, Mosby.
Ex 7A 5 From Batterbury M, et al: *Ophthalmology: an illustrated colour text*, ed 4, St. Louis, 2019, Elsevier, Ltd.
Ex 7A 6 From Zitelli BJ, David HW: *Atlas of pediatric physical diagnosis*, ed 2, St. Louis, 1992, Mosby.
Ex 9B 1 From Seidel H, et al: *Mosby's guide to physical examination*, ed 5, St. Louis, 2003, Mosby.
Ex 9B 3 From Seidel H, et al: *Mosby's guide to physical examination*, ed 5, St. Louis, 2003, Mosby.
Ex 9B 4 From Swartz M: *Textbook of physical diagnosis*, ed 5, Philadelphia, 2006, Saunders.
Ex 9B 5 From Newell FW: *Ophthalmology*, ed 7, St. Louis, 1992, Mosby.
Ex 9B 6 From Bedford MA: *Ophthalmological diagnosis*, London, 1986, Wolfe.
Ex 9B 7 From iStock.com/Zarina Lukash.
Ex 9B 8 From Batterbury M, et al: *Ophthalmology: an illustrated colour text*, ed 4, St. Louis, 2019, Elsevier, Ltd.

Ex 9B 9 From Cote CJ, et al: *A practice of anesthesia for infants and children*, ed 6, Philadelphia, 2019, Elsevier.
Ex 9B 11 From iStock.com/ TefiM.
Ex 9B 12 From iStock.com/sruilk.
Fig. 12.7A and B, From iStock.com/bubaone.
Ex 12B 1 From Black J, Hawks J: *Medical-surgical nursing*, ed 8, St. Louis, 2009, Elsevier.
Ex 12B 2 From Azar DT: *Refractive surgery*, ed 3, 2020, Elsevier.
Ex 12B 3 From Kanski JJ, Bowling B: *Kanski's clinical ophthalmology: a systematic approach*, ed 8, 2016, Elsevier.
Ex 13A 1 From iStock.com/bubaone.
Ex 13A 2 From iStock.com/bubaone.
Ex 13A 4 From Batterbury M, et al: *Ophthalmology: an illustrated colour text*, ed 4, St. Louis, 2019, Elsevier.
Ex 16B 1 From Wilkerson CP, et al: *Ryan's retina*, ed 6, 2018, Elsevier.
Ex 16B 2 From iStock.com/dolgachov.
Ex 16B 3 From Jarvis C: *Physical examination and health assessment*, ed 5, Philadelphia, 2008, Saunders.
Ex 16B 4 From Jarvis C: *Physical examination and health assessment*, ed 5, Philadelphia, 2008, Saunders.
Ex 17A 1 From iStock.com/asikkk.
Ex 17A 2 From Batterbury M, et al: *Ophthalmology: an illustrated colour text*, ed 4, St. Louis, 2019, Elsevier, Ltd.
Ex 17A 3 From iStock.com/TefiM.
Ex 17A 4 From iStock.com/IPGGutenbergUKLtd.
Ex 20B 1 From iStock.com/roberthyrons.
Ex 20B 2 From Zitelli BJ, David HW: *Atlas of pediatric physical diagnosis*, ed 2, St. Louis, 1992, Mosby.
Ex 20B 3 From iStock.com/onepony.
Ex 20B 4 From Batterbury M, et al: *Ophthalmology: an illustrated colour text*, ed 4, St. Louis, 2019, Elsevier, Ltd.
Ex 20B 5 From Batterbury M, et al: *Ophthalmology: an illustrated colour text*, ed 4, St. Louis, 2019, Elsevier, Ltd.
Ex 20B 6 From iStock.com/loonger.
Ex 21A 1 From iStock.com/Ivan-balvan.
Ex 21A 2 From iStock.com/Ivan-balvan.
Ex 21A 3 From iStock.com/coddy.
Ex 21A 4 From iStock.com/joruba.
Ex 24 From iStock.com/100rehanphoto.

Chapter 13

Fg. 13.3 Courtesy Richard A. Buckingham, Clinical Professor, Otolaryngology, Abraham Lincoln School of Medicine, University of Illinois, Chicago. From Barkauskas VH et al: *Health and physical assessment*, ed 3, St. Louis, Mosby, 2002, pp. 278, 290.
Ex 6A 1 From *Zitelli and Davis' atlas of pediatric physical diagnosis*, ed 7, St. Louis, 2017, Elsevier.
Ex 6A 2 From Zitelli BJ, McIntire SC, Nowalk AJ, eds: *Atlas of pediatric physical diagnosis*, ed 6, Philadelphia, 2012, Saunders.

Fig. 13.3 From Barkauskas VH, et al: *Health and physical assessment*, ed 3, St. Louis, 2002, Mosby.
Ex 8B 1 From Brooks A, Krabak BJ: *The young athlete: a practitioner's guide to providing comprehensive sports medicine care*, St. Louis, 2023, Elsevier Inc.
Ex 8B 2 Courtesy Richard A. Buckingham, Clinical Professor, Otolaryngology, Abraham Lincoln School of Medicine, University of Illinois, Chicago. From Barkauskas VH et al: *Health and physical assessment*, ed 3, St. Louis, Mosby, 2002, pp. 278, 290.
Ex 8B 3 From Richardson M, et al: *Cummings otolaryngology—head and neck surgery*, ed 5, St. Louis, 2010, Mosby.
Ex 13B 4 From Swartz MH: *Textbook of physical diagnosis*, ed 8, St. Louis, 2019, Elsevier.
Ex 17A 1 From Sliwa LS, et al: a comparison of audiometric and objective methods in hearing screening of school children: a preliminary study, *International Journal of Pediatric Otorhinolaryngology (sic)*; April 2011 75(4) Elsevier, 483-488.
Ex 17A 2 From Klieger R, et al: *Nelson textbook of pediatrics*, ed 18, St. Louis, 2008, Saunders.
Ex 17A 3 From Jarvis C: *Physical examination and health assessment*, ed 5, Philadelphia, 2008, Saunders.
Ex 17A 4 Amplivox Limited, Eynsham, Oxfordshire, United Kingdom.
Ex 21A 1 From iStock.com/Oga Vasilyeva.
Ex 21A 1 From iStock.com/InsideCreative House.
Ex 21A 1 From iStock.com/kentarus.
Ex 24 From iStock.com/sdominick.

Chapter 14

Fig.14.8 From Thibideau GA, Patton KT: *Anatomy and physiology*, ed 5, St. Louis, 2003, Mosby.
Fig.14.9A From Bontrager KL, Lampignano JP: *Radiographic positioning and related anatomy*, ed 8, St. Louis, 2014, Mosby.
Fig.14.9B From Magee D: *Orthopedic physical assessment*, ed 5, St. Louis, 2008, Saunders.
Fig.14.9C From Manaster BJ: *I*, ed 3, St. Louis, 2007, Mosby.
Fig.14.10 From Kowalczyk N: *Radiographic pathology for technologists*, ed 7, St. Louis, 2018, Elsevier Inc.
Ex 8A 4 From Canale ST, Beaty JH: *Campbell's operative orthopaedics*, ed 11, Philadelphia, 2008, Mosby/Elsevier.
Ex 8A 5 From iStock.com/Stock-PhotosArt.
Ex 11. 1 From Bontrager K, Lampignano NJ: *Textbook of radiographic positioning and related anatomy*, ed 6, St. Louis, 2005, Mosby.
Ex 11.2 From Seidel H: *Mosby's guide to physical examination*, ed 7, St. Louis, 2011, Mosby.
Ex 11.5 From iStock.com/MediaProduction.
Ex 11.6 From Patton KT, Thibodeau GA: *Anthony's texbook of anatomy & physiology*, ed 19, St. Louis, 2010, Mosby.
Ex 11.7 From Mercier LR: *Practical orthopedics*, ed 4, St. Louis, 1995, Mosby.

Ex 11.8 Stone D: *Atlas of infectious diseases*, Philadelphia, 1999, WB Saunders.
Ex 11.12 From iStock.com/AboutnuyLove.
Ex 11.13 From iStock.com/sefa ozel.
Ex 11.14 From iStock.com/33karen33.
Table 14.1 (1) From Long BW, et al: *Merrill's atlas of radiographic positions and radiologic procedures*, ed 13, St. Louis, 2016, Elsevier.
Table 14.1 (3) From Canale S, Beaty J: *Campbell's operative orthopaedics*, ed 12, St. Louis, 2013, Elsevier.
Table 14.1 (5) From Fucentese SF, et al: Total shoulder arthroplasty with an uncemented soft-metal-backed glenoid component, *J Shoulder Elbow Surg* 19: 624-631, 2010.
Ex 16A 2 From Long BW, et al: *Merrill's atlas of radiographic positions and radiologic procedures*, ed 13, St. Louis, 2016, Elsevier.
Ex 16A 3 From iStock.com/undefined undefined.
Ex 16A 4 From iStock.com/Jan-Otto.
Ex 16A 5 From iStock.com/SetsukoN.
Ex 16A 6 From iStock.com/silkfactory.
Fig.14.11A From Taylor J: *Skeletal imaging: Atlas of the spine and extremities*, Philadelphia, 2000, WB Saunders.
Fig.14.11B From Bontrager KL, Lampignano JP: *Radiographic positioning and related anatomy*, ed 8, St. Louis, 2014, Mosby.
Fig.14.12 From Ballinger PW, Frank ED: *Merrill's atlas of radiographic positions and radiologic procedures*, ed 10, St. Louis, 2003, Mosby.
Fig.14.13 From Mercier LR: *Pracitcal orthopedics*, ed 4, St. Louis, 1995, Mosby.
Ex 19C 1 From Lewis SM, Collier IC, Heitkemper MM: *Medical-surgical nursing: assessment and management of clinical problems*, ed 4, St. Louis, 1996, Mosby.
Ex 19C 2 From *Mosby's dictionary of medicine, nursing, and health professions*, ed 9, St. Louis, 2013, Mosby.
Ex 20B 1 From Bontrager KL, Lampignano JP: *Radiographic positioning and related anatomy*, ed 8, St. Louis, 2014, Mosby.
Ex 20B 2 From iStock.com/FatCamera.
Ex 20B 3 From iStock.com/Ivan-balvan.
Ex 20B 4 From iStock.com/Africa Studio.
Ex 14.26B 1 From iStock.com/SDI Productions.
Ex 14.26B 2 From iStock.com/Manuel-F-O.
Ex 14.26B 3 From iStock.com/AlexRaths.
Ex 14.26B 4 From iStock.com/alenkadr.
Ex 14.26B 5 From iStock.com/AJ_Watt.
Ex 14.26B 6 From iStock.com/AzmanJaka.
Ex 31 From Thinkstock.com.

Chapter 15
Fig.15.1 From Thibodeau GA, Patton KT: *Anatomy and physiology*, ed 5, St. Louis, 2003, Mosby.
Fig.15.2 From Thibodeau GA, Patton KT: *Anatomy and physiology*, ed 5, St. Louis, 2003, Mosby.
Ex 7A 1 From iStock.com/maska82.
Ex 7A 3 From Waldman S: *Atlas of common pain syndrome*, ed 2, Philadelphia, 2008, Saunders.
Ex 7A 4 From Kowalcyzk N: *Radiographic pathology for technologists*, ed 6, St. Louis, 2014, Mosby/Elsevier.
Ex 10.8 From Perkin GD, Hotchberg FH, Miller D: *The atlas of clinical neurology*, St. Louis, 1986, Mosby.
Ex 17B 1 From Ballinger PW, Frank ED: *Merrill's atlas of radiographic positions and related anatomy*, ed 6, St. Louis, 2002, Mosby.
Ex 17B 2 From Adam A, et al: *Grainger and Allsion's diagnostic radiology*, ed 5, London, 2008, Churchill Livingstone.
Ex 18B 1 From Aminoff M: *Neurology and general medicine*, ed 4, 2008, Elsevier.
Ex 18B 3 From iStock.com/9632290_400.
Ex 18B 4 From Bontrager KL: *Texbtook of radiographic positioning and related anatomy*, ed 6, St. Louis, 2002, Mosby.
Ex 22B 3 From iStock.com/SDI Productions.
Ex 22B 4 From iStock.com/g-stockstudio.
Ex 22B 5 From iStock.com/magicmine.
Ex 22B 6 From iStock.com/monkeybusinessimages.
Ex 24A 2 From iStock.com/SDI Productions.
Ex 24A 3 From iStock.com/Tunatura.
Ex 24A 4 From iStock.com/SDI Productions.
Ex 24A 5 From iStock.com/wanderluster.
Ex 24A 6 From iStock.com/Claudiad.
Ex 34 From Thinkstock.com/Yasuno Sakata.

Chapter 16
Ex 4B 1 From iStock.com/Pavel1964.
Ex 7A 1 From Mendoloff A, Smith DE: Acromegaly, diabetes, hypermetabolism, proteinuria and heart failure, *The American Journal of Medicine* 20(1): 33, 1956.
Ex 7A 2 From iStock.com/bluebeat 76.
Ex 7A 3 From iStock.com/MarkHatfield.
Ex 11B 1 From Sainani GS, Joshi VR, Sainani RG: *Manual of clinical & practical medicine*, New Delhi, 2010, Elsevier India.
Ex 11B 3 From Goljan E: *Rapid review pathology*, St. Louis, 2004, Mosby.
Ex 11B 4 From Seidel H, et al: *Mosby's guide to physical examination*, ed 5, St. Louis, 2003, Mosby.
Ex 11B 5 From Zitelli BJ, Davis HW: *Atlas of pediatric physical diagnosis*, ed 5, St. Louis, 2007 Mosby.
Ex 11B 7 From Damjanov I: *Pathology for the health professions*, ed 4, Philadelphia, 2011, Saunders.
Ex 11B 8 From Kliegman R, et al: *Nelson textbook of pediatrics*, ed 20, St. Louis, 2016, Elsevier.
Ex 18A 1 From Henningsen C, et al: *Clinical guide to sonography: Exercises for critical thinking*, ed 2, St. Louis, 2014, Elsevier.
Ex 18A 2 From Kowalczyk N: *Radiographic pathology for technologists*, ed 7, St. Louis, 2017, Elsevier.
Ex 18A 3 From Carver E, Carver B: *Medical Imaging: Techniques, Reflection & Evaluation*, ed 2, 2012, Churchill Livingstone-Elsevier Ltd.

Ex 18A 4 From Hagen-Ansert S: *Textbook of diagnostic ultrasonography*, ed 7, St. Louis, 2012, Mosby.
Ex 22B 1 From iStock.com/Shidlovski.
Ex 22B 2 From iStock.com/Foremniakowski.
Ex 22B 3 From iStock.com/mjp.
Ex 22B 4 From iStock.com/fotostorm.
Ex 23B 1 From Swartz MH: *Textbook of physical diagnosis: history and examination*, ed 3, Philadelphia, 1998, Saunders.
Ex 23B 2 From Paul W. Ladenson, MD, The Johns Hopkins University and Hospital, Baltimore, Md.
Ex 26 From iStock.com.

Index

A

-a, 52*t*, 97, 316, 545
a-, 138, 192, 233, 271, 421, 469, 545, 598
AAA (abdominal aortic aneurysm), 377*f*
AB (abortion), 320, 348
abbreviations
   for blood, 405–406
   for cardiovascular system, 405–406
   for digestive system, 455
   for ear, 526
   for endocrine system, 664
   for eye, 497–498
   for female reproductive system, 303–304
   for immune system, 405–406
   for integumentary system, 126
   for lymphatic system, 405–406
   for male reproductive system, 258–259
   for musculoskeletal system, 584
   for neonatology, 348
   for nervous system, 630–631
   for obstetrics, 348
   for oncology, 53
   for respiratory system, 178–180
   for urinary system, 222
abdomen, 419
abdominal aortic aneurysm (AAA), 377*f*
abdominal cavity, 19
abdominal sonography, 445, 445*f*, 445*t*
abdomin/o, 420
abdominocentesis (paracentesis), 434
abdominopelvic cavity, 19
abdominopelvic quadrants, 86, 86*f*
abdominopelvic regions, 71, 72*f*
abdominoperineal resection (APR), 439, 455
abdominoplasty, 434
abduction, 580, 580*f*
ABGs (arterial blood gases), 166, 179
ablation, 247, 288, 380, 380*f*
abnormal uterine bleeding (AUB), 279, 303
abortion (AB), 320, 348
abrasion, 104
abruptio placentae, 320, 321*f*
abscess, 104
absorption, 417, 418
-ac, 421, 545
A1c test, 657
acapnia, 170
-aces, 52*t*
acetabulum, 539
acid-fast bacilli smear (AFB), 166, 179
acne, 104
acoustic nerve, 509
acoustic neuroma, 515
acquired immunity, 403
acquired immunodeficiency syndrome (AIDS), 402
   esophageal candidiasis with, 105
   Kaposi sarcoma with, 106
acr/o, 643
acromegaly, 647, 651
acromion process, 536
acronyms, 3, 3*f*, 14
ACS (acute coronary syndrome), 376, 405

ACTH (adrenocorticotropic hormone), 641, 664
actinic keratosis, 104
activated partial thromboplastin time (aPTT), 394, 406
active surveillance, for prostate cancer, 240*t*
acute, 49, 150
acute coronary syndrome (ACS), 376, 405
acute infection, 49
acute kidney injury (AKI), 201, 222
acute leukemia, 393*t*
acute lymphocytic leukemia (ALL), 393*t*
acute myelogenous leukemia (AML), 393*t*
acute otitis media (AOM), 515*f*, 526
acute renal failure (ARF), 201, 222
acute respiratory distress syndrome (ARDS), 150, 178
acute urinary retention (ADR), 222
AD (Alzheimer disease), 3, 608, 609*t*, 630
Adam's apple, 135
Addison, Thomas, 650
Addison disease, 650
adduction, 580, 580*f*
aden/o, 20, 97
adenocarcinoma, 32
   of lung, 146*f*
adenohypophysis (anterior lobe), of pituitary gland, 641
adenoidectomy, 156
adenoiditis, 145
adenoid/o, 138
adenoids (pharyngeal tonsils), 135–136
adenoma, 32
adenomyosis, 279
ADH (antidiuretic hormone), 641, 664
ADHD (attention deficit/hyperactivity disorder), 628, 630
adhesiolysis, 430
adhesion, 430
adhesiotomy, 430
adjuvant chemotherapy, 37
ADR (acute urinary retention), 222
adrenal cortex, 642
adrenal glands, 642
adrenal medulla, 642
adrenalectomy, 656
adrenaline (epinephrine), 642
adrenalitis, 647
adrenal/o, 643
adren/o, 643
adrenocorticohyperplasia, 659
adrenocorticotropic hormone (ACTH), 641, 664
adrenomegaly, 647
-ae, 52*t*
AFB (acid-fast bacilli smear), 166, 179
afebrile, 48
AFib (atrial fibrillation), 378, 378*f*, 405
afterbirth (placenta), 314
age-associated memory impairment, 623*t*
age-related macular degeneration (AMD), 479*f*, 497
AICD (automatic implantable cardiac defibrillator), 380, 406

AIDS (acquired immunodeficiency syndrome), 402
   esophageal candidiasis with, 105
   Kaposi sarcoma with, 106
airway, 175
AKI (acute kidney injury), 201, 222
-al, 21, 62, 97, 139, 192, 271, 316, 421, 469, 510, 545, 599, 644
albinism, 105
albumin/o, 192
albuminuria, 214
aldosterone, 642
-algia, 233, 271, 469, 510, 545, 599
ALL (acute lymphocytic leukemia), 393*t*
allergen, 402
allergist, 402
allergy, 402
alopecia, 121
ALS (amyotrophic lateral sclerosis), 608, 630
alveolar, 171
alveoli, 136–137
alveolitis, 145
alveol/o, 138
Alzheimer disease (AD), 3, 608, 609*t*, 630
amblyopia (lazy eye), 477
AMD (age-related macular degeneration), 479*f*, 497
amenorrhea, 298
AML (acute myelogenous leukemia), 393*t*
amni/o, 315
amniocentesis, 334, 334*f*
amnion, 315
amnionic fluid (amniotic fluid), 315
amnionic sac (amniotic sac), 314
amnionitis, 320
amnion/o, 315
amniorrhea, 338
amniorrhexis, 338
-amnios, 316
amniotic fluid (amnionic fluid), 315
amniotic sac (amnionic sac, bag of waters), 314
amniotomy, 331
amyotrophic lateral sclerosis (ALS, Lou Gehrig disease), 608, 630
an-, 138, 192, 233, 469, 598
anal, 449
analyzing, 4, 9
anaphylactic shock, 402
anaphylaxis, 402
anastomosis, 439, 440*f*
anatomic planes, 74, 74*f*
anatomic position, 61, 61*f*
anatomy
   for neonatology, 314–315
   for obstetrics, 314–315
   of body, 17–20
   of cardiovascular system, 358
   of digestive system, 416–420
   of ear, 507*f*, 507–509
   of endocrine system, 640–643
   of eye, 466–468, 467*f*
   of female reproductive system, 267*f*, 267–270

Note: Page numbers followed by "*f*" refer to illustrations; page numbers followed by "*t*" refer to tables; page numbers followed by "*b*" refer to boxes.

773

Index

anatomy *(Continued)*
  of integumentary system, 95–96
  of large intestine, 417f
  of male reproductive system, 231–232
  of musculoskeletal system, 534–543
  of nervous system, 594–597
  of respiratory system, 135–137
  of urinary system, 189–191
andr/o, 233
andropathy, 236
anemia, 361, 393, 393t
anesthesia, 619
aneurysm, 376
  abdominal aortic, 377f
  cerebral, 608
angina pectoris, 376
angi/o, 364, 469, 598
angiography, 371
  cerebral, 614
  computed tomography, 371t
  coronary, 371t
  digital subtraction, 371t, 381, 406
  magnetic resonance, 371t
angioma, 369
angioplasty, 370
angioscopy, 371
angiostenosis, 369
anisocoria, 492
anisometropia, 477
ankyl/o, 545
ankylosing spondylitis (rheumatoid spondylitis, Strümpell-Marie disease), 558
ankylosis, 552
an/o, 420
anoplasty, 434
anorchism, 236
anorexia nervosa, 628
anovulation, 299
anoxia, 170
ant (anterior), 66, 68t, 85
  of muscles, 541f
  of skeleton, 537f
ante-, 316
antepartum, 338
anterior (ant), 66, 68t, 85
  of muscles, 541f
  of skeleton, 537f
anterior and posterior colporrhaphy (A&P repair), 288, 303
anterior lobe (adenohypophysis), of pituitary gland, 641
anter/o, 61
anteroposterior (AP), 66, 85
antibiotic-associated colitis, 426
antibody (immunoglobulin), 403
anticoagulant, 395
antidiuretic hormone (ADH), 641, 664
antigen, 403
antrectomy, 434
antr/o, 420
antrum, 418
anuria, 214
anus, 418
anvil (incus), 508
anxiety disorder, 628
AOM (acute otitis media), 515f, 526
aorta, 359–360
aortic stenosis, 369
aortic valve, 359–360
aort/o, 364
aortogram, 371
AP (anteroposterior), 66, 85
A&P repair (anterior and posterior colporrhaphy), 288, 303
Apgar, Virginia, 3, 335
Apgar score, 335, 335f

aphagia, 449
aphakia, 474
aphasia, 619
-apheresis, 364
aphonia, 170
aplastic anemia, 361
apnea, 170
aponeurosis, 540
appendages of the skin, 96
appendectomy, 434
appendicitis, 426
appendic/o, 420
appendix, 419
append/o, 420
APR (abdominoperineal resection), 439, 455
aPTT (activated partial thromboplastin time), 394, 406
aqueous humor, 466
-ar, 139, 364, 469, 510, 545
arachnoid, 596, 596f
ARDS (acute respiratory distress syndrome), 150, 178
areola, 270
ARF (acute renal failure), 201, 222
Aristotle, 2
arrhythmia, 377
ART (assisted reproductive technology), 331, 332f
arterial blood gases (ABGs), 166, 179
arteries
  CAD, 377, 405
  PAD, 379, 405
  pulmonary, 359–360
  UAE, 289, 303
arteri/o, 364
arteriogram, 371
arterioles, 359–360
arteriosclerosis, 369
arthralgia, 575
arthritis, 552. *See also* osteoarthritis; rheumatoid arthritis
  of knee, 553f
arthr/o, 544
arthrocentesis, 565
arthrodesis (joint fusion), 565
arthrography, 570
arthroplasty, 565
  hip resurfacing, 566f, 566t
  shoulder, 566f, 566t
  total hip, 566f, 566t, 584
  total knee, 566f, 566t, 584
arthroscopy, 570
articulations (joints), 539
  of knee, 540f
artificial cardiac pacemaker, 380
artificial insemination, 256
-ary, 139, 192, 469, 545
ascites, 451
ASD (autism spectrum disorders), 628, 630
aspermia, 255
asphyxia, 150
aspirate, 175
assisted reproductive technology (ART), 331, 332f
Ast (astigmatism), 477, 478f, 497
-asthenia, 545
asthma, 150
astigmatism (Ast), 477, 478f, 497
ataxia, 622
atelectasis, 145–146
atel/o, 138
atherectomy, 370
ather/o, 364
atherosclerosis, 369
athlete's foot (tinea pedis), 107t, 109
atrial fibrillation (AFib), 378, 378f, 405

atrial septum, 359
atri/o, 364
atrioventricular (AV), 372, 406
atrioventricular valves, 359–360
atrophy, 575
attention deficit/hyperactivity disorder (ADHD), 628, 630
AUB (abnormal uterine bleeding), 279, 303
audi/o, 509
audiogram, 521
audiologist, 523
audiology, 523
audiometer, 521
audiometry, 521
auditory nerve, 509
aural, 523
aur/i, 509
auricle (pinna), 508
auscultation, 166
autism, 628
autism spectrum disorders (ASD), 628, 630
aut/o, 21
autoimmune disease, 402
automatic implantable cardiac defibrillator (AICD), 380, 406
autopsy, 41
AV (atrioventricular), 372, 406
-ax, 52t
axial, 74, 74f
azoospermia, 256
azotemia, 198, 214
azot/o, 192

B

bacteria, 49
bacterial infection, 107t
bacterial vaginosis (vaginosis), 276
bacterium, 49
bag of waters (amniotic sac), 314
balance, inner ear for, 507
balanitis, 236
balan/o, 233
balanoplasty, 243
balanorrhea, 255
balloon angioplasty (percutaneous transluminal coronary angioplasty, PTCA), 380, 406
bariatric surgery, 439
barium enema (BE), 445, 446f, 455
barium swallow, 441
Barrett esophagus, 430
Bartholin, Caspar, 270
Bartholin glands, 270
basal cell carcinoma (BCC), 105, 105f, 126
basophils, 361f
BC (birth control, contraception), 299, 303
BCC (basal cell carcinoma), 105, 105f, 126
BE (barium enema), 445, 446f, 455
bedsore (pressure injury), 108, 108f
behavioral health, 593–636
  terms not from word parts, 628–629
  word parts for, 626
Bell palsy, 608
benign, 36–37
benign paroxysmal positional vertigo (BPPV), 515, 526
benign prostatic hyperplasia (BPH), 236, 236f, 258
  surgical treatments for, 250t
benign prostatic hypertrophy, 236
benign tumors, 31, 37f
bi-, 62
bilateral, 66
bile ducts, 419
bilevel positive airway pressure (BiPAP), 180

Index

biliary tract, 419
bin-, 469
binocular, 492
bi/o, 21
biochemical testing, 40t
biological response modifiers (BRM), 36
biological therapy, 36, 37
biomarker, 382
biopsy (bx), 53
   cone, 288
   definition of, 41
   of bone marrow, 394
   of breasts, 292, 293f
   sentinel lymph node, 292, 293f
   with transrectal ultrasound, 240t
   wire localization, 292
biotherapy, 36
BiPAP (bilevel positive airway pressure), 180
bipolar disorder, 628
birth control (BC, contraception), 299, 303
birthmarks, 327
bladder outlet obstruction (BOO), 258
blast/o, 192, 469, 598
bleeding disorder, 393
bleeding profile, 394
blepharitis, 474
blephar/o, 468
blepharoplasty, 483
blepharoptosis (ptosis), 474
blood, 360–361
   abbreviations for, 405–406
   cells of, 360–361
   combining forms for, 364
   composition of, 360f, 361
   diagnostic terms not from word parts for, 394
   disease and disorder terms from word parts for, 390
   disease and disorder terms not from word parts for, 393
   function of, 360
   laboratory tests for, 394–395
   medical terms for, 390–397
   surgical terms not from words parts for, 393
blood chemistry studies, 40t
blood coagulation, 394
blood dyscrasia, 395
blood pressure (BP), 381, 406
blood urea nitrogen (BUN), 210, 222
blood vessels, 359–360, 360f
BMI (body mass index), 651
BMT (bone marrow transplant), 395, 406
body. *See also* direction
   anatomy of, 17–20
   cavities of, 19, 19f
   cells of, 17, 17f
   combining forms for, 20, 21
   complementary terms from word parts for, 45
   complementary terms not from word parts for, 36–37, 48–49
   medical terms for, 28–53
   of stomach, 418
   prefixes for, 21
   suffixes for, 21
   systems of, 17, 18t
   word parts for, 20–27, 28–31
body mass index (BMI), 651
body positions, 76–77
boil (furuncle), 106
bone densitometry, 570, 571t
bone density test, 570
bone markers, 572
bone marrow, 535
   aspiration, 394
   biopsy of, 394

bone marrow transplant (BMT), 395, 406
bone scan, 571f
bone structure, 534f, 534–535
BOO (bladder outlet obstruction), 258
Borrelia burgdorferi, 559
botulism, 608
BP (blood pressure), 381, 406
BPH (benign prostatic hyperplasia), 236, 236f, 258
   surgical treatments for, 250t
BPPV (benign paroxysmal positional vertigo), 515, 526
brachytherapy, 37
brady-, 364, 545
bradycardia, 370
bradykinesia, 575
brain, 595f, 595–596
brainstem, 596
breast(s), 270, 270f
   biopsy of, 292, 293f
   cancer of, 279, 279f
   reconstruction of, 286t
   surgical reconstruction of, 285f
breast conserving surgery (lumpectomy), 286t
breathing (respiration), 135
breech presentation, 339
BRM (biological response modifiers), 36
bronchial tree (bronchus), 135–136
bronchiectasis, 145
bronchi/o, 138
bronchioles, 135–136
bronchitis, 145
bronch/o, 138
bronchoalveolar, 171
bronchoconstrictor, 174
bronchodilator, 174
bronchogenic carcinoma (lung cancer), 145, 146f
bronchoplasty, 156
bronchopneumonia, 145
bronchoscope, 161, 162f
bronchoscopy, 161, 162f
bronchospasm, 145
bronchus (bronchial tree), 135–136
bruise (contusion), 105
bruit, 382
building, 4, 9
bulimia nervosa, 628
BUN (blood urea nitrogen), 210, 222
bunion, 558
bursa, 539
bursectomy, 565
bursitis, 552, 559
burs/o, 544
bx (biopsy), 53
   cone, 288
   definition of, 41
   of bone marrow, 394
   of breasts, 292, 293f
   sentinel lymph node, 292, 293f
   with transrectal ultrasound, 240t
   wire localization, 292

C

CA-125 (cancer antigen-125 tumor marker), 294
CA (carcinoma), 32, 37f, 53
CABG (coronary artery bypass graft), 380, 406
CAD (coronary artery disease), 377, 405
calcaneus, 539
calc/i, 643
CA-MRSA (community-associated MRSA), 126

cancellous (spongy) bone, 534
cancer. *See also* oncology
   breast, 279, 279f
   cervical, 279
   endometrial, 279f, 280
   lung, 145, 146f
   ovarian, 280
   prostate, 240, 240t
   testicular, 240
   therapy for, 37
   TNM staging system of, 33
cancer antigen-125 tumor marker (CA-125), 294
cancer/o, 21
cancerous, 45
Candida albicans, 105
candidiasis (thrush), 104
CAP (community-associated pneumonia), 178
capillaries, 135, 359–360
capn/o, 138
capnometer, 162
capsule endoscopy (camera endoscopy), 441, 441f
carbon dioxide (CO_2), 135, 179
carbuncle, 105
carcin/o, 21, 138, 316
carcinogen, 45
carcinogenic, 45
carcinoid, 45
carcinoma (CA), 32, 37f, 53. *See also* oncology
   basal cell, 105, 126
   bronchogenic, 145, 146f
   squamous cell, 105f, 108, 126, 146f
carcinoma in situ, 36, 37f
cardia, 418
cardiac arrest, 377
cardiac catheterization, 371t, 381
cardiac muscle, 540, 543f
cardiac tamponade, 377
cardi/o, 364
cardiogenic, 372
cardiologist, 372
cardiology, 372
cardiomegaly, 370
cardiomyopathy, 370
cardiopulmonary resuscitation (CPR), 383, 406
cardiovascular system, 18t, 358f
   abbreviations for, 405–406
   anatomy of, 358
   combining forms for, 364
   diagnostic procedures and tests for, 371, 381
   diagnostic terms from word parts for, 372
   diagnostic terms not from word parts for, 381
   disease and disorder terms from word parts for, 369–371
   disease and disorder terms not from word parts for, 376–383
   function of, 358
   laboratory tests for, 382
   medical terms for, 369–389
   organs and anatomical structures of, 359–360
   prefixes for, 364
   suffixes for, 364–365
   surgical terms from word parts for, 370–371
   surgical terms not from words parts for, 380
carotid endarterectomy, 370
carpal, 575
carpal bones, 536

carpal tunnel syndrome (CTS), 558–559, 584
carpectomy, 565
carp/o, 544
cartilage, 539
castration, 243
cataract, 477, 478f
catheter ablation, 380, 380f
catheter (cath), 218–219, 222
caudal, 66, 68t
caud/o, 61
cauterization (cautery), 114
cautery (cauterization), 114
cavities
　abdominal, 19
　abdominopelvic, 19
　cranial, 19
　oral, 417f
　pelvic, 19
　spinal, 19
　thoracic, 19, 136–137
CBC (complete blood count), 394
CBC with diff (complete blood count with differential), 41, 53, 406
C1-C7 (cervical vertebrae), 536, 584
CCU (coronary care unit), 406
cec/o, 420
cecum, 418
-cele, 139, 192, 271, 316, 421, 599
celiac, 449
celiac disease (gluten enteropathy), 430
celi/o, 420
celiotomy (laparotomy), 435
cell(s). *See also* red blood cells; white blood cells
　growth progression for, 37f
　of blood, 361
　of body, 17, 17f
cell membrane, 17
cellulitis, 105
-centesis, 139, 316, 364, 421, 545
central nervous system (CNS), 594, 631
central vision loss, 479f
cephalgia (cephalalgia), 619
cephalic, 66, 68t
cephalic presentation, 339
cephal/o, 61, 316, 598
cerebellitis, 603
cerebell/o, 598
cerebellum (hindbrain), 596
cerebral aneurysm, 608
cerebral angiography, 614
cerebral embolism, 603
cerebral palsy (CP), 608, 630
cerebral thrombosis, 603
cerebr/o, 598
cerebrospinal fluid (CSF), 595–596, 631
cerebrovascular accident (CVA), 609, 630
cerebrum, 595
cervical cancer, 279
cervical cerclage, 331
cervical vertebrae (C1-C7), 536, 584
cervicectomy (trachelectomy), 285
cervicitis, 275
cervic/o, 270
cervix (Cx), 268, 304
cesarean section (CS, C-section), 331, 348
CF (cystic fibrosis), 151, 178
chalazion (meibomian cyst), 477
cheilitis, 426
cheil/o, 420
cheiloplasty, 434
chemical stress testing, 381
chemistry panel, 41
chemotherapy (chemo), 36, 53
　for prostate cancer, 240t
chest physiotherapy (CPT), 180

chest x-ray (chest radiograph), 166, 179
CHF (congestive heart failure), 378
chiropractic, 579
chiropractor, 579
chlamydia, 255
chloasma, 315
cholangi/o, 420
cholangiogram, 441
cholangiography, 441
cholangioma, 426
cholecystectomy, 434
cholecystitis, 426
choledoch/o, 420
choledocholithiasis, 426
choledocholithotomy, 434
cholelithiasis (gallstones), 426
cholesteatoma, 515
cholesterol, 382t
chondrectomy, 565
chondr/o, 544
chondromalacia, 552
chondroplasty, 565
chondros, 71
chondrosarcoma, 552
chori/o, 315
chorioamnionitis, 320
choriocarcinoma, 320
chorion, 314
chorionic villus sampling (CVS), 335, 336f, 348
choroid, 466
chromosomes, 17
chronic, 49, 150
chronic atrial fibrillation, 378
chronic GERD (Barrett esophagus), 430
chronic infection, 49
chronic kidney disease (CKD), 201, 201t–202t, 222
chronic leukemia, 393t
chronic lymphocytic leukemia (CLL), 393t
chronic myelogenous leukemia (CML), 393t
chronic obstructive pulmonary disease (COPD), 150, 150f, 178
chronic renal failure (CRF), 201, 222
chronic traumatic encephalopathy (CTE), 608, 630
chronic urinary retention (CUR), 222
ciliary body, 466
circumcision, 247
cirrhosis, 430
CKD (chronic kidney disease), 201, 201t–202t, 222
clavicle, 536
clavicular, 575
clavicul/o, 544
cleft lip or palate, 326, 327f
-cleisis, 271
clinical depression, 628
CLL (chronic lymphocytic leukemia), 393t
Clostridium difficile, 426
cluster headache, 619
CML (chronic myelogenous leukemia), 393t
CMV (cytomegalovirus), 348
CNS (central nervous system), 594, 631
CO_2 (carbon dioxide), 135, 179
coagulation, 394
coarctation of the aorta, 326
-cocci, 97, 178
coccidioidomycosis, 150–151, 178
-coccus, 97
coccyx, 536, 536f
cochlea, 509
cochlear, 523
cochlear implant, 518
cochlear nerve, 509
cochle/o, 509

cognitive, 623
cognitive impairment, 623t
cold (upper respiratory infection, URI), 152, 178
colectomy, 434
colitis, 426
collection sample, 41
col/o, 420
colon, 418
colon cancer, 442f
colon polyp, 442f
colon/o, 420
colonography, 441
colonoscope, 442
　for polypectomy, 435f
colonoscopy, 442, 442f
color, combining forms for, 21
colorectal, 449
colostomy, 434
colostrum, 339
colovaginal fistula, 281t
colp/o, 270
colpocleisis, 284
colpoperineorrhaphy, 284
colpoplasty, 284
colporrhaphy, 284
colposcope, 292
colposcopy, 292
coma, 622
combining forms, 7, 8t
　for blood, 364
　for body, 20, 21
　for cardiovascular system, 364
　for color, 21
　for diagnostic imaging, 61
　for digestive system, 420
　for direction, 61
　for ear, 509
　for endocrine system, 643
　for eye, 468–469
　for female reproductive system, 270–271
　for integumentary system, 96–97
　for lymphatic system, 364
　for male reproductive system, 233
　for musculoskeletal system, 544–545
　for neonatology, 315–316
　for nervous system, 598
　for obstetrics, 315–316
　for respiratory system, 138
　for urinary system, 192
combining vowels, 4, 6–7, 7t
common bile duct, 419, 419f
community-associated MRSA (CA-MRSA), 126
community-associated pneumonia (CAP), 178
compact bone, 534
compartment syndrome, 558
complementary terms from word parts
　for body, 45
　for digestive system, 449
　for ear, 523
　for endocrine system, 659–660
　for eye, 492–493
　for female reproductive system, 298–299
　for integumentary system, 116–117
　for male reproductive system, 255
　for musculoskeletal system, 575–576
　for neonatology, 344
　for nervous system, 619
　for obstetrics, 331, 334
　for respiratory system, 170–171
　for urinary system, 214–215
complementary terms not from word parts
　for body, 36–37, 48–49
　for digestive system, 451–452

complementary terms not from word parts
(Continued)
  for eye, 492
  for female reproductive system, 299–300
  for male reproductive system, 256
  for musculoskeletal system, 579–580
  for neonatology, 344
  for nervous system, 622–623
  for obstetrics, 331
  for respiratory system, 174–175
  for urinary system, 218–219
complete blood count (CBC), 394
complete blood count with differential (CBC with diff), 41, 53, 406
comprehensive metabolic panel, 41
compression fractures, from osteoporosis, 567t
computed tomography (CT), 80, 80t, 85
  colonography, 441
  definition of, 81
  of chest, 166
  of kidney, 209f
  SPECT, 381, 406
computed tomography angiography (CTA), 371t
computed tomography (CT) myelography, 614
conception (fertilization), 314, 314f
concussion, 622
conditions, suffixes for, 5
condom, 256
cone biopsy (conization), 288
congenital anomaly, 344
congenital cytomegalovirus (CMV) infection, 326
congenital dermal melanocytosis, 327
congenital heart disease, 326
congenital hypothyroidism, 650
congestive heart failure (CHF), 378
coni/o, 138
conization (cone biopsy), 288
conjunctiva, 466
conjunctivitis (pink eye), 474
conjunctiv/o, 468
connective tissue, 17
conscious, 623
contact dermatitis, 101f
continuous positive airway pressure (CPAP), 175f, 179
  for OSA, 152f
contraception (birth control, BC), 299, 303
contusion (bruise), 105
convulsion, 622
COPD (chronic obstructive pulmonary disease), 150, 150f, 178
cor pulmonale, 377
cornea, 466
corneal, 492
corne/o, 468
cor/o, 468
coronal (frontal), 74, 74f
coronary, 377
coronary artery bypass graft (CABG), 380, 406
coronary artery disease (CAD), 377, 405
coronary care unit (CCU), 406
coronary stent, 380
coronavirus disease (COVID-19), 151, 178
corpus, 268
cortical, 660
cortic/o, 643
cortisol (hydrocortisone), 642
costectomy, 565
cost/o, 544
COVID-19 (coronavirus disease), 151, 178
CP (cerebral palsy), 608, 630

CPAP (continuous positive airway pressure), 175f, 179
  for OSA, 152f
CPK (creatine phosphokinase), 382, 406
CPR (cardiopulmonary resuscitation), 383, 406
CPT (chest physiotherapy), 180
crackles (rales), 174
cranial, 575
cranial cavity, 19
cranial nerves, 597f
crani/o, 544, 598
craniocerebral, 619
cranioplasty, 565
cranioschisis, 552
craniotomy, 565
C-reactive protein (CRP), 382, 406
creatine phosphokinase (CPK), 382, 406
creatinine, 210
crepitation (crepitus), 579
crepitus (crepitation), 579
CRF (chronic renal failure), 201, 222
Crohn disease, 430
cross-eyed (strabismus), 479
croup (laryngotracheobronchitis), 145, 151, 178
CRP (C-reactive protein), 382, 406
cry/o, 469
cryoretinopexy, 483
cryosurgery, 114, 114f
cryotherapy, 240t
crypt/o, 21, 97, 233
cryptorchidism, 236, 236f
CS (cesarean section), 331, 348
C&S (culture and sensitivity), 40, 41, 53
C-section (cesarean section), 331, 348
CSF (cerebrospinal fluid), 595–596, 631
CT (computed tomography), 80, 80t, 85
  colonography, 441
  definition of, 81
  of chest, 166
  of kidney, 209f
  single-photon emission, 381, 406
CT (computed tomography) myelography, 614
CTA (computed tomography angiography), 371t
CTE (chronic traumatic encephalopathy), 608, 630
CTS (carpal tunnel syndrome), 558–559, 584
culture and sensitivity (C&S), 40, 41, 53
CUR (chronic urinary retention), 222
Cushing, Harvey Williams, 651
Cushing syndrome, 651
cutane/o, 96
cutaneous, 117
CVA (cerebrovascular accident), 609, 630
CVS (chorionic villus sampling), 335, 336f, 348
Cx (cervix), 268, 304
CXR (chest radiograph), 166, 179
cyan/o, 21
cyanosis, 45
cyberchondria, 71
-cyesis, 316
cyst, 121, 122t
  ganglion, 559
  meibomian, 477
  pilonidal, 106, 106f
cystectomy, 203
cystic duct, 419, 419f
cystic fibrosis (CF), 151, 178
cystitis, 197, 197f
cyst/o, 192, 233, 420, 469
cystocele, 197

cystogram, 209
cystography, 209
cystolith, 197
cystolithotomy, 203
cystoscope, 209
cystoscopy, 209
cystostomy, 203
-cyte, 21
cyt/o, 20, 364
cytogenic, 28
cytology, 28
cytomegalovirus (CMV), 326, 348
cytopathology, 41
cytoplasm, 17

D

dacr/o, 469
dacry/o, 468, 469
dacryocystitis, 474
dacryocystorhinostomy, 483
date of birth (DOB), 349
D&C (dilation and curettage), 288, 289f, 303
DC (Doctor of Chiropractic), 584
debridement, 114
decubitus position (recumbent position), 76, 77t
decubitus ulcer (pressure injury), 108, 108f
deep tendon reflexes (DTR), 615, 631
deep vein thrombosis (DVT), 377, 394, 405
defibrillation, 383, 383f
defining, 9
delirium, 623t
dementia, 608, 609t
deoxyribonucleic acid (DNA), 17
derm (dermatology), 117, 126
dermabrasion, 114
dermatitis, 101
dermat/o, 96
dermatofibroma, 101
dermatologist, 117
dermatology (derm), 117, 126
dermatoplasty, 113
dermis, 96
derm/o, 96
-desis, 139, 545
deviated septum, 151
DEXA (dual-energy X-ray absorptiometry), 570, 571t, 584
DI (diabetes insipidus), 651, 664
dia-, 21
diabetes insipidus (DI), 651, 664
diabetes mellitus (DM), 651, 652t, 664
diabetic ketoacidosis (DKA), 664
diabetic retinopathy, 474
diagnosis (Dx), 45, 53
diagnostic imaging. See also specific imaging modalities
  combining forms, 61
  for endocrine system, 657
  for eye, 487–488
  for female reproductive system, 291–292
  for musculoskeletal system, 570, 571t
  for nervous system, 614–615
  for urinary system, 210
  word parts for, 81, 161–162
diagnostic procedures and tests, 161–162. See also laboratory tests
  for cardiovascular system, 371, 381
  for nervous system, 615
diagnostic terms from word parts
  for cardiovascular system, 372
  for digestive system, 441–442
  for ear, 521
  for eye, 487–488

778 Index

diagnostic terms from word parts *(Continued)*
   for female reproductive system, 291–292
   for musculoskeletal system, 570
   for nervous system, 614–615
   for obstetrics, 331
   for respiratory system, 161–162
   for urinary system, 209
diagnostic terms not from word parts
   for blood, 394
   for cardiovascular system, 381
   for digestive system, 445–446
   for endocrine system, 657
   for male reproductive system, 253
   for nervous system, 615
   for pulmonary function, 166
   for respiratory system, 166–167
   for urinary system, 210
diaphoresis, 121
diaphragm, 136–137
diaphragmatic, 171
diaphragmat/o, 138
diaphragmatocele, 145
diaphysis, 535
diarrhea, 451
diastole, 381
diastolic pressure, 381
differential count (Diff), 394, 406
digestion, 417, 418
digestive system, 18t, 415–461
   abbreviations for, 454
   anatomy of, 416–420
   combining forms for, 420
   complementary terms from word parts for, 449
   complementary terms not from word parts for, 451–452
   diagnostic terms from word parts for, 441–442
   diagnostic terms not from word parts for, 445–446
   disease and disorder terms from word parts for, 426–427
   disease and disorder terms not from word parts for, 430–431
   food pathway in, 419f
   function of, 417
   laboratory tests for, 446
   medical terms for, 426–455
   organs of, 416f–417f, 417–419
   prefixes for, 421
   suffixes for, 421
   surgical terms from word parts for, 434–435
   surgical terms not from words parts for, 439
   word parts for, 420–426
digital mammography (mammography), 292
digital rectal examination (DRE), 240t, 253, 259
digital subtraction angiography (DSA), 371t, 381, 406
dilation and curettage (D&C), 288, 289f, 303
diphtheria, 151
dipl/o, 469
diplopia, 474
dips/o, 643
direction
   anatomic position and, 61, 61f
   combining forms for, 61
   medical terms for, 60–91
   prefixes for, 5, 62
   suffixes for, 62
discectomy, 565
discitis, 552
disc/o, 544

disease and disorder terms from word parts
   for blood, 393
   for cardiovascular system, 369–371
   for digestive system, 426–427
   for ear, 513
   for endocrine system, 647–648
   for eye, 474
   for female reproductive system, 275–276
   for lymphatic system, 398
   for male reproductive system, 236–237
   for musculoskeletal system, 552–554
   for neonatology, 326
   for nervous system, 603–604
   for obstetrics, 320
   for respiratory system, 145–147
   for urinary system, 197–198
disease and disorder terms not from word parts
   for blood, 393
   for cardiovascular system, 376–383
   for digestive system, 430–431
   for ear, 515
   for endocrine system, 650–651
   for eye, 477–479
   for female reproductive system, 279–280
   for lymphatic disease, 399
   for male reproductive system, 239–241
   for neonatology, 326–327
   for nervous system, 608–610
   for obstetrics, 320–321
   for respiratory system, 150–152
   for urinary system, 201
dislocation, 559
disorientation, 622
distal, 66
distended, 219
dist/o, 61
diuretic, 218
diurnal enuresis, 218
diverticula, of large intestine, 421f
diverticulectomy, 434
diverticulitis, 426
diverticul/o, 420
diverticulosis, 426, 442f
DKA (diabetic ketoacidosis), 664
DM (diabetes mellitus), 651, 652t, 664
DNA (deoxyribonucleic acid), 17
DO (osteopath), 579
DOB (date of birth), 349
Doctor of Chiropractic (DC), 584
doctor of optometry (OD), 493
Doppler ultrasound, 381
dorsal, 66, 68t
dorsal recumbent position (supine position), 77, 77t
dors/o, 61
doula, 339
Down syndrome (trisomy 21), 326, 327f
DPI (dry powder inhaler), 180
DRE (digital rectal examination), 240t, 253, 259
-drome, 644
drusen, 477
dry macular degeneration, 479f
dry powder inhaler (DPI), 180
DSA (digital subtraction angiography), 371t, 381, 406
DTR (deep tendon reflexes), 615, 631
dual X-ray absorptiometry (DXA), 570–571, 571f, 584
dual-energy X-ray absorptiometry (DEXA), 570, 584
duct(s)
   common bile, 419, 419f
   cystic, 419, 419f
   hepatic, 419, 419f

ductless glands, 640
ductus deferens (vas deferens), 232
duodenal, 449
duodenal ulcer, 431
duoden/o, 420
duodenum, 418
dura mater, 596, 596f
duritis, 603
dur/o, 598
DVT (deep vein thrombosis), 377, 394, 405
Dx (diagnosis), 45, 53
DXA (dual X-ray absorptiometry), 571f, 571t, 584
dys-, 21, 138, 192, 271, 316, 421, 545, 598
dysarthria, 622
dyscrasia, 395
dysentery, 426
dysesthesia, 619
dyskinesia (movement disorders), 575
dysmenorrhea, 298
dyspareunia, 299
dyspepsia, 449
dysphagia, 449
dysphasia, 619
dysphonia, 170
dysplasia, 28, 37f
dyspnea, 170
dystocia, 320
dystrophy, 575
dysuria, 214

E

-e, 316
-eal, 139, 421, 469, 545
ear, 506–530
   abbreviations for, 526
   anatomy of, 507f, 507–509
   combining forms for, 509
   complementary terms from word parts for, 523
   diagnostic terms from word parts for, 521
   disease and disorder terms from word parts for, 513
   disease and disorder terms not from word parts for, 515
   function of, 507
   medical terms for, 513–526
   organs of, 508–509
   sound perception by, 508f
   suffixes for, 510
   surgical terms from word parts for, 518
   word parts for, 509–510
ear, nose, and throat (ENT), 523, 526
eardrum (tympanic membrane), 507–508
ecchymosis, 121, 123f
ECG (electrocardiogram), 372, 406
ech/o, 364
echocardiogram (ECHO), 372, 406
eclampsia, 321
-ectasis, 139
-ectomy, 97, 139, 192, 233, 271, 364, 421, 469, 510, 545, 599, 644
ectopic pregnancy, 321, 321f
eczema, 105
ED (erectile dysfunction), 239, 258
EDD (expected date of delivery), 349
edema, 121, 152
EEG (electroencephalogram), 615, 631
effusion, 174
EGD (esophagogastroduodenoscopy), 442, 455
ejaculation, 256
EKG (electrocardiogram), 372, 406

electr/o, 364, 509, 545
electrocardiogram (ECG, EKG), 372, 406
electrocardiography, 372, 381
electrocochleography, 521
electroencephalogram (EEG), 615, 631
electroencephalograph, 615
electroencephalography, 615
electrolytes, 219
electromyogram (EMG), 570, 584
electrophysiologist, 372
elimination, 417
ellipsis, 28
Em (emmetropia), 492, 497
embolectomy, 370
embolism
   cerebral, 603
   pulmonary, 152, 152f, 178
embol/o, 364, 598
embryo, 314, 315f
emesis, 451
EMG (electromyogram), 570, 584
-emia, 139, 192, 365, 644
emmetropia (Em), 492, 497
emphysema, 151
encapsulated, 36
encephalitis, 603
encephal/o, 598
encephalomalacia, 603
encephalomyeloradiculitis, 603
encephalopathy, 603
endarterectomy, 370
endo-, 138, 271, 364, 469
endocarditis, 370
endocervical, 299
endocrine glands, 640–643
endocrine system, 18t, 639–670, 640f
   abbreviations for, 664
   anatomy of, 640–643
   combining forms for, 643
   complementary terms from word parts for, 659–660
   diagnostic imaging for, 657
   diagnostic terms not from word parts for, 657
   disease and disorder terms from word parts for, 647–648
   disease and disorder terms not from word parts for, 650–651
   function of, 640
   laboratory tests for, 657
   prefixes for, 643
   suffixes for, 644
   surgical terms from word parts for, 656
   word parts for, 643–644
endocrin/o, 643
endocrinologist, 660
endocrinology, 660
endocrinopathy, 647
endograft, 377f
endometrial ablation, 288, 289f
endometrial cancer, 279f, 280
endometri/o, 270
endometriosis, 275, 276f
endometritis, 275
endometrium, 268
endophthalmitis, 474
endoscope, 162
endoscopic, 162
endoscopic retrograde cholangiopancreatography (ERCP), 445, 455
endoscopic ultrasound (EUS), 445, 455
endoscopy, 161–162
   capsule, 441, 441f
endosteum, 534
endotracheal, 171

endovascular stenting, 377f
end-stage kidney disease (ESKD), 222
end-stage renal disease (ESRD), 201, 222
ENT (ear, nose, and throat; otolaryngologist), 523, 526
enteritis, 426
enter/o, 420
enteropathy, 426
enterorrhaphy, 434
enucleation, 247, 483
enuresis, 218
eosinophils, 361f
EP studies (evoked potential studies), 615, 631
epi-, 97
epicardium, 359
epidermal, 117
epidermis, 96
epididymectomy, 243
epididymis, 231
epididymitis, 236
epididym/o, 233
epigastric region, 71
epiglottis, 135–136
epiglottitis, 145
epiglott/o, 138
epilepsy, 608
epinephrine (adrenaline), 642
epiphysis, 535
episi/o, 270, 316
episiorrhaphy, 284
episiotomy (perineotomy), 331, 331f
epispadias, 201
epistaxis (rhinorrhagia), 147, 151
epithelial, 28
epithelial tissue, 17
epitheli/o, 20
epithelioma, 32
eponyms, 3, 3f, 14
Erasistratus, 596
ERCP (endoscopic retrograde cholangiopancreatography), 445, 455
erectile dysfunction (ED), 239, 258
erythema, 48
erythr/o, 21, 97, 364
erythroblastosis fetalis, 326
erythrocyte sedimentation rate (ESR), 402, 406
erythrocytes (red blood cells, RBCs), 28, 53, 361, 406
erythrocytopenia, 390
erythrocytosis, 28
erythroderma, 116
-es, 52t
ESKD (end-stage kidney disease), 222
esophageal, 449
esophageal atresia, 326
esophageal candidiasis, with AIDS, 105
esophagitis, 426
esophag/o, 316, 420
esophagogastroduodenoscopy (EGD), 442, 455
esophagogastroplasty, 435
esophagogram, 441
esophagoscopy, 442
esophagus, 418
ESR (erythrocyte sedimentation rate), 402, 406
ESRD (end-stage renal disease), 201, 222
esthesi/o, 598
ESWL (extracorporeal shock wave lithotripsy), 204, 222
eti/o, 21
etiology, 45
eu-, 138, 643
euglycemia, 659

eupnea, 170
EUS (endoscopic ultrasound), 445, 455
eustachian tube, 508
euthyroid, 660
eversion, 580, 580f
evoked potential studies (EP studies), 615, 631
exacerbation, 49
excision, 114
exercise stress test, 381
exhalation (expiration), 135, 137f
exocrine glands, 640
exophthalmos, 660
exostosis (spur), 559
expected date of delivery (EDD), 349
expiration (exhalation), 135, 137f
extension, 580, 580f
external auditory canal (external auditory meatus), 507–508
external ear, 507–508
external respiration, 135
extracorporeal, 204
extracorporeal shock wave lithotripsy (ESWL), 204, 222
extravasation, 395
extrinsic factors, 394
eye, 465–502
   abbreviations for, 497–498
   anatomy of, 466–468, 467f
   combining forms for, 468–469
   complementary terms from word parts for, 492–493
   complementary terms not from word parts for, 492–493
   diagnostic imaging for, 487–488
   diagnostic terms from word parts for, 487–488
   disease and disorder terms from word parts for, 474
   disease and disorder terms not from word parts for, 477–479
   function of, 466
   light pathway in, 468f
   medical terms for, 474–477
   ophthalmic evaluation of, 487–488
   organs of, 466
   prefixes for, 469
   suffixes for, 469
   surgical terms from word parts for, 483
   surgical terms not from words parts for, 483
   word parts for, 468–473
eyelids, 466

F

FA (fluorescein angiography), 487, 497
facelift (rhytidectomy), 113
fallopian tubes (uterine tubes), 268
Fallopius, Gabriele, 268
familial polyposis, 427
farsightedness (hyperopia), 478, 478f
FAS (fetal alcohol syndrome), 326, 348
fascia, 540
fasciitis, 553
fasci/o, 544
fasciotomy, 565
fasting blood sugar (FBS), 657, 664
fatigue, 48
FCC (fibrocystic breast changes), 280, 303
febrile, 48
fecal immunochemical test (FIT), 446, 447f, 455
fecal occult blood test (gFOBT), guaiac-based, 446, 455
feces, 452

female reproductive system, 266–309
  abbreviations for, 303–304
  anatomy of, 267f, 267–270
  combining forms for, 270–271
  complementary terms from word parts for, 298–299
  complementary terms not from word parts for, 299–300
  diagnostic imaging for, 291–292
  diagnostic terms from word parts for, 291–292
  disease and disorder terms from word parts for, 275–276
  disease and disorder terms not from word parts for, 279–280
  external structures of, 268
  function of, 267
  glands of, 270
  laboratory tests for, 294
  medical terms for, 275–304
  organs and anatomical structures of, 268–269
  prefixes for, 271
  suffixes for, 271
  surgical terms from word parts for, 284–285
  surgical terms not from words parts for, 288–289
  word parts for, 270–275
female surgical sterilization (tubal ligation), 289, 289f
female urinary system, 191f
femoral, 575
femor/o, 544
femoropopliteal bypass, 380
femur, 539
fertilization (conception), 314, 314f
fetal, 344
fetal alcohol syndrome (FAS), 326, 348
fet/o, 315
fetus, 314, 314f
fever, 363
fibrillation, 378
fibr/o, 20
fibrocystic breast changes (FCC), 280, 303
fibroma, 32
fibromyalgia, 553
fibrosarcoma, 32
fibula, 539
fibular, 575
fibul/o, 544
fimbria, 268
fine needle aspiration (FNA), 657, 664
fissure, 106
fistula, 299
FIT (fecal immunochemical test), 446, 447f, 455
flap reconstruction mammoplasty, 284
flatus, 451
flexion, 580, 580f
floating kidney (nephroptosis), 198
flu (influenza), 151, 178
fluorescein angiography (FA), 487, 497
fluoroscopy, 80t, 81
FNA (fine needle aspiration), 657, 664
follicle-stimulating hormone (FSH), 641, 664
food pathway, in digestive system, 419f
formed elements, 361
Fowler position, 76
fracture (fx), 559, 584
frontal (coronal), 74, 74f
frontotemporal dementia (Pick disease), 609t
FSH (follicle-stimulating hormone), 641, 664

FTSG (full-thickness skin graft), 126
fulguration, for urinary bladder, 204, 205f
full-thickness skin graft (FTSG), 126
fundoscopy, 488
fundus, 268, 418
fungal infections, 107t
fungi, 49
fungus, 49
furuncle (boil), 106
fx (fracture), 559, 584

G

gait, 623
gallbladder, 419, 419f
gallstones (cholelithiasis), 426
gamete, 314
gangliectomy (ganglionectomy), 612
gangliitis, 603
gangli/o, 598
ganglion, 597
ganglion cyst, 559
ganglionectomy (ganglionectomy), 612
ganglion/o, 598
gangrene, 106
gastrectomy, 435
gastric gavage, 344
gastric ulcer, 431
gastritis, 426
gastr/o, 420
gastroenteritis, 426
gastroenterologist, 449
gastroenterology, 449
gastroesophageal reflux disease (GERD), 430, 455
gastrointestinal (GI), 455. See also digestive system
gastrojejunostomy, 435
gastroplasty, 435
gastroschisis, 326
gastroscope, 442
gastroscopy, 442
gastrostomy, 435
gavage, 344
-gen, 21, 316
gene therapy, 18
genes, 17
genetic testing, 41
-genic, 21, 97, 139, 316, 365, 599
genital herpes, 255
genital warts, 255
genitalia, 232
genome, 18
genomics, 18
GERD (gastroesophageal reflux disease), 430, 455
gestation period, 314
gestation (pregnancy), 314
  medical terms for, 314–315
  skin in, 315
gFOBT (guaiac-based fecal occult blood test), 446, 455
GFR (glomerular filtration rate), 202, 210, 222
GH (growth hormone), 641, 664
GI (gastrointestinal), 455. See also digestive system
gigantism, 651
gingivectomy, 435
gingivitis, 426
gingiv/o, 420
glands
  adrenal, 642
  Bartholin, 270
  ductless, 640
  endocrine, 640–643

glands (Continued)
  meibomian, 466
  of female reproductive system, 270
  parathyroid, 642, 642f
  pineal, 642f
  pituitary. See pituitary gland
  prostate, 232
  salivary, 419
  sebaceous, 96
  sudoriferous glands, 96
  thymus, 362
  thyroid, 642, 642f
glans penis, 232
glaucoma, 478
glia, 597
gli/o, 598
glioblastoma, 603
glioma, 603
glomerular filtration rate (GFR), 202, 210, 222
glomerul/o, 192
glomerulonephritis, 197
glomerulus, 189
glossitis, 426
gloss/o, 420
glossorrhaphy, 435
gluten enteropathy (celiac disease), 430
glycemia, 660
glyc/o, 643
glycos/o, 192
glycosuria, 214
glycosylated hemoglobin (HbA1C), 657, 664
gno/o, 21
goiter, 660
gonadotropic hormones, 641
gonads, 232
gonorrhea, 255
gout, 559
Graaf, Reinier de, 268
graafian follicles, 268
-gram, 62, 192, 271, 365, 421, 510, 545
-graph, 62
-graphy, 62, 192, 271, 316, 365, 421, 469, 510, 545, 599
Graves disease, 651
gravida, 338
gravid/o, 315, 338t
gravidopuerperal, 338
gray matter, 595
Greek, medical terms from, 2–3, 14
growth hormone (GH), 641, 664
guaiac-based fecal occult blood test (gFOBT), 446, 455
GYN (gynecology), 299, 303
gynec/o, 271
gynecologic laparoscopy (pelviscopy), 292
gynecologic surgery, 281
gynecologist, 299
gynecology (GYN), 299, 303

H

H. pylori (Helicobacter pylori), 455
  antibodies test, 446
hair, 96
hairy cell leukemia (HCL), 393t
hallux valgus, 558
hammer (malleus), 508
HA-MRSA (healthcare-associated MRSA), 126
HAP (hospital-acquired pneumonia), 178
hard of hearing (HOH), 526
hard palate, 417
Hashimoto thyroiditis, 651
HbA1C (glycosylated hemoglobin), 657, 664

Index

HCL (hairy cell leukemia), 393t
Hct (hematocrit), 394, 406
HD (hemodialysis), 204, 218, 219f, 222
HDL (high-density lipoprotein), 382t
headaches, 619
healthcare-associated MRSA (HA-MRSA), 126
heart, 359–360
    congestive heart failure, 378
    hypertensive heart disease, 378, 405
    interior of, 360f
    myocardial infarction of, 378, 405
    rheumatic disease of, 379
heart attack (myocardial infarction), 370, 378, 405
heart failure (HF), 378, 405
heat/moisture exchanger (HME), 180
Helicobacter pylori (*H. pylori*), 455
    antibodies test, 446
hemangiomas, 327
hemarthrosis, 575
hematemesis, 452
hemat/o, 20, 271, 364, 598
hematochezia, 452
hematocrit (Hct), 394, 406
hematologist, 390
hematology, 41
hematology studies, 40t
hematoma, 390
    subdural, 604
hematopoiesis, 360
hematopoietic stem cells, 361
hematosalpinx, 275
hematuria, 214
hemi-, 421, 598
hemicolectomy, 435
hemiparesis, 619
hemiplegia, 619
hem/o, 138, 192, 364, 545, 598
hemochromatosis, 430
hemodialysis (HD), 204, 218, 219f, 222
hemoglobin (Hgb), 395, 406
hemolysis, 390
hemolytic disease of the newborn, 326
hemophilia, 393, 394
hemoptysis, 170
hemorrhage, 390
hemorrhagic stroke, 609–610
hemorrhoidectomy, 439
hemorrhoids, 430
hemostasis, 390
hemothorax, 145
hepatic duct, 419, 419f
hepatitis, 426
hepat/o, 420
hepatoma, 426
hepatomegaly, 449
hernia, 139, 420, 421f
herniated disk (slipped disk, ruptured disk, herniated intervertebral disk), 559
herniated nucleus pulposus (HNP), 559, 584
herni/o, 420
herniorrhaphy, 435
herpes, 106, 255
herpes zoster (shingles), 107t, 609
    postherpetic neuralgia and, 609
HF (heart failure), 378, 405
Hgb (hemoglobin), 395, 406
HHD (hypertensive heart disease), 378, 405
hiatal hernia, 421f
hidradenitis, 101
hidr/o, 96
high-density lipoprotein (HDL), 382t
hilum, 189
hindbrain (cerebellum), 596

hip resurfacing arthroplasty (HRA), 566f, 566t
Hippocrates, 2, 27, 45, 608
hist/o, 20
histology, 28
histopathology, 41
HIV (human immunodeficiency virus), 255, 258
    dementia and, 609t
hives (urticaria), 109
HME (heat/moisture exchanger), 180
HNP (herniated nucleus pulposus), 559, 584
Hodgkin lymphoma, 398
HOH (hard of hearing), 526
holmium laser enucleation of the prostate gland (HoLEP), 247, 248f, 250t, 259
hordeolum (sty), 479
hormone(s), 640–643, 660
    adrenocorticotropic, 641, 664
    antidiuretic, 641, 664
    follicle stimulating, 641, 664
    growth, 641, 664
    luteinizing, 641, 664
    parathyroid, 642, 664
    pituitary gland, 641f, 641–642
    thyroid-stimulating, 657, 664
hormone therapy, 240t, 299
hospice, 36
hospital-acquired pneumonia (HAP), 178
HPV (human papillomavirus)
    description of, 255, 258
    test, 294, 295t
    vaccine for, 279
HRA (hip resurfacing arthroplasty), 566f, 566t
HRT (hormone replacement therapy), 299, 303
HSG (hysterosalpingogram), 291, 303
HTN (hypertension), 383, 405
human immunodeficiency virus (HIV), 255, 258
    dementia and, 609t
human papillomavirus (HPV)
    description of, 255, 258
    test for, 294, 295t
    vaccine for, 279
humeral, 575
humer/o, 544
humerus, 536
humpback (kyphosis), 554
hunchback (kyphosis), 554
hyaline membrane disease, 327
hydramnios (polyhydramnios), 320
hydr/o, 192, 271, 316, 598
hydrocele, 239
hydrocelectomy, 247
hydrocephalus, 603
hydrocortisone (cortisol), 642
hydronephrosis, 197
hydrosalpinx, 275
hymen, 268
hymen/o, 271
hymenotomy, 284
hyper-, 21, 97, 138, 233, 545, 598, 643
hypercalcemia, 647
hypercapnia, 170
hypercholesterolemia, 383
hyperesthesia, 619
hyperglycemia, 647
hyperkalemia, 647
hyperkinesia, 575
hyperlipidemia, 383
hyperopia (farsightedness), 478, 478f
hyperparathyroidism, 647
hyperpituitarism, 647

hyperplasia, 28, 37f
hyperpnea, 170
hypersensitivity, 403
hypertension (HTN), 383, 405
hypertensive heart disease (HHD), 378, 405
hyperthyroidism, 647
hypertrichosis, 116
hypertriglyceridemia, 383
hypertrophy, 575
hyperventilation, 174
hyphema, 478
hyphemia, 478
hypo-, 21, 71, 97, 138, 643
hypocalcemia, 648
hypocapnia, 170
hypochondriac, 71
hypochondriac regions, 71
hypodermic, 117
hypodermis, 96
hypogastric region, 71
hypoglycemia, 648
hypokalemia, 648
hyponatremia, 648
hypophysis cerebri, 641
hypopituitarism, 648
hypoplasia, 28
hypopnea, 170
hypospadias, 201
hypotension, 383
hypothalamus, 642
hypoventilation, 174
hypoxemia, 170
hypoxia, 170
hysterectomy, 284, 285t
hyster/o, 271, 316
hysteropexy, 284
hysterorrhexis, 320
hysterosalpingogram (HSG), 291, 303
hysteroscope, 292
hysteroscopy, 292
hysterosonography (sonohysterography, SHG), 292, 303

I

-i, 52t
-ia, 97, 139, 233, 365, 421, 469, 545, 599, 644
-iasis, 192, 421
-iatrist, 599
iatr/o, 21
iatrogenic, 45
-iatry, 599
IBS (irritable bowel syndrome), 431, 455
-ic, 21, 62, 97, 139, 233, 271, 316, 365, 421, 469, 545
-ices, 52t
-ictal, 599
icterus (jaundice), 121
ID (intradermal), 117, 126
I&D (incision and drainage), 114, 126
IDDM (insulin-dependent diabetes mellitus), 652t
idiopathic, 49
idiopathic pulmonary fibrosis (IPF), 151, 178
-ies, 52t
ile/o, 420
ileocecal, 449
ileostomy, 435
ileum, 418, 544
ileus, 430
iliac, 575
iliac regions, 71
ili/o, 544
ilium, 539, 544

Index

immune deficiency disorders. *See also*
    acquired immunodeficiency syndrome;
    human immunodeficiency virus
immune system, 363, 363f
    abbreviations for, 405–406
    complementary terms not from word
        parts for, 402–403
    function of, 18t, 363
    medical terms for, 401–405
immunity, 403
immun/o, 364
immunodeficiency, 402
immunoglobulin (antibody), 403
immunologist, 401
immunology, 401
immunosuppression, 403
immunotherapy, 36, 240t
impetigo, 106, 107t
implant mammoplasty, 284
implantation, 314, 314f
impotence, 239
in situ, 36
in vitro, 339
in vitro fertilization (IVF), 331, 332f, 348
in vivo, 339
incision, 114
incision and drainage (I&D), 114, 126
incoherent, 623
incontinence, 218
incretins, 660
incus (anvil), 508
induration, 121
inf (inferior), 66, 68t, 85
infection
    definition of, 49
    nosocomial, 175
    opportunistic, 402
    sexually transmitted, 258
    skin, 106, 107t
    types of, 107t
    upper respiratory, 152, 178
    urinary tract, 197f, 201, 222
infectious mononucleosis, 399
inferior (inf), 66, 68t, 85
inferior vena cava, 359–360
infer/o, 61
infertility, 240
inflammation, 48, 363
influenza (flu), 151, 178
ingestion, 417
inguinal hernia, 421f
inguinal regions, 71
inhalation (inspiration), 135, 137f
inherited immunity, 403
inner ear, 507–508
    for balance, 507
INR (international normalized ratio), 395
insidious, 150
inspiration (inhalation), 135, 137f
insulin resistance syndrome (metabolic
    syndrome), 651
insulin-dependent diabetes mellitus
    (IDDM), 652t
integumentary system, 18t, 94–131.
    See also skin
    abbreviations for, 126
    anatomy of, 95–96
    combining forms for, 96–97
    complementary terms from word parts
        for, 116–117
    medical terms for, 101–127
    medical terms not from word parts for,
        104–109
    prefixes for, 97
    suffixes for, 97
    surgical terms from word parts for, 113–116

integumentary system (Continued)
    surgical terms not from words parts for,
        113–114
    word parts for, 96–101
inter-, 545, 598
intercostal, 575
interferons, 37t, 363
interictal, 619
intermittent claudication, 378
intermittent positive-pressure breathing
    (IPPB), 180
international normalized ratio (INR), 395
interventional radiologists, 81
intervertebral, 575
intervertebral disk, 539
intra-, 97, 138, 192, 316, 364, 469,
    545, 598
intracerebral hemorrhage, 603
intracranial, 575
intradermal (ID), 117
intraocular, 492
intraocular lens (IOL), 493
intraocular pressure (IOP), 497
intrapartum, 338
intrapleural, 171
intrauterine device (IUD), 300f, 303
intrauterine system (IUS), 303
intravenous (IV), 372, 406
intravenous (IV) therapy, 372
intravenous urogram (IVU), 210f
intravesical, 215
intrinsic factors, 394
intussusception, 430
inversion, 580, 580f
IOL (intraocular lens), 493
IOP (intraocular pressure), 497
-ior, 62
IPF (idiopathic pulmonary fibrosis),
    151, 178
IPPB (intermittent positive-pressure
    breathing), 180
iridectomy, 483
irid/o, 468
iridoplegia, 474
iridotomy, 483
iris, 466
iritis, 474
ir/o, 468
irritable bowel syndrome (IBS), 431, 455
-is, 52t, 545
ischemia, 370
ischemic stroke, 609
ischial, 575
ischi/o, 544
ischium, 539
isch/o, 364
islets of Langerhans, 642, 643f
-ism, 233, 365, 599, 644
is/o, 469
isocoria, 492
-itis, 97, 139, 192, 233, 271, 316, 365, 421,
    469, 510, 545, 599, 644
IUD (intrauterine device), 300f, 303
IUS (intrauterine system), 303
IV (intravenous), 372, 406
IV (intravenous) therapy, 372
IVF (in vitro fertilization), 331, 332f, 348
IVU (intravenous urogram), 210f
-ix, 52t

J

jaundice (icterus), 121
jejun/o, 420
jejunum, 418
joint fusion (arthrodesis), 565

joints (articulations)
    of knee, 540f
    of musculoskeletal system, 539–540

K

kal/i, 643
Kaposi sarcoma, 106
keloid, 106
keratin, 96
keratitis, 474
kerat/o, 96, 468
keratoconus, 478
keratogenic, 117
keratomalacia, 474
keratometer, 487
keratoplasty, 483
keratosis, 101
ketoacidosis, 651
kidney, 189
    chronic kidney disease, 201, 222
    computed tomography of, 209f
    polycystic kidney disease, 201
kidney, ureter, and bladder (KUB), 210, 222
kidney stones (nephrolithiasis), 197
kidney transplant (renal transplant), 204,
    205f
kinesi/o, 545
knee
    arthritis of, 553f
    joint of, 540f
KUB (kidney, ureter, and bladder), 210, 222
kyph/o, 545
kyphoplasty, 567t
kyphosis (hunchback, humpback), 554

L

laboratory tests
    for blood, 394–395
    for cardiovascular system, 382
    for digestive system, 446
    for endocrine system, 657
    for female reproductive system, 294
    from word parts, 41
    for male reproductive system, 253
    not from word parts, 41
    types of, 40t
    for urinary system, 210
labyrinth, 508
labyrinthectomy, 518
labyrinthitis, 513
labyrinth/o, 509
laceration, 106
lacrimal, 492
lacrimal apparatus, 466, 467f
lacrim/o, 468
lactation, 339
lact/o, 315
lactogenic, 338
lactorrhea, 338
lamina, 536
laminectomy, 565
lamin/o, 544
lapar/o, 420
laparoscope, 442
laparoscopic cholecystectomy, 434, 434f
laparoscopic radical prostatectomy, 243t
laparoscopically assisted vaginal
    hysterectomy (LAVH), 285f, 303
laparoscopy, 442
    gynecologic, 292
laparotomy (celiotomy), 435
large cell carcinoma, of lung, 146f
large intestine, 418
    anatomy of, 417f
    diverticula of, 421f

laryngeal, 171
laryngectomy, 156
laryngitis, 145
laryng/o, 138
laryngomalacia, 326
laryngoplasty, 156
laryngoscope, 162
laryngoscopy, 162
laryngospasm, 145
laryngostomy, 156
laryngotracheobronchitis (LTB, croup), 145, 151, 178
laryngotracheotomy, 156
larynx (voice box), 135–136
laser surgery, 114, 247
laser-assisted in situ keratomileusis (LASIK), 483, 484f, 498
last menstrual period (LMP), 349
lateral (lat), 66, 85
lateral position, 76
lateral recumbent position, 76
later/o, 61
Latin, medical terms from, 2–3, 14
LAVH (laparoscopically assisted vaginal hysterectomy), 285f, 303
lazy eye (amblyopia), 477
LDL (low-density lipoprotein), 382t
LEEP (loop electrosurgical excision procedure), 303
left atrium, 359–360
left eye (OS), 498
left lateral decubitus position, 77t
left lateral recumbent position, 77t
left lower lobe (LLL), 179
left lower quadrant (LLQ), 85–86
left semiprone position, 77t
left upper lobe (LUL), 179
left upper quadrant (LUQ), 85–86
left ventricle, 359–360
lei/o, 21
leiomyoma, 32
　uterine fibroid as, 280
leiomyosarcoma, 32
lens, 466
lesions, 121
leukemia, 361, 393, 393t
leuk/o, 21, 97, 271, 364, 469
leukocoria, 492
leukocytes (white blood cells, WBC), 28, 53, 361, 361f, 406
leukocytopenia (leukopenia), 390
leukocytosis, 28
leukopenia (leukocytopenia), 390
leukoplakia, 121
leukorrhea, 299
Lewy body dementia, 609t
LH (luteinizing hormone), 641, 664
ligament, 540
light pathway, in eye, 468f
linea nigra, 315
lingu/o, 420
lipid profile, 382, 382t
lip/o, 20
lipoid, 28
lipoma, 32
liposarcoma, 32
-lith, 192, 233, 421
lith/o, 192, 233, 420
lithotomy position, 76
lithotripsy, 203
liver, 419, 419f
L1-L5 (lumbar vertebrae), 536, 584
LLL (left lower lobe), 179
LLQ (left lower quadrant), 85–86
LMP (last menstrual period), 349
lobar pneumonia, 145

lobe, 138
lobectomy, 157, 157f
lob/o, 138
lochia, 339
-logist, 21, 27, 62, 97, 139, 192, 271, 316, 365, 421, 469, 510, 599, 644
-logy, 21, 62, 97, 139, 192, 271, 316, 365, 421, 469, 510, 599, 644
loop electrosurgical excision procedure (LEEP), 303
lord/o, 545
lordosis (swayback), 554
Lou Gehrig disease (amyotrophic lateral sclerosis), 608, 630
low sperm count, 255
low-density lipoprotein (LDL), 382t
lower GI series (barium enema), 446f
lower respiratory infection, 153f
lower urinary tract symptoms (LUTS), 258
LP (lumbar puncture), 615, 631
LTB (laryngotracheobronchitis), 145, 151, 178
LUL (left upper lobe), 179
lumbar, 575
lumbar puncture (LP, spinal tap), 615, 631
lumbar region, 71
lumbar vertebrae (L1-L5), 536, 584
lumb/o, 544
lumpectomy (partial mastectomy, breast-conserving surgery), 286t
lung(s), 135–137
　resection of, 157f
lung cancer (bronchogenic carcinoma), 145, 146f
lung ventilation/perfusion scan (V/Q scan), 166, 179
LUQ (left upper quadrant), 85–86
luteinizing hormone (LH), 641, 664
LUTS (lower urinary tract symptoms), 258
luxation, 559
Lyme disease, 559
lymph, 362
lymph nodes, 362, 367
lymphadenitis, 398
lymphaden/o, 364, 367
lymphadenopathy, 398
lymphangiography, 398
lymphangitis, 398
lymphatic system, 361, 362f
　abbreviations for, 405–406
　combining forms for, 364
　disease and disorder terms from word parts for, 398
　disease and disorder terms not from word parts for, 399
　function of, 18t, 361
　medical terms for, 398–401
　organs and anatomical structures of, 362
　surgical terms from word parts for, 370–371
lymphatic vessels, 362
lymphedema, 399
lymph/o, 364
lymphocytes, 361f, 362, 401
lymphocytic leukemia, 393t
lymphocytosis, 390
lymphoma, 361, 398
-lysis, 192, 365, 599

M

-ma, 52t
macula, 466, 478
macular degeneration, 478
macule, 121, 122t
magnetic resonance (MR), 85

magnetic resonance angiography (MRA), 371t
magnetic resonance imaging (MRI), 80t, 85, 240t
　definition of, 81
　multiparametric, 253
　for musculoskeletal system, 570, 571f, 571t
magnetic resonance imaging–transrectal ultrasound (MRI-TRUS), 253
major depression, 628
malabsorption, 452
-malacia, 97, 316, 469, 545, 599
male reproductive system, 230–263
　abbreviations for, 258–259
　anatomy of, 231–232
　combining forms for, 233
　complementary terms from word parts for, 255
　complementary terms not from word parts for, 256
　diagnostic terms not from word parts for, 253
　disease and disorder terms from word parts for, 236–237
　disease and disorder terms not from word parts for, 239–241
　function of, 231
　medical terms for, 236–263
　organs and anatomical structures of, 231f, 231–232
　prefixes for, 233
　suffixes for, 233
　surgical terms from word parts for, 243
　surgical terms not from words parts for, 247–248
　word parts for, 233–235
male urinary bladder, 191f
male urinary system, 191f
malignant, 36–37
malignant tumors, 31, 37f
　breast, surgeries for, 286t
　connective tissue, 32
malleus (hammer), 508
mammary papilla, 270
mamm/o, 271
mammogram, 291
mammography (digital mammography), 292
mammoplasty, 284
mandible, 535
mandibul/o, 544
mastalgia, 299
mastectomy, 285
mastitis, 275
mast/o, 271
mastoid bone (mastoid process), 509
mastoid process (mastoid bone), 509
mastoidectomy, 518
mastoiditis, 513
mastoid/o, 509
mastoidotomy, 518
mastopexy, 285
-mata, 52t
maxilla, 535
maxillectomy, 565
maxill/o, 544
MBS (modified barium swallow), 445, 455
MCI (mild cognitive impairment), 623t
MD (muscular dystrophy), 559, 584
MDI (metered-dose inhaler), 180
measles, 106
meatal, 215
meat/o, 192
meatotomy, 203
meatus, 189
meconium, 344

Index

med (medial), 66, 85
MED (microendoscopic discectomy), 565
medial (med), 66, 85
mediastinal, 171
mediastin/o, 138
mediastinoscopy, 162
mediastinum, 136–137
medical genomics, 18
medical language, 2
   origins of, 2–3
medical terms
   analyzing, 9, 12*t*
   for blood, 390–397
   for body, 28–53
   building, 9, 11, 12*t*
   for cardiovascular system, 369–389
   categories of, 4, 4*t*
   defining, 9–11, 12*t*
   for diagnostic procedures and tests, 161–162, 166
   for digestive system, 426–455
   for direction, 60–91
   for ear, 513–526
   for eye, 474–477
   for female reproductive system, 275–304
   from Greek and Latin, 2–3, 14
   from word parts, 4–13
      learning techniques for, 12*t*
   for immune system, 401–405
   for integumentary system, 101–127, 104–109
   for lymphatic system, 398–401
   for male reproductive system, 236–263
   for musculoskeletal system, 552–584
   for neonatology, 320–349
   for nervous system, 603–631
   not from word parts, 14
   for obstetrics, 320–349
   for oncology, 31–32
   plural endings for, 51, 52*t*
   for pregnancy, 314–315
   for pulmonary function, 166
   for respiratory system, 145–185
   suffixes for, 5
   for urinary system, 197–222
medi/o, 61
mediolateral, 66
medulla oblongata, 596
-megaly, 21, 192, 365, 421, 644
meibomian cyst (chalazion), 477
meibomian glands, 466
melanin, 96
melan/o, 21
melanoma, 32, 105*f*
melena, 452
menarche, 300
Ménière disease, 515
meninges, 596, 596*f*
meningi/o, 598
meningioma, 603
meningitis, 603
mening/o, 598
meningocele, 604
meningomyelocele (myelomeningocele), 327*f*, 604
meniscectomy, 565
meniscitis, 554
menisc/o, 544
meniscus, 539
men/o, 271
menometrorrhagia, 275
menopause, 300
menorrhagia, 275
mental, 619
ment/o, 598
MET (metastasis), 32

meta-, 21
metabolic syndrome (syndrome X, insulin resistance syndrome), 651
metabolism, 660
metacarpus (metacarpal bones), 536
metastases (METS), 53
metastasis (MET), 32, 32*f*
metatarsal bones, 539
-meter, 139, 469, 510
metered-dose inhaler (MDI), 180
methicillin-resistant *Staphylococcus aureus* (MRSA), 106, 126
metr/o, 271
metrorrhagia, 275
-metry, 139, 469, 510
METS (metastases), 53
MG (myasthenia gravis), 559, 584
MI (myocardial infarction), 370, 378, 405
micro-, 21, 316, 545
microbiology, 41
microbiology studies, 40*t*
microcephalus, 326
microdiscectomy, 565
microendoscopic discectomy (MED), 565
microorganism, 49
microscopy, 40*t*
midbrain, 596
middle ear, 507*f*, 507–508
midline, 74
midsagittal, 74*f*, 74–75
midwife, 339
midwifery, 339
migraine, 608, 619
mild cognitive impairment (MCI), 623*t*
minimally invasive surgical treatments (MISTs), 248, 249*f*, 250*t*, 259
miotic, 493
MISTs (minimally invasive surgical treatments), 248, 249*f*, 250*t*, 259
mitral valve, 359–360
   stenosis, 378
modern language, 3, 3*f*, 14
modified barium swallow (MBS), 445, 455
modified radical mastectomy, 286*t*
modified Trendelenburg position, 77
Mohs, Frederic E., 114
Mohs surgery, 114
mole (nevus), 121
mon/o, 598
monocytes, 361*f*, 362
mononeuropathy, 604
monoparesis, 619
monoplegia, 619
mood disorder, 628
morcellation, 248
mother, 345*t*
mouth, 417
movement disorders (dyskinesia), 575
MR (magnetic resonance), 85
MRA (magnetic resonance angiography), 371*t*
MRI (magnetic resonance imaging), 80*t*, 85, 240*t*
   definition of, 81
   multiparametric, 253
   for musculoskeletal system, 570, 571*f*, 571*t*
MRI ultrasound fusion biopsy, 253
MRI-TRUS (magnetic resonance imaging-transrectal ultrasound), 253
MRSA (methicillin-resistant *Staphylococcus aureus*), 106, 126
MS (multiple sclerosis), 608, 630
MSR (muscle stretch reflexes), 615
muc/o, 138
mucoid, 171

mucopurulent, 175
mucous, 171
mucus, 175
mucus membranes, 135
multi-, 316
multigravida, 338
multipara (multip), 338, 348
multiparametric MRI, 253
multiple infarct dementia, 609*t*
multiple myeloma, 390
   thalidomide for, 37*t*
multiple sclerosis (MS), 608, 630
murmur, 383
muscle
   anatomy of, 541*f*–543*f*
   cardiac, 540, 543*f*
   definition of, 540
   skeletal, 540, 543*f*
   smooth, 540, 543*f*
muscle biopsy, 572
muscle stretch reflexes (MSR), 615
muscle tissue, 17
muscular dystrophy (MD), 559, 584
musculoskeletal system, 18*t*, 533–589
   abbreviations for, 584
   anatomy of, 534–543
   body movement types, 580, 580*f*
   bone structure, 534*f*, 534–535
   combining forms for, 544–545
   complementary terms from word parts for, 575–576
   complementary terms not from word parts for, 579–580
   diagnostic imaging for, 570, 571*t*
   diagnostic terms from word parts for, 570
   diagnostic terms not from word parts for, 570–571
   disease and disorder terms from word parts for, 552–554
   functions of, 534
   joints of, 539–540
   medical terms for, 552–584
   muscles of, 540, 541*f*–543*f*
   prefixes for, 545
   skeletal bones of, 535–539, 537*f*–538*f*
   suffixes for, 545
   surgical terms from word parts for, 565
   word parts for, 544–552
myalgia, 575
myasthenia, 575
myasthenia gravis (MG), 559, 584
myc/o, 97, 138, 469, 509
mydriatic, 493
myelitis, 604
myel/o, 364, 598
myelogenous leukemia, 393*t*
myelography, CT, 614
myeloma, 554
myelomalacia, 604
myelomeningocele (meningomyelocele), 327*f*, 604
my/o, 20, 271, 364, 544
myocardial infarction (MI, heart attack), 370, 378, 405
myocardial ischemia, 370
myocarditis, 370
myocardium, 359–360, 540
myoma, 32
   of uterus, 280
myomectomy, 289
myometritis, 276
myometrium, 268
myopathy, 28
myopia (nearsightedness), 478, 478*f*
myorrhaphy, 565

Index

myos/o, 544
myringitis, 513
myring/o, 509
myringoplasty, 518
myringotomy, 518
myxedema, 651

N

NAFLD (nonalcoholic fatty liver disease), 455
nails, 96
nasal polyp, 431f
nasal septum, 135–136
NASH (nonalcoholic steatohepatitis), 431, 455
nas/o, 138, 420, 469
nasogastric, 449
nasolacrimal, 492
nasopharyngeal, 171
nasopharyngitis, 145
natal, 344
nat/o, 315
natr/o, 643
natural killer (NK) cells, 363
nausea, 452
nausea and vomiting (N&V), 455
NB (newborn, neonate), 344, 345t, 348
nearsightedness (myopia), 478, 478f
nebulizer, 175
necr/o, 21, 545
necrosis, 28
negation, prefixes for, 5
neo-, 21, 138, 316
neoadjuvant therapy, 37t
neonate (newborn, NB), 344, 345t, 348
neonatologist, 344
neonatology, 313–353
    abbreviations for, 348
    anatomy for, 314–315
    combining forms for, 315–316
    complementary terms from word parts for, 344
    complementary terms not from word parts for, 344
    disease and disorder terms from word parts for, 326
    disease and disorder terms not from word parts for, 326–327
    medical terms for, 320–349
    prefixes for, 316
    suffixes for, 316
    word parts for, 315–320, 344
neoplasm, 32
nephrectomy, 203
nephritis, 197
nephr/o, 192
nephroblastoma (Wilms tumor), 197
nephrolithiasis (kidney stones), 197
nephrolithotomy, 204, 204f
nephrolithotripsy, 204, 204f
nephrologist, 215
nephrology, 215
nephrolysis, 204
nephroma, 197
nephromegaly, 198
nephron, 189
nephropexy, 204
nephroptosis (floating kidney), 198
nephroscopy, 209
nephrosonography, 209
nephrostomy, 204
nerve(s), 597
    cranial, 597f
    optic, 466
nerve tissue, 17

nervous system, 18t, 593–636, 594f
    abbreviations for, 630–631
    anatomy of, 594–597
    combining forms for, 598
    complementary terms from word parts for, 619
    complementary terms not from word parts for, 622–623
    diagnostic imaging for, 614–615
    diagnostic procedures and tests for, 615
    diagnostic terms from word parts for, 614–615
    diagnostic terms not from word parts for, 615
    disease and disorder terms from word parts for, 603–604
    disease and disorder terms not from word parts for, 608–610
    function of, 594
    medical terms for, 603–631
    organs of, 595–597
    suffixes for, 599
    surgical terms from word parts for, 612
neuralgia, 604
neurectomy, 612
neuritis, 604
neur/o, 20, 598
neuroblastoma, 651
neuroglia, 597
neurohypophysis, 641
neurologist, 619
neurology, 619
neurolysis, 612
neuroma, 32
neuron, 597
neuropathy, 28, 604
neuroplasty, 612
neurorrhaphy, 612
neurotomy, 612
neutrophils, 361f
nevus flammeus (port-wine stain), 327
nevus (mole), 121
newborn (NB, neonate), 344, 345t, 348
-nges, 52t
NIDDM (noninsulin-dependent diabetes mellitus), 652t
night blindness (nyctalopia), 478
nipple-sparing mastectomy (subcutaneous mastectomy), 286t
NIPPV (noninvasive positive-pressure ventilator), 180
NK (natural killer) cells, 363
NM (nuclear medicine), 85
    bone scan, 571t
    definition of, 81
noct/i, 192
nocturia, 214
nocturnal enuresis, 218
nodule, 122, 122t
nonalcoholic fatty liver disease (NAFLD), 455
nonalcoholic steatohepatitis (NASH), 431, 455
non-Hodgkin lymphoma, 398
noninsulin-dependent diabetes mellitus (NIDDM), 652t
noninvasive positive-pressure ventilator (NIPPV), 180
nonobstructive azoospermia, 256
norepinephrine (noradrenaline), 642
normal pressure hydrocephalus, 609t
nose, 135–136
nuchal translucency screening, 335
nuclear medicine (NM), 85
    bone scan, 571t
    definition of, 81

nuclear medicine scanning, 381
nucleus, 17
nulli-, 316
nulligravida, 338
nullipara, 338
numbers, prefixes for, 5
N&V (nausea and vomiting), 455
-nx, 52t
nyctalopia (night blindness), 478
nystagmus, 478

O

O_2 (oxygen), 135, 141, 179
OA (osteoarthritis), 2, 554, 584
    of knee, 2f, 553f
OAB (overactive bladder), 222
OB (obstetrics), 313–353
    abbreviations for, 348
    anatomy for, 314–315
    combining forms for, 315–316
    complementary terms from word parts for, 334
    complementary terms not from word parts for, 339
    diagnostic terms from word parts for, 331
    disease and disorder terms from word parts for, 320
    disease and disorder terms not from word parts for, 320–321
    medical terms for, 320–349
    prefixes for, 316
    suffixes for, 316
    surgical terms from word parts for, 331
    word parts for, 315–320
obesity, 651
oblique, 74
obsessive-compulsive disorder (OCD), 629–630
obstetric ultrasonography (pelvic sonography), 334, 334f
obstetrician, 339
obstetrics (OB), 313–353
    abbreviations for, 348
    anatomy for, 314–315
    combining forms for, 315–316
    complementary terms from word parts for, 334
    complementary terms not from word parts for, 339
    diagnostic terms from word parts for, 331
    disease and disorder terms from word parts for, 320
    disease and disorder terms not from word parts for, 320–321
    medical terms for, 320–349
    prefixes for, 316
    suffixes for, 316
    surgical terms from word parts for, 331
    word parts for, 315–320
obstructive azoospermia, 256
obstructive sleep apnea (OSA), 151, 152f, 175f, 178
occlusion, 383
OCD (obsessive-compulsive disorder), 629–630
OCT (optical coherence tomography), 488, 497
ocul/o, 468
oculomycosis, 474
OD (doctor of optometry), 493
OD (right eye), 498
OE (otitis externa), 515, 526
-oid, 21, 139
olecranon process, 536
olig/o, 192, 233, 271, 316

Index

oligohydramnios, 320
oligomenorrhea, 299
oligoovulation, 299
oligospermia, 255
oliguria, 214
OM (otitis media), 515, 526
-oma, 21, 97, 139, 193, 316, 365, 421, 469, 545, 599, 644
omphalitis, 326
omphal/o, 315
omphalocele, 326
-on, 52t
onc/o, 21
oncogenic, 45
oncologist, 27, 45
oncology. *see also* cancer
   abbreviations for, 53
   complementary terms from word parts for, 45
   definition of, 31, 45
   medical terms from word parts for, 32
   medical terms not from word parts for, 36–37
onych/o, 96
onychocryptosis, 101
onychomalacia, 101
onychomycosis, 101
onychophagia, 101
oophorectomy, 285
oophoritis, 276
oophor/o, 271
Ophth (ophthalmology), 492, 498
ophthalmalgia, 474
ophthalmic, 492
ophthalm/o, 469
ophthalmologist, 492
ophthalmology (Ophth), 492, 498
ophthalmopathy, 474
ophthalmoplegia, 474
ophthalmoscope, 487
ophthalmoscopy, 487
   of retina, 468f
-opia, 469
opportunistic infections, 402
-opsy, 21
optic, 492
optic nerve, 466
optical coherence tomography (OCT), 488, 497
optician, 493
opt/o, 469
optometrist, 493
optometry, 487
oral, 449
oral cancer screening, 460f
oral cavity, 417f
orbit, 466
orchialgia, 255
orchidectomy, 243
orchiditis, 236
orchid/o, 233
orchidopexy, 243
orchidotomy, 243
orchiectomy, 240t, 243
orchiepididymitis, 236
orchi/o, 233
orchiopexy, 243
orchioplasty, 243
orchiotomy, 243
orchitis, 236
orch/o, 233
organ/o, 20
organomegaly, 28
organs
   combining forms of, 420
   defined, 18

organs *(Continued)*
   of cardiovascular system, 359–360
   of digestive system, 416f–417f, 417–419
   of ear, 508–509
   of eye, 466
   of female reproductive system, 268–269
   of lymphatic system, 362
   of male reproductive system, 231f, 231–232
   of nervous system, 595–597
   of respiratory system, 135–137, 136f
   of urinary system, 189
orgasm, 256
or/o, 420
orth/o, 138
orthopedics (ortho), 579, 584
   rheumatology and, 579
orthopedist, 579
orthopnea, 170
orthopnea position (orthopneic position), 76
orthotics, 579
orthotist, 579
OS (left eye), 498
OSA (obstructive sleep apnea), 151, 152f, 175f, 178
-osis, 21, 97, 139, 193, 271, 365, 421, 469, 510, 545, 599
ossicles, 507–508
osteitis, 554
osteoarthritis (OA), 2, 554, 584
   of knee, 2f, 553f
osteochondritis, 554
osteochondroma, 554
osteomalacia, 554
osteomyelitis, 554
osteonecrosis, 554
osteopath (DO), 579
osteopathy, 579
osteopenia, 554
osteopetrosis, 554
osteoporosis, 559
   compression fractures from, 567t
osteosarcoma, 32, 554
osteotomy, 565
otalgia, 513
otitis externa (OE), 515, 526
otitis media (OM), 515, 526
ot/o, 509
otolaryngologist (ear, nose, and throat; ENT), 523, 526
otolaryngology, 523
otomycosis, 513
otoplasty, 518
otopyorrhea, 513
otorhinolaryngologist, 523
otorhinolaryngology, 523
otorrhea, 513
otosclerosis, 513
otoscope, 521
otoscopy, 521
ototoxicity, 515
OU (both eyes), 498
-ous, 21, 97, 139, 365
oval window, 508
ovarian cancer, 280
ovaries, 268
   PCOS, 280, 303
overactive bladder (OAB), 222
overweight, 651
ovulation, 314f
ovum, 268
ox/i, 138
oximeter, 162
oxygen (O$_2$), 135, 141, 179
oxytocin, 641

P

P (pulse), 381, 406
PA (posteroanterior), 66, 85
pachyderma, 101
pachy/o, 97
PAD (peripheral artery disease), 379, 405
PAF (paroxysmal atrial fibrillation), 378
palatal, 449
palate, 417
palat/o, 420
palatoplasty, 435
palliative, 36
pallor, 122
palpate, 452
pan-, 364, 643
pancreas, 419, 419f, 642f–643f
pancreatectomy, 435
pancreatic, 449
pancreatitis, 427
pancreat/o, 420
pancytopenia, 390
panhypopituitarism, 648
panic attack, 629
Pap smear (Papanicolaou test), 294, 295t
Papanicolaou, George N., 294
Papanicolaou test (Pap smear), 294, 295t
papule, 122, 122t
para, 338
para-, 97, 598
par/a, 338t
paracentesis (abdominocentesis), 434
paranasal sinuses, 135–136
paraplegia, 622
parasagittal, 74–75
parasite, 49
parasitic infections, 107t
parathyroid glands, 642, 642f
parathyroid hormone (PTH), 642, 664
parathyroidectomy, 656
parathyroid/o, 643
parathyroidoma, 648
-paresis, 599
paresthesia, 619
Parkinson, James, 609
Parkinson dementia, 609t
Parkinson disease (PD), 609, 630
parkinsonism, 609
par/o, 315
paronychia, 101
paroxysm, 174
paroxysmal atrial fibrillation (PAF), 378
partial mastectomy (lumpectomy), 286t
part/o, 315
parturition, 339
PAS (placenta accreta spectrum), 321, 322f
patella, 539
patellar, 575
patell/o, 544
patellofemoral, 575
patent, 175
path/o, 21
pathogenic, 45
pathologist, 45
pathology, 45
-pathy, 21, 27, 233, 365, 421, 469, 599, 644
PBSCT (peripheral blood stem cell transplant), 395, 406
PCI (percutaneous coronary intervention), 406
PCOS (polycystic ovary syndrome), 280, 303
PCR (polymerase chain reaction), 40t
PD (Parkinson disease), 609, 630
PE (pulmonary embolism), 152, 152f, 178
peak flow meter (PFM), 166, 178

pediculosis, 106
PEG (percutaneous endoscopic gastrostomy), 455
pelv/i, 271, 316, 544
pelvic, 299
pelvic bones, 539
pelvic cavity, 19
pelvic inflammatory disease (PID), 280, 280f, 303
pelvic ultrasound (pelvic sonography), 334, 334f
pelvis, 539
pelviscopic, 292
pelviscopy (gynecologic laparoscopy), 292
-penia, 365, 545
penis, 232
PEP (positive expiratory pressure), 180
-pepsia, 421
peptic ulcer, 431, 431f
per-, 97
percussion, 166
percutaneous, 117
percutaneous coronary intervention (PCI), 406
percutaneous endoscopic gastrostomy (PEG), 455
percutaneous transluminal coronary angioplasty (PTCA, balloon angioplasty), 380, 406
percutaneous vertebroplasty (PV), 567f, 567t
perfusionist, 395
peri-, 271, 364
pericardiocentesis, 370
pericarditis, 370, 371f
pericardium, 359–360
perimetritis, 276
perimetrium, 268
perine/o, 271
perineorrhaphy, 285
perineotomy (episiotomy), 331, 331f
perineum, 269
periosteum, 534
peripheral artery disease (PAD), 379, 405
peripheral blood stem cell transplant (PBSCT), 395, 406
peripheral nervous system (PNS), 594, 631
peripheral neuropathy, 604
peripheral vascular disease (PVD), 379
peristalsis, 418
peritoneal, 449
peritoneal dialysis, 204, 218, 219f
peritone/o, 420
peritoneum, 419
peritonitis, 427
pertussis (whooping cough), 151
PET (positron emission tomography), 80t, 631
 for nervous system, 615
petechia, 123, 123f
petr/o, 545
-pexy, 193, 233, 271, 469
PFM (peak flow meter), 166, 178
PFTs (pulmonary function tests), 166, 178
phac/o, 469
phacoemulsification (PHACO), 483, 498
phacomalacia, 474
phag/o, 97, 420
phagocytosis, 363
phak/o, 469
phalangeal, 575
phalangectomy, 565
phalang/o, 544
phalanx, 539
pharyngeal tonsils (adenoids), 135–136
pharyngitis, 145

pharyng/o, 138, 420
pharynx (throat), 135–136, 417
phas/o, 598
pheochromocytoma, 651
phimosis, 240
phlebectomy, 371
phlebitis, 370
phleb/o, 364
phlebotomist, 395
phlebotomy, 390
phlegm, 175
phobia, 629
-phobia, 469
phon/o, 138
phoropter, 488
phot/o, 469
photophobia, 492
photorefractive keratectomy (PRK), 483, 484f, 498
photoselective vaporization of the prostate gland (PVP), 247, 250t, 259
pia mater, 596, 596f
pica, 629
Pick disease (frontotemporal dementia), 609t
PID (pelvic inflammatory disease), 280, 280f, 303
pilonidal cyst, 106, 106f
pineal glands, 642f
pinguecula, 478
pink eye (conjunctivitis), 474
pinna (auricle), 508
pituitar/o, 643
pituitary gland, 642f
 hormones of, 641, 641f, 641–642
PKD (polycystic kidney disease), 222
placenta accreta, 322f
placenta accreta spectrum (PAS), 321, 322f
placenta (afterbirth), 314
placenta increta, 322f
placenta percreta, 322f
placenta previa, 321, 321f
placental abruption, 320
plantar fasciitis, 559
-plasia, 21, 233, 644
-plasm, 21, 139
plasma, 361
plasmapheresis, 390
plasm/o, 364
-plasty, 97, 139, 193, 233, 271, 365, 421, 469, 510, 545, 599
platelets (thrombocytes), 361
-plegia, 469, 599
pleura, 136–137
pleural effusion, 151
pleurisy, 145
pleuritis, 145
pleur/o, 138
pleurodesis, 157
plural endings, for medical terms, 51, 52t
PM (polymyositis), 554, 584
PMS (premenstrual syndrome), 280, 303
-pnea, 76, 139
pneum/o, 138
pneumoconiosis, 145
pneumonectomy, 157, 157f
pneumonia, 145
 community-acquired, 178
 hospital-acquired, 178
pneumonitis, 145
pneumon/o, 138
pneumothorax, 147
PNS (peripheral nervous system), 594, 631
podiatrist, 579
poli/o, 598
poliomyelitis (polio), 604, 630

poly-, 138, 192, 316, 364, 545, 598, 643
polyarteritis, 370
polycystic kidney disease (PKD), 201, 222
polycystic ovary syndrome (PCOS), 280, 303
polydipsia, 660
polyhydramnios (hydramnios), 320
polymerase chain reaction (PCR), 40t
polymyositis (PM), 554, 584
polyneuritis, 604
polyneuropathy, 604
polyp(s), 431, 431f, 442f
polypectomy, 435
 colonoscope for, 435f
polyp/o, 420
polyposis, 427
polysomnography (PSG), 152f, 162, 179
polyuria, 214
pons, 596
port-wine stain (nevus flammeus), 327
position. See also specific positions
 anatomic, 61, 61f
 of body, 76–77
 prefixes for, 5
positive expiratory pressure (PEP), 180
positron emission tomography (PET), 80t, 631
 for nervous system, 615
post-, 316, 598
posterior, 66, 68t
 of muscles, 542f
 of skeleton, 538f
posterior capsulotomy, 483
posterior lobe (neurohypophysis), of pituitary gland, 641
poster/o, 61
posteroanterior (PA), 66, 85
postherpetic neuralgia, 609
postictal, 619
postnatal, 344
postoperative cholangiography, 441
postpartum, 338
post-traumatic stress disorder (PTSD), 629, 630
PPD (purified protein derivative skin test), 167
pre-, 316, 598
preeclampsia, 321
prefixes
 for blood, 364
 for body, 21
 for cardiovascular system, 364
 defined, 5
 for digestive system, 421
 for direction, 5, 62
 for endocrine system, 643
 for eye, 469
 for female reproductive system, 271
 for immune system, 364
 for integumentary system, 97
 for lymphatic system, 364
 for male reproductive system, 233
 for musculoskeletal system, 545
 for negation, 5
 for neonatology, 316
 for numbers, 5
 for obstetrics, 316
 for position, 5
 for time, 5
pregnancy (gestation), 314–315. See also obstetrics
 medical terms for, 314–315
 skin in, 315
preictal, 619
premature infant, 344
premenstrual syndrome (PMS), 280, 303

prenatal, 344
prepuce, 232
presbycusis, 515
presbyopia, 478
pressure injury (bedsore, decubitus ulcer), 108, 108f
preterm infant, 344
priapism, 240
prim/i, 316
primigravida, 338
primipara (primip), 338, 348
PRK (photorefractive keratectomy), 483, 484f, 498
PRL (prolactin), 641, 664
pro-, 21
procedures. *See also* diagnostic procedures and tests
   suffixes for, 5
proctitis, 427
proct/o, 420
proctoscope, 442
proctoscopy, 442
prognosis (Px), 45, 53
prolactin (PRL), 641, 664
prolapse, 218
pronation, 580, 580f
prone position (ventral recumbent position), 76, 77t
prostate cancer, 240, 240t
prostate gland, 232
prostatectomy, 243, 243t, 250t
prostate-specific antigen (PSA), 240t, 253, 259
prostatic urethral lift (PUL), 248, 249f, 250t, 259
prostatitis, 236
prostat/o, 233
prostatocystitis, 236
prostatocystotomy, 243
prostatolith, 236
prostatolithotomy, 243
prostatorrhea, 237
prostatovesiculectomy, 244
prostatovesiculitis, 237
prosthesis, 579
prothrombin time (PT), 395, 406
proximal, 66
proxim/o, 61
pruritus, 123
PSA (prostate-specific antigen), 240t, 253, 259
pseud/o, 316, 469
pseudocyesis, 320
pseudodementia, 623t
pseudophakia, 492
PSG (polysomnography), 152f, 162, 179
psoriasis, 108
psychiatrist, 626
psychiatry, 626
psych/o, 598
psychogenic, 626
psychologist, 27, 626
psychology, 626
psychopathy, 626
psychosis, 626
psychosomatic, 626
PT (prothrombin time), 395, 406
PTCA (percutaneous transluminal coronary angioplasty), 380, 406
pterygium, 478
PTH (parathyroid hormone), 642, 664
-ptosis, 193, 218, 469
ptosis (blepharoptosis), 474
PTSD (post-traumatic stress disorder), 629, 630
-ptysis, 139

puberty, 256
pubic, 575
pubic symphysis, 539
pubis, 539
pub/o, 544
puerperal, 338
puerperium, 339
puerper/o, 315
PUL (prostatic urethral lift), 248, 249f, 250t, 259
pulmonary, 171
pulmonary artery, 359–360
pulmonary edema, 151
pulmonary embolism (PE), 152, 152f, 178
pulmonary function
   diagnostic procedures and tests for, 166
   word parts for, 162
pulmonary function tests (PFTs), 166, 179
pulmonary neoplasm, 147
pulmonary valve, 359–360
pulmon/o, 138
pulmonologist, 170
pulmonology, 170
pulse oximetry, 166
pulse (P), 381, 406
pupil, 466
pupillary, 492
pupill/o, 469
pupillometer, 487
pupilloscope, 488
purified protein derivative skin test (PPD), 167
purpura, 123, 123f
pustule, 122t, 123
PV (percutaneous vertebroplasty), 567f, 567t
PVD (peripheral vascular disease), 379
PVP (photoselective vaporization of the prostate gland), 247, 250t, 259
Px (prognosis), 45, 53
pyelitis, 198
pyel/o, 192
pyelolithotomy, 204
pyelonephritis, 198, 198f
pyeloplasty, 204
pyelos, 192
pyloric sphincter, 418
pyloric stenosis, 326
pylor/o, 316, 420
pyloroplasty, 435
pylorus, 316, 418
py/o, 138, 271, 509
pyosalpinx, 276
pyothorax, 147
pyuria, 214

Q

quad screen, 335
quadrantectomy (segmental mastectomy), 286t
quadr/i, 598
quadriplegia, 619
quickening, 339

R

RA (rheumatoid arthritis), 402, 559, 579, 584
   of knee, 553f
rachi/o, 544
rachiotomy, 565
rachischisis (spina bifida), 327, 327f, 554
RAD (reactive airway disease), 150
radial, 575
radial keratotomy (RK), 484f
radiation oncology, 37

radiation therapy (XRT), 37, 53
   for prostate cancer, 240t
radical hysterectomy, 285t
radical mastectomy, 286t
radical prostatectomy (RP), 240t, 243t, 259
radical retropubic prostatectomy, 243t
radiculitis, 604
radicul/o, 598
radiculopathy, 604
radi/o, 61, 544
radioactive iodine uptake (RAIU), 657, 664
radiograph, 80–81
radiography (x-ray)
   chest, 166, 179
   definition of, 81
   discovery of, 80
   for musculoskeletal system, 571t
radiologist, 81
radiology, 80–81
radiotherapy, 37
radius, 536
RAIU (radioactive iodine uptake), 657, 664
rales (crackles), 174
RALRP (robotic-assisted laparoscopic radical prostatectomy), 249f
RARP (robot-assisted radical prostatectomy), 259
RASP (robot-assisted simple prostatectomy), 259
Raynaud, Maurice, 379
Raynaud phenomenon, 379
RBCs (red blood cells, erythrocytes), 28, 53, 361, 406
RDS (respiratory distress syndrome), 327, 348
reactive airway disease (RAD), 150
rectal, 449
rectal polyp, 431f
rect/o, 420
rectocele, 427
rectovaginal fistula, 281t
rectum, 418
recumbent position (decubitus position), 76, 77t
red blood cells (RBCs, erythrocytes), 28, 53, 361, 406
red marrow, 535
reflux, 198, 452
regional enteritis, 430
regional ileitis, 430
remission, 37
renal calculus, 201
renal failure, 201
renal function replacement therapies, 204
renal hypertension, 201
renal pelvis, 189
renal scan, nephrogram (renogram), 209
renal transplant (kidney transplant), 204, 205f
ren/o, 192
renogram (renal scan, nephrogram), 209
repetitive strain injury (RSI), 559, 584
reproductive system, 18t. *See also* female reproductive system; male reproductive system
respiration (breathing, ventilation), 135
respiratory distress syndrome (RDS), 327, 348
respiratory syncytial virus (RSV), 178
respiratory system, 18t, 134–185
   abbreviations for, 178–180
   anatomy of, 135–137
   combining forms for, 138
   complementary terms from word parts for, 170–171
   complementary terms not from word parts for, 174–175

respiratory system (Continued)
    disease and disorder terms not from word parts for, 150–152
    diseases and disorders of, 145–147
    function of, 135
    medical terms for, 145–185
    organs of, 135–137, 136f
    prefixes for, 138
    suffixes for, 139
    surgical terms from word parts for, 156–157
    word parts for, 138–144
respiratory therapist (RT), 180
retina, 466
    ophthalmoscopy of, 468f
retinal, 492
retinal detachment, 478, 479f
retinal photocoagulation, 483
retinitis pigmentosa, 479
retin/o, 469
retinoblastoma, 474
retinopathy, 474
retinoscopy, 488
retinosis pigmentosa (RP), 497
retrograde urogram, 209
reverse Trendelenburg position, 77
rhabd/o, 21, 545
rhabdomyolysis, 554
rhabdomyoma, 32
rhabdomyosarcoma, 32
rheumatic fever, 379
rheumatic heart disease, 379
rheumatoid arthritis (RA), 402, 559, 579, 584
    of knee, 553f
rheumatoid spondylitis (ankylosing spondylitis), 558
rheumatologist, 579
rheumatology, 579
    orthopedics and, 579
rhinitis, 147
rhin/o, 138, 469
rhinomycosis, 147
rhinoplasty, 157
rhinorrhagia (epistaxis), 147, 151
rhinorrhea, 170
rhiz/o, 598
rhizomeningomyelitis, 604
rhizotomy, 612
rhonchi, 174
rhytidectomy (facelift), 113
rhytid/o, 97
right atrium, 359–360
right eye (OD), 498
right lateral decubitus position, 77t
right lateral recumbent position, 77t
right lower lobe (RLL), 179
right lower quadrant (RLQ), 85–86
right middle lobe (RML), 179
right semiprone position, 77t
right upper lobe (RUL), 179
right upper quadrant (RUQ), 85–86
right ventricle, 359–360
ringworm (tinea), 107t, 109
rituximab (Rituxan), 37t
RK (radial keratotomy), 484f
RLL (right lower lobe), 179
RLQ (right lower quadrant), 85–86
RML (right middle lobe), 179
robot-assisted radical prostatectomy (RARP), 259
robot-assisted simple prostatectomy (RASP), 259
robotic surgery, 248, 249f
robotic-assisted laparoscopic radical prostatectomy (RALRP), 249f

rosacea, 108
rotation, 580, 580f
rotator cuff disease, 559
RP (radical prostatectomy), 240t, 243t, 259
RP (retinosis pigmentosa), 497
-rraphy, 271
-rrhage, 139, 365, 599
-rrhagia, 139, 271, 365
-rrhaphy, 365, 421, 545, 599
-rrhea, 97, 139, 233, 271, 316, 421, 510
-rrhexis, 316
RSI (repetitive strain injury), 559, 584
RSV (respiratory syncytial virus), 178
RT (respiratory therapist), 180
RUL (right upper lobe), 179
ruptured disk (herniated disk), 559
RUQ (right upper quadrant), 85–86

S

sacral, 575
sacr/o, 544
sacrum, 536
sagittal, 74–75
SAH (subarachnoid hemorrhage), 610, 630
salivary glands, 419
salpingectomy, 285
salpingitis, 276
salping/o, 271
salpingocele, 276
salpingo-oophorectomy, 285
salpingostomy, 285
-salpinx, 271, 271f
sarc/o, 20, 545
sarcoidosis, 402
sarcoma, 32
-sarcoma, 21, 545
sarcopenia, 554
scabies, 107t, 108
scan, 81
scapula, 536
scapular, 575
scapul/o, 544
-schisis, 545
schizophrenia, 629
sciatica, 609
sclera, 466
scleral buckling, 483
scleritis, 474
scler/o, 97, 469
scleroderma, 101
scleromalacia, 474
-sclerosis, 365, 510
sclerotomy, 483
scoli/o, 545
scoliosis, 554, 555f
-scope, 139, 162t, 193, 271, 421, 469, 510
-scopic, 139, 162t, 271
-scopy, 139, 162t, 193, 271, 365, 421, 469, 510, 545
scrotum, 231–232
sebaceous glands, 96
seb/o, 96
seborrhea, 101
seborrheic, 101
sed rate, 402
segmental mastectomy (quadrantectomy), 286t
segmental resection, 157f
seizure, 622
semen, 232
semen analysis, 253
semicircular canals and vestibule, 509
semilunar valves, 359–360
seminal vesicles, 232
seminiferous tubules, 231

semiprone position, 77t
semisitting position, 76
sentinel lymph node biopsy, 292, 293f
sepsis, 394
septal, 171
sept/o, 138
septoplasty, 157
septum, 138
    atrial, 359
    deviated, 151
    nasal, 135–136
    ventricular, 359
serology tests, 40t
serum, 361
-ses, 52t
sestamibi parathyroid scan, 657
sestamibi test, 381
sexually transmitted disease (STD), 255, 258
sexually transmitted infection (STI), 255, 258
SG (specific gravity), 210, 222
SHG (sonohysterography, hysterosonography), 292, 303
shingles (herpes zoster), 107t, 609
    postherpetic neuralgia and, 609
shock wave lithotripsy (SWL), 204
shortness of breath (SOB), 179
shoulder arthroplasty, 566f, 566t
shunt, 622
SIADH (syndrome of inappropriate ADH), 664
sial/o, 420
sialolith, 427
sickle cell disease, 394
side-lying position, 76
sigmoid/o, 420
sigmoidoscopy, 442, 442f
sign, 45
sildenafil (Viagra), 239
silent STD, 255
simple mastectomy, 286t
simple prostatectomy, 243t, 250t
single-photon emission computed tomography (SPECT), 80t, 381, 406
    for musculoskeletal system, 571t
sinus node, 380
sinusitis, 147
sinus/o, 138
sinusotomy, 157
-sis, 21, 52t
sitting position, 77
situ, 36
skeletal bones, 535–539, 537f–538f
skeletal muscle, 540, 543f
skeletal system, 534. See also musculoskeletal system
skin, 95
    function of, 95
    infections of, 107t
    in pregnancy, 315
    structure of, 95f
    vitamin D and, 95
skin graft, 114, 126
skin-sparing mastectomy, 286t
SLE (systemic lupus erythematosus), 108, 126, 402
slipped disk (herniated disk), 559
slit lamp, 488
small cell cancer, of lung, 146f
small intestine, 418
small-volume nebulizer (SVN), 180
smooth muscle, 540, 543f
SOB (shortness of breath), 179
soft palate, 417
somatic, 28
somat/o, 21

somatoform disorders, 629
somatogenic, 28
somn/o, 138
son/o, 61, 192, 316
sonogram, 81
sonography (ultrasound), 80t, 81
   abdominal, 445, 445f, 445t
   Doppler, 381
   MRI ultrasound fusion biopsy, 253
   MRI-TRUS, 253
   nephrosonography, 209
   of thyroid, 657f
   pelvic, 334, 334f
   TRUS, 240t, 253, 259
   TVS, 292, 293f, 303
sonohysterography (SHG, hysterosonography), 292, 303
sound perception, by ear, 508f
-spasm, 139
spasticity, 622
specific gravity (SG), 210, 222
specific immunity, 363
SPECT (single-photon emission computed tomography), 80t, 381, 406
speculum, 300
sperm count, 253
sperm (spermatozoa), 231
   origination and transportation of, 232f
sperm test, 253
spermatic cord, 232
spermat/o, 233
spermatocele, 240
spermatozoa (sperm), 231
   origination and transportation of, 232f
spermicide, 256
sperm/o, 233
sphygmomanometer, 381
spina bifida (rachischisis), 327, 327f, 554
spinal cavity, 19
spinal cord, 595f, 596
spinal fusion (spondylosyndesis), 565
spinal stenosis, 559
spinal tap (lumbar puncture), 615, 631
spir/o, 138
spirometer, 162
spirometry, 162
spit (sputum), 175
spleen, 362
splenectomy, 398
splen/o, 364
splenomegaly, 398
splenorrhaphy, 398
split-thickness skin graft (STSG), 126
spondylarthritis (spondyloarthritis), 554
spondyl/o, 544
spondyloarthritis (spondylarthritis), 554
spondylolisthesis, 560
spondylosis, 554
spondylosyndesis (spinal fusion), 565
spongy bone (cancellous), 534
sprain, 560
spur (exostosis), 559
sputum (spit), 175
squamous cell carcinoma (SCC), 105f, 108, 126, 146f
   of lung, 146f
staining, 40t
stapedectomy, 518, 518f
staped/o, 509
stapes (stirrup), 508, 513
staph (staphylococcus), 117, 126
staphyl/o, 97
staphylococcus (staph), 117, 126
-stasis, 21, 365
STD (sexually transmitted disease), 255, 258
steat/o, 420

steatohepatitis, 427
steatorrhea, 449
steatosis, 449
stem cells, 361
stenosis
   mitral, 378
   pyloric, 326
   spinal, 559
-stenosis, 139, 193, 365
stent, 380
stereotactic breast biopsy, 292, 293f
sterilization, 248
sternal, 575
stern/o, 544
sternum, 536
stethoscope, 162t, 167
STI (sexually transmitted infection), 255, 258
stillborn, 344
stirrup (stapes), 508
stoma, 434–435, 452
stomach, 418
stomatitis, 427
stomat/o, 420
-stomy, 139, 193, 233, 421, 469, 510
strabismus (cross-eyed), 479
strain, 560
strep (streptococcus), 117, 126
strept/o, 97
streptococcus (strep), 117, 126
striae gravidarum, 315
striated muscles, 540
stricture, 218
stridor, 174
stroke
   hemorrhagic, 609–610
   ischemic, 609
Strümpell, Adolf von, 558
Strümpell-Marie disease (ankylosing spondylitis), 558
STSG (split-thickness skin graft), 126
sty (hordeolum), 479
sub-, 97, 545, 598
subacute, 150
subacute infection, 49
subarachnoid hemorrhage (SAH), 610, 630
subarachnoid space, 596
subcutaneous layer, 96
subcutaneous mastectomy (nipple-sparing mastectomy), 286t
subcutaneous (subcut), 117, 126
subdural hematoma, 604
sublingual, 449
subluxation, 560
submandibular, 576
submaxillary, 576
substernal, 576
subtotal hysterectomy (supracervical hysterectomy), 285t
subungual, 117
sudoriferous glands (sweat glands), 96
suffixes
   for body, 21
   for conditions, 5
   defined, 5
   for digestive system, 421
   for direction, 62
   for diseases, 5
   for ear, 510
   for endocrine system, 644
   for eye, 469
   for female reproductive system, 271
   for integumentary system, 97
   for male reproductive system, 233
   for musculoskeletal system, 545
   for neonatology, 316

suffixes (Continued)
   for nervous system, 599
   for obstetrics, 316
   for procedures, 5
   for respiratory system, 139
   for urinary system, 192–193
superior (sup), 66, 68t, 85
superior vena cava, 359–360
super/o, 61
supination, 580, 580f
supine position (dorsal recumbent position), 77, 77t
supra-, 545
supracervical hysterectomy (subtotal hysterectomy), 285t
supraclavicular, 576
suprapatellar, 576
surgical breast biopsy, 292
surgical terms from word parts
   for cardiovascular system, 370–371
   for digestive system, 434–435
   for ear, 518
   for endocrine system, 656
   for eye, 483
   for female reproductive system, 284–285
   for integumentary system, 113–116
   for lymphatic system, 398
   for male reproductive system, 243
   for musculoskeletal system, 565
   for nervous system, 612
   for obstetrics, 331
   for respiratory system, 156–157
   for urinary system, 203–204
surgical terms not from words parts
   for cardiovascular system, 380
   for digestive system, 439
   for eye, 483
   for female reproductive system, 288–289
   for integumentary system, 113–114
   for male reproductive system, 247–248
   for urinary system, 204
suturing, 114, 114f
SVN (small-volume nebulizer), 180
swayback (lordosis), 554
sweat glands (sudoriferous glands), 96
SWL (shock wave lithotripsy), 204
symptom, 45
syn-, 545, 643
syncope, 622
syndrome, 660. See also specific syndromes
syndrome of inappropriate ADH (SIADH), 664
syndrome X (metabolic syndrome), 651
synovectomy, 565
synovia, 539
synovi/o, 544
synoviosarcoma, 554
syphilis, 256, 256f
   dementia and, 609t
system(s). See also specific systems
   defined, 18
   of body, 18, 18t
systemic, 28
systemic infection, 49
systemic lupus erythematosus (SLE), 108, 126, 402
system/o, 20
systole, 381
systolic pressure, 381

T

T4 (thyroxine), 642, 664
   blood test for, 657
T3 (triiodothyronine), 642
tachy-, 138, 364

tachycardia, 370
tachypnea, 170
TAH/BSO (total abdominal hysterectomy/
    bilateral salpingo-oophorectomy), 303
tarsal, 576
tarsal bones, 539
tarsal glands, 466
tarsal tunnel syndrome, 560
tarsectomy, 565
tars/o, 544
TB (tuberculosis), 152, 178
    dementia and, 609t
TBI (traumatic brain injury), 622, 630
TD (transdermal), 117, 126
T1DM (type 1 diabetes mellitus), 664
T2DM (type 2 diabetes mellitus), 664
TEE (transesophageal echocardiogram),
    381, 406
tendinitis (tendonitis), 554, 559
tendin/o, 544
tendon, 540
tendonitis (tendinitis), 554, 559
ten/o, 544
tenomyoplasty, 565
tenorrhaphy, 565
tenosynovitis, 554, 559
tension headache, 619
terat/o, 316
teratogen, 344
teratogenic, 344
teratology, 344
testalgia, 255
testicular cancer, 240
testicular torsion, 241
testis, 231
testosterone, 231
tetany, 660
TGs (triglycerides), 382t
THA (total hip arthroplasty), 566f, 566t,
    584
thalassemia, 394
thalidomide, for multiple myeloma, 37t
therapy
    biological, 37, 37t
    brachytherapy, 37t
    for cancer, 37t
    gene, 18
    hormone, for prostate cancer, 240t
    hormone replacement, 299, 303
    neoadjuvant, 37t
    radiation, 37, 53
        for prostate cancer, 240t
    thrombolytic, 380
thoracentesis (thoracocentesis), 157
thoracic, 171
thoracic cavity, 19, 136–137
thoracic vertebrae (T1-T12), 536, 584
thorac/o, 138
thoracocentesis (thoracentesis), 157
thoracoscope, 157f, 162
thoracoscopy, 162
thoracotomy, 157, 157f
thorax, 136–137
-thorax, 139
throat (pharynx), 135–136, 417
thromb/o, 364, 598
thrombocytes (platelets), 361
thrombocytopenia, 390
thrombolysis, 390
thrombolytic therapy, 380
thrombophlebitis, 370
thrombosis, 390
    cerebral, 603
    deep vein, 377, 394, 405
thrombus, 390
thrush (candidiasis), 105

thulium laser enucleation of the prostate
    gland (ThuLEP), 250t
thymectomy, 398
thym/o, 364
thymoma, 398
thymus gland, 362
thyroid gland, 642, 642f
thyroid sonography, 657
thyroidectomy, 656
thyroiditis, 648
thyroid/o, 643
thyroid-stimulating hormone (TSH), 641,
    664
    blood test for, 657
thyrotoxicosis, 651
thyroxine (T4), 642, 664
    blood test for, 657
TIA (transient ischemic attack), 610, 630
tibia, 539
tibial, 576
tibi/o, 544
time, prefixes for, 5
tinea pedis (athlete's foot), 107t
tinea (ringworm), 107t, 109
tinnitus, 515
tissue, 17
TKA (total knee arthroplasty), 566f, 566t,
    584
TLH (total laparoscopic hysterectomy), 303
TNM staging system of cancer, 33
-tocia, 316
tom/o, 61
tomography, 81
-tomy, 139, 193, 233, 271, 316, 421, 469,
    510, 545, 599
tongue, 417
ton/o, 469
tonometer, 488
tonometry, 488
tonsil(s), 135–136
tonsillectomy, 157
tonsillitis, 147
tonsill/o, 138
total abdominal hysterectomy/bilateral
    salpingooophorectomy (TAH/BSO),
    303
total cholesterol, 382t
total hip arthroplasty (THA), 566f, 566t,
    584
total hysterectomy, 285t
total knee arthroplasty (TKA), 566f, 566t,
    584
total laparoscopic hysterectomy (TLH), 303
total mastectomy, 286t
total testosterone, 253
toxic shock syndrome (TSS), 280, 303
trabeculectomy, 483
trachea (windpipe), 135–136
tracheitis, 147
trachelectomy (cervicectomy), 285
trachel/o, 271
trache/o, 138, 316
tracheoesophageal fistula, 326
tracheoplasty, 157
tracheostenosis, 147
tracheostomy, 157, 158f
tracheotomy, 157, 158f
trans-, 97, 192
transdermal (TD), 117, 126
transesophageal echocardiogram (TEE),
    381, 406
transient ischemic attack (TIA), 610, 630
transplantation
    of bone marrow, 395
    of kidneys, 204, 205f

transrectal ultrasound (TRUS), 240t, 253,
    259
transurethral, 215
transurethral incision of the prostate gland
    (TUIP), 248, 249t, 259
transurethral resection of the prostate gland
    (TURP), 248, 249f, 249t, 259
transvaginal sonography (TVS), 292, 293f,
    303
traumatic brain injury (TBI), 622, 630
Trendelenburg position, 77
trich/o, 96
trichomoniasis, 256
tricuspid valve, 359–360
triglycerides (TGs), 382t
triiodothyronine (T3), 642
-tripsy, 193
trisomy 21 (Down syndrome), 326, 327f
-trophy, 545
troponin, 382
TRUS (transrectal ultrasound), 240t, 253,
    259
TSH (thyroid-stimulating hormone), 664
    blood test for, 657
TSS (toxic shock syndrome), 280, 303
T1-T12 (thoracic vertebrae), 536, 584
T-tube cholangiography, 441
tubal ligation (tubal sterilization, female
    surgical sterilization), 289, 289f
tuberculosis (TB), 152, 178
    dementia and, 609t
TUIP (transurethral incision of the prostate
    gland), 248, 249t, 259
tumors
    benign, 31, 37f
    dementia and, 609t
    malignant, 31, 37f
        breast, 286t
        connective tissue, 32
    Wilms, 197
TURP (transurethral resection of the
    prostate gland), 248, 249f, 249t, 259
TVS (transvaginal sonography), 292, 293f,
    303
tympanic membrane (eardrum), 507–508
tympan/o, 509
tympanometer, 521
tympanometry, 521
tympanoplasty, 518
tympanostomy, 518
type 1 diabetes mellitus (T1DM), 664
type 2 diabetes mellitus (T2DM), 664

U

UA (urinalysis), 210, 222
UAE (uterine artery embolization), 289, 303
UC (ulcerative colitis), 431, 455
UGI (upper gastrointestinal), 455
ulcer, 123
ulcerative colitis (UC), 431, 455
ulna, 536
ulnar, 576
uln/o, 544
ultrasound (ultrasonography, sonography),
    85
    abdominal, 445, 445f, 445t
    Doppler, 381
    MRI ultrasound fusion biopsy, 253
    MRI-TRUS, 253
    nephrosonography, 209
    of thyroid, 657
    pelvic, 334, 334f
    TRUS, 240t, 253, 259
    TVS, 292, 293f, 303
-um, 52t, 316

Index

umbilical hernia, 421f
umbilical region, 71
umbilicus, 71, 315
umbo, 71
unconsciousness, 622
undescended testicle, 236
ungual, 117
ungu/o, 96
uni-, 62
unilateral, 66
unstriated muscles, 540
upper gastrointestinal (UGI), 455
upper GI series, 446
upper respiratory infection (URI, cold), 152, 153f, 178
UPPP (uvulopalatopharyngoplasty), 152f, 435, 455
uremia (azotemia), 198
uremic syndrome, 198
ureter(s), 189
ureterectomy, 204
ureteritis, 198
ureter/o, 192
ureterocele, 198
ureterolithiasis, 198
ureteroscopy, 209
ureterostenosis, 198
ureterostomy, 204
urethra, 189
urethritis, 198
urethr/o, 192
urethrocystitis, 198
urethroplasty, 204
URI (upper respiratory infection), 152, 153f, 178
-uria, 193
urinal, 219
urinalysis (UA), 210, 222
urinary, 215
urinary bladder, 189, 191f
    fulguration for, 204, 205f
urinary catheterization, 218
urinary incontinence, 218
urinary meatus, 189
urinary retention, 201
urinary system, 18t, 188–226, 190f
    abbreviations for, 222
    anatomy of, 189–191
    combining forms for, 192
    complementary terms from word parts for, 214–215
    complementary terms not from word parts for, 218–219
    diagnostic imaging for, 210
    diagnostic terms from word parts for, 209
    diagnostic terms not from word parts for, 210
    disease and disorder terms from word parts for, 197–198
    disease and disorder terms not from word parts for, 201
    female, 191f
    function of, 189
    laboratory tests for, 210
    male, 191f
    medical terms for, 197–222
    organs and structures of, 189
    prefixes for, 192
    suffixes for, 192–193
    surgical terms from word parts for, 203–204
    surgical terms not from words parts for, 204
    word parts for, 192–196
urinary tract infection (UTI), 197f, 201, 222
urine, 191f

urine culture and sensitivity, 210
urine studies, 40t
urin/o, 192
ur/o, 192
urodynamics, 210
urogram, 209
urologist, 215
urology, 215
urostomy, 204
urticaria (hives), 109
-us, 52t, 316, 365, 599
uterine artery embolization (UAE, uterine fibroid embolization), 289, 303
uterine fibroid, 280
uterine fibroid embolization (uterine artery embolization), 289, 303
uterine tubes (fallopian tubes), 268
uterovaginal prolapse, 280
uterus, 268
UTI (urinary tract infection), 197f, 201, 222
uvea, 466
uveitis, 474
uveoscleritis, 474
uvula, 417
uvulectomy, 435
uvulitis, 427
uvul/o, 420
uvulopalatopharyngoplasty (UPPP), 152f, 435, 455

V

VA (visual acuity), 492, 497
vaccine, 279, 403
vagina, 268
vaginal, 299
vaginal birth after cesarean section (VBAC), 348
vaginal fistula, 280, 281t
vaginal hysterectomy (VH), 303
vaginitis, 276
vagin/o, 271
vaginosis (bacterial vaginosis), 276
vagotomy, 439
valley fever, 150
valvulitis, 370
valvul/o, 364
valvuloplasty, 371
VAP (ventilator-associated pneumonia), 180
varicocele, 241
varicose veins, 379, 379f
vas deferens (ductus deferens), 232
vascular dementia, 609t
vasectomy, 244
vas/o, 233
vasoconstrictor, 383
vasodilator, 383
vasovasostomy, 244
VATS (video-assisted thoracic surgery), 157f
VBAC (vaginal birth after cesarean section), 348
VBG (venous blood gas), 179
VCUG (voiding cystourethrography), 209, 210f, 222
veins, 359–360
    deep vein thrombosis, 377, 394, 405
    varicose, 379, 379f
venae cavae, 359–360
venipuncture, 395
ven/o, 364
venogram, 371
venous blood gas (VBG), 179
ventilation (respiration), 135
ventilator, 175, 175f
ventilator-associated pneumonia (VAP), 180
ventral, 66, 68t

ventral recumbent position (prone position), 76, 77t
ventricles, 595
ventricular fibrillation (VF, VFib), 378, 405
ventricular septum, 359
ventricul/o, 364
ventr/o, 61
venules, 359–360
vermiform appendix, 419
verruca (wart), 123
vertebral, 576
vertebral column, 535f, 536
vertebr/o, 544
vertebroplasty, 565
vertigo, 515
very-low-density lipoprotein (VLDL), 382t
vesicle (blister), 122t, 123
vesic/o, 192
vesicoureteral reflux (VUR), 198, 222
vesicourethral suspension, 204
vesicovaginal, 299
vesicovaginal fistula, 281t
vesiculectomy, 244
vesicul/o, 233
vestibular, 523
vestibular nerve, 509
vestibul/o, 509
vestibulocochlear, 523
vestibulocochlear nerves, 509
VF (ventricular fibrillation), 378, 405
VFib (ventricular fibrillation), 405
VH (vaginal hysterectomy), 303
Viagra (sildenafil), 239
video-assisted thoracic surgery (VATS), 157f
villi, 418
viral infections, 107t
Virchow, Rudolph, 597
vir/o, 21
virology, 41
virtual colonoscopy, 441
virus, 49
viscera, 18
visceral, 28
viscer/o, 20
visual acuity (VA), 492, 497
vitamin D, 95
vitiligo, 109
vitrectomy, 483
vitreous humor, 466
VLDL (very-low-density lipoprotein), 382t
voice box (larynx), 135–136
void, 219
voiding cystourethrography (VCUG), 209, 210f, 222
volvulus, 431
vowels, combining, 4, 6–7, 7t
V/Q scan (lung ventilation/perfusion scan), 166, 179
vulva, 269
vulvectomy, 285
vulv/o, 271
vulvovaginal, 299
vulvovaginitis, 276
VUR (vesicoureteral reflux), 198, 222

W

wart (verruca), 123
water vapor thermal therapy (WVTT), 248, 250f, 250t, 259
WBC (white blood cells, leukocytes), 53, 361, 361f, 406
wedge resection, 157f
Wernicke-Korsakoff syndrome, 609t
wet macular degeneration, 479f
wheal, 122t, 123

Index

wheeze, 174
white blood cells (WBC, leukocytes), 53, 361, 361f, 406
white matter, 595
white of the eye, 466
whooping cough (pertussis), 151
Wilms tumor (nephroblastoma), 197
windpipe (trachea), 135–136
wire localization biopsy, 292
word parts, 8t
  for behavioral health, 626
  for blood, 390
  for body, 20–27
  for cardiovascular system, 369–371, 376–383
  for diagnostic imaging, 161–162
  for digestive system, 420–426
  for ear, 509–510
  for endocrine system, 643–644
  for eye, 468–473
  for female reproductive system, 270–275
  for immune system, 402–403
  for integumentary system, 96–101

word parts *(Continued)*
  for laboratory tests, 41
  list of, 10t
  for lymphatic system, 398–399
  for male reproductive system, 233–235
  medical terms from, learning techniques for, 12t
  for musculoskeletal system, 544–552
  for neonatology, 315–320, 344
  for obstetrics, 315–320
  for pulmonary function, 162
  for respiratory system, 138–144
  for urinary system, 192–196
Word root, 5
wrong-sided surgery, 72
WVTT (water vapor thermal therapy), 248, 250f, 250t, 259

X

xanth/o, 21, 97
xanthoderma, 116
xanthoma, 101

xanthosis, 45
xer/o, 97, 469
xeroderma, 101
xerophthalmia, 474
xerosis, 116
xiphoid process, 536
x-ray (radiography)
  CXR, 166, 179
  definition of, 81
  discovery of, 80
  for musculoskeletal system, 571t
XRT (radiation therapy), 37, 53
  for prostate cancer, 240t

Y

-y, 52t, 421
YAG laser capsulotomy, 483
yellow marrow, 535

Z

zygote, 314